Nolen-Hoeksema's
Abnormal Psychology

Nolen-Hoeksema's
Abnormal Psychology

Ninth Edition

Heather Jennings

Mc Graw Hill

ABNORMAL PSYCHOLOGY, NINTH EDITION

Published by McGraw Hill LLC, 1325 Avenue of the Americas, New York, NY 10019. Copyright © 2023 by McGraw Hill LLC. All rights reserved. Printed in the United States of America. Previous editions © 2020, 2017, and 2014. No part of this publication may be reproduced or distributed in any form or by any means, or stored in a database or retrieval system, without the prior written consent of McGraw Hill LLC, including, but not limited to, in any network or other electronic storage or transmission, or broadcast for distance learning.

Some ancillaries, including electronic and print components, may not be available to customers outside the United States.

This book is printed on acid-free paper.

1 2 3 4 5 6 7 8 9 LWI 27 26 25 24 23 22

ISBN 978-1-265-31603-7 (bound edition)
MHID 1-265-31603-1 (bound edition)

ISBN 978-1-266-56819-0 (loose-leaf edition)
MHID 1-266-56819-0 (loose-leaf edition)

Senior Portfolio Manager: *Ryan Treat*
Product Development Manager: *Dawn Groundwater*
Marketing Manager: *Olivia Kaiser*
Lead Content Project Managers: *Lisa Bruflodt; Katie Reuter*
Senior Buyer: *Laura Fuller*
Senior Content Licensing Specialist: *Carrie Burger*
Cover Image: *Kirasolly/Shutterstock*
Compositor: *Aptara®, Inc.*

All credits appearing on page or at the end of the book are considered to be an extension of the copyright page.

Library of Congress Cataloging-in-Publication Data

Names: Nolen-Hoeksema, Susan, 1959-2013, author. | Jennings, Heather,
    author.
Title: Abnormal psychology / Susan Nolen- Hoeksema, Heather Jennings.
Description: Ninth edition. | New York, NY : McGraw Hill, [2023] | Includes
    index.
Identifiers: LCCN 2021029365 (print) | LCCN 2021029366 (ebook) | ISBN
    9781265316037 (hardcover) | ISBN 9781266568190 (spiral bound) | ISBN
    9781266568909 (ebook) | ISBN 9781266568039 (ebook other)
Subjects: LCSH: Psychology, Pathological–Textbooks. | Mental
    illness–Textbooks.
Classification: LCC RC454 .N64 2023 (print) | LCC RC454 (ebook) | DDC
    616.89–dc23
LC record available at https://lccn.loc.gov/2021029365
LC ebook record available at https://lccn.loc.gov/2021029366

The Internet addresses listed in the text were accurate at the time of publication. The inclusion of a website does not indicate an endorsement by the authors or McGraw Hill LLC, and McGraw Hill LLC does not guarantee the accuracy of the information presented at these sites.

ABOUT THE AUTHOR

Courtesy of Morgan Avery Jennings

Heather Jennings is a professor of psychology at Mercer County Community College in West Windsor, New Jersey, where her teaching career spans almost 20 years. Dr. Jennings is passionate about teaching, student success, and engaging students in thinking critically about psychological concepts. As a community college graduate, Dr. Jennings embraces this valuable system that provides educational access to many first-generation, under-represented, and underserved college students.

Dr. Jennings completed her Masters of Arts degree in Clinical Psychology from Columbia University, Teachers College and spent several years working in psychiatric emergency screening services as well as home-based, shelter-based, and school-based therapy programs before earning her PhD in Educational Psychology from Temple University. Dr. Jennings' research interests include the psychological variables that impact academic success among community college students.

Dr. Jennings is also an animal advocate and has run a non-profit dog rescue for more than 10 years that provides rescue, rehabilitation, and re-homing for dogs in need. A native of the Jersey Shore, Dr. Jennings loves the beach and spending time on her farm with family, friends, dogs, and chickens. In her spare time, she enjoys refinishing furniture and is usually covered in paint.

BRIEF CONTENTS

Mc Graw Hill **connect** McGraw Hill Psychology's APA Documentation Style Guide

CONTENTS

5 Anxiety, Obsessive-Compulsive, Trauma, and Stressor-Related Disorders   106

6 Somatic Symptom and Dissociative Disorders   158

7 Mood Disorders and Suicide   184

8 Schizophrenia Spectrum and Other Psychotic Disorders   238

9 Personality Disorders   280

10 Neurodevelopmental and Neurocognitive Disorders   316

11 Disruptive, Impulse-Control, and Conduct Disorders   354

15 Health Psychology   472

16 Mental Health and the Law   506

Mc Graw Hill **connect** McGraw Hill Psychology's APA
Documentation Style Guide

GUIDE TO DIVERSITY, EQUITY, AND INCLUSION

Global changes included specifying mini-cases in terms of gender identity, preferred pronouns, and sexual orientation as appropriate to the case. Additionally, sources were cited from researchers publishing in such journals as

- *Journal of Gay & Lesbian Mental Health*
- *World Journal of Psychiatry*
- *World Psychiatry: Official Journal of the World Psychiatric Association (WPA)*
- *Journal of Cross-Cultural Psychology*
- *Culture and Psychology*
- *International Journal of Emergency Mental Health*
- *International Journal of Women's Dermatology*
- *Journal of Interpersonal Violence*
- *Psychology of Popular Media Culture*
- *Journal of Black Studies*
- *Journal of College Student Development*
- *Archives of Sexual Behavior*
- *Body image*
- *Social Media + Society*
- *International Journal of Advanced Studies in Sexology*
- *International Journal for Equity in Health*
- *AIDS Care*
- *Global Social Sciences Review*

Citations of studies and researchers representing diverse and international samples and issues appear throughout the book.

Chapter 1: Looking at Abnormality

- Expanded coverage of how cultural norms help define abnormality.
- Revised coverage of how cultural relativism relates to definitions of abnormality.
- Expanded coverage of how women throughout history were subject to "diagnoses" of disorder and through them had their behavior controlled, cited in Kapsalis (2017). Coverage of "hysteria" and the wandering womb is expanded.
- Coverage provided on culture and its effect on therapeutic treatment.
- Ancient theories of abnormality across cultures and over time are presented.
- Prehistoric views and treatments of abnormality are given.
- Coverage on ancient Chinese treatment of abnormality: balancing yin and yang.
- Theories and treatments of abnormality from ancient Egypt, Greece, and Rome are provided.
- Updated coverage on contemporary treatment regarding racial disparities and solutions.

- Shades of Gray box shows how sociocultural gender biases affect diagnosis of disorders in women versus men.

Chapter 2: Theories and Treatment of Abnormality

- Coverage provided on socioeconomic disadvantages as transdiagnostic risk factors.
- Significantly expanded coverage of the stigmatization and mental health risks experienced by LGBTQI+ people, citing research by Casey, Wootton, & McAloon (2020).
- New coverage of social media and its impact on bias and the development of echo-chambers that separate social groups often in term of misinformation, citing Wang, Sirianni, Tang, Zheng, & Fu, 2020 and Chou, Oh, & Klein (2018).
- Analysis of cross-cultural issues in treatment: individualistic versus collectivistic cultures.
- New coverage given on multiculturalism and the clinician's need to integrate and embrace cultural difference citing Jones-Smith (2019).
- Added content on innovative mental health interventions, such as synchronous telehealth treatments, because of COVID-19, which highlight the disparities among underserved populations, ethnic minorities and people of color, citing Reay, Looi, & Keightly (2020).
- Coverage of the influence of perceived social group membership on how society views socio-demographic groups, citing D. W. Sue, D. Sue, Neville, & Smith (2019).
- Coverage provided on culturally responsive treatment.
- Revised case study of a Hong Kong immigrant to the United States.
- Coverage on cross-cultural competencies.
- Cultural differences in treating children.
- Culturally specific therapies: Native American and Hispanic examples.
- Prevention programs: focus on social determinants of mental health issues.
- Added content on laws and social policies that affect mental health outcomes for sexually marginalized groups.

Chapter 3: Assessing and Diagnosing Abnormality

- Coverage of the cultural factors in assessing children and adolescents.
- Evaluating individuals across cultures, drawing on research by Soto, et al. (2018); Dominguez (2017), Alegria, Nakash, & Johnson (2018), and others.

- New coverage of the cultural factors in parental assessment of their children, highlighting Asian parenting and citing Nguyen & McAloon (2018).
- Disparities in quality of mental health care across cultures.
- Impact on treatment of cultural differences between therapist and client
- Coverage of *DSM-5* and cultural issues

Chapter 4: The Research Endeavor

- Cross-cultural research on problems in generalizing results of research conducted on white middle-class college students to all social and cultural groups.
- Investigating similarities and differences among cultural groups.
- Different manifestations of disorders across cultures and their impact on research.
- New coverage of the impact of high global migration rates and language differences on conducting research, citing Squires, Sadarangani, & Jones (2020).

Chapter 5: Anxiety, Obsessive-Compulsive, Trauma and Stressor-Related Disorders

- Coverage of the sociocultural factors related to separation anxiety.
- Changed Case Study participants to Navaho family members.
- Coverage of cross-national similarities and differences regarding generalized anxiety disorder
- Cultural and global differences regarding social anxiety disorders, citing Yli-Länttä (2020).
- Coverage of gender differences as they relate to social anxiety disorders.
- Transnational comparisons of phobias.
- World prevalence rates regarding obsessive compulsive disorder.
- Gender differences associated with body dysmorphic disorder, citing Ryding & Kuss (2020).
- World-wide research on trauma and PTSD.
- Coverage of social factors relating to PTSD.
- Hate crimes against Latinx and LGBTQ people and other acts of terror resulting in PTSD, citing Yu-Ru & Wen-Ting (2020) and Mclaughlin & Kar (2019).
- Keira's Story, a box about Keira and her friend Justine at the gay nightclub, Pulse, the night of a mass shooting. The box describes Keira's subsequent PTSD.
- Gender and cross-cultural differences regarding PTSD.
- Racial differences and PTSD.
- Ethnic identity and PTSD, citing Nikulina, Bautista, & Brown (2019).
- Coverage of ethnic identity as a protective factor regarding the possible development of certain psychological disorders.

Chapter 6: Somatic Symptom and Dissociative Disorders

- Clinical use of cultural traditions to treat somatic symptom disorder.

- Global research on diagnosis of dissociative identity disorder (DID).
- Cultural oppression and DID prevalence.
- Revision of the *DSM* to make diagnosis of DID more applicable to diverse cultural groups.
- Latinx population and DID versus *ataque de nervios*.

Chapter 7: Mood Disorders and Suicide

- New Extraordinary People box featuring Dwayne "The Rock" Johnson and his experience with depression.
- International research on unipolar mania.
- US and global prevalence rates of bipolar disorder.
- Cohort effects (age difference) and depression.
- Gender and depression: gender difference, socialization, biological and sociocultural factors.
- Ethnicity, race and depression: focus on Latinx, African American, and Asian American experiences.
- New coverage of major depressive disorder rates among Black, indigenous, and people of color (BIPOC), citing Coman and Wu (2018).
- New coverage of resilience, lower rates of depression, gender, and minority racial groups, citing Laird, et al, 2019.
- New Profiles box on Kanye West and bipolar disorder, citing Lane (2020).
- New coverage on cross-national prevalence rates of unipolar mania, citing Jules, Ajdacic-Gross, & Rossler (2020).
- US and international suicide prevalence rates of bipolar disorder.
- US regional suicide prevalence rates: higher rural rates.
- Gender differences and suicide.
- Ethnic and cross-cultural differences regarding suicidality prevalence rates (Non-Hispanic whites, American Indian/ Alaska Native, African American, Latinx).
- Racial and ethnic factors in suicidality.
- Global comparisons of suicide rates.
- Ethnic and racial factors of suicide and children.
- Substantial new coverage of suicide and LGBTQI+ people: adolescent, young adult, and adult populations, citing the National LGBT Health Education Center (2018) and Hayes (2019).
- Suicide and older adults.
- Global comparisons of suicide and stress.
- Expanded coverage of social media, gender, and suicide, citing Poland, Lieberman, & Niznik (2019) and Yildiz, Orak, Walker, & Solakogluidiz (2019).

Chapter 8: Schizophrenia Spectrum and Other Psychotic Disorders

- Global prevalence rates of schizophrenia: developed versus less-developed countries.
- Gender differences, citing Häfner (2019).
- Cultural influences on epidemiology, phenomenology, outcome, and treatment.
- Psychosocial perspectives on socioeconomic factors, deprived urban settings, social drift.

- US and international findings on Immigration, stress and schizophrenia:.
- Cross-cultural perspectives: traditional beliefs and practices: Case of a Javanese woman
- Culturally appropriate tools to improve the effectiveness of family interventions in multicultural settings, citing Driscoll, Sener, Angmark, & Shaikh (2019).
- Schizophrenia and stigma, citing Mannarini & Rossi (2019) and Fox, Earnshaw, Taverna, & Vogt (2018).

Chapter 9: Personality Disorders

- Global comparisons of paranoid personality disorder.
- African American experience and social and environmental risk factors regarding paranoid personality disorder.
- Comparative global prevalence rates on schizotypal personality disorder.
- Coverage on race and gender on paranoid personality disorder:
- Racial difference and borderline personality disorder (Hispanic, white, African American, East Asian prevalence rates and sociocultural factors), citing Haliczer et al. (2019).
- Gender and borderline personality disorder.
- Gender differences and narcissistic personality disorder.
- Racial differences and narcissistic personality disorder.
- Gender differences and avoidant personality disorder.
- Gender differences and dependent personality disorder.
- Changed Case Study on dependent disorder to feature a gay couple.
- Gender differences and obsessive-compulsive personality disorder.
- Racial and ethnic differences and obsessive-compulsive personality disorder.

Chapter 10: Attention-Deficit/Hyperactivity Disorder

- Sex and gender differences and Attention-Deficit/ hyperactivity disorder (ADHD), citing Mowlem, Agnew-Blais, Taylor, & Asherson (2019).
- Global comparisons of fetal alcohol syndrome prevalence rates.
- The impact diverse socioeconomic backgrounds on intellectual disability.
- The impact of gender, culture, and education on neuro-cognitive disorder.
- African American and Caribbean Hispanics: experience with neurocognitive disorder.
- Institutionalization versus family care: European American, Asian American, Hispanic examples.

Chapter 11: Disruptive, Impulse-Control and Conduct Disorders

- Gender differences and conduct disorders.
- Racial differences and conduct disorders, citing Patel, et al. (2018).

- Racial and socioeconomic differences regarding conduct disorders and hospitalization.
- Gender differences and antisocial personality disorder, citing Azevedo, Vieira-Coehlo, Castelo-Branco, Coehlo, & Figueiredo-Braga (2020).

Chapter 12: Eating Disorders

- Updated coverage of gender and eating disorders (ED), citing Allen, Robson, & Laborde, 2020.
- Updated coverage of gender differences and anorexia nervosa, citing Murray, Quintana, Loeb, Griffiths, & Le Grange (2019).
- Provided coverage ethnic differences and anorexia nervosa.
- Case study of a Chinese woman with anorexia nervosa.
- Presented coverage of gender differences and bulimia nervosa.
- Included coverage of cultural, ethnic and racial differences regarding bulimia nervosa.
- Presented coverage of gender differences and binge-eating disorder.
- Updated coverage of ethnic and racial differences in obesity, Centers for Disease Control and Prevention (2018).
- Updated coverage of global comparisons of obesity, citing Centers for Disease Control and Prevention (2018) and the World Health Organization (2018).
- Provided coverage of gender differences and obesity.
- Social pressure and cultural norms impacting eating disorders.
- Changed Case Study on anorexia from cis-girl to trans-girl.
- Updated coverage "Western" and "non-Western" eating disorders, citing Ioannou, et al. (2020).

Chapter 13: Sexual Disorders and Gender Diversity

- Extraordinary People: *David Reimer, The Boy Who Was Raised as a Girl*.
- Presented extended coverage of female sexual interest/ arousal disorder.
- Updated coverage of male erectile disorder, citing Retzler, 2019 and Kessler, Sollie, Challacombe, Briggs, & Van Hemelrijck (2019).
- Updated global cultural factors related to sexual disfunction, citing Santana, et al. (2019) and Vaishnav, Saha, Mukherji, & Vaishnav (2020).
- Updated considerations for LGBTQ people: stress from prejudice on sexual function, citing Kerckhof et al (2019).
- Transgender: specified stressors (such as violence and transphobia), citing Cocchetti et al. (2021) and Flores, Mallory, & Conron (2020).
- Treating LGBTQ people: therapist training and sensitivity.
- Coverage of the professional disavowal of "conversion" therapy, citing, American Psychological Association, 2019 and Flores, Mallory, & Cannon (2020).

- Included diversity of sexual expression versus paraphilic disorders, citing Thibaut (2020).
- Updated coverage of controversies regarding gender dysphoria and gender diversity.
- Updated coverage of treatments for gender dysphoria, citing Bizic (2018).
- Coverage of gender dysphoria versus transgender experience.

Chapter 14: Substance Use and Gambling Disorder

- Updated coverage of gender differences and alcohol use disorder, citing Krieger, Young, Anthenien, & Neighbors (2018).
- Updated coverage of racial differences and alcohol use disorder, citing Tucker, Chandler, & Witkiewitz (2020).
- Updated coverage of age differences and alcohol use disorder, citing Tucker, et al. (2020).
- Included information on cultural differences and alcohol use.
- New coverage of transnational comparisons of use of Ecstasy (MDMA), citing van Amsterdam, Pennings, & van den Brink (2020).
- Included coverage of sociocultural factors relating to substance abuse, citing Moustafa et al. (2020).
- Updated coverage of gender and substance abuse, citing White, 2020 and Guinle & Sinha (2020).
- Included coverage of older adults and substance abuse.

Chapter 15: Health Psychology

- Updated coverage of gender and stress, citing Robert, Virpi, & John (2019).
- Presented coverage on the impact of minority status, socioeconomic status and culture on stress.
- Highlighted coverage of African American experience and stress.
- Presented gender differences and coping strategies.
- Highlighted coverage of cultural differences in coping.
- Updated and expanded coverage of working with people with AIDS and HIV, citing Spann, van Luenen, Garnefski, & Kraaij (2020) and Bhochhibh (2020).
- Presented coverage of gender differences and coronary heart disease.
- Highlighted coverage on racial differences and hypertension (highlighting African American experience).

Chapter 16: Mental Health and the Law

- Updated coverage on racial stereotypes and assumptions about mental illness, citing Kunsst, Myhren, & Onyeador (2018).
- Coverage of racial status and rates of acquittal in cases with insanity defenses.
- Coverage presented on socioeconomic status and incarceration rates.
- Updated coverage on gender, mental illness, and incarceration rates, citing Al-Rousan, (2017).

PREFACE

Welcome to the ninth edition of Nolen-Hoeksema's *Abnormal Psychology!* The foundation of this book is based on the outstanding scholarship of the late, Dr. Susan Nolen-Hoeksema who was an innovative educator and researcher in the field of psychology. I am honored to continue her vision in this new edition and provide students and faculty with a comprehensive survey of psychological disorders that emphasizes the human perspective. As an educator, I approached this new edition with diversity, inclusion, compassion, and student comprehension as my focus. In terms of best teaching practices, I believe that students are the centerpiece of our shared table. With this philosophy in mind, I created content in this edition to enhance student comprehension and engagement by making information about psychological disorders relatable and contemporary. Although psychological disorders are inherently fascinating to discuss, that does not mean students will always understand the complexities and best clinical practices for treatment. Continuing the practices of Susan Nolen-Hoeksema, *Abnormal Psychology* is designed to promote awareness and empathy about mental health issues, best practices for treatments, and cutting-edge psychological research to better understand how to identify, treat and prevent psychological dysfunction.

At the same time, *Abnormal Psychology* connects proven scholarship with student performance. Through Connect for Abnormal Psychology, a digital assignment and assessment platform, students gain the insight they need to study smarter and improve performance. Connect for *Abnormal Psychology* includes assignable and assessable videos, quizzes, exercises, and interactivities, all associated with learning objectives.

connect A PERSONALIZED EXPERIENCE THAT LEADS TO IMPROVED LEARNING AND RESULTS

How many students think they know everything about abnormal psychology but struggle on the first exam? Students study more effectively with Connect and SmartBook.

- Connect's assignments help students contextualize what they've learned through application, so they can better understand the material and think critically.
- Connect reports deliver information regarding performance, study behavior, and effort so instructors can quickly identify students who are having issues or focus on material that the class hasn't mastered.

- SmartBook helps students study more efficiently by highlighting what to focus on in the chapter, asking review questions, and directing them to resources until they understand.
- SmartBook creates a personalized study path customized to individual student needs.

SmartBook is now optimized for mobile phone and tablet and is accessible for students with disabilities. Content-wise, it has been enhanced with improved learning objectives that are measurable and observable to improve student outcomes. SmartBook personalizes learning to individual student needs, continually adapting to pinpoint knowledge gaps and focus learning on topics that need the most attention. Study time is more productive and, as a result, students are better prepared for class and coursework. For instructors, SmartBook tracks student progress and provides insights that can help guide teaching strategies.

SMARTBOOK POWERFUL REPORTING

Whether a class is face-to-face, hybrid, or entirely online, McGraw Hill Connect provides the tools needed to reduce the amount of time and energy instructors spend administering their courses. Easy-to-use course management tools allow instructors to spend less time administering and more time teaching, while reports allow students to monitor their progress and optimize their study time.

- The **At-Risk Student Report** provides instructors with one-click access to a dashboard that identifies students who are at risk of dropping out of the course due to low engagement levels.
- The **Category Analysis Report** details student performance relative to specific learning objectives and goals, including APA learning goals and outcomes and levels of Bloom's taxonomy.
- The **SmartBook Reports** allow instructors and students to easily monitor progress and pinpoint areas of weakness, giving each student a personalized study plan to achieve success.

PREPARING STUDENTS FOR HIGHER-LEVEL THINKING

At the higher-end of Bloom's taxonomy, **Power of Process** guides students through the process of critical reading and analysis. Faculty can select or upload content, such as journal articles, and assign guiding questions to move students toward higher-level thinking and analysis.

Power of Process for
PSYCHOLOGY

New to this edition and found in Connect, **Writing Assignments** offer faculty the ability to assign a full range of writing assignments to students) with just-in-time feedback.

You may set up manually scored assignments in a way that students can

- automatically receive grammar and high-level feedback to improve their writing before they submit a project to you;
- run originality checks and receive feedback on "exact matches" and "possibly altered text" that includes guidance about how to properly paraphrase, quote, and cite sources to improve the academic integrity of their writing before they submit their work to you.

The new writing assignments will also have features that allow you to assign milestone drafts (optional), easily re-use your text and audio comments, build/score with your rubric, and view your own originality report of student's final submission.

Available in Connect, **Faces of Abnormal Psychology** connects students to real people living with psychological disorders. Through its unique video program, Faces of Abnormal Psychology helps students gain a deeper understanding of psychological disorders and provides an opportunity for critical thinking.

Interactive Case Studies help students understand the complexities of psychological disorders. Co-developed with psychologists and students, these immersive cases bring the intricacies of clinical psychology to life in an accessible, gamelike format. Each case is presented from the point of view of a licensed psychologist, a social worker, or a psychiatrist. Students observe sessions with clients and are asked to identify major differentiating characteristics associated with each of the psychological disorders presented. Interactive Case Studies are assignable and assessable through McGraw Hill Education's Connect.

Inform and Engage on Psychological Concepts

At the lower end of Bloom's taxonomy and located in Connect, **NewsFlash** is a multimedia assignment tool that ties current news stories, TedTalks, blogs, and podcasts to key psychological principles and learning objectives. Students interact with relevant news stories and are assessed on their ability to connect the content to the research findings and course material. NewsFlash is updated twice a year and uses expert sources to cover a wide range of topics including: emotion, personality, stress, drugs, COVID-19, disability, social justice, stigma, bias, inclusion, gender, LGBTQA+, and many more.

SUPPORTING INSTRUCTORS WITH TECHNOLOGY

With McGraw Hill Education, you can develop and tailor the course you want to teach.

McGraw Hill Campus (www.mhcampus.com) provides faculty with true single-sign-on access to all of McGraw Hill's course content, digital tools, and other high-quality learning resources from any learning management system. McGraw Hill Campus includes access to McGraw Hill's entire content library, including eBooks, assessment tools, presentation slides, and multimedia content, among other resources, providing faculty open, unlimited access to prepare for class, create tests/quizzes, develop lecture material, integrate interactive content, and more.

With **Tegrity,** you can capture lessons and lectures in a searchable format and use them in traditional, hybrid, "flipped classes," and online courses. With Tegrity's personalized learning features, you can make study time efficient. Its ability to affordably scale brings this benefit to every student on campus. Patented search technology and real-time learning management system (LMS) integrations make Tegrity the market-leading solution and service.

With McGraw Hill Education's **Create,** faculty can easily rearrange chapters, combine material from other content sources, and quickly upload content you have written, such as your course syllabus or teaching notes, using McGraw Hill Education's Create. Find the content you need by searching through thousands of leading McGraw Hill Education textbooks. Arrange your book to fit your teaching style. Create even allows you to personalize your book's appearance by selecting the cover and adding your name, school, and course information. Order a Create book, and you will receive a complimentary print review copy in 3 to 5 business days or a complimentary electronic review copy via email in about an hour. Experience how McGraw Hill Education empowers you to teach your students your way. **http://create.mheducation.com**

TRUSTED SERVICE AND SUPPORT

McGraw Hill Education's Connect offers comprehensive service, support, and training throughout every phase of your implementation. If you're looking for some guidance on how to use Connect, or want to learn tips and tricks from super-users, you can find tutorials as you work. Our Digital Faculty Consultants and Student Ambassadors offer insight into how to achieve the results you want with Connect.

INTEGRATION WITH YOUR LEARNING MANAGEMENT SYSTEM

McGraw Hill integrates your digital products from McGraw Hill Education with your school's learning management system (LMS) for quick and easy access to best-in-class content and learning tools. Build an effective digital course, enroll students with ease, and discover how powerful digital teaching can be.

Available with Connect, integration is a pairing between an institution's LMS and Connect at the assignment level. It shares assignment information, grades, and calendar items from Connect into the LMS automatically, creating an easy-to-manage course for instructors and simple navigation for students. Our assignment-level integration is available with **Blackboard Learn, Canvas by Instructure,** and **Brightspace by D2L,** giving you access to registration, attendance, assignments, grades, and course resources in real time, in one location.

Instructor Supplements

Instructor's Manual. The instructor's manual provides a wide variety of tools and resources for presenting the course, including learning objectives and ideas for lectures and discussions.

Test Bank and **Test Builder.** Organized by chapter, the questions are designed to test factual, conceptual, and applied understanding; all test questions are available within Test Builder.

Available within Connect, Test Builder is a cloud-based tool that enables instructors to format tests that can be printed, administered within a Learning Management System, or exported as a Word document of the test bank. Test Builder offers a modern, streamlined interface for easy content configuration that matches course needs, without requiring a download.

Test Builder allows you to:

- access all test bank content from a particular title
- easily pinpoint the most relevant content through robust filtering options
- manipulate the order of questions or scramble questions and/or answers
- pin questions to a specific location within a test
- determine your preferred treatment of algorithmic questions
- choose the layout and spacing
- add instructions and configure default settings

Test Builder provides a secure interface for better protection of content and allows for just-in-time updates to flow directly into assessments.

PowerPoint Presentations. The PowerPoint presentations, available in both dynamic lecture-ready and accessible WCAG-compliant versions, highlight the key points of the chapter and include supporting visuals. All of the slides can be modified to meet individual needs.

Remote Proctoring and Browser-Locking Capabilities. Remote proctoring and browser-locking capabilities, hosted by Proctorio within Connect, provide control of the assessment environment by enabling security options and verifying the identity of the student.

- Seamlessly integrated within Connect, these services allow instructors to control students' assessment experience by restricting browser activity, recording students' activity, and verifying students are doing their own work.
- Instant and detailed reporting gives instructors an at-a-glance view of potential academic integrity concerns, thereby avoiding personal bias and supporting evidence-based claims.

CHAPTER-BY-CHAPTER CHANGES

Chapter 1: Looking at Abnormality

- Updated and expanded content in Abnormality along the Continuum.
- Revised content on the 4Ds of abnormality.
- Added COVID-19-related content.
- Revised coverage of "hysteria" and the "wandering uterus."
- Revised content on deinstitutionalization and the Mental Retardation Facilities and Community Mental Health Center Construction Act (1963).
- Updated case study on Khloe, a person with extensive long-term hospitalizations.
- Updated and expanded content on the managed health care system and mentally ill individuals and those with substance abuse.
- Added content regarding subpopulations at risk for not receiving mental health treatment, such as minorities, people of color, and underserved populations.
- Updated professional degrees for psychology and counseling professions.

Chapter 2: Theories and Treatment of Abnormality

- Revised content on Phineas Gage.
- Updated and expanded content on frontal lobe function.
- Expanded Down Syndrome content.
- Added content on environmental and genetic factors associated with disease.
- Updated content on medication to treat psychological disorders.
- Updated content on electroconvulsive therapy (ECT).
- Updated content on repetitive transcranial magnetic stimulation (rTMS) and vagus nerve stimulation.

- Removed content on Freud's psychosexual stages of development, fixations, penis envy, Oedipal/Electra complex, etc.
- Expanded content on psychodynamic therapies, including relational psychoanalysis, the relationship between therapist and client, transference, and countertransference.
- Revised content on acceptance and commitment intervention and mindfulness techniques.
- Added content on innovative mental health interventions, such as synchronous telehealth treatments, because of COVID-19, highlighting the disparities among underserved populations, ethnic minorities, and people of color.
- Expanded content related to disasters, social norms, and stigma that impact marginalized groups such as people of color and LGBTQI+.
- Added content on laws and social policies that affect mental health outcomes for sexually marginalized groups.
- Revised content on cross-cultural issues in treatment, including cultural sensitivity, multiculturalism in practice, culturally relevant therapy, and treatment outcomes.
- Revised content and graphic on primary, secondary, and tertiary prevention programs.
- Added content on developing positive therapeutic relationships and related treatment outcomes.

Chapter 3: Assessing and Diagnosing Abnormality

- Updated introduction.
- Added new section, "How are psychological disorders evaluated?"
- Expanded content on the assessment and diagnostic process.
- Revised content on validity, reliability, and standardization, including new graphic.
- Revised clinical interview content including five (5) categories of the mental status exam, types of clinical interviews (structured, unstructured, and semi-structured) and symptom questionnaires (i.e., MMPI-2).
- New content on the modes of self-report assessment and outcomes via smartphone technology.
- Updated and expanded content on intelligence testing.
- Updated information on Rorschach testing to include current research on validity issues.
- Updated and expanded information on the influence of culture, parental self-reports, parental attitudes about mental health services, perceptions about psychological symptoms displayed by their children, and parental history of psychological disorders on treatment access.
- Revised content on barriers to treatment that focus on cultural factors that affect ethnic minorities and people of color.
- Revised information on the evolution of the *DSM* system.
- Updated and expanded content on the *DSM-5* and *ICD 11* classification systems.
- Removed *DSM-IV* description of Axes 1–5.

- Added section entitled, "What Happens after a Diagnosis is Made?" about creating treatment plans and working with mental health professionals.

Chapter 4: The Research Endeavor

- Expanded the introduction on research across the continuum to highlight categorical versus continuum models.
- Added new Extraordinary People section on social media and echo-chambers.
- Updated content on independent and dependent variables.
- Expanded and updated content on case studies to include neurological biomarkers and brain imaging research on DID.
- Expanded and updated content on correlational research.

Chapter 5: Anxiety, Obsessive-Compulsive, Trauma and Stressor-Related Disorders

- Chapter entirely reorganized.
- Revised continuum to reflect feelings of anxiety rather than fear.
- Added new introduction section and clarified typical versus atypical anxiety.
- Updated prevalence rates for anxiety with emphasis on culture and ethnicity related to diagnostic differences among groups.
- Added new section on the impact of COVID-19 on anxiety and mental health.
- Revised introduction to panic disorder and the biological and psychological factors associated with panic disorder.
- Revised content on separation anxiety disorder for children and adults.
- Updated information on genetics and separation anxiety disorder.
- Expanded and updated information on environmental and parenting factors on anxiety disorders.
- Expanded and revised content on treating separation anxiety disorder.
- Added new section on selective mutism.
- Updated content on generalized anxiety disorder (GAD).
- Updated coverage of social anxiety disorder.
- Updated and expanded coverage of specific phobias.
- Added new introduction section on organization of obsessive-compulsive and related disorders based on *DSM-5* standards.
- Added new profile on celebrity soccer player David Beckham and his battle with OCD.
- Added new Case Study (Carl's compulsions) to highlight compulsive behaviors of OCD.
- Revised discussion of OCD symptomatology.
- Updated prevalence rates and course for OCD with emphasis on sex differences across the lifespan.
- Updated prevalence rates for OCD with emphasis on age groups, sex, culture, and ethnicity related to diagnostic differences among groups.

- Added and updated content on Hoarding Disorder.
- Expanded and updated content on Trichotillomania.
- Expanded and updated content on Excoriation.
- Updated and expanded content on Body Dysmorphic Disorder (BDD), including a new section on the influence of social media platforms on body dissatisfaction.
- Added content on BDD specifier "With absent insight/delusional beliefs."
- Revised content on Muscle dysmorphia (MD).
- Updated information on biological contributions to OCD and related disorders.
- Added section on the link between the hypothalamic-pituitary-adrenal (HPA) axis and obsessive-compulsive type disorders.
- Updated section on the role of inflammation and infection in the development of OCD and related disorders.
- Updated content on cognitive behavioral theories related to OCD development.
- Updated and expanded introduction section on trauma.
- Added new PTSD case study: "Keira's story."
- Updated and expanded discussion of PTSD and traumatic experiences highlighting differences between men and women.
- Updated section on symptoms of PTSD and Acute Stress Disorder (ASD).
- Added section on Reactive Attachment Disorder (RAD).
- Added section on Disinhibited Social Engagement Disorder.
- Updated and expanded section on types of traumas.
- Added section about the mass shooting at Pulse nightclub (2016) and research on resiliency through community support and support networks.
- Added research on increased psychological vulnerability for PTSD following exposure to multiple traumatic events.
- Revised coverage of secondary and vicarious trauma, as well as repeated exposure via social media and frequent access to news updates.
- Revised coverage on risk factors and coping mechanisms for PTSD.
- Updated and expanded coverage of ethnic and cultural differences related to trauma exposure and PTSD.
- Added section on ethnic identity as a protective factor vis-a-vis certain psychological disorders.

Chapter 6: Somatic Symptom and Dissociative Disorders

- Revised discussion of the mind-body connection with regard to physical illness symptoms.
- Updated coverage of diagnostic information, comorbidities, and prevalence rates for Somatic Symptom Disorder and Illness Anxiety Disorder.
- Added a section on the influence of COVID-19 on mental health conditions and preoccupations.

- Expanded content on the impact of trauma on somatic symptoms.
- Revised information on the treatment of somatic symptom and illness anxiety disorder.
- Updated somatic symptom disorder case study.
- Revised content on conversion disorder (Functional Neurological Symptom Disorder).
- Revised content on factitious disorder imposed on self; factitious disorder imposed on another; and malingering.
- Added new introduction on dissociative disorders.
- Revised content on consciousness and the impact of trauma on dissociation, brain function, cognitive unconscious, and dissociation.
- Substantially revised coverage of Dissociative Identity Disorder (DID).
- New content on Dissociative Amnesia including prevalence rates and memory failure.
- Updated content on retrograde amnesia.
- Added content on the impact of recovering traumatic memories.
- Revised content on neurological model of repression.
- Updated and expanded content on state-dependent memory retrieval.
- Updated and expanded discussion on the controversies surrounding DID diagnosis.

Chapter 7: Mood Disorders and Suicide

- Updated Mood Disorders along the Continuum.
- Added new Extraordinary People on Dwayne "the Rock" Johnson.
- Revised and expanded section on symptoms of depression.
- Added content on Major Depressive Disorder (MDD), including updated references on course and specifiers for MDD.
- Updated and expanded content on Complex Bereavement Disorder.
- Added new content of Persistent Depressive Disorder.
- Revised significantly content on Premenstrual Dysphoric Disorder (PMDD).
- Revised content on Disruptive Mood Dysregulation Disorder (DMDD).
- Added new coverage of mental health resiliency among Black, indigenous, and people of color (BIPOC) and depressive disorders.
- Added section on MDD in children and adolescents.
- Added new content on the impact of COVID-19 on children and adolescent mental health.
- Added content on suicidality among children and adolescents.
- Expanded and revised introduction on Bipolar Disorders.
- Added new section on mania.

- Added new profile on Kanye West and mania.
- Updated and expanded content on unipolar mania to include impact of culture on diagnosis.
- Revised content on Bipolar I Disorder.
- Updated content on Rapid Cycling Bipolar Disorder.
- Expanded content on bipolar disorders in children and adolescents.
- Expanded content on prevalence rates and course of bipolar disorder (I and II) across the world.
- Expanded and updated genetic factors associated with biological pathways to depressive disorders.
- Added updated content on neural and synaptic plasticity associated with depressive disorders.
- Expanded content on hypothalamic-pituitary-adrenal axis (HPA) activation, chronic stress, and depressive disorders.
- Added content on adverse childhood experiences (ACEs) on depression.
- Added significant coverage on the gut microbiome and the impact of altered gut microbiota composition on stress, anxiety, depressive symptoms, and social behavior.
- Added content on the influence of microorganisms, central nervous system inflammation, immune function, and stress on neurotransmitter function.
- Added content on the association between neuroinflammation and the development of major depressive disorder (MDD).
- Updated content on behavioral theories and learned helplessness theories of depression.
- Updated an expanded content on psychological flexibility as it relates to COVID-19 adaptation.
- Added section on the possible influence of social media and smartphone use on depression.
- Updated and expanded content on generational differences in disclosing depressive disorders.
- Expanded coverage of genetic factors, brain structure, and psychosocial factors associated with bipolar disorder.
- Expanded section on dysregulation of the circadian rhythms on bipolar disorder.
- Revised content on anti-depressant (SSRI) and Norepinephrine-Dopamine Reuptake Inhibitor, and lithium medication.
- Updated content on Electroconvulsive Therapy (ECT).
- Revised content on Vagus Nerve Stimulation (VNS) *and* repetitive transcranial magnetic stimulation (rTMS).
- Updated suicide statistics with data on sex, race/ethnicity, geographic location, and age group.
- Updated content on gender differences in suicidality.
- Added content on racial/ethnic minorities and the influence of culture on suicide.
- Revised section on suicide in children and adolescents.
- Added new section on LGBTQI+ individuals and the associated risk factors for depression and suicide.
- Updated content on college student risk of suicide.

- Added content on the influence of social media, access to streaming media services, and suicide contagion and self-harm among adolescent populations.
- Updated content on gun access and suicidality.

Chapter 8: Schizophrenia Spectrum and Other Psychotic Disorders

- Updated and expanded the introduction.
- Re-ordered presentation of content to symptoms, diagnosis, course, and prognosis of schizophrenia.
- Updated and clarified section on positive symptoms and negative symptoms of schizophrenia.
- Expanded content on delusions.
- Updated research on the impact of worry and rumination on paranoid thinking.
- Added new profile on delusional behavior.
- Updated research on grandiose delusions.
- Updated content on audio-visual hallucinations.
- Updated content on cognitive deficits.
- Updated content on diagnostic content.
- Updated and expanded content on prevalence and course of schizophrenia.
- Added content on early-onset schizophrenia.
- Updated research on gender differences in schizophrenia.
- Added international prevalence data for schizophrenia.
- Revised content on outcomes for individuals with schizophrenia, including rates of relapse, remission, and treatment.
- Revised content on differences between men and women with schizophrenia.
- Updated content on the prevalence, treatment, and prognosis of Delusional Disorder.
- Updated prevalence data and genetic heritability for schizotypal personality disorder.
- Revised content on multifactorial contributions to schizophrenia to include genetic vulnerability and environmental risk factors.
- Revised content on the prevalence of schizophrenia and heredity among biological relatives.
- Updated research on twin studies and adoption studies examining heritability of schizophrenia.
- Added new section titled "Birth Complications" on the perinatal risk factors associated with the development of schizophrenia.
- Added research and figure on the two-hit model of neuro-developmental disturbance.
- Added research on the role of maternal infection during pregnancy and the development of psychotic disorders.
- Added research on maternal and fetal inflammatory responses to infection and the impact on neurodevelopment.
- Added content on the association between maternal immune activation (MIA) and the development of psychiatric disorders such as autism spectrum disorder (ASD) and schizophrenia in offspring.

- Added content on viral pandemics and increased incidences of schizophrenia, which includes recent data on coronaviruses and COVID-19.
- Added content on the association of psychotic disorders with altered gut microbiota composition and microbiota-gut-brain axis.
- Updated content on dopamine theory, the diathesis-stress model, HPA axis, and neural circuit dysfunction.
- Updated research on social drift theory.
- Added section on trauma, childhood adversity, social inequality, and urban living as risk factors for schizophrenia.
- Added content on stressful life events and relapse rates among individuals with psychotic disorders.
- Added section about exposure to household pets as a protective factor associated with reduced risk of developing schizophrenia.
- Updated and expanded content on the family influence, expressed emotion, and relapse rates for those with schizophrenia.
- Added content on cultural differences in the level and presentation of emotional expression and subsequent rates of relapse for those with schizophrenia.
- Added content on the development of culturally appropriate tools to improve the effectiveness of family interventions in multicultural settings.
- Updated content on second generation antipsychotic medications and response rates.
- Updated and expanded research on the use of clozapine which includes efficacy rates, side effects, and treatment outcomes.
- Updated and expanded content on family-oriented interventions, the use of psychoeducation programs, and outcomes in the treatment of schizophrenia.
- Updated and expanded content on Assertive Community Treatment (ACT) programs.
- Added new research on differences in cultural perception of mental illness, stigmatizing attitudes and behaviors, negative stereotypes, adverse treatment in interactions, impact on treatment seeking behaviors, and discrimination.

Chapter 9: Personality Disorders

- Updated Personality along the Continuum personality traits.
- Revised comprehensively the coverage of Paranoid Personality Disorder (PPD).
- Revised descriptive content, international research, comorbidities, and references for Schizoid Personality Disorder.
- Significantly revised coverage of Schizotypal Personality Disorder relating to descriptive traits, family history, adoption, twin studies, comorbidity, course, and international prevalence rates (highlighting ethnic and sex differences), and the impact of childhood adversity and trauma.
- Clarified and expanded descriptive traits of cluster B personality disorders.
- Revised coverage of Borderline Personality Disorder (BPD), including content on increased association of self-harm and suicide attempt; prevalence rates, including research on men, women, and people of color; comorbidity; course for BPD; the impact of BPD caregiving on family members; and treatments.
- Updated and expanded descriptive traits of Histrionic Personality Disorder (HPD).
- Updated and expanded content Narcissistic Personality Disorder (NPD), including clinical traits, comorbidity, course, and prevalence rates (accenting research on minorities and people of color).
- Revised coverage of Avoidant Personality Disorder (AVPD), including prevalence and comorbidity rates and research on the relationship between neglect and emotional abuse by early caregivers.
- Revised content on Dependent Personality Disorder (DPD), including content on comorbidity and symptom overlap between personality disorders by cluster; behavioral and cognitive models of DPD, attachment theory and treatment.
- Revised coverage of Obsessive-Compulsive Personality Disorder (OCPD), including overlap with OCD; comorbidity; ethnic, gender, and racial differences; family, genetic, and neurological studies on OCPD; and treatment outcomes.

Chapter 10: Neurodevelopmental and Neurocognitive Disorders

- Revised introduction on ADHD.
- Updated prevalence estimates and clinical traits of ADHD, including research on gut-brain axis.
- Revised content on Autism Spectrum Disorder (ASD).
- Removed *DSM-IV* content on Pervasive Developmental Disorders (PDDs).
- Added content on the influence of maternal gut microbiome.
- Added content on the impact of maternal immune activation (MIA) and inflammation on neurodevelopmental disorders.
- Added content on the role of immune dysregulation/inflammation and the microbiota-gut-brain axis in the development of ASD behaviors.
- Added content on the role of childhood adversity, stress, and neglect on systemic inflammation.
- Expanded content on ASD treatments.
- Updated content on Down Syndrome.
- Updated content and prevalence data for Fetal Alcohol Syndrome (FAS).
- Updated and expanded content on behavioral strategies and early intervention programs used to help individuals with intellectual disability (ID).
- Revised content on mainstreaming education practices and outcomes for students with ID.
- Revised content on Tourette's disorder and persistent motor or vocal tic disorder (PMVTD).
- Updated content on habit reversal therapy for motor disorders.

- Updated prevalence estimates for major and mild neurocognitive disorders.
- Expanded content on neurocognitive disorder due to Lewy body disease.
- Updated content on HIV-Associated Neurocognitive Disorder (HAND).
- Updated content on traumatic brain injury (TBI).

Chapter 11: Disruptive, Impulse-Control, and Conduct Disorders

- Updated and expanded clinical discussion of conduct disorder which includes prevalence rates for ethnic minorities, as well as diagnostic and treatment disparities for people of color.
- Updated case study on child with opposition defiant disorder (ODD).
- Updated and expanded discussion for ODD, which includes updated references which includes research on impaired emotional and facial recognition as it is related to self-regulation.
- Updated and expanded content on the influence of neurotransmitters on symptoms of ODD.
- Updated and expanded content on childhood risk factors for the development of ODD.
- Updated discussion of antisocial personality disorder (ASPD).
- Updated ASPD prevalence estimates, comorbidity rates, and heritability rates.
- Updated content on adverse childhood experiences and the development of ASPD.
- Updated content on treatment efficacy for ASPD.
- Updated content for the neurological basis of intermittent explosive disorder (IED).

Chapter 12: Eating Disorders

- Added content to the introduction on eating disorders.
- Added and updated content on clinical symptoms and physical consequences of anorexia nervosa.
- Added case study for anorexia nervosa which includes a sexually marginalized individual.
- Clarified distinction between restrictive and purging type of anorexia nervosa (AN).
- Updated prevalence estimates for AN to include new data on mortality rates and men affected with AN and/or disordered eating practices.
- Updated prevalence estimates on bulimia nervosa, including suicidality rates.
- Updated coverage of binge-eating disorder (BED).
- Updated and revised content on the course of BED, as well as gender differences.
- Removed *DSM-IV* content on eating disorder not otherwise specified (EDNOS).
- Updated and expanded content on other specified feeding or eating disorders.

- Updated and expanded content on the influence of neurotransmitters and neurocognitive deficits on the development of eating disorders.
- Added content on the role of gut microbiota and bacteria on the development of eating disorders.
- Added content on social media and the development of body dissatisfaction and the eating disorders.
- Expanded content on the impact of family dynamics and parenting styles on eating disorders.
- Updated content on effective treatments for eating disorder.

Chapter 13: Sexual Disorders and Gender Diversity

- Revised the Sexuality and Gender along the Continuum feature.
- Updated coverage of erectile dysfunction (ED).
- Revised content on sexual dysfunction to include new global research focused on women and psychosocial factors associated with sexual dysfunction.
- Updated and expanded content for sexual dysfunctions among LGBTQ individuals.
- Clarified content on paraphilic disorders regarding typical versus atypical sexual arousal.
- Updated the table, The Kinds of Sexual Practices People Find Appealing.
- Updated and expanded content on paraphilic disorders.
- Revised and updated content on fetishistic and transvestic disorders.
- Revised and updated content for Sexual Sadism and Sexual Masochism.
- Updated coverage of voyeuristic disorder and *exhibitionistic disorder*.
- Updated content on frotteurism, including gender and cultural differences.
- Updated coverage of pedophilic disorder, including material on gender differences.
- Revised case study on pedophilia.
- Updated and expanded on treatments for pedophilia.
- Revised and updated content on treatments for gender dysphoria included new research on gender affirmation surgery (GAS).

Chapter 14: Substance Use and Gambling Disorders

- Revised content on tolerance and substance withdrawal.
- Updated content on the combination of substance abuse and dependence into one disorder called substance use disorder.
- Updated content on alcohol use and alcohol use disorder.
- Update prevalence data for each substance discussed throughout chapter.
- Updated and expanded content on nicotine use to include vaping prevalence and medical consequences.
- Updated content on hallucinogens and PCP.

- Updated and expanded content on cannabis use, prevalence estimates, and the use of medical marijuana.
- Updated content on the use of inhalants.
- Updated and expanded content on the use of Ecstasy (MDMA) and expanded content on the psychological factors that influence substance abuse disorders.
- Updated content on gender differences among men and women with alcohol use disorder (AUD) which includes global data and cultural implications.
- Revised, updated, and expanded content on the use of methadone maintenance programs and treatment outcomes.
- Updated content on cognitive behavioral therapy (CBT) and motivational interviewing (MI) for substance use disorders.
- Added contact on the impact of COVID-19 on access to substance use services and the increased use of telemedicine in response to COVID-19 distancing requirements.
- Added content on the influence of smart phone and gaming apps on gambling disorder.
- Added content on the influence of COVID-19 on gambling behaviors.

Chapter 15: Health Psychology

- Added content on the influence of social media platforms and online health communities that enhance social support.
- Updated content on chronic arousal of the fight-or-flight system for individuals with psychological disorders.

- Expanded coverage of neuroimmunological research and psychological stress, which includes HPA axis and activation of the sympathetic nervous system.
- Added content on guy microbiota, neuroinflammation, and immune response on psychiatric and neurogenerative diseases.
- Updated and expanded content on stress reduction, psychosocial interventions, and improved health for those with cancer.
- Updated content on psychosocial interventions for individuals living with HIV/AIDS which includes program outcomes that increase the use of active antiretroviral therapy (ART), and the impact of stigma on this population.
- Updated and expanded research on gender differences and psychological factors found among those with cardiovascular disease.
- Updated, revised, and expanded content on the influence of personality type (Type A, Type B, Type C, and Type D) on physical health.
- Added content on the influence of COVID-19 pandemic on insomnia.
- Update and expanded content on sleep terror disorder.

Chapter 16: Mental Health and the Law

- Updated content on competence to stand trials and the ability to make medical decisions.
- Expanded content on the rates of incarceration among those with serious mental illness.

Nolen-Hoeksema's
Abnormal Psychology

Chapter 1

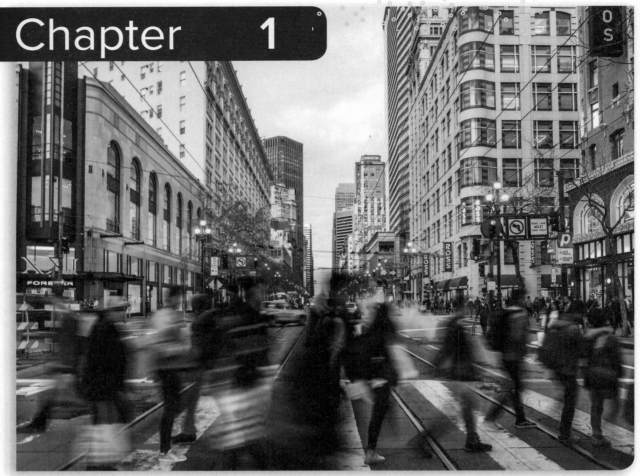

Zeyu Wang/Getty Images

Looking at Abnormality

CHAPTER OUTLINE

Abnormality Along the Continuum

Behaviors, thoughts, and feelings are the following:

- Typical for the social context
- Not distressing to the individual
- Not interfering with social life or work/school
- Not dangerous

(Example: College students who are self-confident and happy, perform to their capacity in school, and have good friends)

Socially established division between normal and abnormal

Behaviors, thoughts, and feelings are one or more of the following:

- Highly unusual for the social context
- The source of significant individual distress
- Significantly interfering with social or occupational functioning
- Highly dangerous to the individual or others

(Example: College students who are hopeless about the future, are self-loathing, chronically abuse drugs, fail courses, and have alienated all their friends)

Normal ———————————————————————————————————— Abnormal

Behaviors, thoughts, and feelings are one or more of the following:

- Somewhat unusual for the social context
- Distressing to the individual
- Interfering with social or occupational functioning
- Dangerous

(Example: College students who are often unsure and self-critical, occasionally abuse prescription drugs, fail some courses, and avoid friends who disapprove of their drug use)

What is normal, anyway? As humans, we often search for a dividing point where normal ends and abnormal behavior suddenly begins. It would make life much easier if this threshold existed; but unfortunately, there is no definitive way to know exactly where *normal* behavior lives within the human experience. Everyday, we are motivated by various thoughts and feelings to behave in ways that others may deem normal or abnormal. However, it's important to recognize that the label we place upon these behaviors (normal vs. abnormal) is related directly to the context in which these behaviors occur, the factors that surround these behaviors, and the culture in which we live. Behaviors considered to be normal in one culture may be considered abnormal in other cultures, and vice versa.

We are each experts in identifying abnormal behavior since we have been socialized in a culture that dictates and defines the behaviors considered acceptable or typical. For example, it would not be unusual to see large groups of people walking around your neighborhood dressed like zombies or killer clowns on Halloween, but if you saw this same group on a random day in the spring, you may quickly turn and run in the other direction. And, you would be wise to run! Prior to the COVID-19 crisis, it may have been unusual to wear a face mask in public. Now, it's become a standard of behavior in a relatively short period of time. You may even remark to another person that you like their face mask!

As human beings, we are all subject to violating these socially defined boundaries of normal behavior. This can lead us to think, feel, or behave in ways that are considered abnormal by others, cause distress to the individual or those around them, or lead to problematic behaviors. For example, it's not uncommon for people to feel hurt or rejected after a relationship ends and it takes time for those feelings to fade. Is it "normal" to keep checking Instagram to see what your ex is doing without you? When does the typical act of checking Instagram or the social media account(s) of your ex-boyfriend or girlfriend become abnormal?

Since there is no way to determine where normal ends and abnormal begins, the *normal-abnormal continuum* is used to illustrate these transitions in behavior. You will see that this **continuum model of abnormality** applies to all the disorders we discuss in this book. In this chapter, we discuss some of the factors that influence how thoughts, emotions, and behaviors are labeled abnormal.

Extraordinary People

My illness began slowly, gradually, when I was between the ages of 15 and 17. I began having visual hallucinations in which people changed into different characters, the change indicating to me their moral value. For example, the mother of a good friend always changed into a witch, and I believed this to be indicative of her evil nature. At the time I didn't know what to make of these changes in my perceptions. On the one hand, I thought they came as a gift from God, but on the other hand, I feared that something was dreadfully wrong. However, I didn't tell anyone what was happening; I was afraid of being called insane.

Source: Anonymous, "First Person Account: Portrait of a Schizophrenic," Schizophrenic Bulletin, 18, 1992. pp. 333–334.

Given the range of human behaviors from common or expectable to strange and even bizarre, abnormal psychology is a very popular subject, how could it not be? This field of study is devoted to understanding, treating, and preventing psychological dysfunction. Abnormal psychology, also known as **psychopathology,** focuses on behaviors that are atypical or unexpected. With this fascinating nature of abnormal psychology, it can be easy for people to become so wrapped up in the terminology, the clusters of symptoms and clinical jargon associated with various psychological disorders that they forget about the people behind the disorder. It is critical to remember that while this topic is very interesting, we must never lose sight of the human perspective. Like any other area of human behavior, psychological disorders are part of the human experience and, as a result, impact us all directly or indirectly. You will learn the symptoms that characterize different psychological disorders, but most importantly, how these symptoms affect the lives of people everyday. It is equally important to realize that while many of the disorders presented in this book seriously influence day-to-day life, they are all treatable, and many are preventable.

The purpose of this book is not only to provide you with information, facts and figures, theories, and research but also to help you understand the experience of people with psychological disorders. The good news is that, thanks to an explosion of research in the past few decades, effective biological and psychological treatments are available for many of the mental health problems we discuss.

DEFINING ABNORMALITY

Once we have determined that a behavior or a person is abnormal we often insert a word to describe this abnormality, sometimes unkindly. Words like crazy or nuts are common in popular culture and easy to use without realizing the unintended consequences. Just like any disparaging label, these words are used to dismiss and dehumanize people who we consider different. What these words also do is reinforce **stigma** among those with mental health issues, which has an impact on how we view those with psychological disorders and how they can see themselves. While difficult to fully define abnormality in all contexts, professionals can use a variety of criteria to assess abnormal function in an individual.

The Four Ds of Abnormality

There is no singular way to define abnormal behavior among professionals. However, modern judgments of abnormality are influenced by the interplay of four dimensions, often called "the four Ds": dysfunction, distress, deviance, and dangerousness. Behaviors, thoughts, and feelings are dysfunctional when they interfere with the person's ability to function in daily life, to hold a job, or to form close relationships. The more dysfunctional behaviors and feelings are, the more likely they are to be considered abnormal by mental health professionals. For example, thinking that is out of touch with reality (such as believing you are Satan and should be punished) makes it difficult to function in everyday life and so is considered dysfunctional.

Behaviors and feelings that cause distress to the individual or those around them are also likely to be considered abnormal. Many of the problems we discuss in this book cause individuals tremendous emotional distress, but how a person's behavior affects those around them is also an important consideration. Imagine in the middle of a lecture a man enters the room wearing nothing but a small bikini bottom, sits down next to you and begins eating a sandwich. This man is engaged in the lecture, he asks questions, and is showing no signs of distress. How do you feel sitting next to this person? Our social norms would dictate very different attire in a classroom setting, particularly in regions where the weather is cold. This violation of our typical classroom practice could cause feelings of distress or discomfort in you, but not to the man wearing only bikini bottoms. In other cases, the person displaying

SHADES OF GRAY DISCUSSION

Consider the following descriptions of two students. In the year between her eighteenth and nineteenth birthdays, Jennifer, who is 5′6″, dropped from a weight of 125 pounds to 105 pounds. The weight loss began when Jennifer had an extended case of the flu and lost 10 pounds. Friends complimented her on being thinner, and Jennifer decided to lose more weight. She cut her intake of food to about 1,200 calories, avoiding carbs as much as possible, and began running a few miles every day. Sometimes she is so hungry she has trouble concentrating on her schoolwork. Jennifer values her new lean look so much, however, that she is terrified of gaining the weight back. Indeed, she'd like to lose a few more pounds so she could fit into a size 2.

Mark is what you might call a "heavy drinker." Although he is only 18, he has ready access to alcohol, and most nights he typically drinks at least five or six beers. He rarely feels drunk after that much alcohol, though, so he might also throw back a few shots, especially when he is out partying on Saturday nights. He's been caught a few times and received tickets for underage drinking, but he proudly displays them on his dorm wall as badges of honor. Mark's grades are not what they could be, but he finds his classes boring and has a hard time doing the work. Do you find Jennifer's or Mark's behaviors abnormal? How would you rate their level of dysfunction, distress, deviance, and danger? (Discussion appears at the end of this chapter.)

abnormal behavior is not in distress but causes others distress through chronic lying, stealing, or violence.

Behavior that deviates from the social norm is another way to assess abnormality since behaviors are influenced by cultural norms and practices within our community. Behaviors that defy our social expectations are easy to spot, but they vary in terms of the culture. It is common to see a person wearing shorts at the gym, but walking outside when it is snowing deviates from the norm. No one criterion defines abnormality, so while wearing shorts in very cold weather is behavior that deviates from the norm, this behavior does not make someone abnormal. Finally, some behaviors and feelings, such as suicidal gestures, are of potential harm to the individual, whereas other behaviors and feelings, such as excessive aggression, could potentially harm others. Such dangerous behaviors and feelings are often seen as abnormal. Once an individual's behaviors or feelings cross that line, we might be justified in suggesting that there is something "wrong" with that person or thinking that a psychological disorder may be present. However, it is important to note that abnormal behavior, even when agreed upon, is not the same as a psychological disorder. The diagnosis of a psychological disorder requires that specific criteria be met after a psychological evaluation is complete. Meaning, displaying abnormal behavior is not necessarily enough to be assigned a psychological diagnosis. We will discuss this topic in depth in Assessing and Diagnosis Abnormality.

The Disease Model of Mental Illness

A common belief is that behaviors, thoughts, or feelings can be viewed as pathological or abnormal if they are symptoms of a *mental illness*. This implies that a disease

process, much like hypertension or diabetes, is present. For example, when many people say that an individual "has schizophrenia" (which is characterized by distorted perceptions and a loss of contact with reality), they imply that he or she has a disease that should show up on some sort of biological test, just as hypertension shows up when a person's blood pressure is taken.

To date, however, no biological test is available to diagnose any of the types of psychological disorder we discuss in this book (Hyman, 2010). This is not just because we do not yet have the right biological tests. In modern conceptualizations, mental disorders are not viewed as singular diseases with a common pathology that can be identified in all people with the disorder. Instead, mental health experts view mental disorders as collections of problems in thinking or cognition, in emotional responding or regulation, and in social behavior (Cuthbert & Insel, 2013; Hyman, 2010). Thus, for example, a person diagnosed with schizophrenia has a collection of problems in behavior, rational thinking, and emotional response in everyday life. It is this collection of problems that we label schizophrenia. It is still possible, and in the case of schizophrenia likely, that biological factors are associated with these problems in thinking, feeling, and behaving. But it is unlikely that a singular disease process underlies the symptoms we call schizophrenia.

Cultural Norms

Consider these behaviors:

1. A man driving a nail through his hand
2. A woman refusing to eat for several days
3. A man barking like a dog and crawling on the floor on his hands and knees

4. A woman building a shrine to her dead husband in her living room and leaving food and gifts for him at the altar

Do you think these behaviors are abnormal? You might reply, "It depends." Several of these behaviors are accepted in certain circumstances. In many religious traditions, for example, refusing to eat for a period of time, or fasting, is a common ritual of cleansing and penitence. You might expect that some of the other behaviors listed, such as driving a nail through one's hand or barking like a dog, are abnormal in all circumstances, yet even these behaviors are accepted in certain situations. In Mexico, some Christians have themselves nailed to crosses on Good Friday to commemorate the crucifixion of Jesus. Among the Yoruba of Africa, traditional healers act like dogs during healing rituals (Murphy, 1976). Thus, the context, or circumstances surrounding a behavior, influences whether the behavior is viewed as abnormal.

Cultural norms play a large role in defining abnormality. A good example is the behaviors people are expected to display when someone they love dies (Rosenblatt, 2008). In cultures dominated by Shinto and Buddhist religions, it is customary to build altars to honor dead loved ones, to offer them food and gifts, and to speak with them as if they were in the room. In cultures dominated by Christian and Jewish religions, such practices would potentially be considered quite abnormal.

Cultures have strong norms for what is considered acceptable behavior for men versus women, and these gender-role expectations also influence the labeling of behaviors as normal or abnormal (Addis, 2008). In many cultures, men who display sadness or anxiety or who choose to stay home to raise their children while their wives work are at risk of being labeled abnormal, while women who are assertive, career-focused, or who don't want to have children are at risk of being labeled abnormal.

Cultural relativism is the view that there are no universal standards or rules for labeling a behavior abnormal; instead, behaviors can be labeled abnormal only relative to cultural norms (Bassett & Baker, 2015; Snowden & Yamada, 2005). The advantage of this perspective is that it honors the norms and traditions of different cultures, rather than imposing the standards of one culture on judgments of abnormality. Yet opponents of cultural relativism argue that dangers arise when cultural norms are allowed to dictate what is normal or abnormal. In particular, psychiatrist Thomas Szasz (1961, 2011) noted that throughout history, societies have labeled individuals and groups abnormal in order to justify controlling or silencing them. Hitler branded Jews abnormal and used this label as one justification for the Holocaust. The

former Soviet Union sometimes branded political dissidents mentally ill and confined them in mental hospitals. When the slave trade was active in the United States, slaves who tried to escape their masters could be diagnosed with a mental disease that was said to cause them to desire freedom; the prescribed treatment for this disease was whipping and hard labor.

Most mental health professionals do not hold an extreme relativist view on abnormality, recognizing the dangers of basing definitions of abnormality solely on cultural norms. Yet even those who reject an extreme cultural-relativist position recognize that culture and gender have a number of influences on the expression of abnormal behaviors and on the way those behaviors are treated. First, culture and gender can influence the ways people express symptoms. People who lose touch with reality may believe that they have divine powers, but whether they believe they are Jesus or Mohammed depends on their religious background.

Second, culture and gender can influence people's willingness to admit to certain types of behaviors or feelings (Snowden & Yamada, 2005). People in Eskimo and Tahitian cultures may be reluctant to admit to feeling anger because of strong cultural norms against the expression of anger. The Kaluli of New Guinea and the Yanomamo of Brazil, however, value the expression of anger and have elaborate and

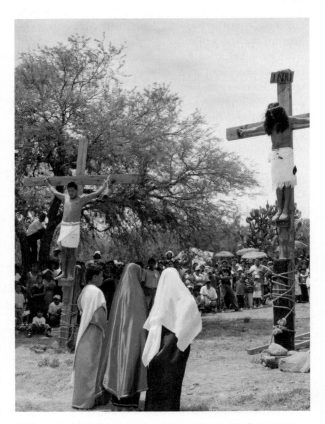

In Mexico, some Christians have themselves nailed to a cross to commemorate the crucifixion of Jesus. *cdrin/Shutterstock*

complex rituals for expressing it (Jenkins, Kleinman, & Good, 1991).

Third, culture and gender can influence the types of treatments deemed acceptable or helpful for people exhibiting abnormal behaviors. Some cultures may view drug therapies for psychopathology as most appropriate, while others may be more willing to accept psychotherapy (Snowden & Yamada, 2005). Throughout this book, we will explore these influences of culture and gender on behaviors labeled abnormal.

HISTORICAL PERSPECTIVES ON ABNORMALITY

Across history, three types of theories have been used to explain abnormal behavior. The **biological theories** have viewed abnormal behavior as similar to physical diseases, caused by the breakdown of systems in the body. The appropriate cure is the restoration of bodily health. The **supernatural theories** have viewed abnormal behavior as a result of divine intervention, curses, demonic possession, and personal sin. To rid the person of the perceived affliction, religious rituals, exorcisms, confessions, and atonement have been prescribed. The **psychological theories** have viewed abnormal behavior as a result of psychological processes, such as beliefs, coping styles, and life events such as trauma, bereavement, or chronic stress. There are a variety of methods to treat abnormal behavior with these theories such as rest, relaxation, or change of environment to improve psychological health. These three types of theories have influenced how people acting abnormally have been regarded in society. A person thought to be abnormal because he or she was a sinner, for example, would be regarded differently from a person thought to be abnormal because of a disease.

Ancient Theories

Our understanding of prehistoric people's conceptions of abnormality is based on inferences from archaeological artifacts—fragments of bones, tools, artwork, and so on—as well as from ancient writings about abnormal behavior. It seems that humans have always viewed abnormality as something needing special explanation.

Driving Away Evil Spirits

Historians speculate that even prehistoric people had a concept of insanity, probably one rooted in supernatural beliefs (Selling, 1940). A person who acted oddly was suspected of being possessed by evil spirits. The typical treatment for abnormality, according to supernatural theories, was exorcism—driving the evil spirits from the body of the suffering person.

When the slave trade was active, slaves who tried to escape were sometimes labeled as having mental illness and were beaten to "cure" them. *Jean Baptiste Debret/Getty Images*

Shamans, or healers, would recite prayers or incantations, try to talk the spirits out of the body, or make the body an uncomfortable place for the spirits to reside—often through extreme measures such as starving or beating the person. At other times, the person thought to be possessed by evil spirits would simply be killed.

One treatment for abnormality during the Stone Age and well into the Middle Ages may have been to drill holes in the skull of a person displaying abnormal behavior to allow the spirits to depart (Tatagiba, Ugarte, & Acioly, 2015). Archaeologists have found skulls dating back to a half-million years ago in which sections of the skull have been drilled or cut away. The tool used for this drilling is called a trephine, and the operation is called **trephination.** Some historians believe that people who were seeing or hearing things that were not real and people who were chronically sad were subjected to this form of brain surgery (Feldman & Goodrich, 2001). Presumably, if the person survived this surgery, the evil spirits would have been released and the person's abnormal behavior would decline. However, we cannot know with certainty that trephination was used to drive away evil spirits. Other historians suggest that it was used primarily for the removal of blood clots caused by stone weapons during warfare and for other medical purposes (W. Maher & B. Maher, 1985).

Some scholars believe that holes found in ancient skulls are from trephination, a crude form of surgery possibly performed on people acting abnormally.
Prisma/UIG via Getty Images

Ancient China: Balancing Yin and Yang

Some of the earliest written sources on abnormality are ancient Chinese medical texts (Tseng, 1973). The *Nei Ching* (Classic of Internal Medicine) was probably written around 2674 BCE by Huang Ti, the legendary third emperor of China.

Ancient Chinese medicine was based on the concept of yin and yang. The human body was said to contain a positive force (yang) and a negative force (yin), which confronted and complemented each other. If the two forces were in balance, the individual was healthy. If not, illness, including insanity, could result. For example, excited insanity was considered the result of an excessive positive force:

> The person suffering from excited insanity initially feels sad, eating and sleeping less; he then becomes grandiose, feeling that he is very smart and noble, talking and scolding day and night, singing, behaving strangely, seeing strange things, hearing strange voices, believing that he can see the devil or gods, etc. As treatment for such an excited condition, withholding food was suggested, because food was considered to be the source of positive force and the patient was thought to be in need of a decrease in such force (Tseng, 1973, p. 570).

Chinese medical philosophy also held that human emotions were controlled by internal organs. When the "vital air" was flowing on one of these organs, an individual experienced a particular emotion. For example, when air flowed on the heart, a person felt joy; when on the lungs, sorrow; when on the liver, anger; when on the spleen, worry; and when on the kidney, fear. This theory encouraged people to live in an orderly and harmonious way so as to maintain the proper movement of vital air.

Although the perspective on psychological symptoms represented by ancient texts was largely a biological one, the rise of Taoism and Buddhism during the Chin and T'ang dynasties (420–618 CE) led to some religious interpretations of abnormal behavior. Evil winds and ghosts were blamed for bewitching people and for inciting people's erratic emotional displays and uncontrolled behavior. Religious theories of abnormality declined in China after this period (Tseng, 1973).

Ancient Egypt, Greece, and Rome: Biological Theories Dominate

Other ancient writings on abnormal behavior are found in the papyri of Egypt and Mesopotamia (Veith, 1965). The oldest of these, a document known as the Kahun Papyrus after the ancient Egyptian city in which it was found, dates from about 1900 BCE. This document lists a number of disorders, each followed

Some of the earliest writings on mental disorders are from ancient Chinese texts. This illustration shows a healer at work.
Chronicle/Alamy Stock Photo

by a physician's judgment of the cause of the disorder and the appropriate treatment.

Several disorders apparently left people with unexplainable aches and pains, sadness or distress, and apathy about life. These disorders were said to occur only in women and were attributed to a "wandering uterus." The uterus was believed to wander around the body like an animal, hungry for semen. It could wander around the body creating various physical ailments, for example, if it wandered the wrong direction and made its way to the throat there would be choking, coughing, or loss of voice, if it got stuck in the the rib cage, there would be chest pain or shortness of breath (Kapsalis, 2017).

Most any symptom that belonged to a female body could be attributed to the wandering uterus. The diagnosis was a catch-all explanation for behavior that afflicted women throughout history and was not only prevalent in the West among mainly white women but it had its prehistory in Ancient Egypt, Greece, Italy, the Far East and Middle East as well. Later, the Greeks named this disorder *hysteria* (from the Greek word *hystera,* which means "uterus"). Various treatments existed within these different cultures for this phenomenon which included vaginal fumigations, bitter potions, balms, fragrances, and vaginal inserts made of wool, that were used to bring the uterus back to its proper place. The triad of marriage, sexual intercourse, and pregnancy was the ultimate treatment for the troublesome womb (Kapsalis, 2017).

These days, the term "hysteria" is outdated and no longer used in reference to physiological symptoms that are the likely result of psychological processes. Hysteria is undoubtedly the first psychological disorder associated with women with over 4,000 years of history. The phenomenon of the wandering uterus is an excellent example of how psychological disorders can be often misunderstood, misinterpreted, and generate pseudo-scientific prejudice and bias (Tasca, Rapetti, Carta, & Fadda, 2012).

Beginning with Homer, the Greeks wrote frequently of people acting abnormally (Wallace & Gach, 2008). The physician Hippocrates (460–377 BCE) described a case of a common phobia: A man could not walk alongside a cliff, pass over a bridge, or jump over even a shallow ditch without feeling unable to control his limbs or his vision becoming impaired.

Most average Greeks and Romans saw abnormal behavior as an affliction from the gods. Those afflicted retreated to temples honoring the god Aesculapius, where priests held healing ceremonies. Plato (423–347 BCE) and Socrates (469–399 BCE) argued that some forms of abnormal behavior were divine and could be the source of great literary and prophetic gifts.

For the most part, however, Greek physicians rejected supernatural explanations of abnormal behavior (Wallace & Gach, 2008). Hippocrates, often regarded as the father of medicine, argued that abnormal behavior was like other diseases of the body. According to Hippocrates, the body was composed of four basic humors: blood, phlegm, yellow bile, and black bile. All diseases, including abnormal behavior, were caused by imbalances in the body's essential humors. Based on careful observation of his many patients, which included listening to their dreams, Hippocrates classified abnormal behavior into four categories: epilepsy, mania, melancholia, and brain fever.

The treatments prescribed by the Greek physicians were intended to restore the balance of the four humors. Sometimes these treatments were physiological and intrusive, such as bleeding a patient to treat disorders that were thought to result from an excess of blood. Other treatments consisted of rest, relaxation, a change of climate or scenery, a change of diet, or living a temperate life. Some nonmedical treatments prescribed by these physicians sound remarkably like those prescribed by modern psychotherapists. Hippocrates, for example, believed that removing a patient from a difficult family could help restore mental health. Plato argued that insanity arose when the rational mind was overcome by impulse, passion, or appetite. Sanity could be regained through a discussion with the individual that was designed to restore rational control over emotions (W. Maher & B. Maher, 1985).

Among the Greeks of Hippocrates' and Plato's time, the relatives of people considered insane were encouraged to confine their afflicted family members to the home. The state claimed no responsibility for insane people; it provided no asylums or institutions, other than the religious temples, to house and care for them. The state could, however, take rights away from people declared insane. Relatives could bring suit against those they considered insane, and the state could award the property of insane people to their relatives. People declared insane could not marry or acquire or dispose of their own property. Poor people who were considered insane were simply left to roam the streets if they were not violent. If they were violent, they were locked away. The general public greatly feared insanity of any form, and many people thought to be insane were shunned or even stoned (W. Maher & B. Maher, 1985).

Medieval Views

The Middle Ages (around 400–1400 CE) are often described as a time of backward thinking dominated by an obsession with supernatural forces, yet even within Europe supernatural theories of abnormal behavior did not dominate until the late Middle Ages, between the eleventh and fifteenth centuries (Neugebauer, 1979). Prior to the eleventh century, witches and witchcraft were accepted as real but were considered mere nuisances, overrated by superstitious people. Severe emotional shock and physical illness or injury most often were seen as the causes of bizarre behaviors. For example, English court records attributed mental health problems to factors such as a "blow received on the head," explained that symptoms were "induced by fear of his father," and noted that "he has lost his reason owing to a long and incurable infirmity" (Neugebauer, 1979, p. 481). While laypeople probably did believe in demons and curses as causes of abnormal behavior, there is strong evidence that physicians and government officials in the early Middle Ages attributed abnormal behavior to physical causes or traumas.

Witchcraft

Beginning in the eleventh century, the power of the Catholic Church in Europe was threatened by the breakdown of feudalism and rebellions. The Church interpreted these threats in terms of heresy and Satanism. The Inquisition was established originally to rid the Earth of religious heretics, but eventually those practicing witchcraft or Satanism also became the focus of hunts. The witch hunts continued long after the Reformation, perhaps reaching their height during the fifteenth to seventeenth centuries—the period known as the Renaissance (Mora, 2008).

Some psychiatric historians have argued that persons accused of witchcraft must have been mentally ill (Veith, 1965; Zilboorg & Henry, 1941). Accused witches sometimes confessed to speaking with the devil, flying on the backs of animals, or engaging in other unusual behaviors. Such people may have been experiencing delusions (false beliefs) or hallucinations (unreal perceptual experiences), which are signs of some psychological disorders. However, confessions of such experiences may have been extracted through torture or in exchange for a stay of execution (Spanos, 1978).

In 1563, Johann Weyer published *The Deception of Dreams*, in which he argued that those accused of being witches were suffering from melancholy (depression) and senility. The Church banned Weyer's writings. Twenty years later, Reginald Scot, in his *Discovery of Witchcraft* (1584), supported Weyer's beliefs: "These women are but diseased wretches suffering from melancholy, and their words, actions, reasoning, and gestures show that sickness has affected their brains and impaired their powers of judgment" (Castiglioni, 1946, p. 253). Again, the Church—joined this time by the state—refuted the arguments and banned Scot's writings.

As is often the case, change came from within. In the sixteenth century, Teresa of Avila, a Spanish nun who was later canonized, explained that the mass hysteria that had broken out among a group of nuns was not the work of the devil but was the result of infirmities or sickness. She argued that these nuns were *comas enfermas,* or "as if sick." She sought out natural causes for the nuns' strange behaviors and concluded that they were due to melancholy, a weak imagination, or drowsiness and sleepiness (Sarbin & Juhasz, 1967).

The culture so completely accepted the existence of witches and witchcraft that some perfectly sane people may have self-identified as witches. In addition, most writings of medieval and Renaissance times, as well as writings from the witch hunt period in Salem, Massachusetts, clearly distinguish between people who were mad and people who were witches. The distinction between madness and witchcraft continues to this day in cultures that believe in witchcraft.

Psychic Epidemics

Psychic epidemics are defined as a phenomenon in which large numbers of people engage in unusual behaviors that appear to have a psychological origin. During the Middle Ages, reports of dance frenzies or manias were frequent. A monk, Peter of Herental, described a rash of dance frenzies that broke out over a 4-month period in 1374 in Germany:

> Both men and women were abused by the devil to such a degree that they danced in their homes, in the churches and in the streets, holding each other's hands and leaping in the air. While they danced they called out the names of demons, such as Friskes and others, but they were unaware of this nor did they pay attention to modesty even though people watched them. At the end of the dance, they felt such pains in the chest, that if their friends did not tie linen clothes tightly around their waists, they cried out like madmen that they were dying (Cited in Rosen, 1968, pp. 196–197).

Other instances of dance frenzy were reported in 1428 during the feast of Saint Vitus, at Schaffhausen, at which a monk danced himself to death. In 1518 a large epidemic of uncontrolled dance frenzy occurred at the chapel of Saint Vitus at Hohlenstein, near Zabern. According to one account, more than 400 people danced during the 4 weeks the frenzy lasted. Some writers of the time began to call the frenzied dancing Saint Vitus' dance.

A similar phenomenon, *tarantism,* was noted in Italy as early as the fourteenth century and became prominent in the seventeenth century. People suddenly developed an acute pain, which they attributed to the bite of a tarantula. They jumped around and danced wildly in the streets, tearing at their clothes and beating each other with whips. Some people dug holes in the earth and rolled on the ground; others howled and made obscene gestures. At the time, many

Some people burned at the stake as witches may have had mental disorders that caused them to act abnormally. *Bettmann/Getty Images*

people interpreted dance frenzies and tarantism as the results of possession by the devil. The behaviors may have been the remnants of ancient rituals performed by people worshiping the Greek god Dionysus.

We see episodes of psychic epidemics in modern times. On February 8, 1991, a number of students and teachers in a high school in Rhode Island thought they smelled noxious fumes coming from the ventilation system. The first person to detect these fumes, a 14-year-old girl, fell to the floor, crying and saying that her stomach hurt and her eyes stung. Other students and the teacher in that room then began to experience symptoms. They were moved into the hallway with a great deal of commotion. Soon students and teachers from adjacent rooms, who could see clearly into the hallway, began to experience symptoms. Eventually, 21 people (17 students and 4 teachers) were admitted to the local hospital emergency room. All were hyperventilating, and most complained of dizziness, headache, and nausea. Although some initially showed symptoms of mild carbon monoxide intoxication in blood tests, no evidence of toxic gas in the school could be found. The physicians treating the children and teachers concluded that the outbreak was a case of mass hysteria prompted by the fear of chemical warfare during the Persian Gulf War (Rockney & Lemke, 1992).

Psychic epidemics are no longer viewed as the result of spirit possession or the bite of a tarantula. Rather, psychologists attempt to understand them through research from social psychology on the influence of others on individuals' self-perceptions. The social context can affect even our perceptions of our own bodies, as we will see when we discuss people's differing reactions to psychoactive substances such as marijuana (see the chapter "Substance Use and Gambling Disorders") and people's interpretations of their physical sensations (see the chapter "Somatic Symptom and Dissociative Disorders").

The Spread of Asylums

As early as the twelfth century, many towns in Europe took some responsibility for housing and caring for people considered mentally ill (Kroll, 1973). Remarkable among these towns was Gheel, Belgium, where townspeople regularly took into their homes the mentally ill who were visiting the shrine of Saint Dymphna for cures.

In about the eleventh or twelfth century, general hospitals began to include special rooms or facilities for people exhibiting abnormal behavior. The mentally ill were little more than inmates in these early hospitals, housed against their will, often in extremely harsh conditions. One of the most famous of these hospitals was the Hospital of Saint Mary of Bethlehem,

Bedlam—the Hospital of Saint Mary of Bethlehem in London—was famous for the chaotic and deplorable conditions in which people with mental disorders were kept. *SOTK2011/Alamy Stock Photo*

in London, which officially became a mental hospital in 1547. This hospital, nicknamed Bedlam, was famous for its deplorable conditions. At Bedlam and other mental hospitals established in Europe in the sixteenth, seventeenth, and eighteenth centuries, patients were exhibited to the public for a fee. They lived in filth and confinement, often chained to the wall or locked inside small boxes. The following description of the treatment of patients in La Bicêtre Hospital, an asylum for male patients in Paris, provides an example of typical care:

> The patients were ordinarily shackled to the walls of their dark, unlighted cells by iron collars which held them flat against the wall and permitted little movement. Often there were also iron hoops around the waists of the patients and both their hands and feet were chained. Although these chains usually permitted enough movement that the patients could feed themselves out of bowls, they often kept them from being able to lie down at night. Since little was known about dietetics, and the patients were presumed to be animals anyway, little attention was paid to whether they were adequately fed or whether the food was good or bad. The cells were furnished only with straw and were never swept or cleaned; the patient remained in the midst of all the accumulated ordure. No one visited the cells except at feeding time, no provision was made for warmth, and even the most elementary gestures of humanity were lacking. (Adapted from Selling, 1940, pp. 54–55)

The laws regarding the confinement of the mentally ill in Europe and the United States were concerned with the protection of the public and the ill person's relatives (Busfield, 1986; Scull, 1993). For example, Dalton's 1618 edition of *Common Law* states that "it is lawful for the parents, kinsmen or other friends of a man that is mad, or frantic . . . to take him and put him into a house, to bind or chain him, and to beat him with rods, and to do any other forcible act to reclaim him, or to keep him so he shall do no hurt" (Alldderidge, 1979).

The first Act for Regulating Madhouses in England was passed in 1774, with the intention of cleaning up the deplorable conditions in hospitals and madhouses and protecting people from being unjustly jailed for insanity. This act provided for the licensing and inspection of madhouses and required that a physician, a surgeon, or an apothecary sign a certificate before a patient could be admitted. The act's provisions applied only to paying patients in private madhouses, however, and not to the poor people confined to workhouses.

These asylums typically were established and run by people who thought that abnormal behaviors were medical illnesses. For example, Benjamin Rush (1745–1813), one of the founders of American psychiatry, believed that abnormal behavior was caused by excessive blood in the brain and prescribed bleeding the patient, or drawing huge amounts of blood from the body. Thus, although the supernatural

In the medieval and early modern periods, doctors used bleeding to treat people with mental disorders and many other ailments.
Photo Researchers/Science History Images/Alamy Stock Photo

theories of the Middle Ages have often been decried as leading to brutal treatment of people with mental illnesses, the medical theories of those times and of the next couple of centuries did not always lead to better treatment.

Moral Treatment in the Eighteenth and Nineteenth Centuries

The eighteenth and nineteenth centuries saw the growth of a more humane treatment of people with mental health problems, a period known as the **mental hygiene movement.** This new treatment was based on the psychological view that people developed problems because they had become separated from nature and had succumbed to the stresses imposed by the rapid social changes of the period (Rosen, 1968). The prescribed treatment, including prayers and incantations, was rest and relaxation in a serene and physically appealing place.

A leader of the movement for **moral treatment** of people with abnormality was Philippe Pinel (1745–1826), a French physician who took charge of La Bicêtre in Paris in 1793. Pinel argued, "To detain maniacs in constant seclusion and to load them with chains; to leave them defenceless, to the brutality of underlings . . . in a word, to rule them with a rod of iron . . . is a system of superintendence, more distinguished for its convenience than for its humanity or success" (Grob, 1994, p. 27). Pinel believed that many forms of abnormality could be cured by restoring patients' dignity and tranquility.

Pinel ordered that patients be allowed to walk freely around the asylum. They were provided with clean and sunny rooms, comfortable sleeping quarters, and good food. Nurses and professional therapists were trained to work with the patients to help them regain their sense of tranquility and engage in planned social activities. Although many physicians thought Pinel himself was mad for releasing the patients from confinement, his approach was remarkably successful. Many people who had been locked away in darkness for decades became able to control their behavior and reengage in life. Some improved so much that they could be released from the asylum. Pinel later successfully reformed La Salpêtrière Hospital, a mental hospital for female patients in Paris (Grob, 1994).

In 1796 the Quaker William Tuke (1732–1822) opened an asylum in England, called The Retreat, in direct response to the brutal treatment he saw being delivered at other facilities to people with abnormal behavior. Tuke's treatment was designed to restore patients' self-restraint by treating them with respect and dignity and encouraging them to exercise self-control (Grob, 1994).

One of the most militant crusaders for moral treatment of the insane was Dorothea Dix (1802–1887). A retired schoolteacher living in Boston, Dix visited a jail on a cold Sunday morning in 1841 to teach a Sunday school class to women inmates. There she discovered the negligence and brutality that characterized the treatment of poor people exhibiting abnormal behavior, many of whom were simply warehoused in jails.

That encounter began Dix's tireless quest to improve the treatment of people with mental health problems. Dix's lobbying efforts led to the passage of laws and appropriations to fund the cleanup of mental hospitals and the training of mental health professionals dedicated to the moral treatment of patients. Between 1841 and 1881, Dix personally helped establish more than 30 mental institutions in the United States, Canada, Newfoundland, and Scotland. Hundreds more public hospitals for the insane established during this period by others were run according to humanitarian perspectives.

Unfortunately, the moral treatment movement grew too fast. As more asylums were built and more people went into them, the capacity of the asylums to recruit mental health professionals and to maintain a humane, individual approach to each patient declined (Grob, 1994; Scull, 1993). The physicians, nurses, and other caretakers simply did not have enough time to give each patient the calm and dedicated attention needed. The fantastic successes of the early moral treatment movement gave way to more modest successes, and to many outright failures, as patients remained impaired or their condition worsened. Even some patients who received the best moral treatment could not benefit from it because their problems were not due to a loss of dignity or tranquility. With so many patients receiving moral treatment, the number of patients who failed to benefit from it increased, and questions about its effectiveness grew louder (Grob, 1994).

At the same time, the rapid pace of immigration into the United States in the late nineteenth century meant that an increasing percentage of its asylum patients were from different cultures and often from the lower socioeconomic classes. Prejudice against these "foreigners," combined with increasing attention to the failures of moral treatment, led to declines in public support for funding such institutions. Reduced funding led to even greater declines in the quality of care. At the turn of the twentieth century, many public hospitals were no better than warehouses (Grob, 1994; McGovern, 1985; Scull, 1993).

Effective treatments for most major mental health problems were not developed until well into the twentieth century. Until then, patients who could not afford private care were warehoused in large, overcrowded,

Philippe Pinel, a leader in the moral movement in France, helped free mental patients from the horrible conditions of the hospitals. *GL Archive/Alamy Stock Photo*

physically isolated state institutions that did not offer treatment (Deutsch, 1937).

THE EMERGENCE OF MODERN PERSPECTIVES

Although the treatment of people who exhibited abnormal behavior unfortunately deteriorated at the turn of the twentieth century, this period of time also saw tremendous advances in the scientific study of disorders. These advances laid the groundwork for the biological, psychological, and social theories of abnormality that now dominate psychology and psychiatry.

The Beginnings of Modern Biological Perspectives

Basic knowledge of the anatomy, physiology, neurology, and chemistry of the body increased rapidly in the late nineteenth century. With the advancement of this basic knowledge came an increasing focus on biological causes of abnormality. In 1845, German psychiatrist Wilhelm Griesinger (1817–1868) published *The Pathology and Therapy of Psychic Disorders,* presenting a systematic argument that all psychological disorders can be

Dorothea Dix fought for the moral treatment of mental patients in the United States. *Library of Congress Prints and Photographs Division [LC-USZ62-9797]*

Emil Kraepelin (1856–1926) developed a classification system for mental disorders that remains influential today.
Hulton Archives/Getty Images

explained in terms of brain pathology. In 1883 one of Griesinger's followers, Emil Kraepelin (1856-1926), also published a text emphasizing the importance of brain pathology in psychological disorders. More important, Kraepelin developed a scheme for classifying symptoms into discrete disorders that is the basis for our modern classification systems (Kendler & Engstrom, 2016), as we will discuss in the chapter "Assessing and Diagnosing Abnormality." Having a good classification system gives investigators a common set of terms for various disorders, as well as, a set of criteria for distinguishing between them, contributing immensely to the advancement of the scientific study of the disorders.

One of the most important discoveries underpinning modern biological theories of abnormality was the discovery of the cause of **general paresis,** a disease that leads to paralysis, insanity, and eventually death (Duffy, 1995). In the mid-1800s, reports that patients with paresis also had a history of syphilis led to the suspicion that syphilis might be a cause of paresis. In 1897, Viennese psychiatrist Richard Krafft-Ebing injected paretic patients with matter from syphilitic sores. None of the patients developed syphilis, and Krafft-Ebing concluded that they must already have been infected with it. The discovery that syphilis is the cause of one form of insanity lent great weight to the idea that biological factors can cause abnormal behaviors (Duffy, 1995).

As we will discuss in more detail in the chapter "Theories and Treatment of Abnormality," modern biological theories of the psychological disorders have focused on the role of genetics, structural and functional abnormalities in the brain, and biochemical imbalances. The advances in our understanding of the biological aspects of psychological disorders have contributed to the development of therapeutic medications.

The Psychoanalytic Perspective

The development of psychoanalytic theory begins with the odd story of Franz Anton Mesmer (1734–1815), an Austrian physician who believed that people have a magnetic fluid in the body that must be distributed in a particular pattern in order to maintain health. The distribution of magnetic fluid in one person could be influenced by the magnetic forces of other people, as well as by the alignments of the planets. In 1778 Mesmer opened a clinic in Paris to treat all sorts of diseases by applying animal magnetism.

The psychological disorders that were the focus of much of Mesmer's treatment were the hysterical disorders, in which people lose functioning or feeling in some part of the body for no apparent physiological reason. His patients sat in darkness around a tub containing various chemicals, and the affected areas of their bodies were prodded by iron rods emerging from the tub. With music playing, Mesmer emerged wearing an elaborate robe, touching each patient as he passed by, supposedly realigning people's magnetic fluids through his own powerful magnetic force. This process, Mesmer said, cured illness, including psychological disorders.

Mesmer eventually was labeled a charlatan by a scientific review committee that included Benjamin Franklin. Yet his methods, known as **mesmerism,** continued to fuel debate long after he had faded into obscurity. The "cures" Mesmer effected in his psychiatric patients were attributed to the trancelike state that Mesmer seemed to induce in his patients. Later this state was labeled hypnosis. Under hypnosis, Mesmer's patients appeared very suggestible, and the mere suggestion that their ailments would disappear seemed enough to make them actually disappear.

The connection between hypnosis and hysteria fascinated several leading scientists of the time, although not all scientists accepted this connection. In particular, Jean Charcot (1825–1893), head of La Salpêtrière Hospital in Paris and the leading neurologist of his time, argued that hysteria (now known as *functional neurological symptom disorder*) was caused by degeneration in the brain. The work of two physicians practicing in the French town of Nancy, Hippolyte-Marie Bernheim (1840–1919) and Ambroise-Auguste Liebault (1823–1904), eventually won over Charcot, however. Bernheim and Liebault showed that they could induce the symptoms of hysteria, such as paralysis in an arm or the loss of feeling in a leg, by suggesting these symptoms to patients who were hypnotized. Fortunately, they could also remove these symptoms under hypnosis. Charcot was so impressed by the evidence that hysteria has psychological roots that he became a leading researcher of the psychological causes of abnormal behavior. The experiments of Bernheim and Liebault, along with the leadership of Charcot, did a great deal to advance psychological perspectives on abnormality.

One of Charcot's students was Sigmund Freud (1856–1939), a Viennese neurologist who went to study with Charcot in 1885. In the course of this work, Freud became convinced that much of the mental life of an individual remains hidden from consciousness. This view was further supported by

Freud's interactions with Pierre Janet (1859–1947) in Paris. Janet was investigating multiple personality disorder, in which people appear to have multiple, distinct personalities, each of which operates independently of the others, often not knowing the others exist (Matarazzo, 1985).

When he returned to Vienna, Freud worked with Josef Breuer (1842–1925), another physician interested in hypnosis and in the unconscious processes behind psychological problems. Breuer had discovered that encouraging patients to talk about their problems while under hypnosis led to a great upwelling and release of emotion, which eventually was called catharsis. The patient's discussion of his or her problems under hypnosis was less censored than conscious discussion, allowing the therapist to elicit important psychological material more easily.

Breuer and Freud collaborated on a paper published in 1893 as *On the Psychical Mechanisms of Hysterical Phenomena,* which laid out their discoveries about hypnosis, the unconscious, and the therapeutic value of catharsis. This paper proved to be a foundation stone in the development of **psychoanalysis,** the study of the unconscious. Freud introduced his ideas to America in 1909 in a series of lectures at Clark University in Worcester, Massachusetts, at the invitation of G. Stanley Hall, one of the founders of American psychology.

Freud wrote dozens of papers and books on his theory of psychoanalysis (discussed in detail in the chapter "Theories and Treatment of Abnormality"), and he became one of the best-known figures in psychiatry and psychology. The impact of Freud's theories on the development of psychology over the next century cannot be overstated. Freudian ideas not only influenced the professional literature on psychopathology but also are used heavily in literary theory, anthropology, and other humanities. They pervade popular notions of psychological processes to this day.

The Roots of Behaviorism

In what now seems like a parallel universe, while psychoanalytic theory was being born, the roots of behaviorism were being planted first in Europe and then in the United States. Ivan Pavlov (1849–1936), a Russian physiologist, developed methods and theories for understanding behavior in terms of stimuli and responses rather than in terms of the internal workings of the unconscious mind. He discovered that dogs could be conditioned to salivate when presented with stimuli other than food if the food was paired with these other stimuli—a process later called **classical conditioning.** Pavlov's discoveries inspired American John Watson (1878–1958) to study

important human behaviors, such as phobias, in terms of classical conditioning (see the chapter "Obsessive-Compulsive, Trauma and Stressor-Related Disorders"). Watson rejected psychoanalytic and biological theories of abnormal behaviors such as phobias and explained them entirely on the basis of the individual's history of conditioning. Watson (1930) went so far as to boast that he could train any healthy child to become any kind of adult he wished:

> Give me a dozen healthy infants, well-formed, and my own specified world to bring them up in, and I'll guarantee to take any one at random and train him to be any type of specialist I might select—doctor, lawyer, artist, merchant-chief, and yes, even beggar-man and thief, regardless of his talents, penchants, tendencies, abilities, vocations, and the race of his ancestors (p. 104).

At the same time, two other psychologists, E. L. Thorndike (1874–1949) and B. F. Skinner (1904–1990), were studying how the consequences of behaviors shape their likelihood of recurrence. They argued that behaviors followed by positive consequences are more likely to be repeated than are behaviors followed by negative consequences. This process came to be known as operant, or instrumental, conditioning. This idea may seem simple to us now (one sign of how much it has influenced thinking over the past century), but at the time it was considered radical to argue that even complex behaviors, such as violence against others, can be explained by the reinforcement or punishment these behaviors have received in the past.

Behaviorism—the study of the impact of reinforcements and punishments on behavior—has had as profound an impact on psychology and on our common knowledge of psychology, as has psychoanalytic theory. Behavioral theories have led to many of the effective psychological treatments for disorders that we will discuss in this book.

The Cognitive Revolution

In the 1950s, some psychologists argued that behaviorism was limited in its explanatory power by its refusal to look at internal thought processes that mediate the relationship between stimulus and response. It wasn't until the 1970s that psychology shifted its focus substantially to the study of **cognitions.** Cognitions are thought processes—like attention, interpretation of events, and beliefs—that influence behavior and emotion. The cognitive revolution shifted perspectives toward such internal processes. An important pioneer in this cognitive revolution was Albert Bandura, a clinical psychologist trained in behaviorism who had contributed a great deal to the application of behaviorism to psychopathology (see the chapters "Theories and Treatment of Abnormality" and "Obsessive-Compulsive, Trauma and Stressor-Related Disorders"). Bandura argued that people's beliefs about their ability to execute the behaviors necessary to control important events—which he called **self-efficacy beliefs**—are crucial in determining people's well-being. Again, this idea seems obvious to us now, but only because it took hold in both professional psychology and lay notions of psychology.

Another key figure in cognitive perspectives was Albert Ellis, who argued that people prone to psychological disorders are plagued by irrational negative assumptions about themselves and the world. Ellis developed a therapy for emotional problems based on his theory called rational-emotive therapy. This therapy was controversial because it required therapists to challenge, sometimes harshly, their patients' irrational belief systems. It became very popular, however, and moved psychology into the study of the thought processes behind serious emotional problems. Another therapy, developed by Aaron Beck, focused on the irrational thoughts of people with psychological problems. Beck's cognitive therapy has become one of the most widely used therapies for many disorders (see the chapter "Theories and Treatment of Abnormality"). Since the 1970s, theorists have continued to emphasize cognitive factors in psychopathology, although behavioral theories have remained strong as interpersonal theories, which we examine in the chapter "Theories and Treatment of Abnormality," have become more prominent.

MODERN MENTAL HEALTH CARE

Halfway through the twentieth century, major breakthroughs were made in drug treatments for some of the major forms of abnormality. In particular, the discovery of a class of drugs that can reduce hallucinations and delusions, known as the phenothiazines (see the chapter "Theories and Treatment of Abnormality"), made it possible for many people who had been institutionalized for years to be released from asylums and hospitals. Since then, there has been an explosion of new drug therapies for psychopathology. The biomedical approach has revolutionized the way we understand and treat mental disorders as biological phenomena. In addition, as we will discuss in the chapter "Theories and Treatment of Abnormality," several types of psychotherapy have been developed that have proven effective in treating a wide range of psychological problems. However, there are still significant problems in the

delivery of mental health care, some of which began with the deinstitutionalization movement of the mid-twentieth century.

Deinstitutionalization

By 1960 a large and vocal movement known as the **patients' rights movement** had emerged. Patients' rights advocates argued that mental patients can recover more fully or live more satisfying lives if they are integrated into the community, with the support of community-based treatment facilities—a process known as **deinstitutionalization.** While many of these patients would continue to need around-the-clock care, it could be given in treatment centers based within the community rather than in large institutions where conditions were often poor. In the United States, the **community mental health movement** was officially launched in 1963 by President John Kennedy as a "bold new approach" to mental health care. *The Mental Retardation Facilities and Community Mental Health Center Construction Act* (1963) promoted the release of psychiatric patients from long-term care facilities to short-term and community mental health centers. A direct result of this legislation resulted in the mass closures of psychiatric institutions and long-term care facilities across the United States. The goal of this movement was to offer less restrictive, more humane treatment options and provide coordinated mental health services to people in **community mental health centers,** a move that had both positive and negative consequences.

The deinstitutionalization movement had a massive effect on the lives of people with serious psychological problems. Between 1955 and 2016, the number of patients in state psychiatric hospitals in the United States declined from a high of 559,000 to about 38,000 despite overall population growth, resulting in a rate lower than that before the moral treatment movement (Allison et al., 2018; Fuller, Sinclair, Geller, Quanbeck, & Snook, 2016; Lamb & Weinberger, 2016). Parallel trends were also seen in Europe. Many former psychiatric patients who lived for years in cold, sterile facilities, receiving little useful care, experienced improvements in their quality of life upon their release. Most importantly, these clients were now able to integrate back into the community with support services in place. Rather than living in highly restrictive conditions, deinstitutionalization promoted community-based interventions and better quality of life for those with mental illness.

Several types of community-based treatment facilities were created as part of deinstitutionalization and continue to serve people with mental health problems today. Community mental health centers often include teams of social workers, therapists, and physicians who coordinate care for services within the community, rather than long-term inpatient hospitals. **Halfway houses** offer people with long-term mental health problems the opportunity to live in a structured, supportive environment as they try to reestablish working relationships with family and friends. **Day treatment centers,** which are also known as partial hospitalization programs (PHP), provide more intensive therapy to those in need. Clients in these programs receive approximately 25 hours of psychiatric, occupational, and rehabilitative therapies during the day while residing at home during recovery. These programs are less intensive than inpatient or residential programs, in which participants live at the treatment facility. There are a variety of treatment sites which offer varying levels of care for people in need (Khawaja & Westermeyer, 2010; Ruffalo, 2018).

While the goal is to provide the least restrictive methods of care to those with mental illness, there are times in which hospitalization is necessary. People who experience acute psychiatric symptoms that require hospitalization may go to inpatient units of general hospitals or specialized psychiatric hospitals for treatment. Unlike institutionalization, inpatient hospitalizations are considerably shorter. The average length of stay for an inpatient psychiatric admission is approximately 3 to 10 days. Once their acute problems have subsided, however, they often are released back to a community-based treatment center to continue their care, rather than remaining in a psychiatric hospital. Brief hospitalizations, referred to as *micro-admissions,* and the practice of short-term care reflects one goal of deinstitutionalization, but it has also led to a less effective treatment with poor outcomes for many clients. In reality, the effective treatment of serious mental health issues require time. These brief hospitalizations are often not long enough for treatment to begin working before the client is released. Many of the chronically ill are hospitalized and rehospitalized every few weeks which has created a revolving door within acute crisis and inpatient units (Ruffalo, 2019; Allison et al., 2018).

The results of community mental health movement have significantly impacted the treatment methods for those with psychological disorders in both positive and negative ways. Deinstitutionalization was designed to enhance the quality of life for people in public psychiatric hospitals, but in reality many people left institutions only to find a life of poverty and neglect on the outside due, in part, to underfunding of community mental health programs. Although deinstitutionalization was well intended, it has been criticized for failing to live up to its expectations. Unfortunately, the resources to care for all the psychiatric patients released from institutions have never been adequate. There were not enough halfway houses built or community mental health centers funded to serve the thousands of men and women who formerly were institutionalized or would have been institutionalized if the movement had not taken place (Figure 1). Meanwhile, the state psychiatric hospitals to which former patients would have retreated were closed down by the hundreds. The community mental health movement spread to Europe, with similar consequences. Twenty-eight percent of European countries have few or no community-based services for people with serious mental health problems (Semrau, Barley, Law, & Thornicroft, 2011; WHO World Mental Health Survey Consortium, 2004).

Men and women released from psychiatric institutions began living in nursing homes and other types of group homes, where they received little mental health treatment, or with their families, many of whom were unprepared to handle the challenges of serious mental illness (Lamb & Weinberger, 2016). An unforeseen consequence of deinstitutionalization, was the significant increase in homelessness among discharged psychiatric patients. Certainly not all homeless people are mentally ill, but according to the White House Council of Economic Advisors (2019), 20 percent (111,122 people) of the homeless in the United States had a severe mental illness (SMI) and 86,647 homeless people (16 percent) suffered from chronic substance abuse.

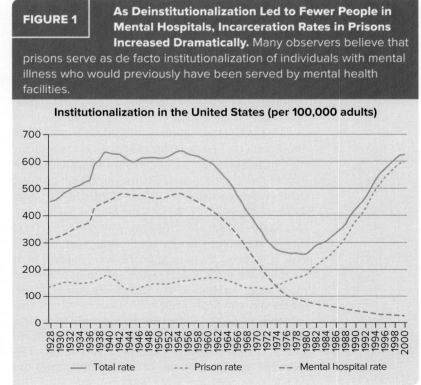

FIGURE 1 **As Deinstitutionalization Led to Fewer People in Mental Hospitals, Incarceration Rates in Prisons Increased Dramatically.** Many observers believe that prisons serve as de facto institutionalization of individuals with mental illness who would previously have been served by mental health facilities.

Institutionalization in the United States (per 100,000 adults)

— Total rate   - - - Prison rate   — — Mental hospital rate

Although estimates of the prevalence of mental illness vary, studies examining mental illness in the homeless population have generally found a high prevalence of psychological disorders. Various research studies suggest that approximately 20 to 50 percent of the homeless population suffer from SMI and the most common disorders may be alcohol and drug dependence (Balasuriya, Buelt, & Tsai, 2020; Center for Substance Abuse Treatment, 2013; Tinland et al., 2020). Some researchers estimate that up to four-fifths of all long-term homeless adults in the United States and Europe have a major mental disorder, a severe substance use disorder (such as alcohol use disorder), or both (WHO World Mental Health Survey Consortium, 2004). Homelessness and mental illness are intricately connected, and each contributes to the existence of the other. This reciprocal phenomenon forces victims to live in a vicious cycle from which an escape is difficult. People with SMI across the world may become homeless as a direct result of the symptoms of their illness, or as the consequence of eroded social and economic networks, or both. In turn, the experience of homelessness can both precipitate and exacerbate symptoms of mental illness (Moorkath, Vranda, & Naveenkumar, 2018; Smartt et al., 2019).

Deinstitutionalization resulted in the closures of most US public psychiatric hospitals and the reduction in acute general psychiatric beds over recent decades which directly impacts the amount of services available today. These closures have led to a crisis in mental health treatment, as the overall inpatient capacity has not kept pace with the needs of patients with psychiatric disorders (Bastiampillai, Sharfstein, & Allison, 2016). Due to the lack of accessible treatment, many people with SMI may end up in hospitals for short periods of time which operate at a reduced capacity and may not be able to provide adequate treatment. Alternatively, people with mental illness often become part of the criminal justice system.

Unprecedented numbers of people with mental illness are now housed in jails and prisons throughout the United States and around the world in lieu of more humane and appropriate facilities in which to treat them (Bastiampillai et al., 2016; Haney, 2017; Lamb & Weinberger, 2017). Across the United States, correctional facilities are struggling with the reality that they have become the nation's de facto mental health care providers, even though these facilities are ill equipped for the job. The prison system has replaced psychiatric hospitals as the largest institutions housing people with SMI. The criminal justice system now contends with tens of thousands of people with mental illness who, by some counts, make up as much as half of their inmate populations (Roth, 2018). Despite the good intentions of deinstitutionalization, people with SMI are being transinstitutionalized to the criminal justice system. This limited access to inpatient treatment is also associated with higher suicide risk, premature mortality, homelessness, violent crime, and incarceration. People with mental illness are among the most disadvantaged members of our society, and when they end up in the criminal justice system, they tend to fare worse than others (Allison et al., 2018).

Studies of prison inmates suggest that two-thirds had experienced some form of diagnosable mental disorder in their lifetime. Serious mental illness affects men and women in jail at rates four to six times higher than in the general population and 60 percent of jail inmates reported having had symptoms of a mental health disorder in the 12 months prior to incarceration. Despite these high rates of psychological disorders among inmates, 83 percent did not receive mental health care after admission, according to recent studies (Heis, Swavola, & Kang-Brown, 2015; Trestman, Ford, Zhang, & Wiesbrock, 2007).

Thus, although deinstitutionalization began with commendable goals designed to enhance the lives of people with psychological disorders, many of these goals were never fully reached. As a result, deinstitutionalization impacted the mental health care system in profound ways that have not adequately served a majority of people with mental illness. In recent years, the financial strains on local, state, and federal governments have led to the closing of many community

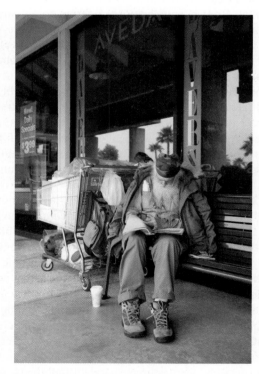

Deinstitutionalization led to a rise in homelessness among people with mental illnesses, who often go untreated.
mikeledray/Shutterstock

mental health centers which has led to less effective and humane care for those in need of mental health services. The overarching goal for those reading this book, who hope to become part of this system, must be to help create a new and better mental health care system that provides comprehensive and appropriate levels of care for people with psychological disorders.

Managed Care

The entire system of private insurance for health care in the United States underwent a revolution in the second half of the twentieth century, when managed care emerged as the dominant means for organizing health care. **Managed care** is a collection of methods for coordinating care that ranges from simple monitoring to total control over what care can be provided and paid for. The goals are to coordinate services for an existing medical problem and to prevent future medical problems. Often, health care providers are given a set amount of money per member (patient) per month and then must determine how best to serve each patient.

Managed care can address some of the problems created by deinstitutionalization. For example, instead of leaving it up to people with a serious psychological problem, or their families, to find appropriate care, the primary provider might find this care and ensure that patients have access to it. Suppose an individual patient reported to his physician that he was hearing voices when no one was around. The physician might refer the patient to a psychiatrist for an evaluation to determine if the patient might be suffering from schizophrenia. In some cases, the primary care physician might coordinate care offered by other providers, such as drug treatments, psychotherapy, and rehabilitation services. The primary provider also might ensure continuity of care so that patients do not "fall through the cracks." Thus, theoretically, managed care can have tremendous benefits for people with long-term, serious mental health problems. For people with less severe psychological problems, the availability of mental health care through managed care systems and other private insurance systems has led to a large increase in the number of people seeking psychotherapy and other types of mental health care.

In the past, there was a significant disparity for those who needed mental health care as compared to those in need to traditional medical care. Even now, depending upon one's insurance coverage, mental health services many not be fully covered by insurance plans, and many people do not have health insurance in the United States. Laws have been passed in recent years that are intended to increase the availability of coverage for mental health services, but these laws are currently being contested. The Affordable Care Act

(ACA), passed in 2010, requires insurance plans to cover mental health and substance abuse treatment, and acknowledges the increasing role of primary care providers in psychiatric treatment. The ACA expanded mental health care access in the United States for those already insured, and it is estimated that millions of severely mentally ill people will newly acquire coverage. Prior to the ACA, most behavioral health insurance benefits were separate and unequal compared with benefits for treatment of general medical and surgical conditions. Lack of equity raised the risk of bankruptcy or financial hardship due to mental health expenditures (Druss & Goldman, 2018; Mechanic & Olfson, 2016). However, the current mental health system has yet to fully adjust to sweeping changes, and health care policy remains a complex, controversial, and shifting political territory with clear implications for people with mental disorders. Mental health services are expensive. Because mental health problems are sometimes chronic, mental health treatment can take a long time.

CASE STUDY

Khloe needs long-term care

Fifty-four-year-old, Khloe has a long history psychological dysfunction that has resulted in multiple hospitalizations throughout her adult life. Since her early twenties, Khloe has battled severe symptoms of major depressive disorder that have significantly disrupted her ability to function. Khloe would often engage in self-injury and suicide attempts during depressive episodes, which routinely put her life in danger. As a young adolescent who lacked appropriate coping skills, Khloe would often engage in self-harm, such as cutting her thighs and upper arms, when she felt emotionally unstable. Upon her recent admission to the psychiatric crisis unit of the local hospital, Khloe had attempted suicide by drinking small amounts of a household cleaning product and cut both wrists. This attempt was serious enough to require sutures on her wrists and the contents of her stomach to be pumped out to save her life.

When assessed by the psychiatric crisis team, Khloe reported that she had intended to end her life due to the depressive feelings she was experiencing and if given the opportunity to leave the hospital she would "finish the job" and attempt suicide again. Due to the severity of her symptoms and concern about her safety, the psychiatric crisis team recommended that Khloe be admitted for inpatient treatment. During her assessment in the crisis unit, Khloe expressed

(continued)

the desire to improve, despite her suicidal ideation, and agreed to go into the hospital for help. During the process to admit her for inpatient services, the screener was unable to get insurance authorization for her care since she had already been hospitalized that year. Khloe's insurance provider suggested that she be placed in an outpatient program, rather than the intensive inpatient treatment she needed. Despite the insurance company's request, Khloe received inpatient treatment for major depression and suicidal ideation.

After 8 days of treatment, Khloe was released from the hospital and referred to an intensive outpatient clinic to continue her therapy and manage her medication. While Khloe did improve during her inpatient stay, she was not fully stabilized before she left the program and shortly after her discharge, she stopped taking her medication and slipped further into a depressive episode. Within only a few weeks of her last visit to the psychiatric crisis unit, Khloe returned after another suicide attempt. However, during this attempt, Khloe ingested large amounts of household cleaning products which caused extensive internal damage resulting in multi-system organ failure. Despite best interventions, the injury inflicted was too serious for her recover.

Since deinstitutionalization was passed, there are many people in need of long-term mental health care. In an effort to reduce restrictive care for many, a system of short-term care was created that does not always adequately address the needs of people living with serious mental illness, like Khloe.

The Medicaid program, which covers one-quarter of all mental health care spending in the United States, has been a target for reductions in recent years, even as the number of people seeking mental health care has risen. Many states have reduced or restricted eligibility and benefits for mental health care, increased co-payments, controlled drug costs, and reduced or frozen payments to providers (Shirk, 2008). At the same time, reductions in state and city welfare programs and other community services targeted at the poor have made daily life more difficult for poor people in general, and in particular for people with serious mental disorders, who often have exhausted their financial resources. In the Medicaid managed care context, states have employed various tools to promote equal access to treatment for mental illness including benefit mandates, risk adjustment, insurance coverage appeals, reporting requirements, and behavioral health carve-outs. Careful assessment, development, and implementation of such tools is essential in addressing undertreatment for behavioral

health issues, including mental illness and substance use disorder (Lawrence, 2020).

Mental illnesses, including substance use disorder, routinely go untreated or undertreated, with tragic results. Research suggests that a substantial number of adults with psychological disorders do not receive treatment for their condition, despite overall increases in the rates of treatment in the past 20 years. The National Comorbidity Survey Replication (2015), reported that only 33 percent of adults with any mental illness and 41 percent of adults with serious mental illness reported receiving mental health treatment in the previous year. People who are less likely to receive treatment tend to be male, Black or Hispanic, younger, uninsured, and of low socioeconomic status (Walker et al., 2015). Other studies suggest that only 50 to 60 percent of people in the United States with serious psychological problems receive stable mental health treatment, with much lower percentages receiving care in less-developed and poorer countries (Kessler et al., 2001; Lawrence, 2020; Wang et al., 2007). For example, in wealthier countries in Europe, such as Finland and Belgium, have more than 20 mental health experts per 100,000 people, whereas poorer countries such as Turkey and Tajikistan have fewer than 2 mental health experts per 100,000 people (Semrau et al., 2011).

Low rates of treatment and unmet needs are persistent among adults with mental illness. Sometimes, people refuse care that might help them, but other times they fall through holes in the health care safety net because of bureaucratic rules designed to shift the burden of mental health care costs from one agency to another, as in the case of Khloe. Recent research suggests that there are many barriers to mental health treatment which include structural barriers, such as cost, lack of insurance or insufficient coverage for services, and not knowing where to go for help or not being able to get an appointment, and attitudinal barriers, such as perceived stigma and perceiving treatments to be ineffective (Walker et al., 2015).

It is also important to consider subpopulations at risk for not receiving mental health treatment. Studies suggest that Black and Hispanic respondents were less likely than non-Hispanic whites to receive treatment. Regardless of insurance status, there are differences among racial groups in terms of seeking out treatment. Distrust of health care providers, low perceived efficacy of treatment, internalized stigma of mental disorders, and loss of income due to taking time off from work for appointments are key reasons among minorities for not seeking mental health treatment. Culturally tailored interventions may be helpful in overcoming barriers to mental health services. In order to improve access to mental health services, additional strategies to reduce both structural barriers, such as cost and insurance coverage, and attitudinal barriers are needed (Walker et al., 2015).

As we discuss the research showing the effectiveness of various treatments for specific disorders throughout the remainder of the book, it is important to keep in mind that those treatments can work only if people have access to them.

Professions Within Abnormal Psychology

There are a number of professional opportunities for those interested in working to improve the quality of life for people with psychological disorders. *Psychiatrists* have an MD degree and have received specialized training in the treatment of psychological disorders. This medical doctor could have become a cardiologist, for example, but selected psychiatric medicine as a specialty. Psychiatrists can prescribe medications for the treatment of these problems and have been trained to conduct psychotherapies as well.

Clinical psychologists typically have a PhD in psychology, with a specialization in treating and researching psychopathology. Another option is a PsyD degree which is a doctoral degree from a graduate program that emphasizes clinical training more than research training. Clinical psychologists conduct various forms of psychotherapy, but in most states they do not currently prescribe medications. (They do have limited prescription privileges in some states, and psychologists are lobbying for prescription privileges in many others.)

There are many master's-level career options which include *marriage and family therapists (MFT)* who specialize in helping families, couples, and children overcome problems that are interfering with their well-being. *Clinical social workers* have a master's degree in social work (MSW) and often focus on helping people with psychological problems overcome social conditions that are contributing to their problems, such as joblessness or homelessness. Some states have *licensed mental health counselors,* individuals who have graduate training in counseling beyond the bachelor's degree in counseling but have not obtained a PhD. These professionals have completed required course work and passed a licensing exam. *Psychiatric nurses* have a degree in nursing, with a specialization in the treatment of people with severe psychological problems. They often work on inpatient psychiatric wards in hospitals, delivering medical care and certain forms of psychotherapy, such as group therapy to increase patients' contacts with one another. In some states, they have privileges to write prescriptions for psychotherapeutic drugs.

Each of these professions has its rewards and limitations. Students who are interested in one or more of these professions often find it helpful to volunteer as a research assistant in studies of psychological problems or for work in a psychiatric clinic or hospital. Some students find tremendous gratification working with people with psychological problems, whereas others find it more gratifying to conduct research that might answer important questions about these problems. Many mental health professionals of all types combine clinical practice and research in their careers.

CHAPTER INTEGRATION

Although the biological, psychological, and social theories of abnormality have traditionally been viewed as competing with one another to explain psychological disorders, many clinicians and researchers now believe that theories that integrate biological, psychological, and social perspectives on abnormality will prove most useful (Figure 2). For example, in the chapter "Obsessive-Compulsive, Trauma and Stressor-Related Disorders," we discuss theories of anxiety disorders that take into account individuals' genetic and biochemical vulnerabilities, the impact of stressful events, and the role of cognition in explaining why some people suffer debilitating anxiety. Throughout this book, we will emphasize how biological, psychological, and social factors interact with and influence one another to produce and maintain mental health problems. In other words, we will present an integrationist approach to psychological problems.

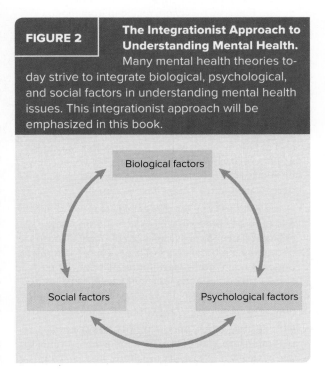

FIGURE 2 **The Integrationist Approach to Understanding Mental Health.** Many mental health theories today strive to integrate biological, psychological, and social factors in understanding mental health issues. This integrationist approach will be emphasized in this book.

SHADES OF GRAY   DISCUSSION

Our society highly values extreme thinness in women, and Jennifer has received substantial reinforcement for her weight loss. Thus, we see her behaviors as not very deviant. Her dieting causes her some dysfunction and distress: She is having trouble concentrating in school and is terrified of gaining weight. But her weight loss is also bringing her social benefits. Are her behaviors dangerous? Extremely thin women risk medical complications such as reduced bone density and heart arrhythmias (see the chapter "Eating Disorders"). So Jennifer's behaviors are somewhat dysfunctional, distressing, and dangerous, but they are so typical of women her age that people will differ in whether they believe her behaviors qualify as abnormal.

Mark's behaviors also seem familiar, because drinking is considered a "rite of passage" by some students. Mark drinks considerably more than most young men (see the chapter "Substance Use and Gambling Disorders"), so his level of drinking is deviant. He also has experienced some dysfunction as a result of his drinking: He has gotten in legal trouble and his grades are low. Mark certainly doesn't seem distressed about his drinking. Mark's behaviors are dangerous: He is more likely to be involved in accidents while drunk and risks alcohol poisoning from the volume he consumes. So Mark's behaviors might be considered more abnormal than Jennifer's behaviors, but people will differ on the degree of abnormality.

Would your judgments of the abnormality of these behaviors change if it were Jennifer who was drinking heavily and Mark who was dieting excessively to lose weight? Cultural norms for thinness and for drinking alcohol differ significantly for women and men. Gender strongly influences our views of normality and abnormality.

CHAPTER SUMMARY

- Cultural relativists argue that the norms of a society must be used to determine the normality of a behavior. Others have suggested that unusual behaviors, or behaviors that cause subjective distress in a person, should be labeled abnormal. Still others have suggested that only behaviors resulting from mental illness or disease are abnormal. All these criteria have serious limitations, however.

- The current consensus among professionals is that behaviors that cause a person to suffer distress, prevent him or her from functioning in daily life, are unusual or deviant, and pose a threat to the person or others are abnormal. These criteria can be remembered as the four Ds: dysfunction, distress, deviance, and dangerousness. Abnormal behaviors fall along a continuum from adaptive to maladaptive, and the location of the line designating behaviors as disordered is based on a subjective decision.

- Historically, theories of abnormality have fallen into one of three categories. Biological theories saw psychological disorders as similar to physical diseases, caused by the breakdown of a system of the body. Supernatural theories saw abnormal behavior as a result of divine intervention, curses, demonic possession, and personal sin. Psychological theories saw abnormal behavior as being a result of stress.

- In prehistoric times, people probably had largely supernatural theories of abnormal behavior, attributing it to demons or ghosts. In the Stone Age, drilling holes in the skull to allow demons to depart, a procedure known as trephination, might have been a treatment for abnormality.

- Ancient Chinese, Egyptian, and Greek texts suggest that these cultures took a biological view of abnormal behavior, although references to supernatural and psychological theories also can be found.

- During the Middle Ages, abnormal behavior may have been interpreted as being due to witchcraft.

- In psychic epidemics and mass hysterias, groups of people show similar psychological and behavioral symptoms. Usually, these have been attributed to common stresses or beliefs.

- Even well into the nineteenth and twentieth centuries, many people who acted abnormally were shut away in prisonlike conditions, tortured, starved, or ignored.

- As part of the mental hygiene movement, the moral management of mental hospitals became more widespread. Patients in these hospitals were treated with kindness and given the best biological treatments available. However, effective biological treatments for most psychological problems were not available until the mid-twentieth century.

- Modern biological perspectives on psychological disorders were advanced by Kraepelin's development of a classification system and the discovery that general paresis is caused by a syphilis infection.

- The psychoanalytic perspective began with the work of Anton Mesmer. It grew as Jean Charcot, and eventually Sigmund Freud, became interested in the role of the unconscious in producing abnormality.

- Behaviorist views on abnormal behavior began with John Watson and B. F. Skinner, who used principles of classical and operant conditioning to explain normal and abnormal behavior.

- Cognitive theorists such as Albert Ellis, Albert Bandura, and Aaron Beck focused on the role of thinking processes in abnormality.

- The deinstitutionalization movement attempted to move mental patients from mental health facilities to community-based mental health centers. Unfortunately, community-based mental health centers have never been fully funded or supported, leaving many former mental patients with few resources in the community.

- Managed care systems are meant to provide coordinated, comprehensive medical care to patients. They can be a great asset to people with long-term, serious psychological disorders.

- The professions within abnormal psychology include psychiatrists, psychologists, marriage and family therapists, clinical social workers, licensed mental health counselors, and psychiatric nurses.

KEY TERMS

continuum model of abnormality

psychopathology

stigma

cultural relativism

biological theories

supernatural theories

psychological theories

trephination

psychic epidemics

mental hygiene movement

moral treatment

general paresis

mesmerism

psychoanalysis

classical conditioning

behaviorism

cognitions

self-efficacy beliefs

patients' rights movement

deinstitutionalization

community mental health movement

community mental health centers

halfway houses

day treatment centers

managed care

Chapter 2

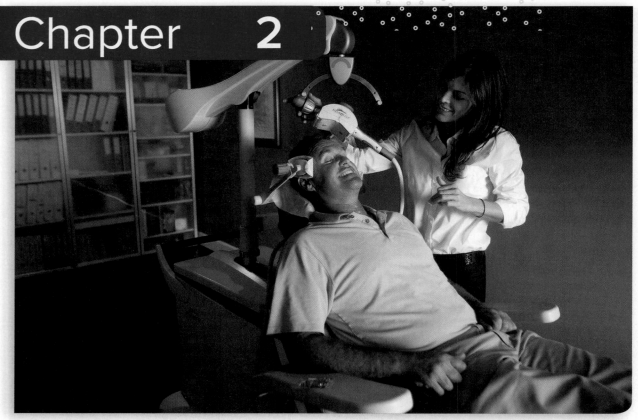

Bruce R. Bennett/The Palm Beach Post/ZUMAPRESS/Alamy Stock Photo

Theories and Treatment of Abnormality

CHAPTER OUTLINE

Approaches Along the Continuum

Extraordinary People: Steven Hayes

Biological Approaches

Psychological Approaches

Shades of Gray

Sociocultural Approaches

Prevention Programs

Common Elements in Effective Treatments

Chapter Integration

Shades of Gray Discussion

Chapter Summary

Key Terms

Approaches Along the Continuum

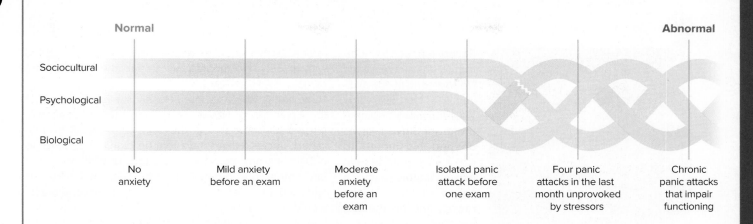

Normal					Abnormal
No anxiety	Mild anxiety before an exam	Moderate anxiety before an exam	Isolated panic attack before one exam	Four panic attacks in the last month unprovoked by stressors	Chronic panic attacks that impair functioning

Sociocultural
Psychological
Biological

In this chapter, we discuss three general approaches to understanding psychological disorders. The **sociocultural approach** views these disorders as the result of environmental conditions and cultural norms. The **biological approach** views disorders as the result of abnormal genes or neurobiological dysfunction. The **psychological approach** views disorders as the result of thinking processes, personality styles, emotions, and conditioning.

People who favor a sociocultural approach generally view psychological disorders as falling along a continuum because they do not view these disorders as vastly different from normal functioning. Instead, they think of psychological disorders as labels that society puts on people whose behaviors and feelings differ from social and cultural norms (Chu & Leino, 2017). While they agree that these behaviors may be dysfunctional, distressing, deviant, and dangerous, they see them as understandable consequences of social stress in the individuals' lives.

A decade ago, proponents of the biological approach generally did not accept a continuum model of abnormality. Instead, they viewed psychological disorders as either present or absent—much the way they viewed medical or physical disorders (such as cancer). In recent years, however, proponents of biological approaches have embraced a continuum perspective on abnormality, seeing disorders as collections of deficits in fundamental neurobiological processes (Beauchaine & Constantino, 2017; Cuthbert & Insel, 2013; Hyman, 2010). For example, the symptoms of schizophrenia are increasingly viewed as problems in cognition and emotional processing that are due to deficits in specific areas of the brain. These problems in cognition and emotional processing can range from very mild to very severe, causing symptoms that also vary along a continuum from mild to severe. In other words, a person can have "a little bit of schizophrenia" or can exhibit significantly more symptoms, to the point of qualifying for a diagnosis of schizophrenia.

Psychological approaches to disorders have also been moving toward a continuum model of psychopathology in recent years (Clark, Cuthbert, Lewis-Fernández, Narrow, & Reed, 2017). According to these approaches, psychological processes such as cognition, learning, and emotional control also fall along a continuum that ranges from very typical to highly dysfunctional. Minor learning difficulties, for example, would be placed on the more "typical" end of the continuum, and severe intellectual disabilities on the "dysfunctional" end. Likewise, problems in emotional control might range from feeling blue (typical) to feeling severely depressed with suicidal intentions (dysfunctional). A continuum perspective would suggest that people on the less severe end of the spectrum (who do not meet the criteria for the disorder) give us insight into the behavior of those on the more severe end (those who do meet the criteria).

As we discuss in this chapter, the sociocultural, biological, and psychological approaches are increasingly being integrated into a biopsychosocial approach to mental disorders. This integrative approach suggests that factors along the continua of biological dysfunction, psychological dysfunction, and sociocultural risks interweave to create the problems we call mental disorders.

Extraordinary People

Steven Hayes

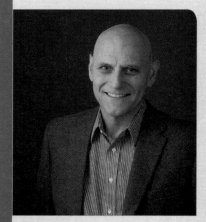

Photo by Drew Altizer, Courtesy of Steven C. Hayes

Sitting in a faculty meeting in the Psychology Department at the University of North Carolina at Greensboro, assistant professor Steven Hayes opened his mouth to make a point and found himself unable to utter a sound. His heart began racing, and he thought he might be having a heart attack. He was only 29. The episode passed, but a week later he had a similar experience in another meeting. Over the next 2 years, his attacks of absolute panic became more frequent and began dominating his life. He had great difficulty lecturing and couldn't be in an enclosed place, such as a movie theater or an elevator, without being engulfed with anxiety. He thought his career and his life were over.

Now, nearly 30 years later, Hayes is a full professor at the University of Nevada and one of the most accomplished psychologists in the field, with over 300 published articles. Hayes says that he didn't overcome his debilitating anxiety with medications or with any of the psychotherapies prominent in the 1980s, when he was suffering the most. Instead, he learned to accept that he would have anxiety attacks and to stop fighting them. Out of his experiences, he developed a new form of psychological therapy, called *acceptance and commitment therapy* or *ACT*. This therapy teaches individuals with psychological problems to be more accepting and compassionate toward themselves, to commit to their values, and to use meditation practices that help them live more in the present moment. ACT is one of the hottest of the *third-wave approaches* to psychotherapy, which we discuss later in this chapter.

Steven Hayes was able to integrate his personal experiences with his training in psychology to develop a new theory and therapy of his own. A **theory** is a set of ideas that provides a framework for asking questions about a phenomenon and for gathering and interpreting information about that phenomenon. A *therapy* is a treatment, usually based on a theory of a phenomenon, that addresses those factors the theory says cause the phenomenon.

Hayes believed that his anxiety attacks were due to the inability to accept his symptoms, but other theories suggest alternative causes. If you took a biological approach to abnormality, you would suspect that Hayes' symptoms were caused by a biological factor, such as a genetic vulnerability to anxiety, inherited from his parents. The psychological approach, like Hayes' approach, looks for the causes of abnormality in people's beliefs, life experiences, and relationships. Finally, if you took a sociocultural approach, you would consider the ways Hayes' cultural values or social environment might affect his anxiety.

Traditionally, these different approaches have been seen as incompatible. People frequently ask, "Is the cause of these symptoms biological *or* psychological *or* environmental?" This question is often called the nature-nurture question: Is the cause of psychological problems something in the nature or biology of the person, or is it in the person's nurturing or history of events to which the person was exposed? This question implies that such problems must have a single cause, rather than multiple causes. Indeed, most theories of psychological problems over history have searched for the one factor—the one gene, the one traumatic experience, the one personality trait—that causes people to develop a particular set of symptoms.

Many contemporary theorists, however, take a **biopsychosocial approach,** recognizing that the development of psychological symptoms often results from a combination of biological, psychological, and sociocultural factors. These factors are often referred to as *risk factors,* because they increase the risk of psychological problems. Risk factors can be biological, such as a genetic predisposition. They may also be psychological, such as difficulty remaining calm in stressful situations. Or they may be sociocultural, such as growing up with the stress of discrimination based on ethnicity or race.

Certain risk factors may lead to specific types of symptoms; for example, a specific gene, known as DISC1, appears to substantially increase the risk of developing schizophrenia, bipolar disorder, and depression. However, there is some debate among researchers about its significance as a proven etiological

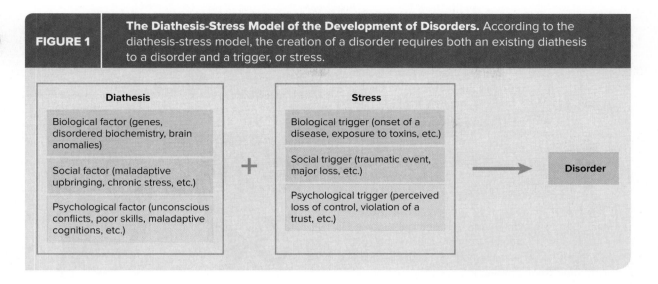

FIGURE 1

The Diathesis-Stress Model of the Development of Disorders. According to the diathesis-stress model, the creation of a disorder requires both an existing diathesis to a disorder and a trigger, or stress.

Diathesis

Biological factor (genes, disordered biochemistry, brain anomalies)

Social factor (maladaptive upbringing, chronic stress, etc.)

Psychological factor (unconscious conflicts, poor skills, maladaptive cognitions, etc.)

Stress

Biological trigger (onset of a disease, exposure to toxins, etc.)

Social trigger (traumatic event, major loss, etc.)

Psychological trigger (perceived loss of control, violation of a trust, etc.)

Disorder

factor (Cannon et al., 2005; Sullivan, 2013; Thompson et al., 2013). More commonly, however, risk factors create increased risk for a number of different problems. For instance, severe stress, such as being the victim of childhood abuse, is associated with increased risk of developing a wide range of psychopathologies (Keyes et al., 2012). Factors that increase risk for multiple types of psychological problems are referred to as *transdiagnostic risk factors* (Krueger, & Eaton, 2015; Nolen-Hoeksema & Watkins, 2011). We will discuss several biological, psychological, and sociocultural transdiagnostic risk factors in this book.

In many cases, a risk factor may not be enough to lead a person to develop severe psychological symptoms. It may take some other experience or trigger for psychopathology to develop. Again, this trigger can be biological, such as an illness that changes a person's hormone levels. Or the trigger can be psychological or social, such as a traumatic event. Only when the risk factor and the trigger or stress come together in the same individual does the full-blown disorder emerge. This situation is often referred to as a **diathesis-stress model** (*diathesis* is another term for risk factor) (Figure 1). Although Hayes may indeed have had a genetic or personality vulnerability to anxiety (his diathesis), it may have been only when he experienced particular stressors that he developed significant anxiety.

Each of the different approaches to abnormality has led to treatments meant to relieve the symptoms people suffer. Proponents of biological theories of mental disorders most often prescribe medication, although several other types of biological treatments are discussed in this book. Proponents of psychological and some sociocultural approaches to abnormality most often prescribe psychotherapy. There are

many forms of psychotherapy, but most involve a therapist (psychiatrist, psychologist, clinical social worker, or counselor) talking with the person suffering from psychological problems (typically called a patient or client) about their symptoms and what is contributing to these symptoms. The specific topic of these conversations depends on the therapist's theoretical approach. Both medications and psychotherapy have proven effective in the treatment of many types of psychological symptoms. Medications and psychotherapy are often used together in an integrated approach, although use of medications alone has increased in recent years (Weissman & Cuijpers, 2017). Proponents of sociocultural approaches also may work to change social policies or the social conditions of vulnerable individuals so as to improve their mental health.

In this chapter, we introduce the major theories of abnormality that have dominated the field in its modern history, along with the treatments that derive from these theories. We present the theories and treatments one at a time to make them easier to understand. Keep in mind, however, that most mental health professionals now take an integrated biopsychosocial approach to understanding mental health problems, viewing them as the result of a combination of biological, psychological, and social risk factors and stresses that come together and feed off one another. We will discuss these integrated biopsychosocial approaches throughout this book.

BIOLOGICAL APPROACHES

Consider the story of Phineas Gage, one of the most dramatic examples of the effect of biological factors on psychological functioning.

CASE STUDY

On September 13, 1848, Phineas P. Gage, a 25-year-old construction foreman for the Rutland and Burlington Railroad in New England, became the victim of a bizarre accident. On the fateful day, an accident led to a powerful explosion that sent a fine-pointed tamping iron which was 3½ feet long, 1.25 inches in diameter, and weighing 13 lbs, hurling, rocketlike, through Gage's face, skull, and brain. The force of the explosion caused the tamping iron to rocket out of the top of Phineas' skull landing about 80 feet away. Gage was momentarily stunned but regained full consciousness immediately after. He was able to talk and even walk with the help of his men.

Phineas Gage not only survived the momentous injury, in itself enough to earn him a place in the annals of medicine, but he survived as a different man. Gage had been a responsible, intelligent, and socially well-adapted individual, a favorite with peers and elders. He had made progress and showed promise. The signs of a profound change in personality were already evident during his convalescence under the care of his physician, John Harlow. But as the months passed, it became apparent that the transformation was not only radical but difficult to comprehend. In some respects Gage was fully recovered. He remained as able-bodied and appeared to be as intelligent as before the accident, he had no impairment of movement or speech, new learning was intact, and neither memory nor intelligence in the conventional sense had been affected. However, he had become irreverent and capricious. His respect for the social conventions by which he once abided had vanished. His abundant use of profanity offended those around him. Perhaps most troubling, he had taken leave of his sense of responsibility. He could not be trusted to honor his commitments. His employers had deemed him "the most efficient and capable" man in their employ but now they had to dismiss him. In the words of his physician, "the equilibrium or balance, so to speak, between his intellectual faculty and animal propensities" had been destroyed. In the words of his friends and acquaintances, "Gage was no longer Gage." (Adapted from Damasio, Grabowski, Frank, Galaburda, & Damasio, 1994, p. 1102)

This accident destroyed much of Gage's left frontal lobe of the cerebral cortex and basic elements of his personality were noted to have changed. Gage was transformed from a responsible, well-liked, and socially competent man into an impulsive, emotional, and socially inappropriate man after the brain injury.

FIGURE 2   Phineas Gage's Brain Injury. Modern neuroimaging techniques have helped identify the precise location of damage to Phineas Gage's brain.

Photo Researchers/Science History Images/Alamy Stock Photo

It has been suggested that many of these symptoms were temporary and his function improved with time which supports the idea that Gage's brain recovered, to some degree.

Recent research suggests that the basis of recovery stems from neuroplasticity, which is the ability of neuronal circuits to adapt and modify connections on both a structural and functional level, ranging from molecular, synaptic, and cellular changes to more global network changes (García-Molina, 2012; Sophie Su, Veeravagu, & Grant, 2018; Turolla, Venneri, Farina, Cagnin, & Cheung, 2018). Almost 150 years later, researchers using modern neuroimaging techniques on Gage's preserved skull and a computer simulation of the tamping-iron accident determined the precise location of the damage to Gage's brain (Figure 2).

Injury to the frontal lobe can result in disruptions to the brain's executive functions which represent higher level cognitive abilities. Attention, inhibition, social cognition and interpersonal behavior, the ability to infer others' mental states are just some of the functions associated with the frontal cortex. Damage to this area of the brain can result in problems with planning, organizing, and prioritizing; problems with attention, exhibit poor judgment, and an inability to monitor and adapt behavior consistent with changing social circumstances. The frontal lobe plays an essential role in contextual adjustment and social interactions, as in those conditions in which it is required to focus on a specific behavior despite distractions or temptations; to make a plan for the future; or to voluntarily switch from one activity to another (Puglisi et al., 2018; Wood & Worthington, 2017).

The damage Gage suffered caused areas of his brain to not function properly. *Brain dysfunction* is one of three causes of abnormality on which biological approaches often focus. The other two are biochemical imbalances and genetic abnormalities. Brain dysfunction, biochemical imbalances, and genetic abnormalities can all influence one another. For example, brain dysfunction may be the result of genetic factors and may cause biochemical imbalances. We explore these three biological causes of abnormality in this section.

Brain Dysfunction

Like Phineas Gage, people whose brains do not function properly often show problems in psychological functioning. The brain can be divided into three main regions: the hindbrain, which includes all the structures located in the hind (posterior) part of the brain, closest to the spinal cord; the midbrain, located in the middle of the brain; and the forebrain, which includes

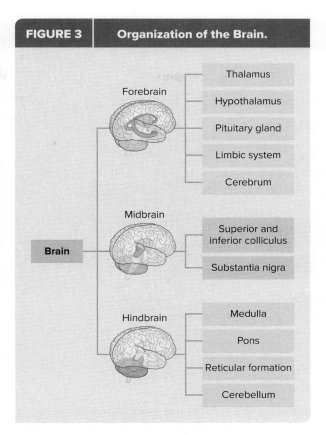

FIGURE 3 | Organization of the Brain.

the structures located in the front (anterior) part of the brain (Figures 3 and 4). The hindbrain sits on top of the spinal cord and is crucial for basic life functions. It contains the medulla, which helps control

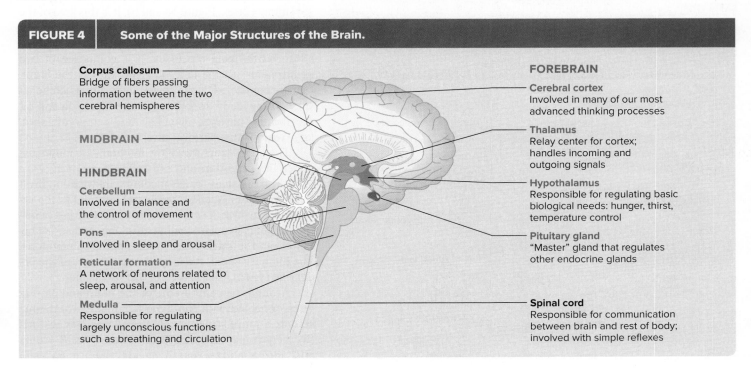

FIGURE 4 | Some of the Major Structures of the Brain.

Corpus callosum
Bridge of fibers passing information between the two cerebral hemispheres

MIDBRAIN

HINDBRAIN

Cerebellum
Involved in balance and the control of movement

Pons
Involved in sleep and arousal

Reticular formation
A network of neurons related to sleep, arousal, and attention

Medulla
Responsible for regulating largely unconscious functions such as breathing and circulation

FOREBRAIN

Cerebral cortex
Involved in many of our most advanced thinking processes

Thalamus
Relay center for cortex; handles incoming and outgoing signals

Hypothalamus
Responsible for regulating basic biological needs: hunger, thirst, temperature control

Pituitary gland
"Master" gland that regulates other endocrine glands

Spinal cord
Responsible for communication between brain and rest of body; involved with simple reflexes

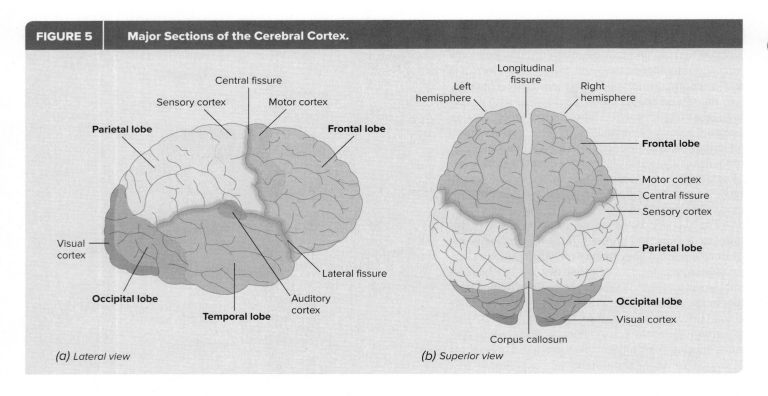

FIGURE 5 | **Major Sections of the Cerebral Cortex.**

(a) Lateral view

(b) Superior view

breathing and reflexes; the pons, which is important for attentiveness and the timing of sleep; the reticular formation, a network of neurons that control arousal and attention to stimuli; and the cerebellum, which is concerned primarily with the coordination

of movement. The midbrain contains the superior colliculus and inferior colliculus, which relay sensory information and control movement, and the substantia nigra, a crucial part of the pathway that regulates responses to reward.

The human forebrain is relatively large and developed compared to that of other organisms. The outer layer of the cerebrum is called the **cerebral cortex** (or simply cortex; Figure 5a and b); it is this area of the brain that was damaged in Phineas Gage's accident. The cerebral cortex is involved in many of our most advanced thinking processes. It is composed of two hemispheres, on the left and right sides of the brain, that are connected by the corpus callosum. Each hemisphere is divided into four lobes (see Figure 5a and b): the frontal, parietal, occipital, and temporal lobes, large regions that perform diverse functions.

The other structures of the forebrain are found just under the cerebrum and are called *subcortical structures*. The **thalamus** directs incoming information from sense receptors (such as vision and hearing) to the cerebrum. The **hypothalamus,** a small structure just below the thalamus, regulates eating, drinking, and sexual behavior, and is involved in processing basic emotions. The pituitary gland, the most important part of the endocrine system, is discussed in the next section.

Around the central core of the brain and closely interconnected with the hypothalamus is the **limbic system,** a set of structures that regulate many instinctive behaviors, such as reactions to stressful events and eating and sexual behavior (Figure 6). The

FIGURE 6 | **Structures of the Limbic System.** The limbic system is a collection of structures that are closely interconnected with the hypothalamus. They appear to exert additional control over some of the instinctive behaviors regulated by the hypothalamus, such as eating, sexual behavior, and reaction to stressful situations.

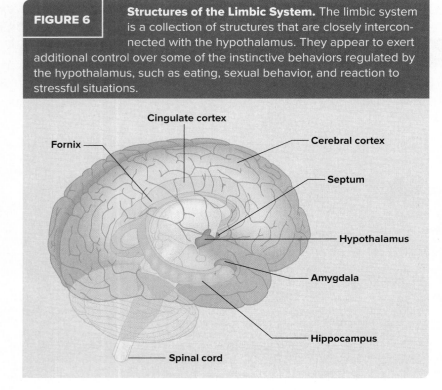

amygdala is a structure of the limbic system that is critical in emotions such as fear. Monkeys with damage to the limbic system sometimes become chronically aggressive, reacting with rage to the slightest provocation. At other times, they become exceptionally passive, not reacting at all to real threats. The hippocampus is a part of the limbic system that plays a role in memory.

Brain dysfunction can result from injury, such as a head injury from a car accident, or from diseases that cause brain deterioration, such as Alzheimer's disease. In this book you will see that certain areas of the brain are associated with a wide range of psychological functions. For example, alterations in the size or activity of the frontal cortex are associated with schizophrenia, a severe disorder in which people have hallucinations (unreal perceptual experiences) and delusions (unreal beliefs); with depression; and with attention-deficit/hyperactivity disorder (ADHD), among other disorders. We will also consider examples of how environmental and psychological factors can change brain functioning. For example, a number of studies have shown that psychotherapy alone, without drug therapy, can change brain activity (Barsaglini, Sartori, Benetti, Pettersson-Yeo, & Mechelli, 2014; Malhotra & Sahoo, 2017).

Biochemical Imbalances

The brain requires a number of biochemicals in order to work efficiently and effectively. These chemicals include neurotransmitters and hormones, the latter produced by the endocrine system.

Neurotransmitters

Neurotransmitters are biochemicals that act as messengers carrying impulses from one neuron, or nerve cell, to another in the brain and in other parts of the nervous system (Figure 7). Each neuron has a cell body and a number of short branches, called dendrites. The dendrites and cell body receive impulses from adjacent neurons. The impulse then travels down the length of a slender, tubelike extension, called an axon, to small swellings at the end of the axon, called synaptic terminals. Here the impulse stimulates the release of neurotransmitters.

The synaptic terminals do not actually touch the adjacent neurons. There is a slight gap between the synaptic terminals and the adjacent neurons, called the *synaptic gap* or synapse. The neurotransmitter is released into the synapse. It then binds to special receptors—molecules on the membrane of adjacent neurons. This binding works somewhat the way a key fits into a lock. The binding stimulates the adjacent neuron to initiate the impulse, which then runs through its dendrites and cell body and down its axon to cause the release of more neurotransmitters between it and other neurons.

Many biochemical theories of psychopathology suggest that the amount of certain neurotransmitters in the synapses is associated with specific types of psychopathology. The amount of a neurotransmitter available in the synapse can be affected by two processes. The process of reuptake occurs when the initial neuron releasing the neurotransmitter into the synapse reabsorbs the neurotransmitter, decreasing the amount left in the synapse. Another process, degradation, occurs when the receiving neuron releases an enzyme into the synapse that breaks down the neurotransmitter into other biochemicals. Degradation also occurs when the releasing neuron provides an enzyme. The reuptake and degradation of neurotransmitters happen naturally. When one or both of these processes malfunction, abnormally high or low levels of neurotransmitter in the synapse result.

FIGURE 7   **Neurotransmitters and the Synapse.** The neurotransmitter is released into the synaptic gap. There it may bind with the receptors on the postsynaptic membrane.

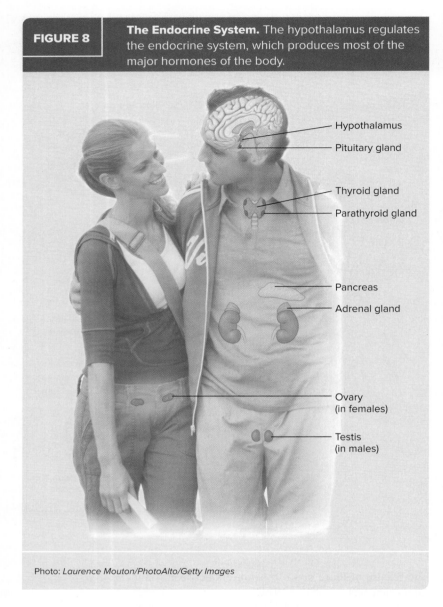

FIGURE 8 **The Endocrine System.** The hypothalamus regulates the endocrine system, which produces most of the major hormones of the body.

Hypothalamus
Pituitary gland
Thyroid gland
Parathyroid gland
Pancreas
Adrenal gland
Ovary (in females)
Testis (in males)

Photo: *Laurence Mouton/PhotoAlto/Getty Images*

Scientists have identified more than 100 different neurotransmitters. *Serotonin* is a neurotransmitter that travels through many key areas of the brain, affecting the function of those areas. You will see throughout this book that dysfunction in the system regulating serotonin is a transdiagnostic risk factor, associated with several different types of psychopathology. It plays an important and complicated role in emotional well-being, particularly in depression and anxiety, and in dysfunctional behaviors, such as aggressive impulses (Albert, Benkelfat, & Descarries, 2012).

Dopamine is a prominent neurotransmitter in those areas of the brain associated with our experience of reinforcements or rewards, and it is affected by substances, such as alcohol, that we find rewarding (Volkow, Wise, & Baler, 2017). Dopamine also is important to the functioning of muscle systems and plays a role in disorders involving control over muscles, such as Parkinson's disease. Thus, dopamine dysfunction is also a transdiagnostic risk factor.

Norepinephrine (also known as noradrenaline) is a neurotransmitter produced mainly by neurons in the brain stem. Two well-known drugs, cocaine and amphetamine, prolong the action of norepinephrine by slowing its reuptake process. Because of the delay in reuptake, the receiving neurons are activated for a longer period of time, which causes the stimulating psychological effects of these drugs, Conversely, when there is too little norepinephrine in the brain, the person's mood is depressed. Another prominent neurotransmitter is gamma-aminobutyric acid, or GABA, which inhibits the action of other neurotransmitters. Certain drugs have a tranquilizing effect because they increase the inhibitory activity of GABA. GABA is thought to play an important role in anxiety symptoms, so one contributor to Steven Hayes' anxiety could be a dysfunction in his GABA system.

The Endocrine System

Other biochemical theories of psychopathology focus on the body's **endocrine system** (Figure 8). This system of glands produces chemicals called hormones, which are released directly into the blood. A **hormone** carries messages throughout the body, potentially affecting a person's mood, level of energy, and reaction to stress. One of the major endocrine glands, the **pituitary,** has been called the *master gland* because it produces the largest number of different hormones and controls the secretion of other endocrine glands. It lies just below the hypothalamus.

The relationship between the pituitary gland and the hypothalamus illustrates the complex interactions between the endocrine and central nervous systems. For example, in response to stress (fear, anxiety, pain, and so forth), neurons in the hypothalamus secrete a

Psychological symptoms may also be associated with the number and functioning of the receptors for neurotransmitters on the dendrites. If there are too few receptors or if the receptors are not sensitive enough, the neuron will not be able to make adequate use of the neurotransmitter available in the synapse. If there are too many receptors or if they are too sensitive, the neuron may be overexposed to the neurotransmitter that is in the synapse. Within the neuron, a complex system of biochemical changes takes place as the result of the presence or absence of neurotransmitters. Psychological symptoms may be the consequence of malfunctioning in neurotransmitter systems; also, psychological experiences may cause changes in neurotransmitter system functioning.

substance called corticotropin-release factor (CRF). CRF is carried from the hypothalamus to the pituitary through a channel-like structure. The CRF stimulates the pituitary to release the body's major stress hormone, adrenocorticotrophic hormone (ACTH). ACTH, in turn, is carried by the bloodstream to the adrenal glands and to various other organs of the body, causing the release of about 30 hormones, each of which plays a role in the body's adjustment to emergency situations.

As we will discuss in the chapters "Trauma, Anxiety, Obsessive-Compulsive, and Related Disorders" and "Mood Disorders and Suicide," some theories of anxiety and depression suggest that these disorders result from dysregulation, or malfunctioning, of a system called the *hypothalamic-pituitary-adrenal axis* (or HPA axis). People who have a dysregulated HPA axis may have abnormal physiological reactions to stress that make it more difficult for them to cope with the stress, resulting in symptoms of anxiety and depression.

The proper working of the neurotransmitter and endocrine systems requires a delicate balance, and many forces can upset this balance. For example, chronic stress can cause dysregulation in neurotransmitter and endocrine systems that persists even after the stress has subsided.

Genetic Abnormalities

Behavioral genetics, the study of the genetics of personality and abnormality, is concerned with the extent to which behaviors or behavioral tendencies inherited and identifying the processes by which genes affect behavior (Loehlin, 2009).

Let us begin by reviewing the basics of genetics. At conception, the normal fertilized embryo has 46 chromosomes, 23 from the female egg and 23 from the male sperm, making up 23 pairs of chromosomes. One of these pairs is referred to as the sex chromosomes because it determines the sex of the embryo: The XX combination results in a female embryo, and the XY combination results in a male embryo. The mother of an embryo always contributes an X chromosome, and the father can contribute either an X or a Y.

Alterations in the structure or number of chromosomes can cause major defects. Down syndrome results when an extra chromosome is present on the 21st pair. Rather than the expected two chromosomes in this spot, there are three which produce very specific characteristics among all people with Down syndrome such as intellectual disabilities, heart malformations, and facial features such as a flat face, a small nose, protruding lips and tongue, and slanted eyes.

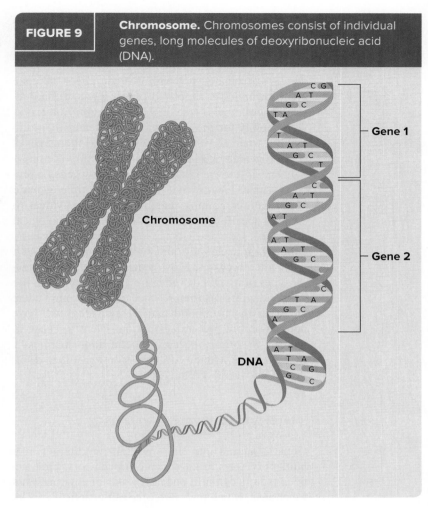

FIGURE 9 | **Chromosome.** Chromosomes consist of individual genes, long molecules of deoxyribonucleic acid (DNA).

Chromosomes contain individual genes, which are segments of long molecules of deoxyribonucleic acid (DNA; Figure 9). Genes give coded instructions to cells to perform certain functions, usually to manufacture certain proteins. Genes, like chromosomes, come in pairs. One half of the pair comes from the mother, and the other half from the father. Abnormalities in genes are much more common than major abnormalities in the structure or number of chromosomes.

For example, as noted earlier, the neurotransmitter serotonin appears to play a role in depression. One gene that influences the functioning of serotonin systems in the brain is the serotonin transporter gene. Every gene has two alleles, or coding sequences. Alleles for the serotonin transporter gene can be either short (s) or long (l). Thus, any given individual could have two short alleles (s/s genotype), two long alleles (l/l genotype), or one short and one long allele (s/l genotype). Some studies have suggested that the presence of at least one s allele on the serotonin transporter gene may increase an individual's chance of developing depression (Levinson, 2006; Starr, Hammen, Brennan, & Najman, 2012).

Although you may often hear of scientists having discovered "the gene" for a major disorder, most disorders are associated not with a single abnormal gene but with multiple abnormal genes. Each of these altered genes might make only a partial contribution to vulnerability for the disorder, some greater than others. But when a critical number of these altered genes come together, the individual may develop the disorder. This is known as a **polygenic** ("many genes") process which means that it takes multiple genetic abnormalities coming together in one individual to create a specific disorder. A number of physiological disorders, such as diabetes, coronary heart disease, epilepsy, and cleft lip and palate, result from such polygenic processes. Most genetic models of the major types of mental disorder are also polygenic. In the case of depression, the presence of at least one s allele increases the likelihood that an individual will have depression but probably is not sufficient to cause it. Rather, a combination of genetic abnormalities is thought to contribute to depression and other disorders (Geschwind & Flint, 2015).

Interactions Between Genes and Environment

Genetic factors and the environment interact in a number of ways to influence our behaviors. First, genetic factors can influence the kinds of environments we choose, which then reinforce our genetically influenced personalities and interests. Consider a startling example that involves identical twins, who have 100 percent of their genes in common. Jim Lewis and Jim Springer were identical twins reunited at the age of 39 after being separated since infancy (Holden, 1980). To their shock, both had married and later divorced women named Linda. Their second wives were both named Betty. Both had sons named James Allan and dogs named Toy. Both chain-smoked Salem cigarettes, worked as sheriffs' deputies, drove Chevrolets, chewed their fingernails, enjoyed stock car racing, had basement workshops, and had built circular white benches around trees in their yards.

Could there possibly be genes for marrying women named Betty or for having basement workshops that account for the similarities between these twins, who had never before met each other? Genetic researchers think not. Instead, people with identical genes may have similar temperaments and talents that cause them to choose similar environments (Vukasović & Bratko, 2015). For example, both of the Jim twins may have woodworking talent that causes them to build workshops in their basements and circular benches in their yards.

Most examples of genes influencing our choices of environment are not as startling as in the case of the Jim twins, but such influences may be important in producing psychological symptoms. For example, children with tendencies toward aggression and impulsive behavior, both of which appear to be influenced by genetic factors, tend to choose friends who encourage their aggressive and impulsive behaviors and provide opportunities to engage in antisocial acts. It is suggested that not all individuals will be affected to the same degree by experiences and exposures, and that genetic predispositions may have different effects depending on the environment. (Dishion & Patterson, 1997; Tuvblad, & Baker, 2011).

Second, the environment may act as a catalyst for a genetic tendency. For example, as noted earlier, the presence of at least one s allele on the serotonin transporter gene may increase an individual's chance of developing depression, but it does not determine whether the individual will develop depression. Caspi et al. (2003) found that individuals who carried at least one s allele for the serotonin transporter gene were at increased risk for depression as adults only if they had a history of being maltreated as young children (Figure 10). Among individuals with no history of maltreatment, their genotype for the serotonin transporter gene had no relationship to depression. Those with the s/l genotype showed a greater probability of depression if they had been maltreated, and those with the s/s genotype showed an even greater probability of depression if they had been maltreated. Some subsequent

Studies of identical twins reared apart offer researchers many opportunities to study the relationship of genes and environment. Lily McLeod and Gillian Shaw were born in China but raised by different adoptive families in Canada where researchers are exploring these factors. In their case, the girls continue to be raised by different parents—who have agreed to let them grow up together as sisters, thereby creating a new form of blended family arrangement. *Carlos Osorio/Toronto Star/Getty Images*

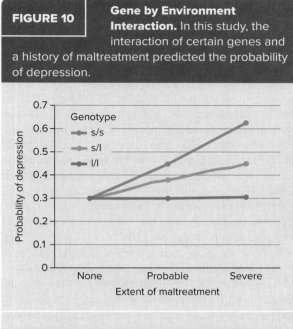

FIGURE 10 | **Gene by Environment Interaction.** In this study, the interaction of certain genes and a history of maltreatment predicted the probability of depression.

Source: Adapted from **Caspi, A., Sugden, K., Moffitt, T. E., Taylor, A., Craig, I. W., Harrington, H., . . . & Poulton, R.** (2003). Influence of life stress on depression: Moderation by a polymorphism in the 5-HTT gene. *Science, 301,* 386–389.

development. Epigenetics is the study of heritable changes in the expression of genes without change in the gene sequence.

During the course of human life, we are exposed to an environment with limitless and dynamic experiences capable of triggering chemical changes that activate or silence genes. There is constant interaction between the external and internal environments that are required for normal development. Some interactions provide a benefit to us while others might be harmful, perhaps manifesting as a disease or psychological disorder. Factors such as diet, exercise, microbiome (beneficial intestinal bacteria) seasonal changes, financial status, psychological state, social interactions, therapeutic drugs, and disease exposure might have beneficial or harmful effects depending on the specific nature of the influence (Kanherkar, Bhatia-Dey, & Csoka, 2014).

The role of epigenetics in psychopathology in humans is in its early stages, but it likely is very important (Barker, Walton, & Cecil, 2018). For example, epigenetic processes could help explain how identical twins who share the same DNA sequence could differ in their expression of a disorder. Both twins may carry genes that increase their risk for a disorder, but if the environments of the twins differ during fetal development or in critical stages of development after birth, the expression of these genes may differ, leading one twin but not the other to develop the disorder (see the chapter "Schizophrenia Spectrum and Other Psychotic Disorders").

Drug Therapies

The standard first-line treatments for psychiatric disorders include medications, as well as psychotherapy (Table 1). These drugs are thought to relieve psychological symptoms by improving the functioning of

studies have failed to replicate the findings of Caspi and colleagues (see Halldorsdottir & Binder, 2017), but this intriguing study inspired many other researchers to search for gene–environment interactions.

Third, the fascinating line of research called **epigenetics** indicates that environmental conditions can affect the expression of genes. DNA can be chemically modified by different environmental conditions, resulting in genes being turned on or off. As a result, cells, tissues, and organs are altered in their

TABLE 1   Drug Therapies for Psychological Disorders

These are the major types of drugs used to treat several kinds of mental disorders.

Type of Drug	Purpose	Examples
Antipsychotic drugs	Reduce symptoms of psychosis (loss of reality testing, hallucinations, delusions)	Thorazine (a phenothiazine) Haldol (a butyrophenone) Clozaril (an atypical antipsychotic)
Antidepressant drugs	Reduce symptoms of depression (sadness, loss of appetite, sleep disturbances)	Parnate (an MAO inhibitor) Elavil (a tricyclic) Prozac (a selective serotonin reuptake inhibitor)
Lithium	Reduces symptoms of mania (agitation, excitement, grandiosity)	Lithobid Cibalith-S
Antianxiety drugs	Reduce symptoms of anxiety (fearfulness, worry, tension)	Nembutal (a barbiturate) Valium (a benzodiazepine)

neurotransmitter systems. Studies show that there is significant overlap among psychiatric disorders and the medications used in treatment, which strongly suggests that these disorders most likely involve widespread and shared circuitry and/or neurotransmitters (Gao, Kemp, Wu, & Calabrese, 2015; Staudt, Herring, Gao, Miller, & Sweet, 2019).

Antipsychotic drugs help reduce the symptoms of psychosis, which include hallucinations (false perceptions) and delusions (false beliefs). The first group of antipsychotic drugs was the *phenothiazines*. These drugs have been extremely helpful in reducing psychotic symptoms, but they carry a number of dangerous side effects. These side effects include severe sedation, visual disturbances, and *tardive dyskinesia,* a neurological disorder characterized by involuntary movements of the tongue, face, mouth, or jaw (see the chapter "Schizophrenia Spectrum and Other Psychotic Disorders"). Fortunately, newer medications, referred to as the atypical antipsychotics, seem to be effective in treating psychosis without inducing some of the same side effects (see the chapter "Schizophrenia Spectrum and Other Psychotic Disorders").

Antidepressant drugs reduce symptoms of depression (sadness, low motivation, and sleep and appetite disturbance). The most frequently used antidepressants, the *selective serotonin reuptake inhibitors* (SSRIs; see the chapter "Mood Disorders and Suicide"), affect the serotonin neurotransmitter system. Some of the newest antidepressant drugs, *selective serotonin-norepinephrine reuptake inhibitors* (SNRIs; see the chapter "Mood Disorders and Suicide"), are designed to target both serotonin and norepinephrine. Common side effects of SSRIs and SNRIs include nausea, diarrhea, headache, tremor, daytime sedation, sexual dysfunction, and agitation. Older classes of antidepressants include the *tricyclic antidepressants* and the monoamine oxidase inhibitors (see the chapter "Mood Disorders and Suicide").

Lithium is widely used as a mood stabilizer and has been an effective treatment for bipolar disorder for more than 60 years. Lithium is successful in the prevention and treatment of mania which involves elevated mood, irritability, grandiosity with the alternation of depressive episodes. Lithium is regarded as the only substance that prevents both new depressive and new manic episodes, as well as reduces suicidal thoughts.

Media stories about so-called wonder drugs, including Prozac, often tout their ability to alleviate a wide range of problems beyond the treatment of serious psychological disorders. *Alex Segre/Alamy Stock Photo*

Lithium is a naturally occurring salt that can be found in rocks and in the waters of many mineral springs. Although the exact mechanism of lithium is unknown, it alters the metabolism of neurotransmitters, specifically catecholamines and serotonin. Despite the positive effects of lithium, the rate of prescriptions has declined in recent past which could be, in part, due to the side effects and the fact that patients need close monitoring. There are many side effects to this medication such as, nausea, vomiting and diarrhea, blurred vision, tremors, and concerns about toxicity and organ damage (Chokhawala, 2020; Won & Kim, 2017) (see the chapter "Mood Disorders and Suicide"). Other drugs, known as the **anticonvulsants,** are also used in the treatment of mania (see details in the chapter "Mood Disorders and Suicide") and have fewer side effects than lithium.

The first group of **antianxiety drugs** was the *barbiturates*, introduced at the beginning of the twentieth century. Although these drugs are effective in inducing relaxation and sleep, they are highly addictive, and withdrawal from them can cause life-threatening symptoms such as increased heart rate, delirium, and convulsions.

The other major class of anxiety-reducing drugs, the *benzodiazepines* (tranquilizers) are a large class of drugs that are used to treat anxiety, as well as other conditions including insomnia, seizures, and neuropathic pain. There are various benzodiazepines that are prescribed annually, such as, alprazolam (Xanax), clonazepam (Klonopin), diazepam (Valium), and lorazepam (Ativan). About 14 million adults receive prescriptions for benzodiazepines each year in the United States, a dramatic increase from past years. Recent research has found that the rate of benzodiazepine prescriptions nearly doubled from 2003 to 2015 from 3.8 percent to 7.4 percent, with primary care physicians accounting for about half of all of these prescriptions (Agarwal & Landon, 2019; Bachhuber, Hennessy, Cunningham, & Starrels, 2016). While the this class of drugs are effective in treating various disorders, they are also highly addictive. Up to 80 percent of people who take them for 6 weeks or longer show withdrawal symptoms, including heart rate acceleration, irritability, and profuse sweating. Benzodiazepines also carry risks of fatal overdose, and have increasingly figured into the United States' crisis of drug overdoses (Bachhuber et al., 2016).

Electroconvulsive Therapy and Newer Brain Stimulation Techniques

An alternative to drug therapies in the treatment of some disorders is **electroconvulsive therapy,** or **ECT.**

This convulsive therapy was introduced in the early twentieth century and is now most commonly used for treating severe mood disorders.

The history of ECT is filled with controversy that has created a significant amount of stigma that surrounds this form of therapy. This treatment is often referred to as "shock therapy" and conjures dark images from its early use in psychiatric hospitals fueled by often incorrect portrayals in movies and media. Once viewed as inhumane and torturous, ECT fell out of favor in the 1960s and 1970s, but it made a resurgence in the 1980s. Today, it is a widely accepted treatment for serious mental disorders and is administered at hospitals throughout the world. It is estimated that 1 million people receive ECT annually (Leiknes, Schweder, & Høie, 2012).

ECT consists of a series of treatments in which a seizure is induced by passing electrical current through the patient's brain. Anesthesia and muscle relaxants are administered at the start of the procedure to make this process more comfortable for the patient and reduce the risk of injury. Electrodes are applied to the head, and a current of 70 to 150 volts is passed through the brain for about ½ second. Patients typically experience a seizure that lasts about 1 minute. The full series of treatments typically consists of 6 to 12 sessions.

Aside from these advantages that helped make ECT a more tolerable experience, ECT proved early on to be a very effective treatment for certain forms of mental illness, including depression. ECT is very effective in treatment-resistant depressive disorders, with 50 to 80 percent of patients achieving remission which makes this one of the most effective treatments for major depressive disorder (Bewernick & Schlaepfer, 2015), bipolar disorder (Perugi et al., 2017), and may also be beneficial for OCD but additional studies are needed (Fontenelle et al., 2015).The negative perception of this therapy resulted in a decreased use of ECT in the developed world and a reduction in access to ECT, which many see as a violation of psychiatric patients' right to access an effective treatment (Gazdag & Ungvari, 2019).

Although the mechanisms of ECT's effects are not totally clear, they may involve structural changes to the parts of the brain implicated in mood disorders (Dukart et al., 2014). Various theories suggest that ECT changes the function of neurotransmitters, such as serotonin and dopamine, reduces brain inflammation, and promotes restructuring of the brain. Recent studies also identified ECT as a strong stimulator of neurogenesis by promoting the proliferation of stem cells (Gazdag & Ungvari, 2019).

More recently, researchers have been developing alternative techniques for stimulating the brain that can be more targeted and that have fewer side effects (Lerner, Wassermann, & Tamir, 2019; Slotema, Blom, Hoek, & Sommer, 2010). One procedure, known as *repetitive transcranial magnetic stimulation (rTMS)*, non-invasively exposes patients to repeated, high-intensity magnetic pulses focused on particular brain structures. In the procedure known as *deep brain stimulation*, electrodes are surgically implanted in specific areas of the brain. These electrodes are then connected to a pulse generator placed under the skin that delivers stimulation to the specific brain areas. In contrast to ECT, no general anesthesia is required and patients should wear earplugs during rTMS. Usually, 10 to 30 treatment sessions of 15 to 45 minutes are administered daily in an outpatient setting. Studies suggest that this form of treatment is an effective and safe treatment for patients with treatment-resistant depression (Bewernick & Schlaepfer, 2015).Recent research supports that is this form of therapy is an effective intervention for various neuropsychiatric diseases (Imori et al., 2019).

*Vagus Nerve Stimulation (*VNS) is an invasive brain stimulation method where electrodes are surgically implanted at the vagus nerve, a part of the nervous system that carries information to several areas of the brain, including the hypothalamus and amygdala. These electrodes are connected to a pulse generator that delivers stimulation to the vagus nerve, which in turn travels to targeted areas of brain. The results of a 5-year longitudinal study of clients treated with VNS resulted in superior outcomes in both effectiveness and mortality for patients with a chronic, severe, and treatment-resistant depression, but it is often difficult to receive this treatment since there is limited coverage from insurance providers which is a financial deterrent for many hospitals (Aaronson et al., 2017; Bewernick & Schlaepfer, 2015).

Some studies have suggested that these newer brain stimulation techniques can help relieve the symptoms of depression and auditory hallucinations (hearing voices that aren't there) in patients (Berry et al., 2013; Slotema et al., 2010). Electrical stimulation of neurons can result in long-term changes in neurotransmission across synapses. Patients who receive these newer brain stimulation treatments report few side effects—usually only minor headaches treatable by aspirin. Thus, there is a great deal of hope that these techniques will be effective and safe alternative therapies, particularly for people who do not respond to drug therapies and may not be able to tolerate ECT. Researchers continue to explore how these treatments affect symptoms across a wide range of disorders, and when they are better or worse treatment options (Coles, Kozak, & George, 2018).

Psychosurgery

Developing effective treatments for psychological disorders that facilitate optimal care has always been a challenge to the clinical community and requires a multidisciplinary approach. The neurosurgical treatment of psychiatric disorders, or "psychosurgery," has been present throughout human history as a potential method of influencing behavior and alleviating psychological dysfunction. However, the mention of such treatment often invokes controversy, as the widespread and indiscriminate use of the lobotomy in the mid-twentieth century resulted in profound ethical ramifications that persist to this day (Staudt, et al., 2019).

In the chapter "Looking at Abnormality" we describe theories suggesting that prehistoric peoples performed crude brain surgery, called **trephination,** on people with mental disorders in order to release the evil spirits causing the disorders. In modern times, brain surgery did not become a mode of treatment for mental disorders until the early twentieth century. A Portuguese neurologist, Antonio de Egas Moniz, introduced a procedure in 1935 in which the frontal lobes of the brain are severed from the lower centers of the brain in people with psychosis. This procedure eventually developed into the procedure known as prefrontal lobotomy. Although Moniz won the Nobel Prize for his work, prefrontal lobotomies eventually were criticized as a cruel and ineffective means of treating psychosis. Patients often would experience severe and permanent side effects, including either an inability to control impulses or an inability to initiate activity, extreme listlessness and loss of emotions, seizures, and sometimes even death (Staudt, et al., 2019).

By the late 1950s, the use of **psychosurgery** had declined dramatically, especially in countries outside the United States. Today psychosurgery is used rarely, and only with people who have severe disorders that do not respond to other forms of treatment. Modern neurological assessment and surgical techniques make psychosurgery more precise and safer than it was formerly, although it remains highly controversial, even among professionals (Tatagiba, Ugarte, & Acioly, 2015). Neurosurgeons attempt to lesion, or destroy, minute areas of the brain thought to be involved in a patient's symptoms. One of the greatest remaining problems in psychosurgery, however, is that we do not yet know what areas of the brain are involved in producing most psychiatric symptoms, and it is likely that many areas of the brain are involved in any given disorder.

Assessing Biological Approaches

The biological therapies have revolutionized the treatment of people with psychological disorders. We entered the twentieth century able only to house and comfort people with severe psychological disturbances. In the twenty-first century, we are able to treat many of these people so successfully that they can lead productive lives, thanks in part to the biological therapies that have been developed in recent decades. Overall, biological approaches have been remarkably effective.

Many people find biological theories appealing because they seem to erase any blame or responsibility that might be placed on the sufferer of a disorder. Indeed, many organizations that advocate for people with mental disorders argue that mental disorders should be seen as medical diseases, just like diabetes or high blood pressure. They argue that people who suffer from these disorders simply must accept that they have a disease and obtain the appropriate medical treatment.

Despite their current popularity, however, the biological therapies are not a universal cure-all and they do not work for everyone. Indeed, some people with psychological disorders do not respond to any of the drugs or other biological treatments currently available. In addition, for some disorders, such as phobias (see the chapter "Trauma, Anxiety, Obsessive-Compulsive, and Related Disorders"), psychotherapy works better than drug therapies in alleviating symptoms (Bandelow, Michaelis, & Wedekind, 2017).

Most of the biological therapies have significant side effects, as other chapters of this book will describe. Often these side effects are tolerable, and people endure them because the drugs offer relief from their psychological disorder. For some people, however, the side effects are worse than the disorder itself. For yet others, the side effects can be dangerous or even deadly.

Some critics of biological theories and drug therapies worry that people will rely on these medications rather than deal with the issues in their lives that are contributing to their psychological problems. Critics also argue that biological theories often ignore the role of environmental and psychological processes in biological functioning. Finally, recent research suggests that individuals who attribute their mental health problems to biological causes are more pessimistic about their prognosis for recovery than are individuals who attribute their mental health problems to nonbiological causes (Lebowitz & Ahn, 2012).

PSYCHOLOGICAL APPROACHES

We turn now to a discussion of different psychological approaches to understanding and treating abnormality. We begin with behavioral and cognitive approaches, which are the focus of much research in psychopathology. We then discuss psychodynamic and humanistic approaches, family systems approaches, and third-wave approaches.

Behavioral Approaches

Behavioral approaches focus on how our environment influences and shapes human behavior through the experiences of reinforcement and punishment. According to behaviorism, classical conditioning, operant conditioning, and observational learning are common processes through which learning occurs.

Classical Conditioning

Around the turn of the twentieth century, Ivan Pavlov, a Russian physiologist, was conducting experiments on the salivary glands of dogs when he made discoveries that would revolutionize psychological theory. Not surprisingly, his dogs would salivate when Pavlov or an assistant put food in their mouths. Pavlov noticed that, after a while, the dogs would salivate when he or his assistant simply walked into the room.

Pavlov had paired a previously neutral stimulus which does not naturally produce a response (himself) with a stimulus that does naturally produce a response (the dish of food, which produces salivation); eventually the neutral stimulus (Pavlov) was able to elicit that response (salivation). This learning process is called **classical conditioning.** The stimulus that naturally produces a response is the **unconditioned stimulus (US),** and the response created by the US is the **unconditioned response (UR).**

Thus, in Pavlov's experiments, the dish of food was the US, and salivation in response to this food was the UR. The previously neutral stimulus becomes the **conditioned stimulus (CS),** and the response that it elicits is the **conditioned response (CR).** Thus, Pavlov was the CS, and when the dogs salivated in response to seeing him, this salivation became the CR (Figure 11).

Classical conditioning has been used to explain people's seemingly irrational responses to a host of neutral stimuli. Just as Pavlov's dog did not choose to salivate in response to a CS, it is common for people to display behaviors that appear almost reflexively. For example, a college student who previously failed a test in a particular classroom may break out in a cold sweat when he enters that room again. This response is the result of classical conditioning. The room has become a CS, eliciting a response of anxiety, because it was paired with a US (failing an exam) that elicited anxiety.

Operant Conditioning

E. L. Thorndike observed that behaviors that are followed by a reward are strengthened, whereas behaviors that are followed by a punishment are weakened. This simple but important observation, which Thorndike labeled the *law of effect,* led to the development of the principles of **operant conditioning**—the shaping of behaviors by providing rewards for desired behaviors and providing punishments for undesired behaviors.

In the 1930s, B. F. Skinner showed that a pigeon will learn to press on a bar if pressing it is associated

FIGURE 11   **Stimulus and Response in Classical Conditioning.** Classical conditioning is a major way abnormal behaviors are learned, according to behavioral theories.

Unconditioned stimulus (US): stimulus that naturally produces a desired response

Conditioned stimulus (CS): previously neutral stimulus paired with the unconditioned stimulus

Unconditioned response (UR): response naturally occurring in the presence of the unconditioned stimulus

Conditioned response (CR): response occurring in the presence of the conditioned stimulus with the delivery of food (reinforcer) and will learn to avoid pressing another bar if pressing it is associated with an electric shock (punisher). Similarly, a child will learn to make his bed if he receives a hug and a kiss from his mother each time he makes the bed, and he will learn to stop hitting his brother if he doesn't get to watch his favorite television show every time he hits his brother.

In operant conditioning, behaviors will be learned most quickly if they are paired with the reward or punishment every time the behavior is emitted. This consistent response is called a *continuous reinforcement schedule*. Behaviors can be learned and maintained, however, on a *partial reinforcement schedule,* in which the reward or punishment occurs only sometimes in response to the behavior. *Extinction*—eliminating a learned behavior—is more difficult when the behavior was learned through a partial reinforcement schedule than when the behavior was learned through a continuous reinforcement schedule. This is because the behavior was learned under conditions of occasional reward, so a constant reward is not needed to maintain the behavior. A good example is gambling behavior. People who frequently gamble are seldom rewarded, but they continue to gamble in anticipation of that occasional, unpredictable win.

Hobart Mowrer's (1939) two-factor model suggests that combinations of classical and operant conditioning can explain the persistence of fears. Initially, people develop fear responses to previously neutral stimuli through classical conditioning. Then, through operant conditioning, they develop behaviors designed to avoid triggers for that fear. For example, a woman may have a fear of bridges developed through classical conditioning: She fell off a bridge into icy waters as a child, and now any time she nears a bridge she feels very anxious. This woman then develops elaborate means of getting around her hometown without having to cross any bridges. Avoiding the bridges reduces her anxiety, and thus her avoidant behavior is reinforced. This woman has developed a *conditioned avoidance response* through operant conditioning. As a result, however, she never exposes herself to a bridge and never has the opportunity to extinguish her initial fear of bridges. As we shall see, many of the therapeutic techniques developed by behavioral theorists are designed to extinguish conditioned avoidance

Gambling is reinforced by wins only occasionally, but this makes it more difficult to extinguish the behavior. *Eric Raptosh Photography/Getty Images*

responses, which can interfere greatly with a person's ability to function in everyday life.

Modeling and Observational Learning

Skinner and other "pure" behaviorists argued that humans and animals learn behaviors only by directly experiencing rewards or punishments for the behaviors. In the 1950s, however, psychologist Albert Bandura argued that people also learn behaviors by watching other people, a view that came to be known as *social learning theory*. First, in **modeling,** people learn new behaviors from imitating the behaviors modeled by important people in their lives, such as their parents. Learning through modeling is more likely to occur when the person modeling the behavior is seen as an authority figure or is perceived to be like oneself. For example, Bandura (1969) argued that children are most likely to imitate the behaviors modeled by their same-sex parent, because this parent is an authority figure and because their same-sex parent seems more similar to them than does their opposite-sex parent.

Second, **observational learning** takes place when a person observes the rewards and punishments that another person receives for his or her behavior and then behaves in accordance with those rewards and punishments. Like modeling, observational learning involves observing others, but it emphasizes observing the consequences of another's behavior, as opposed to simply the behavior of an important person. For example, a child who views her sibling being punished for dropping food on the floor will learn, through observation, the negative consequences of dropping food on the floor and will be less likely to engage in this behavior herself. Some theorists argue that even extremely negative behaviors, such as violence and criminal activity are the result of observational learning (Allen, Anderson, & Bushman, 2018).

Behavioral Therapies

Behavioral therapies focus on identifying those reinforcements and punishments that contribute to a person's maladaptive behaviors and on changing specific behaviors. The foundation for behavioral therapy is the *behavioral assessment* of the client's problem. The therapist works with the client to identify the specific circumstances that seem to elicit the client's unwanted behavior or emotional responses: What situations seem to trigger anxiety symptoms? When is the client most likely to begin heavy drinking? What types of interactions with other people make the client feel most distressed?

There are many specific techniques for behavior change (Table 2). A mainstay of behavior therapy is

Behavioral therapy is very effective for treating phobias.
Vicki Beaver/Alamy Stock Photo

systematic desensitization therapy, a gradual method for extinguishing anxiety responses to stimuli and the maladaptive behavior that often accompanies this anxiety. This process teaches the client to remain deeply relaxed while visualizing a series of increasingly fearsome scenes. The client first learns relaxation exercises and then develops a hierarchy of feared stimuli, ranging from stimuli that would cause them only mild anxiety to stimuli that would cause severe anxiety or panic. A person with a snake phobia might put at the bottom of their hierarchy "imagining a snake in a closed container across the room." A little further up on the hierarchy might be "watching someone else handle a snake." At the top of their hierarchy might be "touching a snake myself."

Then the therapist would help them proceed through this hierarchy, starting with the least-feared stimulus. They would be instructed to vividly imagine the feared stimulus, or even be exposed to the feared stimulus for a short period, while implementing relaxation exercises to control the anxiety. When they gets to the point where they can imagine or experience the least-feared stimulus without feeling anxious, they move on to the next-most-feared stimulus, imagining or experiencing it while implementing relaxation exercises. This process continues until they reach the most-feared stimulus on the list and are able to experience this stimulus without anxiety. Thus, by the end of systematic desensitization therapy, a person with a snake phobia should be able to pick up and handle a large snake without becoming anxious. Systematic Desensitization is supported as an effective treatment for various psychological disorders, anxiety disorders in particular (Sajadi, Goudarzi, Khosravi, Farmahini-Farahani, & Mohammadbeig, 2017; Bulantika, Wibowo & Jafar; 2018).

Often, systematic desensitization therapy is combined with modeling—the client might watch as the therapist picks up a snake, pets it, and plays with it, observing that the therapist is not afraid, is not bitten or choked, and seems to enjoy playing with the snake. Eventually the client is encouraged to imitate the therapist's behaviors with and reactions to the snake. In some cases, people undergoing systematic desensitization are asked only to imagine experiencing the feared stimuli. In other cases, they are asked to experience these stimuli directly—actually touching and holding

TABLE 2   Behavior Change Techniques

These are some of the methods used in behavior therapy.

Label	Description
Removal of reinforcements	Removes the individual from the reinforcing situation or environment
Aversion therapy	Makes the situation or stimulus that was once reinforcing no longer reinforcing
Relaxation exercises	Help the individual voluntarily control physiological manifestations of anxiety
Distraction techniques	Help the individual temporarily distract from anxiety-producing situations; divert attention from physiological manifestations of anxiety
Flooding, or implosive, therapy	Exposes the individual to the dreaded or feared stimulus while preventing avoidant behavior
Systematic desensitization	Pairs the implementation of relaxation techniques with hierarchical exposure to the aversive stimulus
Response shaping through operant conditioning	Pairs rewards with desired behaviors conditioning
Behavioral contracting	Provides rewards for reaching proximal goals
Modeling and observational learning	Models desired behaviors, so that the client can learn through observation

the snake, for example. This latter method, known as in vivo exposure, generally has stronger results than exposure only in the client's imagination (Foa & McLean, 2016).

Assessing Behavioral Approaches

Behavioral theorists set the standard for scientifically testing hypotheses about how normal and abnormal behaviors develop. The hypotheses developed from these theories are precise, and the studies that have been done to test these hypotheses are rigorously controlled and exact. As we will see in other chapters, these studies have provided strong support for behavioral explanations of many types of abnormal behavior, particularly anxiety disorders such as phobias and panic disorder. Similarly, the effectiveness of behavior therapies has been extensively and systematically supported in controlled studies (Foa & MacLean, 2016).

The behavioral theories do have limitations. How behavioral principles could account for some disorders, such as schizophrenia, is unclear. Also, most evidence for behavioral theories is from laboratory studies, but, as we discuss in the chapter "The Research Endeavor," lab results do not always apply to the complexity of the real world. Further, the behavioral theories have been criticized for not recognizing free will in people's behaviors—the active choices people make to defy the external forces acting on them.

Cognitive Approaches

Cognitive theories argue that it is not simply rewards and punishments that motivate human behavior. Instead, our **cognitions**—thoughts or beliefs—shape our behavior and the emotions we experience (Beck & Bredemeier, 2016). The cognitive model suggests that people's emotions and behaviors are influenced by perceptions of events. Meaning, it is not a the actual event that determines what people feel but rather the way in which they perceive or interpret that situation (Fenn & Byrne, 2013).

When something happens to us, we ask ourselves why that event happened (Abramson, Metalsky, & Alloy, 1989; Abramson, Seligman, & Teasdale, 1978). The answer to this "why" question is our **causal attribution** for the event. The attributions

Aaron Beck is one of the founders of cognitive theories of psychopathology.
Courtesy of Aaron Beck

we make for events can influence our behavior because they impact the meaning we give to events and our expectations for similar events in the future.

The attributions we make for our own behavior can affect our emotions and self-concept. For example, if we act rudely toward another person and attribute this behavior to situational factors (we were having a stressful day), we may not feel very guilty. However, if we attribute our rude behavior to personality factors (I am a rude person), then we may feel quite guilty.

In addition to making attributions for specific events, we have broad beliefs about ourselves, our relationships, and the world. These can be either positive and helpful to us or negative and destructive. These broad beliefs are called **global assumptions.** Two prominent proponents of this view are Albert Ellis and Aaron Beck. They argued that most negative emotions or maladaptive behaviors are the result of one or more of the dysfunctional global assumptions that guide a person's life. Dysfunctional assumptions are rigid, conditional "rules for living" that people adopt. These may be unrealistic and therefore maladaptive. For example, one may live by the rule that "It's better not to try than to risk failing" (Fenn & Byrne, 2013). Some of the most common dysfunctional assumptions are these:

1. I should be loved by everyone for everything I do.
2. It is better to avoid problems than to face them.
3. I should be completely competent, intelligent, and achieving in all I do.
4. I must have perfect self-control.

People who hold such beliefs often will react to situations with irrational thoughts and behaviors and negative emotions. For example, someone who believes that **they must be completely competent, intelligent, and achieving in all areas of their life will be extremely upset by even minor failures or unpleasant events. If they** were to score poorly on an exam, they may have thoughts such as "I am a total failure. I will never amount to anything. I should have gotten a perfect score on that exam." (Fenn & Byrne, 2013)

Cognitive Therapies

Cognitive therapies help clients identify and challenge their negative thoughts and dysfunctional belief systems. A principal goal for cognitive therapists is to collaborate with clients to define problems and teach them more effective problem-solving techniques for dealing with the concrete problems in their lives (Fenn & Byrne, 2013). Cognitive therapy is designed to be short-term, on the order of 12 to 20 weeks in

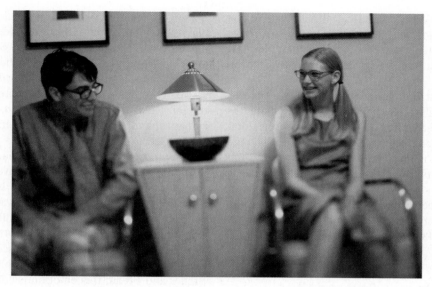

A socially anxious client may be given the behavioral assignment to talk with a stranger at a party. *Ingram Publishing*

duration, with one or two sessions per week (Beck, Rush, Shaw, & Emery, 1979). There are three main goals in cognitive therapy (Beck, 1976):

1. Assist clients in identifying their irrational and maladaptive thoughts. A client might be asked to keep a diary of thoughts they have whenever they feel anxious.

2. Teach clients to challenge their irrational or maladaptive thoughts and to consider alternative ways of thinking. A client might be asked to evaluate the evidence for a belief or to consider how other people might think about a difficult situation.

3. Encourage clients to face their worst fears about a situation and recognize ways they could cope.

Cognitive techniques are often combined with behavioral techniques in what is known as **cognitive-behavioral therapy, or CBT.** The focus of CBT is problem-oriented, with an emphasis on the present. Unlike other forms of psychotherapy, it focuses on the 'here and now' problems and difficulties. Rather than focusing on the causes of distress or experiences in the past, it looks for ways to improve a client's current state of mind (Fenn & Byrne, 2013). The therapist may use behavioral assignments to help the client gather evidence concerning his or her beliefs, to test alternative viewpoints about a situation, and to try new methods of coping with different situations. These assignments are presented to the client as ways of testing hypotheses and gathering information that will be useful in therapy regardless of the outcome. The assignments can also involve trying out new skills,

such as skill in communicating more effectively, between therapy sessions.

The following case study illustrates how a therapist might use behavioral assignments to provide a depressed student with opportunities to practice new skills and to gather information about thoughts that contribute to negative emotions.

Assessing Cognitive Approaches

Particularly in studies of mood disorders and anxiety disorders, and increasingly in studies of sexual disorders, eating disorders, and substance use disorders,

CASE STUDY

A student was unable to complete her degree because she feared meeting with a professor to discuss an incomplete grade she had received in a course. She was quite convinced that the professor would "scream at her," and she had been unable to complete a homework assignment to call the professor's secretary to arrange a meeting. An in vivo task was agreed on in which she called the professor from her therapist's office. Her thoughts and feelings before, during, and after the call were carefully examined. As might be expected, the professor was quite glad to hear from his former student and was pleased to accept her final paper. She was able to see that her beliefs were both maladaptive and erroneous. (Adapted from Freeman & Reinecke, 1995, pp. 203–204) evidence demonstrates the effect of maladaptive cognitions (Joormann & Vanderlind, 2014). Further, as we will see in other chapters, cognitive therapies have proven useful in the treatment of these disorders (Craske, 2017).

The greatest limitation of the cognitive theories has been the difficulty of proving that maladaptive cognitions precede and cause disorders, rather than being the symptoms or consequences of the disorders. For example, it is clear that depressed people think negative thoughts. But do negative thoughts cause depression, or does depression cause negative thoughts? It turns out to be harder than you might think to answer this question definitively, and to clearly delineate which aspects of cognitive therapy lead to effects (e.g., Lemmens et al., 2017).

Psychodynamic Approaches

The **psychodynamic theories** of abnormality suggest that all behaviors, thoughts, and emotions, whether normal or abnormal, are influenced to a large extent by unconscious processes (McWilliams, 2011). The psychodynamic theories began with Sigmund Freud in the late nineteenth century and have expanded to include several newer theories. These theories accept many of Freud's basic assumptions about the workings of the human mind but emphasize processes different from those that Freud emphasized.

Freud developed **psychoanalysis,** which refers to (1) a theory of personality and psychopathology, (2) a method of investigating the mind, and (3) a form of treatment for psychopathology (McWilliams, 2011). As we note in the chapter "Looking at Abnormality," Freud was a Viennese neurologist who became interested in unconscious processes while working with Jean Charcot in Paris in the late nineteenth century. He then returned to Vienna and worked with physician Josef Breuer, most notably on the case of "Anna O."

Anna O. had extensive symptoms of hysteria—physical ailments with no apparent physical cause—including paralysis of the legs and right arm, deafness, and disorganized speech. Breuer attempted to hypnotize Anna O., hoping he could cure her symptoms by suggestion.

Sigmund Freud believed that normal and abnormal behaviors are motivated by needs and drives, most of which are unconscious. *Library of Congress, Prints & Photographs Division, Reproduction number LC-USZ62-139124 (b&w film copy neg.)*

Anna O. began to talk about painful memories from her past, which apparently were tied to the development of her hysterical symptoms. She expressed a great deal of distress about these memories, but following the recounting of the memories under hypnosis, many of her symptoms went away. Breuer labeled the release of emotions connected to these memories **catharsis,** and Anna O. labeled the entire process her "talking cure."

Breuer and Freud suggested that hysteria is the result of traumatic memories that have been repressed from consciousness because they are too painful. They defined **repression** as the motivated forgetting of a difficult experience, such as being abused as a child, or of an unacceptable wish, such as the desire to hurt someone. Repression does not dissolve the emotion associated with the memory or wish. Instead, argued Breuer and Freud, this emotion is "dammed up" and emerges as symptoms.

Psychodynamic Theories

Freud's psychoanalytic theory argued that the nurturance a child receives from their early caregivers strongly influences personality development. Many of Freud's followers modified his original psychoanalytic theory, leading to a group of theories collectively referred to as *psychodynamic theories*. Anna Freud extended her work on defense mechanisms to help develop the field of **ego psychology,** emphasizing the importance of the individual's ability to regulate defenses in ways that allow healthy functioning within the realities of society. Other theorists also focused on the role of the ego as an independent force striving for mastery and competence (e.g., Jacobson, 1964; Mahler, 1968).

The **object relations** perspective integrated significant aspects of Sigmund Freud's drive theory with the role of early relationships in the development of self-concept and personality. According to proponents of this perspective—such as Melanie Klein, Margaret Mahler, and Otto Kernberg—our early relationships create unconscious mental images, or representations, of ourselves and others. We carry these mental representations throughout adulthood, and they affect all our subsequent relationships. For example, our early experiences with caregivers set up our expectations for future romantic partners. More contemporary types of psychoanalysis include **self psychology** and **relational psychoanalysis,** which emphasize the unconscious dimensions of our relationships with one another from pregnancy and infancy throughout all of life. In relational psychoanalysis, the goal is less to see how the past affects the present than to show how current unconscious forces influence the relationship between the therapist and the client. While the past of both the client and the therapist remains influential, the present-day therapeutic relationship is seen as a model for other client relationships, including more troubling aspects of them. By using their own relationship the therapist can help the client see how she or he relates with others, how problems emerge, and how typical defenses block symptom relief and self-awareness.

Carl Jung, who was a student of Freud, rejected many of Freud's ideas about the importance of sexuality in development. He argued that spiritual and religious drives were as important as sexual drives, and he suggested that the wisdom accumulated by a society over hundreds of years of human existence is stored in the memories of individuals. He referred to this wisdom as the **collective unconscious.**

Psychodynamic Therapies

Therapies based on Freud's classical psychoanalytic theory and on later psychodynamic theories focus on uncovering and resolving the unconscious processes that are thought to drive psychological symptoms. The goal of **psychodynamic therapies** is to help clients recognize their maladaptive coping strategies and the sources of their unconscious conflicts. The resulting insights are thought to free clients from the grip of the past and give them a sense of agency in making changes in the present (Safran, 2012).

Freud and others developed the method of **free association,** in which a client is taught to talk about whatever comes to mind, trying not to censor any thoughts. The therapist notices what themes seem to recur in a client's free associations, exactly how one thought seems to lead to another, and the specific memories that a client recalls.

The material the client is reluctant to talk about during psychotherapy—that is, the client's **resistance** to certain material—is an important clue to the client's central unconscious conflicts, because the most threatening conflicts are those the ego tries hardest to repress. The therapist eventually puts together these pieces of the puzzle to form a suggestion or an interpretation of a conflict the client might be facing and then voices this interpretation to the client. Sometimes the client accepts the interpretation as a revelation. At other times the client is resistant to the interpretation. The therapist might interpret resistance as a good indication that the interpretation has identified an important issue in the client's unconscious.

Both clients and therapists can experience intensive emotional reactions toward each other during this process. Strong emotional memories can be triggered in therapy which evokes the feelings tied to those past events. These process of therapy can not only elicit memories but it can also cause the client to respond as they did in the past (Vyskocilova & Prasko, 2014). **Transference** occurs when the client reacts to the ther-

apist as if the therapist were an important person in the client's early development, such as his or her father or mother. For example, a client may find himself reacting with rage or extreme fear when a therapist is just a few minutes late for an appointment, a reaction that might stem from his feelings of having been emotionally abandoned by a parent during childhood. The client's transference to the therapist is also a clue to unconscious conflicts and needs. The therapist might point out the ways the client behaves that represent transference and might then help the client explore the roots of this behavior in the client's relationships with significant others.

Countertransference is an equally important construct in therapy that describes the feelings a therapist may develop for clients they are working with during the course of therapy (Jenks & Oka, 2020). Transference and countertransference can be significant sources of insight about the client and therapist's inner worlds and are seen as a valuable tool in psychotherapy. However, unconscious parts of countertransference may compromise the success of the therapy particularly if the therapist unintentionally needs to solve their own problems at the detriment of the client. Attention to these processes in the therapist's own training and supervision is critical (Vyskocilova & Prasko, 2014).

By **working through,** or going over and over, painful memories and difficult issues, clients are able to understand them and weave them into their self-definition in acceptable ways. This allows them to move forward in their lives. Psychodynamic therapists believe that *catharsis,* or the expression of emotions connected to memories and conflicts, is also central to the healing processes in therapy. Catharsis unleashes the energy bound in unconscious memories and conflicts, allowing this material to be incorporated into a more adaptive self-view. However, while catharsis can have a positive impact, it is not the only emotional aspect of psychoanalytic/dynamic treatment. For decades, the emphasis has been on the healing aspects of the therapeutic relationship itself. Analytic therapists do not necessarily expect an "Ah ha!" moment in which all is revealed through interpretation, but additionally work toward developing a relationship with the client that intensifies trust and a sense of mutuality that touches all of a client's emotional life leading to change.

What is the difference between classical psychoanalysis and modern psychodynamic therapy? Classical (Freudian) psychoanalysis typically involves three or four sessions per week over a period of many years. The focus of psychoanalysis is primarily on the interpretation of dream content, transferences, and resistances, as well as on experiences in the client's past (Luborsky & Barrett, 2006). More modern psychodynamic therapy also may go on for years, but it can be as short as 12 weeks (Leichsenring & Steinert, 2018). Transferences, resistances, and the client's relationships with early caregivers are also the focus of psychodynamic therapy, but psychodynamic therapists, compared with psychoanalysts, may focus more on current situations in the client's life and tends to focus more on symptom relief than deeper self-insight.

Interpersonal therapy, or IPT, emerged out of modern psychodynamic theories of psychopathology, which shifted the focus from the unconscious conflicts of the individual to the client's pattern of relationships with important people in their life (Klerman, Weissman, Rounsaville, & Chevron, 1984; Weissman, Markowitz, & Klerman, 2017). IPT differs from psychodynamic therapies in that the therapist is much more structuring and directive in the therapy, offering interpretations much earlier and focusing on how to change current relationships. IPT is designed to be a short-term therapy, often lasting only about 12 weeks.

Assessing Psychodynamic Approaches

Psychodynamic theories dominated the field of psychology for decades and are often still referenced in popular culture. However, these theories often failed to provide a sharp distinction between "normal and abnormal" functioning despite their use in treating psychological conditions. nonetheless, psychodynamic theories have played a major role in shaping psychology and psychiatry over the past century.

Psychodynamic theories have been widely criticized for many limitations and weaknesses. Among the most critical is the lack of scientific data and the inability to test their fundamental assumptions with valid and reliable research methods (Erdelyi, 1992; but see Shedler, 2010; Westen, 1998). The processes described by these theories are abstract and difficult to measure (e.g., the Oedipus complex). Because the key factors thought to be influencing behavior are unconscious and unobservable, it is easy to provide explanations for why a particular prediction might not be borne out in a particular circumstance. Additionally, Freud's theories are based on a limit sample of upper-class Austrian women living in the early 1900s which limit the ability to generalize these constructs to other populations (Tummala-Narra, et al., 2018).

As for psychodynamic therapy, its long-term, intensive nature makes it unaffordable for many people, especially given insurance company restrictions on number of sessions. This is a challenge for many types of therapy, but partly for this reason, modern psychodynamic therapists have developed some shorter-term, more structured versions of psychodynamic therapy (Leichsenring & Steinert, 2018). Studies conducted on the effectiveness of these short-term therapies suggest that they can result in significant improvement in symptoms for people with psychological problems (Driessen et al., 2017; Leichsenring & Steinert, 2018).

This book focuses on those theories of specific disorders, and the therapies for these disorders, that have received substantial scientific support. Because psychodynamic theories and therapies have had much less empirical support than many newer psychological theories and therapies, we will not discuss them in detail in reviewing the research on most disorders.

Humanistic Approaches

Humanistic theories are based on the assumption that humans have an innate capacity for goodness and for living a full life (Rogers, 1951). Pressure from society to conform to certain norms rather than to seek one's most-developed self interferes with the fulfillment of this capacity. The humanistic theorists recognized that we often are not aware of the forces shaping our behavior and that the environment can play a large role in our happiness or unhappiness. But they were optimistic that once people recognized these forces and became freer to direct their own lives, they would naturally make good choices and be happier.

Carl Rogers (1951) developed the most widely known version of humanistic theory. Rogers believed that, without undue pressure from others, individuals naturally move toward personal growth, self-acceptance, and self-actualization—the fulfillment of their potential for love, creativity, and meaning. Under pressure from society and family, however, people can develop rigid and distorted perspectives of the self. People often experience conflict due to differences between their true self, the ideal self they wish to be, and the self they feel they ought to be to please others. This conflict can lead to emotional distress, unhealthy behaviors, and even the loss of touch with reality.

Humanistic Therapy

The stated goal of humanistic therapy is to help clients discover their greatest potential through self-exploration (Krug, 2016). The job of the therapist in humanistic therapy is not to act as an authority who provides healing to the client but rather to provide the optimal conditions for the client to heal themselves. Humanistic therapists do not push clients to uncover repressed painful memories or unconscious conflicts. Instead, they believe that when clients are supported and empowered to grow, the clients eventually will face the

Carl Rogers (January 8, 1902–February 4, 1987) was one of the founders of the humanistic approach (or client-centered approach) to psychology.
Bettmann/Getty Images

SHADES OF GRAY

A student comes into a therapist's office to discuss her feelings about her schoolwork and career. She says, "I'm feeling so lost in my career. Every time I seem to be getting close to doing something really good, like acing a class, I somehow manage to screw it up. I never feel like I am really using my potential. There is a block there" (Bohart, 1995, p. 101).

How might a humanistic therapist versus a psychodynamic therapist respond to this student's concerns? (Discussion appears at the end of this chapter.)

past when doing so becomes necessary for their further development (Krug, 2016).

The best known of these therapies is Carl Rogers' **client-centered therapy** (**CCT**) (Rogers, 1951). In CCT, the therapist communicates a genuineness in their role as helper to the client, which he termed *congruence*, acting as an authentic person rather than an authority figure. The therapist also shows unconditional positive regard for the client (giving the client a sense that they are inherently valued) and communicates an empathic understanding of the client's underlying feelings and search for self.

The main strategy for accomplishing these goals is the use of reflection. **Reflection** is a method of response in which the therapist expresses an attempt to understand what the client is experiencing and trying to communicate (Krug, 2016). The therapist does not attempt to interpret the unconscious aspects of the client's experience for the patient, but rather tries to communicate an understanding of the client and explicitly checks with the client about the accuracy of this understanding.

Assessing Humanistic Approaches

The humanistic theories struck a positive chord in the 1960s and still have many proponents, especially among self-help groups and peer-counseling programs. The optimism and attribution of free will of these theories are a refreshing change from the emphasis on pathology and external forces of other theories. Humanistic theories shift the focus from what is wrong with people to questions about how people can be helped to achieve their greatest potential. These theories have been criticized, however, for being vague and not subject to scientific testing.

Client-centered therapy has been used to treat people with a wide range of problems, including depression, alcoholism, schizophrenia, anxiety disorders, and personality disorders. Although some studies have shown that CCT results in better outcomes than comparison therapies, other studies have not (Csillik, 2015; Elliott, Greenberg, & Lietaer, 2004). Some therapists believe that CCT may be appropriate for people

who are moderately distressed but insufficient for people who are seriously distressed.

Family Systems Approaches

Family systems theories see the family as a complex interpersonal system, with its own hierarchy and rules that govern family members' behavior. The family system can function well and promote the well-being of its members, supporting their growth and accepting their change. Or the family system can be dysfunctional, creating and maintaining psychopathology in one or more members (Prochaska & Norcross, 2014).

When a member of the family has a psychological disorder, family systems theorists see it not as a problem within the individual but as an indication of a dysfunctional family system. The particular form that any individual's psychopathology takes depends on the complex interactions among the family's cohesiveness, adaptability to change, and communication style (Prochaska & Norcross, 2014).

For example, an inflexible family is resistant to and isolated from all forces outside the family and does not adapt well to changes within the family, such as a child moving into adolescence. In an enmeshed family, each member is overly involved in the lives of the others, to the point that individuals do not have personal autonomy and can feel controlled. A disengaged family, in contrast, is one in which the members pay no attention to each other and operate as independent units isolated from other family members. And in pathological triangular relationships, parents avoid dealing with conflicts with each other by always keeping their children involved in their conversations and activities (Prochaska & Norcross, 2014). So a family theorist trying to understand Steven Hayes' anxiety would examine how his family functioned as he was growing up and how that continues to influence him as an adult.

Some of the research on family systems theories of psychopathology has focused on disorders presented by the children in the family, particularly eating disorders (Treasure & Cardi, 2017). This research suggests that many young girls who develop eating disorders are members of enmeshed families. The parents of these girls are overly controlling and over-invested in their children's success, and in turn the children feel smothered and dependent on their parents. Anorexia nervosa, a disorder in which an individual refuses to eat and becomes emaciated, may be a girl's way of claiming some control over her life. The family system of these girls supports the anorexia rather than helping them overcome it. The anorexia becomes a focal point and excuse for the family's enmeshment. (See also the chapter "Eating Disorders.")

Family systems therapy is based on the belief that an individual's problems are always rooted in interpersonal systems, particularly family systems. According to this viewpoint, you cannot help an individual without treating the entire family system that created and is maintaining the individual's problems. In fact, these theorists argue that the individual may not even have a problem but rather has become the "identified patient" in the family, carrying the responsibility or blame for the dysfunction of the family system (Prochaska & Norcross, 2014).

Behavioral family systems therapy (BFST) targets family communication and problem solving, those beliefs of parents and adolescents that impede communication, and systemic barriers to problem solving. Behavioral and cognitive methods are used to teach problem-solving and communication skills and to challenge the unhelpful beliefs of parents and teens. Therapists also address dysfunctional family system characteristics, such as weak coalitions between parents. Therapists actively provide instructions, feedback, and opportunities for the rehearsal of skills and role playing.

Family therapists work with the entire family rather than with only the "identified patient."
Prostock-studio/Shutterstock

Assessing Family Systems Approaches

Family systems theories have led to therapeutic approaches that have proven useful for treating some types of disorders. Family systems therapies may be particularly appropriate in the treatment of children, because children are so much more entwined in their families than are adults. Although the details of many family systems theories have not been thoroughly tested in research, it is clear that families can contribute to or help diminish the psychological symptoms of their members (e.g., Carr, 2014). However, much more research on family systems theories and therapies is needed. Such research is difficult to carry out, because it usually involves observing people in the context of their relationships, which are difficult to capture in a laboratory setting.

Third-Wave Approaches

In recent years, a group of psychotherapeutic approaches known as **third-wave approaches** (the first wave was behavioral approaches, and the second wave was cognitive approaches) has become prominent in the theory and treatment of psychological disorders. Several of these approaches view poor regulation of emotions as a transdiagnostic risk factor at the core of many forms of psychopathology, including depression, anxiety, substance abuse, and most personality disorders (Barlow et al., 2018; Kring & Sloan, 2009). They combine techniques from behavioral and cognitive therapy with mindfulness meditation practices derived from Zen Buddhism to help individuals accept, understand, and better regulate their emotions.

The most-established third-wave approach is *dialectical behavior therapy* (DBT) (Linehan, 1999). The term *dialectical* in DBT refers to the constant tension between conflicting images or emotions in people prone to certain forms of psychopathology. DBT focuses on difficulties in managing negative emotions and in controlling impulsive behaviors. The therapy involves a number of behavioral and cognitive techniques and mindfulness exercises aimed at increasing problem-solving skills, interpersonal skills, and skill at managing negative emotions. DBT originally was developed by Marsha Linehan to treat people with borderline personality disorder who were suicidal, and studies comparing this therapy to control conditions suggest that it can reduce suicidal behavior and nonsuicidal self-injury (e.g., P. Panos, Jackson, Hasan, & A. Panos, 2014). Reflecting its transdiagnostic relevance, DBT has been adapted for the treatment of eating disorders (Safer, Telch, & Chen, 2009), mood disorders (Van Dijk, Jeffrey, & Katz, 2013), and other problems of emotional regulation and impulse control (Neacsiu, Eberle, Kramer,

Marsha Linehan originally developed Dialectical Behavior Therapy (DBT), one of the third wave therapies, to treat women experiencing emotion regulation problems and who had attempted suicide. *Peter Yates/The New York Times/Redux*

Wiesmann, & Linehan, 2014), including in children (Perepletchikova et al., 2017), and research in these areas is ongoing.

Steven Hayes, whom we met in the Extraordinary People feature at the beginning of this chapter, is the founder of *acceptance and commitment therapy* (ACT), which assumes that *experiential avoidance*—that is, avoidance of painful thoughts, memories, and feelings—is at the heart of many mental health problems. ACT focuses on recognizing participants' own thoughts and emotions, as well as their connections to concrete behavior. More specifically, acceptance and commitment intervention models combine mindfulness and acceptance with behavioral principles and an understanding of personal values. **Mindfulness** refers to a state of consciousness in which attention is focused on present-moment phenomena, and acceptance refers to a willingness to experience all mental events (e.g., thoughts, emotions, and sensations) without changing, avoiding, or controlling them (Puolakanaho et. al., 2019).

Accepting one's feelings, thoughts, and past history and learning to be present in the moment are key to achieving positive change. ACT uses a variety of techniques to help individuals accept their emotions, be present in the moment, relate to their thoughts differently (e.g., watching them as external objects), and commit to changing their behaviors in accord with their goals and values (Hayes et al., 2006). Randomized controlled trials of ACT have supported its efficacy in treating a wide variety of problems, especially in anxiety, substance abuse, and physical health (A-Tjak et al., 2015; Puolakanaho et al., 2019).

Assessing Third-Wave Approaches

The third-wave approaches have their roots in well-established behavioral and cognitive theories and techniques, but they draw innovative ideas and techniques from spiritual and philosophical traditions, such as Buddhism, and theories of adaptive emotion regulation. Existing studies of the effectiveness of therapies based on emotion-focused approaches suggest that these therapies may be helpful in the treatment of a wide range of mental health problems. Much more research is needed, however, particularly into claims of how and why these therapies may help individuals change their behaviors and emotional reactions, and how they compare to other efficacious treatments (Dimidjian et al., 2016; Öst, 2014). An additional therapy, developed by David Barlow and colleagues, is called the Unified Protocol (UP) for emotional disorders (Barlow et al., 2018). The UP directly targets transdiagnostic processes of psychopathology, integrating techniques that have shown efficacy across other treatments for mood and anxiety disorders. The UP simplifies and organizes treatment by targeting processes common across multiple disorders (e.g., tolerating emotional distress). This approach aligns well with current continuum and transdiagnostic models of psychopathology, and a recent randomized controlled trial showed equivalent symptom reduction compared to disorder-specific treatments (Barlow et al., 2017).

Using New Technology to Deliver Treatment

The burden of mental health problems in the world is much greater than the availability of mental health professionals trained to deliver the interventions described (Kazdin & Blase, 2011). For example, recent estimates by the World Health Organization derived from studies done in 17 nations suggest that 12 to 47 percent of individuals will have symptoms that meet the criteria for diagnosis of a mental disorder in their lifetime (Kessler et al., 2009; Tucci & Moukaddam, 2017). In the United States, lifetime rates of mental disorders are estimated at 50 percent, with 25 percent of the population meeting the criteria for a diagnosis in any given year (Kessler & Wang, 2008). That amounts to about 75 million people—when there are only about 700,000 mental health professionals in the United States (Kazdin & Blase, 2011). The rate of mental health problems is especially high within disadvantaged ethnic minority groups (Alegria et al., 2008), but individuals in these groups tend to have less access to mental health services than individuals in majority groups (Cook et al., 2014). In addition, because mental health care providers tend to be concentrated in urban areas of developed countries, people living in rural areas of the United States and in developing areas of the world often have very little access to mental health care. Increasingly, new technology, including the Internet and smartphone applications, is being used to deliver mental health care, with promising effectiveness, including among children and adolescents (Andersson, 2016; Vigerland et al., 2016).

The COVID-19 pandemic has led to a major transformation in the way mental health interventions are delivered. With limited ability to meet in-person, mental health clinicians and services had to rapidly transition to largely telehealth delivery to ensure continuity of care to patients and families. This has provided an opportunity to provide psychological services to traditionally underserved populations. Telepsychology can help reduce the disparities that exist in accessing mental health services that are associated with race, ethnicity, low socioeconomic status, rural locations, immigration status, and other social determinants. Additionally, the integration of telepractice with in-person practice has the potential to enhance the quality of services provided through both mediums (Cooper, Campbell, & Barnwell, 2019; Muñoz et al., 2016).

The increased need for telemental health services due to the COVID-19 pandemic has provided more information which support decades of research on the efficacy of this form of treatment. There is substantial evidence for the effectiveness and acceptability of Internet-delivered treatments delivered to children, adolescents, and adults. Recent research has found telemental health provided to children, young people, and adults demonstrates that interventions are feasible, acceptable, and as effective as in-person services with common mental health disorders (e.g., depression, anxiety, posttraumatic stress disorder, and adjustment disorder) (Reay, Looi, & Keightley, 2020).

Telemental health is available in many forms and often consists of online lessons, printable summaries, homework assignments, emails, texts messages, private forums, phone, videoconferencing, or in-person sessions. There is also good evidence for the efficacy of online-delivered interpersonal psychotherapy, ACT, and psychodynamic approaches. Although these approaches can be self-guided, the degree to which the therapist provides support makes a substantial difference in terms of adherence, completion and efficacy (Reay et al., 2020).

The delivery of interventions through new technologies is a vibrant area of research in mental health, and has also thrived in the field of health psychology, as we discuss in the chapter "Health Psychology." Several studies have shown that interventions delivered through the Internet, smart phones, regular phones, and even fictional television and radio shows have improved people's diets, leading to lower levels of obesity and diabetes; decreased levels of smoking; and increased the use of condoms to prevent sexually transmitted diseases (see the chapter "Health Psychology"; Kazdin & Blase, 2011).

SOCIOCULTURAL APPROACHES

Sociocultural approaches suggest that we need to look beyond the individual or even the family to the larger society in order to understand the needs of the individual. It is important to recognize that each of us is born into a cultural matrix of beliefs, values, rules, and social practices. By virtue of social, cultural, and political distinctions made in our society, perceived group membership exerts a powerful influence over how society views socio-demographic groups and how its members view themselves and others (D. W. Sue, D. Sue, Neville, & Smith, 2019). As such, there are various transdiagnostic risk factors that apply to this construct that impact the mental health of an individual.

Socioeconomic disadvantage is a transdiagnostic risk factor for a wide range of mental health problems (Snowden, 2014). Individuals living at or below the poverty line tend to live in neighborhoods in which they are exposed to violence, inadequate schools, fewer resources for everyday living (such as grocery stores), and little cohesion among neighbors. In turn, people living in poverty-stricken neighborhoods experience more substance abuse, juvenile delinquency, depression, and anxiety (Belle & Doucet, 2003; Freedman & Woods, 2013).

The upheaval and disintegration of societies due to war, famine, and natural disaster are potent transdiagnostic risk factors for mental health problems. Research has shown that disaster, not only disrupts the quality of life but also creates a significant burden of mental health conditions on an individual and the community. In addition to the social and economic losses, individuals and communities often experience mental instability following a disaster which might precipitate posttraumatic stress disorder (PTSD), anxiety, and depression in the population (Makwana, 2019). As we discuss in the chapter "Trauma, Anxiety, Obsessive-Compulsive, and Related Disorders," individuals who live in countries ravaged by war or who must flee their homelands and live as refugees show often high rates of posttraumatic stress disorder and other mental health problems.

Social norms and policies that stigmatize and marginalize certain groups put these individuals at increased risk for mental health problems, even if they do not suffer socioeconomic stress. For example, gay, lesbian, bisexual, and transgender individuals suffer higher rates of depression, anxiety, substance use, and suicidality as compared to heterosexuals (Hatzenbuehler, 2009; Meyer, 2003; Rhoades et al, 2018; Russell & Fish, 2016). Research has found that lesbian, gay, bisexual, transgender, and queer (LGBTQ) individuals are also more likely to have psychiatric diagnoses and family problems prior to their suicidality that contributed to their deaths (Ream, 2019). These disparities are the consequence of long-standing discrimination and marginalization of sexual minorities in our society. These higher rates have been linked to the experience of discrimination based on sexual orientation and to social policies that disadvantage sexual minorities (Hatzenbuehler, 2016; Meyer, 2003; Sutter & Perrin, 2016).

Laws and social policies that impact sexually marginalized groups are inextricably linked with mental health outcomes. For example, multiple epidemiological studies indicate that marriage equality legislation is associated with improved mental health outcomes for LGBTQ people. Studies have shown significant increases in psychiatric disorders experienced by LGB respondents residing in states that passed marriage denial amendment. Conversely, there were no significant increases identified in heterosexual people living in the same states, or LGB people living in other states. This research suggests that marriage denial legislation may have a negative impact on the mental health of LGB people living in these particular states. Historically, these surveys have failed to incorporate transgender populations. Similarly, data from the U.S. Youth Risk Behavior Surveillance System from 1999 to 2015 (N = 762,678) indicated a 7 percent reduction in suicide attempts made by sexual minority youth (i.e., youth who

were lesbian, gay, bisexual, or questioning) in states that passed marriage equality legislation relative to states that did not. It is also important to note that the enactment of legislation regarding the human rights of LGBTQ persons improves mental health outcomes, but the public debate that often precedes such legislation may exacerbate psychological distress, stigma, and minority stress (Casey, Wootton, & McAloon, 2020).

Although definitions of culture vary, the common themes include knowledge and meaning within a group that is transmitted from one generation to the next that involves shared beliefs, values, behaviors, and ways of life. These shared beliefs impact the way in which psychological disorders are identified and understood (Tan, 2018). Societies may influence the types of psychopathology their members show by having implicit or explicit rules about what types of abnormal behavior are acceptable (Chu & Leino, 2017). Throughout this book, we will see that the rates of disorders vary from one culture or ethnic group to another and between males and females. In addition, the particular manifestations of disorders seem to vary from one culture to another.

The influence of social media has changed the way we receive, process, and accept information. In earlier times, our real world community was a large source of information and we could seek out and find opinions and information that both support and deny our personal beliefs. However, today with the widespread use of social media, we are more likely to accept information that supports our existing beliefs. People are also more likely to seek out individuals with similar beliefs. This use of confirmation bias and selective exposure often creates polarized and like-minded clusters of opinion, commonly referred to as *echo chambers*. This practice of opinion-based confirmation bias found within the echo-chamber of social media reduces the likelihood for exchanging differing points of view. This can also strengthen rumors and fake news and intensify the segregation of their believers. This new age of misinformation has profound outcomes for our culture and how we understand and explain issues like mental illness. Social media feeds are personally curated and tailored to individual beliefs, partisan bias, and identity creating information silos (Wang, Sirianni, Tang, Zheng, & Fu, 2020). We live in a time with more information than ever before, but there is a trend of scientific rejection and support of unfounded beliefs like, conspiracy theories, magic, superstition, and the supernatural. According to a 2013 poll, 37 percent of Americans believe that global warming is a hoax, 21 percent believe that a UFO crashed in Roswell, 20 percent think vaccines cause autism, and 15 percent believe that the medical and pharmaceutical industry create new diseases to sell the cure to the public (Stahl & Van Prooijen, 2018). Just like the social media industry, members of the medical field are also challenged to find ways to reduce the spread of false and incomplete health information. Online discourse via social media can be filled with misinformation about alternative therapies or skepticism about medical practices which can create adverse effects on public health. This misinformation may be abundant on social media and some evidence has linked the sharing of misinformation with health-related knowledge, attitudes, and beliefs (Chou, Oh & Klein, 2018).

Indeed, some disorders appear to be specific to certain cultures (Alarcon et al., 2009). In Japan, there is a disorder called *taijin kyofusho*, in which individuals have intense fears that their body displeases, embarrasses, or is offensive to other people (Vriends, Pfaltz, Novianti, & Hadiyono, 2013). Throughout Latin American and Mediterranean cultures, *ataque de nervios* is a common reaction to stress. People may feel out of control, displaying uncontrollable shouting, crying, and trembling and verbal or physical aggression. We will discuss the influence of culture on the manifestation of distress further in the chapter "Assessing and Diagnosing Abnormality."

Cross-Cultural Issues in Treatment

For the most part, people from diverse cultures who seek psychotherapy are treated with the types of psychotherapy described in this chapter, with little adaptation of these approaches to specific cultures (Chu & Leino, 2017). A number of the assumptions inherent in mainstream psychological therapies, however, can clash with the values and norms of people in certain cultures. Therefore, therapists must take a culturally sensitive approach to their clients (Chu, Leino, Pflum, & Sue, 2016; Snowden & Yamada, 2005).

Most psychotherapies are focused on the individual—the individual's dysfunction, problematic ways of thinking, unconscious conflicts, and/or maladaptive patterns of behavior. In contrast, many cultures focus on the group, or collective, rather than on the individual. In these cultures, the identity of the individual is not seen apart from the groups to which that individual belongs—his or her family, community, ethnic group, and religion. It is crucial that therapists address and embrace a multicultural approach when working with clients from various backgrounds since culture guides our behavior and provides the framework for observing and identifying problems. Cultural sensitivity on the part of therapists will also help to identify their own blind spots and biases in working with clients from backgrounds different from their own.

In the context of therapy, **multiculturalism** refers to a clinician's efforts to integrate and embrace cultural differences of their clients, while also acknowledging the influence of their culture on how they perceive and respond to their clients. This process involves the inclusion of of cultural factors, such as client and counselor world views, ethnicity/race, gender, sexual orientation, religion, and social justice while providing counseling services. Culture is an unavoidable silent partner in counseling which necessitates that this process be culture-specific. Culturally relevant therapy helps clients develop a strong therapeutic alliance with their therapist. Developing this cohesive relationship in therapy can create stronger bonds which is associated with higher levels of client engagement and participation. A strong therapeutic bond in treatment is always associated with persistence in therapy and client reports of higher levels of satisfaction. Culturally responsive therapy can be conducted using a variety of theoretical approaches, such as cognitive therapy, person-centered therapy, or psychodynamic therapy (Daniels, Holdsworth & Tramontano, 2017; Jones-Smith, 2019).

Psychotherapies value the expression of emotions and the disclosure of personal concerns, whereas many cultures, for example, Japanese culture, value restraint with regard to emotions and personal concerns (D. W. Sue & D. Sue, 2003). Some counselors may view this restraint as a problem and try to encourage their clients to become more expressive. Again, this effort can clash with the self-concepts of clients and with the norms of their culture. Studies suggest that culture influences the meaning that individuals assign their symptom, the causes, and the impact of their personal difficulties. For example, in Italian and Jewish families, members may use emotional expressiveness to share personal suffering, while those from Scandinavian, Asian, and Native American backgrounds may be inclined to withdraw and not discuss their feelings (Jones-Smith, 2019).

It is often expected, in many psychotherapies, that clients take the initiative in communicating their concerns and desires to the therapist and in generating ideas about what is causing their symptoms and what changes they might want to make. These expectations can clash with cultural norms that require deference to people in authority (D.W. Sue & D. Sue, 2003). A client from a culture in which one speaks only when spoken to and never challenges an elder or an authority figure may be extremely uncomfortable with a therapist who does not directly tell the client what is wrong and how to fix it. The American Psychological Association maintains that psychologists have an ethical obligation to develop cross-cultural competencies when working with clients who are culturally different from themselves, and it is considered unethical to provide therapy to a culturally diverse client if they have not developed these cultural competencies (Jones-Smith, 2019).

CASE STUDY

Mae C. . . . began experiencing problems in her marriage 6 months ago when her husband brought over his parents from Hong Kong . . . After the parents arrived . . . the mother-in-law expected Mae to cook and serve dinner, to wash all the clothes, and to do other chores . . . Mae would occasionally complain to her husband . . . but he supported his parents.

Mae's therapist attempted to reduce her guilt over her perceived failure to be the perfect daughter-in-law . . . However, Mae was fearful that her family might find out that she had sought psychotherapy . . . Since Chinese often use third-party intermediaries to resolve conflicts, Mae called her uncle who came for dinner and spoke with Mae's mother-in-law. He told her that Mae looked unhappy, that she was working too hard, and that she needed a little more praise for the work that she was doing . . . The mother-in-law was surprised about Mae's unhappiness and agreed that Mae was doing a fine job. After this interaction, her mother-in-law's criticisms did noticeably diminish and she had even begun to help Mae with the chores.

Adapted from Sue & Zane, 1987, pp. 42–43.

If Mae's therapist had not been sensitive to Mae's cultural beliefs about her role as a daughter-in-law and had suggested some of the solutions put forward by his colleagues in the case conference, Mae might even have dropped out of therapy. People from ethnic minority groups in the United States are much more likely than European Americans to utilize therapy less, attend fewer sessions, and ultimately drop out of therapy sooner (D. W. Sue, D. Sue, Neville, & Smith, 2019; Snowden & Yamada, 2005). Because Mae's therapist was able to work within the constraints of her cultural beliefs, he and Mae found a solution to her situation that was acceptable to her.

In treating children, cultural norms about childrearing practices and the proper role of doctors can make it difficult to include the family in a child's treatment. For example, in a study of behavior therapy for children, Hong Kong Chinese parents were very reluctant to be trained to engage in behavioral techniques, such as responding with praise or ignoring certain behaviors. Such techniques violated the parents' views of appropriate childrearing practices and their expectations that the therapist should be the person "curing" the child. However, several clinicians argue that family-based therapies are more appropriate than individual therapy in cultures that are highly family-oriented, including Native American, Hispanic, African American, and Asian American cultures (Miranda et al., 2005).

Jeannette Rosselló and Guillermo Bernal (2005) adapted both cognitive-behavioral therapy and interpersonal therapy to be more culturally sensitive in the treatment of depressed Puerto Rican adolescents. The Puerto Rican value of *familism*, a strong attachment to family, was incorporated into the therapy. Issues of the balance between dependence and independence were explicitly discussed in family groups. The adapted therapies proved effective in treating the adolescents' depression. In general, such culturally adapted treatments retain the key characteristics of established treatments, but seek to improve effectiveness by adding specific skills, incorporating culturally specific themes, or addressing client engagement (Chu & Leino, 2017).

Must a therapist come from the same culture as the client to fully understand the client? Research suggests that ethnic matching is not an important predictor of therapy outcome, but may affect clients' preferences and treatment attendance (Chu et al., 2016). A therapist's being from the same ethnic or racial group as the client does not mean that therapist and client share the same value system. For example, a fourth-generation Japanese American who has fully adopted the competitive and individualistic values of Americans may clash with a recent immigrant from Japan who subscribes to the self-sacrificing, community-oriented values of Japanese culture. Value differences among people of the same ethnic/racial group may explain why studies show that matching the ethnicity, race, or gender of the therapist and the client does not necessarily lead to a better outcome for the client. What matters more is therapists' "cultural competence," meaning understanding of and respect for cultural factors in treatment. Cultural competence and sensitivity can be acquired through training and experience (Chu & Leino, 2017), and they are now required elements of therapist training, partially addressing many of the issues discussed here.

Historically, studies testing treatments essentially have ignored the question of whether the effectiveness of treatments varies by cultural group or ethnicity (Miranda et al., 2005). In recent years this pattern is changing, with increased emphasis on identifying how treatments may work differently depending on culture and ethnicity, and how they can be improved (Chu & Leino, 2017).

As for gender, there is little evidence that women or men do better in therapy with a therapist of the same gender, despite a good deal of research (Bhati, 2014). Women and men do tend to report that they prefer a therapist of the same gender, however (Wintersteen, Mensinger, & Diamond, 2005). Because the client's comfort with a therapist is an important contributor to a client's seeking therapy and continuing it for an entire course, gender matching may be important in therapy (Wintersteen, Mensinger, & Diamond, 2005).

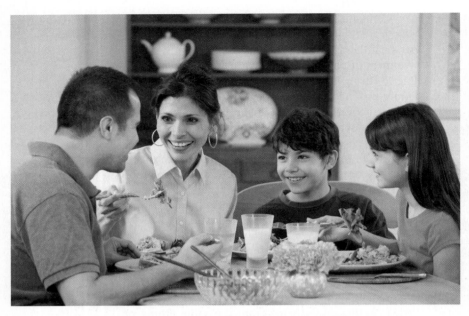

Therapy adapted for Puerto Rican families may incorporate the values of familism.
Ariel Skelley/Blend Images/Getty Images

Culturally Specific Therapies

Our review of the relationships between culture or gender and therapy has focused on those forms of therapy most often practiced in modern, industrialized cultures, such as behavioral, cognitive, and psychodynamic therapies. Even within modern, industrialized countries, however, cultural groups often have their own forms of therapy for distressed people (Hall, 2001; Koss-Chioino, 2000). Let us examine two of these culturally specific therapies.

Native American healing processes focus simultaneously on the physiology, psychology, and religious practices of the individual. "Clients" are encouraged to transcend the self, to experience the self as embedded in the community and as an expression of the community. Family and friends are brought together with the individual in traditional ceremonies involving prayers, songs, and dances that emphasize Native American cultural heritage and the reintegration of the individual into the cultural network. These ceremonies may be supplemented by a variety of herbal medicines that have been used for hundreds of years to treat people exhibiting physical and psychological symptoms (Gone, 2010).

Hispanics in the southwestern United States and Mexico suffering from psychological problems may consult folk healers, known as *curanderos* or *curanderas* (Valdez, 2014). Curanderos use religion-based rituals, including prayers and incantations, to overcome the folk illnesses believed to cause psychological and physical problems. Curanderos also may apply healing ointments or oils and prescribe herbal medicines.

Native Americans and Hispanics often seek help from both folk healers and mental health professionals who practice the therapies described in this chapter. Mental health professionals need to be aware of the practices and beliefs of folk healing when they treat clients from these cultural groups, keeping in mind the possibility that clients will combine the different forms of therapy and follow some recommendations of both types of healers (Chu & Leino, 2017; Valdez, 2014).

Assessing Sociocultural Approaches

The sociocultural approaches to abnormality argue that we should analyze the larger social and cultural forces that may influence people's behavior. It is not enough to look only at what is going on within individuals or their immediate surroundings. A strength of sociocultural approaches is that they avoid "blaming the victim," as other theories seem to do by placing the responsibility for psychopathology within the individual. The sociocultural approaches also raise our consciousness about our responsibility as a society to change the social conditions that put some individuals at risk for psychopathology. Community psychology and social work are two professions focused on empowering individuals to change their social conditions in order to help them improve their psychological well-being and quality of life.

The sociocultural theories can be criticized, however, for being vague about exactly how social and cultural forces lead to psychological disturbance in individuals. In what ways does social change or stress lead to depression, schizophrenia, and so on? Why do most people who are exposed to social stress and change develop no psychological disturbance at all?

PREVENTION PROGRAMS

Preventing people from developing psychopathology in the first place is better than waiting to treat it once it develops and prevention programs are designed to reduce this likelihood. Classifying the type of prevention is based on when during the course of disease the intervention is provided (Figure 12). Stopping the development of disorders before they start is called **primary prevention** (Muñoz, Cuijpers, Smit, Barrera, & Leykin, 2010). Some primary prevention strategies for reducing drug abuse and delinquency might include changing neighborhood characteristics that seem to contribute to drug use or delinquency. **Secondary prevention** is focused on detecting a disorder at its earliest stages and thereby preventing the development of the full-blown disorder. A goal of secondary prevention is early identification through screening as well as providing interventions to prevent the illness from advancing. Secondary prevention often involves screening for early signs of a disorder, for example, administering a questionnaire to detect mild symptoms of depression (Compton & Shim, 2020). An intervention might be administered to individuals with mild symptoms to prevent them from developing depressive disorders. Several studies have shown that administering a cognitive-behavioral intervention to an individual with mild depressive symptoms can significantly reduce the individual's chances of developing a depressive disorder (Cuijpers, van Straten, van Oppen, & Andersson, 2008). **Tertiary prevention** focuses on people who already have a disorder and these are implemented after symptoms are established. This form of intervention seeks to prevent relapse and reduce the impact of the disorder on the person's quality of life. Medical treatments delivered during the course of diseases can be considered tertiary prevention which is the bulk of the work carried out by both medical and mental health professionals (Compton & Shim, 2020). As we discuss in the chapter "Schizophrenia Spectrum and Other Psychotic Disorders," programs that provide job-skills training and social support to people with schizophrenia can help prevent the recurrence of psychotic episodes (Liberman, Glynn, Blair, Ross, & Marder, 2002).

This preventive care model focuses the social determinants of mental health which are societal problems that affect large segments of the population and interfere with optimal mental health both directly and indirectly. These environmental conditions are typically manifestations of social injustice such as exposure to violence, war, forced migration, involvement in the criminal justice system, and inequities that relate to educational, employment, and financial opportunities. Poverty and poor access to stable housing, high-quality diet, health care, or health insurance, and other adversities are also factors assessed in this system of prevention. All of these factors affect a wide range of health risks and outcomes that guide prevention programs. This system also requires changing public policies and social norms to be fully effective (Compton & Shim, 2020; Muñoz et al., 2010).

COMMON ELEMENTS IN EFFECTIVE TREATMENTS

On the surface, the different types of therapy described in this chapter may seem radically different. It is important to note that there is no "one-size-fits-all" approach to mental health services which means that while some therapies may be very effective for some individuals, they are not the right fit for all. The wide variety of therapeutic options for clients is critical and reflects the complex nature of human behavior. With

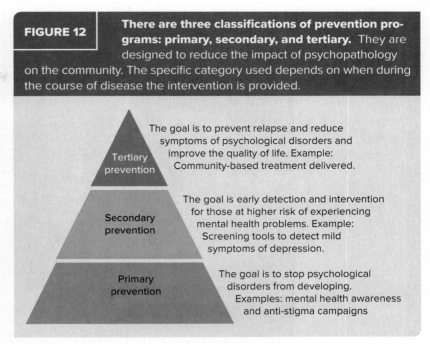

FIGURE 12 **There are three classifications of prevention programs: primary, secondary, and tertiary.** They are designed to reduce the impact of psychopathology on the community. The specific category used depends on when during the course of disease the intervention is provided.

Tertiary prevention — The goal is to prevent relapse and reduce symptoms of psychological disorders and improve the quality of life. Example: Community-based treatment delivered.

Secondary prevention — The goal is early detection and intervention for those at higher risk of experiencing mental health problems. Example: Screening tools to detect mild symptoms of depression.

Primary prevention — The goal is to stop psychological disorders from developing. Examples: mental health awareness and anti-stigma campaigns

so many available options for psychological treatment, there must be something that helps ensure the highest likelihood of success. There is evidence that successful therapies share some common components, even when the specific techniques of the therapies differ greatly. Several common elements seem to play a key role in treatment process and outcome (Norcross & Lambert, 2019; Wampold, 2015).

The development of a positive therapeutic relationship between the client and the therapist is a critical component since therapy is an intensely interpersonal and deeply emotional experience (Norcross, 2002; Norcross & Lambert, 2019). This involves clients trusting their therapist and believing that the therapist understands them. Clients who experience positive relationships are more willing to reveal important information, engage in homework assignments, and try new skills or coping techniques suggested by the therapist. In addition, simply having a positive relationship with a caring and understanding human being helps people overcome distress and change their behaviors. Authenticity occurs when the therapeutic relationship is genuine and without "front" or façade. The ability to be open about feelings and attitudes as they are expressed in a psychotherapy session has been identified as a factor in successful treatment. Empathy and unconditional positive regard (UPR), through which counselors communicate to their clients that they are accepted for who they are without judgment, are also elements that are common to all forms of successful therapy. (Parrow, Sommers-Flanagan, Cova, & Lungu, 2019; Wampold, 2015).

Research on core conditions includes empirical evidence that authenticity, empathy, and positive

A positive relationship between client and therapist is important to successful treatment. *FilippoBacci/Getty Images*

regard are demonstratively effective. Studies support the idea that the quality of the client–therapist alliance is a reliable predictor of successful outcomes in treatment.Indeed, positive counselor–client relationship may account more for successful treatment than the particular treatment method used by the counselor. However, it is almost impossible to determine which of these factors is more significant, so it must be assumed that both the therapy relationship and the treatment method make consistent contributions to treatment success (Ardito, & Rabellino, 2011; Nienhuis et al., 2018; Norcross & Lambert, 2019).

All therapies provide clients with an *explanation or interpretation* of why they are suffering. For example, cognitive therapists convey to clients that the relationships among thoughts, behaviors, and emotions underlie their difficulties, whereas psychodynamic therapists might describe the role of unconscious conflicts. Simply having a label for painful symptoms and an explanation for those symptoms seems to help many people feel better. In addition, the explanations that therapies provide for symptoms usually are accompanied by a set of recommendations for how to overcome those symptoms, and following the recommendations may provide the main relief from the symptoms. Research suggests that clients who accept the treatment rationale, are more likely to experience faster and more successful psychotherapeutic outcomes than for those who do not agree with the

treatment rationale (Locher, Meier, S., & Gaab, 2019). The client must subscribe to and believe in the therapist's interpretation of their symptoms in order to benefit from the therapy. For example, clients to whom the rationale behind cognitive therapy makes sense engage more actively in therapy and are less depressed after a course of therapy than clients who don't accept the rationale for the therapy from the outset.

The various described therapies are all characterized by empathy, warmth, cooperation, and transparency (Langhoff et al., 2008). However, each type of therapy is distinct in terms of the roles assigned to the client and therapist. In cognitive therapies, for example, therapists assist their clients to construct narratives that correct distorted thoughts to relieve the emotional challenges with which they are associated. In systemic therapy, therapists aim to understand and accept how each member of a system understands reality and which unique narratives describe the current problem, while person-centered therapists promote a shared and empathetic understanding of clients' narratives (Locher, Meier, S., & Gaab, 2019).

Therapies often encourage clients to *confront painful emotions* and use techniques designed to help them become less sensitive to these emotions (Barlow et al., 2018). In behavior therapy, systematic desensitization or flooding might be used. In psychodynamic therapy, clients are encouraged to express painful emotions and thoughts. Whatever technique is used, the goal is to help the client stop denying, avoiding, or repressing the painful emotions and become able to accept, experience, and express emotions without being debilitated by them. The purpose of each kind of therapy is to promote change and enhance psychological health and functioning.

CHAPTER INTEGRATION

As we noted at the beginning of this chapter, many scientists believe that only models that integrate biological, psychological, and social risk factors can provide comprehensive explanations of psychological disorders. Only integrated models can explain why many people with disordered genes or deficiencies in neurotransmitters do not develop painful emotional symptoms or bizarre thoughts. Similarly, only integrated models can suggest how traumatic experiences and toxic interpersonal relationships can cause changes in the basic biochemistry of the brain, which then cause changes in a person's emotions, thoughts, and behaviors.

Figure 13 illustrates how some of the biological, psychological, and social risk factors discussed in this chapter might combine to contribute to symptoms of depression, for example. Initially, some people's genetic characteristics lead to poor functioning of the hypothalamic-pituitary-adrenal axis. Chronic arousal of this axis may lead individuals to be overly responsive to stress. If they tend to interpret their reactions to stress in terms of "I can't cope!" they may develop a negative thinking style. This negative thinking style can then cause them to withdraw socially, leading to fewer positive reinforcements. This in turn could feed negative evaluations of themselves and of the world, further contributing to depression. Then, when they are confronted with new stressors, they might not have good strategies for coping with them and might overreact psychologically as well as

FIGURE 13   How Some Biological, Psychological, and Social Factors Might Interact to Cause Depression.

physiologically. All these processes come together to produce the key symptoms of depression—social withdrawal, an inability to cope with stress, negative thinking, and so on.

SHADES OF GRAY   DISCUSSION

A humanistic therapist would provide a reflection that attempts to accurately restate what the student said and the emotions she expressed, without suggesting any interpretation of her feelings:

> **Reflection:** "It's really frustrating to screw up and kill your chances; and it feels like it's something in you that's making that happen again and again."

A psychodynamic therapist might infer that the student's expressed concerns reflect unconscious conflicts about success. When he or she feels there is enough evidence, an interpretation such as the following might be offered:

A psychodynamic interpretation: "It sounds like every time you get close to success you unconsciously sabotage yourself. Perhaps success means something to you that is troubling or uncomfortable, and you are not aware of what that is."

The psychodynamic interpretation may be true, but the client-centered therapist would view it as inappropriate because it brings to the client's attention something not currently in the client's awareness (adapted from Bohart, 1995, p. 101).

CHAPTER SUMMARY

- Biological theories of psychopathology typically attribute symptoms to structural abnormalities in the brain, disordered biochemistry, or faulty genes.

- Structural abnormalities in the brain can be caused by faulty genes, by disease, or by injury. Which particular area of the brain is damaged influences the symptoms individuals show.

- Many biological theories attribute psychopathology to imbalances in neurotransmitters or to the functioning of receptors for neurotransmitters.

- Genetic theories of abnormality usually suggest that it takes an accumulation of faulty genes to cause a psychopathology.

- Genes can influence the environments people choose, which then influence the expression of genetic tendencies. Epigenetics is the study of how environmental conditions can influence the expression of genes.

- Biological therapies most often involve the use of drugs intended to regulate the functioning of the brain neurotransmitters associated with a psychological disorder or to compensate for structural brain abnormalities or the effects of genetics.

- Antipsychotic medications help reduce unreal perceptual experiences, unreal beliefs, and other symptoms of psychosis. Antidepressant drugs help reduce symptoms of depression. Lithium and anticonvulsants help reduce mania. Barbiturates and benzodiazepines help reduce anxiety.

- Electroconvulsive therapy is used to treat severe depression. Various new methods are being developed to stimulate the brain without using electricity. Psychosurgery is used in rare circumstances.

- The behavioral theories of abnormality reject notions of unconscious conflicts and focus only on the rewards and punishments in the environment that shape and maintain behavior.

- Classical conditioning takes place when a previously neutral stimulus is paired with a stimulus that naturally creates a certain response; eventually the neutral stimulus also elicits the response.

- Operant conditioning involves rewarding desired behaviors and punishing undesired behaviors.

- People also learn by imitating the behaviors modeled by others and by observing the rewards and punishments others receive for their behaviors.

- Behavior therapies focus on changing specific maladaptive behaviors and emotions by changing the reinforcements for them.

- Cognitive theories suggest that people's cognitions (e.g., attributions for events, global assumptions) influence the behaviors and emotions with which they react to situations.

- Cognitive therapies focus on changing the way a client thinks about important situations.

- Psychodynamic theories of psychopathology focus on unconscious conflicts that cause anxiety in the individual and result in maladaptive behavior. Freud argued that these conflicts arise when the impulses of the id clash with the constraints on behavior imposed by the ego and superego.

- People use various types of defense mechanisms to handle their internal conflicts. How caregivers handle a child's transitions through the psychosexual stages determines the concerns or issues the child may become fixated on.

- More recent psychodynamic theorists focus less on the role of unconscious impulses and more on the development of the individual's self-concept in the context of interpersonal relationships. They see a greater role for the environment in shaping personality and have more hope for change during adulthood than Freud had.

- Psychodynamic therapy focuses on unconscious conflicts that lead to maladaptive behaviors and emotions. Interpersonal therapies are based on psychodynamic theories but focus more on current relationships and concerns.

- Humanistic theories suggest that all humans strive to fulfill their potential for good and to self-actualize. The inability to fulfill one's potential arises from the pressures of society to conform to others' expectations and values.

- Humanistic therapies seek to help a client realize his or her potential for self-actualization.

- Family systems theories and therapies see the family as a complex interpersonal system, with its own hierarchy and rules that govern family members' behavior. When a member of the family has a psychological disorder, family systems theorists see it not as a problem within the individual but as an indication of a dysfunctional family system.

- Third-wave approaches generally combine methods and theories from the cognitive and behavioral approaches with practices derived from Buddhist mindfulness meditation to help people accept painful thoughts and emotions and regulate them more healthfully.

- Sociocultural theories suggest that socioeconomic stress, discrimination, and social upheaval can lead to mental health problems in individuals. Cultures also have implicit and explicit rules regarding the types of abnormal behavior they permit.

- Some clients may wish to work with therapists of the same culture or gender, but it is unclear whether matching therapist and client in terms of culture and gender is necessary for therapy to be effective. It is important that therapists be sensitive to the influences of culture and gender on a client's attitudes toward therapy and toward various solutions to problems.

- Prevention programs focus on preventing disorders before they develop, retarding the development of disorders in their early stages, and reducing the impact of disorders on people's functioning.

- Common components of effective therapy seem to be a good therapist-client relationship, an explanation for symptoms, and the confrontation and expression of negative emotions.

KEY TERMS

sociocultural approach

biological approach

psychological approach

theory

biopsychosocial approach

diathesis-stress model

cerebral cortex

thalamus

hypothalamus

limbic system

amygdala

hippocampus

neurotransmitters

synapse

receptors

reuptake

degradation

endocrine system

hormone

pituitary

behavioral genetics

polygenic

epigenetics

antipsychotic drugs

antidepressant drugs

lithium

anticonvulsants

antianxiety drugs

electroconvulsive therapy (ECT)

trephination

psychosurgery

behavioral approaches

classical conditioning

unconditioned stimulus (US)

unconditioned response (UR)

conditioned stimulus (CS)

conditioned response (CR)

operant conditioning

modeling

observational learning

behavioral therapies

systematic desensitization therapy

cognitive theories

cognitions

causal attribution

global assumptions

cognitive therapies

cognitive-behavioral therapy (CBT)

psychodynamic theories

psychoanalysis

catharsis

repression

ego psychology

object relations

self psychology

relational psychoanalysis

collective unconscious

psychodynamic therapies

free association

resistance

transference

working through

interpersonal therapy (IPT)

humanistic theories

self-actualization

humanistic therapy

client-centered therapy (CCT)

reflection

family systems theories

family systems therapy

third-wave approaches

mindfulness

multiculturalism

primary prevention

secondary prevention

tertiary prevention

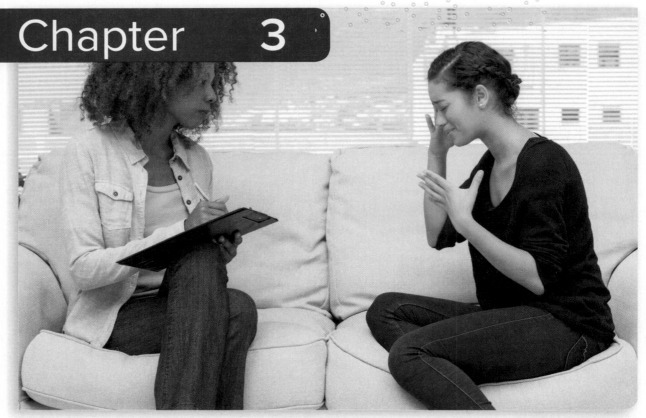

wavebreakmedia/Shutterstock

Assessing and Diagnosing Abnormality

CHAPTER OUTLINE

Assessment and Diagnosis Along the Continuum

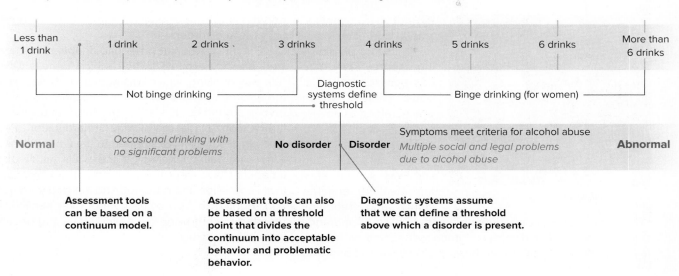

When you drink alcohol, how many drinks do you normally have in one 2-hour period?

| Less than 1 drink | 1 drink | 2 drinks | 3 drinks | 4 drinks | 5 drinks | 6 drinks | More than 6 drinks |

——————— Not binge drinking ———————   Diagnostic systems define threshold   ——————— Binge drinking (for women) ———————

Normal   *Occasional drinking with no significant problems*   **No disorder** **Disorder**   Symptoms meet criteria for alcohol abuse *Multiple social and legal problems due to alcohol abuse*   **Abnormal**

Assessment tools can be based on a continuum model.

Assessment tools can also be based on a threshold point that divides the continuum into acceptable behavior and problematic behavior.

Diagnostic systems assume that we can define a threshold above which a disorder is present.

As a student, you have taken a variety of tests intended to assess your learning in different subjects. Similarly, mental health professionals use various tests or tools to assess mental health. Some assessment tools described in this chapter are based on the assumption that behaviors or feelings lie along a continuum—the task is to determine where an individual's experiences fall along that continuum. For example, a questionnaire that asked you about your drinking behavior might have several options indicating different levels of drinking. The researcher doing a study on predictors of drinking behavior might be interested in what factors predict where people fall along the continuum from little or no drinking to a great deal of drinking. A clinician may be interested in charting how a person's drinking behavior changes over the course of therapy. Other tools, however, are more like true/false tests: They are based on the assumption that there is a threshold for the behaviors they are assessing, and that either people have these behaviors or they do not. For example, some researchers set the threshold for an alcohol "binge" for women at four drinks (see the chapter "Substance Use and Gambling Disorders"). Thus, a person who regularly drinks this amount or more in one sitting would be considered a binge drinker, whereas a person having three drinks would not be considered a binge drinker.

Currently, the guidelines used to determine whether a person has a psychological disorder use a threshold—a specific cutoff point—to make this determination and therefore seem to oppose a continuum model. Increasingly, however, researchers and clinicians are building a continuum perspective into the diagnostic process. For example, the most recent version of the manual used to diagnose disorders in the United States, the *DSM-5,* defines personality disorders at least somewhat in line with a continuum model. For most disorders, however, the *DSM-5* and other diagnostic systems set criteria for when a person's behaviors and feelings cross the line into a disorder, even in the absence of a purely scientific way to draw that line.

There are advantages and disadvantages both to a continuum approach to assessment and diagnosis and to a categorical approach that focuses on thresholds and cutoffs for identifying disorders. The continuum approach captures the nuances in people's behaviors better than does a categorical approach. The continuum approach also does not assume that we know where the cutoff is for problematic behavior. But the continuum approach can make it more difficult to communicate information about people, in part because we often think more in categorical terms. For example, saying that a person is a binge drinker may convey more information to a therapist or researcher than saying that the person drinks moderately to heavily.

Extraordinary People

Marya Hornbacher

STR/AP Photos

By her late twenties, Marya Hornbacher appeared to be an amazing success story. She had published her first book, *Wasted,* which was heralded as an eloquent account of her many years with severe eating disorders, and she was sought after for speaking engagements and readings across the United States and Europe. Apparently cured of her disorder, Hornbacher served as a living testament both to the horrors of bulimia and anorexia nervosa and to a young woman's ability to recover from these disorders.

But those who knew her had doubts that she was well, as she recounts in her book *Madness* (2008). She was drinking, which was nothing new for her. But the volume and ferocity of her drinking surprised everyone around her. Even though she is a petite woman, it took a dozen glasses of wine or hard liquor to even give her a buzz. Marya seemed to have boundless energy and was bouncing off the walls much of the time—that is, except when she went crashing down into depression and retreated into her bed for days on end. Hoping to gain some control over her life, she resorted to controlling her eating again and began to lose weight rapidly.

Marya Hornbacher presents a puzzling picture. Despite periods of time with stable psychological function she showed signs of alcohol abuse, mood swings, and a lingering eating disorder. Why does Marya experience these symptoms and why do they stabilize, but come back? "Why" is often the most common question. And, it is not a question that is easily answered, which is frustrating. There will always be unanswered questions when it comes to psychological dysfunction, but to begin answering these questions we must first understand what disorders are present. These symptoms will qualify Marya for several diagnoses that we will discuss in other chapters, including eating disorders, substance use disorders, and bipolar disorder. However, the first step is to think about how Marya's symptoms impact her ability to function and how to best assess her behaviors. The assessment and diagnosis of symptoms is the focus of this chapter.

How are psychological disorders evaluated?

While working out one day, you twist your ankle and feel a sharp sensation of pain. Your pain increases over the next few hours, the ankle begins to swell and you cannot bear weight to walk. What's the diagnosis? If you went to the emergency room you would not be provided with a diagnosis until the medical doctor ran some tests. However, after an X-ray and examination it's likely that you would be diagnosed with a fractured ankle and a treatment plan would be designed for your care and recovery. Psychological evaluation is not much different in this respect. While we do not have the ability to evaluate psychological symptoms with an X-ray or bloodwork, psychological assessment has the same purpose, which is to collect information, draw conclusions, and develop a treatment plan.

Before a person can be diagnosed with a psychological disorder an assessment is first performed. **Assessment** is the process of evaluating psychological, social, and emotional functioning through a variety of clinical methods. Psychological assessment often includes interviews, observations, psychological and neurological tests to determine the client's **presenting problem** and clinical description. Meaning, a variety of assessment methods are used in combination to determine if a psychological disorder might be present in an individual.

Many types of information are gathered during an assessment, including current symptoms and ways of coping with stress, recent events and physical conditions, drug and alcohol use, personal and family history of psychological disorders, cognitive functioning, and sociocultural background. The information gathered in an assessment is used to determine the appropriate diagnosis for a person's problems. The diagnostic process involves using the assessment data to determine if the pattern of symptoms is consistent with the diagnostic criteria for a specific mental disorder. The criteria used to assign a diagnosis is based on an established classification system, such as the *DSM-5* or *ICD-10,* which we will discuss later in this chapter. Symptoms that cluster together are called a **syndrome.** When symptoms cluster together in specific patterns a **diagnosis** is given that identifies the characteristics of a specific disorder.

Although some clinicians avoid making diagnoses from fear of labeling a person and simplifying their humanity, the process is not about applying a label to a problem–or a person. Instead, it is about understanding the problems experienced by the individual and helping to provide information and effective treatments related to the problem. Various tools of assessment provide important information about the individual's personality characteristics, cognitive function, emotional well-being, and biological functioning. Additionally, we will discuss contemporary classification systems used to diagnose psychological disorders. These standardized diagnostic system enhances effective communication among mental health professionals, facilitates research, and informs the community on best practices for the treatment of psychological disorders.

ASSESSMENT TOOLS

A number of assessment tools have been developed to help clinicians gather information. The assessment process must include tools that are valid, reliable, and standardized. These terms may be unfamiliar, so let's first discuss these important concepts and then look at specific types of assessment tools.

Validity

If you administer a test to determine a person's behaviors and feelings, you want to be sure that the test is accurate. The accuracy of a test in assessing what it is supposed to measure is called its **validity.** For example, when a new test is developed to measure symptoms of depression, its accuracy must be tested to ensure it is a valid instrument. One way to do this is to compare the new test to an existing and proven test, such as the Beck Depression Inventory (BDI). If the new test accurately measures depression, then the outcome of the new test should be similar to or correlate with the results of the BDI. This is an example of *concurrent* (or *convergent*) *validity,* which is the extent to which a test yields the same results as other, established measures of the same behavior, thoughts, or feelings.

As we discuss in the chapter "Looking at Abnormality," there are currently no definitive blood tests, brain scans, or other objective tests for any of the psychological disorders presented in this book. Fortunately, the validity of a test can be estimated in a number of other ways (Figure 1). A test is said to have *face validity* when, on face value, the items seem to measure what the test is intended to measure. For example, a questionnaire for anxiety that asks "Do you feel jittery much of the time?" and "Do you worry

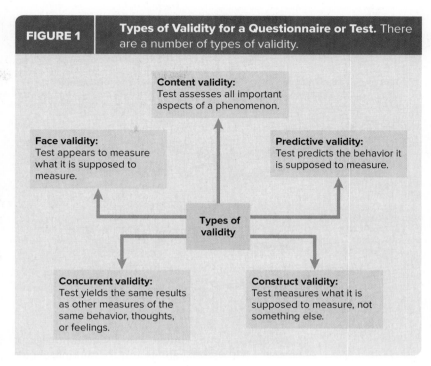

FIGURE 1   **Types of Validity for a Questionnaire or Test.** There are a number of types of validity.

Content validity: Test assesses all important aspects of a phenomenon.

Face validity: Test appears to measure what it is supposed to measure.

Predictive validity: Test predicts the behavior it is supposed to measure.

Types of validity

Concurrent validity: Test yields the same results as other measures of the same behavior, thoughts, or feelings.

Construct validity: Test measures what it is supposed to measure, not something else.

about many things?" has face validity because it seems to assess symptoms of anxiety. If it also meets other standards of validity, researchers are more likely to trust its results.

Content validity is how well an instrument (i.e., a test or questionnaire) appropriately measures the content, theory, or phenomenon being studied. For example, questions on an AP Chemistry exam should be limited to the topics actually taught in that class and unrelated material, like History or French, should not appear. This matching between test questions and the content helps to ensure content validity.

One purpose of research is to make predictions about future behaviors. *Predictive validity* addresses how well an instrument that is used for assessment, like a survey, can predict future behavior. An anxiety measure has good predictive validity if it correctly predicts which people will behave in anxious ways when confronted with stressors in the future.

Construct validity is the extent to which a test measures what it is supposed to measure and not something else altogether (Cronbach & Meehl, 1955). Consider the construct validity of multiple-choice exams in school. They are supposed to measure a student's knowledge and understanding of content. However, they may also measure the student's ability to take multiple-choice tests—that is, their ability to determine the instructor's intent in asking each question and to recognize any obviously incorrect answer choices. For example, if a chemistry exam actually measures a student's understanding of chemistry, the exam can be said to have construct validity; but if it

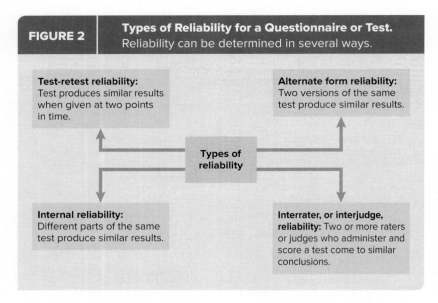

FIGURE 2 | **Types of Reliability for a Questionnaire or Test.** Reliability can be determined in several ways.

Test-retest reliability: Test produces similar results when given at two points in time.

Alternate form reliability: Two versions of the same test produce similar results.

Types of reliability

Internal reliability: Different parts of the same test produce similar results.

Interrater, or interjudge, reliability: Two or more raters or judges who administer and score a test come to similar conclusions.

shows how a clever student with little knowledge of chemistry but a strong ability to take multiple-choice exams, it does not.

Reliability

It is important that a test provides consistent information about a person. The **reliability** of a test indicates its consistency in measuring what it is supposed to measure. As with validity, there are several types of reliability (Figure 2). *Test-retest reliability* describes how consistent the results of a test are over time. If a test supposedly measures an enduring characteristic of a person, then the person's scores on that test should be similar when he or she takes the test at two different points in time. For example, if an anxiety questionnaire is supposed to measure people's general tendencies to be anxious, then their scores should be similar if they complete the questionnaire this week and then again next week. Typically, measures of general and enduring characteristics should have higher test-retest reliability than measures of transient characteristics.

A problem with reliability might arise when people take the same test a second time, they may try to give the same answers so as to seem consistent. For this reason, researchers often will develop two or more forms of a test. When people's answers to different forms of a test are similar, the tests are said to have *alternate form reliability*. Similarly, a researcher may split a test into two or more parts to determine whether people's answers to one part of a test are similar to their answers to another part. When there is similarity in people's answers among different parts of the same test, the test is said to have high *internal reliability*.

Finally, many of the assessments we examine in this chapter are interviews or observational measures that require a clinician or researcher to make judgments about the people being assessed. These tests should have high *interrater,* or *interjudge, reliability.* That is, different raters or judges who administer and score the interview or test should come to similar conclusions when they are evaluating the same people.

Standardization

One important way to improve both validity and reliability is to standardize the administration and interpretation of tests. A standard method of administering a test prevents extraneous factors from affecting a person's response. For example, if the test administrator were to deviate from the written questions, suggesting the "right" answer to the respondents, this would reduce the validity and reliability of the test. In contrast, if the administrator of the test only read aloud the specific questions on the test, this would increase the validity and reliability of the test. Similarly, a standard way of interpreting results (e.g., scores above a certain cutoff are considered extreme) makes the interpretation of the test more valid and reliable. Thus, standardization of both the administration and the interpretation of tests are important to their validity and reliability.

With these concepts in mind, let's explore some commonly used assessment tools.

Clinical Interview

Much of the information for an assessment is gathered in an initial interview, which is the **clinical interview.** This is exactly as the title implies, it's an interview or discussion. A clinical interview is typically a face-to-face conversation between a mental health professional and a client where information is gathered about the client's behavior, attitudes, emotions, life history, and personality. A **mental status exam,** is used to organize the information collected during the interview and systematically evaluate the client through a series of questions. This process helps to determine the client's current mental status. Each part of the mental status examination is designed to look at a different area of mental function to thoroughly capture the objective and subjective aspects of psychological function (Finney, Managar, & Heilman, 2016).

In the mental status exam, the clinician asks various questions that relate to five (5) categories of information. First, the clinician assesses the individual's appearance and behavior, which includes overt physical behaviors, appearance, body language, level of cooperation, and facial expressions. This is something we all do when we meet someone new. Does this person make appropriate eye contact or do they stare a little too long? Is he or she dressed neatly and well groomed, or do they appear disheveled? Do their clothing choices best fit the weather? The ability to care for one's basic grooming indicates how well one is functioning in general. All of these observations help provide insight into the client's behavior.

Second, in a mental status exam a clinician will take note of the individual's thought processes, including how coherently and quickly he or she speaks. Are the client's thoughts linear, organized and goal-directed or disorganized, off-topic and rambling? Third, the clinician will evaluate the individual's mood and affect. Does he or she appear down and depressed, or perhaps elated or euphoric? What mood does the client report feeling and does the outward reflection of this emotion match? It is important to note if the affect is appropriate or inappropriate. Meaning, if the client reports feeling happy, and they appear happy, then the affect is appropriate to mood.

Fourth, the clinician will observe the individual's intellectual functioning, which can be assessed in a variety of ways, including how well the person speaks, responds to questions, and shows any indications of memory or attention difficulty. The last category assesses the client's general awareness to their surrounding and their orientation to time, person, and place, which is called **sensorium.** The clinician will will assess the sensorium by determining whether the individual understands *where they are, when they are, and who they are.* If the individual can provide this information then they are appropriately oriented, or "oriented times three."

The interview can be delivered in a variety of formats, including structured, unstructured, and semistructured. In **structured interviews,** clinicians ask the individual a series of standardized questions about symptoms and use concrete criteria to score responses. Structured interviews offer the benefits of standardization and reliability but lack flexibility to ask client-specific questions (Table 1). An **unstructured interview** is another option for mental health professionals in which open-ended questions are asked and directed by the clinician based on the client's responses. **Semi-structured interviews** combine standardized with open-ended questions that allow clinicians to follow up with specific questions in order to gather more personalized information (Bridley & Daffin, 2018). These interviews help clinicians to determine whether the client's symptoms qualify for a diagnosis. Recently, researchers have sought to develop computerized methods of testing that might retain validity while saving time and resources compared to face-to-face interviews; these methods are not yet widely used (Gibbons, Weiss, Frank, & Kupfer, 2016).

TABLE 1   Sample Structured Interview
ANXIETY DISORDERS
Panic Disorder Questions
Have you ever had a panic attack, when you suddenly felt frightened, anxious, or extremely uncomfortable?
If Yes: Tell me about it. When does that happen? (Have you ever had one that just seemed to come out of the blue?)
If panic attacks took place in expected situations: Did you ever have one of these attacks when you weren't in (EXPECTED SITUATION)?
Have you ever had four attacks like that in a 4-week period?
If No: Did you worry a lot about having another one? (How long did you worry?)
When was the last bad one (EXPECTED OR UNEXPECTED)?
Now I am going to ask you about that attack.
What was the first thing you noticed? Then what?
During the attack . . .
. . . were you short of breath? (have trouble catching your breath?)
. . . did you feel dizzy, unsteady, or as if you might faint?
. . . did your heart race, pound, or skip?
. . . did you tremble or shake?
. . . did you sweat?
. . . did you feel as if you were choking?
. . . did you have nausea, upset stomach, or the feeling that you were going to have diarrhea?
. . . did things around you seem unreal or did you feel detached from things around you or detached from part of your body?

Source: Data from First, Spitzer, Gibbon, & Williams, 1997.

The mental status exam is a useful but subjective assessment. Evaluations can vary significantly between practitioners depending upon their clinical skills level and ability to elicit responses from the client. This process also depends upon practitioners to use their best clinical judgment to combine the interview information with other subjective and objective findings (Norris, Clark, & Shipley, 2016).

Symptom Questionnaires

When clinicians or researchers want a quick way to determine a person's symptoms, often they will ask the person to complete a self-report **symptom questionnaire.** There is no shortage of self-report instruments on the Internet. The clinician might direct a client to a particular example and ask that it be completed before meeting. These questionnaires can be generalized and cover a wide variety of symptoms that represent several disorders or focused on the symptoms of a specific disorder. It is important to note that these instruments are not used to diagnose a psychological disorder and individuals using such Internet-based assessments on their own should consult with a professional.

The BDI-II is one of the most widely used self-report symptom instruments in both research and clinical practice for assessing depression. The most recent form of the BDI has 21 items, each of which describes 4 levels of a given symptom of depression ranging from "I do not feel unhappy" to "I am so unhappy that I can't stand it" measured on a scale of 0 to 3. The respondent is asked to indicate which description best fits how he or she has been feeling in the past week. The items are scored to indicate the level of depressive symptoms the person is experiencing. Cutoff scores have been established to indicate moderate and severe levels of depressive symptoms (A. Beck & R. Beck, 1972; Garcia-Batista, Guerra-Pena, Cano-Vindel, Herrera-Martinez, & Medrano, 2018; Westhoff-Bleck et al., 2019).

Multiple recent studies have found that the first edition of the BDI provides high levels of discrimination for depressive symptomatology and that the BDI-II is an effective screening tool in predicting and detecting major depressive disorder. While the BDI should not be used as a singular diagnostic measure, it is extremely quick and easy to administer and has good test-retest reliability (Westhoff-Bleck et al., 2019).

Clinicians treating depressed people also use the BDI to monitor those individuals' symptom levels from week to week. An individual may be asked to complete the BDI at the beginning of each therapy session, and both the individual and the clinician then have a concrete indicator of any changes in symptoms.

Personality Inventories

Personality inventories are questionnaires designed to assess people's typical ways of thinking, feeling, and behaving. These inventories are used as part of an assessment procedure to obtain information on people's well-being, self-concept, attitudes and beliefs, ways of coping, perceptions of their environment, social resources, and vulnerabilities.

The most widely used personality inventory in professional clinical assessments is the *Minnesota Multiphasic Personality Inventory (MMPI),* which has been translated into more than 150 languages and is used in more than 50 countries (Groth-Marnat & Wright, 2016). The original MMPI was developed in the 1930s by Starke Hathaway and Charnley McKinley. In 1989, an updated version was published as the MMPI-2, followed by the MMPI-2-RF (MMPI-2 Restructured Form) in 2008. The failure to update the test for several decades resulted in disinterest by researchers until the test was restructured in the 2000s (Sellbom, 2019).

This current instrument includes 10 clinical scales that assess 10 major categories of psychological characteristics or problems, such as paranoia, anxiety, social introversion and vulnerability to eating disorders, substance abuse, and poor functioning at work (Sharf, Rogers, Williams, & Henry, 2017). The MMPI presents respondents with sentences describing moral and social attitudes, behaviors, psychological states, and physical conditions, and ask them to respond "true," "false," or "can't say" to each sentence. Here are some examples of items from the MMPI:

> I would rather win than lose in a game.
> I am never happier than when alone.
> My hardest battles are with myself.
> I wish I were not bothered by thoughts about sex.
> I am afraid of losing my mind.
> When I get bored, I like to stir up some excitement.
> People often disappoint me.

The MMPI was developed empirically, meaning that a large group of possible inventory items was given to psychologically "healthy" people and to people with various psychological problems. The items that reliably differentiated groups of people were included in the inventory.

The validity of test interpretation relies heavily on examinees' efforts to be genuine and forthcoming in their responses and can be completely invalidated by feigning or intentional over-reporting or fabrication of symptoms and clinical characteristics. Four validity scales assess the person's general test-taking attitude and whether they answered the items on the test in a truthful and accurate manner. A respondent's scores on each scale are compared with scores from the population, and a profile of the respondent's personality and psychological problems is derived (Sharf et al., 2017). Also, these validity scales determine whether the person responds honestly to the items on the scale or distorts his or her answers in a way that might invalidate the test (Table 2). For example, the Lie Scale measures the respondent's tendency to respond to items in a socially desirable way in order to appear unusually positive or good (Sharf et al., 2017).

Because the items on the MMPI were chosen for their ability to differentiate people with specific types of psychological problems from people without psychological problems, the concurrent validity of the MMPI scales was "built in" during their development. The MMPI may be especially useful as a general screening device for detecting people who are functioning very poorly psychologically.

However, many criticisms have been raised about the use of the MMPI in culturally diverse samples (Groth-Marnat & Wright, 2016). The norms for the

TABLE 2   Clinical and Validity Scales of the Original MMPI

The MMPI is one of the most widely used questionnaires for assessing people's symptoms and personalities. It also includes scales to assess whether respondents are lying or trying to obfuscate their answers.

CLINICAL SCALES

Scale Number	Scale Name	What It Measures
Scale 1	Hypochondriasis	Excessive somatic concern and physical complaints
Scale 2	Depression	Symptomatic depression
Scale 3	Hysteria	Hysterical personality features and tendency to develop physical symptoms under stress
Scale 4	Psychopathic deviate	Antisocial tendencies
Scale 5	Masculinity-femininity	Sex-role conflict
Scale 6	Paranoia	Suspicious, paranoid thinking
Scale 7	Psychasthenia	Anxiety and obsessive behavior
Scale 8	Schizophrenia	Bizarre thoughts and disordered affect
Scale 9	Hypomania	Behavior found in mania
Scale 0	Social introversion	Social anxiety, withdrawal, overcontrol

VALIDITY SCALES

	Scale Name	What It Measures
	Cannot say scale	Total number of unanswered items
	Lie scale	Tendency to present favorable image
	Infrequency scale	Tendency to falsely claim psychological problems
	Defensiveness scale	Tendency to see oneself in unrealistically positive manner

Source: Adapted from Minnesota Multiphasic Personality Inventory (MMPI).

original MMPI—the scores considered "healthy"—were based on samples of people in the United States not drawn from a wide range of ethnic and racial backgrounds, age groups, and social classes. In response to this problem, the publishers of the MMPI established new norms based on more representative samples of eight communities across the United States. Still, concerns persist that the MMPI norms do not reflect variations across cultures in what is considered normal or abnormal. In addition, some question the linguistic accuracy of the translated versions of the MMPI and the comparability of these versions to the English version (Dana, 2005). Ideally, the MMPI-2 should be administered as a part of a battery of psychological tests, so that other testing can either confirm or deny results suggested by the MMPI-2.

Behavioral Observation and Self-Monitoring

Clinicians often will use **behavioral observation** of individuals to assess deficits in their skills or their ways of handling situations. The clinician looks for specific behaviors and what precedes and follows these behaviors. For example, a clinician might watch a child interact with other children to determine what situations provoke aggression in the child. The clinician can then use information from behavioral observation to help the child learn new skills, stop negative habits, and understand and change how he or she reacts to certain situations. A couple seeking marital therapy might be asked to discuss with each other a topic on which they disagree. The clinician would observe this interaction, noting the specific ways the couple handles conflict. For example, one member of the couple may lapse into statements that blame the other member for problems in their marriage, escalating conflict to the boiling point.

Direct behavioral observation has the advantage of not relying on individuals' reporting and interpretation of their own behaviors. Instead, the clinician sees firsthand how the individuals handle important situations. One disadvantage is that individuals may alter their behavior when they are being watched. Another disadvantage is that different observers may draw different conclusions about individuals' skills; that is, direct behavioral observations may have low interrater reliability, especially in the absence of a standard means of making the observations. In addition, any individual rater may miss the details of an interpersonal interaction. For example, two raters watching a child play with others on a playground might focus on different aspects of the child's behaviors or be distracted by the chaos of the playground. For these reasons, when behavioral observation is used in research settings, the situations are highly standardized and observers watch for a set list of behaviors. Finally, direct observation may not be possible in some situations. In that case, a clinician may have a client role-play a situation, such as the client's interactions with an employer.

Since mental health professionals cannot be with clients every day, clinicians may require **self-monitoring** to gather information about the individual's behavior. Traditionally, assessment of psychiatric symptoms relies on the client's retrospective report to a trained interviewer. However, with the emergence of smartphones there are new and innovative ways for client's to self-monitor. For example, recent studies have examined the use of self-monitoring of mood using Patient Reported Outcome Measures (PROMs) which previously was performed by using paper-based and more recently computer-based questionnaires. The widespread access to mobile networks and the rapid evolution of smartphone technology have led to an increased focus on the use of smartphone applications for this process with promising results (Schwartz, Schultz, Rieder, & Saunders, 2016).

Smartphone-based questionnaires are a viable approach that can be effectively used in long-term daily self-monitoring. This approach has advantages because behaviors such as social interaction, physical motion, speech, travel pattern data, and mood states can be reported in real time without the inconvenience of logging to a computer. Studies show high levels of compliance of self-monitoring through smartphone apps which increases the likelihood that self-ratings would be less prone to recall bias. Active real-time monitoring through time-stamped prompts have also been noted; however, there are few validated self-report measures designed for this purpose and more research is needed (Tsanas et al., 2016). Like any self-report assessment, self-monitoring is open to biases about what individuals notice about their behavior and are willing to report. However, individuals can discover the triggers of unwanted behaviors through self-monitoring, which in turn can lead them to change these behaviors.

Smartphone apps are becoming a new and effective way to self-monitor. *Tolgart/iStock/Getty Images*

Intelligence Tests

Assessing an individual's level of intelligence provides mental health professionals with important information that can be used in the diagnostic process. Defining and classifying intelligence is a complicated process and there is no one explanation that is used as a benchmark. Theories of intelligence range from having one general intelligence, such as (g), to certain primary mental abilities, and to multiple category-specific intelligences.

In clinical practice, **intelligence tests** are used to determine an individual's level of cognitive functioning, and consists of a series of tasks that involve both verbal and nonverbal skills (Bridley & Daffin, 2018). Studies on these tests have shown that they are generally reliable and valid tools of measurement. However, these instruments have been criticized as lacking cultural specificity with bias in favor of white, middle-class people. It is hypothesized that this can evoke stereotype threat among people of color due to implied negative stereotypes about a person's ethnicity, gender, or age which causes doubt about his or her abilities, resulting in lower scores. Despite these concerns, when working with children in educational and developmental settings, intelligence testing is still a central component of how children are assessed. The results of such testing are used to inform recommendations for educational and service-based interventions and programming (Forscher et al., 2019; Freeman & Chen, 2019; Ruhl, 2020).

These tests were designed to measure basic intellectual abilities, such as the ability for abstract reasoning, verbal fluency, and spatial memory. The term *IQ,* or *intelligence quotient*, is used to describe a method of comparing an individual's score on an intelligence test with the performance of individuals in the same age group. An IQ score of 100 means that the person performed similarly to the average performance of other people of the same age.

Intelligence tests are controversial in part because there is little consensus as to what is meant by intelligence (Sternberg, 2015). The most widely used intelligence tests assess verbal and analytical abilities but do not assess other talents or skills, such as artistic and musical ability. Some psychologists suggest that success in life is as strongly influenced by social skills and other talents not measured by intelligence tests as it is by verbal and analytic skills. It is further argued that characteristics such as social skill, artistic ability, and physical movement are themselves forms of intelligence. A highly accomplished politician with keen people skills but with limited skills in mathematics, for example, would be considered quite intelligent (Gardner, 2008; Sternberg, 2015).

Another important criticism of intelligence tests is that they are biased in favor of middle- and upper-class, educated individuals because such people are more familiar with the kinds of reasoning assessed on the tests (Sternberg, 2015). In addition, educated European Americans may be more comfortable taking intelligence tests, because testers often are also European Americans and the testing situation resembles testing situations in their educational experience. In contrast, different cultures within the United States and in other countries may emphasize forms of reasoning other than those assessed on intelligence tests, and members of these cultures may not be comfortable with the testing situation.

A "culture-fair" test would have to include items that are equally applicable to all groups or that are different for each culture but psychologically equivalent for the groups being tested. Attempts have been made to develop culture-fair tests, but the results have been disappointing. Even if a universal test were created, making statements about intelligence in different cultures would be difficult because different nations and cultures vary in the emphasis they place on "intellectual achievement."

Neuropsychological Tests

If the clinician suspects neurological impairment in a person, **neuropsychological tests** may be useful in detecting specific cognitive deficits such as a memory problem, as seen in cases of dementia. One frequently used neuropsychological test is the Bender-Gestalt Test (Bender, 1938). This paper-and-pencil test assesses individuals' sensorimotor skills by having them reproduce a set of nine drawings (Figure 3). People with brain damage may rotate or change parts of the drawings or be unable to reproduce the drawings. When asked to remember the drawings after a delay, they may show significant memory deficits. The Bender-Gestalt Test appears to be good at differentiating people with brain damage from those without brain damage, but it does not reliably identify the specific type of brain damage a person has (Groth-Marnat & Wright, 2016).

More extensive batteries of tests have been developed to pinpoint types of brain damage. Two of the most popular batteries are the Halstead-Reitan Test (Reitan & Davidson, 1974) and the Luria-Nebraska Test (Luria, 1973). These batteries contain several tests that provide specific information about an individual's functioning in several skill areas, such as concentration, dexterity, and speed of comprehension.

Brain-Imaging Techniques

Increasingly, neuropsychological tests are being used with brain-imaging techniques to identify specific deficits and possible brain abnormalities. Clinicians use brain imaging to determine if a patient has a brain injury or tumor. Researchers use brain imaging to search for differences in brain activity or structure between people with a psychological disorder and people with no disorder. Let us review existing brain-imaging technologies and what they can tell us now.

FIGURE 3 | **The Bender-Gestalt Test.** On the left are the figures as presented to the clients. On the right are the figures as copied by a child with a brain tumor that is creating perceptual-motor difficulties.

Computerized tomography (CT) is an enhancement of X-ray procedures. In CT, narrow X-ray beams are passed through the person's head in a single plane from a variety of angles. The amount of radiation absorbed by each beam is measured, and from these measurements a computer program constructs an image of a slice of the brain. By taking many such images, the computer can construct a three-dimensional image showing the brain's major structures. A CT scan can reveal brain injury, tumors, and structural abnormalities. The two major limitations of CT technology are that it exposes patients to X-rays, which can be harmful, and that it provides an image of brain structure rather than brain activity.

Positron-emission tomography (PET) can provide a picture of activity in the brain. PET requires injecting the patient with a harmless radioactive isotope, such as fluorodeoxyglucose (FDG). This substance travels through the blood to the brain. The parts of the brain that are active need the glucose in FDG for nutrition, so FDG accumulates in active parts of the brain. Subatomic particles in FDG called positrons are emitted as the isotope decays. These positrons collide with electrons, and both are annihilated and converted to two photons traveling away from each other in opposite directions. The PET scanner detects these photons and the point at which they are annihilated and constructs an image of the brain, showing those areas that are most active. PET scans can be used to show differences in the activity level of specific areas

CT scans can detect structural abnormalities such as brain tumors. *Puwadol Jaturawutthichai/Alamy Stock Photo*

of the brain between people with a psychological disorder and people without a disorder.

Another procedure to assess brain activity is **single photon emission computed tomography,** or **SPECT.** The procedures of SPECT are much like those of PET except that a different tracer substance is injected. It is less accurate than PET but also less expensive.

Magnetic resonance imaging (MRI) has several advantages over CT, PET, and SPECT technology. It does not require exposing the patient to any radiation or injecting radioisotopes, so it can be used repeatedly for the same individual. It provides much more finely detailed pictures of the anatomy of the brain than do other technologies, and it can image the brain at any angle. Structural MRI provides static images of brain structure. Functional MRI (fMRI) provides images of brain activity.

MRI involves creating a magnetic field around the brain that causes a realignment of hydrogen atoms in the brain. When the magnetic field is turned off and on, the hydrogen atoms change position, causing them to emit magnetic signals. These signals are read by a computer, which reconstructs a three-dimensional image of the brain. To assess activity in the brain, many images are taken only milliseconds apart, showing how the brain changes from one moment to the next or in response to some stimulus. Researchers are using MRI to study structural and functional brain abnormalities in almost every psychological disorder.

Psychophysiological Tests

Psychophysiological tests are alternative methods to CT, PET, SPECT, and MRI used to detect changes in the brain and nervous system that reflect emotional and psychological changes. An **electroencephalogram**

(EEG) measures electrical activity along the scalp produced by the firing of specific neurons in the brain. EEG is used most often to detect seizure activity in the brain and can also be used to detect tumors and stroke. EEG patterns recorded over brief periods (such as ½ second) in response to specific stimuli, such as the individual's viewing of an emotional picture, are referred to as *evoked potentials* or *event-related potentials*. Clinicians can compare an individual's response to the standard response of healthy individuals.

Heart rate and respiration are highly responsive to stress and can be easily monitored. Sweat gland activity, known as *electrodermal response* (formerly called *galvanic skin response*), can be assessed with a device that detects electrical conductivity between two points on the skin. Such activity can reflect emotional arousal. Psychophysiological measures are used to assess people's emotional response to specific types of stimuli, such as the responses a veteran with posttraumatic stress disorder might have to scenes of war.

Projective Tests

A **projective test** is based on the assumption that when people are presented with an ambiguous stimulus, such as an oddly shaped inkblot or a captionless picture, they will interpret the stimulus in line with their current concerns and feelings, relationships with others, and conflicts or desires. People are thought to project these issues onto their description of the "content" of the stimulus—hence the name "projective tests." Proponents of these tests argue that they are useful in uncovering the unconscious issues or motives of a person or in cases when the person is resistant or is heavily biasing the information he or she presents to the assessor. Two of the most frequently used projective tests are the *Rorschach Inkblot Test* and the *Thematic Apperception Test (TAT)*.

Upon hearing the word Rorschach, people are likely to think of ambiguous shapes or inkblots. One person may see a bat, while another may see a bird. We've all seen references to the the Rorschach Inkblot Test, commonly referred to as the Rorschach, in movies and media for decades. This test was developed in 1921 by Swiss psychiatrist Hermann Rorschach and consists of 10 cards, each containing a symmetrical inkblot in black, gray, and white in color. The trained examiner tells the respondent something like "People may see many different things in these inkblot pictures; now tell me what you see, what it makes you think of, what it means to you" (Exner et al., 2008). This is a test in which subjects' perceptions of inkblots are recorded and then analyzed using psychological interpretation.

The basic idea behind this test is the client will project unconscious aspects of their personality by giving meaning to ambiguous images. Clinicians are interested in both the content and the style of the individual's responses to the inkblot. In the content of responses, clinicians look for particular themes or concerns, such as frequent mention of aggression or fear of abandonment. Important stylistic features may include the person's tendency to focus on small details of the inkblot rather than the inkblot as a whole or hesitation in responding to certain inkblots (Exner et al., 2008). A meta-analysis of the Rorschach test recently found that the variables that provided the strongest empirical support were those related to perceptual processes (Yazigi et al., 2016).

Since its conception, this test has been surrounded by controversy with researchers questioning whether the Rorschach is a useful and valid tool for clinicians. For some, this method is a sensitive and accurate tool for showing the inner workings of the mind and detecting a range of mental conditions, including latent problems that other tests or direct observation cannot reveal. While some critics refer to this test as pseudoscience that lacks scientific reliability and validity. Psychologists have argued the psychologist administering the test can also project his or her unconsciousness on to the inkblots when interpreting responses, this creating a biased interpretation. For example, if the person being tested sees a bra, a male psychologist might classify this as a sexual response, whereas a female psychologist may classify it as clothing. Critics of the test also suggest a lack of reliability as it is possible for two different testers to create two different personality profiles for the same person. The Rorschach has also been criticized for its validity. Does the test measure what it is supposed to measure? Rorschach was clear that his test measured disordered thinking (as found in schizophrenia) and this has never been disputed. But whether it accurately measures personality as well is up for debate (Searls, 2017).

The results of the Rorschach test are not cut-and-dried, like an IQ or blood test. But, then again, how can the complexities of the human mind ever be reduced to one simple score? Like other assessments, no one tool should be used solely to make diagnostic decisions. These assessments are best used in combination with other instruments and clinical expertise to best service the client.

The TAT consists of a series of pictures. The individual is asked to make up a story about what is happening in the pictures (Murray, 1943). Proponents of the TAT argue that people's stories reflect their concerns and wishes as well as their personality traits and motives. As with the Rorschach, clinicians are interested in both the content and the style of people's responses to the TAT cards. Some cards may stimulate more emotional responses than others or no response at all. These cards are considered to tap the individuals' most important concerns.

Clinicians operating from psychodynamic perspectives value projective tests as tools for assessing the underlying conflicts and concerns that individuals cannot or will not report directly. Clinicians operating from other perspectives question the usefulness of these tests. The validity and reliability of all the projective tests have not proven strong in research (Groth-Marnat & Wright, 2016; Mihura, Meyer, Dumitrascu, & Bombel, 2013). In addition, because these tests rely so greatly on subjective interpretations by clinicians, they are open to a number of biases. Finally, the criteria for interpreting the tests do not take into account an individual's cultural background (Dana, 2005).

CHALLENGES IN ASSESSMENT

Some challenges that arise in assessing psychological problems is the individual's inability or unwillingness to provide information. In addition, special challenges arise when evaluating children and people from cultures different from that of the assessor.

Resistance to Providing Information

One of the greatest challenges to obtaining valid information from an individual can be his or her resistance to providing information. Sometimes the person does not want to be assessed or treated. For example, when a teenager is forced to see a psychologist because of parental concern about his behavior, he may be resistant to providing any information. Because much of the information a clinician needs must come directly from the person being assessed, resistance can present a formidable problem.

Even when a person is not completely resistant to being assessed, he or she may have a strong interest in the outcome of the assessment and therefore may be highly selective in the information he or she provides, may bias his or her presentation of the information, or may even lie to the assessor. Such problems often arise when assessments are part of a legal case, as when parents are fighting for custody of their children in a divorce. When speaking to psychologists who have been appointed to assess fitness for custody of the children, each parent will want to present himself or herself in the best light and also may negatively bias his or her reports on the other parent.

Evaluating Children

Consider the following conversation between a mother and her 5-year-old son, Jonathon, who was sent home from preschool for fighting with another child.

Mom: Jonathon, why did you hit that boy?

Jonathon: I dunno. I just did.

Mom: But I want to understand what happened. Did he do something that made you mad?

Jonathon: Yeah, I guess.

Mom: What did he do? Did he hit you?

Jonathon: Yeah.

Mom: Why did he hit you?

Jonathon: I dunno. He just did. Can I go now?

Mom: I need to know more about what happened. (Silence)

Mom: Can you tell me more about what happened?

Jonathon: No. He just hit me and I just hit him. Can I go now?

Anyone who has tried to have a conversation with a distressed child about why he or she misbehaved has some sense of how difficult it can be to engage a child in a discussion about emotions or behaviors. Even when a child talks readily, his or her understanding of the causes of his or her behaviors or emotions may not be very well developed. Children, particularly preschool-age children, cannot describe their feelings or associated events as easily as adolescents or adults can. Young children cannot express in words whether they feel afraid, overwhelmed, or helpless. However, their behaviors provide parents, families, and professional with important clues about how they are affected. Young children may not differentiate among different types of emotions—often just saying that they feel "bad." When distressed, children may talk about physical aches and pains rather than the emotional pain they are feeling. Or a child might show distress only in nonverbal behavior, such as making a sad face, withdrawing, or behaving aggressively, adolescents may become disruptive, withdrawn, or resistant to authority (NCTSN, 2010; National Scientific Council on the Developing Child, 2005/2014).

These problems with children's self-reporting of emotional and behavioral concerns have led clinicians and researchers to rely on other people, usually adults in the children's lives, to provide information about children's functioning. Parents are often the first source of information about a child's functioning. A clinician may interview a child's parents when the child is taken for treatment, asking the parents about changes in the child's behavior and corresponding events in the child's life. A researcher studying children's functioning may ask parents to complete questionnaires assessing the children's behavior in a variety of settings.

Parental perception and awareness about psychological illness in children and adolescents is an important determinant of early detection and treatment (Abera, Robins, & Tesfaye, 2015). Because parents typically spend more time with their child than any other person does, they potentially have the most complete information about the child's functioning and the best sense of how the child's behavior has or has not changed over time. Unfortunately, however, parents are not always accurate in their assessments of their children's functioning. One study found that in 63 percent of cases, parents and children disagreed on what problems had brought the child to a psychiatric clinic (Yeh & Weisz, 2001). Parents' perceptions of their children's well-being can be influenced by their own symptoms of psychopathology and by their expectations for their children's behavior (Keeton, Teetsel, Dull, & Ginsburg, 2015; Nock & Kazdin, 2001). Indeed, parents sometimes take children for assessment and treatment of psychological problems as a way of seeking treatment for themselves.

Parents may also suffer from a psychological disorder or exhibit psychological dysfunction that can have a direct impact on the behavioral issues displayed by the child. As a result, they may be unwilling to acknowledge or seek help for the child's difficulties. Numerous studies support the notion that parental psychological well-being influences the overall mental health of the child (Breaux, Harvey, & Lugo-Candelas, 2014). For example, the children of anxious parents often display more psychological dysfunction such as, fears or worries, lower perceptions of control, behavioral inhibition, insecure attachments, and social isolation relative to their peers. There is also evidence of deficits in academic and social functioning. Studies that examined parental self-reports suggest that psychopathology symptoms may play a role in the prognosis of behavioral, social, and emotional outcomes of children with behavior problems (Breaux et al., 2014; Keeton et al., 2015).

Parents with mental health issues can not only negatively impact the development of their child's mental health, but also keep them from receiving the assessment, diagnosis, and treatment that they need. Resistance to mental health services is often a reflection of a parental attitudes that has been shown to influence help-seeking decisions. Additionally, beliefs that mental health problems are caused by child's personality or relational issues, negative perceptions of mental health services, and perceived stigma associated with mental health problems have all been associated with reduced help-seeking behavior (Reardon et al., 2017).

Culture is a critical factor when discussing parental assessment of their child's behavior and decision to seek out mental health services since such wide variation exists among different groups. For example, Eastern cultures place a strong emphasis on interdependence and a child's obligation to, and reliance on, his or her family. These various practices among cultures impact how abnormal behavior is defined and can be seen as undesirable in one culture, but very desirable in another. For example, enmeshment between a mother and child is endorsed in Japan, such that overt displays of clinginess and neediness are considered adaptive. Socially anxious behaviors such as being shy, timid, and reserved are viewed favorably in Asian countries, and sleeping with a parent is a common and socially acceptable practice in Vietnam, Thailand, India, Indonesia, Japan, and China. Western mothers attributed a child's proximity-seeking and demanding behaviors to attention seeking and self-interest, whereas Japanese mothers attributed them to a need for security and interdependence. Taken together, these findings suggest that Asian parents may be less likely to pathologize certain behaviors than parents from Western cultures (Nguyen & McAloon, 2018).

Additionally, even if the family believes the child's behaviors is disruptive or unwanted, the decision to seek out services remains influenced by one's culture. Researchers have focused on identifying the factors that best predict access to mental health services since many children and adolescents are still in need of assistance. Family and child characteristics, including ethnicity, family socioeconomic, and insurance status, living in an urban or rural area, and severity of the child's problems have all been implicated in determining the likelihood of service utilization. Overall, studies suggest that being Caucasian, having insurance coverage (in the USA), living in an urban area, and having a child with more severe mental health problems increases the likelihood of a family accessing treatment. Barriers to treatment reported by parents include concerns about the effectiveness or negative consequences of treatment, feeling blamed for the child's issues, the detrimental impact of perceived negative attitudes of others, as well as personal discomfort surrounding mental health (Reardon et al., 2017).

Teachers also provide information about children's functioning. Teachers and other school personnel (such as guidance counselors and coaches) are often the first to recognize that a child has a problem and to initiate an intervention to address the problem. Teachers' assessments of children, however, are often different from the assessments made by other adults, including parents and trained clinicians (De Los Reyes et al., 2015). Such discrepancies may arise because these other adults are providing invalid assessments of the children whereas the teachers are providing valid assessments. The discrepancies may also arise because children function differently in different settings. At home, a child may be well behaved, quiet, and withdrawn, while at school the same child may be impulsive, easily angered, and distractible.

Evaluating Individuals Across Cultures

A number of challenges to assessment arise when there are significant cultural differences between the client and the therapist (Dana, 2005; Paniagua & Yamada, 2013). Mental health treatments have been shown to be more effective when therapists demonstrate multicultural competence and the treatment aligns with their culture (Soto, Smith, Griner, Rodriguez, & Bernal, 2018). Unfortunately, the diversity of clinician identities continues to lag behind the general population, leading to frequent cultural mismatching in patient/clinician relationships. When this occurs, the likelihood for miscommunication and subpar treatment increases, worsening the health disparities that already exist between these minority populations and the dominant cultural groups (Dominguez, 2017). For example, minority clients are less likely than white patients to state concerns, seek information, or feel trust, thereby decreasing the likelihood of improvement in treatment (Alegria, Nakash, & Johnson, 2018). Additionally, research has shown that there is underutilization of mental health care among several racial and ethnic minority groups across the lifespan (Liang, Matheson, & Douglas, 2016).

A lack of culturally competent professionals also leads to disparities in diagnostic rates and ultimately treatments outcomes. Studies have shown that ethic and racial minority children receive poorer quality mental health care than their non-Hispanic and white counterparts. Additionally, recent research found that mental health professionals (psychiatrists, social workers, psychologists) were more likely to assign a diagnosis to a non-Hispanic white youth as compared to African American or Hispanic youth. Ethnic minorities and people of color (POC) more often receive diagnoses of disruptive- or conduct-related disorders than white individuals (Liang et al., 2016). Additional cultural factors, such as symptom presentation and figurative expressions of distress, among others, may influence how parents recognize and report their problems, which may influence diagnoses.

Cultural biases can arise when everyone supposedly is speaking the same language but has a unique cultural background. There is evidence that African

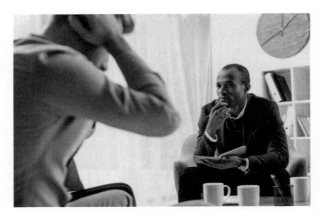

Cultural differences between clients and clinicians can lead to misinterpretations of clients' problems. *LightField Studios/ Shutterstock*

Americans in the United States are over-diagnosed as having symptoms of schizophrenia (Neighbors, Trierweiler, Ford, & Muroff, 2003). Some investigators believe that cultural differences in the presentation of symptoms play a role (Kirmayer, 2001). African Americans may present more intense symptoms than European Americans, and these symptoms then are misunderstood by European American assessors as representing more severe psychopathology. Some European American assessors may be too quick to diagnose psychopathology in African Americans because of negative stereotypes.

Even when clinicians avoid all these biases, they are still left with the fact that people from other cultures often think and talk about their psychological symptoms differently than do members of the clinician's culture. We discuss examples of cultural differences in the presentation of symptoms throughout this book. One of the most pervasive differences is in whether cultures experience and report psychological distress in emotional or somatic (physical) symptoms. European Americans tend to view the body and mind separately, whereas many other cultures do not make sharp distinctions between the experiences of the body and those of the mind (Paniagua & Yamada, 2013). Following a psychologically distressing event, European Americans tend to report that they feel anxious or sad, but members of many other cultures tend to report having physical aches and maladies. To conduct an accurate assessment, clinicians must be aware of cultural differences in the manifestation of disorders and in the presentation of symptoms, and they must use this information correctly in interpreting the symptoms individuals report. Cultural differences are further complicated by the fact that not every member of a culture conforms to what is known about that culture's norms. Within every culture, people differ in their acceptance of cultural norms for behavior.

DIAGNOSIS

Recall that a *diagnosis* is a label we attach to a set of symptoms that tend to occur together. This set of symptoms is called a syndrome. Typically, several symptoms make up a syndrome, but people differ in which of these symptoms will be most prominent. Some of the symptoms that make up the syndrome we call *depression* include sad mood, loss of interest in one's usual activities, sleeplessness, difficulty concentrating, and thoughts of death. But not everyone who becomes depressed experiences all these symptoms—for example, some people lose interest in their usual activities but never really feel sad or blue, and only a subset of depressed people have prominent thoughts of death.

Syndromes are not lists of symptoms that all people have all the time if they have any of the symptoms at all. Rather, they are lists of symptoms that tend to co-occur within individuals. The symptoms of one syndrome may overlap those of another. Figure 4 shows the overlap in the symptoms that make up depression (see the chapter "Mood Disorders and Suicide") and anxiety (see the chapter "Anxiety, Obsessive-Compulsive, Trauma, and Stressor-Related Disorders"). Both syndromes include the symptoms fatigue, sleep disturbances, and concentration problems. However, each syndrome has symptoms more specific to it.

For centuries, people have tried to organize the confusing array of psychological symptoms into a limited set of syndromes. A set of syndromes and the

| FIGURE 4 | **Syndromes as Clusters of Symptoms.** Syndromes are clusters of symptoms that frequently co-occur. The symptoms of one syndrome, such as symptoms of depression, can overlap the symptoms of another syndrome, such as symptoms of anxiety. |

Symptoms of depression

Depressed mood
Loss of interest
Weight loss
Worthlessness, guilt
Suicidal thoughts

Fatigue
Sleep disturbances
Concentration problems

Symptoms of anxiety

Excessive worry
Restlessness
Irritability
Muscle tension

rules for determining whether an individual's symptoms are part of one of these syndromes constitute a **classification system.**

One of the first classification systems for psychological symptoms was proposed by Hippocrates in the fourth century BCE. Hippocrates divided all mental disorders into mania (states of abnormal excitement), melancholia (states of abnormal depression), paranoia, and epilepsy. In 1883, Emil Kraepelin published the first modern classification system, which is the basis of our current systems. Current systems divide the world of psychological symptoms into a much larger number of syndromes than did Hippocrates. We will focus on the classification system most widely used in the United States, the *Diagnostic and Statistical Manual of Mental Disorders,* or *DSM.* The classification system used in Europe and much of the rest of the world, the *International Classification of Disease (ICD),* has many similarities to the most recent editions of the *DSM* (Clark, Cuthbert, Lewis-Fernández, Narrow, & Reed, 2017).

Diagnostic and Statistical Manual of Mental Disorders (DSM)

For more than 60 years, the official manual for diagnosing psychological disorders in the United States has been the *Diagnostic and Statistical Manual of Mental Disorders* of the American Psychiatric Association (APA) now in the fifth edition (2013), known as *DSM-5.* The development of a classification system was motivated by professionals to improve communication about the types of patients that were cared for in hospitals during this time. The *DSM* has drastically changed since the first edition which was published in 1952 and contained the 60 psychological disorders. The *DSM* has evolved since that time through four major revisions into the classification system for psychiatrists, physicians and mental health professionals that describe the critical features of mental disorders (American Psychiatric Association, 2013).

This classification system will always reflect the time in which is it designed and utilized. This also makes it a system that will never be complete and revisions are a necessity. Early editions of this system (*DSM-I* and *DSM-II*) reflect the heavy influence of the psychoanalytic theory, which was widely popular at that time. As subsequent research learned more about mental illness, these criteria became seen as inadequate. For example, the diagnosis of anxiety neurosis could be manifested in a great variety of behaviors and emotions. The key to the diagnosis was whether the clinician believed that unconscious conflicts were causing the individual to experience anxiety. Although the *DSM-II,* published in 1968, included revisions of existing disorders the theoretical framework remained resulting in the low reliability of the diagnoses. For example, one study found that four experienced clinicians using the first edition of the *DSM* to diagnose 153 patients agreed on their diagnoses only 54 percent of the time (Beck, Ward, Mendelson, Moch, & Erbaugh, 1962). This low reliability eventually led psychiatrists and psychologists to call for a radically new system of diagnosing mental disorders.

DSM-III, DSM-IIIR, DSM-IV, DSM-IV-TR, and DSM-5

In response to the concerns about the reliability of disorders outlined in *DSM-I* and *DSM-II,* the American Psychiatric Association published the *DSM-III in 1980.* This third edition was followed in 1987 by a revised third edition, known as *DSM-III-R,* and in 1994 by a fourth edition, known as *DSM-IV,* revised as *DSM-IV-TR* in 2000. These newer editions improved diagnosis by replacing the vague descriptions of disorders with specific and concrete criteria for each disorder. These criteria are in the form of behaviors people must show or experience, or feelings they must report, in order to be given a diagnosis.

The *DSM* authors focused on making the criteria for each disorder as descriptive as possible for professionals to best identify symptoms of these various disorders. As a result, each disorder is defined by a set of diagnostic criteria and text containing information about the disorder. A good example is the diagnostic criteria for panic disorder, which are given in Table 3. A person must have 4 of 13 possible symptoms as well as meet other criteria in order to be diagnosed with panic disorder. These criteria reflect the fact that not all the symptoms of panic disorder are present in every individual.

There are two other elements that distinguish the latter editions of the *DSM* from their predecessors. First, the later editions specify how long a person must show symptoms of the disorder in order to be given the diagnosis (see Table 3, item B). Second, the criteria for most disorders require that symptoms interfere with occupational or social functioning. This emphasis on symptoms that are long-lasting and severe reflects the consensus among psychiatrists and psychologists that abnormality should be defined in terms of the impact of behaviors on the individual's ability to function and on his or her sense of well-being (see the chapter "Looking at Abnormality"). While the *DSM* attempts to precisely define the threshold between normality and abnormality, remember that the setting of the threshold along the continuum is a subjective judgment.

In 1999, the APA created work groups to evaluate the strengths and weaknesses of the *DSM* in preparation of its fifth major revision. This process included

TABLE 3   *DSM-5* Criteria for Panic Disorder

A. Recurrent unexpected panic attacks, defined as an abrupt surge of intense fear or intense discomfort that reaches a peak within minutes, and during which time four or more of the following symptoms occur. (*Note:* The abrupt surge can occur from a calm state or an anxious state.)
  1. Palpitations, pounding heart, or accelerated heart rate
  2. Sweating
  3. Trembling or shaking
  4. Sensations of shortness of breath or smothering
  5. Feelings of choking
  6. Chest pain or discomfort
  7. Nausea or abdominal distress
  8. Feeling dizzy, unsteady, lightheaded, or faint
  9. Chills or heat sensations
  10. Paresthesias (numbness or tingling sensations)
  11. Derealization (feelings of unreality) or depersonalization (being detached from oneself)
  12. Fear of losing control or going crazy
  13. Fear of dying
B. At least one of the attacks has been followed by 1 month (or more) of one or both of the following:
  1. Persistent concern or worry about additional panic attacks or their consequences (e.g., losing control, having a heart attack, "going crazy")
  2. Significant maladaptive change in behavior related to the attacks (e.g., behaviors designed to avoid having panic attacks, such as avoidance of exercise or unfamiliar situations)
C. The disturbance is not attributable to the direct physiological effects of a substance (e.g., a drug of abuse, a medication) or another medical condition (e.g., hyperthyroidism, cardiopulmonary disorders).
D. The disturbance is not better accounted for by another mental disorder (e.g., the panic attacks do not occur only in response to feared social situations in social anxiety disorder, circumscribed phobic objects or situations in specific phobia, obsessions in obsessive-compulsive disorder, reminders of traumatic events in posttraumatic stress disorder, or separation from attachment figures in separation anxiety disorder).

extensive "literature reviews and secondary analyses, publishing research reports in scientific journals, developing draft diagnostic criteria, posting preliminary drafts on the *DSM-5* website for public comment, presenting preliminary findings at professional meetings, performing field trials, and revisiting criteria and text"(American Psychiatric Association, 2013). The result of this effort provided the professional community with a summary of the current science relevant to psychiatric diagnosis and identified where gaps existed in the current research. Additionally, this evaluation produced a more universal language among professionals to better communicate about the diagnosis of psychological disorders.

The extensive research that was performed in anticipation of the *DSM-5* contributed to the modification and development of the clinical criteria for all existing psychological disorders. This new edition removed, added, and modified as necessary the existing criteria for other disorders. This information will continue to be modified as new evidence is gathered in future research. To represent the *DSM* as a "living document," the APA replaced the roman numeral in the title with an Arabic one that can be updated as research develops, as in *DSM 5.1, 5.2,* and so on.

When the *DSM-5* was finalized, some disorders that had been evaluated were not included within the main body of the document because there was not enough scientific evidence to support their widespread clinical use. However, these disorders are included in Section III under "Conditions for Further Study" to "highlight the evolution and direction of scientific advances in these areas to stimulate further research" (American Psychiatric Association, 2013). In addition, the authors of the *DSM-5* attempted to incorporate a continuum or dimensional perspective, much like that described in the chapter "Looking at Abnormality," into the diagnosis of several disorders, particularly autism and the personality disorders (Clark, Cuthbert, Lewis-Fernandez, Narrow, & Reed, 2017), which was a departure from the previous categorical assessment.

While the *DSM* is the most used classification system in the United States, the *ICD*, published by the World Health Organization (WHO), is used worldwide. The *ICD-11* is the global standard for

SHADES OF GRAY

As you read the following case study, compare Mark's symptoms to the criteria in Table 3. Do Mark's symptoms meet the criteria for panic disorder? *(Discussion appears at the end of this chapter.)*

When Mark went to an appointment with his physician, he looked pale and visibly nervous. He told his doctor that twice in the last month he had had an episode in which his heart suddenly started racing, he felt short of breath and cold all over, and he trembled uncontrollably. He was sure, when these feelings were happening, that he was dying of a heart attack. The symptoms lasted about 10 minutes and then subsided. His doctor asked Mark where he was when these symptoms began. Mark said the first time he felt this way was when he was about to give a presentation in an important class. The second time was when he was on his way to meet his parents for dinner.

diagnostic health information. A shared goal between the authors of the *DSM-5* and *ICD-11* was to harmonize these two classifications systems to reflect the globalization of mental health research and the desire for a similar diagnostic system. Aligning these two systems will enhance the consistency of *DSM* and *ICD* revisions for clinical guidance, provide a more accurate collection of national health statistics, support the design and dissemination of research, and help enhance diagnostic agreement (Regier, Kuhl, & Kupfer, 2013).

Continuing Debates About the *DSM*

Is this system perfect? Of course it's not. Just because this is a widely implemented system doesn't make it without flaws and criticisms. Substantial controversy has surrounded the development of the *DSM-5* (Frances & Widiger, 2012) focused on the empirical justification for the inclusion and exclusion of disorders, claims that the process of developing the *DSM-5* was clouded by secrecy and a disregard for alternative points of view, and concerns about the social impact of some of the new diagnoses (e.g., lowering the threshold for some diagnoses risks pathologizing normal variations in behaviors).

Although the *DSM-5* was meant to reflect developments in our understanding of mental disorders, debates continue over fundamental questions about the classification and diagnosis of disorders. We next consider some of these debates.

For over 60 years the *Diagnostic and Statistical Manual of the Mental Disorders,* or *DSM,* has been the official reference for diagnosing psychological disorders in the United States. The fifth edition was published in 2013. *Murat Sarica/Getty Images*

Reifying Diagnoses. Once a diagnosis is defined in any classification system, people tend to reify it. That means seeing the diagnosis as real and true rather than as the product of a set of judgments about how symptoms tend to occur together (Hyman, 2010). These clinical judgments are made by experts and based on the best empirical science of the time, but they are imperfect and reflect the social constructions of our society's current views of mental disorders. Moreover, as noted in the chapter "Looking at Abnormality," it's increasingly clear that certain problems in biological, psychological, and social functioning cut across many disorders (Cuthbert & Insel, 2013; Sanislow et al., 2011). The reification of diagnoses can impede progress in research and treatment as researchers focus on understanding the causes of and treatments for the diagnosis rather than on the biological, psychological, and social problems that underlie the disorder and related disorders (Hyman, 2010). Indeed, it can be difficult for researchers to obtain funding to study problems that are not official diagnoses in the *DSM* and for clinicians to be reimbursed by insurance companies to treat them.

Category or Continuum. The *DSM-IV-TR* and its predecessors were *categorical* diagnostic systems, meaning that their diagnostic criteria defined where normality ends and psychopathology begins. The *DSM-5* retains the categorical system for most diagnoses, but it introduces a continuum or dimensional perspective for a number of disorders, such as the autism spectrum disorders, personality disorders, and substance use disorders. Further, a number of dimensional assessment scales for rating a person's symptoms and functioning have been added to the *DSM-5*. These moves toward a more dimensional model of diagnosis reflect the growing consensus that all behaviors fall along a continuum and that most disorders represent extremes along this continuum (Clark et al., 2017).

Yet questions have been raised about whether a continuum perspective is practical for real-world use (First, 2010). Busy clinicians have to make a multitude of decisions every day, and it may be easier to think in terms of categories than continuums. Prior versions of the *DSM* had some dimensions along which clinicians could rate patients' functioning, but there is evidence that most clinicians did not use them (First, 2010). So although in reality mental health and mental disorders may exist along continuums or dimensions, the human mind may be constructed to think more in terms of categories to determine the presence or absence of disorders.

Differentiating Mental Disorders from One Another. A frequent complaint with the *DSM-IV* and *DSM-IV-TR* was the difficulty in differentiating the mental disorders from one another (Watson, 2009). Most people who were diagnosed with one disorder also met the criteria for at least one other disorder, a situation referred to as **comorbidity.** This overlap occurs, in part, because certain symptoms show up in the criteria for several different disorders. For example, irritability or agitation can be part of depression, mania, anxiety, schizophrenia, some of the personality disorders, and some of the childhood disorders. Some changes in the *DSM-5* were made to try to correct the problem of comorbidity. For example, many of the diagnoses of the personality disorders (see the chapter "Personality Disorders") were revised to reduce the amount of overlap in the criteria for different disorders.

Although we might want to make the diagnostic criteria for disorders more distinct, recent research suggests that much of the comorbidity among disorders exists because it reflects problems in fundamental cognitive, emotional, and behavioral processes that cut across many disorders, such as sleep problems, depressed or anxious mood, and substance use (Sanislow et al., 2011). Some experts believe that diagnostic systems of the future will specify how these dimensions come together to create different types of psychopathology, as well as how and why these psychopathologies are related (Cuthbert & Insel, 2013). The authors of the *DSM-5* developed a set of instruments to assess variations in cognitive, emotional, and behavioral processes. These instruments are not part of the *DSM-5* but are available for use by researchers and clinicians to obtain ratings for important dimensions regardless of the specific disorder with which an individual might be diagnosed in Section III of the manual (Helzer et al., 2008).

In the meantime, however, most people who are given one diagnosis of a mental disorder will also meet the criteria for at least one other diagnosis (Kessler et al., 2005). This leads to many questions, such as which diagnosis should be considered the primary diagnosis and which the secondary diagnosis, which diagnosis should be treated first, whether people with diagnoses A and B are fundamentally different from or similar to people with diagnoses A and C, and so on.

Addressing Cultural Issues. Different cultures have distinct ways of conceptualizing mental disorders. Some disorders that are defined in one culture do not seem to occur in others. Table 4 describes some of these culture-bound syndromes. In addition, there is cultural variation in the presentation of symptoms. For example, there are differences among cultures in the content of delusions (beliefs out of touch with reality) in schizophrenia. The *DSM-5* and its predecessors provide guidelines for considering cultural

TABLE 4   Culture-Bound Syndromes

Certain syndromes appear to occur only in some cultures.

Syndrome	Cultures Where Found	Symptoms
Amok	Malaysia, Laos, Philippines, Polynesia, Papua New Guinea, Puerto Rico	Brooding followed by an outburst of violent, aggressive, or homicidal behavior
Ataque de nervios	Latin America and Latin Mediterranean cultures	Uncontrollable shouting, attacks of crying, trembling, heat in the chest rising into the head, verbal or physical aggression, a sense of being out of control
Dhat	India, Sri Lanka, China	Severe anxiety about the discharge of semen, whitish discoloration of the urine, feelings of weakness and exhaustion
Ghost sickness	Native American cultures	Preoccupation with death and the deceased, manifested in dreams and in severe anxiety
Koro	Malaysia, China, Thailand	Episode of sudden and intense anxiety that the penis (or, in women, the vulva and nipples) will recede into the body and possibly cause death
Mal de ojo	Mediterranean cultures	Fitful sleep, crying without apparent cause, diarrhea, vomiting, fever
Shinjingshuairuo	China	Physical and mental fatigue, dizziness, headaches, other pains, concentration difficulties, sleep disturbance, memory loss
Susto	U.S. Latinos, Mexico, Central America, South America	Appetite disturbances, sleep problems, sadness, lack of motivation, low self-worth, aches and pains; follows a frightening experience
Taijin kyofusho	Japan	Intense fear that one's body displeases, embarrasses, or is offensive to other people

issues such as the kinds of symptoms acceptable in the individual's culture. Some critics do not believe these guidelines have gone far enough in recognizing cultural variation in what behaviors, thoughts, and feelings are considered healthy or unhealthy (Kirmayer, 2001). Throughout the remainder of this book, we will comment on cultural variations in the experience and prevalence of each disorder recognized by the *DSM*.

The Social-Psychological Dangers of Diagnosis

We noted earlier that once a diagnosis is given, people tend to see it as real rather than as a judgment. This can make people oblivious to the biases that may influence diagnoses. One influential critic of psychiatry, Thomas Szasz (1920–2012), argued that so many biases are inherent in determining who is labeled as having a mental disorder that the entire system of diagnosis is corrupt and should be abandoned. Szasz (1961) believed that people in power use psychiatric diagnoses to label and isolate people who do not "fit in." He suggested that mental disorders do not really exist and that people who seem to be suffering from mental disorders are oppressed by a society that does not accept their alternative ways of behaving and looking at the world.

Even psychiatrists and psychologists who do not fully agree with Szasz' perspective recognize that giving a person a diagnosis leads to certain judgments and expectations of them that can have unintended consequences. This point was made in a classic study of the effects of diagnoses by psychologist David Rosenhan (1973). He and seven colleagues had themselves admitted to 12 different mental hospitals by reporting to hospital staff that they had been hearing voices saying the words "empty," "hollow," and "thud." When they were questioned by hospital personnel, they told the truth about every other aspects of their lives, including the fact that they had never experienced mental health problems before. All eight were admitted to the hospitals, all but one with a diagnosis of schizophrenia (see the chapter "Schizophrenia Spectrum and Other Psychotic Disorders").

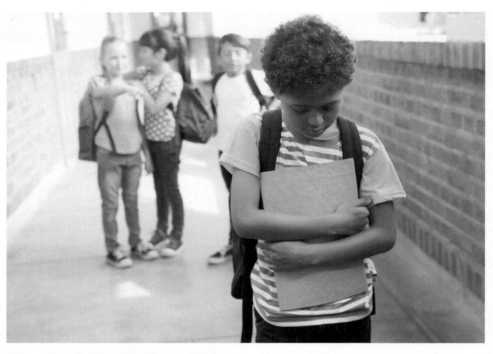

Children who are labeled as different can be ostracized by other children. *Wavebreakmedia/Getty Images*

Once they were admitted to the hospitals, the pseudopatients stopped reporting that they were hearing voices and behaved as normally as they usually did. When asked how they were doing by hospital staff, the pseudopatients said they felt fine and no longer heard voices. They cooperated in activities. The only thing they did differently from other patients was to write down their observations on notepads occasionally during the day.

Nevertheless, not one of the pseudopatients was ever detected as normal by hospital staff, although they remained in the hospitals for an average of 19 days. Several of the other patients in the mental hospitals detected the pseudopatients' normality, however, making comments such as "You're not crazy, you're a journalist, or a professor [referring to the continual note taking]. You're checking up on the hospital" (Rosenhan, 1973). When the pseudopatients were discharged, they were given the diagnosis of schizophrenia in remission, meaning that the physicians still believed the pseudopatients had schizophrenia but the symptoms had subsided for the time being.

Rosenhan (1973) concluded, "It is clear that we cannot distinguish the sane from the insane in psychiatric hospitals. The hospital itself imposes a special environment in which the meanings of behavior can be easily misunderstood." He also noted that, if even mental health professionals cannot distinguish sanity from insanity, the dangers of diagnostic labels are even greater in the hands of nonprofessionals: "Such labels, conferred by mental health professionals, are as influential on the patient as they are on his relatives and friends, and it should not surprise anyone that the diagnosis acts on all of them as a self-fulfilling prophecy. Eventually, the patient himself accepts the diagnosis, with all of its surplus meanings and expectations, and behaves accordingly."

Not surprisingly, Rosenhan's study created a furor in the mental health community. How could seasoned professionals have made such mistakes—admitting mentally healthy people to psychiatric hospitals on the basis of one symptom (hearing voices), not recognizing the pseudopatients' behavior as normal, allowing them to be discharged carrying a diagnosis that suggested they still had schizophrenia? Even today, Rosenhan's study is held up as an example of the abuses of the power to label people as sane or insane, normal or abnormal, good or bad. Not only do clinicians and the public begin to view the person as his or her disorder (e.g., he is a schizophrenic, she is a depressive), but people with disorders also take on the role of a disordered person, a role they may carry for the rest of their lives.

So, should we avoid psychiatric diagnoses altogether? Probably not. Despite the potential dangers of diagnostic systems, they serve vital functions. The primary role of diagnostic systems is to organize the confusing array of psychological symptoms in an agreed-upon manner. This organization facilitates communication from one clinician to another and across time.

For example, if Dr. Jones reads in a patient's history that he was diagnosed with schizophrenia according to the *DSM-5*, she knows what criteria were used to make that diagnosis and can compare the patient's diagnosis then with his symptoms now. Such information can assist Dr. Jones in making an accurate assessment of the patient's current symptoms and in determining the proper treatment for his symptoms. For example, if the patient's current symptoms also suggest schizophrenia and the patient responded to Drug X when he had schizophrenia a few years ago, this history indicates that he might respond well to Drug X now.

Having a standard diagnostic system also greatly facilitates research on psychological disorders. For example, if a researcher at University A is using the *DSM-5* criteria to identify people with obsessive-compulsive disorder and a researcher at University B is using the same criteria for the same purpose, the two researchers will be better able to compare the results of their research than if they were using different criteria to diagnose obsessive-compulsive disorder. Standardization can lead to faster advances in our understanding of the causes of and effective treatments for disorders.

What Happens after a Diagnosis Is Made?

Assigning a diagnosis is the easy part. The work that the client and therapist will perform to address the symptoms of the disorder is much harder. Once a client has completed the diagnostic process they must now work with their therapist (psychiatrist, psychologist, counselor, social worker, etc.) to develop a comprehensive treatment plan specially designed to meet the client's needs and improve psychological function. The treatment plan will be designed to establish clear goals and objectives to help provide the most appropriate treatment for the client. The treatment plan is used by the mental health professional to organize treatment goals, track the progress of the client, and keep a record of patient care. The clinician should triage this process and focus the treatment on the most

FIGURE 5 | Integration of Biological, Psychological, and Social Factors in Assessment and Diagnosis.

critical psychological issues, such as suicidal ideation or inability to take care of one's self. Once the crisis is addressed, the therapist can then address problems in the near future and finally issues that require extensive work well into the future.

CHAPTER INTEGRATION

Assessment is inherently a process of biopsychosocial integration of pieces of information about an individual. After clinicians administer a battery of assessment tests to a person, they must then integrate the information gathered from these tests to form a coherent picture of the person's characteristics, symptoms, strengths, and weaknesses. This picture weaves together information on biological functioning (major illnesses, possible genetic vulnerability to psychopathology), psychological functioning (personality, coping skills, intellectual strengths), and social functioning (support networks, work relationships, social skills) (Figure 5).

SHADES OF GRAY DISCUSSION

If you determined that Mark has experienced panic attacks, you are correct. The *DSM-5* requires four symptoms for diagnosis of a panic attack (see criterion A), and Mark reports five: rapid heartbeat, shortness of breath, chills, trembling, and feeling as though he was going to die. Further, these symptoms seem to have developed suddenly and to have increased in intensity within minutes, meeting criterion A in Table 3.

It is less clear whether Mark's symptoms meet the criterion that they are "unexpected," because his panic attacks occurred before giving an important presentation and before meeting his parents and may often (or

expectedly) occur in these situations. In addition, criterion B requires him to have been persistently fearful of another panic attack or to have made significant maladaptive changes in his behavior related to panic attacks for at least a month. We cannot tell whether either of these conditions has been met. We also cannot rule out the possibility of an organic factor, such as too much coffee, or another mental disorder having caused his panic attacks, so we do not know if he meets criteria C and D. Thus, although it appears that Mark has experienced some panic attacks, we cannot currently diagnose him with panic disorder.

CHAPTER SUMMARY

- Assessment is the process of gathering information about people's symptoms and the causes of these symptoms. Diagnosis is a label we attach to symptoms that tend to co-occur.

- The validity and reliability of assessment tools indicate their quality. Validity is the accuracy of a test in assessing what it is supposed to assess. Five types of validity are face validity, content validity, concurrent validity, predictive validity, and construct validity. Reliability is the consistency of a test. Types of reliability include test-retest reliability, alternate form reliability, internal reliability, and interrater reliability. Standardization of the implementation and interpretation of an assessment tool can increase both validity and reliability.

- In a mental status exam, the clinician assesses the individual's (a) appearance and behavior, (b) thought processes, (c) mood and affect, (d) intellectual functioning, and (e) orientation.

- To assess emotional and behavioral functioning, clinicians use structured clinical interviews, symptom questionnaires, personality inventories, behavioral observation, and self-monitoring.

- Paper-and-pencil neuropsychological tests can assess specific cognitive deficits that may be related to brain damage in patients. Intelligence tests provide a more general measure of verbal and analytical skills.

- Brain-imaging techniques such as CT, PET, SPECT, and MRI scans currently are being used primarily for research purposes, but in the future they may contribute to the diagnosis and assessment of psychological disorders.

- Psychophysiological tests, including the electroencephalogram (EEG) and electrodermal responses, assess brain and nervous system activity detectable on the periphery of the body (such as on the scalp and skin).

- Projective tests present individuals with ambiguous stimuli. Clinicians interpret individuals' reactions to the stimuli. Both the validity and the reliability of these tests are low.

- During the assessment procedure, many problems and biases can be introduced. Individuals may be resistant to being assessed and thus distort the information they provide. They may be too impaired by cognitive deficits, distress, or lack of development of verbal skills to provide information. Further, many biases can arise when the clinician and the individual are from different cultures.

- A classification system is a set of definitions of syndromes and rules for determining when a person's symptoms are part of each syndrome. In the United States, the predominant classification system for psychological problems is the *Diagnostic and Statistical Manual of Mental Disorders (DSM)* of the American Psychiatric Association. Its most recent editions provide specific criteria for diagnosing each of the recognized psychological disorders, as well as information on the course and prevalence of disorders.

- The explicit criteria in the *DSM* have increased the reliability of diagnoses, but there is still room for improvement.

- The *DSM-5* provides three axes on which clinicians can assess individuals. On Axis I, major clinical syndromes and any medical conditions individuals have are noted. On Axis II, psychosocial and environmental stressors are noted. On Axis III, individuals' general levels of functioning are assessed.

- Critics point to many dangers in labeling people as having psychiatric disorders, including the danger of stigmatization. Diagnosis is important, however, to communication among clinicians and researchers. Only when a system of definitions of disorders is agreed on can communication about disorders be improved.

KEY TERMS

assessment

presenting problem

syndrome

diagnosis

validity

reliability

clinical interview

mental status exam

sensorium

structured interview

unstructured interview

Semi-structured interviews

symptom questionnaire

personality inventories

behavioral observation

self-monitoring

intelligence tests

neuropsychological tests

computerized tomography (CT)

positron-emission tomography (PET)

single photon emission computed tomography (SPECT)

magnetic resonance imaging (MRI)

psychophysiological tests

electroencephalogram (EEG)

projective test

classification system

Diagnostic and Statistical Manual of Mental Disorders (DSM)

comorbidity

Chapter 4

MachineHead/Getty Images

The Research Endeavor

CHAPTER OUTLINE

Research Along the Continuum

Research with Continuum Approach

Studies focus on people with symptoms that range in severity from the everyday *(occasional sad mood)* to the highly impairing and likely to meet criteria for a disorder *(paralyzing depression)*.

Research with Threshold Approach

Studies focus on people with diagnosed disorders of various severities *(adjustment disorder with depressed mood, major depressive disorder)* or on comparisons of people with diagnosed disorders and people without disorders.

Depressive symptoms:
| *No symptoms* | *Low symptoms* | *Moderate symptoms* | *Severe symptoms meeting diagnostic criteria* |

This textbook is designed to help you understand psychopathology using a continuum model which remains a hot topic for debate in the field of abnormal psychology. Researchers disagree on whether studies should be based on a continuum or a categorical model of psychopathology (Lilienfeld & Treadway, 2016). The difference lies mainly in how researchers view people who have some symptoms of a disorder but do not meet all the criteria for diagnosis.

Researchers who favor continuum models believe that they provide valuable insights into people who have diagnosable disorders. The continuum model takes into consideration the positive aspects of mental health, rather than just the dysfunction to provide a well-rounded view of psychological health (Angst et al., 2007).

Researchers who do not support continuum models argue that people who fall short of a diagnosable disorder are inherently different from those who have a disorder and that therefore studies of these people cannot be applied to those who have a disorder. Many researchers focus on cut-off points to determine where one behavior ends and a disorder begins. Much of psychological research on mental illness views clinical pathology through a lens of normal versus abnormal function (Gibbons et al., 2013; Maurer, Raymond, & Davis, 2018). Much of psychological research on mental illness views clinical pathology through a lens of normal versus abnormal function despite the difficulties in establishing one from the other. Indeed, there are very few widely accepted ideas in the field of psychopathology research.

The debate continues, with evidence supporting both points of view. Some research methods use a continuum model, such as a study of the relationship between how many stressors individuals have experienced and how many depressive symptoms they report. In contrast, investigators who are interested only in differences between people with diagnosed disorders and people who do not meet diagnostic criteria would be more likely to compare these two groups on the number of stressors they have experienced. We explore several research methods in this chapter.

It is important to remember that research is a cumulative process. No one study can definitively answer complex questions about the causes of and best treatments for mental disorders. Too often, individual studies generate a great deal of media attention, with headlines such as "Scientists Find the Gene for Schizophrenia" or "Study Shows Antidepressant Medications Do Not Work." The public can be given false hopes for breakthroughs that are dashed by future studies, leading to cynicism and reduced funding of mental health science. People with mental health problems can also come to believe that they should discontinue some treatment because one study raised doubts about its effectiveness. Only with the accumulation of evidence from multiple studies using multiple methods can we begin to have faith in the answer to a question about the causes of or appropriate treatments for a disorder.

Extraordinary People

Communication in the Time of Social Media

Momentum Fotograh/Shutterstock

The influence of social media has changed the way we receive, process, and accept information. In earlier times, our real world community was a large source of information and we could seek out and find opinions and information that both support and deny our personal beliefs. However, today with the widespread use of social media, we are more likely to accept information that supports our existing beliefs. People are also more likely to seek out individuals with similar beliefs. This use of confirmation bias and selective exposure often creates polarized and like-minded clusters of opinion, commonly referred to as *echo chambers*. This practice of opinion-based confirmation bias found within the echo-chamber of social media reduces the likelihood for exchanging differing points of view. This can also strengthen rumors and fake news and intensify the segregation of their believers. This new age of misinformation has profound outcomes for our culture and how we understand and explain issues like mental illness. Social media feeds are personally curated and tailored to individual beliefs, partisan bias, and identity creating information silos (Wang, Sirianni, Tang, Zheng, & Fu, 2020).

We live in a time with more information than ever before, but there is a trend of scientific rejection and support of unfounded beliefs like, conspiracy theories, magic, superstition, and the supernatural. According to a 2013 poll, 37 percent of Americans believe that global warming is a hoax, 21 percent believe that a UFO crashed in Roswell, 20 percent think vaccines cause autism, and 15 percent believe that the medical and pharmaceutical industry create new diseases to sell the cure to the public (Stahl & Van Prooijen, 2018). Just like the social media industry, members of the medical field are also challenged to find ways to reduce the spread of false and incomplete health information. Online discourse via social media can be filled with misinformation about alternative therapies or skepticism about medical practices which can create adverse effects on public health. This misinformation may be abundant on social media and some evidence has linked the sharing of misinformation with health-related knowledge, attitudes, and beliefs (Chou, Oh, & Klein, 2018).

Although research in abnormal psychology in many ways resembles research in other fields, the study of psychopathology presents some special challenges. One challenge is accurately measuring abnormal behaviors and feelings. We cannot see, hear, or feel other people's emotions and thoughts. Researchers often must rely on people's own accounts, or self-reports, of their internal states and experiences. Self-reports can be distorted in a number of ways, intentionally or unintentionally. Similarly, relying on an observer's assessments of a person has its own pitfalls. The observer's assessments can be biased by stereotypes involving gender and culture, idiosyncratic biases, and lack of information. A second challenge is the difficulty of obtaining the participation of populations of interest, such as people experiencing paranoia in which they believe there is a conspiracy against them or hallucinations, such as hearing voices that no one else can.

A third challenge, mentioned in the Research Along the Continuum feature, is that most forms of abnormality probably have multiple causes. Unless a single study can capture all the biological, psychological, and social causes of the psychopathology of interest, it cannot fully explain the causes of that abnormality. Rarely can a single study accomplish so much. Instead, we usually are left with partial answers to the question of what causes a certain disorder or symptom, and we must piece together the partial answers from several studies to get a complete picture.

Despite these challenges, researchers have made tremendous strides in understanding many forms of abnormality in the past 50 years or so. They have overcome many of the challenges of researching psychopathology by using a multimethod approach—that is, using different methods to study the same issue. Each different research method may have some limitations, but taken together the methods can provide convincing evidence concerning an abnormality.

In this chapter, we discuss the most common methods of mental health research. In our discussion, we will use various research methods to test the idea that stress contributes to depression. Of course, these research methods are also used to test many other ideas.

THE SCIENTIFIC METHOD

Any research project involves a basic series of steps designed to obtain and evaluate, in a systematic way, information relevant to a problem. This process is often called the **scientific method.**

First, researchers must select and define a problem. In our case, the problem is to determine the relationship between stress and depression. Then a **hypothesis,** or testable statement of what we predict will happen in our study, must be formulated. Next, the method for testing the hypothesis must be chosen and implemented. Once the data have been collected and analyzed, the researcher draws the appropriate conclusions and documents the results in a research report.

Defining the Problem and Stating a Hypothesis

Throughout this chapter, we will examine the idea that stress causes depression. This simple idea is too broad and abstract to test directly. Thus, we must state a hypothesis, or a testable prediction of what relationship between stress and depression we expect to find in our study.

To generate a hypothesis, we might ask, "What kind of evidence would support the idea that stress causes depression?" If we find that people who have recently experienced stress are more likely to be depressed than people who have not recently experienced stress, this evidence would support our idea. One hypothesis, then, is that people who have recently been under stress are more likely to be depressed than people who have not. We can test this hypothesis by a number of research methods.

The alternative to our hypothesis is that people who experience stress are not more likely to develop depression than people who do not experience stress. This prediction that there is no relationship between the phenomena we are studying—in this case, stress and depression—is called the **null hypothesis.** Results often support the null hypothesis instead of the researcher's primary hypothesis.

Does support for the null hypothesis mean that the underlying idea has been disproved? No. The null hypothesis can be supported for many reasons, including flaws in the study design. Researchers often will continue to test their primary hypothesis, using a variety of methodologies. If the null hypothesis continues to get much more support than the primary hypothe-

sis, the researchers eventually either modify or drop the primary hypothesis.

Choosing and Implementing a Method

Once we have stated a hypothesis, the next step in testing our idea that stress leads to depression is to choose how we are going to define the phenomena we are studying.

A **variable** is a factor or characteristic that can vary within an individual or between individuals. Weight, mood, and attitudes toward one's mother are all factors that can vary over time, so they are considered variables. Characteristics such as sex and ethnicity do not vary for an individual over time, but because they vary from one individual to another, they too can be considered variables. An **independent variable** is the factor that is manipulated to see if it has any effect. For example, the independent variable is the amount of stress an individual has experienced. A **dependent variable** is the factor that is measured to predict an outcome in the study. Meaning, in this study, the amount of stress the person experiences (IV) influences whether or not depression develops (DV). The amount of stress is manipulated and the behaviors associated with depression are observed, which provides a cause and effect relationship in this type of research.

In order to research depression and stress, we must first define what we mean by these terms. As we discuss in the chapter "Mood Disorders and Suicide," depression is a syndrome or a collection of the following symptoms: sadness, loss of interest in one's usual activities, weight loss or gain, changes in sleep, physical agitation or slowing down, fatigue and loss of energy, feelings of worthlessness or excessive guilt, problems in concentration or indecisiveness, and suicidal thoughts (American Psychiatric Association, 2013). Researchers who adopt a continuum model of depression focus on the full range of depressive symptoms, from no symptoms to moderate symptoms to the most severe symptoms. Researchers who do not accept a continuum model would not consider anyone who has some of these symptoms to be depressed because they do not meet the full diagnostic criteria.

Stress is more difficult to define, because the term has been used in so many ways in research and in the popular press. Many researchers consider stressful events to be events that are uncontrollable, unpredictable, and challenging to the limits of people's abilities to cope (see the chapter "Health Psychology").

Operationalization refers to the way we measure or manipulate the variables in a study. Our definitions of depression and stress will influence how we

SHADES OF GRAY

Imagine that you are the student member of the human participants committee that is considering the ethics of research at your school. A researcher proposes a study in which participants would believe they were taking a test that indicated their intellectual ability. In truth, half the participants would be randomly assigned to receive feedback that they had done poorly on the test, and half would be randomly assigned to receive feedback that they had done well on the test. The researcher would measure participants' moods before and after taking the test and receiving the feedback.

At a minimum, what would you require of the researcher in order to consider this study ethical? (Discussion appears at the end of this chapter.)

measure these variables. For example, if we define depression as a diagnosable depressive disorder, then we will measure depression in terms of the diagnostic criteria for a depressive disorder. If we define depression as symptoms along the entire range of severity, then we might measure depression as scores on a depression questionnaire.

In measuring stress, we might assess how often a person has encountered events that most people would consider stressful. Or we might devise a way of manipulating or creating stress so that we can then examine people's depression in response to this stress. In the remaining sections of this chapter, we will discuss different methods for testing hypotheses, as well as the conclusions that can and cannot be drawn from these methods.

Ethical Issues in Research

Any research, whether experimental or otherwise, must be evaluated to ensure it is ethical. All colleges and universities have *human participants committees* (often referred to as human subjects committees, institutional review boards, or ethics committees). These committees review the procedures of studies done with humans to ensure that the benefits of the study substantially outweigh any risks to the participants and that the risks to the participants have been minimized. The committees ensure that each research study includes certain basic rights for all participants:

1. *Understanding the study.* Participants have the right to understand the nature of the research they are participating in, particularly any factors that might influence their willingness to participate. For example, if they are likely to experience discomfort (psychological or physical) as a result of participating in the study or if the study entails any risk to their well-being, the researcher should explain this in plain language to the participants. Individuals not capable of understanding the risks of a study, such as young children or adults with cognitive impairments, must have a parent, guardian, or other responsible adult make the judgment about their participation in the study.

2. *Confidentiality.* Participants should expect their identity and any information gathered from them in the course of the study to be held in strict confidence. Researchers usually report data aggregated across participants rather than data gathered from individual participants. Researchers who intend to report data gathered from individuals should obtain their explicit permission.

3. *Right to refuse or withdraw participation.* Participants should be allowed to refuse to participate in the study or to withdraw from participation once the study has begun without suffering adverse consequences. If students are participating in a study as a course requirement or as an opportunity for extra credit for a class, they should be given the choice of equitable alternative activities if they wish not to participate. Payment or other inducements for being in a study should not be so great that individuals essentially cannot afford to refuse to participate.

4. *Informed consent.* Usually, participants' consent to participate in the study should be documented in writing. In some cases, a written informed consent document is not used, as when participants are filling out an anonymous survey (in this case, their willingness to complete the survey is taken as their consent to participate). Also, if obtaining written documentation of participants' consent could put them at risk, the researcher sometimes is allowed to obtain only verbal consent. Examples of when this would be permitted include research being done in countries where a civil war is ongoing or an oppressive regime is in power, in which case participants might be at risk if it is discovered they have talked with researchers.

5. *Deception.* Researchers should use deception in studies only when doing so is absolutely essential and justified by the study's potential contributions.

Participants should not be deceived about those aspects of the research that might affect their willingness to participate, such as physical risks, discomfort, or unpleasant emotional experiences. If deception is necessary, researchers should explain the deception to the participants after the research is completed.

6. *Debriefing.* At the end of the study, researchers should explain the purpose of the research and answer participants' questions. Although these rights may seem straightforward, human participants committees must make judgment calls as to whether a given study adequately protects participants' rights and whether the potential benefits of the study outweigh any risks to the participants.

Case studies can provide very detailed information about a person with a unique condition, but lack generalizability to other groups. *Tom M Johnson/Blend Images/Getty Images*

CASE STUDIES

Throughout this book, you will see **case studies**—detailed histories of unique individuals who have some form of psychological disorder. Case studies have been used for centuries as a way to understand the experiences of individuals and to make more general inferences about the sources of psychopathology.

If we wanted to use a case study to test our idea that stress causes depression, we would focus on an individual, interviewing him or her at length to discover the links between periods of depression and stressful events in his or her life. We might also interview close friends and family to obtain additional information. Based on the information we gathered, we would create a detailed description of the causes of their depressive episodes, with emphasis on the role of stressful events in these episodes.

Evaluating Case Studies

Case studies are a time-honored method of research, for several reasons. No other method captures the uniqueness of the individual as much as a case study. The nuances of an individual's life and experiences can be detailed, and the individual's own words can be used to describe these experiences. Exploring the unique experiences of individuals and honoring their perspectives on these experiences are important goals for many researchers, and in-depth case studies of individual lives have become even more popular in recent years.

Case studies can be the only way to study rare problems, because there simply are not enough people with such problems to study through another method. For example, much of the research on people with Dissociative Identity Disorder (DID), who have multiple alters, has come from case studies, because this form of psychopathology historically has been quite rare. Case studies help researchers perform exploratory studies that can help generate new ideas that will be tested by other methods. The rich and detailed qualitative information that is produced in a case study can help guide future studies. For example, a case study of a person with DID cannot be generalized to a non-DID population. However, the neurological testing of this one individual can provide valuable information about the areas of the brain that are associated with identity switching. As a result of this case study, future studies about the neurological biomarkers for people with DID can be developed. The information gathered from one case study can inspire other research studies that explore the biological basis for identifying people with DID (Reinders et. al., 2019).

Case studies have drawbacks, however. The first involves **generalizability**—the ability to apply what we have learned to other individuals or groups. The conclusions drawn from the study of an individual may not apply to many other individuals. This limitation is especially obvious when case studies focus on people whose experiences may have been dramatic but unusual. For example, the circumstances leading to the deaths of such celebrities as Amy Winehouse, Kurt Cobain, or Phillip Seymour Hoffman may be interesting and relevant, but they may not tell us much about why other people commit suicide or engage in self-harming behaviors that might result in death.

The other drawback of case studies is that they can lack objectivity. This lack of objectivity can be on the part of both the individuals telling their stories and the therapists or researchers listening to the stories. People might have biased recollections of their pasts and may selectively report events that happen in the present. Moreover, the therapists or researchers might selectively remember parts of the stories that support their beliefs and assumptions about the causes of human behavior and forget parts that do not align with their theories. Thus, two case studies of the same person conducted by two different researchers may lead to different conclusions about the motivations and key events in that person's life.

CORRELATIONAL STUDIES

Correlational studies examine the relationship between an independent variable and a dependent variable without manipulating either variable. Correlational studies are the most common type of study in psychology and medicine. For example, you will often read about studies of the link between television watching and violence, smoking and heart disease, and social media use and depression in which researchers have examined the naturally occurring relationships between variables.

There are many kinds of correlational studies. The most common type of correlational study in abnormal psychology is a study of two or more continuous variables. A **continuous variable** is measured along a continuum. For example, on a scale measuring severity of depression, scores might fall along a continuum from 0 (no depression) to 100 (extreme depression). On a scale measuring number of recent stressors, scores might fall along a continuum from 0 (no stressors) to 20 (20 or more recent stressors). If we measured severity of depression and number of recent stressors in the same group of people and then looked at the relationship between these two continuous variables, we would be doing a continuous variable correlational study. For example, we might find that people who experience more stressors also report more depressive symptoms.

Another type of correlational study is a **group comparison study.** In this type of study, researchers are interested in the relationship between people's membership in a particular group and their scores on some other variable. For example, we might be interested in the relationship between depression and whether people have experienced a specific type of stress, such as failing a test. In this case, the groups of interest are students who failed a test and students who did not. We would find people who represented these two groups, then measure depression in both groups. This is still a correlational study because we are only observing the relationship between two variables—test failure and depression—and are not manipulating any variable. In this type of study, however, at least one of the variables—group membership—is not a continuous variable.

Both continuous variable studies and group comparison studies can be either **cross-sectional**—observing people at only one point in time—or **longitudinal**—observing people on two or more occasions over time.

Longitudinal studies have a major advantage over cross-sectional studies, because they can show that the independent variable precedes and predicts changes in the dependent variable over time. For example, a longitudinal study of stress and depression can show that people who are not depressed at the beginning of the study are much more likely to be depressed later in the study if they have experienced a stressful event in the interim than if they have not.

Measuring the Relationship Between Variables

In most correlational studies, the relationship between the variables is indicated by a correlation coefficient. Let us review what this statistic is and how to interpret it.

Correlation Coefficient

A **correlation coefficient** is a statistic used to represent the relationship between variables, usually denoted by the symbol r. A correlation coefficient can fall between -1.00 and $+1.00$. A positive correlation coefficient indicates that as values of the independent variable increase, values of the dependent variable also increase (Figure 1a). For example, a positive correlation between stress and depression would mean that people who report more stressors have higher levels of depression.

A negative correlation coefficient indicates that as values of the independent variable increase, values of the dependent variable decrease (Figure 1b). If we were measuring stressors and depression, a negative correlation would mean that people who report more stressors actually have lower levels of depression. This is an unlikely scenario, but there are many instances of negative correlations between variables. For example, people who receive more positive social support from others typically have lower levels of depression.

The magnitude (size) of a correlation is the degree to which the variables move in tandem with each other. It is indicated by how close the correlation coefficient is to either $+1.00$ or -1.00. A correlation (r) of 0 indicates no relationship between the variables (Figure 1c). A value of r of $+1.00$ or -1.00 indicates a perfect relationship between the two variables (as illustrated in Figure 1a and b)—the value of one variable is perfectly predicted by the value of the other variable; for example, every time people experience stress they become depressed.

Seldom do we see perfect correlations in psychological research. Instead, correlations often are in the low to moderate range (for example, 0.2 to 0.5), indicating some relationship between the two variables but a far from perfect relationship (Figure 1d). Many relationships between variables happen by chance and

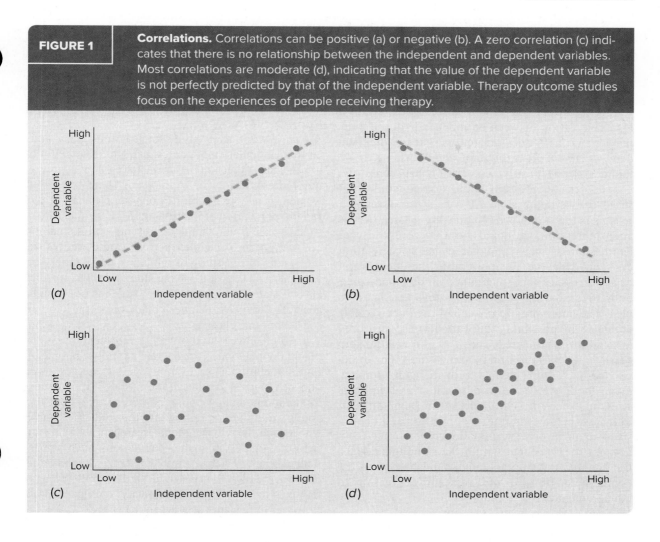

FIGURE 1

Correlations. Correlations can be positive (a) or negative (b). A zero correlation (c) indicates that there is no relationship between the independent and dependent variables. Most correlations are moderate (d), indicating that the value of the dependent variable is not perfectly predicted by that of the independent variable. Therapy outcome studies focus on the experiences of people receiving therapy.

are not meaningful. Scientists evaluate the importance of a correlation coefficient by examining its statistical significance.

Statistical Significance

The **statistical significance** of a result, such as a correlation coefficient, is an index of how likely it is that the result occurred simply by chance. You will often see statements in research studies such as "The result was statistically significant at $p < 0.05$." This means that the probability (p) is less than 5 in 100 that the result occurred only by chance. Researchers typically accept results at this level of significance ($p < 0.05$) as support of their hypotheses, although the choice of an acceptable significance level is somewhat arbitrary.

Whether a correlation coefficient will be statistically significant at the $p < 0.05$ level is determined by its magnitude and the size of the sample on which it is based. Both larger correlations and larger sample sizes increase the likelihood of achieving statistical significance. A correlation of 0.30 will be significant if it is based on a large sample, say 200 or more, but will not be significant if it is based on a small sample, say 10 or fewer participants. On the other hand, a correlation of 0.90 will be statistically significant even if the sample is as small as 30 people.

A result can be statistically significant but not clinically significant. For example, a study of 10,000 people might find a correlation of 0.15 between the number of stressors people experienced and their scores on a depression questionnaire. This correlation would likely be statistically significant because of the very large sample, but it is so small as to suggest that stress is not a very good predictor of depression. Similarly, two groups may differ in their mean levels of depression to a statistically significant degree because the sample sizes of both groups are very large. But if the two groups actually differ only by 1 or 2 points on a depression questionnaire in which scores can range from 0 to 60, the clinical significance of the difference in the two groups would be questionable. Increasingly, research is being examined for whether an effect is not only statistically significant but also clinically significant.

Correlation Is Not Causation

A very important fact about correlations is that a high correlation between an independent and a dependent variable does not tell us that the independent variable *caused* the dependent variable. If we found a strong positive correlation between stress and depression, we still could not conclude that stress causes depression. All a positive correlation tells us is that there is a relationship between stress and depression. It could be that stress causes depression—as we hypothesized—but a correlation does not rule out the possibility that depression causes stress, or that some other variable may cause both stress and depression (like poverty, for example). The latter situation is called the **third variable problem**—the possibility that variables not measured in a study are the real cause of the relationship between the variables that are measured. For example, perhaps some people with difficult temperaments both are prone to depression and generate stressful experiences in their lives by being difficult to live with. If we measured only stress and depression, we might observe a relationship between them because they co-occur within the same individuals. But this relationship actually would be due to the common relationship of stress and depression to temperament.

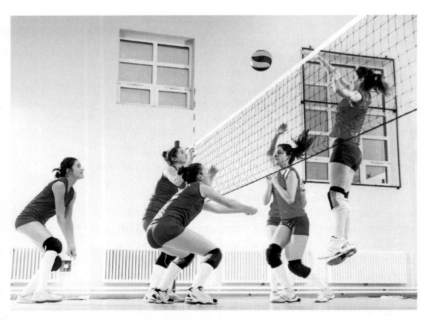

A study of depression in student athletes might need to include a comparison group of students who are not athletes. *kristian sekulic/Getty Images*

Selecting a Sample

A critical choice in a correlational study is the choice of the sample. A **sample** is a group of people taken from the population we want to study.

Representativeness

A *representative sample* is a sample that is highly similar to the population of interest in terms of sex, ethnicity, age, and other important variables. If a sample is not representative—for example, if there are fewer women or people of color in our sample than in the general population of interest—then the sample is said to have *bias*. If our sample represents only a small or unusual group of people, then we cannot generalize the results of our study to the larger population. For example, if all the people in our study are white, middle-class females, we cannot know whether our results generalize to males, people of color, or people in other socioeconomic classes.

An effective way to obtain a representative sample of a population is to generate a random sample of that population. For example, some studies have obtained random samples of the entire U.S. population by randomly dialing phone numbers throughout the country and then recruiting into the study the people who answer the phone. Often, researchers can settle for random samples of smaller populations, such as particular cities. When a sample is truly random, the chances are high that it will be similar to the population of interest in terms of ethnicity, sex, age, and all the other important variables in the study.

Selection of a Comparison Group

A group comparison study compares the experiences of one group with those of another group. For example, we may be interested in the depression levels of students who are athletes and students who are not athletes. We might begin by recruiting our sample of student athletes, attempting to make this sample as representative as possible of student athletes at our university.

Our comparison group of nonathletes should match our group of athletes on any variable (other than stress) that might influence levels of depression. If the two groups are not as similar as possible, then any differences in their levels of depression could be attributable to other variables. For example, women generally are more likely to be depressed than men. If we had more women in our athlete group than in our nonathlete group, then higher levels of depression in the athlete group might be attributable to a third variable—the fact that there are more women in that group—rather than to the effects of participation in athletics. For this reason, our athlete and nonathlete groups should be alike on all third variables that might influence our dependent variable, depression.

Evaluating Correlational Studies

Correlational studies have provided much important information for abnormal psychology. One major advantage of correlational studies is that many of them focus on situations occurring in the real world, rather than those manipulated in a laboratory. This gives them relatively good **external validity,** the extent to which a study's results can be generalized to real-life phenomena. The results of these studies may be generalizable to wider populations and to people's actual life experiences.

Longitudinal correlational studies have several advantages over cross-sectional correlational studies. In longitudinal correlational studies, researchers can determine whether there are differences between the groups before the event of interest occurs. If there are no differences before the event but significant differences after the event, then researchers can have more confidence that it was the event that actually led to the differences between the groups. Longitudinal designs also allow researchers to follow groups long enough to assess both short-term and long-term reactions to the event. The factors that predict the onset of various psychological disorders are always of great interest to researchers. Using longitudinal correlation research has been able to identify protective factors that decrease the onset of major depression in adolescent populations. Social bonding, resiliency, emotional competence, and positive self-perceptions predicted less depressive symptoms over time (Zhou, Shek, Zhu, & Dou, 2020).

Longitudinal studies can be time consuming and expensive to run. Some of these studies have been going on for more than 25 years and have cost millions of dollars. They are producing extremely valuable data, but at a high cost in both researchers' time and research dollars. The greatest disadvantage of all correlational studies is that they cannot indicate what is a cause and what is a consequence. For example, many stressful events that depressed people report may be the consequences of their depression rather than the causes (Hammen, 2018). The symptoms of depression can cause stress by impairing interpersonal skills, interfering with concentration on the job, and causing insomnia. The same problem exists for studies of many types of psychopathology. For example, the symptoms of schizophrenia can disrupt social relationships, alcohol abuse can lead to unemployment, and so on. A correlational study linking the two variables would not be sufficient evidence to conclude that disrupted social relationships *cause* schizophrenia,

or that unemployment leads to substance abuse, because either direction is possible.

Finally, all correlational studies suffer from the third variable problem. Researchers seldom can measure all possible influences on participants' levels of depression or other psychopathologies. Third variable problems are one of the major reasons why researchers turn to experimental studies.

EPIDEMIOLOGICAL STUDIES

Epidemiology is the study of the frequency and distribution of a disorder, or a group of disorders, in a population. An epidemiological study asks how many people in a population have the disorder and how this number varies across important groups within the population, such as men and women or people with high and low incomes.

Epidemiological research focuses on three types of data. First, research may focus on the **prevalence** of a disorder, or the proportion of the population that has the disorder at a given point or period in time. For example, a study might report the lifetime prevalence of a disorder, or the number of people who will have the disorder at some time in their life. The 12-month prevalence of a disorder would be the proportion of the population who will be diagnosed with the disorder in any 12-month period.

Table 1 shows the lifetime and 12-month prevalence of one of the more severe forms of depression—major depressive disorder—from a nationwide epidemiological study conducted in the United States (Hasin et al., 2018). Not surprisingly, the proportion of the population who will be diagnosed with major depressive disorder at some time in their life is larger than the proportion who will be diagnosed with the disorder in any 12-month period.

Table 1 illustrates the fact, mentioned earlier, that the prevalence of major depression is greater for

TABLE 1 Lifetime and 12-Month Prevalence of Major Depressive Disorder

	Lifetime Prevalence (%)	12-Month Prevalence (%)
Males	14.7	7.2
Females	26.1	13.4
Total	20.6	10.4

Source: Hasin, D., Sarvet, A., Meyers, J., Saha, T., Ruan, J., Stohl, M., & Grant, B. (2018). Epidemiology of adult *DSM-5* major depressive disorder and Its specifiers in the United States. *JAMA Psychiatry, 75*(4):336–346.

women than for men. As we discuss in the chapter "Mood Disorders and Suicide," this fact, revealed by many epidemiological studies, has been an important focus of research into depression.

Second, epidemiological research seeks to determine the **incidence** of a disorder, or the number of new cases of the disorder that develop during a specified period of time. The 1-year incidence of a disorder is the number of people who develop the disorder during a 1-year period.

Third, epidemiological research is concerned with the **risk factors** for a disorder—those conditions or variables that are associated with a higher risk of having the disorder. If women are more likely than men to have a disorder, then being a woman is a risk factor for the disorder. In terms of our interest in the relationship between stress and depression, an epidemiological study might show that people who live in high-stress areas of a city are more likely to have depression than people who live in low-stress areas of the city.

How do researchers determine the prevalence, incidence, and risk factors for a disorder? Epidemiological researchers first identify the population of interest and next identify a random sample of that population, for example, by randomly phoning residential telephone numbers. They then use structured clinical interviews that ask specific questions of participants to assess whether they have the symptoms that make up the disorder and the risk factors, such as gender or socioeconomic status, being studied. (Recall our discussion of structured clinical interviews in the chapter "Assessing and Diagnosing Abnormality.") From these data, epidemiologists estimate how many people in different categories of risk factors have the disorder.

Evaluating Epidemiological Studies

Epidemiological studies have provided valuable information on the prevalence, incidence, and risk factors for disorders, and we discuss evidence gathered from some major nationwide and international epidemiological studies throughout this book. This research can give us important clues as to who is at highest risk for a disorder. In turn, we can use this information to test hypotheses about why those people are at higher risk.

Epidemiological studies are affected by many of the same limitations as correlational studies. First and foremost, they cannot establish that any risk factor causes a disorder. While a study may show that people living in higher-stress neighborhoods are more likely to have a disorder, this does not mean that the high-stress environment caused the disorder. Also, as in

correlational studies, third variables may explain the relationship between any risk factor and the rates of a disorder.

EXPERIMENTAL STUDIES

The hallmark of **experimental studies** is control. Researchers attempt to control the independent variable and any potentially problematic third variables rather than simply observing them as they occur naturally. There are various types of experimental studies we could do to investigate whether stress leads to depression. We will examine four types in particular.

Human Laboratory Studies

To test our hypothesis that stress leads to depression, we could expose participants to a stressor in the laboratory and then determine whether it causes an increase in depressed mood. This method is known as a **human laboratory study.**

Several ground-breaking studies of this type have been done to induce stress and create learned helplessness which is associated with feelings of powerlessness after persistent failure to succeed. Learned helplessness is thought to be an underlying factor in onset of depression (Hiroto & Seligman,1975; Peterson & Seligman, 1984). The stressor that is often used in this type of study is an unsolvable task or puzzle, such as an unsolvable anagram. In our fictional study, our index of stress is participants' exposure to unsolvable anagrams. Because we are manipulating stress, not simply measuring it, we have the advantage of knowing precisely what type of stress participants are exposed to and when. We cannot create in the laboratory many of the types of stress that may cause depression in the real world, such as the destruction of a person's home in a hurricane or continual physical abuse. Instead, we create analogues—situations that capture some key characteristics of these real-world events, such as their uncontrollability and unpredictability.

Internal Validity

We want to ensure that our experiment has **internal validity,** meaning that changes in the dependent variable can confidently be attributed to our manipulation of the independent variable and not to other factors. For example, people who participate in our experiment using anagrams might become more depressed over the course of the experiment simply because participating in an experiment is a difficult experience, not because the anagrams are unsolvable. This threat to internal validity is basically the same type of third variable problem encountered in correlational and epidemiological studies.

To control third variables, researchers create a **control group** or control condition, in which participants have all the same experiences as the group of main interest in the study except that they do not receive the key manipulation—in our example, the stressor of the unsolvable puzzles. The control group for our study could be given similar but solvable anagrams. Thus, the control group's experience would be identical to that of the other group—the **experimental group** or experimental condition—except for receiving the unsolvable puzzles.

Another threat to internal validity can arise if the participants in the experimental group (the group given the unsolvable anagrams) and in the control group (the group given the solvable anagrams) differ in important ways before beginning the experiment. If such differences exist, we cannot be sure that our manipulation is the cause of any changes in the dependent variable. Internal validity requires **random assignment,** which means that each participant must have an equal chance of being in the experimental group or the control group. Often, a researcher will use a table of random numbers to assign participants to groups.

Yet another threat to internal validity is the presence of **demand characteristics**—situations that cause participants to guess the purpose of the study and thus change their behavior. For example, if our measure of depression is too obvious, participants might guess what hypothesis we are testing and respond differently, consciously or unconsciously. To avoid the presence of demand characteristics, we could use subtler measures of depression embedded in other tests— often called *filler measures*—to obscure the real purpose of our study. Researchers also often use *cover stories,* telling participants a false story to prevent them from guessing the true purpose of the experiment. After the study, participants should be debriefed about the deception they were exposed to in the study, as well as its true purpose.

Participants' behavior in the study can be affected if they know what group they are in ahead of time. Similarly, if experimenters know what condition a participant is in, they might inadvertently behave in ways that affect how the participant responds to the manipulations. In order to reduce these demand characteristics, both the participants and the experimenters who interact with them should be unaware of whether participants are in the experimental condition or the control condition. This situation is referred to as a **double-blind experiment.**

We have instituted a number of safeguards to ensure internal validity in our study. Participants have been randomly selected and assigned, and our participants and experimenters are unaware of which condition participants are in. Now we can conduct the

Researchers may give participants an unsolvable puzzle in order to observe the effects of stress on mental health.
Gary He/McGraw Hill

study. When our data are collected and analyzed, we find that, as we predicted, participants given the unsolvable anagrams showed greater increases in depressed mood than did participants given the solvable anagrams.

What can we conclude about our idea of depression, based on this study? Our experimental controls have helped us rule out third variable explanations, so we can be relatively confident that it was the experience of the uncontrollable stressor that led to the increases in depression in the experimental group. Thus, we can say that our study supports our hypothesis that people exposed to uncontrollable stress will show more depressed mood than will people not exposed to such stress.

Evaluating Human Laboratory Studies

The primary advantage of human laboratory studies is control. Researchers have more control over third variables, the independent variable, and the dependent variable in these studies than they do in any other type of study they can do with humans.

Yet human laboratory studies also have their limitations. Because we cannot know if our results generalize to what happens outside the laboratory, their external validity can be low. Is being exposed to unsolvable anagrams anything like being exposed to major, real-world uncontrollable stressors, such as the death of a loved one? Clearly, the severity of the two types of experiences differs, but is this the only important difference? Similarly, do the increases in depressed mood in the participants in our study, which probably were small, tell us anything about why some people develop extremely severe, debilitating episodes of depression? Experimental studies such as this have been criticized for their lack of generalizability to major psychopathologies that occurs in real life, as opposed to what we can capture in the laboratory.

Apart from posing problems of generalizability, human laboratory studies sometimes pose serious ethical concerns. Is it ethical to deliberately induce distress, even mild distress, in people? Different people will give different answers to this question.

Therapy Outcome Studies

Therapy outcome studies are experimental studies designed to test whether a specific therapy—a psychological therapy or a biological therapy—reduces psychopathology in individuals who receive it. Because therapies target supposed causes of psychopathology, therapy outcome studies can produce evidence that reducing these causes reduces psychopathology, which in turn supports the hypothesis that these factors played a role in creating the psychopathology in the first place.

Control Groups

Sometimes, people simply get better with time. Thus, to see whether our participants' improvement actually has anything to do with our therapy, we need to compare the experiences of people who receive our experimental therapy with those of a control group made up of people who do not receive the therapy. Sometimes, researchers use a **simple control group** consisting of participants who do not receive the experimental therapy but are tracked for the same period of time as the participants who do receive the therapy.

A variation on this simple control group is the **wait list control group.** The participants in this type of group do not receive the therapy when the experimental group does but instead are put on a wait list to receive the intervention at a later date, when the study is completed. Both groups of participants are assessed at the beginning and end of the study, but only the experimental group receives the therapy as part of the study.

Another type of control group, the **placebo control group,** is used most often in studies of the effectiveness of drugs. The participants in this group have the same interactions with experimenters as the participants in the experimental group, but they take pills that are placebos (inactive substances) rather than the drug being studied. In psychotherapy studies, the placebo control group might receive an "inactive" treatment, such as a weekly check-in that does not include the therapy. Usually, to prevent demand effects, both the participants and the experimenters in these studies are unaware of which group the participants are in; thus, this type of experiment is double-blind.

Evaluating Therapy Outcome Research

Although therapy outcome studies might seem the most ethical way of conducting research on people in distress, they have their own methodological

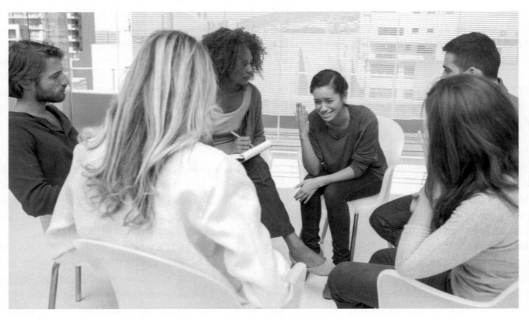

Photo of group therapy with diverse participants. *wavebreakmediamicro/123RF*

challenges and ethical issues. Most psychological therapies involve a package of techniques for responding to people's problems. For example, depressed people in an experimental therapy group might be taught assertiveness skills, social problem-solving skills, and skills in changing self-defeating thinking. Which of these skills was most responsible for alleviating their depression? Even when a therapy works, researchers often cannot know exactly what it is about the therapy that works.

Ethical problems arise in using all three types of control groups—simple control groups, wait list control groups, and placebo control groups—in therapy outcome research. Some researchers believe it is unethical to withhold treatment or to provide a treatment believed to be ineffective for people in distress. For example, many depressed participants assigned to a control group may be in severe distress or in danger of harming themselves and therefore may need immediate treatment.

In response to this concern, many therapy outcome studies now compare the effectiveness of two or more therapies expected to have positive effects. These studies basically are a competition between rival therapies and the theories behind them. The idea is that all the participants in such studies benefit, while at the same time researchers gain useful information about the most effective type of therapy for the pathology. Regardless of which type of control or comparison group experimenters use in a therapy outcome study, participants must be informed of the types of groups the study involves and of the fact that they will be randomly assigned to one group or another (and thus run the risk of not receiving useful treatment as part of the study).

Another ethical issue concerns the obligation of the therapist to respond to the needs of the patient. How much can a therapy be modified to respond to a specific participant's needs without compromising the scientific integrity of the study? Therapists may feel the need to vary the dosage of a drug or to deviate from a study's procedure for psychological intervention. Departing too much from the standard therapy, however, will lead to significant variation in the therapy received by participants in the intervention, which could compromise the results of the study.

A related methodological issue has to do with generalizing results from therapy outcome studies to the real world. In these studies, the therapeutic intervention usually is delivered to patients in a controlled, high-quality atmosphere by the most competent therapists. Patients usually are screened so that they fit a narrow set of criteria for being included in the study, and often only patients who stick with the therapy to its end are included in the final analyses.

In the real world, mental health services are not always delivered in controlled, high-quality atmospheres by the most competent therapists. Patients are who they are, and their complicated symptom presentations and lives may not fit neatly into the criteria for an "optimal patient." Also, patients often leave and return to therapy and may not receive a full trial of the therapy before dropping out for financial or personal reasons.

Therapy outcome research that tests how well a therapy works in highly controlled settings with a narrowly defined group of people is said to test the **efficacy** of a therapy. In contrast, therapy outcome research that tests how well a therapy works in real-world settings, with all the complications mentioned, is said to test the **effectiveness** of a therapy.

Single-Case Experimental Designs

Another type of experimental study is the **single-case experimental design,** in which a single individual or a small number of individuals are studied intensively. Unlike the case studies discussed earlier, a single-case experimental design exposes the individual to some manipulation or intervention, and his or her behavior is examined before and after the intervention to determine the effects. In addition, in a single-case experimental design, the participant's behaviors are measured repeatedly over time through some standard method, whereas a case study often is based on the researcher's impressions of the participant and the factors affecting his or her behaviors, thoughts, and emotions.

ABAB Design

A specific type of single-case experimental design is the **ABAB design,** or **reversal design,** in which an intervention is introduced, withdrawn, and then reinstated and the behavior of the participant is examined both on and off the treatment. For example, in the study of the effects of a drug for depression, an individual depressed participant might be assessed for her level of depression each day for 4 weeks. This is the baseline assessment (A; Figure 2). Then the participant would be given the drug for 4 weeks (B), and her level of depression would be assessed each day during that period. The drug then would be withdrawn for 4 weeks (A), and, again, her level of depression would be assessed each day. Finally, the drug would be reinstated for 4 weeks (B) and her level of depression assessed each day during that period. If the participant's levels of depression followed the pattern seen in Figure 2, this result would suggest that her depression level was much lower when she was taking the drug (B) than when she was not taking the drug (A).

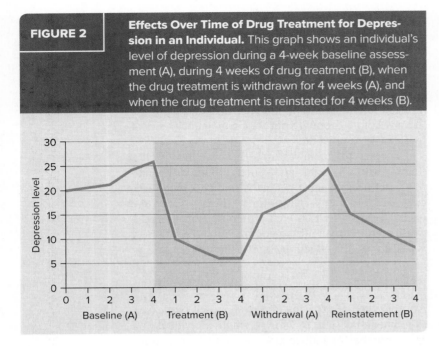

FIGURE 2 | **Effects Over Time of Drug Treatment for Depression in an Individual.** This graph shows an individual's level of depression during a 4-week baseline assessment (A), during 4 weeks of drug treatment (B), when the drug treatment is withdrawn for 4 weeks (A), and when the drug treatment is reinstated for 4 weeks (B).

Multiple Baseline Designs

In a **multiple baseline design,** an intervention might be given to the same individual but in different settings, or to different individuals at different points in time. To test whether a meditation exercise reduces depression, a researcher might teach a depressed person how to use the exercise while at work when they feel depressed. If the participant's depression decreased at work but not at home, where they did not use the meditation exercise, the researcher has some evidence that the exercise was responsible for the reduction in depression. If the participant were then told to use the meditation exercise at home and depression decreased in this setting also, this would be further evidence of the exercise's utility.

Similarly, the researcher might teach the meditation exercise to multiple individuals, but at different points in time when their experiences are likely to be different. For example, the researcher might teach the meditation exercise to one depressed college student during the first week of classes, to another student during spring break, and to still another during exam week. If all the students experienced relief of their depression symptoms after learning the meditation exercise, despite their different levels of stress, this would be evidence that the effects of the meditation exercise were generalizable across individuals and settings.

Evaluating Single-Case Experimental Designs

A major advantage of single-case experimental designs is that they allow much more intensive assessment of participants than might be possible if there were more participants. For example, an individual child could be observed for hours each day as the child was put on and then taken off a treatment. This intensity of assessment can allow researchers to pinpoint the types of behaviors that are and are not affected by the treatment.

The major disadvantage of single-case experimental designs is that their results may not be generalizable to the wider population. One individual's experience on or off a treatment may not be the same as other individuals' experiences. In addition, not all hypotheses can be tested with single-case experimental designs. Some treatments have lingering effects after they end. For example, if a person is taught new skills for coping with stress during the treatment, these skills will continue to be present even after the treatment is withdrawn.

Animal Studies

Researchers sometimes try to avoid the ethical issues involved in experimental studies with humans by conducting the studies with animals. Animal research has its own set of ethical issues, but many researchers feel it is acceptable to expose animals to situations in the laboratory that it would not be ethical to impose on humans. **Animal studies** thus provide researchers with even more control over laboratory conditions and third variables than is possible in human laboratory studies.

In a well-known series of animal studies designed to investigate depression (discussed in the chapter "Mood Disorders and Suicide"), Martin Seligman, Bruce Overmier, Steven Maier, and their colleagues subjected dogs to an uncontrollable stressor in the laboratory (Overmier & Seligman, 1967; Seligman & Maier, 1967). The experimental group of dogs received a series of uncontrollable electric shocks. Let us call this Group E, for experimental.

In addition, there were two control groups. One control group of dogs received shocks but could control them by jumping over a barrier (Figure 3). Let us call this Group J, for jump. The dogs in Groups E and J received the same number and duration of shocks. The only difference between the groups was that the dogs in Group E could not control the shocks, whereas the dogs in Group J could. The second control group of dogs received no shock. Let us call this Group N, for none.

Dogs in Group E initially responded to the shocks by jumping around their cages. Soon, however, the majority became passive. Later, when the researchers provided the dogs with an opportunity to escape the shock by jumping over a barrier, these dogs did not learn to do so. It seemed that they had learned they could not control the shock, so they did not recognize

FIGURE 3 **Shuttle Box for Learned Helplessness Experiments.** Researchers used an apparatus like this to deliver controllable or uncontrollable shocks to dogs in order to investigate the phenomenon of learned helplessness.

drugs, animals often are given the drugs to determine their effects on different bodily systems and behaviors. Sometimes the animals are killed after receiving the drugs, to enable detailed physiological analyses of their effects. Obviously, such studies could not be done with humans. Animal studies of drugs are particularly useful in the early stages of research, when the possible side effects of the drugs are unknown.

Evaluating Animal Studies

There clearly are problems with animal studies. First, some people believe it is no more ethical to conduct painful, dangerous, or fatal experiments with animals than it is to do so with humans. Second, from a scientific vantage point, we must ask whether we can generalize the results of experiments with animals to humans. Are learned helplessness deficits in dogs really analogous to human depression? The debate over the ethical and scientific issues of animal research continues. Particularly with regard to research on drug effectiveness, however, animal research may be crucial to the advancement of our knowledge of how to help people overcome psychopathology.

GENETIC STUDIES

Identifying genetic factors associated with psychopathology involves a variety of research methods. Researchers investigate the degree to which genes play a role in a particular disorder, or its heritability, through three types of genetic studies: family history studies, twin studies, and adoption studies. To investigate specific genes that may be involved in a disorder, they may use molecular genetic studies (also called association studies) or linkage analyses.

Family History Studies

Disorders that are genetically transmitted should, on average, show up more often in families of people who have the disorder than they do in families of people who do not have the disorder. This is true whether the disorder is associated with one or with many genes. To conduct a **family history study,** scientists first identify people who clearly have the disorder in question. This group is called the *probands.* The researchers also identify a control group of people who clearly do not have the disorder. They then trace the family pedigrees, or family trees, of individuals in these two groups and determine how many of their relatives have the disorder. Researchers are most interested in first-degree relatives, such as full siblings, parents, or children, because these relatives are most genetically similar to the subjects (unless they have an identical twin, who will be genetically identical to them).

opportunities for control when offered. The researchers labeled this set of behaviors *learned helplessness deficits.*

The dogs in the controllable shock group, Group J, learned to control the shock and did not develop learned helplessness deficits. The fact that the two groups of dogs experienced the same number and duration of shocks suggests that lack of control, not the shocks alone, led to the learned helplessness deficits in the experimental group. The dogs in Group N, which received no shocks, also did not develop learned helplessness deficits.

Seligman and colleagues likened the learned helplessness deficits shown by their dogs to the symptoms of depression in humans: apathy, low initiation of behavior, and the inability to see opportunities to improve one's environment (see Seligman, 1975). They argued that many human depressions result from people learning that they have no control over important outcomes in their lives. This learned helplessness theory of depression seems helpful in explaining the depression and passivity seen in chronically oppressed groups, such as battered spouses and some people who grow up in poverty.

Another type of animal study is similar to therapy outcome studies. In studies of the effectiveness of

FIGURE 4

Degrees of Genetic Relationship.
People with whom you share 50 percent of your genes are your first-degree relatives. People with whom you share 25 percent of your genes are your second-degree relatives. People with whom you share 12.5 percent of your genes are your third-degree relatives.

Percent of genes in common

Identical (monozygotic) twins — 100%

Parent–child
Full siblings (both parents in common)
Nonidentical (dizygotic) twins

50%

Grandparent–grandchild
Uncle/aunt–nephew/niece
Half-siblings (one parent in common)

25%

Great-grandparent–great-grandchild — 12.5%
Great-uncle/aunt–grandnephew/niece
First cousins

Figure 4 illustrates the degree of genetic relationship between an individual and various categories of relatives. This figure gives you an idea of why the risk of inheriting the genes for a disorder quickly decreases as the relationship between an individual and the relative with the disorder becomes more distant. The percentage of genes the individual and the relative with the disorder have in common decreases greatly with distance.

Although family history studies provide very useful information about the possible genetic transmission of a disorder, they have their problems. The most obvious is that families share not only genes but also environment. Several members of a family might have a disorder because they share the same environmental stresses. Family history studies cannot tease apart the genetic and environmental contributions to a disorder. Researchers often turn to twin studies to do this.

Twin Studies

Notice in Figure 4 that identical twins, or **monozygotic (MZ) twins,** share 100 percent of their genes. This is because they come from a single fertilized egg, which splits into two identical parts. In contrast, nonidentical twins, or **dizygotic (DZ) twins,** share, on average, 50 percent of their genes because they come from two separate eggs fertilized by separate sperm, no different than non-twin siblings.

Researchers have capitalized on this difference between MZ and DZ twins to conduct **twin studies** on the contribution of genetics to many disorders. If a disorder is determined entirely by genetics, then when one member of a MZ twin pair has a disorder, the other member of the pair should always have the disorder. This probability that both twins will have the disorder if one twin has it is called the **concordance rate** for the disorder. Thus, if a disorder is entirely determined by genes, the concordance rate among MZ twins should be close to 100 percent. The concordance rate for the disorder among DZ twins will be much lower than 100 percent. Even when a disorder is transmitted only partially by genes, the concordance rate for MZ twins should be considerably higher than the concordance rate for DZ twins, because MZ twins are genetically identical while DZ twins share only about half their genes.

For example, suppose the concordance rate for Disorder X for MZ twins is 48 percent, whereas the concordance rate for DZ twins is 17 percent. These concordance rates tell us two things. First, because the concordance rate for MZ twins is considerably higher than that for DZ twins, we have evidence that Disorder X is genetically transmitted. Second, because the concordance rate for MZ twins is well under 100 percent, we have evidence that a combination of a genetic predisposition and other factors (biological or environmental) causes an individual to develop Disorder X.

Twin studies do not fully separate genetic and environmental factors, because MZ twins may have more similar environments and experiences than do DZ twins. For example, MZ twins typically look alike, whereas DZ twins often do not, and physical appearance can affect other people's reactions to an individual. MZ twins also may be more likely than DZ twins to share talents that influence their opportunities. For instance, MZ twins may both be athletic or talented academically or musically, which can affect their treatment by others and their opportunities in life. Finally, parents may simply treat MZ twins more similarly than they do DZ twins. To address these problems, researchers have turned to a third method for studying heritability, the adoption study.

Adoption Studies

An **adoption study** can be carried out in a number of ways, but they all take advantage of the fact that adopted individuals share genes with biological parents who did not raise them, and do not share genes with the adoptive parents who did raise them. This allows researchers to separate the role of genetics and environment. Most commonly, researchers first identify people who have the disorder of interest who were adopted shortly after birth. They then determine the rates of the disorder in the biological relatives of these adoptees and in the adoptive relatives of the adoptees. If a disorder is strongly influenced by genetics, researchers should see higher rates of the disorder among the biological relatives of the adoptee than among the adoptive relatives. If the disorder is strongly influenced by environment, they should see higher rates of the disorder among the adoptive relatives than among the biological relatives.

Molecular Genetic Studies and Linkage Analyses

The technology for examining human genes has advanced rapidly in recent decades, allowing researchers to search for associations between specific genetic abnormalities (also referred to as genetic markers) and psychopathology in what are called **molecular genetic studies** or **association studies.** A typical study might compare a group of people who have been diagnosed with a particular disorder, such as depression, with people who have no form of psychopathology. DNA from individuals in both groups is obtained either through blood samples or by swabbing the inside of the individuals' cheeks to obtain a small amount of tissue. This DNA is then analyzed (genotyped) to determine whether each individual has a genetic characteristic or marker of interest.

Because the human genome is so vast, researchers may try to narrow down the location of the gene marker associated with a psychological disorder by looking for other characteristics that co-occur with the disorder and have known genetic markers, a process called **linkage analysis.** For example, in the study of mood disorders among the Amish, researchers found that two markers on chromosome 11, one for insulin and one for a known cancer gene, were linked to the presence of mood disorder in one large family (Biron et al., 1987). This suggests that a gene that plays a role in vulnerability to mood disorders may be on chromosome 11. Unfortunately, this linkage has not been replicated in other studies. In the chapter "Schizophrenia Spectrum and Other Psychotic Disorders," we discuss genetic linkage studies that have identified possible genetic markers for schizophrenia.

CROSS-CULTURAL RESEARCH

Not long ago, most psychological research was conducted with college students, most of whom were white and middle- or upper-class. Researchers believed that any results they obtained from these samples could be generalized to any other relevant sample. Only anthropologists and a handful of psychologists and psychiatrists argued that what is true of one ethnic group, culture, or gender is not necessarily true of others.

In the past few decades, however, there has been an explosion of cross-cultural research in abnormal psychology. Researchers are investigating the similarities and differences across culture in the nature, causes, and treatment of psychopathology. These cross-cultural researchers face several special challenges.

First, researchers must be careful in applying theories or concepts that were developed in studies of one culture to another culture (Rogler, 1989). Because the manifestations of disorders can differ across cultures, researchers who insist on narrow definitions of disorders may fail to identify people manifesting disorders in culturally defined ways. Similarly, theoretical variables can have different meanings or manifestations in different cultures.

A good example is the variable known as *expressed emotion.* Families high in expressed emotion are highly critical of and hostile toward other family members and emotionally overinvolved with one another. Several studies of the majority cultures in America and Europe have shown that people with schizophrenia whose families are high in expressed emotion have higher rates of relapse than those whose families are low in expressed emotion (Hooley, 2007). The meaning and manifestation of expressed emotion can differ greatly across cultures, however:

> Criticism within Anglo-American family settings, for example, may focus on allegations of faulty personality traits (e.g., laziness) or psychotic symptom behaviors (e.g., strange ideas). However, in other societies, such as those of Latin America, the same behaviors may not be met with criticism. Among Mexican-descent families, for example, criticism tends to focus on disrespectful or disruptive behaviors that affect the family but not on psychotic symptom behavior and individual personality characteristics. Thus, culture plays a role in creating the content or targets of criticism. Perhaps most importantly, culture is influential in determining whether criticism is a prominent part of the familial emotional atmosphere. (Jenkins & Karno, 1992, p. 10)

Considering the impact of culture is critical in research because it bears upon what all individuals bring into the clinical setting. Today's researchers are more careful to search for culturally specific manifestations of the characteristics of interest in their studies and for the possibility that the characteristics or variables that predict psychopathology in one culture may be irrelevant in other cultures.

In the twenty-first century, global migration rates are at record levels and language barriers present multiple obstacles for conducting cross-language research. With the inclusion of various cultures into the research process, researchers may have difficulty translating their questionnaires or other assessment tools into different languages. Studies suggest that using a client's preferred language when conducting research offers the best opportunity to gather valid results that are representative of their experiences. Research suggests that best practices in cross-language research should include the appropriate use of competent interpreters, systematic planning for how to address the language barrier between participant and researcher and the use of reliably and validly translated survey instruments (Squires, Sadarangani, & Jones, 2020).

META-ANALYSIS

Often the research literature contains many studies that have investigated a particular idea (e.g., that stress leads to depression). An investigator may want to know what the overall trend across all studies is—in other words, what the evidence suggests is true when you put it all together. He or she may also want to know what factors might account for some studies supporting their hypothesis and others not. To do this, a researcher could just read over all the studies and draw conclusions about whether most of them support or do not support the hypothesis. However, these conclusions can be biased by the reader's interpretations of the studies.

A more objective way to draw conclusions about a body of research is to conduct a **meta-analysis,** a statistical technique for summarizing results across several studies. The first step in a meta-analysis is to do a thorough literature search, usually by searching scholarly databases using key words (like "depression" and "stress"). Because studies use different methods and measures for testing a hypothesis, the second step of a meta-analysis is to transform the results of each study into a statistic that then allows results to be compared across studies. You can think of this as translating the results of each separate study into a single language, so that they all make sense with respect to one another. This statistic, called the *effect size,* indicates how big the differences are between two groups (such as a group that received a specific form of therapy and one that did not) or how strong the relationship is between two

continuous variables (such as the correlation between levels of stress and levels of depression). Researchers can then examine the average effect size across studies to make a conclusion about what the research literature has to say across multiple studies. They can also relate the effect size to characteristics of the study, such as the year it was published, the type of measure used, or the age or gender of the participants, to see whether those factors might play a role in differing results. For example, a meta-analysis of studies of children's depression levels found that studies done in more recent years tend to find lower levels of depression than studies done previously (Twenge & Nolen-Hoeksema, 2002). This finding raises the possibility that levels of depression among children may be decreasing.

Evaluating Meta-Analysis

Meta-analysis can overcome some of the problems resulting from small numbers of participants in an individual study because they pool the data from thousands of study participants, thereby providing more power to find significant effects. For example, the studies examined by Twenge and Nolen-Hoeksema (2002) generally had small numbers of ethnic minority children, making it difficult for each individual study to compare their depression scores with those of nonminority children. By pooling studies, however, the overall sample sizes of Hispanic and African American children were large enough to allow comparisons by race/ethnicity. The meta-analysis found that Hispanic children generally had higher depression scores than African American or white children. This is an example of a finding that meta-analyses can provide what single studies often cannot.

Meta-analyses have their problems, however. First, some published studies have methodological flaws. These flawed studies may be included in a meta-analysis along with methodologically stronger studies, influencing the overall results. Second, there is a *file drawer effect*—studies that do not support the hypothesis they are designed to test are less likely to get published than studies that do (and instead are "filed away," thus the name). For example, a study that finds that a psychotherapy is not any more effective than a wait list control is less likely to get published than a study that finds that the same psychotherapy is more effective than the wait list control. The bias toward publishing studies with positive results means that many perfectly good studies that fail to find the expected effects do not get published and therefore do not end up in meta-analyses. This file drawer effect biases the results of meta-analyses toward finding an overall positive effect of a treatment or of some other difference between groups.

CHAPTER INTEGRATION

We noted in the chapter "Theories and Treatment of Abnormality" that theories or models of psychopathology are increasingly based on the integration of concepts from biological, psychological, and social approaches. These concepts often are viewed from a vulnerability-stress perspective. The characteristics that make a person more vulnerable to abnormality might include biological characteristics, such as a genetic predisposition, or psychological characteristics, such as a maladaptive style of thinking about the world. These personal characteristics must interact with characteristics of the situation or environment to create the abnormality. For example, a woman with a genetic predisposition to depression may never develop the disorder in its full form if she has a supportive family and never faces major stressors.

Conducting research that reflects this integrationist perspective on abnormality is not easy. Researchers must gather information about people's biological, psychological, and social vulnerabilities and strengths. This work may require specialized equipment or expertise. It also may require following participants longitudinally to observe what happens when people with vulnerabilities face stressors that may trigger episodes of their disorder.

Increasingly, researchers work together in teams to share both their expertise in specialized research methods and their available resources, making multidisciplinary longitudinal research possible. Researchers also train in multiple disciplines and methods. For example, some psychologists use magnetic resonance imaging (MRI), positron-emission tomography (PET) scans, and other advanced biological methods in their investigations of abnormality.

A new and prominent movement in the area of abnormal psychology research, called the Research Domain Criteria (RDoC), encourages researches to integrate across such methods (Cuthbert & Insel, 2013). In addition to advocating the biopsychosocial approach, this initiative from the National Institute of Mental Health also directly reflects issues highlighted in the previous chapters, including increased emphasis on the continuum model of abnormality, the role of common mechanisms underlying multiple disorders, and the limitations of diagnostic categories (Clark, Cuthbert, Lewis-Fernández, Narrow, & Reed, 2017; Lilienfeld & Treadway, 2016).

If you pursue a career in researching abnormality, you might integrate methods from psychology (which have been the focus of this chapter), sociology, and biology to create the most comprehensive picture of the disorder you are investigating. This task may seem daunting, but an interactionist approach holds out the possibility of producing breakthroughs that can greatly improve the lives of people vulnerable to psychopathology.

SHADES OF GRAY   DISCUSSION

Your greatest challenge in deciding the ethics of this particular study is that the study involves deception. Some ethics committees would never accept a study in which students were deceived about their results on an intelligence test. Other committees might approve this study if it ensured all or most of the basic rights discussed in the section "Ethical Issues in Research." Participants must be made aware that they may experience psychological distress as a result of participating. They must know that they may decline participation or withdraw at any point. Usually, these statements must appear in an informed consent document that individuals should read before deciding to participate. This document should also tell participants how confidential their responses in the study will be. In this case, there is no reason why participants' responses should not be confidential.

If the researcher told participants before the study began that the feedback they will receive is bogus, this clearly would affect participants' responses to the feedback. The researcher would argue that participants cannot be told in the informed consent document that the study involves deception. Your ethics committee then must decide whether the potential benefits of the information obtained in this study warrant the deception.

Following the study, the researcher should reveal the nature of the deception and the justification for using it. Many participants, especially college students, continue to believe negative feedback they receive in an experiment even after being told that they were deceived. The researchers who discovered this phenomenon recommended conducting a *process debriefing* (Ross, Lepper, & Hubbard, 1975). In such a debriefing, experimenters discuss at length the purposes and procedures of the experiment, explaining that the feedback was not a reflection of participants' abilities.

CHAPTER SUMMARY

- A hypothesis is a testable statement of what we predict will happen in a study.

- The dependent variable is the factor the study aims to predict. The independent variable is the factor used or manipulated to predict the dependent variable.

- A sample is a group taken from the population of interest to participate in the study. The sample for the study must be representative of the population of interest, and the research must be generalizable to the population of interest.

- A control group consists of people who are similar in most ways to the primary group of interest but who do not experience the variable the theory hypothesizes causes changes in the dependent variable. Matching the control group to the group of primary interest can help control third variables, which are variables unrelated to the theory that still may have some effect on the dependent variable.

- The basic rights of participants in studies include being told the risks of participation, having their information kept confidential, having the right to refuse participation or withdraw from the study, giving informed consent, not being exposed to deception unless it is well justified, and being debriefed following the study.

- Case studies of individuals provide detailed information about their subjects. They are helpful in generating new ideas and in studying rare problems. They suffer from problems in generalizability and in the subjectivity of both the person being studied and the person conducting the study.

- Correlational studies examine the relationship between two variables without manipulating the variables. A correlation coefficient is an index of the relationship between two variables. It can range from −1.00 to +1.00. The magnitude of the correlation indicates how strong the relationship between the variables is.

- A positive correlation indicates that as values of one variable increase, values of the other variable increase. A negative correlation indicates that as values of one variable increase, values of the other variable decrease.

- A result is said to be statistically significant if it is unlikely to have happened by chance. The convention in psychological research is to accept results for which there is a probability of less than 5 in 100 that they happened by chance.

- A correlational study can show that two variables are related, but it cannot show that one variable causes the other. All correlational studies have the third variable problem—the possibility that variables not measured in the study actually account for the relationship between the variables measured in the study.

- Continuous variable studies evaluate the relationship between two variables that vary along a continuum.

- A representative sample resembles the population of interest on all important variables. One way to generate a representative sample is to obtain a random sample.

- Whereas cross-sectional studies assess a sample at one point in time, longitudinal studies assess a sample at multiple points in time. A longitudinal study often assesses a sample that is expected to experience some key event in the future both before and after the event, then examines changes that occurred in the sample. Group comparison studies evaluate differences between key groups, such as a group that experienced a certain stressor and a matched comparison group that did not.

- Epidemiological studies look at the frequency and distribution of a disorder in a population. The prevalence of a disorder is the proportion of the population that has the disorder at a given point or period in time. The incidence of a disorder is the number of new cases of the disorder that develop during a specific period of time. Risk factors for a disorder are conditions or variables associated with a higher risk of having the disorder.

- Experimental studies can provide evidence that a given variable causes psychopathology. A human laboratory study has the goal of inducing the conditions that we hypothesize will lead to our outcome of interest (e.g., increasing stress to cause depression) in people in a controlled setting. Participants are randomly assigned to either the experimental group, which receives a manipulation, or a control group, which does not.

- Generalizing experimental studies to real-world phenomena sometimes is not possible. In addition, manipulating people who are in distress in an experimental study can create ethical problems.

- A therapy outcome study allows researchers to test a hypothesis about the causes of a psychopathology while providing a service to participants.

- In therapy outcome studies, researchers sometimes use wait list control groups, in which control participants wait to receive the interventions until after the studies are completed. Alternatively, researchers may try to construct placebo control groups, in which participants receive the general support of therapists but none of the elements of the therapy thought to be active. Both types of control groups have practical and ethical limitations.

- Difficult issues associated with therapy outcome studies include problems in knowing what elements of therapy were effective, questions about the appropriate control groups to use, questions about whether to allow modifications of the therapy to fit individual participants' needs, and the lack of generalizability of the results of these studies to the real world.

- Single-case experimental designs involve the intensive investigation of single individuals or small groups of individuals before and after a manipulation or intervention. In an ABAB, or reversal, design, an intervention is introduced, withdrawn, and then reinstated, and the behavior of a participant on and off the treatment is examined.

- In multiple baseline designs, an individual is given a treatment in different settings or multiple individuals are given a treatment at different times across different settings, and the effects of the treatment are systematically observed.

- Animal studies allow researchers to manipulate their subjects in ways that are not ethically permissible with human participants, although many people feel that such animal studies are equally unethical. Animal studies raise questions about their generalizability to humans.

- Genetic studies include a variety of research methods. Family history studies determine whether biological relatives of someone with a disorder are more likely to have it than are people not related to someone with the disorder. Adoption studies determine whether the biological family members of adoptees with a disorder are more likely to have the disorder than are the adoptive family members. Twin studies determine whether monozygotic twins are more alike in the presence or absence of a disorder than are dizygotic twins. Molecular genetic (or association) studies look for specific genes associated with a disorder. Linkage analyses investigate the relationship between a biological characteristic for which the genes are known and a psychological disorder for which they are not.

- Cross-cultural research poses challenges. Theories and concepts that make sense in one culture may not be applicable to other cultures. Questionnaires and other assessment tools must be translated accurately. Also, culture can affect how people respond to the social demands of research. Finally, researchers must be careful not to build into their research any assumptions that one culture is normal and another is deviant.

- Meta-analysis is a statistical technique for summarizing results across several studies. In a meta-analysis, the results of individual studies are standardized by use of a statistic called the effect size. Then the magnitude of the effect size and its relationship to characteristics of the study are examined.

- Meta-analyses reduce bias that can occur when investigators draw conclusions across studies in a more subjective manner, but they can include studies that have poor methods or exclude good studies that did not get published because they did not find significant effects.

KEY TERMS

scientific method

hypothesis

null hypothesis

variable

dependent variable

independent variable

operationalization

case studies

generalizability

correlational studies

continuous variable

group comparison study

cross-sectional

longitudinal

correlation coefficient

statistical significance

third variable problem

sample

external validity

epidemiology

prevalence

incidence

risk factors

experimental studies

human laboratory study

internal validity

control group

experimental group

random assignment

demand characteristics

double-blind experiment

therapy outcome studies

simple control group

wait list control group

placebo control group

efficacy

effectiveness

single-case experimental design

ABAB (reversal) design

multiple baseline design

animal studies

family history study

monozygotic (MZ) twins

dizygotic (DZ) twins

twin studies

concordance rate

adoption study

molecular genetic studies

association studies

linkage analysis

meta-analysis

Chapter 5

Peter Dazeley/Getty Images

Anxiety, Obsessive-Compulsive, Trauma, and Stressor-Related Disorders

CHAPTER OUTLINE

Fear and Anxiety Along the Continuum

- Fear is in response to **objectively threatening** events *(fearing you will fail a class after failing the midterm)*
- Fear is of **appropriate severity** given the threat *(being concerned because you need this class to graduate)*
- Fear **subsides when threat has passed** *(relaxing when you learn there was a grading error and you actually did well)*
- Fear leads to **adaptive behaviors** to confront or avoid threat *(asking your instructor if you can improve your grade with extra work)*

Potentially meets diagnostic criteria for an anxiety disorder:

- Anxiety is **moderately unrealistic** *(anxietying a car accident if you drive on Friday the 13th)*
- Anxiety is **definitely more than is warranted** given the severity of the threat *(being very nervous when forced to drive on Friday the 13th)*
- Anxiety **persists for quite a while after the threat has passed** *(worrying about the next Friday the 13th)*
- Anxiety leads to **behaviors that are potentially dangerous or impairing** *(skipping class to avoid driving on Friday the 13th)*

Functional ———————————————————————————— **Dysfunctional**

- Anxiety may be **somewhat unrealistic** *(anxiety of appearing foolish when giving a presentation in class)*
- Anxiety may be **somewhat more than is warranted** given the severity of the threat *(being unable to sleep the night before a presentation)*
- Anxiety **persists after the threat has passed** *(after you give the presentation, analyzing it and worrying about what people thought)*
- Anxiety **leads to behaviors that may be somewhat inappropriate** *(taking a tranquilizer before the presentation to relax)*

Likely meets diagnostic criteria for an anxiety disorder:

- Anxieties are **completely unrealistic** *(anxieting that every ache or pain is a sign of terminal illness)*
- Anxieties are **excessive** given the objective threat *(thinking one is dying when one feels pain)*
- Anxieties **persist long after the threat has passed,** and chronic anticipatory anxiety exists *(believing one has a terminal illness despite physician reassurance)*
- Anxiety **leads to dangerous behavior or impairment** *(seeking out surgery to cure the terminal illness your physician says you do not have)*

We have all experienced feelings of anxiety. Why? Because as human beings we each have moments when we are filled with doubt or insecurity. Think of a time when you felt anxious or worried, perhaps on your first day of college. Chances are you felt a bit tense or jittery, you worried about what you might encounter, and there were times you wished you could just retreat back to familiar surroundings and people. This is a typical response to a new and potentially threatening situation—here, the threat is that you might not like these new experiences of college. You may not like the new people at your college, you might feel like you do not belong or fit in, or you might not do well in your classes. Replace first day of college with any other scenario like, meeting the parents of a new love interest, interviewing for a job that you really want, or taking a cross-fit class for the first time, and the response can be the same—we worry. Humans are exceptional in our ability to think about the future and, in this case, worry about things that have not yet happened, which produces anxiety. Anxiety is an interesting emotional state that has an immediate impact on the body. Your chest tightens as you enter the classroom for the first time, your hands are sweaty before the job interview, and your heart beats faster than normal as you open the door for your first date.

Although anxiety is typically discussed in negative terms, it is important to recognize that anxiety is a normal reaction to stress and can be helpful in many situations. Return to the scenarios above—how could feelings of anxiety benefit you? Anxiety can help us prepare for those new experiences, force us to pay attention to what's happening around us, and alert us to potential dangers. These typical feelings of nervousness or worry differ from anxiety disorders, which involve excessive fear or anxiety.

Fears and anxiety exist along a continuum that ranges from typical to pathological, and are influenced simultaneously by environmental and individual factors.

Anxiety is a future-oriented apprehension, tension, or sense of dread while fear is an immediate emotional response to danger or perceived threat in the environment. For example, after binge-watching Criminal Minds, you may feel anxious while walking to your car alone at night worried that something dangerous is waiting for you, but when your friend sneaks up behind you and screams "Boo!" as you enter your car you are suddenly filled with fear, even if it's just for a moment. In daily language, anxiety and fear are often indistinguishable to most people; however, they are separate mechanisms of the brain with distinct neurobiology. As with all emotions, both fear and anxiety are rooted in evolution and influenced by our perception of experiences that we label as "threatening" or "non-threatening" which are cultivated over the course of the lifespan. Even though our nervous system is designed to respond to threats in ways that help ensure survival, some individuals too often experience intense or frequent bouts of anxiety that are maladaptive and can interfere with one's ability to function. This clinical significance is what separates typical feelings of anxiety from an anxiety disorder.

FIGURE 1

The Fight-or-Flight Response. The body's fight-or-flight response is initiated by the part of the brain known as the hypothalamus. The hypothalamus stimulates the sympathetic division of the autonomic nervous system, which acts on smooth muscles and internal organs to produce the bodily changes shown in the figure. The hypothalamus also releases corticotropin-release factor (CRF), which triggers the pituitary gland to release adrenocorticotropic hormone (ACTH). In turn, ACTH stimulates the adrenal glands to release about 30 other hormones. The hormones act on organs and muscles to prepare the body to fight or flee.

When we face any type of threat or stressor, our body mobilizes to handle it. Over evolutionary history, humans have developed a characteristic fight-or-flight response, a set of physical and psychological responses that help us fight a threat or flee from it. The physiological changes of the **fight-or-flight** response result from the activation of two systems controlled by the hypothalamus, as seen in Figure 1: the **autonomic nervous system** (in particular, the sympathetic division of this system) and the **adrenal-cortical system** (a hormone-releasing system; see the chapter "Theories and Treatment of Abnormality").

When we experience a perceived threat, the hypothalamus first activates the sympathetic division of the autonomic nervous system. This system acts directly on the smooth muscles and internal organs to produce key bodily changes: The liver releases extra sugar (glucose) to fuel the muscles, and the body's metabolism increases in preparation for expending energy on physical action. Heart rate, blood pressure, and breathing rate increase, and the muscles tense. Less essential activities, such as digestion, are curtailed. Saliva and mucus dry up, increasing the size of the air passages to the lungs. The body secretes endorphins, which are natural painkillers, and the surface blood vessels constrict to reduce bleeding in case of injury. The spleen releases more red blood cells to help carry oxygen.

In addition to the autonomic nervous system, the hypothalamus activates the adrenal-cortical system. It does this by releasing corticotropin-release factor (CRF), which signals the pituitary gland to secrete adrenocorticotropic hormone (ACTH), the body's major stress hormone. ACTH stimulates the outer layer of the adrenal glands (the adrenal cortex), releasing a group of hormones, the major one being cortisol. The amount of cortisol in blood or urine samples is often used as a measure of stress. ACTH also signals the adrenal glands to release about 30 other hormones, each of which plays a role in the body's adjustment to emergency situations. Eventually, when the threatening stimulus has passed, the hippocampus, a part of the brain that helps regulate emotions, turns off this physiological cascade. The fight-or-flight system thus has its own feedback loop that normally regulates the level of physiological arousal we experience in response to a stressor. In many of the disorders we discuss in this chapter, the normal response becomes abnormal, and the fight-or-flight system becomes dysregulated.

In response to a stressor or threat, humans have specific physiological responses to danger as well as emotional, cognitive, and behavioral responses (Table 1). Emotionally, we experience feelings of dread or apprehension, which can cause irritability or restlessness. In terms of cognition, we both consciously and unconsciously evaluate a stimulus to determine the degree of the potential threat. The noise that woke you in the middle of night was momentarily threatening until you cognitively recognized that it was your roommate coming home late from work. Once you interpret this event as non-threatening, the fear subsides. Behaviorally, we seek to confront the threat or escape from it. In anxiety and related disorders, these responses may persist in the absence of any objective threat.

The COVID-19 pandemic proved to be an excellent example of how life events can rapidly and profoundly influence our psychological and emotional health. This global pandemic quickly became a significant source of anxiety and stress for millions of people around the world and provided an opportunity for us to examine the psychological effects of the coronavirus. Historically, public health crises cause massive disruptions to the day-to-day behavior and psychological well-being of many in the population.

The COVID-19 health crisis has affected every part of daily life and generated valuable research on the impact of various psychological factors, such as social distancing, stay-at-home requirements, mask-wearing, health concerns, and disruption of our typical practices,

TABLE 1 Responses to Threat

These characteristic responses to threat can also be symptoms of an anxiety disorder.

Somatic	Emotional	Cognitive	Behavioral
Tense muscles	Sense of dread	Anticipation of harm	Escape
Increased heart rate	Terror	Exaggeration of danger	Avoidance
Changes in respiration	Restlessness	Problems in concentrating	Aggression
Dilated pupils	Irritability	Hypervigilance	Freezing
Increased perspiration		Worried, ruminative thinking	
Adrenaline secretion		Fear of losing control	
Inhibited stomach acid		Fear of dying	
Decreased salivation		Sense of unreality	
Bladder relaxation			

on the development of anxiety. Research on previous global disease outbreaks has shown that people suffering from pandemic-related anxiety tend to exhibit elevated levels of posttraumatic stress, general stress, anxiety, health anxiety, and suicidality. Anxiety related to COVID-19, referred to as *coronaphobia*, involves feelings of anxiety that are not limited to typical impairment and distress (Asmundson & Taylor, 2020).

Recent research has found significant increases in anxiety related to the coronavirus outbreak, as well as positive correlations with coronavirus diagnosis, coronavirus fear, impairment, alcohol and drug coping, religious coping, hopelessness, suicidal ideation, as well as social attitudes and avoiding Chinese food and products (Asmundson & Taylor, 2020; Lee, 2020; Lee, Mathis, Jobe, & Pappalardo, 2020). These phenomena have a pervasive influence on all aspects of the individual's life from coping skills to social attitudes. Research on the psychological reactions to previous epidemics and pandemics suggests that various psychological vulnerability factors may play a role in coronaphobia, including individual difference variables such as the intolerance of uncertainty, perceived vulnerability to disease, and anxiety proneness. The tremendous impact of the COVID-19 pandemic on society highlights the multifactorial influence of situational events on mental health.

This chapter will discuss numerous anxiety disorders, each with varying characteristics, behaviors, and symptoms. While these disorders are all distinct, anxiety is a key component in each because it causes clinically significant distress and impairment in daily function. Some of these disorder involve periods of anxiety that are acute and more or less specific to certain objects, thoughts, or situations, while other disorders involve a more general and constant experience of anxiety.

PANIC DISORDER

"I think I am having a heart attack, please help me . . . I need to go to the emergency room . . . . I can't breathe, I'm dizzy . . . . I might be dying." These are common words for someone having a panic attack because the symptoms of this disorder often look like a medical emergency, rather than what actually is: a psychological experience. **Panic attacks,** short but intense periods during which one experiences many symptoms of anxiety such as: heart palpitations, trembling, shortness of breath, dizziness, intense dread, and the fear of dying (Table 2). Celia suffers from panic attacks, which are described in the following case summary.

Celia's panic attacks appear to come "out of the blue," in the absence of any environmental trigger. Simply handing a customer a hamburger should not cause such terror, but this is a common feature of panic attacks that is not fully understood. Just like Celia's experience, some panic attacks can appear without explanation while others can be triggered by specific situations or events. Someone with a social anxiety disorder, for instance, may have a panic attack when forced into a social situation (Craske et al., 2010). Most commonly, panic attacks arise in certain situations but not every time. In all cases, however, they are terrifying experiences, causing a person intense fear or discomfort, the physiological symptoms of anxiety, and the feeling of losing control, "going crazy," or dying (American Psychiatric Association, 2013). As with many other psychological disorders, a *specifier* can be added to panic disorder which allows for a more specific diagnosis. For example, major depressive disorder with peripartum onset specifier is assigned to allow to clarify that the symptoms of depression have occurred within or during the 4 weeks following pregnancy.

As many as 28 percent of adults have occasional panic attacks, especially during times of stress (Kessler et al., 2006). For most, the attacks are inconvenient but isolated events that do not change how they live their lives. A diagnosis of **panic disorder** is only made when the panic attacks are more problematic (See Table 2). This includes when they become a common occurrence, when they are not usually provoked by any particular situation but are unexpected, and when a person begins to worry about having them and changes their behavior as a result of this worry.

Some people with panic disorder have many episodes in a short period of time, such as every day for a week, and then go weeks or months without any episodes, followed by another period of frequent attacks. Other people have attacks less frequently but more regularly, such as once every week for months.

"I MIGHT BE DYING!" THE CASE OF CELIA

The first time Celia had a panic attack, two days before her twentieth birthday, she was working at McDonald's. As she was handing a customer a Big Mac, the earth seemed to open up beneath her. Her heart began to pound, she felt she was suffocating, she broke into a sweat, and she was sure she was going to have a heart attack and die. After about 20 minutes of terror, the panic subsided. Trembling, she got in her car, raced home, and barely left the house for the next 3 months.

Since that time, Celia has had about three attacks a month. She does not know when they are coming. During them she feels dread, searing chest pain, suffocating and choking, dizziness, and shakiness. She sometimes thinks this is all not real and she is going crazy. She also thinks she is going to die.

(Source: Adapted from Seligman, 1993, p. 61)

TABLE 2 DSM-5 Diagnostic Criteria for Panic Disorder

A. Recurrent unexpected panic attacks. A panic attack is an abrupt surge of intense fear or intense discomfort that reaches a peak within minutes, and during which time four (or more) of the following symptoms occur:

Note: The abrupt surge can occur from a calm state or an anxious state.

1. Palpitations, pounding heart, or accelerated heart rate
2. Sweating
3. Trembling or shaking
4. Sensations of shortness of breath or smothering
5. Feelings of choking
6. Chest pain or discomfort
7. Nausea or abdominal distress
8. Feeling dizzy, unsteady, light-headed, or faint
9. Chills or heat sensations
10. Paresthesias (numbness or tingling sensations)
11. Derealization (feelings of unreality) or depersonalization (being detached from oneself)
12. Fear of losing control or "going crazy"
13. Fear of dying

Note: Culture-specific symptoms (e.g., tinnitus, neck soreness, headache, uncontrollable screaming or crying) may be seen. Such symptoms should not count as one of the four required symptoms.

B. At least one of the attacks has been followed by one month (or more) of one or both of the following:

1. Persistent concern or worry about additional panic attacks or their consequences (e.g., losing control, having a heart attack, "going crazy").
2. A significant maladaptive change in behavior related to the attacks (e.g., behaviors designed to avoid having panic attacks, such as avoidance of exercise or unfamiliar situations).

C. The disturbance is not attributable to the physiological effects of a substance (e.g., a drug of abuse, a medication) or another medical condition (e.g., hyperthyroidism, cardiopulmonary disorders).

D. The disturbance is not better explained by another mental disorder (e.g., the panic attacks do not occur only in response to feared social situations, as in social anxiety disorder; in response to circumscribed phobic objects or situations, as in specific phobia; in response to obsessions, as in obsessive-compulsive disorder; in response to reminders of traumatic events, as in posttraumatic stress disorder; or in response to separation from attachment figures, as in separation anxiety disorder).

Between full-blown attacks, they might experience minor bouts of panic.

People with panic disorder often believe that they are experiencing a life-threatening illness and they are more likely to have a personal or family history of serious chronic illness. Even after such an illness is ruled out, they may continue to believe they are about to die of a heart attack, seizure, or other physical crises. Another common but erroneous belief is that they are "going crazy" or "losing control." Many people with panic disorder feel ashamed and try to hide it from others. If left untreated, people with panic disorder may become demoralized and depressed (Craske & Waters, 2005).

About 3 to 5 percent of people will develop panic disorder at some time (Craske & Waters, 2005; Kessler et al., 2005), usually between late adolescence and the mid-thirties. It is more common in women and tends to be chronic. There is some evidence that panic disorder—as well as social anxiety disorder—may have a more chronic course among African Americans compared to Caucasians (Sibrava et al., 2013). Panic disorder can be debilitating. Many sufferers also show chronic generalized anxiety, depression, and alcohol abuse (Wilson & Hayward, 2005). Those with panic disorder who are depressed or who abuse alcohol may be at an increased risk for suicide attempts (Craske et al., 2010).

Theories of Panic Disorder

Biological and cognitive theories present various explanations and identify factors that create vulnerability to panic disorder.

Biological Factors

Panic disorder and generalized anxiety disorder both have a high lifetime prevalence but it is unclear how mechanisms of the brain contribute to these persistent symptoms. Panic disorder clearly runs in families (Hettema, Neale, & Kendler, 2001), and family history and twin studies suggest that the heritability of panic disorder is about 43 to 48 percent (Wittchen et al., 2010). No specific genes have been consistently identified as causing panic disorder.

The fight-or-flight response appears to be poorly regulated in people who develop panic disorder, perhaps due to poor regulation of several neurotransmitters, including norepinephrine, serotonin, gamma-aminobutyric acid (GABA), and cholecystokinin (CCK; Charney et al., 2000). Panic attacks can easily be triggered in sufferers of panic disorder if they hyperventilate, inhale a small amount of carbon dioxide, ingest caffeine, breathe into a paper bag, or take infusions of sodium lactate, a substance that resembles the lactate produced during exercise (Craske & Barlow, 2014; Wittchen et al., 2010). These activities initiate the physiological changes of the fight-or-flight response. People without a history of panic attacks may experience some physical discomfort during these activities, but rarely a full-blown attack.

Neuroimaging studies show differences between people with panic disorder and those without panic disorder in several areas of the limbic system involved in the stress response, including the amygdala, hypothalamus, and hippocampus (Duval, Javanbakht, & Liberzon, 2015). Research by Cui et. al. (2016) suggests that abnormalities involving the somatosensory cortex and

FIGURE 2 **Areas of the Brain Involved in Panic Disorder.** Several areas of the limbic system shown here, along with the locus ceruleus, may be involved in panic attacks.

Amygdala

Hypothalamus

Hippocampus

Periaqueductal gray

Locus ceruleus

thalamus may best explain the development of the symptoms of panic disorder, since these areas relate to how people interpret sensations within their body. Dysregulation of norepinephrine systems in an area of the brain stem called the **locus ceruleus** (see Figure 2) have also been linked to panic disorder. The locus ceruleus has well-defined pathways to the limbic system. Poor regulation in the locus ceruleus may cause panic attacks, which then stimulate the limbic system, lowering the threshold for the activation of diffuse and chronic anxiety (Rappaport et al., 2017). This anticipatory anxiety may, in turn, increase the likelihood of dysregulation of the locus ceruleus and thus of another panic attack.

Some women with panic disorder report increased anxiety symptoms during premenstrual periods and postpartum (Maeng & Milad, 2015). The hormone progesterone can affect the activity of both the serotonin and GABA neurotransmitter systems. Fluctuations in progesterone levels with the menstrual cycle or postpartum might lead to an imbalance or dysfunction of the serotonin or GABA systems, thereby influencing susceptibility. Increases in progesterone also can induce mild chronic hyperventilation. In women prone to panic attacks, this may be enough to induce a full-blown attack.

Cognitive Factors

Although many people with panic disorder may have a biological vulnerability to it, psychological factors also appear to help determine who develops the disorder. Cognitive theorists argue that people prone to panic attacks tend to (1) pay very close attention to their bodily sensations, (2) misinterpret these sensations in a negative way, and (3) engage in snowballing catastrophic thinking, exaggerating symptoms and their consequences (Barlow, 2011; Craske & Barlow, 2014). For example, a person not prone to panic disorder might feel a bit dizzy after standing up quickly and think "I'm feeling dizzy; I guess I stood up too quickly," and leave it at that. But a person prone to panic disorder might think, "I'm really dizzy. I think I'm going to faint. Maybe I'm having a seizure. Oh God, what's happening?" This kind of thinking increases the subjective sense of anxiety as well as physiological changes such as increased heart rate. The person interprets these feelings catastrophically and is on the way to a full panic attack. Between attacks, the person is hypervigilant for any bodily sensations, worrying about his or her health generally and about having more panic attacks specifically. This constant arousal makes further attacks more likely (Craske & Barlow, 2014).

The unfounded belief that bodily symptoms have harmful consequences is labeled **anxiety sensitivity** (McNally, 2002). People high in anxiety sensitivity are more likely than people low in it to have panic disorder, to have more frequent panic attacks, or to develop panic attacks over time (Hayward, Killen, Kraemer, & Taylor, 2000; Olatunji & Wolitzky-Taylor, 2009).

Those prone to panic attacks also appear to have increased **interoceptive awareness**—a heightened awareness of bodily cues (such as slight sensations of arousal or anxiety) that may signal a coming panic attack (Razran, 1961). These bodily cues have occurred at the beginning of previous panic attacks and have become conditioned stimuli signaling new attacks, a process called **interoceptive conditioning** (Bouton, Mineka, & Barlow, 2001). Thus, slight increases in anxiety, even if not consciously recognized, can elicit conditioned fear that grows into a full panic attack. If the individual doesn't recognize this process, the attack seems to come from nowhere. This interplay between physiological and cognitive factors also plays a role in elevated comorbidity between panic disorder and medical illnesses (Meuret, Kroll, & Ritz, 2017).

Beliefs about the controllability of symptoms appear to be important to the development of panic attacks. In one study, two groups of people with panic disorder were asked to wear breathing masks, which delivered air slightly enriched with carbon dioxide. Participants were warned that inhaling carbon dioxide could induce an attack. One group was told they could not control the amount of carbon dioxide that came through their masks. The other group was told they could control it by turning a knob. Actually, neither group had any control over the amount of carbon dioxide, and both groups inhaled the same amount. However, 80 percent of the people who believed they had no control experienced a panic attack, compared to 20 percent of those who believed they had control (Sanderson, Rapee, & Barlow, 1989). In summary, a number of cognitive factors contribute to panic disorder, including biased thoughts, anxiety sensitivity, high interoceptive awareness, interoceptive conditioning (learning), and beliefs about controllability.

An Integrated Model

The biological and psychological factors of panic disorder have been integrated into the model illustrated in Figure 3 (Bouton et al., 2001; Craske & Waters, 2005). Many people who develop panic disorder seem to have a biological vulnerability to a hypersensitive fight-or-flight response. Presented with only a mild stimulus, their heart begins to race, their breathing becomes rapid, and their palms begin to sweat.

These people typically will not develop frequent panic attacks or a panic disorder, however, unless they engage in catastrophizing thinking about their physiological symptoms. Such cognitions increase the intensity of initially mild physiological symptoms to the point of a panic attack. They also make the individuals hypervigilant for signs of another panic attack, putting them at a constant mild to moderate level of anxiety. This anxiety increases the probability that they will become panicked again, and the cycle continues.

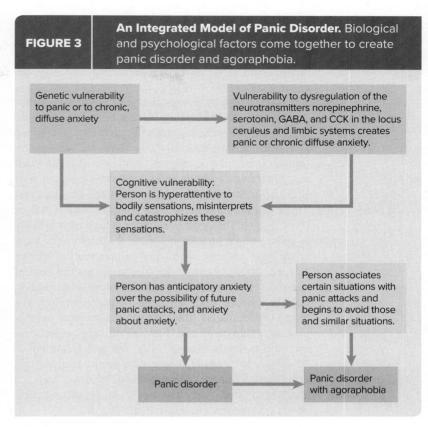

FIGURE 3 **An Integrated Model of Panic Disorder.** Biological and psychological factors come together to create panic disorder and agoraphobia.

Some people then begin to associate certain situations with symptoms of panic and may begin to feel them again if they return to the situations. By avoiding these places, they reduce their symptoms, thereby reinforcing their avoidance behavior. This process is known as a **conditioned avoidance response** (Mowrer, 1939). Thus, a man who has a panic attack while sitting in a theater may later associate the theater with his symptoms and begin to feel anxious whenever he is near it. By avoiding it, he can reduce his anxiety. He may associate other places, such as his home or a specific room, with lowered anxiety levels, so being in these places is reinforcing. Eventually, he confines himself to his safe places and avoids a wide range of places he feels are unsafe. Thus he develops agoraphobia, which frequently co-occurs with panic disorder. According to Neueder, Andreatta, & Pauli (2019), these types of contextual conditioning and generalization processes may be the basis for developing panic disorder and agoraphobia since they may cause anxiety in and avoidance of various contexts (e.g., shopping malls, crowded spaces), and may motivate withdrawal to safety contexts (e.g., the home).

Treatments for Panic Disorder

Effective biological and psychological treatments for panic disorder are available to help people suffering from this disorder. As with any treatment method, there is no "one-size-fits-all" approach, but there are many treatment options such as antidepressant drugs and cognitive-behavioral therapies that are successful in reducing symptoms and preventing relapse.

Biological Treatments

The most common biological treatment for panic disorder is medication affecting serotonin and norepinephrine systems, including selective serotonin reuptake inhibitors (SSRIs, such as Paxil, Prozac, Zoloft), serotonin-norepinephrine reuptake inhibitors (SNRIs, such as Effexor), and tricyclic antidepressants (Batelaan, Van Balkom, & Stein, 2012; see the chapter "Theories and Treatment of Abnormality" for common side effects of these drugs). The benzodiazepines, which work quickly to reduce panic attacks and general symptoms of anxiety in most patients, are also often prescribed (Susman & Klee, 2005). Benzodiazepines suppress the central nervous system and influence functioning in the GABA, norepinephrine, and serotonin neurotransmitter systems. Unfortunately, they are physically (and psychologically) addictive and have significant withdrawal symptoms (see the chapter "Theories and Treatment of Abnormality"). Most people with panic disorder will experience a relapse of symptoms when drug therapies are discontinued if they have not also received cognitive-behavioral therapy (Batelaan et al., 2012).

Cognitive-Behavioral Therapy

Similar to treatment for other anxiety disorders such as PTSD and phobias, cognitive-behavioral therapy for panic disorder has clients confront the situations or thoughts that arouse anxiety. Confrontation seems to help in two ways: It allows clients to challenge and change irrational thoughts about these situations, and it helps them extinguish anxious behaviors.

Cognitive-behavioral interventions have multiple components (Craske & Barlow, 2014). First, clients are taught relaxation and breathing exercises, which impart some control over symptoms and permit clients to engage in the other components of the therapy. Second, the clinician guides clients in identifying the catastrophizing cognitions they have about changes in bodily sensations. Clients may keep diaries of their thoughts about their bodies on days between sessions, particularly at times when they begin to feel they are going to panic. Figure 4 shows one man's panic thoughts diary. He noted mild symptoms of panic at work but more severe symptoms while riding the subway home. In both situations, he had thoughts about feeling trapped, suffocating, and fainting.

Many clients, too overwhelmed while having symptoms to pay attention to their thoughts, need to experience panic symptoms in the presence of their therapist in order to identify their catastrophizing cognitions (Craske & Barlow, 2014). The therapist may try to induce symptoms during sessions by having clients exercise to elevate their heart rate, spin to get dizzy, or put their head between their knees and then stand up quickly to get light-headed (due to sudden changes in blood pressure). None of these activities is dangerous, but all are likely to produce the kind of symptoms clients catastrophize. As clients experience these symptoms and their catastrophizing cognitions, the therapist helps them collect their thoughts.

Third, clients practice relaxation and breathing exercises while experiencing panic symptoms during the session. If attacks occur during sessions, the therapist talks to clients through them, coaching them in the use of relaxation and breathing techniques, suggesting ways to improve their skills, and noting clients' success in using the skills to stop the attacks.

Fourth, the therapist challenges clients' catastrophizing thoughts about their bodily sensations and teaches them to challenge these thoughts themselves, using the cognitive techniques described in the chapter "Theories and Treatment of Abnormality." The therapist might help clients reinterpret the sensations accurately. For example, the client whose thoughts are listed in Figure 6 frequently felt as if he were choking. His therapist might explore whether his choking sensation might be due to the stuffiness of a small office or a subway on a warm summer day. If he interprets the increase in his heart rate as a heart attack, the

FIGURE 4	**A Panic Thoughts Diary.** This man recorded the thoughts he had had during panic attacks and then worked on these thoughts in cognitive therapy.

SITUATION	SYMPTOMS AND SEVERITY	THOUGHTS
Office at work	Choking (mild)	Oh, I can't have an attack here. People will see me and I might get fired. I'm suffocating! I'm going to faint.
	Dizziness (mild)	
	Heart racing (mild)	
Riding subway home	Sweating (severe)	I can't stand this! I've got to get out of here. I'm going to choke to death. I'm trapped. I'm going to faint!
	Choking (severe)	
	Shaking (severe)	
	Heart racing (severe)	
	Dizziness (severe)	
At home	Sweating (mild)	I can't believe I made it home.
	Heart still racing (moderate)	
	A little faintness	

therapist might have him collect evidence from his physician that he is in perfect cardiac health. The therapist might also explore the client's expectations that he will die of a heart attack because a relative did. If relaxation techniques allow a client to reduce panic symptoms during a therapy session, the therapist will challenge the client's belief that the symptoms are uncontrollable (Craske & Barlow, 2014).

Fifth, the therapist uses systematic desensitization therapy to expose clients gradually to the situations they fear most while helping them maintain control over their symptoms (Craske & Barlow, 2014). The client and therapist begin by listing panic-inducing situations, from most to least threatening. Then, after learning relaxation and breathing skills and perhaps gaining some control over panic symptoms induced during therapy sessions, clients begin to expose themselves to their panic-inducing situations, starting with the least threatening. The therapist might accompany clients in this exercise, coaching them in their relaxation and breathing skills and in how to challenge catastrophic cognitions that arise.

A large-scale, multisite study compared tricyclic antidepressants to cognitive-behavioral therapy (CBT) in the treatment of 312 people with panic disorder and found them equally effective in eliminating symptoms (Barlow, Gorman, Shear, & Woods, 2000). Several other studies have found that 85 to 90 percent of panic disorder patients treated with CBT experienced complete relief from their panic attacks within 12 weeks (Craske & Barlow, 2014; Schmidt & Keough, 2010). In follow-up studies of patients receiving CBT, nearly 90 percent were panic-free more than 2 years after treatment. Cognitive-behavioral therapy appears to be considerably better than antidepressants at preventing relapse after treatment ends, probably because this therapy teaches people strategies to prevent the recurrence of panic symptoms.

SEPARATION ANXIETY DISORDER

Children, like adults, can suffer from posttraumatic stress disorder, panic attacks, phobias, social anxiety disorder, and generalized anxiety disorder. One anxiety disorder is especially associated with childhood onset: **separation anxiety disorder** (see the *DSM-5* criteria in Table 3). Many infants become anxious and upset if they are separated from their primary caregivers. With development, however, most come to understand that their caregivers will return, and they find ways to comfort themselves while their caregivers are away.

However, some children continue to be extremely anxious when they are separated from their caregivers, even into later childhood and adolescence, which causes significant emotional distress and is not developmentally appropriate. They may be very shy, sensitive, and demanding of adults. They may refuse to go to school because they fear separation, and they may experience stomachaches, headaches, nausea, and

---

TABLE 3   *DSM-5* Criteria for Separation Anxiety Disorder

A. Developmentally inappropriate and excessive fear or anxiety concerning separation from those to whom the individual is attached, as evidenced by at least three of the following:

   1. Recurrent excessive distress when anticipating or experiencing separation from home or major attachment figures.

   2. Persistent and excessive worry about losing major attachment figures or possible harm to them, such as illness, injury, disasters, or death.

   3. Persistent and excessive worry about experiencing an untoward event (e.g., getting lost, being kidnapped, having an accident, becoming ill) that causes separation from a major attachment figure.

   4. Persistent reluctance or refusal to go out, away from home, to school, to work, or elsewhere because of fear of separation.

   5. Persistent and excessive fear or reluctance about being alone or without major attachment figures at home or in other settings.

   6. Persistent reluctance or refusal to sleep away from home or to go to sleep without being near a major attachment figure.

   7. Repeated nightmares involving the theme of separation.

   8. Repeated complaints of physical symptoms (e.g., headaches, stomachaches, nausea, vomiting) when separation from major attachment figures occurs or is anticipated.

B. The fear, anxiety, or avoidance is persistent, lasting at least 4 weeks in children and adolescents and typically 6 months or more in adults.

C. The disturbance causes clinically significant distress or impairment in social, academic, occupational, or other important areas of functioning.

D. The disturbance is not better explained by another mental disorder, such as refusing to leave home because of excessive resistance to change in autism spectrum disorder; delusions or hallucinations concerning separation in psychotic disorders; refusal to go outside without a trusted companion in agoraphobia; worries about ill health or other harm befalling significant others in generalized anxiety disorder; or concerns about having an illness in illness anxiety disorder.

vomiting if forced to leave their caregivers. They may follow their caregivers around the house, have nightmares with themes of separation, and be unable to sleep at night unless they are with their caregivers. When separated from their caregivers, they worry that something bad will happen to the caregivers and harbor exaggerated fears of natural disasters, kidnappings, and accidents. Younger children may cry inconsolably. Older children may demonstrate school refusal and avoid activities, such as being on a baseball team, that might take them away from their caregivers. Regardless of the variation, the symptoms of separation anxiety disorder all include emotional distress caused by the possibility of being separated from their caregivers.

Following a trauma or significant life event, such as loss of a pet, getting lost in a shopping mall, or seeing a parent hospitalized for a sudden illness, it is not uncommon for children to display symptoms of separation anxiety. It is important to recognize that separation anxiety disorder is not diagnosed unless symptoms persist for at least 4 weeks and significantly impair the child's functioning. Separation anxiety disorder occurs in about 4 to 10 percent of children and is equally common in boys and girls (Scarpa & Wilson, 2017). Left untreated, the disorder can continue throughout childhood and adolescence, significantly interfering with academic progress and peer relationships.

In past versions of the *DSM,* separation anxiety disorder was classified among disorders limited to children and adolescents, but authors of the *DSM-5* now acknowledge separation anxiety disorder as a condition that may span the entire life, and begin at any age, which led to its inclusion among anxiety disorders. Remarkably, recent research suggests the prevalence of separation anxiety disorder may be greater among adults than in children and adolescents, with adults displaying fewer somatic and more cognitive and emotional symptoms. Adults with separation anxiety disorder may have difficulties with change such as moving or getting married. They may focus their concerns on parents or children; and to maintain attachment they may make frequent phone calls, adhere to rigid routines, talk excessively, or fear being alone. Contrary to previous theories, it appears that the vast majority of persons classified as having separation anxiety disorder report first onset in adulthood, with a peak of onset in the early twenties (Carmassi, Gesi, Massimetti, Shear, & Dell'Osso, 2015; Starcevic & Castle, 2016). Research by Bandelow and Michaelis (2015) suggests that the lifetime prevalence rate for separation anxiety among adolescents (13 to 17 years) is 7.7 percent, and 6.6 percent among adults (18 to 64 years) with over half reporting onset of symptoms in adulthood, as opposed to symptoms continuing from childhood onset. Worldwide, it is estimated that separation anxiety disorder affects 5.3 percent of the population and half of those people also developing initial symptoms in adulthood (Carmassi et al., 2015; Silove et al., 2015).

Separation anxiety disorder among adults is highly comorbid with other mental disorders and is associated with substantial impairment in functioning. Recent studies have found a significant correlation with internalizing disorders (e.g., major depression, bipolar disorder, specific and social phobias, panic disorder, generalized anxiety disorder, and posttraumatic stress disorder), and externalizing disorders (e.g., ADHD, oppositional defiant disorder, and conduct disorder). This evidence supports the notion that the presence of separation anxiety disorder may represent a vulnerability for a wide range of common psychiatric conditions (Bögels, Knappe, & Clark, 2013; Carmassi et al., 2015; Pini et al., 2010).

Theories of Separation Anxiety Disorder

Researchers have tended to focus on biological, psychological, and sociological theories to explain separation anxiety disorder.

Biological Factors

Children with separation anxiety disorder tend to have family histories of anxiety and depressive disorders (Biederman et al., 2001; Manicavasagar, Silove, Rapee, Waters, & Momartin, 2001). There is also evidence of a genetic component, with some research demonstrating heritability estimates around 70 percent, but further studies are needed to better ascertain prevalence, gender distribution, and demographic correlates (Carmassi et al., 2015; Starcevic & Castle, 2016). Twin studies suggest that the tendency toward anxiety is heritable, more so in girls than in boys. However, it is not clear that a specific tendency toward separation anxiety is heritable (Rapee, Schniering, & Hudson, 2009). What may be inherited is a tendency toward a trait known as **behavioral inhibition.** Children high on behavioral inhibition are shy, fearful, and irritable as toddlers and cautious, quiet, and introverted as school-age children. These children tend to avoid or withdraw from novel situations, are clingy with their parents, and become excessively aroused in unfamiliar situations. Behavioral inhibition appears to be a risk factor for developing all types of anxiety disorders in childhood (Caspi et al., 2003; Smoller, Cerrato, & Weatherall, 2015, Paulus et al., 2015).

These children tend to avoid or withdraw from novel situations, are clingy with their parents, and become excessively aroused in unfamiliar situations. Behavioral inhibition appears to be a risk factor for developing anxiety disorders in childhood (Caspi et al., 2003; Smoller et al., 2015).

Psychological and Sociocultural Factors

Observational studies of interactions between anxious children and their parents show that the parents tend to be more controlling and intrusive both behaviorally and emotionally, and also more critical and negative in their communications with their children (Drake & Ginsburg, 2012). Some of this behavior may be in response to the children's anxious behaviors, but many parents of anxious children are themselves anxious or depressed. Research suggests that despite the possibility the anxiety is genetically contributed the environment may be more influential in terms of separation anxiety. Elay et al. (2015) twin-studies suggests that learning through modeling is a more significant contributor to the development of anxiety than genetics. Children learn to be anxious by modeling the behaviors of their anxious parents.

Additional evidence that environmental and parenting factors can influence the development of anxiety disorders in youngsters comes from studies of primates (Mineka, Gunnar, & Champoux, 1986; Suomi, 1999). Susan Mineka and colleagues found that rhesus monkeys who, from ages 2 to 6 months, were given adequate food and water but could not control their access to them became fearful and inhibited. Other monkeys given the same amount of food and water but under conditions that allowed them to exert some control did not become fearful. This result suggests that human children raised in conditions over which they have little control may develop anxiety symptoms. Recent research on relationship between separation anxiety and parenting style suggests that over-permissive parenting positively predicts adult separation anxiety symptoms by distorting how the children feel about themselves (Başbuğ, Cesur, & Durak Batıgün, 2017). Parental interaction is likely influenced the parent's level of anxiety or neuroticism which may affect the likelihood of developing separation anxiety. An overprotective parenting style has been identified as a significant factor in the relationship between levels of maternal anxiety and child separation anxiety. Mothers with higher trait anxiety, and those younger in age, were more likely to use an overprotective, punitive, or less assertive parenting style that is linked to higher rates of separation anxiety (Orgilés, Penosa, Morales, Fernandez-Martinez, & Espada, 2018). Additionally, children who perceive their parents as strict or highly controlling were significantly more anxious than children whose parents encourage independence while maintaining boundaries (Yaffe, 2018).

Children may learn to be anxious from their parents or as an understandable response to their environment (Rapee et al., 2009). In some cases, such as in the following case study, separation anxiety disorder develops after a traumatic event.

Children with separation anxiety disorder often cling desperately to their parents. *A3pfamily/Shutterstock*

CASE STUDY

In the early morning hours, 7-year-old Maria was abruptly awakened by a loud rumbling and violent shaking. She sat upright in bed and called out to her 10-year-old sister, Rosemary, who was leaping out of her own bed 3 feet away. The two girls ran for their mother's bedroom as their toys and books plummeted from shelves and dresser tops. The china hutch in the hallway teetered in front of them and then fell forward with a crash, blocking their path to their mother's room. Mrs. Marshall called out to them to go back and stay in their doorway. They huddled there together until the shaking finally stopped. Mrs. Marshall climbed over the hutch and broken china to her daughters. Although they were all very scared, they were unhurt.

Two weeks later, Maria began to complain every morning of stomachaches, headaches, and dizziness, asking to stay home with her mother. After 4 days, when a medical examination revealed no physical problems, Maria was told she must return to school. She protested tearfully, but her mother insisted, and Rosemary promised to hold her hand all the way to school. In the classroom, Maria could not concentrate on her schoolwork and was often out of her seat, looking out the window in the direction of home. She told her teacher she needed to go home to see whether her mother was okay. When told she couldn't go home, she began to cry and tremble so violently that the school nurse called Mrs. Marshall, who picked Maria up and took her home.

The next morning, Maria's protests grew stronger and she refused to go to school until her mother promised to go with her and sit in her classroom for the first hour. When Mrs. Marshall began to leave, Maria clung to her, crying, pleading for her not to

(continued)

leave, and following her into the hallway. The next day, Maria refused to leave the house for her Brownie meeting and her dancing lessons or even to play in the front yard. She followed her mother around the house and insisted on sleeping with her at night. "I need to be with you, Mommy, in case something happens," she declared.

Treatments for Separation Anxiety Disorder

Although there are many treatment options for both children and adults with this disorder, pharmacotherapy and cognitive-behavioral therapy (CBT) have received the most empirical support. CBT is designed to create changes in thinking and behavioral patterns that can help reduce vulnerability to anxiety and decrease the chances that symptoms return after therapy has ended. Modifications of CBT, such as mindfulness-based therapy and acceptance and commitment therapy have also demonstrated efficacy (Starcevic & Castle, 2016). Studies suggest that children benefit most from CBT as they are taught new skills for coping and for challenging cognitions that feed their anxiety. In this form of therapy, they might learn relaxation exercises to practice when they are separated from their parents. Their fears about separation are challenged, and they are taught to use self-talk to calm themselves when they become anxious (Kendall, Crawford, Kagan, Furr, & Podell, 2017).

As therapy progresses, the number and duration of periods of separation from their parents are increased. Parents must be willing to participate in therapy and to cope with their children's (and their own) reactions to increased periods of separation. Parents may need to be taught to model nonanxious reactions to separations from their children and to reinforce nonanxious behavior in their children.

Controlled clinical trials of this type of therapy show that it can be effective in the short term and maintain its effects over the long term (Rapee et al., 2009; Shortt, Barrett, & Fox, 2001; Velting, Setzer, & Albano, 2004). Philip Kendall and his colleagues (Kendall, Hudson, Gosch, Flannery-Schroeder, & Suveg, 2008) tested three treatments: individualized CBT to anxious children, family-based CBT to anxious children and their parents, and simple education and support. At the end of therapy, the children in both the individualized and the family-based CBT treatment showed substantial declines in anxiety symptoms, while the children who received only education and support showed less improvement. With all three treatments, the declines in anxiety symptoms were sustained over a 1-year follow-up period.

Consider how Maria was treated for her separation anxiety in her case study below:

CASE STUDY

Mrs. Benally was instructed to take Yanaha to school and leave four times during the period she was there. Initially, Mrs. Benally left for 30 seconds each time. Over time, she gradually increased the amount of time and distance she was away while Yanaha remained in the classroom. Yanaha was given a sticker at the end of the school day for each time she remained in her seat while her mother was out of the room. In addition, she was praised by her teacher and her mother, and positive self-statements ("My mommy will be okay; I'm a big girl and I can stay at school") were encouraged. No response was made when Yanaha failed to stay in her chair. Yanaha could exchange her stickers for prizes at the end of each week.

At home, Mrs. Benally was instructed to give minimal attention to Yanaha's inquiries about her well-being and to ignore excessive, inappropriate crying. Eventually, Yanaha was given a sticker and praise each morning for sleeping in her own bed.

The first few times Mrs. Benally left the classroom, Yanaha followed her out. Soon, however, she began to stay in her chair and receive stickers. At home, she remained in her own bed the first night, even though she was told she had to stay only 2 hours to earn her sticker. At her own request, she returned to Brownie meetings and attended summer camp.

Drugs used to treat separation anxiety disorders include antidepressants; antianxiety drugs, such as the benzodiazepines; stimulants; and antihistamines. The selective serotonin reuptake inhibitors, such as fluoxetine and sertraline, are used most frequently and have been shown to be most consistent in effectively reducing anxiety symptoms in children. Pharmacological and psychological treatments are often combined in clinical practice and there is some evidence to support this approach (Starcevic & Castle, 2016; Strawn, Welge, Wehry, Keeshin, & Rynn, 2015; Walkup et al., 2008).

SELECTIVE MUTISM

My friend James is a little shy with new people, but once he gets to know you we can't get him to stop talking! It is not uncommon for people to speak less when they are in a new situation that makes them uncomfortable. However, this behavior is typically temporary and will pass as the person becomes less anxious in the situation. These momentary periods of reduced speech should not be confused with the clinical disorder, selective mutism (SM) which involves the failure to speak in specific social situations. Studies over the past 20 years have consistently demonstrated a strong

Mikael Vaisanen/Getty Images

The most common feature associated with GAD is generalized worry that impacts daily life. fizkes/Shutterstock

relationship between SM and anxiety, most notably social phobia. These findings have led to the recent reclassification of SM as an anxiety disorder in the *DSM-5* (Hua & Major, 2016).

Selective mutism (SM) is an anxiety disorder that typically emerges in early childhood and can last into adulthood if untreated. Children with SM are capable of typical, age-appropriate language but remain silent in situations that provoke anxiety, such as a school setting. Since persons with SM can produce speech in certain situations (e.g., at home), this failure to speak cannot be attributed to a disturbance of language development. Nonetheless, this lack of speech may produce significant interference with social, occupational, and academic activities, which makes SM a debilitating disorder (Driessen, Blom, Muris, Blashfield, & Molendijk, 2020; Hua & Major, 2016; Koskela et al., 2020).

The development of SM appears to result from the interaction of various genetic, temperamental, environmental, and developmental factors. The mean age of onset of SM is between 2.7 and 4.6 years, and appears to be slightly more common in girls than in boys although the condition may go unnoticed until the child enters elementary school. Most attempts to estimate the prevalence of SM have been conducted in school-based communities and prevalence rates range between 0.03 and 0.79 percent. Therefore, SM is considered a relatively rare psychiatric disorder (Koskela et al., 2020).

GENERALIZED ANXIETY DISORDER

Some people experience anxiety that is comparable to carrying around a bucket of worry that weighs them down and trickles into almost every area of their life.

It's not specific to any one event or situation. It's everywhere; it's generalized. In this section, we will discuss other anxiety disorders that are associated with factors that have almost laser-point specificity or concentration, but unlike those disorders, **generalized anxiety disorder (GAD)** (Table 4) is not very discriminating and the defining feature is uncontrollable worry (American Psychiatric Association, 2013). People with this disorder are often referred to as "worrywarts" since this anxiety is a constant feature of a person's day-to-day existence. People with GAD worry about many things in their lives, and the lives of others they know, as Claire describes in the following profile (Ruscio, Stein, Chiu, & Kessler, 2017).

PROFILE ON CLAIRE: "I WORRY ALL THE TIME."

I just feel anxious and tense all the time. It started in high school. I was a straight-A student, and I worried constantly about my grades, whether the other kids and the teachers liked me, being prompt for classes—things like that. . . . Now I vacuum four times a week and clean the bathrooms every day. There have even been times when I've backed out of going out to dinner with my husband because the house needed to be cleaned.

I get so upset and irritated over minor things. . . . I still worry about being on time to church and to appointments. Now I find I worry a lot about my husband. He's been doing a tremendous amount of traveling for his job, some of it by car, but most of it by plane. Because he works on the northeastern seaboard, and because he frequently has to travel in the winter, I worry that he'll be stuck in bad weather and get into an accident or, God forbid, a plane crash.

(continued)

Oh, and I worry about my son. He just started playing on the varsity football team, so he's bound to get an injury some time. It's so nerve-wracking to watch him play that I've stopped going to his games. I'm sure my son must be disappointed . . . , but it's simply too much for me to take. (Brown, T. A., O'Leary, T. A., & Barlow, D. H. [2001]. *Generalized Anxiety Disorder, Clinical Handbook of Psychological Disorders: A Step-By-Step Treatment Manual* [3rd ed.]. Guilford Press, 193–194. Copyright ©2001 Guilford Press. Reprinted with permission. Permission conveyed through Copyright Clearance Center)

People with GAD typically experience excessive anxiety about ordinary, everyday situations. The anxiety is intrusive, causes distress or functional impairment, and often encompasses multiple domains such as work and health. People with GAD may worry about their performance on the job, their relationships, their health, and finances. The focus of their worries may shift frequently, and they tend to worry about many things instead of focusing on only one issue of concern (Andrews et al., 2010). The anxiety is often associated with physical symptoms, such as sleep disturbance, chronic restlessness, muscle tension, gastrointestinal symptoms, and chronic headaches. GAD is a relatively common psychological disorder that affects 2.9 percent of U.S. adults (18 to 64 years) in any given year. In this population, the lifetime prevalence is 7.7 percent in women and 4.6 percent in men. This disorder is not limited to adult sufferers and children and adolescents can experience symptoms of GAD. While GAD can occur at any age, many individuals with the disorder report feeling anxious all their lives (Locke, Kirst & Schultz, 2015; Ruscio et al., 2017).

As with most areas of study, we still have a lot to learn about this disorder. In comparison to other anxiety disorders, GAD is less understood and the degree to which this disorder affects personal function is commonly debated. Previous studies on GAD were typically limited to affluent, industrialized nations and less attention was given to other parts of the world, which likely skewed our understanding of GAD. However, a recent study by Ruscio et al. (2017) provides new insight into GAD by examining 147,261 adults, ranging in age from 18 to 99 years from 26 different countries across the world. Results of this study suggests that GAD is a common disorder associated with considerable comorbidity and functional impairment.

TABLE 4   *DSM-5* Criteria for Generalized Anxiety Disorder

A. Excessive anxiety and worry (apprehensive expectation), occurring more days than not for at least 6 months, about a number of events or activities (such as work or school performance).

B. The individual finds it difficult to control the worry.

C. The anxiety and worry are associated with three (or more) of the following six symptoms (with at least some symptoms having been present for more days than not for the past 6 months):

   1. Restlessness or feeling keyed up or on edge

   2. Being easily fatigued

   3. Difficulty concentrating or mind going blank

   4. Irritability

   5. Muscle tension

   6. Sleep disturbance (difficulty falling or staying asleep, or restless, unsatisfying sleep)

D. The anxiety, worry, or physical symptoms cause clinically significant distress or impairment in social, occupational, or other important areas of functioning.

E. The disturbance is not attributable to the direct physiological effects of a substance (e.g., a drug of abuse, a medication) or another medical condition (e.g., hyperthyroidism).

F. The disturbance is not better explained by another mental disorder (e.g., anxiety or worry about having panic attacks in panic disorder, negative evaluation in social anxiety disorder [social phobia], contamination or other obsessions in obsessive-compulsive disorder, separation from attachment figures in separation anxiety disorder, reminders of traumatic events in posttraumatic stress disorder, gaining weight in anorexia nervosa, physical complaints in somatic symptom disorder, perceived appearance flaws in body dysmorphic disorder, having a serious illness in illness anxiety disorder, or the content of delusional beliefs in schizophrenia or delusional disorder).

Researchers also found a significant increase in prevalence rates among participants in this study that suggest GAD affects more people each year around the globe than previously noted. Significant increases in the rates of comorbidity was found with more than 80 percent of people with lifetime GAD experiencing another lifetime disorder, most often major depressive disorder. Differences in the level of severity among those with GAD was found as well as a significant positive correlation found between high-income countries and GAD-related impairment. Those persons with GAD from high-income countries had significantly higher levels of impairment than those from middle- and low-income countries. Generalized anxiety disorder was also a more disabling disorder in some countries than others, with severe impairment reported by a small minority of persons with GAD in China (17.3 percent in Shenzhen, 21.8 percent in Beijing/Shanghai) and Mexico (28.7 percent) but by a large majority of those with GAD in the Netherlands (80.3 percent) and Romania (82.3 percent). These findings suggest that there are differences exist across the world in terms of GAD prevalence, course, and impairment. These differences may be associated with culture, but more research is needed (Ruscio et. al., 2017).

Theories of Generalized Anxiety Disorder

Much time has been devoted to understanding the roots of generalized anxiety disorder. While we do not have universal agreement, researchers have explored various emotional, cognitive, and biological dimensions of GAD. Each section below focuses on a set of factors that best explains the disorder. In reality, the best explanation is likely a combination of many of these factors.

Emotional and Cognitive Factors

People with GAD report experiencing more intense negative emotions, even compared to people with major depression (Aldao, Mennin, Linardatos, & Fresco, 2010), and are highly reactive to negative events (Tan et al., 2012). They report feeling that their emotions are not controllable or manageable (Newman, Llera, Erickson, Przeworski, & Castonguay, 2013). These emotional disturbances occur alongside cognitive disturbances. Cognitively, people with GAD make a number of maladaptive assumptions, such as "It's always best to expect the worst" and "I must anticipate and prepare myself at all times for any possible danger" (Beck & Emery, 1985; Ellis, 1997). Many of these assumptions reflect concerns about losing control or being unable to tolerate uncertainty. Their maladaptive assumptions lead people with GAD to respond to situations with automatic thoughts that stir up anxiety,

cause them to be hypervigilant, and lead them to overreact (S. Gautam, Jain, M. Gautam, Vahia, & A. Gautam, 2016). For example, when facing an exam, a person with GAD might reactively think, "I don't think I can do this," "I'll fall apart if I fail this test," and "I can't predict what will be on the test, so I have to stay up all night re-reading everything in the book in case it's on there."

Even the unconscious cognitions of people with GAD appear to focus on detecting possible threats in the environment (Mathews & MacLeod, 2005). In the Stroop color-naming task, participants are presented with words printed in color on a computer screen (Figure 5). Their role is to say what color the word is printed in. In general, people are slower in naming the color of words that have special significance to them (such as disease or failure for people with chronic anxiety) than in naming the color of nonsignificant words. Presumably, they are paying more attention to the content of those words than to the colors (Mathews & MacLeod, 2005).

Why do some people become hypervigilant for signs of threat? One theory is that they have experienced stressors or traumas that were uncontrollable and came without warning, particularly an interpersonal trauma such as a rejection or a loss. People who have had unpredictable and uncontrollable life experiences—such as an abusive parent—also may develop chronic anxiety (Newman et al., 2013). Other influences during childhood and adolescence may include negative parental behaviors, such as being overly controlling, demanding, protective, or rejecting.

What function does the characteristic worry of GAD serve? People with GAD say that worrying helps them avoid bad events by motivating them to engage in problem solving (Abasi et. al., 2018). Yet, they seldom get to the problem solving. Thomas Borkovec (Borkovec, Alcaine, & Behar, 2004), in his

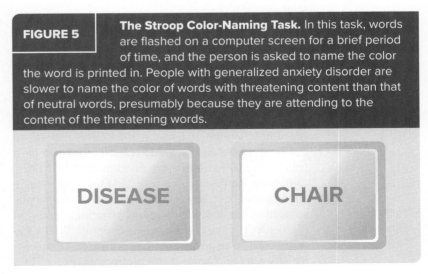

FIGURE 5 The Stroop Color-Naming Task. In this task, words are flashed on a computer screen for a brief period of time, and the person is asked to name the color the word is printed in. People with generalized anxiety disorder are slower to name the color of words with threatening content than that of neutral words, presumably because they are attending to the content of the threatening words.

DISEASE   CHAIR

People with GAD maintain a constant level of anxiety. This level of distress may explain why such people sometimes display maladaptive behavior, including hostility, which in turn may exacerbate the GAD symptoms. *Dmytro Zinkevych/Shutterstock*

cognitive avoidance model of GAD, argues that worrying actually triggers people with GAD to avoid awareness of internal and external threats and thus helps reduce their reactivity to unavoidable negative events. Michelle Newman and Sandra Llera (2011) extended the cognitive avoidance model to suggest that by worrying about possible threats, people with GAD maintain a constant level of anxiety that is more tolerable than leaving themselves open to sudden sharp increases in negative emotion. That is, they prefer a chronic but familiar state of distress to anticipating sudden shifts in response to specific negative events, so using worry in this way is reinforced. This constant state of distress and hypervigilance may also explain why people with GAD sometimes display maladaptive interpersonal behavior—such as appearing cold, intrusive, or even hostile—which can exacerbate interpersonal problems and GAD symptoms (Crouch, Lewis, Erickson, & Newman, 2017; Przeworski et al., 2011).

Biological Factors

We've already noted that people with GAD show heightened activity of their sympathetic nervous system and greater reactivity to emotional stimuli in the amygdala, a part of the brain's limbic system. This greater activity may be associated with abnormalities in the GABA neurotransmitter system, which plays an important role in many areas of the brain, including the limbic system (Charney, 2004; Hölzelab et. al, 2013). It is posited that GAD results, at least in part, from disrupted coordination of brain activity. In neuroimaging studies, people with GAD showed heightened reactivity to emotional stimuli in the amygdala, an area of the brain involved in processing emotion (Schienle, Hettema, Caceda, & Nemeroff, 2011). Recent research also suggests that decreased connectivity between the amygdala and prefrontal cortex (PFC)

is present among those with the diagnosis of GAD which can be seen across adolescence and adulthood (Patriquin & Mathew, 2017). Physiologically, they show chronically elevated activity of their sympathetic nervous systems and hyperreactivity to threatening stimuli (Brosschot, Van Dijk, & Thayer, 2007; Pieper, Brosschot, van der Leeden, & Thayer, 2010).

When GABA binds to a neuronal receptor, it prevents the neuron from firing. One theory is that people with generalized anxiety disorder have a deficiency of GABA or of GABA receptors, which results in excessive firing of neurons through many areas of the brain, particularly the limbic system. As a result of excessive and chronic neuronal activity, the person experiences chronic, diffuse symptoms of anxiety. Recent research also supports the idea that dysfunctional activity of GABA receptors in the motor cortex may play a key role in pathological anxiety (Cheng-Ta et al., 2017). Genetic studies suggest that GAD, as a specific disorder, has a modest heritability (Andrews et al., 2010). The more general trait of anxiety is much more clearly heritable and puts individuals at risk for GAD (Craske & Waters, 2005).

Treatments for Generalized Anxiety Disorder

Cognitive-Behavioral Treatments

Cognitive-behavioral treatments focus on helping people with GAD confront the issues they worry about most; challenge their negative, catastrophizing thoughts; and develop coping strategies. In the following profile, a cognitive-behavioral therapist helps Claire challenge her tendency to overestimate the probability that her son will be injured while playing football.

TREATING CLAIRE WITH CBT

Therapist: Claire, you wrote that you were afraid about your son playing in his football game. What specifically were you worried about?

Claire: That he'd get seriously hurt. His team was playing last year's state champions, so you know that those boys are big and strong.

Therapist: How specifically do you imagine your son getting hurt?

Claire: Getting a broken back or neck. Something that will result in paralysis or death. It happened to two NFL players this past year, remember?

Therapist: What happened to your son when he played in the game?

Claire: Nothing, really. He came home that afternoon with a sore thumb, but that went away after a while. He said he scored a touchdown and had an interception. I guess he played really well.

Therapist: So you had predicted that he would be injured during the game, but that didn't happen. When we're anxious, we tend to commit a common cognitive error, called "probability overestimation." In other words, we overestimate the likelihood of an unlikely event. While you were feeling anxious and worried, what was the probability in your mind that your son would be hurt, from 0 to 100 percent?

Claire: About 75 percent.

Therapist: And now what would you rate the probability of your son getting hurt in a future game?

Claire: Well, if you put it that way, I suppose around a 50 percent chance of him getting injured.

Therapist: So that means for every two times that your son plays football, he gets hurt once. Is that correct?

Claire: Umm, no. I don't think it's that high. Maybe about 30 percent.

Therapist: That would be one out of every three times that your son gets hurt. What evidence can you provide from your son's playing history to account for your belief that he'll get hurt one out of every three games?

Claire: Well, none. He had a sprained ankle during summer training, but that's it.

Therapist: So what you're saying is that you don't have very much evidence at all to prove that your son has a 30 percent chance of getting hurt in a game.

Claire: Gee, I never thought of it that way.

(Brown, T. A., O'Leary, T. A., & Barlow, D. H. [2001]. *Generalized Anxiety Disorder, Clinical Handbook of Psychological Disorders: A Step-By-Step Treatment Manual* [3rd ed.]. Guilford Press, 193–194. Copyright ©2001 Guilford Press. Reprinted with permission. Permission conveyed through Copyright Clearance Center)

Overall, CBT for GAD appears equally effective as benzodiazepine therapy in the short term, and superior to placebos or nondirective supportive therapy (Borkovec, Newman, & Castonguay, 2003; Borkovec & Ruscio, 2001; Siev & Chambless, 2007). In one follow-up study, its positive effects remained after 2 years (Borkovec, Newman, Pincus, & Lytle, 2002). CBT for

GAD also has effects on depression, which is important because GAD and depression often co-occur, and because anxiety can often precede the onset of depressive episodes (Cuijpers et al., 2014). This is a good example of how targeting common processes, like emotion dysregulation and negative thinking, can ameliorate symptoms of multiple disorders. A newer therapy, emotion regulation therapy (ERT), focuses on emotional awareness and regulation, and trials suggest it is efficacious in treating GAD with and without comorbid depression (Mennin, Fresco, O'Toole, & Heimberg, 2018).

Biological Treatments

The benzodiazepine drugs (such as Xanax, Librium, Valium, and Serax) provide short-term relief from anxiety symptoms (Gorman, 2003). However, their side effects and addictiveness preclude long-term use. Once people discontinue the drugs, their anxiety symptoms return (Davidson, 2001). Antidepressant medications, including SSRI and SNRI classes are an effective option for persons with GAD. Examples of antidepressants used to treat GAD include escitalopram (Lexapro), duloxetine (Cymbalta), venlafaxine (Effexor XR), and paroxetine (Paxil, Pexeva). Meta-analyses support these types of biological treatments for GAD and a combination of drug treatment and CBT may substantially improve quality of life in GAD patients (Bandelow, Michaelis, & Wedekind, 2017).

SOCIAL ANXIETY DISORDER

Most of us don't like to be embarrassed in front of others or rejected by other people. One of the most common social fears is public speaking (see Table 5). Nearly half of college students identify themselves as

TABLE 5   Lifetime Prevalence of Social Fears in a National Survey

Social Fear	Percentage of People Saying They Experienced the Fear in Their Lifetime (%)
Public speaking	30.2
Talking in front of a small group	15.2
Talking with others	13.7
Using a toilet away from home	6.6
Writing while someone watches	6.4
Eating or drinking in public	2.7
Any social fear	38.6

Source: Kessler, Stein, & Berglund, 1998, p. 614.

"shy" and say they get nervous meeting new people or encountering unfamiliar social situations (Heiser, Turner, & Beidel, 2003). Such concerns are normal but people with **social anxiety disorder** become so anxious in social situations and are so afraid of being rejected, judged, or humiliated in public that they are preoccupied with worries about such events to the point that their lives may become focused on avoiding social encounters (see the *DSM-5* criteria in Table 6). Socially anxious individuals are more likely to experience heightened fear, anxiety, and avoidance of social interactions and situations associated with potential social scrutiny. Symptoms of social anxiety disorder fall on a continuum that can range from mild to debilitating, causing significant impairment. Social anxiety disorder is among the most prevalent mental illnesses; contributes to the development of other psychiatric disorders, such as depression; and is challenging to treat (Hur et al., 2020; Ruscio, 2019). Research suggests that the development of close friendships and other kinds of social support reduce the risk of developing social anxiety symptoms in adolescence and early adulthood. Likewise, for those in treatment for social anxiety, higher levels of perceived social support are associated with a more favorable prognosis (Hur et al., 2020). Consider the inner pain Malcolm, in the case study, experiences and the way he has organized his life to avoid social situations.

TABLE 6   *DSM-5* Criteria for Social Anxiety Disorder

A. Marked fear or anxiety about one or more social situations in which the individual is exposed to possible scrutiny by others. Examples include social interactions (e.g., having a conversation, meeting unfamiliar people), being observed (e.g., eating or drinking), and performing in front of others (e.g., giving a speech).

B. The individual fears that he or she will act in a way or show anxiety symptoms that will be negatively evaluated (i.e., will be humiliating or embarrassing; will lead to rejection or offend others).

C. The social situations almost always provoke fear or anxiety.

D. The social situations are avoided or endured with intense fear or anxiety.

E. The fear or anxiety is out of proportion to the actual threat posed by the social situation and to the sociocultural context.

F. The fear, anxiety, or avoidance is persistent, typically lasting for 6 months or more.

G. The fear, anxiety, or avoidance causes clinically significant distress or impairment in social, occupational, or other important areas of functioning.

H. The fear, anxiety, or avoidance is not attributable to the physiological effects of a substance (e.g., a drug of abuse, a medication) or another medical condition.

I. The fear, anxiety, or avoidance is not better explained by the symptoms of another mental disorder, such as panic disorder, body dysmorphic disorder, or autism spectrum disorder.

J. If another medical condition (e.g., Parkinson's disease, obesity, disfigurement from burns or injury) is present, the fear, anxiety, or avoidance is clearly unrelated or is excessive.

Specify if:
Performance only: If the fear is restricted to speaking or performing in public.

CASE STUDY

Malcolm was a computer expert who worked for a large software firm. One of the things he hated most was to ride the elevator at his office when there were other people riding it. He felt that everyone was watching him, commenting silently on his rumpled clothes, and noticing every time he moved. He held his breath for almost the entire elevator ride, afraid that he might say something or make an embarrassing sound. Often, he walked up the eight flights of stairs to his office rather than risk that someone might get on the elevator with him.

Malcolm rarely went anywhere except to work and home. He hated even to go to the grocery store for fear that he would run his cart into someone or say something stupid to a clerk. He found a grocery store and several restaurants that took orders online for food to be delivered to customers' homes. He liked this service because he could avoid even talking to someone over the phone to place an order.

In the past, Malcolm's job had allowed him to remain quietly in his office all day, without interacting with other people. Recently, however, his company was reorganized and took on a number of projects. Malcolm's supervisor said that everyone in Malcolm's group needed to begin working together more closely to develop new products. Malcolm was supposed to make a presentation to his group about some software he was developing, but he called in sick the day of the presentation because he could not face the situation. Malcolm was thinking that he had to change jobs and perhaps go into private consulting, so he could work from his home and avoid having to work with anyone else.

In social situations, people with social anxiety disorder may tremble and perspire, feel confused and dizzy, have heart palpitations, and eventually have a full panic attack. Like Malcolm in the case study, they think others see their nervousness and judge them as inarticulate, weak, stupid, or crazy. Malcolm avoided speaking in public and having conversations with others for fear of being judged. People with social anxiety disorder may avoid eating or drinking in public, for fear that they will make noises when they eat, drop food, or otherwise embarrass themselves. They may avoid writing in public, afraid that others will see their hands tremble. Men with social anxiety disorder often avoid urinating in public bathrooms. The key characteristic of social anxiety disorder is that the feared situations are social in nature.

Social anxiety disorder is the most common anxiety disorder and the third most common mental health problem with a lifetime prevalence of about 12 percent in the United States (Kessler et al., 2005; Yli-Länttä, 2020) and 1 to 7 percent internationally (Stein et al., 2017). Multiple studies show that women are somewhat more likely than men to develop this disorder (Asher, Asnaani, & Aderka, 2017; Xu et al., 2012). Women with social anxiety disorder tend to have more severe social fears than men, particularly with regard to performance situations (such as giving a presentation), but men seek treatment more often, possibly because their fears often include dating situations (Asher et al., 2017).

Social anxiety disorder tends to develop in either the early preschool years or adolescence. This is when many people become self-conscious and concerned about others' opinions of them (Blöte, Miers, Heyne, & Westenberg, 2015; Bögels et al., 2010). Over 90 percent of adults with social anxiety disorder report humiliating experiences earlier in their lives that contributed to their symptoms, such as extreme teasing as a child (McCabe, Antony, Summerfeldt, Liss, & Swinson, 2003). Others report feeling uncomfortable in social situations as far back as they can remember. Social anxiety disorder often co-occurs with mood disorders and other anxiety disorders. Once it develops, social anxiety disorder tends to be chronic if left untreated, and most people do not seek treatment (Kessler, 2003).

In Japan, the term *taijinkyofu-sho* describes an intense fear of interpersonal relations. Taijinkyofu-sho is characterized by shame about and persistent fear of causing others offense, embarrassment, or even harm through one's personal inadequacies. It is most frequently encountered, at least in treatment settings, among young men. People with this disorder may fear blushing, emitting body odor, displaying unsightly body parts, speaking their thoughts aloud, or irritating others (see Lewis-Fernandez et al., 2010). This concern is in line with the emphasis in Japan on deference to others (Kirmayer, 2001).

Theories of Social Anxiety Disorder

Social anxiety, or more generally shyness, runs in families, and twin studies suggest it has a genetic basis (Scaini, Belotti, & Ogliari, 2014). Genetic factors appear to lead, not specifically to anxiety about social situations, however, but instead to a more general tendency toward the anxiety disorders (Shimada-Sugimoto, Otowa, & Hettema, 2015), possibly via their role in the brain areas of the amygdala, hippocampus, and prefrontal cortex (Bas-Hoogendam et al., 2016).

Cognitive perspectives on social anxiety disorder have dominated psychological theories (Heimberg, Brozovich, & Rapee, 2010; Morrison & Heimberg, 2013). According to these perspectives, people with social anxiety disorder have excessively high standards for their social performance—for example, they believe they should be liked by everyone. They also focus on negative aspects of social interactions and evaluate their own behavior harshly. They tend to notice potentially threatening social cues (such as a grimace on the face of the person they are speaking to), misinterpret them in self-defeating ways, and overvalue social evaluation (Wong & Rapee, 2016). They are exquisitely attuned to their self-presentation and their internal feelings and tend to assume that, if they feel anxious, it is because the social interaction is not going well (Clark & Wells, 1995). They engage in a number of "safety behaviors" to reduce their anxiety. For example, they may avoid eye contact, or social interactions altogether; excessively rehearse what they will say in an interaction; and fail to self-disclose, thereby reducing the quality of the social interaction and the impression they actually leave with others (Morrison & Heimberg, 2013). After a social interaction, they ruminate excessively about their performance and the other person's reactions.

The popular singer-songwriter Sia, who often hides her face in public performances, has described paralyzing social anxiety that led to depression, substance abuse, and thoughts of suicide before she developed coping strategies.
Frederick M. Brown/Getty Images

What creates these behavioral habits and cognitive biases? Adults with social anxiety disorder often describe their parents as having been overprotective and controlling but also critical and negative (Bögels et al., 2010). Such retrospective accounts could be incorrect. Some prospective and experimental studies support the notion that such family environments, and parents' modeling of socially anxious behavior, can lead to the development of social anxiety disorder, especially for children temperamentally prone to shyness (Spence & Rapee, 2016; Wong & Rapee, 2016).

Treatments for Social Anxiety Disorder

SSRIs and SNRIs have been shown to be efficacious in reducing symptoms of social anxiety (see meta-analysis by Mayo-Wilson et al., 2014). Symptoms tend to return when individuals stop taking these medications, however.

Cognitive-behavioral therapy (CBT) seems particularly useful for treating social anxiety (Mayo-Wilson et al., 2014; Morrison & Heimberg, 2013). The behavioral component of this therapy involves exposing clients to social situations that make them anxious, starting with the least anxiety-producing situations and working up to the more anxiety-producing situations. Therapists may role-play situations with clients (e.g., having a conversation with a store clerk), accompany clients in social situations to coach them as they engage in social encounters, and assign clients homework to carry out "experiments" in which they attempt a social interaction they believe they can't tolerate. They may teach them relaxation techniques to quell their anxiety in these situations or skills that can help them interact more effectively with others, for example, in starting conversations. They also help them recognize and eliminate their safety behaviors (e.g., avoiding eye contact). The cognitive component of therapy involves identifying negative cognitions clients have about themselves and about social situations and teaching them how to dispute these cognitions. CBT for social anxiety can be administered in a group setting in which group members form an audience for one another, providing exposure to the very situation each member fears. Individuals can practice their feared behaviors in front of the others while the therapist coaches them in the use of relaxation techniques to calm their anxiety. The group can also help the individual challenge any negative, catastrophizing thoughts about their behavior, as in the following excerpt from a group cognitive therapy session with Gina.

PROFILES

Therapist: So your automatic thought is, "I don't know how to have a conversation," is that right?

Gina: Yeah, I always screw it up.

Therapist: All right, let's ask the rest of the group what they think about that. Who has had a conversation with Gina or noticed her talking with someone else?

Ed: We walked out to our cars together last week and talked in the parking lot for a while. [Several other group members mention similar conversations.]

Therapist: So it sounds like you have had a number of conversations with the rest of the group.

Gina: I guess so.

Therapist: Group, how did she do? How did the conversations go?

Sally: It was fine. She was asking me about my car, because she has been looking for a new one, so we talked mostly about that. [Other group members provide similar answers.]

Therapist: Well, Gina, the rest of the group doesn't seem to agree that you don't know how to have conversations.

Gina: I guess I've always been so nervous that I never stopped to think that sometimes the conversations go OK.

(Source: Adapted from Turk, Heimberg, & Hope, 2001, pp. 124–125)

A number of meta-analyses have found that CBT is an effective treatment for social anxiety disorder, is just as effective as antidepressants in reducing symptoms over the course of therapy, and is much more effective in preventing relapse following therapy (see; Mayo-Wilson et al., 2014; Morrison & Heimberg, 2013). Mindfulness-based interventions also can prove helpful for people with social anxiety disorder (Goldin & Gross, 2010). These interventions teach individuals to be less judgmental about their own thoughts and reactions and more focused on, and relaxed in, the present moment. Therapies such as acceptance and commitment therapy (ACT)—which builds on CBT techniques to emphasize mindfulness, acceptance, and values—are similar to CBT in effectiveness for social anxiety disorder (Craske et al., 2014).

A variety of effective smartphone apps are now being used to deliver treatment for social anxiety disorder. Postmodern Studio/ Alamy Stock Photo

In addition to individual therapy for social anxiety disorder, cognitive-behavioral therapies delivered in a group format have also been shown to be about equally effective (Mayo-Wilson et al., 2014; Wersebe, Sijbrandij, & Cuijpers, 2013). As you might imagine, group settings allow a natural way to engage patients in social situations, increasing exposure while also building social skills (Herbert et al., 2005), though for some clients, individual therapy is preferred. New treatments that use virtual reality technology to present a "social" scenario in individual treatment appear to have some effectiveness as well (Anderson et al., 2013), but research in this area is in its earlier stages.

The use of internet-based cognitive–behavioral treatments (ICBT) have shown promise for various psychological disorders, including social anxiety disorder. Most of these treatments have been delivered on computers, but more recently the use of social anxiety apps are being explored. Research on the use of smartphone-based interventions suggest these are a useful and effective alternative method for delivering treatment to those with social anxiety disorder. Considering the significant amount of smartphone use, 77 percent of U.S. adults, and 94 percent of U.S. adults aged 18 to 29, this form of treatment may be better utilized as people are more likely to integrate treatment program into their daily routines. The use of smartphone apps to treat this disorder have the potential to overcome barriers to accessing services as many people with social anxiety disorder may be unable or unwilling to use traditional treatment delivery methods (Dagoo et al., 2016; Ruscio, 2019; Stolz et al., 2018).

SPECIFIC PHOBIAS AND AGORAPHOBIA

People can develop irrational fears of many objects and situations. The *DSM-5* divides phobias into *specific phobias,* which focus on particular objects or animals (e.g., snakes) or places (e.g., heights), and *agoraphobia,* which is a generalized fear of situations in which the person might not be able to escape or get help if needed.

Specific Phobias

We all have things we fear and that we may even go out of our way to avoid. Things that make your skin crawl at the mere thought, like those creepy-long-legged things that come out in the dark! Or, perhaps it's the thought of encountering clowns, small spaces . . . or small spaces with clowns! That is extra scary. It's very common for people to relate their own personal fears to this disorder, but it is extremely important to remember that phobias are psychological disorders that should not be confused with "normal" fears.

Specific phobias are unreasonable or irrational fears of specific objects or situations (LeBeau et al., 2010). The *DSM-5* groups specific phobias into five categories: *animal type, natural environment type, situational type, blood-injection-injury type,* and *other* (Table 7). The key symptoms of specific phobia include a marked fear or anxiety about a specific object or situation that is disproportionate to the actual danger. The diagnostic criteria also include the individual actively avoiding the object or situation, or enduring it with intense fear or anxiety. These symptoms have to last for at least 6 months, cause clinical distress or impairment, and cannot be better attributed to another mental or physical disorder (American Psychiatric Association, 2013). When people with these phobias encounter their feared object or situation, their anxiety is immediate and intense, sometimes producing a panic attack. They also become anxious over the possibility of encountering the object or situation and will go to great lengths to avoid it.

Most phobias develop during childhood but will persist across the lifespan if untreated. Adults with phobias recognize that their anxieties are unreasonable, although children may not. In the course of a given year, phobias affect about 8 percent of the U.S. population but, as many as 13 percent, will have a specific phobia at some time in their lives, making phobias one of the most common psychological disorders (Kessler et al., 2005). According to recent epidemiological studies, the median lifetime prevalence for specific phobias worldwide is 7.2 percent with differences noted among various nations such as, 1.5 percent in Florence, Italy, 2.6 percent in China to 14·4 percent in Oslo, Norway. Although some of this variation is likely to be due to the use of different assessment procedures, these studies indicate that the lifetime prevalence of specific phobias around the world ranges from 3 to 15 percent, with fears and phobias concerning heights and animals being the most common. Rather than treating their phobia, most

TABLE 7 *DSM-5* Criteria for Specific Phobia

A. Marked fear or anxiety about a specific object or situation (e.g., flying, heights, animals, receiving an injection, seeing blood).

B. The phobic object or situation almost always provokes immediate fear or anxiety.

C. The phobic object or situation is actively avoided or endured with intense fear or anxiety.

D. The fear or anxiety is out of proportion to the actual danger posed by the specific object or situation and to the sociocultural context.

E. The fear, anxiety, or avoidance is persistent, typically lasting 6 months or more.

F. The fear, anxiety, or avoidance causes clinically significant distress or impairment in social, occupational, or other important areas of functioning.

G. The disturbance is not better explained by the symptoms of another mental disorder, including fear, anxiety, and avoidance of situations associated with panic-like symptoms or other incapacitating symptoms (as in agoraphobia); objects or situations related to obsessions (as in obsessive-compulsive disorder); reminders of traumatic events (as in PTSD); separation from home or attachment figures (as in separation anxiety disorder); or social situations (as in social anxiety disorder).

Specify if:

Code based on the phobic stimulus:

300.29 (F40.218) Animal (e.g., spiders, insects, dogs).
300.29 (F40.228) Natural environment (e.g., heights, storms, water).
300.29 (F40.23x) Blood-injection-injury (e.g., needles, invasive medical procedures).

> **Coding note:** Select specific *ICD-10-CM* code as follows: **F40.230** fear of blood; **F40.231** fear of injections and transfusions; **F40.232** fear of other medical care; or **F40.233** fear of injury.

300.29 (F40.248) Situational (e.g., airplanes, elevators, enclosed places).
300.29 (F40.298) Other (e.g., situations that may lead to choking or vomiting; in children, e.g., loud sounds or costumed characters).

Coding note: When more than one phobic stimulus is present, code all *ICD-10-CM* codes that apply (e.g., for fear of snakes and flying, F40.218 specific phobia, animal, and F40.248 specific phobia, situational).

adapt their lives to avoid coming into contact with the item or event so only the most severe cases tend to seek treatment (Eaton, Bienvenu & Miloyan, 2018).

Animal-type phobias focus on specific animals or insects, such as dogs, cats, snakes, or spiders. Snakes and spiders are the most common objects of animal phobias, probably because it has been adaptive over evolutionary history to fear these dangerous objects (Jacobi et al., 2004). While most people who come across a feared animal or insect will startle and move away quickly, they would not be diagnosed with a phobia because they do not live in terror of encountering a snake or spider or organize their lives around avoiding them.

Natural environment type phobias, which are also extremely common (LeBeau et al., 2010), focus on events or situations in the natural environment, such as storms, heights, or water. Mild to moderate fears of these natural events or situations are extremely common and are adaptive in that they help us avoid danger. A diagnosis of phobia is warranted only when people reorganize their lives to avoid the feared situations or have severe anxiety attacks when confronted with them.

Situational type phobias usually involve fear of public transportation, tunnels, bridges, elevators, flying, or driving. Claustrophobia, or fear of enclosed spaces, is a common situational phobia. One prominent person with a situational phobia is John Madden, the former coach and sports announcer. Madden is so afraid of flying that he travels over 60,000 miles a year on his personal bus to get to sports events around the United States.

Former Super Bowl–winning coach and sports television commentator John Madden. His fear of flying leads him to travel to sports events by luxury RV coach. *G. Paul Burnett/AP Photo*

Blood-injection-injury type phobias are diagnosed in people who fear seeing blood or an injury. Whereas people with another type of specific phobia typically experience increases in heart rate, blood pressure, and other fight-or-flight responses when confronted with their feared object or situation, people with blood-injection-injury type phobia experience significant drops in heart rate and blood pressure and are likely to faint. This type of phobia runs more strongly in families than do the other types (LeBeau et al., 2010).

Agoraphobia

The term *agoraphobia* comes from the Greek for "fear of the marketplace." People with **agoraphobia** fear places where they might have trouble escaping or getting help if they become anxious. This often includes public transportation (being on a bus, train, plane, or boat), open spaces (such as a parking lot), being in shops or theaters, being in crowded places, or being alone anywhere outside their home. People with agoraphobia also often fear that they will embarrass themselves if others notice their symptoms or their efforts to escape during an attack. Actually, other people can rarely tell when a person is anxious (Craske & Barlow, 2014).

About 50 percent of people with agoraphobia have a history of panic attacks (described below) that preceded the development of the agoraphobia (Wittchen, Gloster, Beesdo-Baum, Fava, & Craske, 2010). The remaining people with agoraphobia typically have a history of another anxiety disorder, a somatic symptoms disorder (see the chapter "Somatic Symptom and Dissociative Disorders"), or depression (Wittchen et al., 2010). Agoraphobia most often begins when people are in their early twenties and is more common in women than in men.

People with agoraphobia often reach the point where they will not leave their homes alone. Sometimes, they are able to venture out with a close family member who makes them feel safe. However, family and friends may not be willing to chaperone them everywhere they go. When people with agoraphobia force themselves to enter situations that frighten them, they experience persistent and intense anxiety, causing many to retreat to their homes. Some turn to alcohol or another substance to dampen their anxiety symptoms (Wittchen et al., 2010).

Theories of Phobias

Behavioral Theories

The behavioral theories have been very successful in explaining the development of phobias. According to Mowrer's (1939) two-factor theory, classical conditioning leads to the fear of the phobic object, and operant conditioning helps maintain it. As discussed in the chapter "Theories and Treatment of Abnormality," in

Little Albert, shown in this photo, developed a fear of white rats through classical conditioning. *Prof. Ben Harris*

classical conditioning a previously neutral object (the conditioned stimulus) is paired with an object that naturally elicits a reaction (an unconditioned stimulus [US] that elicits an unconditioned response [UR]) until the previously neutral object elicits the same reaction (now called the conditioned response [CR]). When a tone is paired with an electric shock, the conditioned stimulus is the tone, the US is the electric shock, the UR is anxiety in response to the shock, and the CR is anxiety in response to the tone.

The first application of these theories to phobias came in a series of studies done almost 100 years ago by John Watson and Rosalie Raynor (1920). Watson and Raynor placed a white rat in front of an 11-month-old boy named Little Albert. As Little Albert reached for the white rat, they banged a metal bar loudly just above his head. Naturally, Little Albert was startled and began to cry. After several more pairings of the white rat with the loud noise from the metal bar, Little Albert would have nothing to do with the rat. When presented with it, he retreated and showed distress. Little Albert's fear also generalized to other white furry animals—he would not approach white rabbits either.

Although by today's standards this experiment would raise serious ethical questions, it showed the creation of a phobia through classical UR was Little Albert's startle response to the noise. The CS was the white rat, and the CR was the startle-and-fear response to the white rat (Figure 6). If Little Albert had later been presented with the white rat several times without the noise, his fear of white rats should have been extinguished.

Most people who develop a phobia, however, try to avoid being exposed to their feared object, thus avoiding what could extinguish the phobia. If they are suddenly confronted with their feared object, they experience extreme anxiety and run away as quickly as possible. Running away reduces their anxiety; thus, their avoidance of the feared object is reinforced by the

FIGURE 6

The Behavioral Account of Little Albert's Phobia. The pairing of the banged bar (the US), which naturally leads to a startle response (the UR), and the white rat (the CS) eventually leads to the white rat producing the same startle response (now referred to as the CR).

reduction of their anxiety—an operant conditioning process known as **negative reinforcement** (Mowrer, 1939). Thereafter, they avoid the feared object. Some theorists argue that phobias can develop through observational learning as well as through direct classical conditioning (see Mineka & Zinbarg, 2006). For example, small children may learn to fear snakes if their parents show severe fright when they see a snake (Bandura, 1969; Mineka, Davidson, Cook, & Keir, 1984).

An extension of the behavioral theory of phobias may answer the question of why humans develop phobias of some objects or situations and not others (deSilva, Rachman, & Seligman, 1977; Mineka, 1985; Seligman, 1970). Phobias of spiders, snakes, and heights are common, but phobias of flowers are not. Many phobic objects appear to be things whose avoidance, over evolutionary history, has been advantageous for humans. Our distant ancestors had many nasty encounters with insects, snakes, heights, loud noises, and strangers. Those who quickly learned to fear and avoid these objects or events were more likely to survive and bear offspring. Thus, evolution may have selected for the rapid conditioning of fear to certain objects or situations. Although these are less likely to cause us harm today, we carry the vestiges of our evolutionary history and are biologically prepared to learn certain associations quickly. This theory is known as **prepared classical conditioning** (Seligman, 1970). Many objects more likely to cause us harm in today's world (such as guns and knives) have not been around long enough, evolutionarily speaking, to be selected for rapid conditioning, so phobias of them should be relatively difficult to create.

To test this idea, researchers presented subjects with pictures of objects that theoretically should be evolutionarily selected for conditioning (snakes and spiders) and objects that should not be so selected (houses, faces, and flowers). They paired the presentation of these pictures with short but painful electric shocks. The subjects developed anxiety reactions to the pictures of snakes and spiders within one or two pairings with shock, but it took four or five pairings of the pictures of houses, faces, or flowers with shock to create a fear reaction. Extinguishing the subjects' anxiety reactions to houses or faces was relatively easy once the pictures were no longer paired with shock, but the anxiety reactions to spiders and snakes were difficult to extinguish (Hugdahl & Ohman, 1977; Ohman, Fredrikson, Hugdahl, & Rimmo, 1976; Ohman & Mineka, 2001).

The behavioral theory seems to provide a compelling explanation for phobias, particularly when we add the principles of observational learning and prepared classical conditioning. It has also led to effective therapies. Its most significant problem is that many people with phobias can identify no traumatic event in their own lives or the lives of people they are close to that triggered their phobias. Without conditioned stimuli, it is hard to argue that they developed their phobias through classical conditioning or observational learning. Some individuals who develop phobias may have a chronic low-level anxiety or reactivity, which makes them more susceptible to the development of phobias given even mildly aversive experiences (Craske & Waters, 2005).

Biological Theories

The first-degree relatives (that is, parents, children, and siblings) of people with phobias are three to four times more likely to have a phobia than the first-degree relatives of people without phobias. Twin studies suggest that this is due, at least in part, to genetics (Hettema, Neale, & Kendler, 2001; Merikangas, Lieb, Wittchen, & Avenevoli, 2003). Some studies suggest that situational and animal phobias are associated with similar genes, while other studies suggest a general tendency toward phobias that is not isolated to one type of phobia (LeBeau et al., 2010).

Treatments for Phobias

A number of behavioral techniques can treat phobias. Some therapists include cognitive techniques and medications.

Behavioral Treatments

Behavioral therapies for phobias use exposure to extinguish the person's fear of the object or situation. These therapies cure the majority of phobias (Hopko, Robertson, Widman, & Lejuez, 2008). Some studies suggest that just one, intensive session of behavior therapy can lead to major reductions in phobic behaviors and anxiety (Ollendick & Davis, 2013). Three basic components of behavior therapy for phobias are systematic desensitization, modeling, and flooding.

As we have already discussed, in systematic desensitization clients formulate lists of situations or objects they fear, ranked from most to least feared. They learn relaxation techniques and begin to expose themselves to the items on their "hierarchy of fears," beginning with the least feared. A person with a severe dog phobia who has "seeing a picture of a dog in a magazine" first on her list might look at a picture of a dog. The therapist will coach her to use relaxation techniques to replace her anxiety with a calm reaction. When she can look at a picture of a dog without experiencing anxiety, she might move on to looking at a dog in a pet store window, again using relaxation techniques to lower her anxiety reaction and replace it with calm. Gradually, the client and therapist will move through the entire list, "relearning" that dogs can lead to neutral or positive consequences, until the client is able to pet a big dog without feeling overwhelming anxiety (Craske, Treanor, Conway, Zbozinek, & Vervliet, 2014).

Blood-injection-injury phobia requires a different approach, because people with this phobia experience severe decreases in heart rate and blood pressure (Öst & Sterner, 1987). Thus, therapists teach them to tense the muscles in their arms, legs, and chest until they feel the warmth of their blood rising in their faces. This **applied tension technique** increases blood pressure and heart rate and can keep people with this type of phobia from fainting when confronted with the feared object. Then systematic desensitization can help extinguish fear of blood, injury, or injections.

Modeling techniques are often adopted in conjunction with systematic desensitization. A therapist treating a person with a snake phobia may model each behavior on the client's hierarchy of fears before asking the client to perform it. The therapist will stand in the room with the snake before asking the client to do so, touch the snake before asking the client to do so, and hold the snake before the client does. Through observational learning, the client associates these behaviors with a calm response in the therapist, which reduces anxiety about engaging in the behaviors. Modeling is as effective as systematic desensitization in reducing phobias (Bandura, 1969). Various recent studies support that reinforced practice and modeling show the greatest degree of empirical support for their efficacy in reducing fearful or phobic reactions to stimuli (Lyndon, Healy, O'Callaghan, Mulhern, & Holloway, 2015).

The therapist shows dead spiders behind glass to this woman as a first step in desensitizing her fear. Next, she will touch pictures of spiders and hold a stuffed toy spider to further the process of desensitization. Eventually, she will hold a live spider without a problematic level of fear. *(All): Zapf/ullstein bild/Getty Images*

Flooding intensively exposes a client to his or her feared object until anxiety is extinguished. In a flooding treatment, a person with claustrophobia might lock themselves in a closet for several hours, and a person with a dog phobia might spend the night in a dog kennel. The therapist typically will prepare clients with relaxation techniques they can use to reduce their fear. Flooding is as effective as systematic desensitization or modeling and often works more quickly. However, it is more difficult to get clients to agree to this type of therapy, because it is frightening to contemplate.

Biological Treatments

Some people use the benzodiazepines to reduce their anxiety when forced to confront their phobic objects; for example, they use Valium before flying or giving a presentation. These drugs produce temporary relief, but the phobia remains (Jefferson, 2001). In fact, this temporary relief provided by benzodiazepines—along with the risk of withdrawal symptoms when they wear off—can lead to benzodiazepine addiction, creating more problems than it solves. In contrast, behavioral techniques can cure most phobias in a few hours (Davis, Ollendick, & Öst, 2009). It is also important to note that although behavioral treatments are quite effective, relapse is not uncommon. Researchers are working to better understand how the extinction of irrational fears can be maintained over the long term (Vervliet, Craske, & Hermans, 2013). For now, it appears that the age-old advice to "confront your fears" through behavior therapy is the best strategy.

OBSESSIVE-COMPULSIVE DISORDER

Authors of the *DSM-5* created a new diagnostic category by grouping several disorders together that share common features, such as obsessive preoccupation and repetitive behaviors, since these disorders share enough similarities to put them in the same diagnostic category but enough differences to identify each as distinctive disorders. Obsessive-compulsive and related disorders (OCRDs) all have an obsessive-compulsive component that connect each disorder in this group. These disorders include obsessive-compulsive disorder (OCD), hoarding disorder, body dysmorphic disorder (BDD), trichotillomania (hair-pulling disorder), and excoriation (skin picking) disorder. These disorders are linked by repetitive behaviors and impaired behavioral inhibition, age of onset and comorbidities, brain circuitry and neurotransmitter abnormalities and responses to treatment. However, the removal of OCD from the anxiety disorder category is not without controversy (Abramowitz & Jacoby, 2015; Hirschtritt, Bloch, & Mathews, 2017).

Obsessive-Compulsive Disorder is one of the most well known psychological disorders in the *DSM-5*, in part due to portrayals of the disorder in movies and TV, but also due to the prevalence of the disorder among people. There are many misconceptions surrounding this disorder that we will clarify in this section, but its name provides a helpful start to this discussion.

OCD (see Table 8) is diagnosed when either obsessions, compulsions, or both are present to a significant degree. **Obsessions** are thoughts, images, ideas, or urges (e.g., to harm oneself) that are persistent, repetitive, intrusive, unwanted, and that usually cause significant anxiety or distress. Obsessions can take many forms and create ritualistic behaviors. Recent suggests that most common obsessions center around several themes. Germs, cleaning, contamination, and illness (*What if the public toilet I used had the COVID virus on it?*); responsibility for causing or failing to prevent harm or bad luck (*What if I hit a pedestrian with my car by mistake?*); forbidden thoughts: aggressive, sexual, and religious (*recurrent pornographic images or worries that they have inadvertently offended God*) and symmetry and order (*The feeling that books have to be arranged "just right" on the shelf*). Most people with OCD display multiple types of obsessions that evoke distress and the development of compulsions created to neutralize these feelings. Although thoughts of this kind occur to most people occasionally, these are thoughts that most of us can dismiss or ignore, but unfortunately, people with OCD cannot (Abramowitz & Jacoby, 2015; Boileau, 2011).

Compulsions are repetitive behaviors or mental acts that an individual feels he or she must perform in an effort to reduce anxiety and distress. People with OCD often create rituals that are deliberate, purposeful, and goal directed, but despite the appearance of organization, these behaviors and/or actions are nonsensical and disproportionate to the obsession they are trying to neutralize. Compulsive rituals can be both covert (mental) and/or overt (behavioral) and tie directly to the obsessive thought, feeling, or urge that increased their distress. Common overt compulsions involve excessive decontamination (e.g., cleaning, washing), counting, repeating routine actions (e.g., flipping the light switch on and off repeatedly before entering a room until an obsession is dismissed), checking/rechecking (e.g., windows, appliances), and repeatedly asking people for reassurance. Mental compulsions may include internally repeating "good" numbers or phrases, or counting the number of e's in every sentence to minimize obsessional thoughts or to reassure oneself (Abramowitz & Jacoby, 2015). Since people with OCD cannot resist the urge to perform compulsions, it is not uncommon for individuals to spend large

Extraordinary People

David Beckham

Photo Works/Shutterstock

Celebrity soccer player, David Beckham, is best known for his extraordinary athletic ability and his marriage to former Spice Girl, Victoria Beckham. This superstar has a life that most would envy, but entwined throughout his exceptional career is the diagnosis of OCD. David Beckham has spoken about his struggles with OCD and his need for order, symmetry, and perfection and how it impacts his life on a daily basis. Wife, Victoria Beckham discusses his need for symmetry and order that can be seen throughout their home ". . . everything has to match. We've got three fridges—food in one, salad in another, and drinks in the third . . . coordinated down either side . . . everything is symmetrical. If there's three cans he'll throw away one because it has to be an even number." Beckham has traveled around the world, playing for top teams including Real Madrid, Manchester United, Los Angeles Galaxy, and AC Milan. Each time he enters a new hotel room, he has to rearrange everything. "I'll go into a hotel room. Before I can relax, I have to move all the leaflets and all the books and put them in a draw. Everything has to be perfect." His teammates on Manchester United knew of his obsessions and compulsiveness and would deliberately rearrange his clothes or move the furniture around his hotel room to infuriate him. When asked if he wanted to stop his obsessive behavior, he said: "I would like to . . . I've tried and can't stop" (Frith, 2009).

TABLE 8   *DSM-5* Criteria for Obsessive-Compulsive Disorder

A. Presence of obsessions, compulsions, or both:

Obsessions are defined by (1) and (2):

1. Recurrent and persistent thoughts, urges, or images that are experienced, at some time during the disturbance, as intrusive and unwanted, and that in most individuals cause marked anxiety or distress.

2. The individual attempts to ignore or suppress such thoughts, urges, or images, or to neutralize them with some other thoughts or actions (i.e., by performing a compulsion).

Compulsions are defined by (1) and (2):

1. Repetitive behaviors (e.g., hand washing, ordering, checking) or mental acts (e.g., praying, counting, repeating words silently) that the individual feels driven to perform in response to an obsession or according to rules that must be applied rigidly.

2. The behaviors or mental acts are aimed at preventing or reducing anxiety or distress, or preventing some dreaded event or situation; however, these behaviors or mental acts are not connected in a realistic way with what they are designed to neutralize or prevent, or are clearly excessive.

B. The obsessions or compulsions are time consuming (e.g., take more than 1 hour per day) or cause clinically significant distress or impairment in social, occupational, or other important areas of functioning.

C. The obsessive-compulsive symptoms are not attributable to the physiological effects of a substance (e.g., a drug of abuse, a medication) or another medical condition.

D. The disturbance is not better explained by the symptoms of another mental disorder (e.g., excessive worries, as in generalized anxiety disorder; preoccupation with appearance, as in body dysmorphic disorder; difficulty discarding or parting with possessions, as in hoarding disorder; hair pulling, as in trichotillomania [hair-pulling disorder]; skin picking, as in excoriation [skin-picking] disorder; stereotypies, as in stereotypic movement disorder; ritualized eating behavior, as in eating disorders; preoccupation with substances or gambling, as in substance-related and addictive disorders; preoccupation with having an illness, as in illness anxiety disorder; sexual urges or fantasies, as in paraphilic disorders; impulses, as in disruptive, impulse-control, and conduct disorders; guilty ruminations, as in major depressive disorder; thought insertion or delusional preoccupations, as in schizophrenia spectrum and other psychotic disorders; or repetitive patterns of behavior, as in autism spectrum disorder).

periods of their day performing these rituals. These activities are time consuming and tend to dominate their daily life, often getting in the way of other things like work or social relationships.

The obsessions and compulsions of some people with OCD, like David Beckham's obsession with orderliness described in the Extraordinary People feature can seem simply quirky. Other patterns of obsessions and compulsions can appear much stranger, or even bizarre, as illustrated by the profile of a young man named Carl who has OCD. The difference between an obsession and a compulsion often confuses students. Obsessions are the thoughts that fuel anxiety and the need to perform compulsive acts, whereas the compulsion is created to reduce the anxiety they feel. Review the case of Carl and take note of his compulsions.

CARL'S COMPULSIONS

22-year-old Carl had struggled with symptoms of OCD since his early adolescence but over the last 2 years his compulsive behaviors had become so time consuming and debilitating that he was unable to leave his room. Since Carl left his bedroom infrequently, he began defecating on paper towels and urinating in paper cups in his bedroom that he would store in the corner of his closet. He also felt compelled to save anything from his body such as fingernail clippings, eyelashes, and skin scrapings. Carl often felt the need to save saliva that he would spit into various containers stored within his room.

Carl's eating habits deteriorated from eating with his family, to eating in a separate room, to now only eating alone in his room. In the last 2 months, Carl had lost 25 pounds and would only eat late at night, when others were asleep to avoid possible contamination. Carl could not resist the urge to count each item of food, such as corn, peas, or rice which had to be in certain quantities that would often fluctuate each day. This counting and recounting behavior was needed to ensure the correct number of food items were present so he could eat. Carl would also limit food options to those that started with letters that coincided with certain "good" numbers. Even numbers were usually considered "good" or "safe" and therefore dictated his food selections. For example, the tenth letter of the alphabet is J which means Carl could only eat foods that started with a J, like Jello, jalapeno, or jelly. Carl also avoided several types of foods that he believed are contaminated or poisonous, like beef, avocados, fish, and chicken.

The worsening of Carl's compulsions led to problems with grooming, hygiene, and his ability to care for himself. When asked about these behaviors Carl would express his frustration and distress, "I know it's crazy, but I still feel like I have to do all these things or else something bad will happen. I'll get contaminated or someone in my family will die. I would give anything for this to stop."

OCD is characterized by irrational beliefs, but ironically, individuals with OCD vary in terms of their insight into these obsessions and compulsions. Some people can acknowledge the irrationality of their obsessive thoughts compulsive behaviors, whereas others are firmly convinced that these behaviors are completely rational. An individual's degree of insight may change over time and can vary among their different obsessions. For example, a woman might recognize her obsessive thoughts about bad luck from uneven numbers as senseless and yet have poor insight into the irrationality of her contamination obsessions (Abramowitz & Jacoby, 2015; Robbins, Vaghi, & Banca, 2019). Often, the link between the obsession and the compulsion is the result of magical thinking. Many people with OCD believe that repeating a behavior a certain number of times will ward off danger to themselves or others. Their rituals often become stereotyped and rigid, and they develop obsessions and compulsions about not performing them correctly. An individual might feel compelled to read a passage in a book 25 times perfectly, fearing that something bad will happen to his family if he does not.

Carl's thoughts and behaviors might seem out of touch with reality. However, an important part of OCD is that people with OCD usually know that their thoughts and behaviors are irrational. They simply cannot control them.

"Did I lock the door? Is the iron turned off? Oh no, I think I left stove on! I have to go back and check." We all have moments when we are not sure if we missed something, like forgetting to turn off the stove or curling iron. That moment creates some distress, which dissipates when we recheck that item . . . and then we tend to move on to other things. Unfortunately, for people with OCD, this checking does not happen only from time-to-time and confirming the door is locked does not provide much relief. "Checking" compulsions, which are extremely common, are tied to obsessional doubts, as illustrated in the following profile. The man's compulsive checking makes some sense, given what he is thinking. However, what he is thinking—that he hit someone on the road without knowing it—is highly improbable. The compulsive checking briefly quells his obsessional thoughts, but they recur with even more force causing dysfunction.

It is important to recognize that these symptoms of OCD cause the individual to suffer from significant distress and individuals go to great lengths to reduce this anxiety. Howie Mandel, comedian and judge on America's Got Talent, has obsessions about germs and contamination that keep him from shaking hands with anyone (Mandel, 2009). He will do a fist bump with contestants but will not shake their hand to avoid feeling contaminated. He also keeps his head shaved because it helps him feel cleaner. Often an individual's compulsion is tied logically to his or her obsession, for example, if Howie Mandel does touch someone's hand or an object he feels is contaminated, he will wash his hands over and over until he feels clean (Mandel, 2009). Prior to the *DSM-5,* OCD was classified as an anxiety disorder because people with OCD experience anxiety as a result of their obsessional thoughts, as well as when they are unable to carry out their compulsive behaviors.

Profiles: I can't stop checking!

I'm driving . . . doing 55 MPH. Out of nowhere my obsessive-compulsive disorder (OCD) strikes. While in reality no one is on the road, I'm intruded by the . . . thought that I *might* have hit someone . . . !

I start ruminating, "Maybe I did hit someone and didn't realize it. . . . Oh, my God! I might have killed somebody! I have to go back and check." Checking is the only way to calm the anxiety. It brings me closer to truth somehow. I can't live with the thought that I actually may have killed someone—I have to check it out.

(Source: Rapoport, 1990, pp. 21–22)

OCD affects approximately 1.2 percent of U.S adults each year and has an estimated lifetime prevalence of 2.3 percent. There are sex differences in terms of the average age of onset occurring earlier for males (6 to 15 years) than for females (20 to 29 years) (Angst et al., 2004). In adulthood, females are affected at a slightly higher rate than males (Ruscio et al., 2010). Symptoms of OCD often begin at a young age, with rate of OCD among children varying between 2 to 4 percent with a mean age of onset between 7.5 and 12.5 years. Interestingly, the sex ratio for OCD is reversed in childhood cases with more males affected than females since boys tend to develop symptoms earlier in life. However, by mid-adolescence the sex ratio is approximately equal before becoming predominantly female in adulthood. Children and adolescents often attempt to hide their symptoms, and as a result, the symptoms can go undetected for years. Although with more severe symptoms, this is not usually possible (Leonard, Ale, Freeman, Garcia, & Ng, 2005; Rapoport et al., 2000).

OCD is typically described as a chronic condition with symptoms that ebb and flow at different periods of time (Leckman et al., 2010; Marcks et al., 2011). People with OCD also have significantly high rates of comorbidity with other psychological disorders. While there is a strong likelihood of anxiety and mood disorders, there is also a strong correlation with impulse-control and substance use disorders as well. Studies suggest the major depressive disorder (MDD) is one of the most comorbid disorders; as many as 66 percent of people with OCD are also diagnosed with depression (Altintaş & Taşkintuna, 2015; Boileau, 2011; Ruscio et. al., 2010).

Worldwide, approximately 1 to 3 percent of people will develop OCD at some time in their lives, and many more people will display symptoms that don't quite meet the diagnostic criteria (Kessler et al., 2005; Leckman et al., 2010). In the United States, European Americans show higher rates of OCD than African Americans or Hispanic Americans. The prevalence of OCD does not seem to differ greatly across countries that have been studied, including the United States, Canada, Mexico, England, Norway, Hong Kong, India, Egypt, Japan, and Korea (Escobar, 1993; Insel, 1984; Kim, 1993).

The man's compulsive checking makes some sense, given what he is thinking. However, what he is thinking—that he hit someone on the road without knowing it—is highly improbable. The compulsive checking briefly quells his obsessional thoughts, but they recur with even more force.

Hoarding is a psychological disorder that involves uncontrollable urges to keep items that have no utility or instrumental value. People with this disorder develop a sentimental attachment to items and have difficulties discarding their possessions even when those items have no apparent purpose. Hoarding is a compulsive behavior that is closely related to OCD but is classified as a separate diagnosis in the *DSM-5* (see Table 9), due to evidence that hoarding has distinct features and may have different biological correlates (Frost, Steketee, & Tolin, 2012; Mataix-Cols et al., 2010).

As displayed on the reality TV show *Hoarding: Buried Alive,* people who hoard cannot throw away their possessions—even things that most of us consider trash, such as newspapers or take-out food containers. They stockpile these items in their homes and cars to the point of creating a hazard, making these spaces unusable. Compulsive hoarders often show emotional attachments to their possessions, equating them with their identity or imbuing them with human characteristics (Frost, Steketee, & Tolin, 2012). For example, one woman bought a half dozen puppets from a TV shopping station because no one else was bidding on them and she didn't want the puppets' feelings to be hurt (Plimpton, Frost, Abbey, & Dorer, 2009). The woman fully realized her behavior wasn't rational, but she still felt bad for the puppets.

TABLE 9   *DSM-5* Criteria for Hoarding Disorder

A. Persistent difficulty discarding or parting with possessions, regardless of their actual value.

B. This difficulty is due to a perceived need to save the items and to distress associated with discarding them.

C. The difficulty discarding possessions results in the accumulation of possessions that congest and clutter active living areas and substantially compromises their intended use. If living areas are uncluttered, it is only because of the interventions of third parties (e.g., family members, cleaners, authorities).

D. The hoarding causes clinically significant distress or impairment in social, occupational, or other important areas of functioning (including maintaining a safe environment for self and others).

E. The hoarding is not attributable to another medical condition (e.g., brain injury, cerebrovascular disease, Prader–Willi syndrome).

F. The hoarding is not better explained by the symptoms of another mental disorder (e.g., obsessions in obsessive-compulsive disorder, decreased energy in major depressive disorder, delusions in schizophrenia or another psychotic disorder, cognitive deficits in major neurocognitive disorder, restricted interests in autism spectrum disorder).

Specify if:
With excessive acquisition: If difficulty discarding possessions is accompanied by excessive acquisition of items that are not needed or for which there is no available space.

Specify if:
With good or fair insight: The individual recognizes that hoarding-related beliefs and behaviors (pertaining to difficulty discarding items, clutter, or excessive acquisition) are problematic.

With poor insight: The individual is mostly convinced that hoarding-related beliefs and behaviors (pertaining to difficulty discarding items, clutter, or excessive acquisition) are not problematic despite evidence to the contrary.

With absent insight/delusional beliefs: The individual is completely convinced that hoarding-related beliefs and behaviors (pertaining to difficulty discarding items, clutter, or excessive acquisition) are not problematic despite evidence to the contrary.

Hoarding differs from OCD in that people with the disorder experience thoughts about their possessions, not as intrusive, unwanted, or distressing, but instead as part of their natural stream of thought

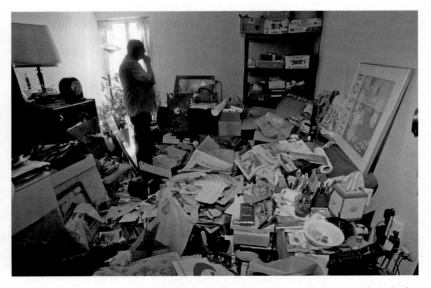

Only a small subset of people who hoard also meet the criteria for OCD, but people with hoarding disorder tend to have high rates of major depression, social anxiety, and generalized anxiety disorder. *Mark Wilson/The Boston Globe/Getty Images*

(Mataix-Cols et al., 2010). People with hoarding disorder tend to create a nest or cocoon with these items which brings them comfort and they do not often report feelings of anxiety over their hoarding. However, they may become extremely anxious, angry, or sad when pressured to get rid of their hoarded possessions by well-intentioned friends or family (Bratiotis, Davidow, Glossner & Steketee, 2016).

Epidemiological studies have estimated that hoarding disorder occurs in up to 5 percent of the U.S. population and is associated with high rates of psychiatric comorbidity (Bratiotis et al., 2016). Only a small subset of people who hoard also meet the criteria for OCD, but these people also tend to have high rates of major depression, social anxiety, and generalized anxiety disorder (Frost et al., 2012; Samuels et al., 2008). People's hoarding behavior often increases as they age (Ayers, Saxena, Golshan, & Wetherell, 2009).

Trichotillomania (hair-pulling disorder) is another obsessive-compulsive type disorder that is characterized by the repetitive pulling out of one's own hair leading to noticeable hair loss and functional impairment. Pulling can occur at any bodily region with hair, but the scalp is the most common site followed by eyebrows, and pubic region. Many people with this disorder report being unaware of their pulling behaviors, at least some of the time, which is referred to as "automatic" pulling. In contrast, "focused" pulling occurs when the person sees or feels a hair that is "not right," or that the hair feels coarse, irregular, or "out of place" (Grant & Chamberlin, 2016; Stein et al., 2010).

Excoriation (skin-picking disorder) is characterized by recurrent picking at one's own skin from any part of the body which often results in skin lesions, scars, and/or infections and causes disruption in daily function. People with excoriation typically pick in multiple sites, most commonly in the face, followed by the hands, fingers, arms, and legs. There does not appear to be a difference in whether the person selects areas of healthy skin or areas with minor skin irregularities. This disorder is associated with an inability to stop picking despite repeated efforts, which can lead to shame, social embarrassment, avoidance of certain situations or activities, anxiety, and depression (Lochner, Roos, & Stein, 2017).

Trichotillomania and excoriation were included in the *DSM-5* category together with OCD and hoarding because they share features of repetitiveness, problems with behavioral inhibition, and comorbidity (Lochner et al., 2017; Woods & Houghton, 2014). Another common feature among these disorders is the tension reported immediately before or while attempting to resist the impulse, and pleasure or relief experienced when giving in to it. The estimated prevalence of trichotillomania disorder is 0.5 to 2.0 percent. In adults, trichotillomania appears to overwhelmingly impact females with a 4:1 ratio, but in childhood, the sex distribution appears to be equal. Trichotillomania typically develops early in life with the average age of onset between 10 and 13 years and the symptoms often present along a continuum from mild to severe (Grant & Chamberlin, 2016). The estimated prevalence of excoriation is 2 to 5 percent, and it most often begins in adolescence, often with a focus on acne lesions (Lochner et al., 2017).

Trichotillomania is the compulsion to pull out one's own hair.
Ryan Jackson/Getty images

Whether it be weight loss, the shape of their nose, breast size, or the amount of desired muscle tone, most people would like to change some aspects of the way they look. However, the common desire to dislike and want to change our physical appearance, should not be confused with the psychological disorder **body dysmorphic disorder (BDD)** which is as an obsessive-compulsive disorder characterized by excessive concern about physical appearance which results in significant distress and the impairment of interpersonal situations (Ryding & Kuss, 2020).

People with BDD are excessively preoccupied with a part of their body that they believe is defective but that others see as normal or only slightly unusual. It's easy to appreciate these feelings since we live in a world where body dissatisfaction is significantly high among men and women. However, we must resist the urge to think about this disorder in terms of typical body dissatisfaction because BDD is a clinical disorder that causes people to have a distorted view of how they look, often thinking of themselves as ugly or disfigured. Concerns among people with BDD range from feeling unattractive to believing they are hideous and they look like a monster (American Psychiatric Association, 2013). This preoccupation with a perceived flaw or defect can involve any body part, but the most common ones are the skin, hair, nose, eyes, eyelids, mouth, lips, jaw, and chin. The obsession can be limited to one body part or can include several at the same time; with an average of four bodily preoccupations (Khanna & Sharma, 2017). People with BDD may complain of a lack of symmetry in an area of the face or body, or they may feel that a particular feature is out of proportion to the rest of the body. Reassurance that the defect is minimal or even nonexistent provides no relief or psychological benefit to people with BDD (Higgins & Wysong, 2017).

Preoccupation with specific body parts is a primary clinical feature among people with BDD, but gender differences have been observed in terms of the areas of concern. For example, women are more likely to focus concerns on their face, weight, stomach, and breasts, whereas men tend to be preoccupied with their body build, genitals, excessive body hair, and thinning hair. It has been posited that these gender differences likely represent extreme versions of societal norms as they relate to perceived attractiveness in women and men. This observation also supports why such differences exist among men and women worldwide in terms of which features are of most concern (Phillips et al., 2010; Ryding & Kuss, 2020).

As a result of their preoccupations, people with BDD may spend a great deal of time checking and re-checking themselves in the mirror, often returning to see if the flaw has changed. These compulsive rituals are performed to manage and reduce the distress that accompanies these appearance concerns, but often strengthen psychological dysfunction. Some of the most common compulsive behaviors in BDD include mirror gazing, touching, checking or inspecting the disliked body areas, excessive grooming, seeking reassurance from others, comparing their features with others, researching potential solutions, and strategically camouflaging their perceived flaw with makeup or clothing. Research suggests that these appearance-related compulsions may help maintain BDD symptoms (Summers & Cougle, 2018; Wilver, Summers & Cougle, 2020). People with BDD spend an average of 3 to 8 hours per day on these preoccupations and they may even seek surgery to correct their perceived flaws (Phillips et al., 2010). This significant amount of time excessively checking on their "defect" negatively impacts their ability to function. If preoccupations with weight and shape are part of an eating disorder (see the chapter "Eating Disorders"), then BDD is not diagnosed.

According to the American Psychiatric Association (American Psychiatric Association, 2013), BDD most often develops in adolescence with the average age of onset at 16. This disorder is likely to become chronic if left untreated. One study reported that more than 70 percent of cases developed symptoms before the age of 18 (Higgins & Wysong, 2017). Research shows that BDD affects men and women almost equally. In the United States, BDD occurs in about 2.5 percent in males, and in 2.2 percent of females. BDD is highly co-morbid with several disorders, including anxiety and depressive disorders, personality disorders, substance use disorders, and especially is associated with OCD (Frías, Palma, Farriols, & González, 2015).

If the areas of preoccupation vary among different cultures, is it possible that this disorder can be influenced by the use of social media within the culture? With the tremendous increase in smartphone and social media usage, researchers are studying the influence on mental health, body dissatisfaction and BDD, in particular. Research suggests that one risk of social media use is the development of a compulsive preoccupation with physical appearance (Zimmer-Gembeck, Hawes, & Pariz, 2020).

Various studies have found that the average time spent on social media platforms, such as Facebook, Instagram, Pinterest, Snapchat, Twitter, and YouTube, has increased drastically over the last decade. For example, 78 percent of 18- to 24-year-olds use Snapchat, and a sizable majority of these users (71 percent) visit the platform multiple times per day (Smith & Anderson, 2018). Social media platforms serve as a place to display and directly compare social circumstances, status, and physical appearance, which results in frequent direct feedback from others about one's appearance, interests, and behavior. Unfortunately, social media use directly links with concerns related to appearance and comparing favorably with peers among adolescents and young adults (Zimmer-Gembeck et al., 2020). Recent research has found the amount of social media usage correlates significantly with age, with 88 percent of young adults (18 to 24 years) reporting more time on social media than older adults, as well as the number of times these platforms are accessed each day. With this increased time spent and preoccupation with social media, research has focused on whether this practice has a detrimental effect on the mental health of these users (Ryding & Kuss, 2020; Smith & Anderson, 2018).

The creation of online communities is associated with novel behaviors such as posting "selfies" to social media platforms. Researchers have identified excessive "selfies" as a factors that influence the course of BDD. While research does not suggest that high amounts of social comparison and social media usage cause the development of BDD, they may be factors that contribute to the development of symptoms. Recent research suggests that exposure to social media increases the likelihood that users will engage in increased appearance comparisons, internalization of ideal thinness, and self-objectification, which contributes to body dissatisfaction. Those who spend more time on social media platforms and engage in appearance comparisons may more negatively evaluate their own appearance which may increase the likelihood of developing BDD (Zimmer-Gembeck et al., 2020).

Individuals with BDD are more likely to compare themselves to others on social media when they consider that person attractive or if that person's physical features are also the ones the BDD individual feels are personally defective. Research suggests that this type of comparison may contribute to the maintenance of BDD symptoms by amplifying overall appearance-related preoccupations or heightening the focus on the specific body parts that the BBD individual experiences as defective in himself or herself. Additionally a relationship between overuse of social media and OCD has also been supported through recent studies. Research has also found that excessive selfie use is used as a safety behavior to manage the distress related to BDD, particularly when the BDD individual has preoccupations that focus on the nose, complexion, and hair. The excessive use of selfies among people with BDD indicates that excessive levels of Internet and smartphone use may play a role in the maintenance of BDD (Khanna & Sharma, 2017; Ryding & Kuss, 2020).

Frequent social media use is a potential risk factor in the development of BDD among young adolescent girls who are more likely to spend more time online. Since many young individuals who engage in high levels of social media use and social comparison are below the diagnostic cutoff for BDD, it could also be suggested that individuals who seek to use social media to compare themselves to others may present subthreshold BDD symptoms, which makes them more vulnerable to the future development of clinical symptoms (Ryding & Kuss, 2020; Zimmer-Gembeck et al., 2020).

The perception of the physical deformities experienced by people with BDD can be so severe that they become out of touch with reality, sometimes displaying delusional thoughts (Phillips, Didie, Feusner, & Wilhelm, 2008). The authors of the *DSM-5* discussed the possibility of labeling BDD as a delusional disorder category since the pathology of this disorder lies in the BDD individual's reacting to a deformity that others cannot perceive. It is recognized in *DSM-5* that these delusions are not the same as those related to psychotic disorders like schizophrenia. For now, those who firmly hold these false beliefs are given the specifier "with absent insight/delusional beliefs." Even if they do not lose touch with reality, some people with the disorder have severe impairment in their functioning. Most people with this disorder avoid social activities because of their "deformity," many become housebound, and many obtain cosmetic surgery. Addressing the perceived defect through cosmetic surgery is not advised and can often worsen the area of preoccupation and create new areas of concern (American Psychiatric Association, 2013).

Muscle dysmorphia (MD) is a subtype of BDD that almost exclusively affects men who view their bodies as very small and weak, even though the person generally possesses an average or above average muscle mass. MD is a specifier that can be assigned to a BDD client with this type of symptomatology and is often described as "reverse anorexia." As a result of this inaccurate perception, individuals with MD obsessively engage in behaviors to increase their muscularity such as weightlifting, dieting, and drug use (Gomes et al., 2020; Ryding & Kuss, 2020).

BDD is a disorder associated with alarmingly high rates of suicidal ideation, suicide attempts, and completed suicide. Recent research indicates that approximately 80 percent of individuals with BDD experience lifetime suicidal ideation and 21.5 to 28 percent have attempted suicide. Although data on completed suicide are limited and preliminary, the suicide rate appears markedly high. It is theorized that factors specific to BDD such as: early onset, symptom severity, poor insight, and the presence of additional psychological disorders increase the risk of suicide attempts or suicidal ideation (Albert et al., 2019; Phillips, 2007).

Theories of OCD and Related Disorders

Biological Theories

OCD is a multifactorial disorder with strong high genetic predispositions (Abdolhosseinzadeh, Sina, Ahmadiani, Asadi, & Shams, 2019). Biological theories of OCRDs have focused on a circuit in the brain involved in motor behavior, cognition, and emotion. OCD has been repeatedly linked to dysfunction in this circuit which projects from specific areas of the frontal cortex to areas of the basal ganglia called the striatum (caudate and putamen), through the basal ganglia to the thalamus, anterior cingulate cortex (ACC), which then loops back to the frontal cortex (Sinopoli et al., 2020) (Figure 7). People with OCD, trichotillomania (hair-pulling disorder), and excoriation (skin-picking disorder) show alterations in the structure and activity level of these areas and in the

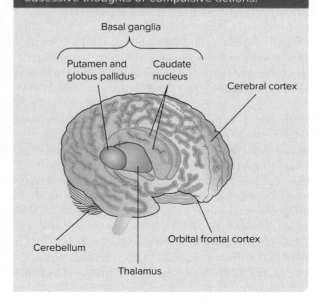

FIGURE 7 **OCD in the Brain.** A three-dimensional view of the human brain (with parts shown as they would look if the overlying cerebral cortex were transparent) clarifies the locations of the orbital frontal cortex and the basal ganglia—areas implicated in obsessive-compulsive disorder. Among the basal ganglia's structures are the caudate nucleus, which filters powerful impulses that arise in the orbital frontal cortex so that only the most powerful ones reach the thalamus. Perhaps the orbital frontal cortex, the caudate nucleus, or both are so active in people with obsessive-compulsive disorder that numerous impulses reach the thalamus, generating obsessive thoughts or compulsive actions.

connections between these areas (Milad & Rauch, 2012). People with hoarding disorder show alterations in other areas of the frontal cortex and the limbic system (Saxena, 2008). The brain activity of people with BDD seems to differ from that of healthy controls when they are processing visual stimuli, including faces (Fang & Wilhelm, 2015).

For people with OCD and related disorders, dysfunction in this circuit may result in the system's inability to turn off the primitive urges (e.g., aggressive urges) or the execution of the stereotyped behaviors. When most of us think our hands are dirty, we engage in a fairly stereotyped form of cleansing: We wash them. People with OCD, however, continue to have the urge to wash their hands because their brains do not shut off their thoughts about dirt or their hand-washing behavior when the behavior is no longer necessary. Proponents of this biological theory point out that many of the obsessions and compulsions of people with OCD have to do with contamination, sex, aggression, and repeated patterns of behavior—all issues with which this brain circuit deals (Milad & Rauch, 2012; Rauch et al., 2003).

Additional studies suggest that the stress-response and the activity of the hypothalamic-pituitary-adrenal (HPA) axis is linked to obsessive-compulsive type disorders. Research theorizes stressful life events may precede the onset of OCD and OCD symptoms typically increase at times of stress (Morgado, Freitas, Bessa, Sousa, & Cerqueira, 2013).

People with OCD and related disorders often get some relief from their symptoms when they take drugs that regulate the neurotransmitter serotonin, which plays an important role in the circuit's proper functioning (Micallef & Blin, 2001; Saxena et al., 2003). Those patients who respond to serotonin-enhancing drugs tend to show a greater reduction in the rate of activity in these brain areas than patients who do not respond well to the drugs (Saxena et al., 2003). Interestingly, people with OCD who respond to behavior therapy also tend to show decreases in the rate of activity in the caudate nucleus and the thalamus (Schwartz, Stoessel, Baxter, Martin, & Phelps, 1996).

Recent research has examined the influence of strep infection in children and the sudden onset of OCD. Various studies have found that those who tested positive for streptococcal infection were more likely to have both OCD and tics (Orefici, Cardona, Cox, & Cunningham, 2016; Vogel, 2018). It is thought that autoimmune processes triggered by the infection affect the areas of the basal ganglia implicated in OCD in some vulnerable children, creating the symptoms of OCD (Leckman et al., 2010) evidence to date for inflammation in the brain in OCD. The demonstration of elevated TSPO V_T in the CSTC circuit addresses a critical gap in the autoimmune/neuroinflammatory theory of OCD. The regional distribution of greater TSPO V_T throughout the CSTC circuit argues for consideration of autoimmune mechanisms beyond the basal ganglia and suggests a new opportunity for repurposing immunomodulatory therapies to treat OCD (Attwells et al., 2017).

Finally, genes may help determine who is vulnerable to OCD (Mundo, Zanoni, & Altamura, 2006). Family history studies clearly show that OCD, hair pulling, and skin picking run in families, and twin studies support a substantial genetic component in obsessive and compulsive behaviors (Eley et al., 2003; Hudziak et al., 2004). Different genes may be involved in vulnerability to OCD and to hoarding or body dysmorphic disorder (Mataix-Cols et al., 2010; Phillips et al., 2010).

Cognitive-Behavioral Theories

Most people, including those without OCD, occasionally have negative, intrusive thoughts which may even include thoughts about harming others or doing something against their moral code (Angst et al., 2004; Leckman et al., 2010). We are all more prone to such thoughts and engaging in rigid, ritualistic behaviors when distressed. Most people can dismiss these unwanted thoughts and attribute them to a period of distress and soon these thoughts subside. Why do people who develop OCD have trouble turning off their thoughts? According to cognitive-behavioral theories of OCD, what differentiates people with OCD from people without the disorder is their inability to turn off these negative, intrusive thoughts (Jacoby, Leonard, Riemann, & Abramowitz, 2016; Salkovskis & Millar, 2016).

First, they may be depressed or generally anxious much of the time so that even minor negative events are likely to invoke intrusive, negative thoughts (Jacoby et al., 2016). Second, people with OCD may have a tendency toward rigid, moralistic thinking (Rachman, 1993; Salkovskis, 1998). That is, they judge their negative, intrusive thoughts as more unacceptable than most people would and become more anxious and guilty about having them. Their anxiety then makes it harder for them to dismiss the thoughts (Salkovskis, 1998). People who feel more responsible for events that happen in their lives and the lives of others will also have more trouble dismissing thoughts such as "Did I hit someone on the road?" and thus might be more likely to develop OCD. Lastly, people with OCD appear to believe that they should be able to control all their thoughts and have trouble accepting that everyone has horrific notions from time to time (Jacoby et al., 2016; Salkovskis & Millar, 2016). They tend to believe that having these thoughts means they are going crazy, or they equate having the thoughts with actually engaging in the behaviors

("If I'm thinking about hurting my child, I'm as guilty as if I actually did"). Of course, this just makes them more anxious when they have the thoughts, making it harder to dismiss the thoughts.

According to these theories, compulsions develop largely through operant conditioning. People with anxiety-provoking obsessions discover that if they engage in certain behaviors, their anxiety is reduced. For example, the new mother might develop rituals (like praying for 5 minutes before touching the baby) to reduce anxiety caused by her intrusive thoughts. Each time the obsessions return and the person uses the behaviors to reduce them, the behaviors are negatively reinforced. Thus, compulsions are born. Research supports the argument put forth by this theory that people with OCD have these rigid and unrealistic beliefs (Salkovskis & Millar, 2016). Also, as we will see, CBTs based on this model have proven quite useful in treating OCD (Foa & McLean, 2016).

People with hoarding disorder also often have an exaggerated sense of responsibility, feeling guilty about wasting things, having an excessive need to "be ready just in case," and feeling responsible for not "hurting" the item (Frost et al., 2012). People who hoard also tend to believe they have a poor memory and therefore need to keep items in sight in order to remember them or to keep control over them. People with body dysmorphic disorder show biases toward appearance-specific stimuli, and overvaluation and negative interpretations of their perceived flaw (Fang & Wilhelm, 2015).

Treatment of OCD and Related Disorders

Both biological and cognitive-behavioral treatments are helpful for people with OCD.

Biological Treatments

In the 1980s, it was fortuitously discovered that antidepressant drugs affecting levels of serotonin helped relieve symptoms of OCD in many patients (Marazziti, Catena, & Pallanti, 2006). Clomipramine (trade name Anafranil) was the first such drug (Rapoport, 1989). Then the SSRIs, including fluoxetine (trade name Prozac), paroxetine (trade name Paxil), sertraline (trade name Zoloft), and fluvoxamine (trade name Luvox), proved effective. Controlled studies suggest that 50 to 80 percent of OCD patients experience decreases in their obsessions and compulsions while on these drugs, compared to only 5 percent of patients on placebos (Hurley, Saxena, Rauch, Hoehn-Saric, & Taber, 2008; Marazziti et al., 2006). These drugs can also be effective with people with hoarding disorder (Mataix-Cols et al., 2010) and body dysmorphic disorder (Phillips et al., 2010).

These drugs are not the complete answer for people with OCD and related disorders, however. A substantial number of OCD sufferers do not respond to the SSRIs. Among those who do, obsessions and compulsions are reduced only 30 to 40 percent, and patients tend to relapse if they discontinue the drugs. Significant side effects, which include drowsiness, constipation, and loss of sexual interest, prevent many people from taking them. Studies suggest that adding an atypical antipsychotic (see the chapter "Schizophrenia Spectrum and Other Psychotic Disorders") can help people who do not respond fully to the SSRIs (Bystritsky et al., 2004).

Cognitive-Behavioral Treatments

Many clinicians believe that drugs must be combined with CBTs that use **exposure and response prevention** to help people recover completely from OCD and related disorders. Exposure and response prevention therapy repeatedly exposes the client to the focus of the obsession and prevents compulsive responses to the resulting anxiety (Foa & McLean, 2016). Repeated exposure to the content of the obsession while preventing the person from engaging in the compulsive behavior extinguishes the client's anxiety about the obsession. The client learns that not engaging in the compulsive behavior does not lead to the terrible result they fear, and that their anxiety can decrease without their engaging in the behavior (Foa & McLean, 2016; Jacoby & Abramowitz, 2016).

Clients may be given homework that helps them confront their obsessions and compulsions. Early in therapy, a client might be assigned simply to refrain from cleaning the house every day and instead to clean it only every 3 days. Later he might be asked to drop a cookie on a dirty kitchen floor and then pick it up and eat it, or to drop the kitchen knives on the floor and then use them to prepare food. Because the client progressively learns to decrease anxiety without acting on compulsions, these behavioral techniques in turn decrease the distress caused by the obsessions.

The cognitive component of CBT for OCD involves challenging the individual's moralistic thoughts and excessive sense of responsibility. For example, a woman with a germ obsession who believes she would be a bad mother if she touched her baby when she wasn't completely sure her hands were clean would be guided through exposure exercises (such as touching her baby with slightly dirty hands) with response prevention (not washing her hands), while being helped to challenge her thoughts that her baby was being harmed (by noticing that the baby was fine after being touched by slightly dirty hands).

These CBTs lead to significant improvement in obsessions and compulsive behavior in 60 to

90 percent of OCD clients (Foa & McLean, 2016; Öst, Havnen, Hansen, & Kvale, 2015). CBT for OCD is at least as effective as pharmacotherapy (e.g., SSRIs), and the combination of CBT with medication is the most effective (Romanelli, Wu, Gamba, Mojtabai, & Segal, 2014). In most clients, the improvement remains for up to 6 years. CBT can also be effective in the treatment of hoarding (Frost et al., 2012), although less research has been conducted on this disorder. Cognitive-behavioral treatment for skin-picking disorder and hair-pulling disorder often focuses on *habit reversal training* (Azrin, Nunn, & Frantz, 1980). This therapy, in which patients are led to become more aware of their behaviors and cues and to replace behaviors with healthier responses, has shown effectiveness for these conditions (Lochner et al., 2017).

CBTs for BDD focus on challenging clients' maladaptive cognitions about their body, exposing them to feared situations concerning their body, extinguishing anxiety about their body parts, and preventing compulsive responses to that anxiety (Fang & Wilhelm, 2015). For example, a client might identify her ears as her deformed body part. The client could develop her hierarchy of things she would fear doing related to her ears, ranging from looking at herself in the mirror with her hair fully covering her ears to going

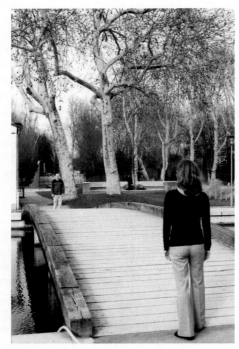

Exposure and response prevention is a treatment for OCD in which therapists help patients to face their fears step by step—in this case, walking across a bridge of planks—without engaging in the problematic compulsions patients have come to rely on for relieving distress, like counting to a certain number, or avoiding stepping on the cracks. *BSIP/UIG/Getty Images*

out in public with her hair pulled back and her ears fully exposed. After learning relaxation techniques, the client would begin to work through the hierarchy and engage in the feared behaviors, beginning with the least feared and using the relaxation techniques to quell her anxiety. Eventually, the client would work up to the most feared situation, exposing her ears in public. At first, the therapist might contract with the client that she could not engage in behaviors intended to hide the body part (such as putting her hair over her ears) for at least 5 minutes after going out in public. The eventual goal in therapy would be for the client's concerns about her ears to diminish totally and no longer affect her behavior or functioning. Empirical studies have supported the efficacy of CBTs in treating BDD (Fang & Wilhelm, 2015).

POSTTRAUMATIC STRESS DISORDER AND ACUTE STRESS DISORDER

What is trauma? In everyday conversations, people refer to a wide range of events as "traumas," ranging from a romantic breakup ("He was traumatized by her leaving him") to horrific tragedies (e.g., being the victim of a mass shooting, losing one's family in a tornado). Traumas are entwined within our life experiences and personally affect our psychological state, and in some cases, lead to psychological dysfunction. Unfortunately, the experience of trauma is relatively common with approximately 70 percent of people reporting trauma in their lifetime (Benjet et al., 2016; Kessler et al., 2017). It is important to note that trauma is very personal and the experience affects everyone differently. After a traumatic experience, some individuals display minimal, short-term effects while others develop pathological symptoms. Two psychological disorders, **posttraumatic stress disorder (PTSD)** and **acute stress disorder (ASD)** are by definition the psychological and physiological consequences of exposure to traumatic event(s). We will explore the development of these two disorders in which symptoms acutely emerge in individuals directly after a traumatic event.

The *DSM-5* constrains the category of traumas to events in which individuals are exposed to actual or threatened death, serious injury, or sexual violation that creates feelings of fear and/or helplessness (Table 10). In addition, the diagnostic criteria for PTSD and ASD, the *DSM-5* requires that individuals either directly experience or witness the traumatic event, learn that the event happened to someone they are close to, or experience repeated or extreme exposure to the details of a traumatic event (as do first responders at a tragedy).

TABLE 10   *DSM-5* Criteria for Posttraumatic Stress Disorder

A. Exposure to actual or threatened death, serious injury, or sexual violence in one (or more) of the following ways:

   1. Directly experiencing the traumatic event(s).

   2. Witnessing, in person, the event(s) as it occurred to others.

   3. Learning that the traumatic event(s) occurred to a close family member or close friend. In cases of actual or threatened death of a family member or friend, the event(s) must have been violent or accidental.

   4. Experiencing repeated or extreme exposure to aversive details of the traumatic event(s) (e.g., first responders collecting human remains; police officers repeatedly exposed to details of child abuse).

      Note: Criterion A4 does not apply to exposure through electronic media, television, movies, or pictures, unless this exposure is work related.

B. Presence of one (or more) of the following intrusion symptoms associated with the traumatic event(s), beginning after the traumatic event(s) occurred:

   1. Recurrent, involuntary, and intrusive distressing memories of the traumatic event(s).

   2. Recurrent distressing dreams in which the content and/or affect of the dream are related to the traumatic event(s).

   3. Dissociative reactions (e.g., flashbacks) in which the individual feels or acts as if the traumatic event(s) were recurring. (Such reactions may occur on a continuum, with the most extreme expression being a complete loss of awareness of present surroundings.)

   4. Intense or prolonged psychological distress at exposure to internal or external cues that symbolize or resemble an aspect of the traumatic event(s).

   5. Marked physiological reactions to internal or external cues that symbolize or resemble an aspect of the traumatic event(s).

C. Persistent avoidance of stimuli associated with the traumatic event(s), beginning after the traumatic event(s) occurred, as evidenced by one or both of the following:

   1. Avoidance of or efforts to avoid distressing memories, thoughts, or feelings about or closely associated with the traumatic event(s).

   2. Avoidance of or efforts to avoid external reminders (people, places, conversations, activities, objects, situations) that arouse distressing memories, thoughts, or feelings about or closely associated with the traumatic event(s).

D. Negative alterations in cognitions and mood associated with the traumatic event(s), beginning or worsening after the traumatic event(s) occurred, as evidenced by two (or more) of the following:

   1. Inability to remember an important aspect of the traumatic event(s) (typically due to dissociative amnesia and not to other factors such as head injury, alcohol, or drugs).

   2. Persistent and exaggerated negative beliefs or expectations about oneself, others, or the world (e.g., "I am bad," "No one can be trusted," "The world is completely dangerous," "My whole nervous system is permanently ruined").

   3. Persistent, distorted cognitions about the cause or consequences of the traumatic event(s) that lead the individual to blame themself or others.

   4. Persistent negative emotional state (e.g., fear, horror, anger, guilt, or shame).

   5. Markedly diminished interest or participation in significant activities.

   6. Feelings of detachment or estrangement from others.

   7. Persistent inability to experience positive emotions (e.g., inability to experience happiness, satisfaction, or loving feelings).

E. Marked alterations in arousal and reactivity associated with the traumatic event(s), beginning or worsening after the traumatic event(s) occurred, as evidenced by two (or more) of the following:

   1. Irritable behavior and angry outbursts (with little or no provocation) typically expressed as verbal or physical aggression toward people or objects.

   2. Reckless or self-destructive behavior.

   3. Hypervigilance.

   4. Exaggerated startle response.

   5. Problems with concentration.

   6. Sleep disturbance (e.g., difficulty falling or staying asleep or restless sleep).

(continued)

TABLE 10   *DSM-5* Criteria for Posttraumatic Stress Disorder (*continued*)

F. Duration of the disturbance (Criteria B, C, D, and E) is more than 1 month.

G. The disturbance causes clinically significant distress or impairment in social, occupational, or other important areas of functioning.

H. The disturbance is not attributable to the physiological effects of a substance (e.g., medication, alcohol) or another medical condition.

Specify whether:

With dissociative symptoms: The individual's symptoms meet the criteria for posttraumatic stress disorder, and in addition, in response to the stressor, the individual experiences persistent or recurrent symptoms of either of the following:

1. **Depersonalization:** Persistent or recurrent experiences of feeling detached from, and as if one were an outside observer of, one's mental processes or body (e.g., feeling as though one were in a dream; feeling a sense of unreality of self or body or of time moving slowly).

2. **Derealization:** Persistent or recurrent experiences of unreality of surroundings (e.g., the world around the individual is experienced as unreal, dreamlike, distant, or distorted).

    Note: To use this subtype, the dissociative symptoms must not be attributable to the physiological effects of a substance (e.g., blackouts, behavior during alcohol intoxication) or another medical condition (e.g., complex partial seizures).

Specify if:

With delayed expression: If the full diagnostic criteria are not met until at least 6 months after the event (although the onset and expression of some symptoms may be immediate).

KEIRA'S STORY: IT WAS SUPPOSED TO BE A FUN NIGHT OUT . . .

The night was a reunion for high school friends, Keira and Justine, who after drifting apart decided to meet at Pulse nightclub, a gay bar that was hosting Latino night. Two old friends spent the night in a swirl of salsa and hip-hop beats on the dance floor. As the night was ending, they apologized for not keeping in touch for so long. They hugged and made plans to have lunch the next day. Then, they heard a noise. Firecrackers? No, those were gunshots. They ran to the nearest bathroom and huddled with a group of people struggling to fit their bodies inside an overcrowded stall, some already injured by the gunman. Keira and Justine heard more gunshots. They heard the gunman screaming and sounds of the gunshots were getting closer. "God forgive me for everything that I've done," Kiera prayed. "Take care of my kids, please . . ."

While Kiera survived this tragic event, her friend Justine did not and the memory of this night continues to haunt her. "I just can't let go of it. Since that night, I don't sleep very well. I try, but just as I'm falling asleep the images of that night come flooding into my mind. Even during the day memories flood my mind and I can still see people injured from gunshots or trying to escape. I see the ones who didn't make it out who were lying dead on the ground.

I smell the gunpowder and I hear the cries for help and those who begged the gunman for their lives. Sometimes it's so real that I feel like I am back in that moment and it scares me."

Many nights, "I cry to the point that my pillow is soaked. During the day, I go to work, but it's often as if my head is in another place and I am living in a fog. At times, someone will say something to me, but I won't hear them and I feel like I am floating around not touching or really seeing anything around me. I am consumed by guilt that Justine was killed that night . . . if she hadn't been there to see me she would be alive today. Most days I drink wine to help me relax, but it doesn't really help."

A wide range of specific events can induce PTSD or ASD, ranging from extraordinary events such as a terrorist attack to common events such as a traffic accident. The experiences qualify as traumas under the *DSM-5* as long as they expose the individual to actual or threatened death, serious injury, or sexual violation. About 7 percent of adults develop PTSD at some time in their lives, with women at greater risk than men. For some, the symptoms can be mild to moderate, permitting normal functioning. For others, however, the symptoms can be immobilizing, causing deterioration in their work, family, and social lives (Kessler et al., 2005). Women are more likely than men to be diagnosed with PTSD, because they may more frequently experience sexual assault, sexual abuse, and rape which are strongly associated with the development of PTSD symptoms. According to research by Snipes, Calton, Green, Perrin, & Benotsch (2017), women reported higher levels of lifetime history of rape than men with approximately 20 percent of women experiencing sexual assault as compared to 10 percent of men. These types of traumatic experiences still involve a significant amount of stigma, which likely decreases the amount of social support they receive increasing their PTSD risk. Men are more likely to report traumas that carry less stigma, such as exposure to war, physical assault, and accidents (Hanson et al., 2008; Roberts, Gilman, J. Breslau, N. Breslau, & Koenen, 2011).

A diagnosis of PTSD requires the presence of four types of symptoms: (1) reexperiencing of the traumatic event, (2) avoidance, (3) negative changes in thought or mood, and (4) hypervigilance or chronic arousal (Table 2). The first involves repeated *reexperiencing* of the traumatic event. PTSD sufferers may experience intrusive images or thoughts, recurring nightmares, or *flashbacks* in which they relive the event. **Flashbacks** are particularly disturbing since these uncontrollable, intense, and repeated episodes force the individual to relive the traumatic experience. Flashbacks are vivid, sensory experiences during which, a person may experience images, sounds, body sensations, tastes, or smells that mirror what they experienced during the traumatic moment (Ehlers, 2010). Experiences in the environment often trigger the onset of a flashback such as hearing a loud noise or smelling a cologne that is linked with that traumatic memory, but sometimes they occur unexpectedly. Flashback experiences typically last only a few seconds, but the emotional aftereffects can linger for hours or longer. These flashbacks are emotionally

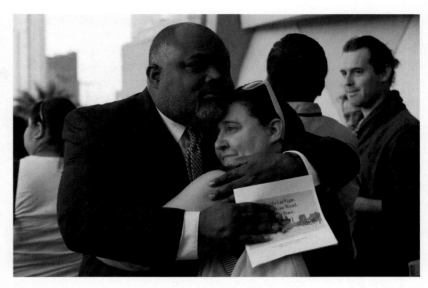

Witnessing traumatic events such as the 2017 Harvest Country Music Festival shooting at which 59 people died and over 500 were injured, can lead to posttraumatic stress.
Denise Truscello/Getty Images News/Getty Images

intrusive memories that are comprised of highly selective neural hotspots which are personally significant to that individual (Clark, Holmes, Woolrich, & Mackay, 2016). These are often more disturbing than an intrusive memory since sufferers often cannot distinguish between the flashback and reality, feeling like the traumatic experience is happening again, in that moment.

Return to the story of Keira who described how her memories of the Pulse nightclub shooting intruded into her consciousness against her will, particularly when she encounters something that reminds her of the event. She also relives her emotional reaction to the event, and she chronically experiences negative emotions that have not diminished with time.

SHADES OF GRAY

Read the following case study.

Last week, Ramón was turning left at a light when another driver sped through the intersection and ran into his car, smashing the entire passenger side. Fortunately, Ramón was physically uninjured, thanks in part to his air bag. He got out of his car screaming at the driver who hit him but then saw that he was unconscious and bleeding. Ramón immediately called 911, and the ambulance came within a few minutes.

Since the accident, Ramón has been having nightmares in which he is in the accident again, only this time his 3-year-old daughter is in the backseat and is seriously injured. He wakes up sweating and sometimes screaming. He has to go into his daughter's bedroom and touch her to convince himself she is okay. His concentration at work is diminished because he is tired from loss of sleep and because he keeps going over the accident, thinking about how he could have prevented it. Today he was at his desk, replaying the accident again in his mind, when his boss came by to ask him a question. Ramón jumped so badly at the sound of his name that he spilled his coffee all over his desk.

Does Ramón meet the criteria for PTSD or acute stress disorder? (Discussion appears at the end of this chapter.)

The second type of symptoms in PTSD involves *persistent avoidance* of situations, thoughts, or memories associated with the trauma. It is very common for survivors of trauma to stay away from activities, places, or other people that remind them of the event. As a result of this persistent avoidance, people with PTSD often isolate from others, which often causes problems in interpersonal relationships, social function, and a diminished interest in activities.

The third group of symptoms involves *negative changes in thought and mood* associated with the event. People may not be able to remember aspects of the trauma. They may unrealistically blame themselves or others for the event and feel permanently damaged. They may report "survivor guilt" about having lived through the traumatic event or about things they had to do to survive. They may be chronically distressed or become emotionally numb and withdrawn, feeling detached from themselves and their ongoing experiences. Dysfunctional attempts to reduce negative feelings is often displayed through self-medication, with drugs and/or alcohol. Research suggests that this method is used as a way to regain emotional control, although it ultimately causes even further emotional dysregulation (Center for Substance Abuse Treatment, 2014).

The fourth type of symptoms includes *hypervigilance and chronic arousal*. Trauma changes the responses in our central nervous system and people suffering from PTSD are physiologically overaroused. People with PTSD are often on guard, focusing their attention on potential threats, displaying hypervigilance. They have an increased startle response, tend to experience elevated levels of irritability and agitation such as heightened emotional reactivity, anger outbursts (Brenner, Köllner, & Bachem, 2019).

Problems with sleep are also common with many people with PTSD experiencing insomnia. Sounds or images that remind them of their trauma can instantly create panic and flight. A war veteran, hearing a car backfire, may jump into a ditch and begin to have flashbacks of the war, reexperiencing the terror they felt on the front lines. Hypervigilance undermines the quality of life as it is extremely stressful and taxing to the individual. People with hypervigilance often feel exhausted as a result and this behavior commonly interferes with interpersonal relationships, work, and one's ability to function on a day-to-day basis. Research by Kimble et al. (2014) suggests that the presence of hypervigilance may be strongly connected to both the development etiology and maintenance of the disorder.

In addition to these symptoms, many people with PTSD experience some symptoms of *dissociation*. Dissociation is a process in which different facets of their sense of self, memories, or consciousness become disconnected from one another. For example, a person could feel like she is not in her own body, or that the world around her feels unreal (see the chapter "Somatic Symptom and Dissociative Disorders"). For some people with PTSD, dissociative symptoms are especially prominent and persistent (see Friedman et al., 2011). These people can be diagnosed with the subtype **PTSD with prominent dissociative (depersonalization/derealization) symptoms.**

Acute stress disorder (ASD) occurs in response to traumatic events but is diagnosed when symptoms arise within 1 month of exposure to the stressor and last no longer than 4 weeks. As in PTSD, the individual with ASD persistently reexperiences the trauma through flashbacks, nightmares, and intrusive thoughts; avoids reminders of the trauma; and is constantly aroused. In ASD, dissociative *symptoms* are common, including numbing or detachment, reduced awareness of surroundings, derealization (experiencing the world as unreal or dreamlike), depersonalization (feeling detached from one's body or mental processes), and an inability to recall important aspects of the trauma. It's not uncommon to see a person wandering around aimlessly immediately following a traffic accident. In that moment, the individual who was just involved in a car accident is disconnected from the event: They are experiencing dissociation. This feature can be present in PTSD, but is extremely common in ASD. Although ASD is defined as a short-term response to trauma, people who experience ASD are at high risk of continuing to experience posttraumatic stress symptoms for many months (Bryant, Friedman, Spiegel, Ursano, & Strain, 2011).

Another trauma- and stress-related diagnosis is **adjustment disorder,** which consists of emotional and behavioral symptoms (depressive symptoms, anxiety symptoms, and/or antisocial behaviors) that arise within 3 months of the experience of a stressor. The stressors that lead to adjustment disorder can be of any severity, while those that lead to PTSD and ASD are, by definition, extreme. Adjustment disorder is a diagnosis for people experiencing emotional and behavioral symptoms following a stressor that does not meet the criteria for a diagnosis of PTSD, ASD, or an anxiety or mood disorder resulting from stressful experience.

Reactive attachment disorder (RAD) occurs as a result of severe neglect, abuse, and maltreatment in early childhood and typically presents between 9 months and 5 years. Affected children have difficulty forming emotional attachments to others, they are emotionally withdrawn and show little positive affect. Children with this disorder suffer from significant interpersonal dysfunction and cannot form attachment relationships with their caregivers. As a result, children with RAD do not seek out or respond to comfort during times of stress. These children have trouble controlling their emotions and experience significant emotional dysregulation (Ellis & Saadabadi, 2020).

Almost the polar opposite of RAD, **disinhibited social engagement disorder** is a disorder where children develop inappropriate and overly familiar behavior with adult strangers. Unlike RAD, these children are very comfortable with and interact indiscriminately with adult strangers. This characteristic makes this group particularly vulnerable to abuse, as they do not experience fear or discomfort with unfamiliar adults. These behaviors violate social norms and are associated with children who have experienced severe neglect (Humphreys, Nelson, Fox, & Zeanah, 2017).

Traumas Leading to PTSD

Despite what we may want to believe, most people will experience one or more traumatic events in the course of their lifetime, making trauma a common occurrence among the majority of people (Kessler et al., 2017). As we already know, exposure to trauma increases the probability of developing PTSD, but there is variability as to which types of trauma are more associated with the onset of this disorder. Sadly, there is no shortage of collective examples of trauma whether it be natural disasters, (like earthquakes, tornadoes, or tsunamis), mass shootings (such as Columbine, Sandy Hook elementary, Pulse nightclub, or the Stoneman Douglas High School shooting), car accidents, or assaults. Since 9/11, there has been an increase in global terrorism, which has resulted in many mass casualty events. The locations of terrorist attacks include airports, concerts, city streets, schools, office buildings, nightclubs, public events such as marathons, and places of worship (Molina, Yegidis, & Jacinto, 2019). And of course, since early 2020, millions around the world have experienced trauma associated with the corona virus and COVID-19 in terms of medical condition or related economic stress.

Across the world, exposure to traumatic events is common, unequally distributed, and inconsistent which makes the risk of developing PTSD variable. The fact that so many people experience trauma at some point in their life, but only a small minority of the population will develop PTSD requires a review of our individual differences in terms of psychological vulnerability to PTSD. One possible explanation is that the risk of developing PTSD varies significantly by trauma type. Research has shown that differences do exist among different types of exposure to trauma with the highest PTSD risk associated with traumas involving interpersonal violence, especially relationship–sexual violence, and/or a history of repeated experiences with violence (Kessler et al., 2017). Various studies support the idea that sexual assault is strongly associated with PTSD, with nearly half (46 percent) of sexual assault survivors developing symptoms of PTSD at some time in their lives. Traumas involving the unexpected death of a loved one, witnessing the death or injury of a loved one, and accidents are very common trauma types and are associated with low individual-level PTSD risk (Alim et al., 2008; Kessler et al., 2017; Zinzow et al., 2012). In addition to the impact of specific traumas on the development of symptoms, there also appears to be a variety of risk factors associated with adverse psychological outcomes such as demographic characteristics, proximity to event and fewer psychosocial resources (Lowe & Galea, 2017).

The shooting at Pulse nightclub in Orlando Florida on June 12, 2016, left 49 dead and 53 others wounded in what has been characterized as both a terrorist attack and hate crime because of the Latinx and gay clientele. This was both the deadliest mass shooting by a single shooter in United States' history until October 1, 2017, when a shooting at a country music festival in Las Vegas left 58 dead and 527 injured (Yu-Ru & Wen-Ting, 2020). As a result of these events, a large number of people reported symptoms of PTSD which included survivors, but also members of their family, mental health professionals, first responders, and community members. Research suggests that mass shooting survivors may be at greater risk for mental health difficulties as compared with those who experience other types of trauma. The National Center for PTSD estimates that 28 percent of people who have witnessed a mass shooting develop PTSD and one-third develop ASD (Mclaughlin & Kar, 2019). Although this exposure can create symptoms of PTSD, it is equally important to recognize that protective factors, such as strong community support that can benefit survivors of trauma, particularly when it is a community-based traumatic event. This community network is a critical factor in reducing psychological distress following a trauma. The Orlando community rallied around the Pulse nightclub survivors and because of existing and well-established community networks, services were mobilized to provide immediate and long-term support. A well-developed support network is a critical factor for individual resiliency (Molina et al., 2019).

Exposure to one traumatic event maybe significant enough to develop symptoms of PTSD, but studies also suggest that multiple exposures to trauma further increase risk of PTSD. Research examined the psychological impact of Superstorm Sandy (also called Hurricane Sandy) which was the deadliest and most destructive hurricane of 2012. This natural disaster is strongly associated with the development of PTSD, particularly among those in the NY and NJ area who were also exposed to the trauma of 9/11. This research suggests that psychological vulnerability for PTSD increases following exposure to multiple traumatic events (Caramanica, Brackbill, Stellman, & Farfel, 2015).

Exposure to trauma is not limited to direct, personal experience. Indirect or vicarious experiences are also associated with the development of a trauma or stressor-related disorder. *Secondary trauma* can occur in those who experience the traumatic event through a firsthand account or narrative. Research suggests that certain occupations associated with high-stress or trauma-exposed fields are more at risk for the development of PTSD, such as social workers, prosecutors, judges, therapists, and health care professionals. Research that focused on first responders suggests that this group is at particular risk for developing this disorder. A meta-analysis of 28 studies of ambulance personnel, firefighters, police, and other first responders across the world found that 10 percent currently experienced PTSD, regardless of whether they had recently responded to a large-scale traumatic event. Ambulance workers had the highest rates of PTSD, presumably because their job involves daily exposure to people who are seriously injured and dying, in a chronically stressful work environment (Berger et al., 2012).

Indirect trauma is not limited to professionals and also affects civilians who do not work in high-trauma fields but are deeply impacted by stories whether through graphic media exposure or by a friend sharing details of their trauma. Media exposure to traumatic events has been shown to influence the development of PTSD. Unfortunately, coverage of large-scale collective traumas (e.g., terrorist attacks and disasters) appear in traditional and social media with increasing frequency. The extensive media coverage that follows collective trauma is often repetitious, graphic, and includes sensationalized descriptions of the events (Thompson, Jones, Holman, & Silver, 2019). Various studies have studied the psychological consequences of media exposure collective community trauma following the Boston Marathon Bombing, the Pulse nightclub shooting, Sandy Hook Elementary School shooting, September 11, 2001 (9/11) terrorist attacks, and Superstorm Sandy.

These studies suggest that repeated exposure to this type of news coverage is associated with acute stress and psychological dysfunction in the immediate aftermath and posttraumatic stress responses over time. Research studies have found live media–based exposure to 9/11, Superstorm Sandy, and the Sandy Hook shooting were positively associated with acute stress responses. The 24-hour news cycle and the widespread use of mobile technologies means that much of the viewing public is habitually plugged into news updates. This frequent access to media coverage of community-based traumas increases distress by broadcasting an event to whole populations that would otherwise have been restricted to local communities. Following exposure to a collective trauma, it is common for individuals to increase their media use, which may exacerbate distress and worry about future events. These postevent responses to a national trauma might sensitize people to news coverage of another tragedy over time making them more vulnerable to psychological dysfunction (Garfin, Holman, & Silver, 2015; Thompson et al., 2019).

Survivors of natural disasters, such as Super Storm Sandy in 2012, may experience posttraumatic stress disorder. *meunierd/Shutterstock*

Theories of PTSD

If traumatic experiences are relatively common then what determines or exacerbates pathology? What kind of trauma is most likely to cause long-term, severe psychological impairment? And, why do some people develop PTSD in the wake of trauma, whereas others do not? Researchers have identified a number of factors that increase the likelihood of developing PTSD. Whether or not an individual develops PTSD is a complex, multifactorial issue. This essentially means we bring our own psychological, biological, and psychosocial vulnerabilities with us to each experience and the greater the vulnerability, the more likely that PTSD will develop.

Environmental and Social Factors

No one factor fully insulates against nor makes one completely vulnerable to PSTD; rather, a variety of factors increase or decrease one's likelihood of developing PSTD symptoms. How an event affects an individual depends on many factors, including the psychological traits of the individual, the characteristics of the trauma(s), the perception of the trauma, and sociocultural factors (Center for Substance Abuse Treatment, 2014).

An important set of risk factors involves the contexts in which people experience trauma. Strong predictors of people's reactions to trauma include its *severity* and *duration* and the individual's *proximity* to the event (Hoge et al., 2004). People who experience more severe and longer-lasting traumas and who are directly affected by a traumatic event are more prone to developing PTSD. For example, veterans are more likely to experience PTSD if they were on the front lines for an extended period (Iversen et al., 2008). People at Ground Zero during the World Trade Center attacks were more likely to develop PTSD than were those who were not at the site (Galea et al., 2002). Rape survivors who were violently and repeatedly raped over an extended period are particularly likely to experience PTSD (Zinzow et al., 2012). Victims of natural disasters who are injured or who lose their homes or loved ones are more likely to experience PTSD than are those whose lives are less severely affected (Galea, Tracy, Norris, & Coffey, 2008). These examples illustrate how contextual factors affect how one person's reaction to traumatic events can differ from another person's.

Another predictor of vulnerability to PTSD is the availability of social support. The relationship between social support and mental health outcomes suggests that a support network can be used to buffer against the development of PTSD. Research suggests that an individual's ability to draw on relationships with others as a resource in times of stress is associated

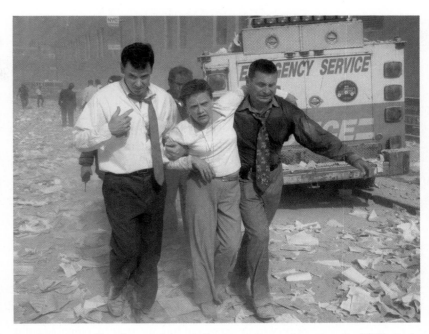

People supported by others during and after traumatic events, such as the 2001 attack on the World Trade Towers, often recover more quickly than those who do not. *Library of Congress Prints and Photographs Division [LC-DIG-ppmsca-01814]*

with decreased risk of psychological dysfunction. Meaning, people who have a stronger support network and the emotional support of others are more likely to recover from trauma than people who do not (Ozbay et. al., 2007). Survivors of Hurricane Katrina who could talk with others about their experiences and who received emotional and practical support were less likely to develop PTSD than were those who did not receive such support (Galea et al., 2008). Search and rescue personnel responding to the 2010 earthquake in Haiti were unlikely to develop PTSD if they had strong social support among their colleagues and in their community (van der Velden, van Loon, Benight, & Eckardt, 2012).

Psychological Factors

Comorbidity may also be a risk factor for developing PTSD. People who already are experiencing symptoms of anxiety or depression before a trauma occurs are more likely to develop PTSD following the trauma (Cardozo, Kaiser, Gotway, & Agani, 2003; Hoge et al., 2004; Mayou, Bryant, & Ehlers, 2001). Children who were anxious prior to Hurricane Katrina were more likely to develop symptoms of PTSD than were those who were not (Weems et al., 2007). War veterans who have psychological distress or poor interpersonal relationships before they enter combat are more likely to develop symptoms of PTSD (Koenen et al., 2002).

Once trauma occurs, one's individual methods of coping may also influence their vulnerability. Several studies have shown that people who use self-destructive or avoidant coping strategies, such as drinking and self-isolation, are more likely to experience PTSD (Merrill, Thomsen, Sinclair, Gold, & Milner, 2001). Another form of coping that may increase the likelihood of PTSD is dissociation, or psychological detachment from the trauma and ongoing traumatic events. People who dissociate may feel that they are in another place, or in someone else's body watching the trauma and its aftermath unfold. Those who dissociate shortly after a trauma are at increased risk of developing PTSD (Cardeña & Carlson, 2011; Friedman et al., 2011).

Finding a sense of purpose or meaning as it relates to a traumatic experience may increase the person's ability to cope with the stress and consequently decrease the chances of developing PTSD. Research suggests that finding purpose may motivate an individual's ability to reframe stressful situations and deal with them more productively, thereby facilitating recovery from stress and trauma. In turn, enhanced ability to recover from negative events may allow a person to achieve or maintain a feeling of greater purpose in life over time. Traumatic events can create feelings of helplessness in those who suffer from PTSD which lowers overall psychological well-being and is correlated with higher rates of depression and emotional dysregulation. Recent research supports the notion that finding purpose or attributing meaning to a traumatic event is an effective resiliency factor associated with better recovery from trauma. Studies on at-risk African American assault survivors, cancer patients, and Pakistani earthquake survivors, found that participants with higher levels of purpose had decreased rates of PTSD after suffering trauma. Purpose in life might be a resilience factor that protects individuals against the development of psychopathologies, such as PTSD and depression, after stress and trauma exposure, or even the repeated minor stresses experienced over the course of a lifetime (Alim et al., 2008; Schaefer et al., 2013).

Gender and Cross-Cultural Differences

Nationwide studies in the United States find that African Americans have higher rates of PTSD compared to whites, Hispanics, and Asian Americans (Roberts, Gilman, Brelau, & Koenen, 2011). Whites reported being exposed to the greatest number of potentially traumatizing events, but African Americans reported more traumas of certain types than did other groups, namely, witnessing domestic violence and being the victim of a violent assault. Asians had the most reports of being a refugee or a civilian in a war zone. All the non-white racial and ethnic minority groups were less likely than whites

to seek treatment for trauma-related symptoms, perhaps due to lower socioeconomic status and less access to health care or to greater stigmatization against seeking mental health treatment (Roberts et al., 2011).

Culture also appears to strongly influence the manifestation of anxiety. People in Latino cultures report a syndrome known as *ataque de nervios* (attack of the nerves) (see Lewis-Fernandez et al., 2010). A typical ataque de nervios might include trembling, heart palpitations, a sense of heat in the chest rising into the head, difficulty moving limbs, loss of consciousness or the mind going blank, memory loss, a sensation of needles in parts of the body (paresthesia), chest tightness, difficulty breathing (dyspnea), dizziness, faintness, and spells. Behaviorally, the person begins to shout, swear, and strike out at others. The person then falls to the ground and either experiences convulsive body movements or lies as if dead. Ataque de nervios is more common among recent trauma victims (Guarnaccia, Rivera, Franco, Neighbors, & Allende-Ramos, 1996).

More chronic anxiety-like symptoms, known as *nervios,* are common in Latino communities, particularly among the poor and uneducated (Guarnaccia et al., 1996). The term nervios (which is more general than ataque de nervios) encompasses a broad array of symptoms, including physical ailments (headaches, stomach problems, dizziness) and emotional symptoms (sadness, irritability, anger, absentmindedness), as well as the presence of intrusive worries or negative thoughts. One study of 942 adults in rural Mexico found that 21 percent of the women and 10 percent of the men had chronic nervios (de Snyder, Diaz-Perez, & Ojeda, 2000). The authors suggest that among the underprivileged, particularly women, nervios expresses the anger and frustration of "being at the bottom" and provides temporary release from the grinding everyday burdens of life (see also Lopez & Guarnaccia, 2000).

Cultural Assets   There are many psychological factors that can make people vulnerable to psychological dysfunction, and those that can provide protection. One such psychological factor is the construct of *ethnic identity* which refers to a person's sense of commitment and belonging to an ethnic group. People with a strongly developed ethnic identity also tend to have positive feelings about the group and display behaviors that indicate membership in this cultural or social group. The process of developing ethnic identity typically begins in adolescence and according to Williams et al. (2012), achieved ethnic identity among adolescents is positively associated with self-esteem, coping, sense of mastery, and optimism. Conversely, research has also shown that loneliness and depression have been negatively related to ethnic identity across the lifespan which suggests that an achieved ethnic identity may serve as a protective factor against psychological distress among adolescents and adults alike. Many studies suggest that ethnic identity is generally stronger and more salient among African Americans and other ethnic minorities than among European Americans. In the United States, "whiteness" is considered normative and as such, European Americans are less likely to be regularly reminded of their race or ethnicity as compared to African Americans and other ethnic minorities.

Research examining ethnic identity development across the lifespan suggests that an achieved ethnic identity may serve as a protective factor against psychological distress among adults as well. Recent studies support the notion that ethnic identity among African Americans provides a protective role against anxiety. Higher levels of ethnic identity are correlated to lower rates of anxiety and depression in African Americans but not European Americans (Hopkins & Shook, 2017; Williams et al, 2012). Additional studies on ethnic identity and response to sexual trauma also suggest that a well-developed sense of ethnic identity can provide protection against psychological dysfunction. It is hypothesized that a strong sense of ethnic identity may moderate the association between negative responses to the first disclosure of sexual victimization and symptoms of PTSD and depression. Research has also shown that a stronger sense of ethnic affiliation may protect women against PTSD when they receive high levels of negative messages about sexual victimization experiences (Nikulina, Bautista, & Brown, 2019).

Biological Factors

The biological responses to threat appear to be different in people with PTSD than in people without the disorder. Genetic factors may predispose victims of threat to these different biological responses. Research on biological factors has focused on three areas: neuroimaging, biochemistry, and genetics.

Neuroimaging studies using positron-emission tomography (PET) and magnetic resonance imaging (MRI; see the chapter "Assessing and Diagnosing Abnormality") have shown differences in brain activity between people with PTSD and those without in response to powerful emotional stimuli. These differences occur in brain areas that regulate emotion, the fight-or-flight response, and memory, including the amygdala, hippocampus, and prefrontal cortex (Britton & Rauch, 2009). The amygdala, which activates when processing emotional material and threat, appears to respond more actively to emotional stimuli in those with PTSD. Further, the medial prefrontal cortex, which modulates the reactivity of the amygdala to emotional stimuli, is less active in people with more severe symptoms of PTSD than among individuals who display less severe symptoms. Thus, the brains of those with severe PTSD may be both more reactive to emotional stimuli and less able to dampen that reactivity when it occurs (Shin et al., 2011).

Some studies also show shrinkage in the hippocampus among PTSD patients, possibly due to overexposure to neurotransmitters and hormones released in the stress response (Britton & Rauch, 2009). The hippocampus functions in memory, and damage to it may result in some of the memory problems reported by PTSD patients. It also helps regulate the body's fear response, as discussed earlier. Thus, damage to the hippocampus may interfere with returning the fear response to a normal level after the threat has passed. Together, these findings about the brain align with the types of symptoms and behaviors seen in PTSD.

Biochemical Findings Recall that one of the major hormones released as part of the fight-or-flight response is **cortisol** and that high levels usually indicate an elevated stress response. Interestingly, resting levels of cortisol among people with PTSD (when not exposed to trauma reminders) tend to be lower than among people without PTSD (Yehuda, Pratchett, & Pelcovitz, 2012). For example, studies that have assessed cortisol levels in people injured in a traffic accident 1 to 2 days previously have found that those with lower cortisol levels are at significantly increased risk for PTSD over the next weeks and months (Ehring, Ehlers, Cleare, & Glucksman, 2008; McFarlane, Barton, Yehuda, & Wittert, 2011). Cortisol acts to reduce sympathetic nervous system activity after stress, so lower levels may result in prolonged activity of the sympathetic nervous system following stress. As a result, some people may more easily develop a conditioned fear of stimuli associated with the trauma and subsequently develop PTSD (Ballenger et al., 2004).

Some other physiological responses to stress are exaggerated in PTSD sufferers, including elevated heart rate and increased secretion of the neurotransmitters epinephrine and norepinephrine (Ballenger et al., 2004; Pole et al., 2007). In people vulnerable to PTSD, different components of the stress response may not be working in sync with one another. The HPA axis may be unable to shut down the response of the sympathetic nervous system by secreting necessary levels of cortisol, resulting in overexposure of the brain to epinephrine, norepinephrine, and other neurochemicals. This overexposure may cause memories of the traumatic event to be "over-consolidated," or planted more firmly in memory (Ballenger et al., 2004; Walderhaug, Krystal, & Neumeister, 2011).

Increasing evidence suggests that exposure to extreme or chronic stress during childhood may permanently alter children's biological stress response, making them more vulnerable to PTSD—as well as to other anxiety disorders and depression—throughout their lives (Cicchetti & Toth, 2005; Nemeroff, 2004). Studies of maltreated (severely neglected or physically, emotionally, or sexually abused) children show abnormal cortisol responses to stressors (Cicchetti & Rogosch, 2001) and a diminished startle response (Klorman, Cicchetti, Thatcher, & Ison, 2003). Adults abused as children continue to have abnormal cortisol responses and elevated startle and anxiety responses to laboratory stressors, even when they no longer show symptoms of PTSD or depression (Heim, Meinlschmidt, & Nemeroff, 2003; Pole et al., 2007). Depressed women who were abused as children show lower volume of the hippocampus than depressed women who were not abused as children (Vythilingam et al., 2002). Thus, early childhood trauma may leave permanent physical and emotional scars that predispose individuals to later psychological problems, including PTSD.

Genetics Vulnerability to PTSD may be inherited (Smoller, 2016). One study of about 4,000 twins who served in the Vietnam War found that if one developed PTSD, the other was much more likely to develop it if the twins were identical rather than fraternal (True et al., 1993; Stein, Jang, Taylor, Vernon, and Livesley, 2002). The adult children of Holocaust survivors with PTSD are over three times more likely to develop it than are matched comparison groups. They also have abnormally low levels of cortisol, whether or not they have ever been exposed to traumatic events or developed PTSD (Yehuda, Blair, Labinsky, & Bierer, 2007). These findings suggest that abnormally low cortisol levels may be one heritable risk factor for PTSD. Other studies have found that the abnormalities in brain responses to emotional stimuli also appear to have a genetic basis (Stevens et al., 2014).

Treatments for PTSD

Psychotherapies for PTSD generally have three goals: exposing clients to what they fear in order to extinguish that fear, challenging distorted cognitions that contribute to symptoms, and helping clients reduce stress in their lives. These goals are addressed in CBT for PTSD and in stress-management therapies. Some

clients also benefit from antianxiety and antidepressant medications.

Cognitive-Behavioral Therapy and Stress Management

CBT has proven effective in the treatment of PTSD (Chard, Shuster, & Resick, 2012; Cusack et al., 2016). A major element is systematic desensitization (see the chapter "Theories and Treatment of Abnormality"). The client identifies thoughts and situations that create anxiety, ranking them from most anxiety-provoking to least. The therapist takes the client through this hierarchy, exposing the client to the trauma cues that elicit fear, avoidance, and other symptoms of PTSD, sometimes using relaxation techniques to quell the anxiety. It usually is impossible to return to the actual traumatic event, so imagining it vividly must replace actual exposure. A combat veteran being treated for PTSD imagines the bloody battles and scenes of killing and death that haunt him; a rape survivor imagines the minute details of the assault. The therapist also watches for unhelpful thinking patterns, such as survivor guilt, and helps the client challenge these thoughts.

Repeatedly and vividly imagining and describing the feared events in the safety of the therapist's office allows the client to habituate to his or her anxiety so that reactions to stimuli become less powerful, and to distinguish memory from present reality. It may also allow the client to integrate the events into his or her concepts of self and of the world (Chard et al., 2012). For example, sexual assault survivors' experience often shatters their prior belief that the world is generally safe, or confirms their previous belief that it is unsafe; CBT can help them process the event in a more balanced and adaptive way. Two specific types of CBT for PTSD include prolonged exposure therapy, which focuses on repeated exposure to trauma

Technology can provide a controlled repetitive exposure to "virtual" trauma to help people, such as this soldier, process their actual trauma. *Ted S. Warren/AP Images*

reminders, and cognitive processing therapy, which focuses on reinterpretation of the trauma (Foa & MacLean, 2016; Resick et al., 2017). Studies of rape survivors, combat veterans, survivors of traffic collisions, and refugees have found that repeated exposure therapy significantly decreases PTSD symptoms and helps prevent relapse (Ehlers et al., 2010; Institute of Medicine, 2008; Resick, Williams, Suvak, Monson, & Gradas, 2012). Studies indicate that the effects of exposure therapies on negative thoughts and beliefs may also decrease symptoms of depression, which commonly co-occurs with PTSD (Schumm, Dickstein, Walter, Owens, & Chard, 2015; Zalta et al., 2014).

Some clients with PTSD cannot tolerate exposure to their traumatic memories. For these clients, **stress-inoculation therapy** may be warranted. Therapists teach clients skills for overcoming problems in their lives that increase their stress and problems that may result from PTSD, such as marital problems or social isolation. Stress-inoculation therapy is an efficacious form of treatment for PTSD, but exposure-based therapies show somewhat more consistent outcomes (Cusack et al., 2016; Foa & MacLean, 2016).

As with many other disorders, the most effective treatments for PTSD may not be available to many individuals. To overcome barriers to PTSD treatment, Internet-based treatments have been developed that show early evidence of effectiveness for some people (Kuester, Niemeyer, & Knaevelsrud, 2016), including some veterans (Hobfoll, Blais, Stevens, Walt, & Gengler, 2016). Researchers are also exploring newer treatment techniques incorporating mindfulness techniques (Hopwood & Schutte, 2017), complementary approaches like yoga and meditation (Gallegos, Crean, Pigeon, & Heffner, 2017), and virtual reality technology for exposure (Rizzo et al., 2017).

Biological Therapies

The SSRIs and, to a lesser extent, the benzodiazepines are used to treat symptoms of PTSD, particularly sleep problems, nightmares, and irritability (Ballenger et al., 2004). Although some people with PTSD benefit from these medications, the evidence for their effectiveness in treating PTSD is mixed (Institute of Medicine, 2008), and some (in particular, the benzodiazepines) can have significant side effects and addictive potential.

ANXIETY DISORDERS IN OLDER ADULTS

Anxiety is one of the most common problems among older adults, with up to 15 percent of people over age 65 experiencing an anxiety disorder (Bryant, Jackson, & Ames, 2008; Reynolds, Pietrzak, El-Gabalawy,

MacKenzie, & Sareen, 2015). Some older people have had anxiety disorders all their lives. For other people, anxiety first arises in old age. It often takes the form of worry about loved ones or about the older person's own health or safety, and it frequently exists together with medical illness and with depression, as with Mrs. Johnson in the following case study.

CASE STUDY

Mrs. Johnson is a 71-year-old female who was referred by a family practice physician working in a nearby town. Mrs. Johnson had become extremely anxious and moderately depressed following a major orthopedic surgery, a total hip replacement. She was a retired office worker.

I was immediately struck by her general level of anxiety. For example, she expressed fears about her ability to get her husband to take her to an appointment and was concerned that she might not be the right type of person for psychological treatment. Her anxiety seemed to interfere with her ability to adequately attend to and process information. For example, she seemed to have difficulty getting down the directions to my office. She stated that she was concerned about being able to find the building and that she would leave her house early in case she got lost.

Mrs. Johnson indicated that she loved all her children but that she worried about two of them. Both had been divorced and she was concerned about their well-being and that of her three grandchildren. She reported not having the desire to eat because her stomach was "fluttery." I asked, "Do you find yourself worrying about things?" to which she responded, "Yes, a lot. I worry that I've begun to be a burden for my husband. I worry about my hip and I worry about not being able to get around. I guess I'm crazy because I worry about being worried so much." I assured her that she was not crazy, just anxious, which can oftentimes make you feel like you are crazy.

(Source: Adapted from Scogin, Floyd, & Forde, 2000, pp. 117–118)

Mrs. Johnson was diagnosed with generalized anxiety disorder. Although rates of mental disorders tend to decrease in older age (Reynolds et al., 2015), older adults may worry more about health and about family issues than do younger adults (Scogin et al., 2000). Too often, their worries about health are dismissed as understandable when in fact these worries indicate that they are suffering from GAD.

Panic disorder is relatively rare in later life (Bryant et al., 2008). One epidemiological study estimated that only 0.5 percent of people over age 65 can be diagnosed with this disorder (Reynolds et al., 2015). Obsessive-compulsive disorder also is quite rare, diagnosed in only 0.8 percent of the older people in this study. The symptoms of PTSD and acute stress disorder, however, are more common among older people, often occurring in response to the loss of a loved one (Bryant et al., 2008).

Very few older adults seek treatment for anxiety disorders, and those who do tend to consult their family physician rather than a mental health professional (Scogin et al., 2000). For those older people who do seek help, CBT has been shown to be effective in treating their anxiety symptoms (Wetherell, Lenze, & Stanley, 2005).

Physicians frequently prescribe an antianxiety drug, such as a benzodiazepine, when an older patient complains of anxiety. With age come changes in drug absorption and distribution, metabolism, and sensitivity to side effects. Side effects such as unsteadiness can lead to falls and bone fractures (Scogin et al., 2000). Also, tolerance can develop with prolonged use of the benzodiazepines, leading to severe withdrawal effects and the rebound of anxiety symptoms when the person discontinues their use. Antidepressant drugs, including buspirone and the SSRIs, are increasingly used to treat anxiety symptoms and have fewer side effects and withdrawal effects than the benzodiazepines. Older adults often are taking several prescription and over-the-counter medications that can interact with psychotropic drugs. All these factors make the management of drug therapy in older adults more complex than in younger adults (Scogin et al., 2000).

CHAPTER INTEGRATION

Biology clearly influences the experience of anxiety. Evolution has prepared our bodies to respond to threatening situations with physiological changes that make it easier for us to flee from or confront a threat. For some people, this natural physiological response may be impaired, leading to overreactivity, chronic arousal, or poorly regulated arousal. These people may be more prone to severe anxiety reactions to threatening stimuli and to anxiety disorders.

Psychological and social factors also clearly play a role in anxiety and the anxiety disorders. Traumatic experiences lead to the development of some anxiety disorders, particularly PTSD. People differ in what they perceive as threatening, leading to differences in the level of anxiety they feel in potentially threatening situations. These differences may be due to specific traumas that some people have experienced or to people's upbringing. A child may develop a phobia of dogs because her mother modeled a fearful response to dogs. Another child may be chronically anxious and may believe they must be perfect because their parents punish them severely if they make any type of mistake.

Vulnerability (diathesis)-stress models (Figure 8) stipulate that people who develop an anxiety disorder have pre-existing biological or psychological vulnerabilities due in part to trauma or severe stress and that these vulnerabilities interact with new stressors to create anxiety disorders. Such models help explain why some people, but not others, experience anxiety so severe and chronic that it develops into a disorder.

FIGURE 8 | **Vulnerability-Stress Models.** Vulnerability-stress models of anxiety disorders describe how biological, psychological, and social factors work together to create these disorders.

SHADES OF GRAY DISCUSSION

Neither PTSD nor acute stress disorder applies to Ramón. Although his recurrent nightmares meet the reexperiencing criterion for PTSD and acute stress disorder, he actively thinks about the accident rather than avoiding thoughts of it. We have no evidence that he displays a lack of interest in activities, feels detached or estranged from others, has restricted affect, or has a sense of a foreshortened future or other negative beliefs or thoughts. We also lack evidence that Ramón has significant arousal symptoms; the exaggerated startle response he had in the interchange with his boss seems to be an isolated incident, and his sleep difficulties are caused primarily by his nightmares.

For now, Ramón appears to be having an understandable, but not diagnosable, reaction to a very frightening event. If you were his psychologist, you would want to check up in a week or two. If his nightmares and thoughts about the accident persist, and if they begin to more significantly impair his functioning, you might then diagnose him with an adjustment disorder.

CHAPTER SUMMARY

- Posttraumatic stress disorder (PTSD) occurs after exposure to actual or threatened death, serious injury, or sexual violation. It manifests four types of symptoms: (1) repeatedly reexperiencing the traumatic event through intrusive images or thoughts, recurring nightmares, flashbacks, and psychological and physiological reactivity to stimuli that remind the person of the traumatic event; (2) avoidance of anything that might arouse memories of the event; (3) negative cognitive and emotional symptoms; and (4) hypervigilance and chronic arousal.

- A subtype of PTSD is characterized by prominent dissociative (depersonalization/derealization) symptoms.

- Acute stress disorder has symptoms similar to those of PTSD but occurs within 1 month of a stressor and usually lasts less than 1 month.

- Social factors appear to influence the risk for PTSD. The more severe and longer-lasting a trauma and the more deeply involved a person is in it, the more likely he or she is to develop PTSD. People with less social support are at increased risk.

- Psychological factors also play a role in PTSD. People who are already depressed or anxious before a trauma or who cope through avoidance or dissociation may be at increased risk.

- The biological factors that increase vulnerability to PTSD may include abnormally low cortisol levels and a genetic risk. People with PTSD show hyperarousal of the amygdala, atrophy in the hippocampus, and exaggerated heart rate responses to stressors.

- Effective treatment for PTSD exposes a person to memories of a trauma through systematic desensitization to extinguish the anxiety these memories elicit. Cognitive techniques that help clients develop more adaptive viewpoints on the trauma are also useful. Some people cannot tolerate such exposure, however, and may do better with stress-inoculation therapy to reduce and prevent stress.

- The benzodiazepines and antidepressant drugs can quell some of the symptoms of PTSD.

- The specific phobias are fears of certain objects or situations. Common categories are animal type, natural environment type, situational type, and blood-injection-injury type.

- Behavioral theories suggest that phobias develop through classical and operant conditioning. The person has learned that avoiding the phobic object reduces fear, so avoidance is reinforced. Phobias also develop through observational learning. It appears that, through prepared classical conditioning, humans more readily develop phobias to objects our distant ancestors had reason to fear, such as snakes.

- Behavioral treatments focus on extinguishing fear responses to phobic objects and have proven effective. People with blood-injection-injury phobias must learn to tense their muscles when they confront their phobic objects to prevent decreases in blood pressure and heart rate. Drug therapies have not proven useful for phobias.

- Social anxiety disorder is fear of being judged or embarrassed.

- Cognitive theories suggest that social anxiety disorder develops in people who have overly high standards for their social performance, assume others will judge them harshly, and give biased attention to signs of social rejection.

- Antidepressant drugs show some effectiveness in the treatment of social anxiety symptoms, and cognitive-behavioral therapy has also been proven effective.

- A panic attack is a short, intense experience of several physiological symptoms of anxiety, plus thoughts that one is going crazy, losing control, or dying. Panic disorder is diagnosed when a person has spontaneous panic attacks frequently, worries about having them, and changes his or her lifestyle as a result.

- One biological theory of panic disorder holds that sufferers have overreactive autonomic nervous systems, putting them into a full fight-or-flight response with little provocation. This reaction may be the result of imbalances in norepinephrine or serotonin in areas of the brain stem and the limbic system. Evidence of genetic contributions to panic disorder also exists.

- Psychological theories of panic disorder suggest that afflicted people pay close attention to bodily sensations, misinterpret these sensations in negative ways, and engage in snowballing or catastrophic thinking, which increases physiological activation and promotes a full panic attack.

- Antidepressants and benzodiazepines are effective in reducing panic attacks and agoraphobic behavior, but people tend to relapse when they discontinue the drugs.

- An effective cognitive-behavioral therapy for panic attacks and agoraphobia teaches clients to use relaxation exercises and to identify and challenge their catastrophic styles of thinking, often during panic attacks induced in therapy sessions. Systematic desensitization techniques reduce agoraphobic behavior.

- People with generalized anxiety disorder (GAD) are chronically anxious in most situations. Cognitive theories argue that people with GAD appear more vigilant toward threatening information, even on an unconscious level.

- Benzodiazepines can produce short-term relief for some people with GAD but are not suitable in long-term treatment. Antidepressants appear helpful in treating GAD.

- Cognitive-behavioral therapies focus on changing the catastrophic thinking styles of people with GAD and have been shown to reduce acute symptoms and prevent relapse in most patients.

- People (mostly children) with separation anxiety disorder become excessively anxious when apart from their attachment figures.

- Separation anxiety disorder may stem from a general biological vulnerability to shyness and behavioral inhibition. The parents of children with separation anxiety have also been shown to be overprotective and controlling.

- Obsessions are thoughts, images, ideas, or impulses that are persistent, intrusive, and distressing. They commonly focus on contamination, sex, violence, and repeated doubts. Compulsions are repetitive behaviors or mental acts the individual feels he or she must perform to dispel obsessions.

- People with hoarding disorder collect objects and have great difficulty giving up their possessions.

- People diagnosed with hair-pulling disorder (trichotillomania) have a history of pulling out their hair, resulting in noticeable hair loss. People with skin-picking disorder recurrently pick at scabs or places on their skin, creating significant lesions that often become infected and cause scars.

- People with body dysmorphic disorder are excessively preoccupied with a part of their body that they believe is defective but that others see as normal or only slightly unusual.

- One biological theory of obsessive-compulsive disorder (OCD) and related disorders speculates that they result from abnormalities in a brain circuit that projects from specific areas of the frontal cortex to areas of the basal ganglia called the striatum, then through the basal ganglia to the thalamus, and then loops back to the frontal cortex. Dysfunction in these areas may result in the system's inability to turn off the primitive urges (e.g., aggressive urges) or the execution of the stereotyped behaviors. These brain areas are rich in the neurotransmitter serotonin. Drugs that regulate serotonin have proven helpful in treatment.

- Cognitive-behavioral theories suggest that people with OCD judge the occasional intrusive thoughts that most people have as unacceptable and believe they should be able to control all their thoughts. Studies further suggest that people with OCD are overly moralistic and prone to feeling excessively responsible for their own and others' well-being. Compulsive behaviors develop through operant conditioning when people are reinforced for behaviors that reduce their anxiety.

- The most effective drug therapies for OCD and related disorders are the SSRIs.

- Exposure and response prevention has also proven to be an effective therapy for OCD and related disorders.

KEY TERMS

anxiety	panic disorder
fight-or-flight	locus coeruleus
autonomic nervous system	anxiety sensitivity
adrenal-cortical system	interoceptive awareness
panic attacks	interoceptive conditioning

conditioned avoidance response

separation anxiety disorder

behavioral inhibition

generalized anxiety disorder (GAD)

social anxiety disorder

specific phobias

animal-type phobias

natural environment type phobias

situational type phobias

blood-injection-injury type phobias

agoraphobia

negative reinforcement

prepared classical conditioning

applied tension technique

obsessive-compulsive disorder

obsessions

compulsions

hoarding

trichotillomania (hair-pulling disorder)

excoriation (skin-picking disorder)

body dysmorphic disorder (BDD)

exposure and response prevention

posttraumatic stress disorder (PTSD)

acute stress disorder (ASD)

flashbacks

PTSD with prominent dissociative (depersonalization/derealization) symptoms

adjustment disorder

reactive attachment disorder (RAD)

disinhibited social engagement disorder

cortisol

stress-inoculation therapy

Chapter 6

PeopleImages/Getty Images

Somatic Symptom and Dissociative Disorders

CHAPTER OUTLINE

Somatic Symptom and Dissociative Disorders Along the Continuum

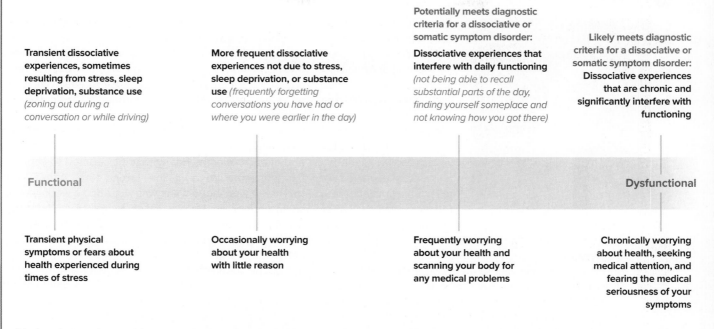

Transient dissociative experiences, sometimes resulting from stress, sleep deprivation, substance use *(zoning out during a conversation or while driving)*

More frequent dissociative experiences not due to stress, sleep deprivation, or substance use *(frequently forgetting conversations you have had or where you were earlier in the day)*

Potentially meets diagnostic criteria for a dissociative or somatic symptom disorder: **Dissociative experiences that interfere with daily functioning** *(not being able to recall substantial parts of the day, finding yourself someplace and not knowing how you got there)*

Likely meets diagnostic criteria for a dissociative or somatic symptom disorder: **Dissociative experiences that are chronic and significantly interfere with functioning**

Functional   **Dysfunctional**

Transient physical symptoms or fears about health experienced during times of stress

Occasionally worrying about your health with little reason

Frequently worrying about your health and scanning your body for any medical problems

Chronically worrying about health, seeking medical attention, and fearing the medical seriousness of your symptoms

You're driving down a highway listening to a favorite song and before you know it that song has been over for a while and you are much farther down the road than you realized! You continued driving at 65 mph and navigated the traffic but you weren't aware of it at the time. Maybe during this short period you were thinking about a loved one, errands you need to run, or that one exceptionally fun night you had with friends. This experience is common to us all and often referred to as daydreaming. Think about where you go when you daydream and what precedes this experience. Were you bored? Stressed? These dissociative moments provide a temporary mental escape.

While in everyday life this is referred to as daydreaming, in clinical terms this same experience is called dissociation. Dissociation is a normal process that provides us with a short escape from reality. What happens when a momentary mental escape becomes less than momentary? How would your life be impacted if you were constantly disconnected from the events surrounding you everyday? Daydreaming is a dissociative experience, but like all behaviors placed on a continuum this experience can become dysfunctional and cause psychological impairment. Some of the disorders presented in this chapter are associated with significant *dissociation,* in which an individual's thoughts, feelings, sensations, identity, memory, or consciousness are disconnected from the psyche.

This category of disorders illustrates the mind-body connection in which our psychological state can influence our body functions. Just as how we can all experience mild symptoms of

dissociation, we can also experience somatic concerns that are brought on by psychological distress. Think about how your own psychological stress can impact your body. During times of distress, it is common to experience physical symptoms or ailments, such as preoccupying aches, pains, and health concerns. Usually these aches and pains subside as our stress subsides, which is why these experiences fall outside of the abnormal continuum. However, for some people, their attention to their perceived aches and pains is chronic which produces clinically significant levels of worry about illness that results in impairment in daily function. These somatic symptom disorders cause excessive concerns about one's physical health, and regardless of whether or not the symptoms are medically explained their suffering is real. This category of psychological disorders all share physical symptoms that may or may not be accountable by a medical condition. Each of these disorders shares the common thread of physical symptoms that often have no physical cause and can directly impact thoughts, feelings, and behaviors that disrupt their everyday lives and cause distress.

Unlike other disorders that can be placed in simpler categories, these disorders are not black or white, but rather shades of gray. As we will discuss in this chapter, both dissociative and somatic disorders are often difficult for students (and professionals) to fully understand since many of the symptoms are hard to fully conceptualize. Both of these types of disorders serve as a reminder that the human mind is very complex and there are many things that we do not fully understand.

Extraordinary People

Anna O., *The Talking Cure*

Sigmund Freud/Ullstein bild/
Getty Images

One of the most famous cases in the annals of psychology and psychiatry was that of Anna O., a young woman whose real name was Bertha Pappenheim. She was born in Vienna in 1859 into a wealthy Orthodox Jewish family. Highly intelligent, she craved intellectual stimulation but rarely received it after leaving school. She was strong-willed and slightly temperamental. In 1880, at age 21, Pappenheim became ill while caring for her father during his serious illness and eventual death. Josef Breuer, a colleague of Freud who treated Pappenheim, noted, "Up to the onset of the disease, the patient showed no sign of nervousness, not even during pubescence. . . .

Upon her father's illness, in rapid succession there seemingly developed a series of new and severe disturbances" (quoted in Edinger, 1963). These new disturbances were a variety of physical ailments that didn't appear to have any physical causes. She experienced head pain, dizziness, and profound visual disturbances, an inability to move her head and neck, and numbness and contractions in her lower-right limbs. Breuer treated Pappenheim by asking her to talk about her symptoms under hypnosis, and after 18 months her symptoms seemed to subside. Pappenheim dubbed this the "talking cure." After Breuer told her that he thought she was well and he would not be seeing her again, he was called to her house later that evening, where she was thrashing around in her bed, going through imaginary childbirth. She claimed that the baby was Breuer's. He calmed her down by hypnotizing her, but he soon fled the house and never saw her again. Breuer collaborated with Sigmund Freud in writing about Anna O., and their descriptions of the talking cure launched psychoanalysis as a form of psychotherapy.

Bertha Pappenheim, or Anna O., appeared to suffer from what the *DSM-5* calls a *somatic symptom disorder*—she experienced physiological symptoms that Breuer argued were the result of painful emotions or memories. In this chapter, we discuss the somatic symptom disorders as well as the *dissociative disorders,* in which people develop multiple separate identities or can have the inability to recall information due to significant dissociation. The somatic symptom disorders and dissociative disorders have historically been thought to result from similar processes—patients cannot confront difficult emotions and stressful experiences, so they unconsciously convert their emotions into physical and psychological symptoms. As seen in the story of Bertha Pappenheim, these phenomena provided the material for much of the early theorizing by Breuer, Freud, and other psychoanalysts. In recent years, these disorders and the idea that people can completely lose conscious access to painful memories and emotions have become controversial. We discuss this controversy at the end of the chapter.

SOMATIC SYMPTOM AND RELATED DISORDERS

As noted throughout this book, drawing sharp distinctions between the body and the mind is becoming increasingly difficult as we better understand how biological and psychological factors are intertwined.

The **somatic symptom disorders** are a prime example of the fluid boundary between mind and body. People with these disorders may experience significant physical symptoms for which there is no apparent organic cause, but rather the result of psychological factors. They are often excessively concerned about their symptoms and spend a great deal of time worrying and seeking medical treatment (American Psychiatric Association, 2013).

One difficulty in diagnosing somatic symptom disorders is the possibility that an individual has a real physical disorder that is difficult to detect or diagnose. Many of us have friends or relatives who have complained for years about symptoms that physicians attributed to "nervousness" or "attention seeking" but that later were determined to be early symptoms of serious disease. The diagnosis of somatic symptom disorder is easier when psychological factors leading to the development of the symptoms can be identified clearly or when physical examination proves that the symptoms are not physiologically possible. For example, when a child is perfectly healthy on weekends but has stomachaches in the morning just before going to school, it is possible that the stomachaches are due to distress over going to school.

Experiencing aches or pains during a time of stress is a very common occurrence but nonetheless, it illustrates the connection that exists between psychological distress and physiological symptoms. Less common but still an example of this phenomenon is *pseudocyesis* which is a rare, but debilitating somatic disorder in which a woman presents with outward signs of pregnancy, although there is no presence of a fetus. In the cases of phantom pregnancy, this false belief of being pregnant is also associated with physical symptoms of pregnancy that may include morning sickness, abdominal enlargement, increased appetite, reduced or cessation of menstrual flow, subjective sensation of fetal movement, nausea, breast engorgement, and labor pains at the expected date of delivery. These physical symptoms of pregnancy are the result of psychological disruption and have no physical cause. Commonly, women of lower socioeconomic status, limited access to health care, and feeling under significant stress to conceive are most at risk for this disorder (Campos & Link, 2016; Yadav & Kataria, 2012). It is clear from the Extraordinary People section that Bertha Pappenheim, known as Anna O. suffered from pseudocyesis.

The category of somatic symptom disorders includes five specific disorders. The first is simply called *somatic symptom disorder*. This disorder is new to the *DSM-5* and combines a number of diagnoses from the *DSM-IV-TR* that were difficult to distinguish. Other disorders in the somatic symptom disorders category are *illness anxiety disorder* (formerly hypochondriasis), *conversion disorder,* and *factitious disorder.* One final diagnosis in this category of disorders is *psychological factors affecting other medical conditions* (sometimes referred to as psychosomatic disorders), in which people have an actual, documented physical illness or defect, such as high blood pressure, that is worsened by psychological factors. For example, depression can exacerbate a number of medical diseases, including cancer, heart disease, diabetes, arthritis, and asthma (Everson-Rose & Lewis, 2005; Katon, 2003). We will discuss the effects of psychological factors on medical conditions in detail in the chapter "Health Psychology." In this chapter, we focus on disorders in which there are distressing somatic symptoms along with abnormal thoughts, feelings, and behaviors in response to these bodily symptoms. Medically unexplained symptoms are present to varying degrees, particularly in conversion disorder where psychological factors are assumed to underlie the symptoms.

Somatic Symptom Disorder and Illness Anxiety Disorder

A person with somatic symptom disorder has one or more distressing physical symptoms and spends a great deal of time and energy thinking about these symptoms and seeking medical care for them. Symptoms often involve complaints, such as pain in different locations of the body, fatigue, heart palpitations, neurological symptoms (e.g., dizziness, tremors), gastrointestinal symptoms (e.g., nausea, diarrhea), and limb weakness. Many clients complain of multiple symptoms concurrently and over time, while others suffer from only one persisting symptom. Although anyone with painful or life-threatening symptoms might be preoccupied with them and seek alternative opinions about their causes and treatments, people with somatic symptom disorder have health concerns that are excessive given their actual physical health, that persist even when they have evidence that they are well, and that interfere with their daily functioning (see Table 1). Suffering is not confined to the experience of bodily complaints; it also entails psychological and behavioral aspects like high health anxiety and checking behavior (Henningsen,

---

TABLE 1 *DSM-5* Diagnostic Criteria for Somatic Symptom Disorder

A. One or more somatic symptoms that are distressing or result in significant disruption of daily life.

B. Excessive thoughts, feelings, or behaviors related to the somatic symptoms or associated health concerns as manifested by at least one of the following:

1. Disproportionate and persistent thoughts about the seriousness of one's symptoms.
2. Persistently high level of anxiety about health or symptoms.
3. Excessive time and energy devoted to these symptoms or health concerns.

C. Although any one symptom may not be continuously present, the state of being symptomatic is persistent (typically more than 6 months).

Specify if:

With predominant pain, for individuals whose somatic symptoms predominantly involve pain.

Persistent: characterized by severe symptoms, marked impairment, and long duration (> 6 months).

Mild (only one Criterion B symptom); **Moderate** (two or more Criterion B symptoms); **Severe** (two or more Criterion B symptoms, and multiple or one very severe somatic complaint).

2018). When they experience a symptom, they may assume the worst—that it is cancer, a heart attack, a stroke, and so on. They may insist on medical procedures—even surgeries—that clearly are unnecessary. They may avoid a wide range of activities, fearing exacerbation of their symptoms, to the point that they become isolated and inactive. For others, their health concerns become a core feature of their identity and dominate their interpersonal relationships. Often, the fears and complaints focus on a particular organ system.

The prevalence of somatic symptom disorder in the general population is an estimated 5 to 7 percent making this one of the most common categories of patient concerns in the primary care setting. These disorders can begin in childhood, adolescence, or adulthood and females tend to present with somatic symptom disorder more often than males, with an estimated female-to-male ratio of 10:1 (Kurlansik & Maffei, 2016). Carlos, in the following case study, was convinced there was a serious gastrointestinal illness causing his symptoms.

Illness anxiety disorder is very similar to somatic symptom disorder. The primary distinction in the *DSM-5* between the two disorders is that people with somatic symptom disorder actually experience physical symptoms and seek help for them, whereas people with illness anxiety disorder worry that they will develop or have a serious illness but do not always experience severe physical symptoms (Table 2). If a physical sign is present, it is typically a normal physical sensation. Formerly called hypochondriasis, people with this disorder have no physical illness, but they are overly preoccupied with the belief that a serious illness is present which adversely affects their daily life (French & Hameed, 2020).

People with illness anxiety disorder tend to misinterpret normal body sensations as a sign of a serious illness which causes significant distress and the

CASE STUDY

Carlos, a married man of 39, came to the clinic complaining, "I have trouble in my bowels and then it gets me in my head. My bowels just spasm on me, I get constipated." The patient's complaints dated back 12 years to an attack of "acute indigestion" in which he seemed to bloat up and pains developed in his abdomen and spread in several directions. He traced some of these pathways with his finger as he spoke. Carlos spent a month in bed at this time and then, based on an interpretation of something the doctor said, rested for another 2 months before working again. Words of reassurance from his doctor failed to take effect. He felt "sick, worried, and scared," feeling that he would never really get well again.

Carlos became very dependent on the woman he married when he was 22 years old. He left most of the decisions to her and showed little interest in sexual relations. His wife was several years older than he and did not seem to mind his totally passive approach to life. His attack of "acute indigestion" followed her death, 5 years after marriage, by 3 months during which he felt lost and hopeless. In time, he moved to a rural area and remarried. His second wife proved less willing to assume major responsibility for him than the first, and she made sexual demands on him that he felt unable to meet. He became more and more preoccupied with his gastrointestinal welfare.

(Source: Adapted from Cameron, N., & Rychlak, J. F. [1985]. *Personality development and psychopathology: A dynamic approach.* Boston: Houghton Mifflin.)

TABLE 2   *DSM-5* Diagnostic Criteria for Illness Anxiety Disorder

A. Preoccupation with having or acquiring a serious illness.

B. Somatic symptoms are not present or, if present, are only mild in intensity. If another medical condition is present or there is a high risk of developing a medical condition (e.g., strong family history is present), the preoccupation is clearly excessive or disproportionate.

C. There is a high level of anxiety about health, and the individual is easily alarmed about personal health status.

D. The individual performs excessive health-related behaviors (e.g., repeatedly checking his or her body for signs of illness) or exhibits maladaptive avoidance (e.g., avoiding doctor appointments and hospitals).

E. Illness preoccupation has been present for at least 6 months, but the specific illness that is feared may change over that period of time.

F. The illness-related preoccupation is not better explained by another mental disorder, such as somatic symptom disorder, panic disorder, generalized anxiety disorder, body dysmorphic disorder, obsessive-compulsive disorder or delusional disorder, somatic type.

Specify whether:

Care-seeking type: Medical care is frequently used.

Care-avoidant type: Medical care is rarely used.

SHADES OF GRAY

Consider this description of a young boy with health worries.

Ben is a 9-year-old whose teachers refer to him as "the worrier." At least once a week, he ends up in the school nurse's office with complaints of a headache or a stomachache, insisting he needs to rest or go home. The school nurse always dutifully takes Ben's temperature, which is always normal. Still, Ben will not go back to class. His frequent absences are causing his grades to decline. Ben's mother has taken him to his pediatrician a number of times, and multiple tests have revealed no medical problems that could be causing his frequent headaches and stomachaches.

Ben's health worries seem to have started about 8 months ago, after he had a serious case of the flu that kept him home in bed for over a week. Shortly after that, his parents separated because of marital conflict that had been escalating for years. When his mother has tried to talk with Ben about the possibility that his aches and pains are connected to his parents' separation, he has acknowledged that this could be true. But within a few days, he has experienced another headache or stomachache, saying "This time it's real, and it really hurts!"

Does Ben appear to have a somatic symptom disorder? If so, which one? (Discussion appears at the end of this chapter.)

tendency to seek immediate medical care. Typical body sensations that all people experience are misinterpreted by people with this disorder. For example, after hitting the all-you-can-eat China Buffet with your friends after studying for exams you leave the restaurant feeling really full . . . too full. For the rest of the night, your stomach is making all sorts of noises, you have heartburn, stomach cramps and gas. How would you interpret these physical symptoms? Most likely, you'd attribute these gastrointestinal symptoms to overeating Chinese food late at night. A person with illness anxiety disorder would likely panic at these body sensations and assume that they have a serious medical issue, like stomach cancer!

The core feature of illness anxiety disorder is the cycle of worry and reassurance- seeking behaviors about health concerns, as opposed to a focus on relief of distress caused by somatic symptoms as in Somatic Symptom Disorder (Scarella, Boland, & Barsky, 2019). People with illness anxiety disorder often consult with multiple physicians for the same medical problem and believe that their previous doctors missed their serious medical condition. People with this disorder often report that they frequently check their bodies for skin lesions, hair loss, or physical changes. These body-checking behaviors and health concerns significantly impact their social and occupational functioning (French & Hameed, 2020). It is important to note that unlike other somatic disorders that we will discuss later in this chapter, people with illness anxiety disorder are not faking these symptoms for or pretending to feel this way for attention. Rather, they become easily alarmed about their health and seek unnecessary medical tests and procedures to rule out or treat their exaggerated or imagined illnesses. This preoccupation with the idea that they are sick creates significant anxiety about health and disease despite reassurance from doctors or negative test results.

People with somatic symptom disorder or illness anxiety disorder may be prone to periods of anxiety and depression. They may express their distress as physical symptoms or mask the distress with alcohol abuse or antisocial behavior (Feder et al., 2001; Katon, Sullivan, & Walker, 2001; Löwe et al., 2008). Their symptoms and health concerns become a large part of their identity. Moreover, changes in their symptoms mirror their emotional well-being: When they are anxious or depressed, they report more physical complaints and worries than when they are not anxious or depressed (Bekhuis, Schoevers, van Borkulo, Rosmalen, & Boschloo, 2016). Recent research has found that people with somatic symptom disorder are more likely than people with illness anxiety disorder to report more severe health anxiety, somatic symptoms, depression, and higher health service use. Persons with somatic symptoms disorder are also more likely to experience higher rates of major depressive disorder, panic disorder, and agoraphobia than people with illness anxiety disorder (Newby, Hobbs, Mahoney, Shiu, Andrews, 2017). Comorbidities with other psychiatric disorders have been found among people with health anxiety (somatic symptoms disorder or illness anxiety disorder) such as generalized anxiety disorder (GAD), panic disorder (PD), and obsessive–compulsive disorder (OCD) are also high for this group (Villadsen et al., 2017).

Increased attention has been given to people infected with COVID-19, frontline health professionals, and to the community effort to reduce the transmission of this virus. A parallel concern has been raised by mental health professionals who hope to bring attention to the fact that the COVID-19 pandemic has created significant challenges for individuals with pre-existing mental health conditions, such as illness anxiety disorder. Recent research has explored the influence of the COVID-19 crisis on those with existing preoccupations related to their health and wellness. Heightened concerns about somatic sensations and fear of infection may be increasing ritualistic behaviors as a way of coping with the worry about becoming ill. The COVID-19 virus has caused profound adjustments to our daily function that can be seen in new precautionary and hygienic practices such as daily health screenings, mask wearing, and cleaning procedures all performed in an effort to reduce infection. For those with somatic symptom and illness anxiety disorder, this new way of life may become a trigger for anxiety, stress, and fear. Often, fear of illness or coming into contact with sick individuals results in high levels of distress and anxiety (Rivera & Carballea, 2020).

It's no surprise that somatic concerns related to personal health have increased during a global pandemic. These health-related concerns put those with somatic symptom disorders more at risk for psychological distress. However, the impact of this pandemic is affecting even those individuals without psychological disorders. Studies have found that general health concerns related to the COVID-19 pandemic have influenced the presence of somatization among the general population. Recently, studies in China have found a high proportion of somatic and anxiety symptoms among a nonclinical population (Huang et al., 2020) meaning that individuals without a clinical history of anxiety and somatic symptom disorders are experiencing an increase in somatic concerns that relate to COVID-19 such as preoccupation with physical symptoms like fatigue or aches and pains.

It is reasonable to speculate that people suffering from pre-existing mental health conditions, such as somatic symptom disorder and illness anxiety disorder, are at higher risk of relapse due to the stress of the COVID-19 pandemic. Due to the emotional impact of the COVID-19 pandemic it is reasonable to speculate that there is a higher risk for relapse among people suffering from a pre-existing mental health condition. Additionally, testing positive for COVID-19 would likely amplify the fears associated with the infection. When COVID-19-like symptoms occur, clinicians may have to differentially diagnose a possible worsening of a pre-existing somatic symptom disorder that has been triggered by the fear of being infected (Colizzi et al., 2020).

Studies find that a large percentage of the population complain of multiple somatic symptoms and health concerns that are not well-explained by a medical condition (Rief & Martin, 2014). For example, one large study of patients seeking care in cardiology, neurology, respiratory, and gastrointestinal clinics found

that nearly 20 percent had excessive illness anxiety (Tyrer et al., 2011), and 1 to 7 percent of the general population experiences severe levels of illness anxiety annually (Hedman & Axelsson, 2017). Multiple symptom complaints and concerns about health are more common in older adults than in middle-aged adults, even after taking into account the increased incidence of medical illness with age (Feder et al., 2001; Ladwig, Martin-Mittag, Lacruz, Henningsen, & Creed, 2010). The cultural norms with which older adults were raised often prohibited admitting to depression or anxiety. For this reason, older adults who are depressed or anxious may be more likely to express their negative emotions in somatic complaints, which are acceptable and expected in old age. Conversely, somatic complaints are often seen in children who may lack the language to express difficult emotions. Multiple studies have shown that high levels of health anxiety symptoms are significantly associated with unspecific somatic complaints (Villadsen et al., 2017).

The experience of multiple somatic symptoms and health concerns tends to be long-term and disabling. One longitudinal study found that people with many health complaints but no diagnosed medical illness were more likely to suffer disability, low income, impaired sleep, and psychological distress (Ladwig et al., 2010). They also were more likely to develop high blood pressure, obesity, and high cholesterol, were hospitalized more often, and were more likely to die in the 12-year follow-up than people with few health complaints.

It is important to note that diagnoses of somatic symptom disorder and illness anxiety disorder are new to the *DSM-5*, and more research is needed to better understand these disorders. Some studies indicate that these diagnoses are improvements on the *DSM-IV*, but it is not yet clear that the two disorders are fundamentally different, beyond the presence of physical symptoms and more functional impairment and psychiatric comorbidity in somatic symptom disorder (Newby, Hobbs, Mahoney, Wong, & Andrews, 2017). Some researchers are concerned that the criteria are too broad, lump too many different syndromes together, and risk mislabeling physical illness as mental illness (Frances, 2013; Rief & Martin, 2014).

Theories of Somatic Symptom Disorder and Illness Anxiety Disorder

Cognitive factors are thought to play a strong role in somatic symptom disorder and illness anxiety disorder (Hedman & Axelsson, 2017; Rief & Martin, 2014). People with these disorders often have dysfunctional beliefs about illness, often assuming that serious illnesses are common, and they tend to misinterpret any physical change in themselves as a sign for concern. They believe they are vulnerable to a wide range of physical illnesses and unable to tolerate pain. People with somatic symptom disorder tend to experience bodily sensations more intensely than other people, to pay more attention than others to physical symptoms and health-related information, and to catastrophize these symptoms (Rief & Martin, 2014; Witthöft et al., 2016). For example, a person with somatic symptom disorder might have generalized stomach pain that is intermittent. They might perceive mild and transient symptoms as severe; for example, they might feel that mild chest pain is a sign of serious cardiac illness. The person's interpretation of their experience may have a direct influence on their physiological processes by increasing their heart rate or blood pressure, thereby maintaining and exacerbating the pain. Further, the perception and cognition the client reports may influence how they present their symptoms to their physician and family. As a result, the physician may prescribe more potent medication or order more diagnostic tests, and family members may express more sympathy, excuse the person from responsibilities, and otherwise encourage passive behavior. Additionally, due to frequent fears of being sick, clients may frequently take leave from work, causing problems within their occupational functioning. Similarly, they might avoid social events for fear of a future "attack" (French & Hameed, 2020). In these cases, the person's misinterpretation and catastrophizing of symptoms reinforces their distorted perceptions, increasing the likelihood that they will interpret future symptoms similarly.

Somatic symptoms for which no sufficient physical causes are found, are frequently reported among those with posttraumatic stress disorder (PTSD), regardless of the traumatic event. Recent research has found that the symptoms of PTSD and somatic symptom disorder relate to each other, which suggests a common psychological factor underlying them both. Research on survivors of disasters has found that PTSD severity was positively correlated with somatization among survivors with PTSD reporting more physical symptoms than those without PTSD, a finding that was also found 14 years after the genocide in Ruanda. Additional studies have found that PTSD increased the risk of developing somatization symptoms but that new PTSD cases were not elevated in people with a somatization disorder. Taken together, it seems that somehow PTSD may mediate the development of somatization following a traumatic event (Morina, et al., 2018).

Various studies have explored the impact of trauma on somatic symptoms and highlight that negative physical or emotional events adversely impact psychological health and well-being. Studies have shown a significant association between childhood and adolescent emotional or sexual abuse and the severity of somatic symptoms (Nelson, Baldwin, & Taylor, 2012; Morina, et al., 2018). One study demonstrated that older women from seven European countries experienced somatic complaints such as fatigue and chronic pain that originated in childhood abuse. Specifically, older women reported somatic complaints, such as fatigue and chronic pain, in a general population sample from seven European countries. Women with a lifetime history of sexual or domestic abuse reported high levels of disabling chronic pain and somatic symptoms. Men with a lifetime history of psychological abuse also reported higher levels of somatic symptoms. A painful event, such as intimate partner violence, may indeed have long-term negative effects on health beyond the time of the violence itself (Eslami et al., 2019).

Treatment of Somatic Symptom Disorder and Illness Anxiety Disorder

Convincing people with these disorders that they need psychological treatment is not easy since the core symptoms relate to bodily complaints that are attributed to physical disease. Also, severity often ranges from mild symptoms that cause little impairment to severely disabling conditions which impact the individual's decision to seek help. Inconsistencies in diagnosis and lack of effective treatments often prolong the client's suffering and increases their frustration. Many patients complain of multiple symptoms concurrently and over time, while others suffer from only one persisting symptom. Suffering is not confined to the experience of bodily complaints; it also entails psychological and behavioral aspects like high health anxiety and checking behavior (Henningsen, 2018).

People with this disorder may insist that they are physically ill despite reassurance from multiple physicians and various medical tests establishing no physical illness. Psychodynamic therapies focus on providing insight into the connections between emotions and physical symptoms by helping people recall events and memories that may have triggered their symptoms. Behavioral therapies attempt to determine the reinforcements individuals receive for their symptoms and health complaints and to eliminate these reinforcements while increasing positive rewards for healthy behavior. Cognitive therapies for these disorders help people learn to interpret their physical symptoms appropriately and to avoid catastrophizing them, similar to the cognitive treatment of panic symptoms (see the chapter "Trauma, Anxiety, Obsessive-Compulsive, and Related Disorders"; Hedman & Axelsson, 2017). Cognitive-behavioral treatments that focus on identifying and challenging illness beliefs and misinterpretations of physical sensations, as well as exposing clients to their anxiety triggers, have shown positive effects (Olatunji et al., 2014). More recent treatments incorporating mindfulness and acceptance skills, including acceptance and commitment therapy, have shown promise as well (Eilenberg, Fink, Jensen, Rief, & Frostholm, 2016), as have trials of Internet-delivered CBT (Newby, et al., 2018).

Some clinicians use the belief systems and cultural traditions of individuals they are treating to motivate them to engage in therapy and help them overcome their physical complaints. Following is a case study that shows the use of cultural beliefs in treating a Hispanic woman with somatic symptom disorder.

CASE STUDY

Ellen was a 45-year-old woman who consulted many doctors for "high fever, vomiting, diarrhea, inability to eat, and rapid weight loss." After numerous negative lab tests, her doctor told her, "I can't go on with you; go to one of the *espiritistas* or a *curandera* (traditional healers)." A cousin then took her to a Spiritist center "for medicine." She was given herbal remedies—some baths and a tea of *molinillo* to take in the morning before eating. But the treatment focused mainly on the appearance of the spirit of a close friend who had died a month earlier from cancer. The spirit was looking for help from Ellen, who had not gone to help during her friend's illness because of her own family problems. Although psychological science can not directly corroborate the efficacy of the spiritual healer's treatment, we can see similarities between how the healer and a CBT therapist might help Ellen to clarify her conscious thinking about her strained circumstances and her somatic symptoms.

(Source: Adapted from Koss, J. D. (1990). Somatization and somatic complaint syndromes among Hispanics: Overview and ethnopsychological perspectives. *Transcultural Psychiatric Research Review, 27,* 5–29.)

The spiritual healer in Ellen's case recognized the cause of her somatic complaints as stress, anger, and guilt; helped her link her physical symptoms to these emotions; and helped her find ways to cope more adaptively with the emotions. The context for this intervention was not cognitive therapy or another type of psychotherapy used by the dominant, non-Hispanic culture but rather the cultural belief system concerning the role of spirits in producing physical symptoms.

Conversion Disorder (Functional Neurological Symptom Disorder)

A dramatic type of somatic symptom disorder is **conversion disorder (Functional Neurological Symptom Disorder)** which is parenthetically referenced in the DSM 5 as *Functional Neurological Symptom Disorder.* This disorder features neurological symptoms that can't be explained by a neurological disease or other medical condition. People with this disorder may lose neurological function in a part of their body that cannot be attributed to a medical cause. Some of the most common conversion symptoms are paralysis, tremors, blindness, mutism, nonepileptic seizures, loss of hearing, severe loss of coordination, difficulty swallowing or feeling "a lump in the throat", pseudocyesis (false pregnancy), and anesthesia in a limb. The diagnostic criteria require at least one symptom of altered motor or sensory function that is not due to recognized neurobiological or medical conditions, and not attributable to another disorder (American Psychiatric Association, 2013). One particularly dramatic conversion symptom is glove anesthesia, in which people lose all feeling in one hand, as if they were wearing a glove that wiped out physical sensation. As Figure 1 shows, however, the nerves in the hand are distributed in a way that makes this pattern of anesthesia highly unlikely. Conversion disorder typically involves one specific symptom, such as blindness or paralysis, but a person can have repeated episodes of conversion involving different parts of the body. The name "conversion disorder" presumes that psychological distress, often over a traumatic event, is "converted" into a physical symptom. Patients and physicians alike often object to this presumption (Stone et al., 2011), which supports the use of the parenthetical label

FIGURE 1   Glove Anesthesia. In the conversion symptom called glove anesthesia, the entire hand from fingertips to wrist becomes numb. Actual physical damage to the ulnar nerve, in contrast, causes anesthesia in the ring finger and little finger and beyond the wrist partway up the arm; damage to the radial nerve causes anesthesia only in parts of the ring, middle, and index fingers and the thumb and partway up the arm.

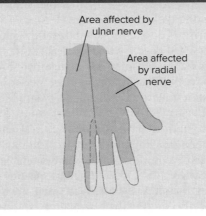

Area affected by ulnar nerve

Area affected by radial nerve

functional neurological symptom disorder, a more neutral name that doesn't presume a psychological cause. Unexplained neurological symptoms are relatively common. It has been estimated that 20 percent of patients in neurological clinics have symptoms with no apparent medical cause (Feinstein, 2011). The number of individuals meeting full criteria for persistent conversion disorder is very low, perhaps around 20 in 100,000 (Feinstein, 2011).

Theories of Conversion Disorder

Freud and his contemporaries viewed conversion symptoms as the result of the transfer of the psychic energy attached to repressed emotions or memories to physical symptoms. The symptoms often symbolized the specific concerns or memories being repressed. The reduction in anxiety was referred to as the *primary gain*. In addition, patients receive attention and concern from others and may be relieved of obligations and expectations, reinforcing the conversion symptoms. Freud called this the *secondary gain*.

Behavioral theories don't infer that conversion symptoms represent transferred unconscious anxiety, but they do emphasize the role conversion symptoms play in alleviating distress by removing the individual from difficult environments and allowing him or her to avoid unwanted responsibilities or situations (Deary, Chalder, & Sharpe, 2007). Behavioral models view these symptoms of conversion disorder as a learned maladaptive behavior that is reinforced by the environment (Marshall, 2017).

Conversion symptoms were quite common during the two world wars, when soldiers inexplicably would become paralyzed or blind and therefore unable to return to the front (Ironside & Batchelor, 1945). Many of the soldiers seemed unconcerned about their paralysis or blindness, a phenomenon called *la belle indifference*. Sometimes, the physical symptoms represented traumas the soldiers had witnessed. For example, a soldier who had shot a civilian in the chest might have chest pains. The impact of traumatic experience has been significantly associated with this disorder.

Children can also have conversion symptoms. Most often, their symptoms mimic those of someone close to them who has a physical illness or impairment (de Gusmão et al., 2014). For example, a child whose cherished grandfather has had a stroke and has lost functioning on his right side may become unable to use his right arm. As demonstrated in other psychological disorders, the experience of trauma can influence physical symptoms, as those displayed in conversion disorder. Various studies have found significant correlations between childhood trauma and the development of conversion disorder. Studies suggest that childhood sexual abuse is significantly associated with poor treatment outcome for physical symptoms in clients with conversion disorder and is associated with higher levels of symptomatology among clients with with nonepileptic seizures. Research supports trauma as a factor in the development of conversion disorder with more than 50 percent of participants in a case study series reporting a history of exposure to physical violence and 25 percent reporting a history of sexual assault in childhood. While a significant relationship between trauma experiences and conversion disorder have been demonstrated, it is also important to mention that traumatic events were not always present among studies exploring the role of trauma and stress in the development of conversion disorder. This is why the DSM 5 criteria for conversion disorder no longer requires the presence of a stressor for diagnosis (American Psychiatric Association, 2013; Van der Feltz-Cornelis et al., 2020).

People with conversion symptoms are highly hypnotizable (Roelofs et al., 2002; Stone et al., 2011). This supports the idea that stressful life events and maltreatment conversion symptoms may result from spontaneous self-hypnosis in which the mind dissociates (or "splits off") sensory or motor functions from conscious awareness. (Ludwig et al., 2018).

Neurological models suggest that conversion symptoms arise when sensory or motor areas of the brain are impaired by anxiety (Aybek & Vuilleumier, 2016). For example, in a case study of a woman with conversion mutism, researchers used functional neuroimaging to show that there was normal activity in speech areas of the brain (the inferior frontal gyrus) when the woman did a vocalization task, but impaired connectivity between these speech areas and areas of the brain that regulate anxiety (specifically the anterior cingulate) (Bryant & Das, 2012). After this woman received cognitive-behavioral therapy that overcame her mutism, connectivity between the speech areas and the areas regulating anxiety was restored, whereas the connectivity between speech areas and areas involved in the experience of anxiety (the amygdala) was reduced. Such studies suggest that conversion disorder does not involve impaired activity in areas of the brain associated specifically with the loss of functioning (such as speech areas in mutism) but instead changes in connectivity between these areas and areas associated with the generation and regulation of anxiety.

Treatment of Conversion Disorder

People with Conversion Disorder can be difficult to treat because they do not believe there is anything wrong with them psychologically, and prognosis is generally poor (Gelauff & Stone, 2016). For some people, the symptoms of conversion disorder may improve with time, even without treatment. However, a 3-year follow-up study of conversion disorder clients showed persistence in abnormal movements in more than 90 percent of the patients (Van der Feltz-Cornelis et al., 2020). This can occur after they receive a diagnosis of the disorder, reassurance that the symptoms aren't caused by an underlying medical problem, and validation that the symptoms are real. Psychoanalytic treatment for conversion disorder focuses on the expression of painful emotions and memories and on insight into the relationship between these and the conversion symptoms (Feinstein, 2011). Cognitive-behavioral treatments focus on relieving the person's anxiety centered on the initial trauma that caused the conversion symptoms and on reducing any benefits the person is receiving from the conversion symptoms (Lehn et al., 2016). For example, Jane, who is a survivor of rape, sought treatment for her conversion symptoms. Treatment for these symptoms and for any secondary gain will be addressed through both systematic desensitization therapy and exposure therapy (see the chapters "Theories and Treatment of Abnormality" and "Trauma, Anxiety, Obsessive-Compulsive, and Related Disorders"). A hierarchy of situations that Jane avoided—mostly situations that reminded her of her rape—was constructed. For the exposure therapy, Jane was aided in approaching those situations that made her feel anxious and in progressing through her hierarchy to increasingly more feared situations while practicing relaxation techniques. During the imagery sessions, Jane recounted the details of the assault first in general terms and later in great detail, including both the details of the situation and the details of her physiological and cognitive reactions to the assault. At first, Jane was able to describe the assault only in a whisper, but she cried at full volume. After crying, Jane's speech became increasingly louder, with occasional words uttered at full volume. Eventually, she regained a full-volume voice. Following treatment, Jane's PTSD symptoms also decreased, and they diminished further over the next year (Rothbaum & Foa, 1991).

Factitious Disorder

The final diagnosis in the *DSM-5* somatic symptom disorder category we will consider is **factitious disorder imposed on self,** in which a person deliberately fakes an illness specifically to gain medical attention in order to become a patient. People with factitious disorders fabricate, simulate, or exaggerate the symptoms of a physical or mental illness through a variety of deceptive methods for the purpose of gaining attention. For example, an individual may contaminate a urine sample with blood to manipulate a laboratory test, ingest a substance to create an abnormal test result or cause an illness by injecting fecal material into themselves to create an infection or

abscess (American Psychiatric Association, 2013). While physical illness is very common, people with this disorder can also fabricate symptoms of psychological disorders, such as depression or psychosis. People with this disorder may make false reports of suicidality and depressive symptoms or take medications to induce psychotic symptoms, like ingesting a hallucinogen like LSD before going to a psychological evaluation.

Factitious disorder is commonly referred to as *Munchhausen's syndrome*. Factitious disorder differs from somatic symptom disorder in that factitious disorder involves evidence that the individual is providing false information or behaving deceptively. Factitious disorder differs from **malingering,** in which people fake a symptom or a disorder in order to avoid an unwanted situation, such as military service, or in order to gain something, such as drugs or money donated through a GoFundMe fundraiser. The major difference between malingering and factitious disorder is the motivation for faking symptoms. In malingering the symptoms provide some practical or concrete external gain, while in factitious disorder the symptoms are intentionally created to gain attention. Malingering is not considered a psychological disorder although it can occur in the context of other mental illnesses, such as antisocial personality disorder (American Psychiatric Association, 2013).

Factitious disorder imposed on another (formerly referred to as *factitious disorder by proxy*) is diagnosed when an individual falsifies illness in another (e.g., child, pet, older adult). For example, parents fake or even create illnesses in their children in order to gain attention for themselves. They act as devoted and long-suffering protectors of their children, drawing praise for their dedicated nursing. Their children are subjected to unnecessary and often dangerous medical procedures and may actually die from their parents' attempts to make them ill.

With factitious disorder imposed on another, one individual fabricates an illness in another for an emotional benefit, such as praise from others for providing care. *kali9/Getty Images*

Seven-year-old Jennifer Bush appeared to be one victim of factitious disorder imposed by another. Jennifer underwent almost 200 hospitalizations and 40 operations in an effort to cure the mysterious array of her medical ailments. Her mother, Kathleen Bush, was with her through it all, consulting with medical professionals and standing by as the family's finances were ruined by Jennifer's medical bills. All the while, however, it seems Kathleen Bush was actually causing her daughter's illnesses by giving her unprescribed drugs, altering her medications, and even putting fecal bacteria in her feeding tube. Jennifer was removed from her mother's care and placed in a hospital for testing during which her health improved immediately. Bush eventually was arrested and convicted of aggravated child abuse and fraud and served 3 years in prison (Toufexis, Blackman, & Drummond, 1996). Almost two decades after this event, Jennifer still defends and supports her mother's claims of innocence (McMahon, 2018).

DISSOCIATIVE DISORDERS

States of consciousness involve an ongoing awareness of oneself and one's environment. Nevertheless, many everyday experiences such as daydreaming, losing track of time, being submerged in a book, and watching YouTube videos or a movie are all typical and temporary dissociations from our consciousness. Getting into, and especially getting out of, these states is typically relatively easy, so they are usually considered to be a normal experience. However, in some individuals, particularly those who have been exposed to psychological trauma, dissociation occurs unconsciously and cannot be controlled. When dissociation falls outside the typical spectrum a **dissociative disorder** can be diagnosed which is characterized by a disruption in the normal integration of memory, identity, consciousness, perception, behavior, and motor control that disrupts one or more aspects of psychological functioning (American Psychiatric Association, 2013; Radulovic, Lee, & Ortony, 2018).

Scientific interest in dissociative disorders has waxed and waned over the past century (Kihlstrom, 2005). There was a great deal of interest in dissociation in nineteenth-century France and in the United States among neurologists and psychologists such as Charcot, Freud, Carl Jung, and William James. French neurologist Pierre Janet viewed **dissociation** as a process in which components of mental experience are disconnected from consciousness but remain accessible through dreams and hypnosis. One case he investigated was that of a woman named Irene, who had no memory of the fact that her mother had died. However, during her sleep, Irene physically dramatized the events surrounding her mother's death.

After about 1910, interest in dissociative phenomena waned, partly because of the rise within psychology of behaviorism and biological approaches, which rejected the concept of repression and the use of techniques such as hypnosis in therapy. Ernest Hilgard (1977/1986) revitalized interest in dissociation in his experiments on the *hidden observer* phenomenon. He argued that there is an active mode to consciousness, which includes our conscious plans and desires and our voluntary actions. In its passive receptive mode, the conscious registers and stores information in memory without being aware that the information has been processed, as if a person has internal hidden observers that watch and record events in that person's life without that person being aware of it. Recent functional neuroimaging studies suggest that hypnosis is a process that can increase or decrease neural activity and change functional connectivity (and in activity) between brain regions. There is increasing evidence that subliminal information processes, problem solving, motivation, decisions mechanisms, or working memory can take place and operate unconsciously. (Csaszar-Nagy, Scholkmann, Kapócs, Bokkon, 2016).

Hilgard and his associates conducted experimental studies in which participants were hypnotized and given a suggestion that they would feel no pain during a painful procedure but would remember the pain when the hypnotist gave them a specific cue. These subjects indeed showed no awareness of pain during the procedure. When cued, they reported memories of the pain in a matter-of-fact fashion, as if a lucid, rational observer of the event had registered the event for the subject. Other research showed that some anesthetized surgical patients could later recall, under hypnosis, specific pieces of music played during the surgery. Again, it was as if a hidden observer was registering the events of the operation even while the patient was completely unconscious under anesthesia (Kihlstrom, 2001; Kihlstrom & Couture, 1992). Recent research on the phenomenon of the "hidden observer" suggests that this process may be due to the self-dissociation of the cognitive unconscious or might be a special state of the cognitive unconscious that emerges principally in highly susceptible individuals (Csaszar-Nagy et al., 2016).

For most people, the active and receptive modes of consciousness weave our experiences together so seamlessly that we do not notice any division between them. People who develop dissociative disorders, however, may have chronic problems integrating their active consciousness with their receptive consciousness (Hilgard, 1992; Lynn, Lilienfeld, Merckelbach, Giesbrecht, & van der Kloet, 2012). That is, the different aspects of consciousness in these people do not integrate with each other in expected ways but instead remain split and operate independently of each other.

We begin our discussion of specific dissociative disorders with dissociative identity disorder (DID), formerly known as multiple personality disorder. We then move to dissociative amnesia and depersonalization/derealization disorder. All these disorders involve frequent experiences in which various aspects of a person's "self" are split off from each other and felt as separate.

CASE STUDY

Eve White was a quiet, proper, and unassuming woman, a full-time homemaker and devoted mother to a young daughter. She sought help from a psychiatrist for painful headaches that were occurring with increasing frequency. The psychiatrist decided that her headaches were related to arguments she was having with her husband over whether to raise their young daughter in the husband's church (which was Catholic) or in her church (which was Baptist). After undergoing some marital therapy, Mrs. White's marriage improved and her headaches subsided for a year or so.

Then, her husband recontacted her therapist, alarmed over changes in his wife's behavior. She had gone to visit a favorite cousin in a town 50 miles away and during the visit had behaved in a much more carefree and reckless manner than she usually did. Mrs. White told her husband over the phone that she was not going to return home, and the two had a terrible fight that ended in an agreement to divorce. When Mrs. White did return home a few days later, however, she said she had no memory of the fight with her husband or, for that matter, of the visit with her cousin.

Shortly thereafter, Mrs. White apparently went shopping and bought hundreds of dollars worth of elaborate clothing, which the couple could not afford. When confronted by her husband about her expenditures, Mrs. White claimed to have no memory of buying the clothing.

At the urging of her husband, Mrs. White made an appointment with the therapist whom she had originally consulted about her headaches. In the session, she admitted that her headaches had returned and were much more severe now than before. Eventually, she also tearfully admitted that she had begun to hear a voice other than her own speaking inside her head and that she feared she was going insane. The therapist asked her more questions about the clothes-buying spree, and Mrs. White became more tense and had difficulty getting words out to discuss the incident. Then, as her therapist reported,

The brooding look in her eyes became almost a stare. Eve seemed momentarily dazed. Suddenly her posture began to change. Her body slowly stiffened until she sat rigidly erect. An alien, inexplicable expression then came over her face. This was suddenly erased into utter blankness. The lines of her countenance seemed to shift in a barely visible, slow, rippling transformation. For a moment there was the impression of something arcane. Closing her eyes, she winced as she put her hands to her temples, pressed hard, and twisted them as if to combat sudden pain. A slight shudder passed over her entire body.

Then the hands lightly dropped. She relaxed easily into an attitude of comfort the physician had never before seen in this patient. A pair of blue eyes popped open. There was a quick reckless smile. In a bright, unfamiliar voice that sparked, the woman said, "Hi, there, Doc!"

Still busy with his own unassimilated surprise, the doctor heard himself say, "How do you feel now?"

"Why just fine—never better! How you doing yourself, Doc? . . . She's been having a real rough time. There's no doubt about that," the girl said carelessly. "I feel right sorry for her sometimes. She's such a damn dope though. . . . What she puts up with from that sorry Ralph White—and all her mooning over that little brat . . . ! To hell with it, I say!" . . .

The doctor asked, "Who is 'she'?"

"Why, Eve White, of course. Your long-suffering, saintly, little patient."

"But aren't you Eve White?" he asked.

"That's for laughs," she exclaimed, a ripple of mirth in her tone. . . . "Why, I'm Eve Black," she said. . . . "I'm me and she's herself," the girl added. "I like to live and she don't. . . . Those dresses—well, I can tell you about them. I got out the other day, and I needed some dresses. I like good clothes. So I just went into town and bought what I wanted. I charged 'em to her husband, too!" She began to laugh softly. "You ought've seen the look on her silly face when he showed her what was in the cupboard!"

(Thigpen, C. H., and Cleckley, H. M., *The Three Faces of Eve*. McGraw-Hill Education, 1957. Used with permission.)

Dissociative Identity Disorder

Even within the realm of abnormal psychology, **Dissociative Identity Disorder (DID)** is one of the most controversial and fascinating disorders. DID has been portrayed on television and in movies for decades, often creating misconceptions and curiosity for this often confusing disorder. DID is a disorder defined by identity disruption marked by the presence of two or more distinct identities or personality states in

The movie *The Three Faces of Eve* depicts the story of a woman with dissociative identity disorder. Here, she has discovered extravagant articles of clothing in her closet that she doesn't remember buying. *Everett Collection*

TABLE 3 *DSM-5* Diagnostic Criteria for Dissociative Identity Disorder

A. Disruption of identity characterized by two or more distinct personality states, which may be described in some cultures as an experience of possession. The disruption in identity involves marked discontinuity in sense of self and sense of agency, accompanied by related alterations in affect, behavior, consciousness, memory, perception, cognition, and/or sensory-motor functioning. These signs and symptoms may be observed by others or reported by the individual.

B. Recurrent gaps in the recall of everyday events, important personal information, and/or traumatic events that are inconsistent with ordinary forgetting.

C. The symptoms cause clinically significant distress or impairment in social, occupational, or other important areas of functioning.

D. The disturbance is not a normal part of a broadly accepted cultural or religious practice. Note: In children, the symptoms are not better explained by imaginary playmates or other fantasy play.

E. The symptoms are not attributable to the direct physiological effects of a substance (e.g., blackouts or chaotic behavior during intoxication) or another medical condition (e.g., complex partial seizures).

Reprinted with permission from the *Diagnostic and Statistical Manual of Mental Disorders,* Fifth Edition. Copyright ©2013 by American Psychiatric Association. All Rights Reserved.

an individual (Table 3). According to the DSM 5, the presence these identities create a pronounced discontinuity in the sense of self, feelings of control over actions, affect, consciousness, and memory in the individual leading to clinically significant distress or impairment of functioning (American Psychiatric Association, 2013).

The presence of multiple, partially independent, identities that co-exist within the individual is referred to as *alters* or alternate identities. Each of these identities has their own first-person perspective or experience of self-consciousness. Consequently, these identities often report their own subjective experiences, memories, and their own sense of agency and will. DID individuals often report being unaware of other identities or report amnesia for experiences that presumably occurred when other identities were in control of the host identity (Sar, Dorahy, & Krüger, 2017). Sometimes people with DID report periods of amnesia during the periods when alters are in control or having one-way amnesia between certain alter identities. In these instances, one alter is aware of what the other is doing, but the second alter is completely amnesic for periods when the first identity is in control. This transition from one alter to another is called a "switch"during which one identity essentially pushes another out of charge (Howell, 2011).

Individuals with DID often experience recurrent memory gaps in personal history and lapses in memory for learned activities such as job skills, computer skills, or driving skills. According to the DSM 5, memory gaps in everyday activities are also common for people with DID such as finding unexplained objects among their possessions, finding unfamiliar drawings or writings they must have created or suddenly "coming to" in the midst of an activity (American Psychiatric Association, 2013). These recurrent memory gaps are not consistent with ordinary forgetting and thought to be a disconnection from consciousness when they are under the control of an alter identity. As with Eve White, people with DID may suddenly discover unknown objects in their home or may lose objects. People they do not recognize might approach them on the street, claiming to know them. They may consistently receive mail addressed to someone with a different first or last name. Verifying reports of amnesia is difficult, but some studies suggest that information and memories tend to transfer between identities, even in individuals who believe that certain identities experience amnesia (Kong, Allen, & Glisky, 2008; Lynn et al., 2012).

Each alter identity has different ways of perceiving and relating to the world, and each takes control over the individual's behavior on a regular basis, which causes significant distress and dysfunction. As was true of Eve White/Black, the alternate identities can be extremely different from one another, with distinct facial expressions, speech characteristics, physiological responses, gestures, interpersonal styles, attitudes. Additionally, these alters are often different ages, gender, sexual orientation with significant differences in physiological response than the host identity. Differences in visual acuity, response to medication, allergic reactions, glucose levels in diabetic patients, heart rate, blood pressure, immune function, and brain activity have been noted in various studies (International Society for the Study of Trauma and Dissociation [ISSTD], 2011). During this time, the individual host may report feeling like a depersonalized observer of their own speech, body, or actions. Despite depictions of DID in movies and TV, these alters are best characterized as a fragmentation or splintering of identity, rather than the growth of separate individual identities. Alters are typically fragments of the host that are created as a way of coping with traumatic experiences. The dissociation that influences the development of alters is done to escape the physical and/or emotional pain of trauma (Brand et al., 2016).

PROFILES

Well, say B. J. hears someone call me names, then he would strike me to do something, like I'd be running at the other kid, but it wouldn't be my legs, I'd be saying to my legs, "no . . . , stop . . . , " but they'd keep going on their own because that's B. J. doing that. Then my arm would be going at the other kid, hitting him, and I could see my arm doing that, but I couldn't stop it, and it wouldn't hurt when my hand hit him, not until later when B. J. goes back in and then my arm is my own arm. Then it starts hurting.
(Source: Hornstein, N. L., & Putnam, F. W. [1992]. Clinical phenomenology of child and adolescent dissociative disorders. *Journal of the American Academy of Child & Adolescent Psychiatry, 31,* 1077–1085.)

Alters can take many different shapes and perform various functions, leading to the classification of various alter types that are created by the host identity for specific purpose. Types like the child, persecutor, helper, opposite gender, memory trace, and suicidal alters are among them (Öztürk & Sar, 2016). Child alters—alters that are young children, who do not age as the individual ages—appear to be the most common type of alter (Ross, 1997). Childhood trauma is often associated with the development of DID. A child alter may be created during a traumatic experience to take on the role of victim in the trauma, while the *host*

personality escapes into the protection of psychological oblivion. Or an alter may be created as a type of big brother or sister to protect the host personality from trauma. When a child alter is "out," or in control of the individual's behavior, the adult may speak and act in a childlike way. Persecutory alters are hostile to the host personality and often originate from the shame and anger related to the traumatic experience and to the perpetrator (Öztürk & Sar, 2016). These alters inflict pain or punishment on the other alters by engaging in self-mutilative behaviors, such as self-cutting or -burning and suicide attempts (Coons & Milstein, 1990; Ross, 1997). A persecutor alter may engage in a dangerous behavior, such as taking an overdose of pills or jumping in front of a truck, and then "go back inside," leaving the host personality to experience the pain. Persecutors may believe that they can harm other personalities without harming themselves. Helper alters display a kind and well-intentioned attitude toward the host (Öztürk & Sar, 2016). The function of this identity is to offer advice to other personalities or perform functions the host personality is unable to perform, such as engaging in sexual relations or hiding from abusive parents. Helpers sometimes control the switching from one identity to another or act as passive observers who can report on the thoughts and intentions of all the other identities (Ross, 1997).

While DID is classified as a dissociative disorder, it is best described as a chronic, complex post-traumatic developmental disorder as various studies have found significant associations with psychological trauma. In cases of DID, adverse experiences that typically begin in early childhood result in significant dissociation and the creation of alter identities. One basic assumption is that alters emerge due to an unsuccessful attempt of the child to process psychological trauma (Öztürk & Sar, 2016). The alters are the result of the child's inability to develop and maintain a unified sense of self since identity is still maturing within the individual. Meaning, as a result of psychological trauma, the dissociations within the individual occur at the level of identity during a period of critical development that leads to fragmentation. A very significant number of people with DID report a history of abuse, and it is widely supported that DID develops when a child is exposed to a chaotic and dysfunctional environment, coercion, and overt severe physical and/or sexual abuse (Şar, Dorahy, & Krüger, 2017).

Trauma may occur as a one-time event, intermittently, or on a continuous and chronic basis. Sexual abuse, physical trauma, and growing up in an environment of domestic violence often serve as triggers to the development of this form of complex trauma. Additionally, vicarious exposure to trauma, such as witnessing an event or watching a loved one undergoing the actual traumatic event(s), is linked to the development of DID. More severe and earlier-onset child abuse appears to differentiate DID from other disorders, like PTSD. Large-scale clinical and epidemiological studies in the United States, Australia, Turkey, Puerto Rico, the Netherlands, Germany, and Canada have consistently found that DID is linked to antecedent chronic abusive experiences in childhood, typically at the hands of an attachment figure or care giver. In most clinical series, childhood abuse and/or neglect is reported by 90 to 100 percent of the patients directly during the study examination. Dissociative amnesia for childhood events may prevent such reports by some people with DID. It is also speculated that the experience of abuse and neglect may activate feelings of alienation, isolation, and loneliness which may compound the impact of trauma and the development and maintenance of DID (Rehan et al., 2017; Şar et al., 2017).

Individuals with DID often feel very isolated and lonely with the belief that they are the only one in the world who is "different" from others and the confusion that stems from not fully understand themselves. As a result, people with DID experience depersonalization and derealization that was likely experienced throughout childhood. Individuals with DID often feel shame, betrayal, self-blame, anger, and fear, but more than anything else, they feel highly alienated. These feelings of alienation are most connected to them feeling alone, disconnected, and different from others (Şar, et al., 2017). The contribution of psychological trauma in the development of dissociative disorders is widely acknowledged among professionals such that the dissociative disorders chapter directly follows the chapter on trauma- and stressor-related disorders in the DSM and a dissociative subtype now exists within the PTSD classification (Ducharme, 2017). Additionally, PTSD is frequently comorbid with DID (Spiegel et al., 2013).

Both adults and children diagnosed with DID exhibit a host of behavioral and emotional problems (Silberg, 2014). Children may have poor or erratic performance in school. They are prone to antisocial behavior, such as stealing, fire setting, and aggression. They may engage in sexual relations and abuse alcohol or illicit drugs at an early age. They tend to show many symptoms of posttraumatic stress disorder (PTSD; see the chapter "Trauma, Anxiety, Obsessive-Compulsive, and Related Disorders"), including hypervigilance, flashbacks to traumas they have endured, traumatic nightmares, and an exaggerated startle response. Their emotions are unstable, alternating among explosive outbursts of anger, deep depression, and severe anxiety.

Self-injurious behavior is common among people with DID and often is the reason they seek or are taken for treatment. Impulsive risk-taking behaviors, self-harm, (such as self-inflicted burns or other injuries, wrist slashing, and drug overdoses) and suicide attempts are common. Recent research suggests that trauma, pathological dissociation, and depersonalization/derealization influence the function of self-harm. Many studies have found a strong association between high levels of dissociation and increased frequency of self-harming behavior. Individuals with dissociative disorders often report emotional numbness feelings shortly self-injury. From this perspective, it is feasible to understand individuals who engage in self-harm as either escaping from uncomfortable dissociative states or experiencing internal conflicts in which one dissociative part of the self is being abusive toward another. Recent research has also found that people with dissociative disorders more frequently engage in self injury and suicide attempt than those who do not dissociate. Individuals with dissociative disorders are also more likely to use multiple methods of self-injury and engage in self-harm at earlier ages (Kılıç, Coşkun, Bozkurt, Kaya, & Zoroğlu, 2017; Nobakht & Dale, 2017;).

While DID is often discussed as a rare disorder mostly diagnosed in North America, recent research has found prevalence of this disorder worldwide. Individuals with DID are consistently identified in outpatient, inpatient, and community samples around the world. A recent prospective study of DID clients from Argentina, Australia, Belgium, Brazil, Canada, Germany, Israel, the Netherlands, New Zealand, Norway, Singapore, Slovakia, South Africa, Sweden, Taiwan, and the United States identified individuals with DID on every continent except Antarctica. It is also posited by researchers that this disorder is underdiagnosed among professionals who may lack the experience to properly identify this disorder early in a client's assessment process (Brand et al., 2016).

DID is often described as an uncommon disorder that affects a very small number of people each year. However, the prevalence rates found among clients in psychiatric inpatient units, psychiatric outpatient units, the general population, and specialized inpatient units for substance dependence suggest otherwise. Based on recent studies, it is more likely that DID is underdiagnosed and consequently undertreated among the general population. DID is found in approximately 1.1 to 1.5 percent of representative community samples. Specifically, in a representative sample of 658 individuals from New York State, 1.5 percent met criteria for DID when assessed and similarly, a large study of community women in Turkey (n = 628) found 1.1 percent of the women had DID. Additional studies have found DID in 0.4 to 6.0 percent of clinical samples. Studies assessing groups with particularly high exposure to trauma or cultural oppression show the highest prevalence rates. For example, 6 percent of consecutive admissions in a highly traumatized, U.S. inner city sample were diagnosed with DID. By contrast, only 2 percent of consecutive psychiatric inpatients received a diagnosis of DID in the Netherlands. The difference in prevalence may partially stem from the very high rates of trauma exposure and oppression in the U.S. inner-city, primarily minority sample (Brand et al., 2016).

While agreement on DID prevalence rates is often difficult, recent additional international studies have led to a consensus that rates of DID are approximately 5 percent among psychiatric inpatients, 2 to 3 percent among outpatients, and 1 percent in the general population. Prevalences appear heightened among adolescent psychiatric outpatients and in the psychiatric emergency units which suggest that acute transient crisis situations may exacerbate underlying DID. These crisis situations usually serve as a diagnostic window for the clinician as it is possible that the core symptoms of DID remain dormant until a stressful event triggers a more prominent manifestation (Sar, et al., 2017). The average DID patient spends years in the mental health system before being correctly diagnosed. These patients have high rates of suicidal and self-destructive behavior, experience significant disability, and often require expensive and restrictive treatments such as inpatient and partial hospitalization (Brand et al., 2016). The vast majority of people diagnosed with this disorder are adult women. People with DID have an increased risk of comorbid psychiatric conditions including PTSD, depression, personality disorders, substance abuse disorders, eating disorders, and conversion or somatoform disorders (Brand et al., 2013; Rehan et al., 2017).

In addition to identity disturbance it is not uncommon for both children and adults, with DID to report hearing voices, a phenomenon most associated with psychotic disorders like schizophrenia. Voice hearing can often occur in trauma spectrum disorders such as PTSD and dissociative disorders although there is no mention in previous or current versions of the DSM (Shinn et al., 2020). Some report awareness that their actions or words are being controlled by other identities. For example, Joe, an 8-year-old boy with DID, described how "a guy inside of me," called B. J. (for Bad Joey), would make him do "bad things." Research on combat trauma has shown that voices could be heard inside or outside the head, frequently commanded self-harm, and were often crying or criticizing in nature. These voices were often those of soldiers whose deaths they had witnessed or someone they killed in combat. Consistent with prior studies, recent research has found that the content of the voices was often symbolically or thematically related

to trauma but that the voices were distinct from the memory of the traumatic events and not attributed to other trauma-related symptoms, such as a flashbacks (Shinn et al., 2020).

Issues in Diagnosis

DID was first included as a diagnostic category in the *DSM-III*, published in 1980. The availability of specific diagnostic criteria for this disorder increased the number of identified cases over the next few decades. At that same time, the diagnostic criteria for schizophrenia were made more specific in the *DSM-III*. These changes may have impacted individuals who would previously have been diagnosed with schizophrenia could now be diagnosed with DID. One final, and important, influence on diagnostic trends was the publication of a series of influential papers by psychiatrists describing persons with DID whom they had treated (Coons, 1980; Greaves, 1980; Rosenbaum, 1980). These cases aroused interest in the disorder within the psychiatric community and often gained popularity among the general population after the appearance of several best-selling books and movies. Even though this disorder has been officially recognized in the DSM since 1980, many people with DID share a long and painful history misdiagnoses, inefficient treatment, and several admissions to psychiatric facilities. To date, many clinicians and scientists still question the validity and even the very existence of DID which has created a significant barrier for those with DID (Reinders et al., 2018).

Although recent research has enhanced our understanding of DID, this disorder is often underdiagnosed and undertreated. Research studies examining mental health professionals suggest that a lack of training, coupled with skepticism, about dissociative disorders seems to contribute to the underrecognition and delayed diagnosis. For example, in a survey of Puerto Rican psychologists only 5 percent reported being knowledgeable about DID, and the majority of those in the sample (73 percent) reported little or no clinical training about DID. It appears that clinicians' skepticism, about DID has increased as their knowledge about the disorder has decreased which directly impacts the ability to effectively treat those suffering with this disorder.

Among U.S. clinicians who reviewed a vignette of an individual presenting with the symptoms of DID, only 60 percent of them accurately diagnosed DID. Clinicians misdiagnosed the patient as most frequently suffering from PTSD, followed by schizophrenia and major depression. Accurate diagnoses are most often made by clinicians with experiencing treating DID and who were not skeptical about the disorder. The inability for individual to receive an accurate DID diagnosis prolongs the amount of time in which that person must suffer with DID symptoms and ineffective treatment. Recent research has found that from the time an individual begins seeking treatment for DID symptoms to the time of an accurate diagnosis clients received an average of four prior other diagnoses and spent 7 to 12 years in mental health services. Overall, current research suggests that DID is significantly underdiagnosed and underrecognized among mental health professionals, despite levels of experience and/or professional degree and this disorder is found around the world, despite claims that this is primarily found in North America (Brand et al., 2016; Reinders et al., 2018).

While the diagnostic criteria for DID had not changed very much since *DSM-III, DSM-5* includes some important changes. *DSM-5* added the words "or an experience of possession" to Criterion A (see Table 4) to make the criteria more applicable to diverse cultural groups by identifying a common presentation of DID in non-Western cultures as well as subgroups in Western cultures (e.g., immigrant and some conservative or fundamentalist religious groups; Spiegel et al., 2013). Many features of DID can be influenced by an individual's cultural background and the fragmented identities may take the form of possessing spirits, deities, demons, animals, or mythical figures considered to be real. In contrast to culturally normative possession states that may be part of a spiritual practice, abnormal possession DID is experienced as involuntary, distressing, and uncontrollable, and often involves conflict between the individual and social, cultural, or religious norms (Criterion D). Research has shown that cases of pathological possession with dissociative symptoms occur in many countries (Cardeña, van Duijl, Weiner, & Terhune, 2009), and one study showed that nearly 60 percent of patients with DID in Western settings felt as if they were possessed (Ross, 2011). Other *DSM-5* changes include that transitions in identity do not have to be directly observed by others but instead could be self-reported (Criterion A), and problems with recall (amnesia) include everyday events and not just traumatic experiences (Criterion B).

Some studies suggest that Latinx people, both within and outside the United States, may be more likely than other ethnic groups to experience dissociative symptoms in response to traumas. For example, a study of Vietnam veterans found that Latinx veterans were more likely than non-Latinx veterans to show dissociative symptoms (Koopman et al., 2001). Another study conducted with Latinx survivors of community violence in the United States found that those who were less acculturated to mainstream U.S. culture were more likely to show dissociative symptoms than were those who were more acculturated (Marshall & Orlando, 2002). Dissociative symptoms may be part of the syndrome *ataque de nervios,* a culturally accepted reaction to stress among Latinx people that involves transient periods of loss of consciousness, convulsive movements, hyperactivity, assaultive behaviors, and impulsive acts (see the chapter "Trauma, Anxiety, Obsessive-Compulsive, and Related Disorders").

Substantial controversy has revolved around claims by some people with dissociative disorders that during adulthood they have recovered memories of severe abuse after years of not remembering the abuse. We discuss this controversy in detail at the end of this chapter.

Theories of Dissociative Identity Disorder

Many theorists who study DID view it as the result of coping strategies used by persons faced with intolerable trauma—most often childhood sexual and/or physical abuse—that they are powerless to escape

---

TABLE 4   *DSM-5* Diagnostic Criteria for Dissociative Amnesia

A. An inability to recall important autobiographical information, usually of a traumatic or stressful nature, that is inconsistent with ordinary forgetting. Note: Dissociative amnesia most often consists of localized or selective amnesia for a specific event or events; or generalized amnesia for identity and life history.

B. The symptoms cause clinically significant distress or impairment in social, occupational, or other important areas of functioning.

C. The disturbance is not attributable to the direct physiological effects of a substance (e.g., alcohol or other drug of abuse, a medication) or a neurological or other medical condition (e.g., partial complex seizures, sequelae of a traumatic brain injury, other neurological condition).

D. The disturbance is not better explained by dissociative identity disorder, posttraumatic stress disorder, acute stress disorder, somatic symptom disorder, or major or mild neurocognitive disorder.

Specify if:

With Dissociative Fugue: Apparently purposeful travel or bewildered wandering that is associated with amnesia for identity or for other important autobiographical information.

(ISSTD, 2011; Putnam, Zahn, & Post, 1990; Schimmenti & Caretti, 2016). As Ellason and Ross (1997, p. 64) describes:

> The little girl being sexually abused by her father at night imagines that the abuse is happening to someone else, as a way to distance herself from the overwhelming emotions she is experiencing. She may float up to the ceiling and watch the abuse in a detached fashion. Now not only is the abuse not happening to her, but she blocks it out of her mind—that other little girl remembers it, not the original self. In this model, DID is an internal divide-and-conquer strategy in which intolerable knowledge and feeling is split up into manageable compartments. These compartments are personified and take on a life of their own.

Indeed, most studies find that the majority of people diagnosed with DID self-report having been a victim of sexual or physical abuse during childhood (Brand et al., 2016; Dorahy et al., 2014; Shinn et al., 2020). In turn, dissociative experiences are commonly reported by survivors of child sexual abuse (Şar et al., 2017; Vonderlin et al., 2018). For example, in a study of 135 persons with DID, 92 percent reported having been sexually abused, and 90 percent reported having been repeatedly physically abused (Ellason, Ross, & Fuchs, 1996; see also Putnam, Guroff, Silberman, & Barban, 1986). Researchers have found similar results in studies in which patients' reports of abuse were corroborated by at least one family member or by emergency room reports (Brand et al., 2016). The abuse most often was carried out by parents or other family members and was chronic over an extended period of childhood. Other types of trauma that have been associated with the development of DID include kidnapping, natural disasters, war, famine, and religious persecution (Ross, 1999). Some people with DID report having been the victim of torture and abuse by cults, human trafficking, multigenerational abusive family systems, and pedophile networks (ISSTD, 2011).

Some evidence indicates that people who develop DID tend to be highly suggestible and hypnotizable and may use self-hypnosis to dissociate and escape their traumas (Dell, 2018; Kihlstrom, Glisky, & Angiulo, 1994). They may create the alternate identities to help them cope with their traumas, much as a child might create imaginary playmates to ease pangs of loneliness. These alters can provide the safety, security, and nurturing that they are not receiving from their caregivers. Retreating into their alternate personalities or using these personalities to perform frightening functions becomes a chronic way of coping with life.

However, not all researchers believe trauma plays the determining role in DID (see Lynn et al., 2012). A contrasting view is the sociocognitive model (Spanos, 1994; Lynn et al., 2012), which argues that the alternate identities are created by patients who adopt the idea or narrative of DID as an explanation that fits their lives. The identities are not true personalities with clear-cut demarcations but rather metaphors used by the patients to understand their subjective experiences. Patients are not faking their multiple identities but rather are playing out a role that helps them deal with stresses in their lives and is reinforced by attention and concern from others, and by cultural narratives, psychotherapy, and media. Both trauma and sociocognitive factors likely play a role in the development of this disorder (Sar, Krüger, Martinez-Taboas, Middleton, & Dorahy, 2013).

Whereas psychosocial explanations of DID include developmental traumatization and sociocognitive conditions, biological factors include trauma-generated neurobiological responses. Meaning, psychological trauma impacts brain function that can directly relate to DID symptoms. At this point, no direct examination of genetics has occurred in DID. However, it is likely to exist, given the genetic link to dissociation in general and in relation to childhood adversity in particular (Şar et al., 2017). A few family history studies suggest that DID may run in some families (Coons, 1984; Dell & Eisenhower, 1990). In addition, studies of twins and of adopted children have found evidence that the tendency to dissociate is substantially affected by genetics (Becker-Blease et al., 2004; Pieper, Out, Bakermans-Kranenburg, & van IJzendoorn, 2011). The ability and tendency to dissociate as a coping response may to some extent be biologically determined.

Early life stressors, such as childhood trauma, have long-lasting detrimental effects on the brain. Research using brain imaging has found that individuals with DID can be accurately differentiated from non-DID individuals based on abnormal brain structures and function. Models of trauma-related dissociation suggest that the cingulate gyrus, medial prefrontal cortex, and superior frontal lobe regions are significantly affected in the dissociation process. Additionally, people with DID have smaller hippocampal volume which seems to be the result of exposure to stress hormones due to early psychological trauma. Although it is currently unknown how early traumatization affects the development of the brain, long-lasting widespread patterns of affected brain regions, most prominently in the frontal grey and white matter regions, have been observed. Applying biomarkers in the process of assessing DID could reduce misdiagnoses, treatment time, treatment costs, and ultimately improve the patient's quality of life (Reinders et al., 2019).

Treatment of Dissociative Identity Disorder

Treating DID can be extremely challenging. Current DID treatment guidelines recommend a three–phase, trauma-focused psychotherapy process. In the first stage, clinicians focus on safety issues, stabilize DID symptoms, and establish a therapeutic alliance (the trusting and cooperative relationship between therapist and client). Failure to stabilize the patient or a premature focus on traumatic memories can result in deterioration in functioning and a diminished sense of safety. In the second stage of treatment, following the ability to regulate affect and manage their symptoms, patients begin processing, grieving, and resolving trauma. In the third and final stage of treatment, patients integrate dissociated self-states and become more socially engaged. The goal of treatment is integrating all the alter identity into one coherent sense of self in which the client is able to develop the capacity for coping with distress and trusting healthy relationships (Brand et al., 2016; Brand, Loewenstein, & Spiegel, 2014; ISSTD, 2011).

This integration is sometimes achieved by "giving voice" to each identity and helping the identities become aware of one another, determining the function or role of each personality, helping each personality confront and work through the traumas that led to the disorder and the concerns each one has or represents, and negotiating with the personalities for unification into one personality who has learned adaptive styles of coping with stress. Building trust and therapeutic alliance is critical, as patients with DID often have experienced traumas that have completely shattered their trust in others. The therapist may interact with each of the alters to engage them in the process of reviewing and understanding the trauma history and integrating their memories and strengths into one coherent personality. Possession-form DID likely requires culturally adapted treatments, perhaps involving indigenous healers (Martinez-Taboas, 2005; Spiegel et al., 2013).

The ultimate goal of DID treatment is not to eliminate the different alters but to have them co-exist in a coordinated way. One of the few studies to empirically evaluate the treatment of DID found that patients who were able to integrate their identities through treatment remained relatively free of symptoms over the subsequent 2 years (Ellason & Ross, 1997). These patients also reported few symptoms of substance abuse or depression and were able to reduce their use of antidepressants and antipsychotic medications. In contrast, patients who had not achieved integration during treatment continued to show symptoms of DID and a number of other disorders. A more recent study (using clinician reports) suggests that DID treatment can improve functioning for as long as 6 years (Myrick et al., 2017). These studies did not compare the outcome of the clients who received therapy with that of patients who did not, nor did they compare different types of therapy.

Dissociative Amnesia

In DID, individuals experience amnesia for those periods of time when their alternate identities are in control. Yet some people have significant periods of amnesia without assuming alternate identities. They cannot remember important facts about their lives and their personal identities and typically are aware of large gaps in their memory or knowledge of themselves. **Dissociative amnesia** (Table 4) is characterized by functional impairment that results from an inability to recall autobiographical information. This amnesia may be localized to a specific event or time period or it can generalized to a person's identity and life history (American Psychiatric Association, 2013; Staniloiu & Markowitsch, 2014) and affected people have an increased and possibly underestimated risk of suicide. Dissociative amnesia affects approximately 1.8% of adults in any given year (1% for males; 2.6% for females). The onset of dissociative amnesia is typically sudden and individuals may report multiple episodes. The duration of memory loss can range from minutes to decades. Some episodes of dissociative amnesia can resolve rapidly whereas other episodes may persist for long periods of time with some individuals gradually recalling the dissociated memories years later (American Psychiatric Association, 2013).

Dissociative amnesia affects memory systems and typically prevents individuals from connecting to the past. Theories on dissociative amnesia suggest that these types of memory failures result from inordinate psychological stress that prevents the integration of traumatic and normal conscious experiences, making trauma-related memories inaccessible. Recent studies similarly describe this phenomenon as a process whereby individuals automatically lose access to memories of an entire traumatic event or details of that event, resulting in significant memory gaps or no memory at all as a result of dissociation. Dissociative amnesia can also generalize to identity and life history, causing clinically significant distress or impairment in social, occupational, affective, and other important areas of functioning. This disorder, as others in this category, is strongly associated with psychological trauma. It has been argued by some that amnesia of traumatic events can be protective, as evidenced in survivors of childhood sexual abuse suffering from dissociative amnesia who had less depression and anxiety than survivors without it (Radulovic et al., 2018).The prevalence of dissociative amnesia and its accompanying clinical features differ substantially across countries, populations, and cultures (Staniloiu & Markowitsch, 2014).

TABLE 5 Differences Between Psychogenic and Organic Amnesia	
There are several important differences between psychogenic amnesia and organic amnesia.	
Psychogenic Amnesia	**Organic Amnesia**
Caused by psychological factors	Caused by biological factors (such as disease, drugs, and blows to the head)
Seldom involves anterograde amnesia (inability to learn new information acquired since onset of amnesia)	Often involves anterograde amnesia
Can involve retrograde amnesia (inability to remember events from the past)	Can involve retrograde amnesia
Retrograde amnesia often only for personal information, not for general information	Retrograde amnesia usually for both personal and general information

Amnesia is considered to be either organic or psychogenic (Table 5). **Organic amnesia** is caused by brain injury resulting from disease, drugs, accidents (such as blows to the head), or surgery. Organic amnesia that involves the inability to remember new information is known as **anterograde amnesia. Psychogenic amnesia** arises in the absence of any brain injury or disease and is thought to have psychological causes. **Retrograde amnesia,** which is most associated with dissociation, involves memory impairments that are mostly limited to memories for past events and personal history. Anterograde dissociative amnesia, where memories for new events are impaired, rarely occurs without significant retrograde memory impairments. Functional neuroimaging studies of dissociative amnesia with retrograde memory impairments show changes in the neural network associated with autobiographical memory (Radulovic et al., 2018).

Amnesias for specific periods of time around traumas appear to be fairly common, but generalized retrograde amnesias for an individual's entire past and identity appear to be very rare. Studies of people in countries that have been the site of attempted genocides, ethnic cleansings, and wars have suggested that the rate of dissociative amnesias in these countries may be elevated. For example, a study of 810 Bhutanese refugees in Nepal found that almost 20 percent of those who had been tortured during conflicts in their countries could be diagnosed with dissociative amnesia (van Ommeren et al., 2001).

CASE STUDY

Some years ago a man was found wandering the streets of Eugene, Oregon, not knowing his name or where he had come from. The police, who were baffled by his inability to identify himself, called in Lester Beck . . . , a psychologist they knew to be familiar with hypnosis, to see if he could be of assistance. He found the man eager to cooperate and by means of hypnosis and other methods was able to reconstruct the man's history. . . .

Following domestic difficulties, the man had gone on a drunken spree completely out of keeping with his earlier social behavior, and he had subsequently suffered deep remorse. His amnesia was motivated in the first place by the desire to exclude from memory the mortifying experiences that had gone on during the guilt-producing episode. He succeeded in forgetting all the events before and after this behavior that reminded him of it. Hence the amnesia spread from the critical incident to events before and after it, and he completely lost his sense of personal identity.

Source: Hilgard, E. R. [1977/1986]. *Divided consciousness: Multiple controls in human thought and action.* New York: Wiley.

While it may seem desirable for a person with dissociative amnesia to remember these missing memories, recent studies suggest that successfully recalling traumatic memories may increase the risk of experiencing higher levels of traumatic symptoms. The successful recall of traumatic memories can be highly stressful and can influence symptoms of PTSD or suicidal urges. Conversely, some individuals who are able to regain access to trauma-related memories experience positive outcomes. For some with dissociative amnesia, the ability to access traumatic memories provide a therapeutic benefit that allows these individuals to better understand how the traumatic experience influenced their memory, how it impacted their life and how to best resolve the trauma to help prevent further trauma-related symptoms (Radulovic et al., 2018). At present, no evidence-based treatments are available for dissociative amnesia and no broad framework exists for its rehabilitation. Research on the neurobiology of DID is needed which will help inform best practices for treatment (Staniloiu & Markowitsch, 2014).

A subtype of dissociative amnesia is a **dissociative fugue,** in which the individual travels to a new place and may assume a new identity with no memory of his or her previous identity. People in a dissociative fugue may behave quite normally in their new environment and not find it odd that they cannot remember anything from their past. Just as suddenly, they may return to their previous identity and home, resuming their life as if nothing had happened, with no memory of what they did during the fugue. The autobiographical memory loss in a dissociative fugue may be especially long-lasting and resistant to "relearning." A fugue may last for days or years, and a person may experience repeated fugue states or a single episode. Dissociative fugue diagnoses are extremely rare.

As in DID, some theorists argue that psychogenic amnesias may be the result of using dissociation as a defense against intolerable memories or stressors (Gleaves, Smith, Butler, & Spiegel, 2004; Öztürk & Sar, 2016). Several theories have been proposed to explain this restricted access to traumatic memories. Historically, the idea was that such unwanted memories are repressed, but how this occurred was unknown. More recently, a neurological model of repression has identified changes in activation levels within in the prefrontal cortex and hippocampus that result in impaired retention of those unwanted memories (Anderson et al., 2004). An alternative view proposes an automatic process where such memories are state-dependent. This theory suggests that memories are more retrievable if observers' emotional states are consistent between encoding and retrieval (Xie & Zhang, 2018). Amnesia for a specific event may occur because individuals were in such a high state of arousal during the event that the memory is encoded and stored very specifically. State dependent retrieval theories suggest that these memories are difficult to recall unless the conditions at encoding and recall are similar. The memories may be accessed if the individual returns to the same state as they were when the event occurred (Radulovic et al., 2018).

People suffering from dissociative amnesia may recover on their own. Psychotherapy involves helping patients recall and understand the trauma that contributed to their dissociation, but there are few empirical studies of psychotherapy's effectiveness for these disorders (Staniloiu & Markowitsch, 2014).

Depersonalization/Derealization Disorder

People with **depersonalization/derealization disorder** have frequent episodes during which they feel detached from their own mental processes or body, as if they are outside observers of themselves (Table 6). Occasional experiences of depersonalization or derealization are common, particularly when people are sleep-deprived or under the influence of drugs (Baker et al., 2003). Approximately half of all adults report having had at least one brief episode of depersonalization or derealization, usually following a significant stressor (American Psychiatric Association, 2013). The worldwide lifetime prevalence of depersonalization/derealization disorder is between 0.8 and 2.8 percent, and is equally common among men and women.

Depersonalization/derealization disorder is diagnosed when episodes are so frequent and distressing that they interfere with the individual's ability to function. One study of people diagnosed with the disorder found that the average age of onset was about 23 years and that two-thirds reported having had chronic experiences of depersonalization/derealization since the onset (Baker et al., 2003). Seventy-nine percent reported impaired social or work functioning, and the majority also had another psychiatric diagnosis, most often depression. People diagnosed with this disorder often report a history of childhood emotional, physical, or sexual abuse (Simeon, Guralnik, Schmeidler, Sirof, & Knutelska, 2001).

Controversies Around the Dissociative Disorders

Skeptics argue that these disorders are artificially created in suggestible clients by clinicians who reinforce

Lorena Bobbit cut off her husband's penis after years of experiencing his abuse. She claimed to have amnesia for the act of cutting it off.
Consolidated News/Getty Images

TABLE 6 *DSM-5* Diagnostic Criteria for Depersonalization/Derealization Disorder

A. The presence of persistent or recurrent experiences of depersonalization, derealization, or both:

1. Depersonalization: Experiences of unreality, detachment, or being an outside observer with respect to one's thoughts, feelings, sensations, body, or actions (e.g., perceptual alterations, distorted sense of time, unreal or absent self, emotional and/or physical numbing).

2. Derealization: Experiences of unreality or detachment with respect to surroundings (e.g., individuals or objects are experienced as unreal, dreamlike, foggy, lifeless, or visually distorted).

B. During the depersonalization or derealization experiences, reality testing remains intact.

C. The symptoms cause clinically significant distress or impairment in social, occupational, or other important areas of functioning.

D. The disturbance is not attributable to the direct physiological effects of a substance (e.g., a drug of abuse, medication) or another medical condition (e.g., seizures).

E. The disturbance is not better explained by another mental disorder, such as schizophrenia, panic disorder, major depressive disorder, acute stress disorder, posttraumatic stress disorder, or another dissociative disorder.

Reprinted with permission from the *Diagnostic and Statistical Manual of Mental Disorders*, Fifth Edition. Copyright ©2013 by American Psychiatric Association. All Rights Reserved.

these clients for creating symptoms of a dissociative disorder and who may even induce symptoms of the disorder through hypnotic suggestion (see Kihlstrom, 2005; Loftus, 2011; Lynn et al., 2012; Spanos, 1994). Controversy over the diagnosis of dissociative amnesia increased in response to claims that some survivors of childhood sexual abuse repressed their memories of the abuse for years and then eventually recalled these memories, often in the context of psychotherapy. These repressed memories represent a form of dissociative amnesia.

Those who believe in repressed memories argue that the clinical evidence for dissociative or psychogenic amnesia is ample and that the empirical evidence is growing (DePrince & Freyd, 2014). Those who do not support the notion of repressed memory argue that the empirical evidence against the validity of dissociative amnesia is ample and that the supportive evidence is biased (Kihlstrom, 2005; Loftus, 2011). They have also raised questions about the methods used in previous studies that may have biased the conclusions of these studies (Kihlstrom, 2005; Loftus, 2003; McNally, 2003). Additionally opponents of repressed memories also cite numerous studies from the literature on eyewitness identification and testimony indicating that people can be made to believe certain events occurred that in fact never happened (Ceci & Bruck, 1995; Frenda, Nichols, & Loftus, 2011; Laney & Loftus, 2013) and that these beliefs can persist for months or years (Zhu et al., 2012). For example, Elizabeth Loftus and her colleagues developed a method for instilling a childhood memory of being lost on a specific occasion at age 5 (Loftus, 2003).

This method involved a trusted family member engaging the subject in a conversation about the time he or she was lost (Loftus, 1993, p. 532):

Chris (14 years old) was convinced by his older brother Jim that he had been lost in a shopping mall when he was 5 years old. Jim told Chris this story as if it were the truth: "It was 1981 or 1982. I remember that Chris was 5. We had gone shopping in the University City shopping mall in Spokane. After some panic, we found Chris being led down the mall by a tall, oldish man (I think he was wearing a flannel shirt). Chris was crying and holding the man's hand. The man explained that he had found Chris walking around crying his eyes out just a few moments before and was trying to help him find his parents." Just two days later, Chris recalled his feelings about being lost: "That day I was so scared that I would never see my family again. I knew that I was in trouble." On the third day, he recalled a conversation with his mother: "I remember Mom telling me never to do that again." On the fourth day: "I also remember that old man's flannel shirt." On the fifth day, he started remembering the mall itself: "I sort of remember the stores." In his last recollection, he could even remember a conversation with the man who found him: "I remember the man asking me if I was lost."... A couple of weeks later, Chris described his false memory and he greatly expanded on it. "I was with you guys for a second and I think I went over to look at the toy store, the Kay-Bee Toy and uh, we got lost and I was looking around and I thought, 'Uh-oh, I'm in trouble now.' You know. And then I . . . I thought I was never going to see my family again. I was really scared you know. And then this old man, I think he was wearing a blue flannel, came up to me. . . . He was kind of old. He was kind of bald on top. . . . He had like a ring of gray hair . . . and he had glasses."

Other studies have found that repeatedly asking adults about childhood events that never actually happened leads perhaps 20 to 40 percent eventually to "remember" these events and even explain them in detail (Frenda et al., 2011; Laney & Loftus, 2013). For example, in one study, 40 percent of a British sample said they had seen footage of a bus exploding in the 2005 London terrorist attacks, when such footage did not exist (Ost, Granhag, Udell, Roos, & Hjelmsater, 2008). Thirty-five percent of these described memories of details that they could not have seen.

The percentage of participants developing false memories of events that never happened can be increased by procedures that mimic some of the psychotherapeutic methods used with people who "recover" repressed memories (Scoboria et al., 2017). For example, family photo albums are sometimes reviewed in psychotherapy to help people remember traumatic events. In false memory experiments, showing participants photographs of themselves or other family members in the context of telling a story of a false memory makes participants more likely to believe the false memory with strong confidence (Lindsay, Hagen, Read, Wade, & Garry, 2004). Simply having a psychologist suggest that an individual's dreams reflect repressed memories of childhood events leads a majority of subjects subsequently to report that the events depicted in their dreams actually happened (Mazzoni & Loftus, 1998).

Critics of this line of work question the application of these studies to claims of repressed memories of sexual abuse (Brewin & Andrews, 2017; Gleaves, Hernandez, & Warner, 2003). They argue that although people might be willing to go along with experimenters who try to convince them that they were lost in a shopping mall as a child, they are unlikely to be willing to go along with a therapist who tries to convince them that they were sexually abused if such abuse did not in fact happen. Abuse is such a terrible thing to remember, and the social consequences of admitting the abuse and confronting the abuser are so negative, that people simply would not claim the memory was true if it was not.

Researchers have used paradigms from cognitive psychology to test hypotheses about the reality of repressed memories. In a series of studies, Richard McNally and colleagues (McNally, 2003; McNally, Clancy, & Schacter, 2001; McNally, Clancy, Schacter, & Pitman, 2000a, 2000b) have found that individuals reporting recovered memories of either childhood sexual abuse or abduction by space aliens have a greater tendency to form false memories during certain laboratory tasks. For example, one task required participants to say whether they recognized words similar to, but not exactly the same as, other words they previously had learned. People who claimed to have recovered memories of alien abductions were more prone than comparison groups to falsely recognize words they had not seen previously (Clancy, Schacter, McNally, & Pitman, 2000; Clancy, McNally, Schacter, Lenzenweger, & Pitman, 2002). The researchers argue that these people are characterized by an information-processing style that may render them more likely to believe they have experienced specific events, such as childhood sexual abuse, when in fact they have experienced other, broadly similar events, such as physical abuse or emotional neglect.

Jennifer Freyd and colleagues have argued that the kinds of cognitive tasks McNally and colleagues used do not tap into the specific cognitive phenomena associated with repressed memories. Specifically, they suggest that individuals who dissociate from, and forget, their abusive experiences are most likely to differ from other individuals in the performance of cognitive tasks that require divided attention—that is, paying attention to more than one thing at a time—because a division of attention is critical to dissociation (DePrince & Freyd, 2014; Freyd, Martorella, Alvarado, Hayes, & Christman, 1998). One divided-attention task requires participants to press a key on a keyboard in response to a secondary task while attending to words on a computer screen and committing them to memory. Under these divided-attention conditions, people who score high on measures of dissociation recall fewer trauma-related words but more neutral words they previously had been instructed to remember, while low-dissociation participants show the opposite pattern. This suggests that people high in dissociation are better able to keep threatening information from their explicit awareness, particularly if they can instead turn their attention to other tasks or other events in their environment.

The repressed memory debate is likely to continue for some time (see Brewin & Andrews, 2017; McNally, 2017). Researchers are striving to apply scientific techniques to support their views, with significant real-world implications. Psychologists are being called on to testify in court cases involving claims of recovered or false memories. Through all the controversy, people trying to understand their distressing symptoms find themselves at the center of this scientific whirlpool.

FIGURE 2   **Mind and Body in the Somatic Symptom and Dissociative Disorders.**

Social factors: trauma, role models who express distress through physical symptoms, reinforcement for physical symptoms

Psychological factors: inability to cope with or express distress, exaggerated physical symptoms

Physical symptoms

CHAPTER INTEGRATION

Philosophers and scientists have long debated the mind-body problem: Does the mind influence bodily processes? Do changes in the body affect a person's sense of "self"? Exactly how do the body and the mind influence each other?

As noted earlier, the dissociative and somatic symptom disorders provide compelling evidence that the mind and the body are complexly interwoven (Figure 2). In conversion disorder, psychological stress causes the person to lose eyesight, hearing, or functioning in another important physiological system. In somatic symptom disorder, a person under psychological stress experiences physiological symptoms, such as severe headaches. An underlying theme of these disorders is that some people find it easier or more acceptable to experience psychological distress through changes in their body than to express it more directly as sadness, fear, or anger, perhaps because of cultural or social norms.

We all somatize our distress to some degree—we feel more aches and pains when we are upset about something than when we are happy. People who develop somatic symptom disorders, and perhaps dissociative disorders, may somatize their distress to an extreme degree. Their tendency to differentiate between what is going on in their mind and what is going on in their body may be minimal, and they may favor an extreme bodily expression of what is going on in their mind.

SHADES OF GRAY   DISCUSSION

Ben's health concerns do seem to be linked to his parents' separation and not to a medical condition. His insistence of real pain and his refusal to return to class signal that he experiences significant physical and emotional distress over his perceived headaches and stomachaches. Therefore, his symptoms are more in line with a somatic symptom disorder than with illness anxiety disorder.

CHAPTER SUMMARY

- The somatic symptom disorders are a group of disorders in which the individual experiences distressing physical symptoms and abnormal thoughts, feelings, and behaviors in response to these symptoms.

- Somatic symptom disorder involves a long history of physical complaints for which an individual has sought treatment. Medically unexplained symptoms are present to various degrees and are a key feature in conversion disorder. People with these disorders show high rates of anxiety and depression.

- People with illness anxiety disorder fear becoming ill, although they may not experience actual symptoms of illness.

- The cognitive theory of the somatic symptom disorders is that affected people believe they are vulnerable to illness, focus excessively on physical symptoms, and catastrophize these symptoms. They are reinforced by the attention and concern they receive from others. Treatment involves helping people have more realistic perspectives on their health, removing reinforcements for illness behavior, and teaching people to cope better with stress.

- In conversion disorder, individuals lose all sensory and/or motor functioning in a part of their body, such as the eyes or the legs. Conversion symptoms often occur after trauma or stress. People with conversion disorder tend to have high rates of depression, anxiety, alcohol abuse, and antisocial personality disorder. Treatment for the disorder focuses on the expression of associated emotions or memories.

- In the dissociative disorders, the individual's identity, memories, and consciousness become separated, or dissociated, from one another. In dissociative identity disorder (DID), the individual develops two or more distinct personalities, which alternate their control over the individual's behavior. Persons with dissociative identity disorder often engage in self-injurious and self-mutilative behaviors.

- The vast majority of diagnosed cases of dissociative identity are women, and they tend to have a history of severe childhood sexual and/or physical abuse. The alternate personalities may have been formed during the traumatic experiences as a way of psychologically managing these experiences, particularly among people who are highly hypnotizable. The treatment of dissociative identity disorder typically involves helping the various personalities become integrated into one functional personality.

- Dissociative, or psychogenic, amnesia involves the loss of memory due to psychological causes. It differs from organic amnesia, which is caused by brain injury and in which a person may have difficulty remembering new information (anterograde amnesia), a rare condition in psychogenic amnesia. In addition, with organic amnesia loss of memory for the past (retrograde amnesia) usually is generalized, whereas with psychogenic amnesia memory loss is limited to personal information.

- Psychogenic amnesia typically occurs following traumatic events. It may be due to motivated forgetting of events, to poor storage of information during events due to hyperarousal, or to avoidance of the emotions experienced during traumatic events and of the memories associated with these events.

- Dissociative fugue is a subtype of dissociative amnesia in which the person suddenly moves away from home and assumes an entirely new identity, with complete amnesia for the previous identity.

- Depersonalization/derealization disorder involves frequent episodes in which individuals feel detached from their mental processes or their body. Transient depersonalization/derealization experiences are common, especially in people who are sleep-deprived or under the influence of drugs.

KEY TERMS

somatic symptom disorders

illness anxiety disorder

conversion disorder (functional neurological symptom disorder)

functional neurological symptom disorder

factitious disorder imposed on self

malingering

factitious disorder imposed on another

dissociative disorder

dissociation

dissociative identity disorder (DID)

dissociative amnesia

organic amnesia

anterograde amnesia

psychogenic amnesia

retrograde amnesia

dissociative fugue

depersonalization/derealization disorder

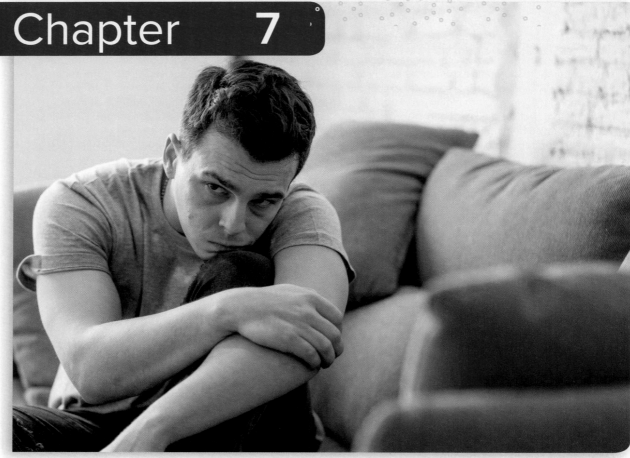

Chapter 7

Sam Wordley/Shutterstock

Mood Disorders and Suicide

CHAPTER OUTLINE

Mood Disorders Along the Continuum

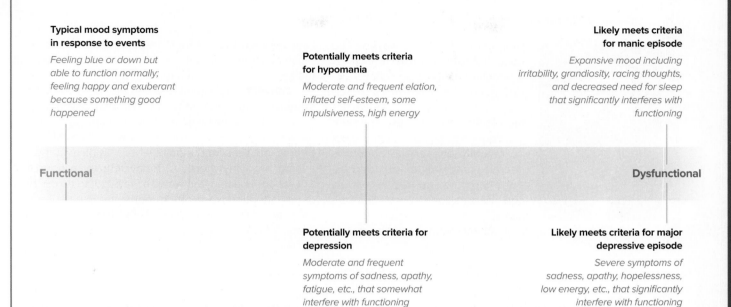

Typical mood symptoms in response to events

Feeling blue or down but able to function normally; feeling happy and exuberant because something good happened

Potentially meets criteria for hypomania

Moderate and frequent elation, inflated self-esteem, some impulsiveness, high energy

Likely meets criteria for manic episode

Expansive mood including irritability, grandiosity, racing thoughts, and decreased need for sleep that significantly interferes with functioning

Functional

Dysfunctional

Potentially meets criteria for depression

Moderate and frequent symptoms of sadness, apathy, fatigue, etc., that somewhat interfere with functioning

Likely meets criteria for major depressive episode

Severe symptoms of sadness, apathy, hopelessness, low energy, etc., that significantly interfere with functioning

We often hear people say things like, "I'm in such a bad mood today!" which we all know means someone is upset for some particular reason. But, what does that actually mean? Think about the range of moods we can experience in just one day. For example, you left your house feeling "fine" but then on your drive to class someone cut you off and almost caused an accident. At that moment you may have yelled at the other driver and perhaps even made a hand gesture to express your anger. However, moments later you hear a favorite song on the radio and feel relaxed and happy. When you arrive on campus you get a great parking spot and see someone you have a crush on parked next to you. You might feel excited and energized to walk to class together. Is it "normal" to experience these fluctuations in mood in such a short time? Yes, it is.

Mood states ebb and flow throughout the day often influenced by events in life that can take us from feeling on top of the world all the way down to the depths of despair. Unlike these typical and temporary variations in mood, some people experience a significant disruption of mood associated with psychological dysfunction. This category of psychological disorders includes depressive and bipolar disorders as disruption of mood is the most common feature. The spectrum of mood includes feelings of sadness and melancholy to feelings of elation and euphoria, and everything in between.

"I'm depressed" is a phrase you may have uttered, perhaps after you didn't do as well as you expected on an exam, you lost a job, or when a relationship has ended. Feelings of depression are very common and such events often sap our energy and motivation, shake our self-esteem, and make us feel down and blue. These common experiences represent feelings of depression and give us an opportunity to empathize with those who battle the psychological disorder we call depression. In this chapter, we will explore a variety of psychological disorders that all impact and disrupt function on the depressed end of the mood spectrum.

Just as we can experience depressive feelings there are times, such as getting into your first-choice college or having a great first date, when our mood becomes elevated. We feel energized, exhilarated, and joyful. While these feelings may have positive attributes, a person who experiences persistently elevated mood may be experiencing the mood disorder called mania. A manic episode goes beyond feeling happy when something good has happened and instead involves high levels of energy, excessive self-confidence, grandiose ideas, and extremely risky or impulsive behaviors that interfere with daily function. In some people depressive and manic moods alternate in a condition called bipolar disorder. This chapter will explore the various depressive and bipolar disorders that impact the mood of many individuals, every day.

Extraordinary People

Dwayne "The Rock" Johnson: The Struggle is Real

Jaguar PS/Shutterstock

Hollywood celebrity Dwayne "The Rock" Johnson first rose to fame as a popular wrestling personality before becoming a box-office superstar. The Rock is best known for his blockbuster movies, muscular physique, and positive attitude, but he recently opened up about his decades-long battle with depression. "Struggle and pain is real . . . and depression never discriminates." Johnson reflected on several painful moments in his life and later tweeted the essential lesson he learned through those hardships. "It took me a long time to realize it but the key is to not be afraid to open up . . ."

Johnson discussed the impact of his mother's struggles with depression on his own psychological health and how he witnessed her attempt suicide when he was only 15. Johnson said, "I was devastated and depressed. I reached a point where I didn't want to do a thing or go anywhere . . ." Today Johnson reports that ". . . we both healed, but we've always got to do our best to pay attention when other people are in pain . . . help them through it and remind them they are not alone" (Izadi, 2018).

The emotional battles described by Dwayne "The Rock" Johnson are indicative of a psychological disorder called major depression which is one disorder listed within the category of **depressive disorders.** We will examine the different symptoms of depressive disorders, as well as bipolar disorders in which depressive symptoms alternate with elevated mood, called mania.

CHARACTERISTICS OF DEPRESSIVE DISORDERS

Let's begin on the depressive end of the spectrum. In depressive disorders, the symptoms of depression affect the whole person which impacts their emotions, behaviors, thinking, and ability to function. Like previous disorders discussed in this book, the intensity of depressive symptoms can vary from low/mild to profound/severe, as well as the duration of time these symptoms impact the individual. Regardless of these individual differences, depressive disorders cause significant distress and impact daily function.

Symptoms of Depression

We've all experienced feelings of depression. Think about how these feelings impact the individual. Life just isn't the same when feelings of depression are present, some may argue that the world has no color, food has no taste, and there's no purpose in anything. These feelings are often found in depressive disorders and many people diagnosed with depression report that they have no joy or pleasure in life. They have no interest in activities that were previously considered fun, a symptom referred to as *anhedonia*. Even when they try to do something enjoyable, they may feel no emotion during the activity and often report that they "just don't care anymore." As Kay Jamison (1995, p. 110) writes, she was "unbearably miserable and seemingly incapable of any kind of joy or enthusiasm."

With the loss of pleasure in daily activities, it is also common that depressive thoughts may contain themes of worthlessness, guilt, hopelessness, and even suicide. This sense of worthlessness or guilt associated with depressive symptoms may involve unrealistically negative self-evaluations or preoccupations with previous failures, that were minor in nature. People with depressive disorders often have trouble concentrating and making decisions. Some people with severe depression lose touch with reality and can experience psychotic symptoms, such as hallucinations (false perceptions) and delusions (false beliefs). When symptoms of depression become this severe it is indicative of severe cognitive impairment that cause significant distress. For example, hallucinations may be in the form of voices that tell the individual that they are a disgusting person and should hurt themselves, possibly commanding the individual to self-injure or attempt suicide (American Psychiatric Association, 2013).

Physical symptoms are also present in depression, such as changes in appetite, sleep, and activity levels. Think about a time you were depressed, how was your appetite and sleep? For some, depression may reduce appetite, while others find themselves eating more, perhaps even binge eating. Typically, these behaviors will directly impact weight and it is common for people with depression to experience significant weight loss or weight gain. These same patterns also exist for sleep. When depression is present, some people may want to crawl into bed, pull the blankets over their head and sleep for days. Whereas, others with depression may feel fatigued but find it difficult to maintain sleep and battle problems with insomnia (American Psychiatric Association, 2013).

Symptoms of depression often involve sustained fatigue and decreased energy that results in a physically slowed appearance known as *psychomotor retardation*. This causes a general slowing in behavior causing people with depression, for example, to walk more slowly, gesture more slowly, think and talk more slowly and quietly. They may have more accidents because they cannot react quickly enough to avoid them. Many people with depressive disorders lack energy and report feeling chronically fatigued. A subset of people, however, exhibit *psychomotor agitation* instead of psychomotor retardation—these people feel physically agitated, cannot sit still, and may move around or fidget aimlessly (American Psychiatric Association, 2013).

Diagnosing Depressive Disorders

There are several depressive disorders that each have varying symptoms, but share the common feature of **dysphoria** (the opposite of euphoria) that is characterized by intense feelings of sadness. **Major depressive disorder (MDD)** involves acute, but time-limited symptoms of depressed mood lasting at least two weeks that significantly impact daily function. The diagnosis of MDD requires that a person experience either depressed mood or loss of interest in usual activities, plus at least four other symptoms of depression, chronically for at least 2 weeks (Table 1).

TABLE 1   *DSM-5* Criteria for Major Depressive Disorder

A. Five (or more) of the following symptoms have been present during the same 2-week period and represent a change from previous functioning; at least one of the symptoms is either (1) depressed mood or (2) loss of interest or pleasure. (Note: Do not include symptoms that are clearly attributable to another medical condition.)

   1. Depressed mood most of the day, nearly every day, as indicated by either subjective report (e.g., feels sad, empty, hopeless) or observation made by others (e.g., appears tearful). (Note: In children and adolescents, can be irritable mood.)

   2. Markedly diminished interest or pleasure in all, or almost all, activities most of the day, nearly every day (as indicated by either subjective account or observation).

   3. Significant weight loss when not dieting or weight gain (e.g., a change of more than 5 percent of body weight in a month), or decrease or increase in appetite nearly every day. (Note: In children, consider failure to make expected weight gain.)

   4. Insomnia or hypersomnia nearly every day.

   5. Psychomotor agitation or retardation nearly every day (observable by others, not merely subjective feelings of restlessness or being slowed down).

   6. Fatigue or loss of energy nearly every day.

   7. Feelings of worthlessness or excessive or inappropriate guilt (which may be delusional) nearly every day (not merely self-reproach or guilt about being sick).

   8. Diminished ability to think or concentrate, or indecisiveness, nearly every day (either by subjective account or as observed by others).

   9. Recurrent thoughts of death (not just fear of dying), recurrent suicidal ideation without a specific plan, or a suicide attempt or a specific plan for committing suicide.

B. The symptoms cause clinically significant distress or impairment in social, occupational, or other important areas of functioning.

C. The episode is not attributable to the physiological effects of a substance or to another medical condition. Note: Criteria A to C represent a major depressive episode.

Note: Responses to a significant loss (e.g., bereavement, financial ruin, losses from a natural disaster, a serious medical illness or disability) may include the feelings of intense sadness, rumination about the loss, insomnia, poor appetite, and weight loss noted in Criterion A, which may resemble a depressive episode. Although such symptoms may be understandable and considered appropriate to the loss, the presence of a major depressive episode in addition to the normal response to a significant loss should be carefully considered. This decision inevitably requires the exercise of clinical judgment based on the individual's history and the cultural norms for the expression of distress in the context of loss.

D. The occurrence of the major depressive episode is not better explained by schizoaffective disorder, schizophrenia, schizophreniform disorder, delusional disorder, or other specified and unspecified schizophrenia spectrum and other psychotic disorders.

E. There has never been a manic episode or a hypomanic episode. Note: This exclusion does not apply if all the manic-like or hypomanic-like episodes are substance induced or are attributable to the physiological effects of another medical condition.

In addition, these symptoms must be severe enough to interfere with the person's ability to function in everyday life.

Depressive episodes are time-limited and if left untreated will resolve during a specific course of time, typically somewhere between 2 weeks and 9 months (Harding, 2019; Mullen, 2018). Meaning, if the depressed individual does not participate in treatment for their symptoms, the depressive episode will eventually resolve without treatment. This is a double-edged sword for many individuals struggling with depression who may believe that this disorder was fleeting, temporary, or that they overcame these symptoms through personal strength and willpower. However, it is more likely than not that people who experience one depressive episode will experience another in the course of their lifetime.

People who experience only one depressive episode receive a diagnosis of *MDD, single episode*. Two or more episodes separated by at least 2 consecutive months without symptoms merit the diagnosis of *MDD, recurrent episode*. Although MDD may be limited to a single episode in some people, it is more likely that the most clients with this disorder will move in and out of depressive symptoms over time. Recent research suggests that the majority of people affected are more likely to have recurrent episodes which makes this a chronic and disabling condition (Verduijn et al., 2017). Research has shown that at least 50 percent of those who recover from a first episode of depression will experience one or more additional episodes in their lifetime. Approximately 80 percent of those with a history of two episodes are likely to experience another recurrence of depression. Meaning, the likelihood of a person experiencing a single episode of depression is rare. Once a first episode has occurred, recurrent episodes will usually begin within 5 years of the initial episode and, on average, individuals with a history of depression will have five to nine separate depressive episodes in their lifetime (Bercusa & Iacono, 2007). The recurrent pattern of MDD often makes this a chronic condition but prior episodes of depression is one of the best predictors of future depression. There are other predictive factors such as severity of symptoms, number of prior episodes, age at onset, and adult psychiatric comorbidity that are all important predictors of future recurrence (Sellers et al., 2016).

More than 70 percent of people diagnosed with major depressive or persistent depressive disorder also have another psychological disorder at some time in their lives. The most common disorders that are comorbid with (occur with) depression are substance abuse, such as alcohol abuse; anxiety disorders, such as panic disorder; and eating disorders (Kessler, 2003).

The *DSM-5* criteria in Table 1 includes a note to clinicians that a "normal and expected" depressive response to a negative event such as a loss should not be diagnosed as an MDD unless other, more atypical symptoms are present, including worthlessness, suicidal ideas, psychomotor retardation, and severe impairment (American PsychiatricAssociation, 2013). Differentiating grief from a major depressive episode requires clinical judgment. It is expected that when individuals experience a significant loss, such as loss of a loved one, financial ruin, or serious illness, they will experience feelings of intense sadness, disrupted sleep, and appetite that resemble a symptoms of a depressive episode. While such symptoms may be appropriate to the loss, the presence of a major depressive episode in addition to the normal response to loss requires careful consideration. Currently, there is no agreement on whether or not grief symptoms can be pathological and *DSM-5* authors placed *Persistent complex bereavement disorder (PCBD)* as a proposed new diagnostic category in section III (conditions for further study) (American Psychiatric Association, 2013). Many argue that the intense, prolonged symptoms of grief, coupled with some form of functional impairment beyond 6 months post–loss constitutes a distinct mental disorder. Numerous studies have demonstrated that symptoms of grief are distinct from symptoms of depression (Maciejewski, Maercker, Boelen, & Prigerson, 2016). PCBD people who show complex bereavement after a loss are more likely to be functioning poorly 2 to 3 years after the loss than are those who show milder grief reactions or those who show only symptoms of MDD (Bonanno et al., 2007; Bonanno, Westphal, & Mancini, 2011).

Although the *DSM-5* criteria determines when to diagnose a major depressive episode, depression can take many different forms and sometimes it is necessary to add a specifier. The *DSM-5* recognizes several specifiers that can be attached to a disorder to provide more explanation or clarity (see Table 2 for their names and key symptoms). The first specifier is depression with *anxious distress*. Anxiety is extremely common in depression (Watson, 2009), and people with this subtype have prominent anxiety symptoms as well as depressive symptoms. The second specifier of depression is with *mixed features*. People with this specifier meet the criteria for an MDD and have at least three symptoms of mania, but they do not meet the full criteria for a manic episode (discussed below in the section on bipolar disorder). The third specifier is depression with *melancholic features*, in which the physiological symptoms of depression are particularly prominent. The fourth specifier is depression with *psychotic features*, in which people experience delusions and hallucinations. The content of delusions and hallucinations may be consistent with typical

TABLE 2   Major Depressive Episode Specifiers

Subtype	Characteristic Symptoms
Anxious distress	Prominent anxiety symptoms
Mixed features	Presence of at least three manic/hypomanic symptoms, but does not meet criteria for a manic episode
Melancholic features	Inability to experience pleasure, distinct depressed mood, depression regularly worse in morning, early morning awakening, marked psychomotor retardation or agitation, significant anorexia or weight loss, excessive guilt
Psychotic features	Presence of mood-congruent or mood-incongruent delusions or hallucinations
Catatonic features	Catatonic behaviors: not actively relating to environment, mutism, posturing, agitation, mimicking another's speech or movements
Atypical features	Positive mood reactions to some events, significant weight gain or increase in appetite, hypersomnia, heavy or leaden feelings in arms or legs, long-standing pattern of sensitivity to interpersonal rejection
Seasonal pattern	History of at least 2 years in which major depressive episodes occur during one season of the year (usually the winter) and remit when the season is over
Peripartum onset	Onset of major depressive episode during pregnancy or in the 4 weeks following delivery

depressive themes of personal inadequacy, guilt, death, or punishment (mood-congruent), or their content is unrelated to depressive themes or mixed (mood-incongruent). In the fifth specifier, depression with *catatonic features*, people show the strange behaviors collectively known as catatonia, which can range from a complete lack of movement to excited agitation. The sixth specifier is depression with *atypical features*—the criteria for this subtype are an odd assortment of symptoms, and are not particularly unusual, as the label would suggest (see Table 2).

The seventh specifier of MDD is depression with *seasonal pattern,* previously referred to as **seasonal affective disorder,** or **SAD.** People with seasonal pattern specifier have a history of at least 2 years of experiencing and fully recovering from major depressive episodes. In most cases, these depressive episodes begin in the fall/winter and resolve in the spring. Meaning, they are more likely to become depressed when the daylight hours are short and recover when the daylight hours are long. In the Northern Hemisphere, this means that people are more likely to experience depressive symptoms from November through February and less symptoms from June through August. The onset and remission of these symptoms at characteristic times of the year cannot be better explained by psychosocial events, such as seasonal unemployment or school schedule (American Psychiatric Association, 2013).

The eighth specifier is depression with **peripartum onset** (previously *postpartum specifier*). This diagnosis is given to women when the onset of a major depressive episode occurs during pregnancy or in the 4 weeks following childbirth. Because 50 percent of "postpartum" major depressive episodes actually begin prior to delivery, *DSM-5* refers to these episodes collectively as peripartum episodes. More rarely,

some women develop mania postpartum and are given the diagnosis of bipolar disorder with peripartum onset. In the first few weeks after giving birth, as many as 30 percent of women experience the postpartum blues—emotional lability (unstable and quickly shifting moods), frequent crying, irritability, and fatigue. For most women, these symptoms cease completely within 2 weeks of the birth. About 1 in 10 women experiences postpartum depression serious enough to warrant a diagnosis of a MDD with peripartum onset (O'Hara & McCabe, 2013). Many of the risk factors for postpartum depression are similar to those for depressive episodes in general, but specific biological factors (like hormonal changes) and psychosocial factors (such as support from partners and parents) relevant to childbirth may play specific roles as well (Yim, Tanner Stapleton, Guardino, Hahn-Holbrook, & Dunkel Schetter, 2015).

Persistent Depressive Disorder

While symptoms of MDD are intense and time-limited, persistent depressive disorder has a more chronic course. **Persistent depressive disorder** (formerly *dysthymic disorder* and *chronic MDD* in *DSM-IV*) has its essential feature depressed mood for most of the day, for more days than not, for at least 2 years. In children and adolescents, persistent depressive disorder requires depressed or irritable mood for a duration of at least 1 year. In addition, its diagnosis requires the presence of two or more of the following symptoms: (a) poor appetite, (b) insomnia or hypersomnia, (c) low energy or fatigue, (d) low self-esteem, (e) poor concentration, and/or (f) hopelessness. During these 2 years (1 year in youth), the person must never have been without symptoms of depression for longer than a 2-month period. When an individual meets diagnostic criteria for MDD for 2 years, they are also given the diagnosis of persistent depressive disorder. *DSM-5* combined the *DSM-IV* categories of dysthymic and chronic MDD because research failed to find a meaningful difference between these two conditions, despite the *DSM-IV* notion that dysthymic disorder was a less severe form of depression. In fact, individuals with persistent depressive disorder show a higher risk for comorbid disorders than those with MDD alone, particularly anxiety and substance use disorders, and tend to experience worse functional consequences (American Psychiatric Association, 2013).

Premenstrual Dysphoric Disorder

Some women regularly experience clinically significant increases in distress during the premenstrual phase of their menstrual cycle, that is not explained by premenstrual syndrome (PMS). **Premenstrual dysphoric disorder (PMDD)** is a severe mood disorder, is characterized by cognitive–affective and physical symptoms that occur in the week before menses. This disorder affects millions of women worldwide and is a new addition to the *DSM* after decades of scientific review. Symptoms of PMDD include perimenstrual pattern of at least five physical, affective, and/or behavioral symptoms, with a requirement of at least one symptom of unstable emotion such as mood swings, tearfulness, or sensitivity to rejection. Individuals with PMDD may display irritability or anger that is often characterized by increased interpersonal conflicts. Significantly depressed mood, hopelessness, or self-deprecating thoughts, anxiety or feeling out of control or on edge are also common (Hantsoo & Epperson, 2015). Symptoms of PMDD are often a mixture of depression, anxiety, and tension, and irritability and anger that present during the week before the onset of menses. Significant distress and/or impairment must be present in the area of work, school, social activities, or relationships with others. These symptoms improve once menses has begun and become minimal or absent in the week post menses. These women also often report physical symptoms such as breast tenderness or swelling, bloating and weight gain, and joint and muscle pain (American Psychiatric Association, 2013).

Although a large majority of women experience mild premenstrual symptoms, approximately 2 to 8 percent suffer from PMDD around the world. Research has found the presence of PMDD in countries throughout the world with consistent prevalence rates, although cultural variation did occur (Chumpalova et al., 2020). These symptoms have been described in diverse cultural settings, even among women who are not generally aware of the disorder. For example, similar rates of the disorder have been reported in Mediterranean countries, the Middle East, Iceland, Kenya,

New Zealand, and Asia (Yonkers & Caser, 2019). Although some have argued that this new diagnostic category pathologizes a typical female experience, recent studies support that PMDD is clinically unique from MDD and may have more irritability and anxiety-like features. Additionally, *DSM-5* authors believe that better diagnosis and treatment will result for women who experience a highly exaggerated mood disturbance prior to their monthly menstrual cycle (American Psychiatric Association, 2013; Hantsoo & Epperson, 2015). Although PMDD can be observed in women without other psychiatric disorders, comorbid conditions are reported in up to 70 percent of cases, especially generalized anxiety disorder, agoraphobia, social phobia, bipolar disorder, posttraumatic stress disorder, major depression, and bipolar disorder (Bezerra de Carvalho et al., 2018; Sepede, Brunetti, & Di Giannantonio, 2020).

Disruptive Mood Dysregulation Disorder

Disruptive mood dysregulation disorder (DMDD) is a new disorder found in the in *DSM-5* characterized by severe and chronic irritability, persistently negative mood (irritable, angry, or sad), and severe temper outbursts among children and adolescents who previously would be misdiagnosed as having bipolar disorder. The initial diagnosis should not be applied to children under the age of 6 or adolescents over the age of 18 (American Psychiatric Association, 2013). This disorder is characterized by chronic, nonepisodic irritability, and temper tantrums that are disproportionate to the situation. These outbursts are typically in response to frustration and are typically manifested in exaggerated verbal rages or behaviorally through acts of physical aggression. Children and adolescents with DMDD exhibit low frustration tolerance and difficulties with emotion regulation, distress tolerance, and behavioral self-control (Ramires, Godinho, & Goodman, 2017). Behavioral outbursts are often displayed as physical aggression against property, self, or other people. These symptoms are associated with severe impairment in childhood and with negative adolescent and adult outcomes.

DMDD is associated with high rates of comorbidity with other psychiatric disorders or neuropsychiatric problems, such as oppositional defiant disorder (ODD), conduct disorder, attention-deficit/hyperactivity disorder, learning difficulties, depression, problems at school, peer relationships, and social issues (Perepletchikova et al., 2017). The severity of these problems only affect the life of their parents, siblings, peers, and teachers. In addition, children and adolescents with DMDD are at an increased risk for developing antisocial personality disorder, alcohol or substance abuse, or other psychiatric illness(es) in their adult lives (Ramires et al., 2017).

Since it is a new diagnostic entity, literature on DMDD prevalence, epidemiology, risk factors, and treatment guidelines, is still sparse and unclear makes DMDD a controversial addition to the *DSM-5*. This lack of empirical data was led many to question the validity of this disorder (Baweja, Mayes, Hameed, & Waxmonsky, 2016; Bruno et al., 2019). Irritable mood among youth receiving mental health services is a common presenting problem in clinical and represents a transdiagnostic trait that is present across various psychiatric disorders and personality dimensions (Moore et al., 2019). Since there appears to be a significant diagnostic overlap with this disorder and other conditions, there is an increasing use of pharmacological treatments in children and adolescents. Intervention strategies for children with disruptive behavior disorders are still under investigation, and common treatments include pharmacological interventions and cognitive–behavioral therapy. Treatments regarded as evidence based include social skills training, parent training, and multisystemic therapy, which fall within the cognitive–behavioral spectrum (Ramires et al., 2017).

Multiple studies on DMDD have consistently found that environmental factors (e.g., peer victimization, parenting) significantly contribute to the irritability that is the core feature of this disorder. To determine the most effective treatment methods it is critical that these environmental associations be properly identified. Targeting these prominent triggers will help develop effective treatments that can teach these individuals to manage and regulate their emotional responses. One such treatment for DMDD youth with severe irritability is exposure therapy, whereby they are repeatedly exposed to frustrating situations designed to increase adaptive coping strategies and frustration tolerance. There is also evidence that a new treatment that incorporates elements of dialectical behavior therapy (DBT) and parent training may help those with DMDD. This type of intervention has been shown to reduce disruptive behaviors through environmental modifications. (Moore et al., 2019). DMDD is common among children and adolescents in mental health clinics and prevalence rates range between 2 and 5 percent, depending upon the age group. This disorder tends to be present among males and school-age children at higher rates than among females and adolescents (American Psychiatric Association, 2013).

Prevalence and Course of Depressive Disorders

MDD is often referred to as the "common cold" of psychiatric conditions since it is among the most common of mental health disorders. This disorder affects a significant number of people around the world every year and is a leading cause of global disability and morbidity. The prevalence of MDD is about 7 percent of the adult population in the United States, which amounts to approximately 17.3 million people. Recent studies suggest that the prevalence of MDD could be a high as 10 percent of the general population, depending upon the culture. Within this group of adults battling major depressive episode, 64 percent report severe impairment which suggests that the majority of people with MDD have very significant symptoms (NIMH, 2017). In Korea, MDD was ranked first among all mental and substance use disorders, and research has found that associated mortality rates which include death from suicide have significantly increased in that country over time (Rhee et al., 2020). Major depression is typically reported at higher rates among adult females (8.7 percent) as compared to adult males (5.3 percent). This gender difference in depression has been found in many countries, in most ethnic groups, and in all adult age groups (Nolen-Hoeksema & Hilt, 2013). We discuss possible reasons for these differences later in the chapter. Among adults diagnosed with MDD, individuals between the ages of 18 and 25 are the group most impacted by this disorder with 13 percent of young adults meeting criteria for major depression (NIMH, 2017). Rates of depression are lowest in people over age 65 (Kessler et al., 2010); however, the rates of depression rise among people over age 85. When it does occur, depression in older people tends to be severe, chronic, and debilitating (Fiske, Wetherell, & Gatz, 2009).

Depression appears to be a long-lasting and recurrent problem. Left untreated, a major depressive episode often improves and remits within 7 to 9 months of symptom onset. Nearly two-thirds of patients receiving clinically effective medications for depression fail to achieve full remission, and there is a substantial risk of relapse among patients who do not achieve remission. Half of patients taking medication for their depression fail to respond at all (Thase et al., 2019). After recovery from one episode of depression, these individuals remain at high risk for relapse with approximately 75 percent experiencing subsequent episodes (Buckman et al., 2018; Burcusa & Iacono, 2007). People with a history of multiple episodes of depression are more likely to remain depressed for long periods of time. On average, people suffering with depression are likely to experience four episodes that last for approximately 14 to 17 weeks per mild episode or 23 weeks when symptoms are severe (Buckman et al., 2018).

As a result of this relapsing course and functional impairment, individuals with depression experience the highest levels of burden worldwide in terms of life-years lost to disability. Depression is a costly disorder, both to the individual and to society. People who have a diagnosis of major depression lose an average of 27 days of work per year because of their symptoms.

Depression in workers costs employers an estimated $37 billion per year in lost productivity alone (not including the cost of treatment) (Buckman et al., 2018; Kessler et al., 2007).

The good news is that when people undergo treatment for their depression, they tend to recover more quickly than without treatment which reduces the risk of relapse. The bad news is that many people with depression either never seek care or wait years after the onset of symptoms before they seek care (Kessler, 2003). We might ask why people experiencing the terrible symptoms of depression don't seek treatment. One reason is that they may lack insurance or the money to pay for care. Often, however, they expect to get over their symptoms on their own. They believe that their symptoms are simply a phase that will pass with time and that won't affect their lives over the long term.

Cultural Assets

The idea that our environment influences our psychological well-being is a well-accepted notion. The neighborhood where we grow up, our family dynamics, experiences with peers, and our group membership all play a role in how we interpret the world and cope with various life stressors. The experiences that we have as members of a certain group can also influence our psychological health, providing both strength or vulnerability to different conditions, such as the development of psychological disorders, like depression. Lower rates of MDD have been found among BIPOC (Black, indigenous, and people of color) in various studies. Research suggests that different racial/ethnic groups may be more or less vulnerable to the same conditions, and the resilience mechanisms that can protect them likely operate differently in each population (Coman & Wu, 2018). Psychological resilience is a complex psychosocial process through which individuals exposed to sustained adversity or potentially traumatic events experience positive psychological adaptation over time. Meaning, despite experiencing severe stress and adversity, people with high levels of resiliency are able to manage and recover from these stressful life experiences which reduces the likelihood of developing depressive disorders (Graber, Pichon, & Carabine, 2015; Llabre et al., 2017).

Studies have found that resilience is a significant factor associated with lower rates of depression among minority racial groups. A recent study of nearly 30,000 older U.S. women found that Black women had a lower risk of late-life depression compared to whites. Another study of 7,690 adults aged 54 to 65 years found that MDD was significantly less prevalent among Blacks than whites, and similarly prevalent among Hispanics and whites. Meaning, there appear to be racial differences in terms of the development of MDD and a factor that may influence this phenomenon is resiliency. Specifically, the notion of "resilience training" postulates that early life exposure to mild-to-moderate adversity often serves as resilience training for later life which is more likely to be experienced by BIPOC individuals (Laird et al., 2019). Studies have also found greater prevalence among Caucasian and Native American adults than among African American, Asian American, and Hispanic adults. Reasons for racial/ethnic differences in MDD remain unclear but do not reduce the importance of treatment for minorities, among whom treatment disparities often remain. MDD is often comorbid with anxiety disorders, particularly panic disorder and generalized anxiety disorder, as well as with PTSD (Hasin et al., 2017).

Major Depressive Disorder in Children and Adolescents

Depression among children and adolescents presents a significant public health concern within the United States. Approximately 3.1 million adolescents (12.8 percent) experience a depressive episode annually with over 70 percent of these episodes causing severe functional impairment. Additionally, rates of MDD among pre-adolescent populations have significantly increased in recent years. The onset of MDD during childhood and adolescence are associated with significant risk factors and subsequent challenges including impaired school performance, interpersonal difficulties, early parenthood, and increased risk of other mental health and substance use disorders. Since adolescents often present symptoms of depression differently than adult suffers it often goes underrecognized and undertreated in this population (Cohen, Thakur, Burkhouse, & Gibb, 2019).

Pediatric depression is often underrecognized and undertreated since many symptoms presented among children and adolescents vary from what is expected among adults. *djedzura/123RF*

As a result of COVID-19, children and adolescents have experienced unprecedented interruptions to their daily routines that may be precipitants of mental illness, including anxiety, depression, and stress-related symptoms (Racine et al., 2020). Due to COVID-related social restrictions, many of the daily activities that provide structure, meaning, and a healthy psychological outlet, such as participating in school, extracurricular activities, social interactions, and physical activity became limited or removed all together. Over a sustained period, these losses may contribute to or worsen depressive symptoms and promote social withdrawal, loss of pleasure (*anhedonia*), and hopelessness. In addition to the environmental conditions that can exacerbate feelings of depression, the COVID-19 pandemic has also impeded the early detection of mood and anxiety disorders among children and adolescents who are now spending more time at home. With less access to mental health services, the pandemic may worsen the already serious problem of identifying children and adolescents with depressive disorders. Clinicians who detect and treat mental illness in the early stages of disorder development are seeing fewer children and youth during the pandemic. Furthermore, behaviors that may otherwise be red flags for emotional distress, such as physical distancing and decreased activity, are promoted as desirable and adaptive during this public health crisis (Courtney, Watson, Battaglia, Mulsant, & Szatmari, 2019).

Pediatric depression has been observed in preschoolers as young as 3 years of age; however, children are often less likely to verbalize their feelings or meet the *DSM-5* criteria for major depression. Depressed children 3 to 8 years of age often present with more somatic complaints, are more irritable, show symptoms of anxiety, and have other behavioral problems. As children become adolescents and then adults, symptom presentation becomes more consistent with the *DSM-5* criteria. In addition, children and adolescents typically experience less hypersomnia, more variations in weight and appetite, and fewer delusions as compared with adults. Teens may also present with fewer complaints of decreased energy or psychomotor slowing as compared to adults with MDD. Pediatric MDD is often underdiagnosed and undertreated with only 50 percent of adolescents diagnosed before reaching adulthood. Just like adults suffering with MDD, this is a common, chronic, recurrent, and debilitating disease that disrupts daily function. The Centers for Disease Control and Prevention estimate the incidence at 0.5 percent in children 3 to 5 years old, 2 percent for 6- to 11-year-olds, and up to 12 percent for 12- to 17-year-olds. During childhood, the diagnosis of MDD in males and females is equal, but after puberty, females are more frequently diagnosed with depression. These sex differences are likely to be multifactorial, but females appear to experience more external risk factors , such as history of family conflicts and abuse, for depression prior to and during puberty (Mullen, 2018).

Among children with MDD, the most common comorbidities include attention-deficit/hyperactivity disorder (ADHD), anxiety disorders, disruptive disorders, substance use disorders, enuresis/encopresis (urinary/fecal incontinence), and separation anxiety disorder. Research suggests that children and adolescents with comorbidities have greater impairment and symptom severity, more chronic course of illness, and decreased response to treatment, as compared to those without another psychological disorder. In addition to problems with social and academic function, untreated depression is also associated with an increased risk of suicidal ideation and attempts. Multiple studies estimate that 12 percent of the adolescent population (12 to 17 years) has been diagnosed with at least one major depressive episode. And, as many as 8 percent of adolescents diagnosed with MDD complete suicide by young adulthood, making suicide the second leading cause of death among adolescents 12 to 17 years of age (Dochnal et al., 2019; Mullen, 2018).

Early intervention is critical to effectively treating depressed children and adolescents. Treatment for pediatric MDD includes a combination of psychotherapy and antidepressant medications, specifically selective serotonin reuptake inhibitors (SSRIs). Prozac (*fluoxetine*) is approved by the Food and Drug Administration (FDA) for children 8 years of age and older, and Lexapro (*escitalopram*) is approved for ages 12 years and older. Prozac (*fluoxetine*) has the strongest evidence for effective use in treating pediatric depression. In 2004, a large-scale meta-analysis of 100,000 participants confirmed an increased rate of suicidal thoughts and behaviors among children, adolescents, and young adults which resulted in the FDA **black box warning** to all antidepressants. Celexa (Citalopram), Luvox (fluvoxamine), Paxil (paroxetine), Prozac (fluoxetine), Zoloft (sertraline), Effexor (venlafaxine), Remeron (mirtazapine), Serzone (nefazodone), and Wellbutrin (bupropion) continue to have this warning attached. As a result of these possible adverse effects, SSRI prescription for adolescents decreased, particularly for those 14 years of age and younger.

Although the risk of suicidality may increase upon initiation of antidepressants, this risk also increases when symptoms of depression remain untreated. This FDA warning impacted the treatment of adults with depression even though the advisory focused on children and adolescents. There was a marked decrease in antidepressant prescriptions (4.61 percent annually) after the black box warning was issued. This was an unintended outcome for a population that was not the target of this warning and for whom there is solid

SHADES OF GRAY

Consider the following case study of a college student, who may resemble someone you know.

Carmen's friends were shocked to find her passed out in her dorm room with an empty bottle of sleeping pills on the floor next to her. Carmen had experienced years of unhappiness, a sense of low self-worth, pessimism, and chronic fatigue. She often told her friends she couldn't remember a time when she was happy for more than a few days at a time. Since the beginning of the winter term, however, Carmen's depressed mood had deepened, and she had spent days on end locked in her bedroom, apparently sleeping. She had said it was no use going to class because she couldn't concentrate. She had been skipping meals and had lost 12 pounds.

Based on the timeframe and symptoms described, what diagnosis would Carmen most likely receive? (Discussion appears at the end of the chapter.)

evidence of a positive effect of antidepressant medication on suicide risk (Friedman, 2014).

Psychotherapy is also an effective method to treat MDD among children and adolescents and some options include individual or group CBT or interpersonal psychotherapy (IPT). Both have been shown to be effective for adolescents but none more effective than the other. Studies have shown that psychotherapy used to treat mild cases of MDD is effective for 62 percent of individuals. Overall, psychotherapy in combination with medication is the most recommended treatment for MDD in children and adolescents with monitoring for increased risk of suicidality. Most children and adolescents (96.4 percent) will successfully recover from a depressive episode but future episodes will likely occur within 2 years (Curry et al., 2011). Seventy percent of children and adolescents who have recovered after treatment will experience symptoms within 5 years of symptoms remission. Although no single variable has been shown to predict the recurrence of MDD in the pediatric population, the earlier age of onset, number of depressive episodes, severity of episodes, and psychosocial stressors may play a role in predicting relapse. In comparison to adult sufferers, children and adolescents are more likely to recover from their episode faster, have a higher rate of recurrence, and have a higher probability of a bipolar disorder diagnosis (Mullen, 2018).

CHARACTERISTICS OF BIPOLAR DISORDERS

The spectrum of mood is best viewed as a vertical pole with depression on the bottom and mania on the top. As we previously discussed, the common thread that connects each disorder in this chapter is a disruption of mood. Unlike characteristics found within depressive disorders where the common feature is a depressed mood state, the opposite is true for mania and mood is elevated. Think of the tell-tale symptoms of major depression and then reverse them. For example, someone with depression has low energy whereas someone with mania has increased (at times, boundless) energy. Depressive thoughts create feelings of worthlessness, but people with mania have an abundance of self-worth. You may think, wait . . . feeling excessively happy with excess energy, and lots of confidence. Where do I get some? While mania may sound like a great time, realize that mania still represents disrupted mood, in this case it is persistently elevated mood that causes psychological dysfunction (Table 3). Variations in manic symptoms can lead to one of four **bipolar disorder** diagnoses which are all defined by fluctuations in mood and activity levels (Stanton & Watson, 2020): *bipolar I disorder, bipolar II disorder, cyclothymic disorder,* and *rapid cycling bipolar disorder* which all involve some degree of alternation between mania and depressive states. The features of each of these bipolar disorders will be discussed within this section.

Mania: The opposite of depression

Manic episodes involve a period of abnormally and persistently elevated or irritable mood with goal-directed activity or energy lasting at least 1 week (American Psychiatric Association, 2013). During a manic episode, people often report feeling euphoric or "high" with some even feeling like they are experiencing a continuous orgasm. It has been noted in multiple studies that statements like, "I've never felt better in my life" is a common and recurring theme during mania. Episodes of mania include boastful, overconfident, and grandiose (inflated) self-esteem, racing thoughts, poor judgment, and decreased impulse control (Kendler, 2017). Similar to severe depressive episodes, psychotic symptoms can develop when mood is significantly disrupted during manic episodes which signifies severe cognitive dysfunction. Meaning, as a person in a manic episode moves further away from a balanced mood state (*euthymia*) their thoughts are

TABLE 3   *DSM-5* Criteria for a Manic Episode

A. A distinct period of abnormally and persistently elevated, expansive, or irritable mood and abnormally and persistently increased goal-directed activity or energy, lasting at least 1 week and present most of the day, nearly every day (or any duration if hospitalization is necessary).

B. During the period of mood disturbance and increased energy or activity, three (or more) of the following symptoms (four if the mood is only irritable) are present to a significant degree, and represent a noticeable change from usual behavior:

   1. Inflated self-esteem or grandiosity

   2. Decreased need for sleep (e.g., feels rested after only 3 hours of sleep)

   3. More talkative than usual or pressure to keep talking

   4. Flight of ideas or subjective experience that thoughts are racing

   5. Distractibility (i.e., attention too easily drawn to unimportant or irrelevant external stimuli), as reported or observed

   6. Increase in goal-directed activity (either socially, at work or school, or sexually) or psychomotor agitation (i.e., purposeless non-goal–directed activity)

   7. Excessive involvement in activities that have a high potential for painful consequences (e.g., engaging in unrestrained buying sprees, sexual indiscretions, or foolish business investments)

C. The mood disturbance is sufficiently severe to cause marked impairment in social or occupational functioning or to necessitate hospitalization to prevent harm to self or others, or there are psychotic features.

D. The episode is not attributable to the direct physiological effects of a substance (e.g., a drug of abuse, a medication, or other treatments), or to another medical condition.

Note: At least one lifetime manic episode is required for the diagnosis of bipolar I disorder.

significantly affected. Grandiose, and often irrational, thoughts that they can cure cancer with a special mixture of Red Bull, hot sauce, and Flintstone vitamins may worsen to delusions that create false beliefs that they have special powers, like the ability to cure the sick through touch.

PROFILES

Kanye West

Kanye West is a Grammy Award-winning rapper, record producer, and fashion designer who is outspoken and prone to controversy. While West has won nearly two dozen Grammy Awards, his award-show theatrics and marriage to Kim Kardashian also keep him in the public eye. West was diagnosed with bipolar disorder in 2016 and during his time in the spotlight, has displayed numerous symptoms of mania. In a 2019 interview in Vogue magazine, his wife, Kim Kardashian-West openly discussed her husband's mental health issues. She said that, in the past, West found it hard to accept that he has bipolar disorder, telling people that he was instead suffering from sleep deprivation, but he has come to terms with his diagnosis. "'I think we're in a pretty good place with it now . . . that shows how you can live a normal life with mental illness . . ." West admitted that during his manic periods he may suffer from racing thoughts, irritability, sleep loss, and paranoia or psychosis. "When you're in this state, you're hyper-paranoid about everything . . . Everything's a conspiracy." (Berman, 2020).

Fiona Spring/ABACAPRESS/Alamy Stock Photo

On July 4, 2020, West announced that he was running for President under a proposed new political party, called the *Birthday Party,* despite missing the

(continued)

deadline to file the required paperwork needed to run for election, having never voted in his lifetime and without any organized campaign in place. A few days after announcing his Presidential run, he did a 4-hour nonsensical interview with *Forbes* magazine and spoke about how he envisions a White House organizational model based on the fictitious country of Wakanda in the "Black Panther" film. West said, ". . . you got Kanye West, one of the most powerful humans—I'm not saying *the* most because you got a lot of alien-level superpowers and it's only collectively that we can set it free. This is not going to be some Nipsey Hussle being murdered, they're doing a documentary, we have so many soldiers that die for our freedom, our freedom of information, that there is a cure for AIDS out there, there is going to be a mix of big pharma and holistic" (Lane, 2020).

Just as anyone with bipolar disorder who is not getting effective treatment, the profile on Kanye West highlights how an individual with mania can function well for a while but eventually symptoms return which disrupt mood and behavior resulting in an inability to function. As symptoms of mania increase, individuals are more likely to exhibit impulsive behaviors, rapid speech, and racing thoughts. The incoherent language displayed by West during his interview is called "*flight of ideas*," which refers to the continuous flow of accelerated speech that is often incoherent as it abruptly shifts from topic to topic (American Psychiatric Association, 2013). People experiencing mania are often flooded with so many rapid and exciting ideas that it's difficult to express them at once. These racing thoughts often make it difficult for others to understand what is being said. This rapid speech and the pressure to speak make it difficult to interrupt a person manifesting this manic symptom.

Increased energy experienced during mania results in a reduced need for sleep and the tendency to awaken very early in the morning after a short sleep feeling refreshed. Decreased appetite and weight loss are also common, and manic individuals often report that they don't have time to eat or eat less due to their many distractions. This hyperactivity and distraction can range from an increased pace of typical daily tasks to disorganized and rapidly shifting behaviors. In more severe episodes, destructive agitation can result in the need for hospitalization Some people may become agitated and irritable, particularly with people they perceive as "getting in the way" of what they believe is an epiphany or sudden and brilliant insight. Manic episodes also include an increase in impulsive behaviors, such as sexual indiscretions or spending sprees. During these episodes, individuals commonly give money away, buy unneeded things, or enter into unsound business ventures. Noticeable changes to typical behaviors can also be seen in personal appearance and behaviors where individuals may dress indiscreetly, become flirtatious and engage in sexual behaviors typically judged to be wildly inappropriate by their families and peers, such as infidelity or indiscriminate sexual encounters with strangers. Catastrophic consequences of mania include problems with law enforcement, financial difficulties, impaired insight, and hyperactivity which might result in involuntary hospitalization or incarceration (American Psychiatric Association, 2013; Kendler, 2017).

Mania is a core criterion for bipolar disorders which are centrally characterized by emotional disturbance that involves alternation of manic and depressive episodes. While it is possible to experience only manic episodes without the alternation with depression (unipolar mood disorder), it is far more likely the individual will fluctuate between manic and depressive episodes (bipolar disorder). In order to be diagnosed with a manic episode, an individual must show an elevated, expansive, or irritable mood for at least 1 week, as well as at least three of the other symptoms listed in Table 3. These symptoms must impair the individual's social or occupational function (American Psychiatric Association, 2013). Currently, none of the worldwide classification systems defines mania as a separate psychological disorder, but various studies have found support that there may be need to qualify mania as an independent psychological disorder. Multiple studies have shown a significant percentage of participants who present with *unipolar mania*, which means manic episodes without the presence of depression. Similar results were reported in other studies on individuals in Africa, India, China, and Tunisia that found a high prevalence of recurrent mania with limited or no depressive episodes. Other studies have found that a majority of people with bipolar disorder from Spain, the United States, and Germany spend more than half of the time in depressive states than in the manic states (Jules, Ajdacic-Gross, & Rossler, 2020).

Bipolar I Disorder

Individuals whose moods alternate between depressive and manic states meet criteria for bipolar disorder, which is a common and disabling mental illness with significant morbidity and mortality. People who experience full manic episodes that alternate with full depressive episodes have **bipolar I disorder.** For some people with bipolar I disorder, depressions are as severe as major depressive episodes, whereas for others the episodes of depression are relatively mild and infrequent. Some people diagnosed with bipolar I disorder have mixed episodes in which they experience the full criteria for manic episodes and at least three key symptoms of major depressive episodes in the same day, every day for at least 1 week (American Psychiatric Association, 2013; Yatham et al., 2018). You have probably heard the phrase "he's so bipolar" to refer to someone who experiences day-to-day moodiness, unpredictability, or emotional reactivity. Although it is true that people with bipolar disorder show some symptoms (like irritability) even between episodes, this loose terminology for subthreshold fluctuations does not truly capture the episodic nature that defines the disorder, and can lead to stigma. Importantly, the episodes in bipolar disorder are periods with multiple symptoms of mania or depression.

Bipolar II Disorder

Whereas people with bipolar I disorder experience mania, people with **bipolar II disorder** experience **hypomania.** Hypomania involves the same symptoms as mania, but the episodes are milder (Table 4). The major difference is that in hypomania these symptoms are not severe enough to interfere with daily functioning, do not involve hallucinations or delusions, and last at least 4 consecutive days (rather than a week). Whereas depression is common in bipolar I disorder but not required for the diagnosis, for bipolar II disorder, in addition to hypomania the person also has to experience major depressive episodes (American Psychiatric Association, 2013).

Cyclothymic Disorder

Cyclothymic disorder is a chronic form of bipolar disorder, characterized by less extreme mood states. A person with **cyclothymic disorder,** alternates between periods of some hypomanic symptoms and periods of some depressive symptoms, chronically over at least a 2-year period. The defining feature is that the hypomanic and depressive symptoms are of insufficient number, severity, or duration to meet full criteria for hypomania or major depressive episode, respectively. During the periods of hypomanic symptoms, the person may be able to function reasonably well. Often, however, the periods of depressive symptoms significantly interfere with daily functioning, although the episodes are less severe than major depressive episodes. People with cyclothymic disorder are at increased risk of developing bipolar disorder. Epidemiological studies suggest that cyclothymic disorder is the most prevalent subtype of bipolar disorder, however, it is rarely diagnosed, particularly among children and adolescents (Van Meter et al., 2017).

Rapid Cycling Bipolar Disorder

About 90 percent of people with bipolar disorder have multiple episodes or cycles during their lifetimes (Merikangas et al., 2007). The length of an individual episode of bipolar disorder varies greatly from one person to the next. Some people are in a manic state for several weeks or months before moving into a depressed state. More rarely, people switch from mania to depression and back within a matter of days or, as noted above, even in the same day. The number of lifetime episodes also varies tremendously from one person to the next, but a relatively common pattern is for episodes to become more frequent and closer together over time. Four or more mood episodes that meet criteria for manic, hypomanic, or major depressive episode within 1 year lead to a diagnosis of **rapid cycling bipolar disorder.** Multiple studies have consistently found that evidence of poorer prognosis and greater disease burden in rapid cycling bipolar disorder (Peters, West, Eisner, Baek, & Deckersbach, 2016). Interestingly, there appears to be a seasonal aspect to bipolar disorder for some people, as in unipolar depression. Some studies show that up to 25 percent of people with bipolar disorder experience their depressive or manic episodes in a seasonal pattern (Geoffroy et al., 2013; Goikolea et al., 2007).

TABLE 4 Criteria for Bipolar I and Bipolar II Disorders

Bipolar I and II disorders differ in the presence of major depressive episodes, episodes meeting the full criteria for mania, and hypomanic episodes.

Criteria	Bipolar I	Bipolar II
Major depressive episodes	Can occur but are not necessary for diagnosis	Are necessary for diagnosis
Episodes meeting full criteria for mania	Are necessary for diagnosis	Cannot be present for diagnosis
Hypomanic episodes	Can occur between episodes of severe mania or major depression but are not necessary for diagnosis	Are necessary for diagnosis

Bipolar Disorder in Children

One area of great interest and controversy is the presence of bipolar disorder in children and adolescents. Various epidemiological, clinical, and high-risk studies suggest that the peak period for bipolar disorder onset spans late adolescence and early adulthood. There is a substantial debate on the existence of a prepubertal form of bipolar disorder that manifests in early childhood. US researchers proposed that chronic, irritability aggression and explosive temper in very young children with comorbid ADHD represented a prepubertal form of bipolar disorder. These behaviors, which are theorized to be a variant of mania, do not adequately fit the diagnostic criteria for DMDD, which is a proposed alternative diagnosis for these children (Duffy, Carlson, Dubicka, & Hillegers, 2020). Increasingly, researchers and clinicians have become interested in identifying early signs of bipolar disorder in children and young teenagers so interventions can be initiated and researchers can investigate the causes and course of the disorder in youth (Brotman, Sharif-Askary, Dickstein, & Leibenluft, 2016).

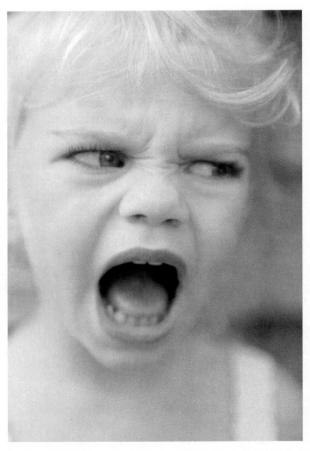

Some children who regularly have consistent and developmentally inappropriate temper tantrums may have disruptive mood dysregulation disorder. *Steve Wisbauer/Digital Vision/Getty Images*

Although some children show the alternating episodes of mania and depression interspersed with periods of normal mood characteristic of bipolar disorder (Birmaher et al., 2006), others show chronic symptoms and rapid mood switches. Individuals in the latter group tend toward severe irritability characterized by frequent temper tantrums or rages. These children are at increased risk of developing anxiety and depressive disorders later in life but do not tend to develop classic bipolar disorder (Stringaris, Cohen, Pine, & Leibenluft, 2009). In addition, it is difficult to distinguish the agitation and risky behavior that accompany mania in youth from the symptoms of ADHD (see the chapter "Neurodevelopmental and Neurocognitive Disorders"), which include hyperactivity, poor judgment, and impulsivity, or from the symptoms of oppositional defiant disorder (see the chapter "Disruptive, Impulse-Control, and Conduct Disorders"), which include chronic irritability and refusal to follow rules. There has been considerable debate as to whether these agitated, irritable children have bipolar disorder, ADHD, or oppositional defiant disorder, none of which seems to fit their symptoms perfectly.

Prevalence and Course of Bipolar Disorder

Bipolar disorder may be less common than depressive disorders but these together affect nearly 6 million adults in the United States. The estimated prevalence of bipolar disorder varies but approximately 2.8 percent of U.S. adults experience bipolar disorder in any given year, whereas, the World Mental Health Survey Initiative reported estimates of 1.5 percent across bipolar I, bipolar II. The total lifetime prevalence internationally is approximately 2.4 percent, while it is estimated that 4.4 percent of U.S. adults experience bipolar disorder at some time in their lives (NIMH, 2017c). Internationally, only 0.6 percent of people will experience bipolar I disorder and only 0.4 percent of people will experience bipolar II disorder in their lifetimes. Men and women seem equally likely to develop the disorder, and there are no consistent differences in the prevalence of the disorder among ethnic groups or across cultures. These facts suggest that biological factors may be more responsible for bipolar disorder than for depressive disorders, which show more variability across cultures. Symptoms of bipolar disorder typically present in late adolescence or early adulthood and the average age of onset is 25 years. Those with an earlier age of onset tend to have a longer delay to treatment, greater depressive symptom severity, and higher levels of comorbid anxiety and substance use (Merikangas et al., 2011; Yatham et al., 2018)

Bipolar disorders have a recurrent course of illness which is associated with poor prognosis. The likelihood that affected individuals will return to their previous level of function diminishes with each recurrent episode. Recurrent episodes of mania and depression do not equally contribute to levels of impairment. Repeated depressive episodes are more likely to negatively impact daily function (Peters et al., 2016). Like people with depressive disorders, people with bipolar disorder often face chronic problems on the job and in their relationships (Marangell, 2004). The majority of people with bipolar disorders also meet the criteria for other psychiatric disorders, most often an anxiety disorder. In addition, people with bipolar disorder often abuse substances such as alcohol and hard drugs, which impairs their control over their disorder, their willingness to take medications, and their functioning. Despite the impairment resulting from their symptoms, most people with bipolar disorder, especially those in developing countries, do not receive any treatment (Merikangas et al., 2011).

Creativity and the Mood Disorders

As noted in Mood Disorders Along the Continuum, some theorists have argued that the symptoms of mania—increased self-esteem, a rush of ideas, and the courage to pursue those ideas, high energy, little need for sleep, excessive optimism, and decisiveness—can actually have benefits in certain settings. In turn, the melancholy of depression is often seen as

Rap artist and actor DMX (aka Earl Simmons) has publicly acknowledged struggling with depression before his death. *hurricanehank/123RF*

inspirational for artists. Indeed, some of the most influential people in history—including political leaders, religious figures, and artists—have suffered, and perhaps benefited, from bipolar disorder or depression (Jamison, 1993).

Political leaders including Abraham Lincoln, Alexander Hamilton, Winston Churchill, Napoleon Bonaparte, and Benito Mussolini and religious leaders including Martin Luther and George Fox (founder of the Society of Friends, or Quakers) have been posthumously diagnosed by psychiatric biographers as having had periods of mania, hypomania, or depression (Jamison, 1993). Although during periods of depression these leaders often were incapacitated, during periods of mania and hypomania they accomplished extraordinary feats. While manic, they devised brilliant and daring strategies for winning wars and solving national problems and had the energy, self-esteem, and persistence to carry out these strategies.

Writers, artists, and composers have a higher-than-normal prevalence of mania and depression. For example, a study of 1,005 famous twentieth-century artists, writers, and other professionals found that the artists and writers experienced two to three times the rate of mood disorders, psychosis, and suicide attempts than comparably successful people in business, science, and public life. The poets in this group were most likely to have been manic (Ludwig, 1992). More recently, actors Jim Carrey, Kirsten Dunst, and Zach Braff, game-show host Drew Carey, rapper DMX, and singers Demi Lovato and Mariah Carey are among the celebrities who have publicized their mood disorder.

Although many creative people with bipolar disorder may have been able to learn from their periods of depression and to exploit their periods of mania, many also have found the highs and lows of the disorder unbearable and have attempted or completed

Winston Churchill had periods of manic symptoms that may have been both an asset and a liability. *Library of Congress Prints and Photographs Division [LC-DIG-npcc-17934]*

suicide. In general, the mood disorders substantially impair thinking and productivity. As Elizabeth Wurtzel (1995, p. 295) notes:

> While it may be true that a great deal of art finds its inspirational wellspring in sorrow, let's not kid ourselves in how much time each of those people wasted and lost by being mired in misery. So many productive hours slipped by as paralyzing despair took over. This is not to say that we should deny sadness its rightful place among the muses of poetry and of all art forms, but let's stop calling it madness, let's stop pretending that the feeling itself is interesting. Let's call it depression and admit that it is very bleak.

THEORIES OF DEPRESSION

Depression is one of the most researched of all the psychological disorders. We will discuss biological, behavioral, cognitive, interpersonal, and sociocultural theories.

Biological Theories of Depression

Depression is a common, complex, and debilitating condition with a lifetime prevalence of 20 percent worldwide (Cai, Choi, & Fried, 2020). A number of different biological processes appear to be involved in depression, including genetics, neurotransmitter systems, structural and functional abnormalities of the brain, and neuroendocrine systems.

Genetic Factors

There are lots of things that people believe "run in the family" and depressive behaviors are one of these ideas. For decades, there has been much focus on attempting to successfully unravel the genetic architecture of depression which can be done through family and twin studies that examine genetic similarities among family members with various conditions, like depression. Family history studies have found that the first-degree relatives of people with major depressive disorder are three to four times more likely to also have depression than are the first-degree relatives of people without the disorder (Howard et al., 2019; Flint & Kendler, 2014). Twin studies of major depression find higher concordance rates for monozygotic twins than for dizygotic twins, implicating genetic processes in the disorder. Meaning, research has found that the more genes you share with someone who has depression, the more likely it is that you will also have depression.

Interestingly, recent large-scale genetic data were collected through the direct-to-consumer genetic testing company 23andMe. In this study, self-report data were provided by 75,607 consumers who reported a history of clinical diagnosis or treatment for major depression and 231,747 individuals who reported no history of depression. This novel approach to psychiatric research produced a high genetic correlation between the results from the 23andMe study and data from one genome-wide association studies (GWAS) which supports a common genetic overlap. Research has shown that depression is a polygenic trait influenced by many genetic variants, each demonstrating a small effect. Therefore, in order to identify the genetic variables most associated with the etiology of depression, a very large sample of individuals must be studied. As sample sizes continue to increase, researchers will be able to uncover more about the genetic architecture of this debilitating disorder (Mullins & Lewis, 2017). Despite robust evidence for a genetic component, identifying these specific genetic variants involved in the development of depression has been a major challenge. But current research suggests that major depressive disorder may consist of various subtypes with different underlying biological pathways and environmental contributions. Future genetic research on depression may find that disorder consists of an entangled web of partly overlapping biopsychosocial constructs, genetic contributions, and underlying biological mechanisms (Cai et al., 2020). In addition to research on the genetic contributions of depression, there is an ever-growing body of evidence that there are shared genetic components between many behavioral and psychiatric disorders. Using meta-analysis, researchers have found evidence of significant genetic correlations for depression with anorexia nervosa, ADHD, schizophrenia, and bipolar disorder were found (Howard et al., 2019).

It is probable that multiple genetic abnormalities contribute to depression. Several studies suggest that the serotonin transporter gene may play a role (Flint & Kendler, 2014; Howard et al., 2019; Saveanu & Nemeroff, 2012). As we will discuss below, serotonin is one of the neurotransmitters implicated in depression. Abnormalities on the serotonin transporter gene could lead to dysfunction in the regulation of serotonin, which in turn could affect the stability of individuals' moods. In a landmark longitudinal study, Av-shalom Caspi and colleagues (Caspi et al., 2003) found that people with abnormalities on the serotonin transporter gene were at increased risk for depression when they faced negative life events (see also Kaufman et al., 2004, 2006). Not all studies have replicated these findings (see Risch et al., 2009), but a recent meta-analysis supported the interaction between the serotonin transporter gene and early stress in the prediction of later depression (Karg, Burmeiester, Shedden, & Sen, 2011). Other genes have been linked with depression and also show evidence of gene-environment interactions (Dunn et al., 2015).

Neurotransmitter Theories

The neurotransmitters that have been implicated most often in depression are the **monoamines,** specifically, **norepinephrine, serotonin,** and, to a lesser extent, **dopamine.** These neurotransmitters are found in large concentrations in the limbic system, a part of the brain associated with the regulation of sleep, appetite, and emotional processes. The early theory of the role of these neurotransmitters in mood disorders was that depression is caused by a reduction in the amount of norepinephrine or serotonin in the synapses between neurons (Glassman, 1969; Schildkraut, 1965).

As our understanding of the functioning of neurotransmitters in the brain has increased, theories of their role in depression have become much more complex (Saveanu & Nemeroff, 2012). A number of processes within brain cells that affect the functioning of neurotransmitters may go awry in depression (Figure 1). For example, serotonin and norepinephrine are synthesized in neurons from tryptophan and tyrosine, respectively, and some studies suggest that abnormalities in this synthesis process may contribute to depression (Howard et al., 2019; Zhang, Beaulieu, Sotnikova, Gainetdinov, & Caron, 2004). Both serotonin and norepinephrine are released by one neuron (referred to as the presynaptic neuron) into the synapse and then bind to receptors on other neurons (referred to as the postsynaptic neurons; see Figure 1). The release process, which is regulated by the serotonin transporter gene, may be abnormal in depression. In addition, the receptors for serotonin and norepinephrine on the postsynaptic neurons may be less sensitive than normal in people with depression, or they may sometimes malfunction (Saveanu & Nemeroff, 2012).

Structural and Functional Brain Abnormalities

Neuroimaging studies have found consistent abnormalities in at least four areas of the brain in people with depression: the prefrontal cortex, anterior cingulate, hippocampus, and amygdala (Figure 2).

Neural plasticity is a fundamental mechanism that allows the nervous system to modify itself, both functionally and structurally, in response to experience and injury (von Bernhardi, Bernhardi, & Eugenín, 2017). Various studies have shown that this adaptive process is disrupted in depression and the changes in neural plasticity that are induced by stress and other negative stimuli play a significant role in the development of depression. An increasing number of clinical research studies have highlighted the correlations between neural plasticity and depression. These studies have found that the effects of depression on neural plasticity are complex pathophysiological processes that involve multiple brain structures, such as the hippocampus, prefrontal cortex, and amygdala (Liu et al., 2017).

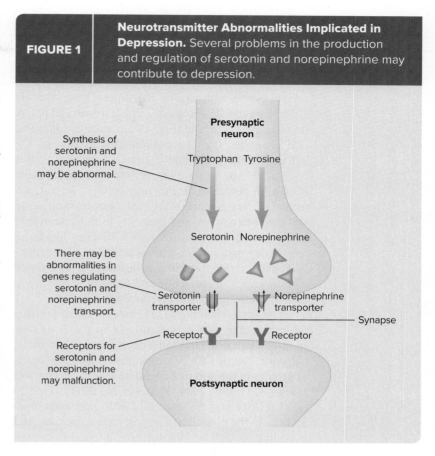

FIGURE 1 **Neurotransmitter Abnormalities Implicated in Depression.** Several problems in the production and regulation of serotonin and norepinephrine may contribute to depression.

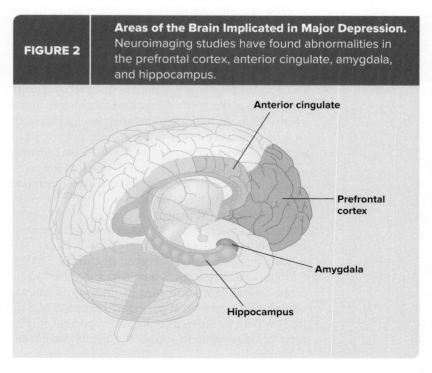

FIGURE 2 **Areas of the Brain Implicated in Major Depression.** Neuroimaging studies have found abnormalities in the prefrontal cortex, anterior cingulate, amygdala, and hippocampus.

Critical functions of the prefrontal cortex include attention, working memory, planning, and novel problem solving. Many studies have shown reduced metabolic activity and a reduction in the volume of gray matter in the prefrontal cortex, particularly on the left side, in people with serious depression (Howard et al., 2019; Saveanu & Nemeroff, 2012; Thase, Hahn, & Berton, 2015). In addition, electroencephalographic (EEG) studies show lower brain-wave activity on the left side of the prefrontal cortex in depressed people compared to nondepressed people (Davidson, Pizzagalli, Nitschke, & Putnam, 2002). The left prefrontal cortex is particularly involved in motivation and goal orientation, and inactivity in this region may be associated with motivational difficulties like those seen in depression. The successful treatment of depression with antidepressant medications is associated with increases in metabolic and brain-wave activity in the left prefrontal cortex (Kennedy et al., 2001).

The anterior cingulate, a subregion of the prefrontal cortex, plays an important role in the body's response to stress, in emotional expression, and in social behavior. People with depression show different levels of activity in the anterior cingulate relative to controls (Singh & Gotlib, 2014; Thase et al., 2015). This altered activity may be associated with problems in attention, in the planning of appropriate responses, and in coping, as well as with anhedonia found in depression. Again, activity normalizes in this region of the brain when people are successfully treated for their depression (Dougherty & Rauch, 2007).

The hippocampus is critical in memory and in fear-related learning. Neuroimaging studies show smaller volume and lower metabolic activity in the hippocampus of people with major depression (Cole, Costafreda, McGuffin, & Fu, 2011; Liu et al., 2017). Damage to the hippocampus could be the result of chronic arousal of the body's stress response. As we will discuss, people with depression show chronically high levels of the hormone cortisol, particularly in response to stress, indicating that their bodies overreact to stress and their levels of cortisol do not return to normal as quickly as those of nondepressed people. The hippocampus contains many receptors for cortisol, and chronically elevated levels of this hormone may kill or inhibit the development of new neurons in the hippocampus (Pittenger & Duman, 2008). Treatment with antidepressants or electroconvulsive therapy results in the growth of new cells in the hippocampus in rats (Pittenger & Duman, 2008). Chronic and severe stress has been shown to impair hippocampus-dependent explicit memory in animal models of depression. Hippocampal synaptic plasticity is widely considered to play an important role in hippocampus-dependent explicit memory formation. Additionally, stress can also decrease neuronal dendrite branching and plasticity in the hippocampus and can trigger the activation of the hypothalamic-pituitary-adrenal axis (HPA), and increase levels of corticosteroids (Liu et al., 2017).

Abnormalities in the structure and functioning of the amygdala also are found in depression (Singh & Gotlib, 2014; Thase et al., 2015). The amygdala helps direct attention to stimuli that are emotionally salient and have major significance for the individual. Studies of people with mood disorders show an enlargement and increased activity in this part of the brain, and activity in the amygdala has been observed to decrease to normal levels in people successfully treated for depression (Singh & Gotlib, 2014; Thase et al., 2015). The effects of overactivity in the amygdala are not yet entirely clear, but the overactivity may bias people toward aversive or emotionally arousing information and lead to rumination over negative memories and negative aspects of the environment (Davidson et al., 2009).

Interestingly, differences in brain function may begin emerging in childhood, even before a depressive episode. Girls who are at high risk for depression (because their mothers have had depression) exhibit decreased neural reactivity to rewarding stimuli, as early as age 9 (Kujawa, Proudfit, & Klein, 2014; Sharp et al., 2014). Such patterns could be due to a number of factors, but they suggest that vulnerability to depression can have neural aspects early in life.

Neuroendocrine Factors

Hormones have long been thought to play a role in mood disorders, especially depression. The neuroendocrine system regulates a number of important hormones, which in turn affect basic functions such as sleep, appetite, sexual drive, and the ability to experience pleasure (to review the neuroendocrine system, see the chapter "Theories and Treatment of Abnormality"). These hormones also help the body respond to environmental stressors.

Three key components of the neuroendocrine system—the hypothalamus, pituitary, and adrenal cortex—work together in a biological feedback system richly interconnected with the amygdala, hippocampus, and cerebral cortex. This system, often referred to as the **hypothalamic-pituitary-adrenal axis,** or **HPA axis,** is involved in the fight-or-flight response (see the chapter "Anxiety, Obsessive-Compulsive, Trauma, and Stressor-Related Disorders"). Activation of the HPA axis causes secretion of glucocorticoids, which act on multiple organ systems to redirect energy resources to meet real or anticipated demand (Herman et al., 2016). Normally, when we are confronted with a stressor, the hypothalamus releases corticotropin-releasing hormone (CRH) onto receptors on the anterior pituitary (Figure 3). This results in secretion of corticotropin into the plasma in the bloodstream,

FIGURE 3 | The Hypothalamic-Pituitary-Adrenal Axis.

The hypothalamus synthesizes corticotropin-releasing hormone (CRH). CRH is transported to the pituitary gland, where it stimulates the synthesis and release of adrenocorticotropic hormone (ACTH), which then circulates to the adrenal glands, producing cortisol. Cortisol then inhibits the production of further ACTH and CRH. Normally, this process prevents too much or too prolonged physiological arousal following a stressor. In major depression, however, people often show abnormal cortisol functioning, suggesting that there is dysregulation in the hypothalamic-pituitary-adrenal (HPA) axis.

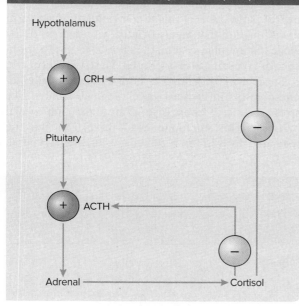

stimulating the adrenal cortex to release cortisol into the blood. This process helps the body fight the stressor or flee from it. The hypothalamus has cortisol receptors that detect when cortisol levels have increased and normally responds by decreasing CRH to regulate the stress response. Thus, this biological feedback loop both helps activate the HPA system during stress and calms the system when the stress is over. There is a well-established relationship between chronic stress and the development of psychological disorders, like depression and PTSD, for example. This relationship illustrates the mechanisms of neurocircuitry that are pinned to underlying physiological and behavioral changes often seen under conditions of prolonged stress exposure (Herman et al., 2016).

People with depression tend to show elevated levels of cortisol and CRH, indicating chronic hyperactivity in the HPA axis and difficulty in the HPA axis's returning to normal functioning following a stressor

(Saveanu & Nemeroff, 2012). In turn, the excess hormones produced by heightened HPA activity seem to have an inhibiting effect on receptors for the monoamine neurotransmitters. One model for the development of depression proposes that people exposed to chronic stress may develop poorly regulated neuroendocrine systems. Then, when they are exposed to even minor stressors later in life, the HPA axis overreacts and does not easily return to baseline. This overreaction changes the functioning of the monoamine neurotransmitters in the brain, and an episode of depression is likely to follow (Southwick, Vythilingam, & Charney, 2005). In addition, chronic excessive exposure to cortisol may account for the volume reductions in several brain areas seen in depressed people, including the hippocampus, the prefrontal cortex, and the amygdala.

Early traumatic stress, such as being the victim of sexual and/or physical abuse, suffering severe neglect, or being exposed to other serious chronic stress, may lead to some of the neuroendocrine abnormalities that predispose people to depression (Southwick et al., 2005). Studies of children who have been abused or neglected show that their biological responses to stress—particularly the response of their HPA axis—often are either exaggerated or blunted (Cicchetti & Toth, 2016). Christine Heim and colleagues (Heim & Nemeroff, 2001; Heim, Plotsky, & Nemeroff, 2004) have found that women who were sexually abused as children show altered HPA responses to stress as adults, even when they are not depressed. Similarly, animal studies show that early stress (such as separation from the mother) promotes exaggerated neurobiological stress reactivity and a vulnerability to depression-like responses to future stressors (Saveanu & Nemeroff, 2012). Notably, these neurobiological vulnerabilities can be reduced in animals by providing them with subsequent supportive maternal care and/or pharmacological interventions.

Adverse childhood experiences (ACEs) are associated with increased risks for a variety of medical, psychological, and behavioral conditions in adulthood. ACEs refer to physical, sexual, or psychological abuse, neglect, or living in a dysfunctional household prior to the age of 18. Research has shown that ACEs are highly associated with chronic conditions such as depression, smoking, and alcohol use. The associations indicate that exposure to an abusive and neglectful family environment in childhood increases the individual's vulnerability to emotional and behavioral pathways that are conducive to chronic diseases (Llabre et al., 2017).

Hormonal factors have often been implicated in women's greater vulnerability to depression (Nolen-Hoeksema & Hilt, 2013). Changes in the ovarian hormones, estrogen and progesterone, affect the serotonin and norepinephrine neurotransmitter systems and thus theoretically could affect mood. Some women show increases in depressed mood when their levels of estrogen and progesterone are in flux, such as during pregnancy and the postpartum period and premenstrually (Epperson et al., 2012; O'Hara & McCabe, 2013). Further, girls show increases in their rate of depression around ages 13 to 15 (Twenge & Nolen-Hoeksema, 2002), possibly because of the hormonal changes of puberty (Angold, Castello, & Worthman, 1998). Findings of a direct link between changes in estrogen and progesterone levels and vulnerability to depression have not been consistent, however. The hormonal changes of puberty, the menstrual cycle, the peripartum period, and menopause may trigger depression only in women with a genetic or other biological vulnerability to the disorder (Steiner, Dunn, & Born, 2003; Young & Korzun, 1999).

The Gut Microbiome and Inflammation

Most people don't associate the bacteria that live in our digestive tract with psychological disorders, like depression. However, recent studies have established that depression is associated with altered gut microbiota composition which influences the brain

(Figure 4). The gut microbiome is made up of the collection of bacteria, fungi, and viruses, harbored in the gastrointestinal tract which has a measurable impact on the brain (Martinez, Leone, & Chang, 2017). Without question, major depressive disorder is viewed as a disease of the brain and effective treatment requires that neurological factors are understood. However, the brain does not exist in isolation and it is embedded within the overall physiology of the individual, and it is undeniable that this disorder directly impacts the body. Depression commonly produces somatic symptoms, such as sleep disturbance, weight loss/gain and psychomotor agitation/retardation in addition to the cognitive symptoms like feelings of sadness, loss of pleasure, difficulties concentrating, and thoughts of death. Some of the possible physiological pathways that might contribute to changes in brain function that are associated with depression include the immune system, the HPA axis, and the presence of preceding illness (Winter, Hart, Charlesworth, & Sharpley, 2018). Studies have shown that the gut microbiome influences psychological factors like stress, anxiety, depressive symptoms, and social behavior. This microbiome–gut–brain axis may be mediated by various mechanisms including neural,

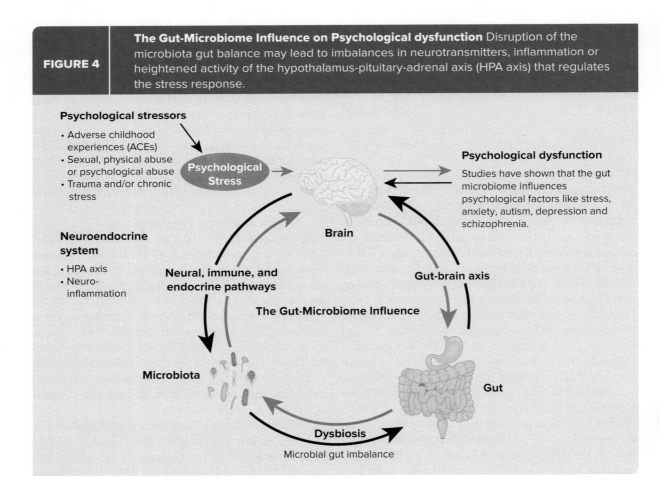

FIGURE 4   **The Gut-Microbiome Influence on Psychological dysfunction** Disruption of the microbiota gut balance may lead to imbalances in neurotransmitters, inflammation or heightened activity of the hypothalamus-pituitary-adrenal axis (HPA axis) that regulates the stress response.

Psychological stressors
- Adverse childhood experiences (ACEs)
- Sexual, physical abuse or psychological abuse
- Trauma and/or chronic stress

Psychological Stress

Neuroendocrine system
- HPA axis
- Neuro-inflammation

Psychological dysfunction

Studies have shown that the gut microbiome influences psychological factors like stress, anxiety, autism, depression and schizophrenia.

Brain

Neural, immune, and endocrine pathways

Gut-brain axis

The Gut-Microbiome Influence

Microbiota

Gut

Dysbiosis
Microbial gut imbalance

immune, and endocrine pathways that are relevant to psychiatric disorders (Johnson, 2020).

It is suggested that these microorganisms can also produce various neuroactive chemicals that modulate neurotransmitter levels. For example, recent research has found that the relative abundance of *bacteroides* is negatively associated with brain signatures of depression, suggesting that bacterially derived GABA may play a role in the microbiome–gut–brain axis. Meaning, gut microbes influence the release serotonin and GABA which are both neurotransmitters associated with depression and other psychological disorders. Additionally, disruption of the microbial gut balance (*dysbiosis*) may lead to imbalances in neurotransmitters, inflammation or heightened activity of the HPA axis that regulates the stress response. This suggests that microbiota may potentially contribute to the levels of these neurotransmitters in the brain as well as in the gut by altering brain functioning in an indirect manner through changes in inflammatory states and immune status (Beurel, Toups, & Nemeroff, 2020; Winter et al., 2018).

The comorbidity of gastrointestinal problems with psychiatric illness also supports the role of the microbiome-gut-brain axis in human biology and psychology. A number of studies report associations between the composition of the gut microbiome and conditions such as autism, depression, and schizophrenia. Research over the last decade provides evidence that the gut microbiome interacts with the central nervous system and these findings have the potential to aid the development of new treatments for conditions such as autism and depression (Johnson, 2020).

Recent research has also found an association between the neurobiology of major depressive disorder and neuroinflammation. **Neuroinflammation** is an inflammatory response within the brain or spinal cord that occurs in response to disease, injury, infection, or stress (DiSabato, Quan, & Godbout, 2016). Studies support the role of inflammation in the moderation of suicidal behavior, as well. Inflammatory processes have been implicated in the pathophysiology of depression, but the specific mechanism still remains unclear (Dong-Bin et al., 2020; Holmes et al., 2018). Dysregulation of the immune system occurs in depressed patients which hinders favorable prognosis, including the response of antidepressant medications. It is likely that inflammation is a critical disease modifier that may promote susceptibility to depressive symptoms. Research suggests that controlling inflammation in MDD clients may provide an overall therapeutic benefit, regardless of whether the inflammation is related to early life trauma, response to acute stressors, microbiome alterations, genetic predispositions, or a combination of factors (Beurel, Toups, & Nemeroff, 2020).

Psychological Theories of Depression

Behavioral theorists have focused on the role of uncontrollable stressors in producing depression. Cognitive theorists have argued that the ways people think can contribute to, and maintain, depression. Interpersonal theorists have considered the role of relationships in causing and maintaining depression. Sociocultural theorists have focused on explanations for the differences in rates of depression among sociodemographic groups.

Behavioral Theories

Depression often arises as a reaction to stressful negative events, such as the breakup of a relationship, the death of a loved one, a job loss, or a serious medical illness (Hammen, 2018; Monroe, 2010). The overwhelming majority of people with depression report a negative life event prior to the onset of their depression, a relationship that has been demonstrated in various studies. In a recent study, 96 percent of clients surveyed had at least one acute critical life event within 6 months prior to first symptoms of a depressive episode. Previous studies have shown that genetic factors influence the risk of a major depressive episode due to increased sensitivity to multiple stressful life events that produces a cumulative depression-inducing effect (Strauss et al., 2018). Additionally, people with depression are more likely than people without depression to have chronic life stressors, such as financial strain or a bad marriage. They also tend to have a history of traumatic life events, particularly events involving loss (Hammen, 2018).

Behavioral theories of depression suggest that life stress leads to depression because it reduces the positive reinforcers in a person's life (Hollon & Dimidjian, 2015; Lewinsohn & Gotlib, 1995). The person begins to withdraw, which results in a further reduction in reinforcers, which leads to more withdrawal, creating a self-perpetuating chain.

For example, a man having difficulty in his marriage may initiate interactions with his wife less often because these interactions are no longer as positively reinforcing as they once were. This only worsens the communication between him and his wife, so the relationship deteriorates. He then withdraws further and becomes depressed about this area of his life. Behavioral theorists suggest that such a pattern is especially likely in people with poor social skills, because they are more likely to experience rejection by others and also more likely to withdraw in response to rejection than to find ways to overcome it (Lewinsohn, 1974). In addition, once a person begins engaging in depressive behaviors, these behaviors are reinforced by the sympathy and attention they engender in others.

Integrating this psychosocial perspective with a biological account, Pizzagalli (2014) has argued that life stress also contributes to the loss of pleasure (*anhedonia*) and behavioral withdrawal of depression by affecting interrelated biological pathways of stress (such as neuroendocrine pathways) and reward processing (such as dopamine systems).

Another behavioral theory—the **learned helplessness theory**—suggests that the type of stressful event most likely to lead to depression is an uncontrollable negative event (Seligman, 1975). Such events, especially if they are frequent or chronic, can lead people to believe they are helpless to control important outcomes in their environment. In turn, this belief in helplessness leads people to lose their motivation and to reduce actions on their part that might control the environment as well as leaving them unable to learn how to control situations that are controllable. These learned helplessness deficits are similar to the symptoms of depression: low motivation, passivity, and indecisiveness (Seligman, 1975). For example, individuals who experience domestic violence may develop the belief that they have no control over this violence or other parts of their lives. No matter what they do, the physical or psychological abuse will continue. Fight, don't fight, argue, don't argue, do something nice for their partner, don't do something nice for their partner . . . these experiences will continue because they believe that they have no control. Learned helplessness is the psychological process giving up and assuming nothing in life will change. This learned helplessness may help explain the likelihood that this individual will experience depression and remain in abusive relationships. The ability to adapt and adjust psychological behaviors in response to situational demands is a factor associated with psychological health and resiliency called *psychological flexibility*. This concept includes a range of inter- and intrapersonal skills and is considered the cornerstone of psychological health.

Recent research has found a significant relationship between learned helplessness and psychological flexibility. When faced with environmental stressors, people with higher levels of psychological flexibility experience less psychological dysfunction. For example, preliminary data suggest the COVID-19 pandemic adversely impacted mental health in approximately a quarter of the general population. In an effort to reduce the rates of COVID-19 transmission, social distancing measures were used in many countries to curb its spread resulting in lengthy lockdowns. Both the pandemic and the lockdown conditions increased psychological distress as it related to concerns about disease and death, economic uncertainty, conflicting information about the virus, the absence of a medical cure, and media saturation about the deaths, infection rates, and overcrowded hospitals. Results show that psychological flexibility moderates the relationship between risk factors associated with the COVID-19 lockdown and mental health outcomes. Conversely, higher psychological inflexibility exacerbates the adverse effects of COVID-19 pandemic and lockdown risk factors on mental health indicating that higher psychological inflexibility predicts psychopathology in a variety of contexts. These results suggest that people with high psychological flexibility are able to mitigate COVID-19 impacts on mental health outcomes which decreases the likelihood of psychopathology (Pakenham et al., 2020).

Specifically, studies have shown that psychological flexibility influences the relationship between learned helplessness and symptoms of depression. Higher psychological flexibility seems to protect against symptoms of depression particularly for those individuals who experience higher levels of learned helplessness. Individuals who are most likely to struggle with learned helplessness are potentially those who could benefit the most from an intervention targeting psychological flexibility as a way to ameliorate depressive symptomatology. (Trindade, Mendes, & Ferreira, 2020).

Cognitive Theories

Aaron Beck (1967) argued that people with depression look at the world through a **negative cognitive triad:** They have negative views of themselves, the world, and the future. They then commit errors in thinking that support their negative cognitive triad, such as ignoring good events and exaggerating negative events. Their negative thinking both causes and perpetuates their depression. Many studies have demonstrated that people with depression show these negative ways of thinking, and some longitudinal studies have shown that these thinking styles predict depression over time (Abramson et al., 2002; Joormann & Vanderlind, 2014). Beck's theory led to one of the most widely used and successful therapies for depression—cognitive-behavioral therapy.

Another cognitive theory of depression, the **reformulated learned helplessness theory,** explains how cognitive factors might influence whether a person becomes helpless and depressed following a negative event (Abramson, Seligman, & Teasdale, 1978; Peterson & Seligman, 1984). This theory focuses on people's causal attributions for events. A causal attribution is an explanation of why an event happened. According to this theory, people who habitually explain negative events by causes that are internal, stable, and global tend to blame themselves for these negative events, expect negative events to recur in the future, and expect to experience negative events in many areas of their lives. In turn, these expectations lead them to experience long-term learned helplessness deficits as well as loss of self-esteem in many areas of their lives.

For example, consider a student who becomes depressed after failing a psychology exam. The reformulated learned helplessness theory would suggest that he has blamed his failure on internal causes (he didn't study hard enough) rather than external causes (the exam was too hard). Further, he has assumed that the failure was due to stable causes, such as a lack of aptitude in psychology, rather than to unstable causes, such as the instructor not allowing enough time. Therefore, he expects to fail again. Finally, he has attributed his failure to a global cause, such as his difficulty learning the material. This global attribution then leads him to expect failure in other academic areas. A related cognitive theory involves *hopelessness depression*. Hopelessness depression develops when people make pessimistic attributions for the most important events in their lives and perceive that they have no way to cope with the consequences of these events (Abramson, Metalsky, & Alloy, 1989). For example, the student above might not only conclude that he didn't study hard enough, but also that there is no way he can ever graduate.

Both the reformulated learned helplessness theory and the hopelessness theory have led to much additional research (Abramson et al., 2002). One of the most definitive studies of the hopelessness theory of depression was a long-term study of college students (Alloy, Abramson, & Francis, 1999). The researchers interviewed first-year students at two universities and identified those with hopeless attributional styles and those with optimistic attributional styles. They then tracked these students for the next 2 years, interviewing them every 6 weeks. Among the students with no history of depression, those with a hopeless attributional style were much more likely to develop a first onset of major depression than were those with an optimistic attributional style (17 percent vs.1 percent). In addition, among students with a history of depression, those with a hopeless style were more likely to have a relapse of depression than were those with an optimistic style (27 percent vs. 6 percent). Thus, a pessimistic attributional style predicted both first onset and relapse of depression. Attributional style, feelings of hopelessness, and symptoms of depression may have shared genetic pathways which suggests that biological explanations may further reinforce this influential theory (Waszczuk, Coulson, Gregory & Eley, 2016).

Another cognitive theory, the ruminative response styles theory, focuses more on the process of thinking than on the content of thinking as a contributor to depression (Nolen-Hoeksema, Wisco, & Lyubomirsky, 2008). Some people, when they are sad, blue, and upset, focus intently on how they feel—their symptoms of

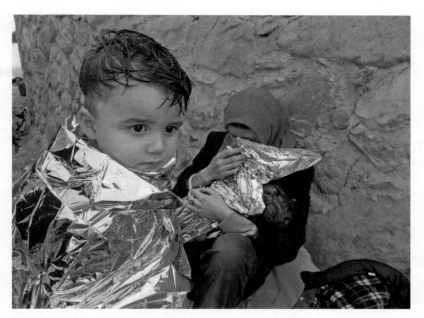

The loss of a loved one can increase the risk of depression. *Anjo Kan/Shutterstock*

People who attribute negative events, such as taking an exam, to internal ("*I*" failed), stable ("I *always* fail), and global causes (I always fail at *everything*") may be at greater risk for depression. *Digital Vision/Getty Images*

fatigue and poor concentration and their sadness and hopelessness—and can identify many possible causes. They do not attempt to do anything about these causes, however, and instead continue to engage in **rumination** about their depression. Several studies have shown that people with this more ruminative coping style are more likely to develop major depression (Nolen-Hoeksema et al., 2008). Ruminative thinking is one way in which, for some people, stressful experiences can give rise to depression (Ruscio et al., 2015). The cognitive phenomenon of rumination has also been linked with genetic, neural, and physiological processes, consistent with the biopsychosocial approach (Mandell, Siegle, Shutt, Feldmiller, & Thase, 2014; Woody, McGeary, & Gibb, 2014).

People who are depressed show a bias toward negative thinking in basic attention and memory processes (Harvey, Watkins, Mansell, & Shafran, 2004; Joormann & Vanderlind, 2014). Depressed people are more likely than nondepressed people to dwell on negative stimuli, such as sad faces (Gotlib, Krasnoperova, Yue, & Joormann, 2004) and to have trouble disengaging their attention from negative stimuli (Joormann, 2004). After learning a list of words and then being surprised with the task of recalling those words, depressed people tend to recall more negative words than positive words, while nondepressed people show the opposite memory bias (Blaney, 1986; Matt, Vasquez, & Campbell, 1992). These biases in attention to and memory for negative information could form the basis of depressed people's tendency to see the world in a negative light and may help maintain this tendency.

In addition, depressed people tend to show overgeneral memory (Williams et al., 2007). When given a simple word cue such as "angry" and asked to describe a memory prompted by that cue, depressed people are more likely than nondepressed people to offer memories that are highly general (e.g., "People who are mean") instead of concrete (e.g., "Jane being rude to me last Friday"). Mark Williams and colleagues (2007) suggest that depressed people develop the tendency to store and recall memories in a general fashion as a way of coping with a traumatic past (Ono, Devilly, & Shum, 2016). Vague, general memories are less emotionally charged and painful than memories that are rich in concrete detail, and thus they help reduce the emotional pain depressed people feel over their past. Interestingly, the one other disorder characterized by overgeneral memory is posttraumatic stress disorder (see the chapter "Anxiety, Obsessive-Compulsive, Trauma, and Stressor-Related Disorders"), which develops specifically in response to traumatic events (Williams et al., 2007).

As far back as the 1930s, research has shown that a substantial proportion of children and adolescents experience psychological distress to various aspects of media content, especially movies, television dramas, and the news. Similarly, with social media, researchers have examined whether exposure to social networking sites can influence psychological dysfunction,

like depression and anxiety, in adolescent populations. The term "social media" refers to the various internet-based networks that enable users to interact with others, verbally and visually. According to the Royal Society for Public Health, & Young Health Movement (2017), the prevalence of anxiety and depression has increased by 70 percent in the past 25 years in young adults and the rate of self-harm in among girls aged 13 to 16 in the United Kingdom has risen by 68 percent over the last 10 years. According to the Pew Research Center (2017), at least 92 percent of teenagers are active on social media. and individuals in the 13 to 17 age group are identified as particularly heavy users of social media. Among this group, 87 percent report having access to a computer, 58 percent to a tablet device and almost three-quarters of adolescents aged 15 to 17 use a smartphone (Keles, McCrae, & Grealish, 2020). This dramatic increase in access to the Internet and social media among adolescents and the amount of time spent online has been studied in terms of its impact on mental health.

A growing body of research confirms the relationship between digital media use and depression. Studies have also found that negative social comparison that results in negative self-evaluation and cyberbullying are strongly associated with poor mental health outcomes, like depression, anxiety, suicidal ideation/attempt, and self-injury. Although there is evidence that greater Internet-based media use is associated with depressive symptoms, there is also evidence that it may be possible to harness the social nature of digital communication to improve mood and to promote health-enhancing strategies. Similarly, not all types of electronic media are expected to worsen symptoms of depression. The increases in the momentary positive affect found in social media use may actually lower some people's risk for depression, making certain types of media use an effective therapeutic. Media use that provides effective distraction, humor, connection to peers, and a wide social network could serve to help adolescents avoid depression and potentially reduce its impact on their functioning (Hoge, Bickham, & Cantor, 2017).

Interpersonal Theories

The interpersonal relationships of people with depression often are fraught with difficulty. The **interpersonal theories of depression** focus on these relationships (Coyne, 1976; Hames, Hagan, & Joiner, 2013). Interpersonal difficulties and losses frequently precede depression and are the stressors most commonly reported as triggering depression (Hammen, 2018; Rudolph, 2008). Depressed people are more likely than nondepressed people to have chronic conflict in their relationships with family, friends, and co-workers (Hammen, 2018).

Depressed people may act in ways that engender interpersonal conflict, in part due to deficits in social and communication skills (Hammen, 2018; Hames et al., 2013). Some depressed people have a heightened need for approval and expressions of support from others (Leadbeater, Kuperminc, Blatt, & Herzog, 1999; Rudolph & Conley, 2005) but at the same time easily perceive rejection by others, a characteristic called **rejection sensitivity** (Downey & Feldman, 1996). They engage in excessive reassurance seeking, constantly looking for assurances from others that they are accepted and loved (Joiner & Timmons, 2009). They never quite believe the affirmations other people give, however, and anxiously keep going back for more. After a while, their family and friends can become weary of this behavior and may become frustrated or hostile. The insecure person picks up on these cues of annoyance and panics over them. The person then feels even more insecure and engages in excessive reassurance seeking. Eventually the person's social support may be withdrawn altogether, leading to increased and longer depression. The self-defeating interpersonal behaviors of depressed individuals may be a result of such various influences as negative thinking patterns, history of maltreatment, and even genetic vulnerabilities (Liu, 2013).

Just as depression is characterized by certain social behaviors, social and interpersonal factors also affect the internal factors of depression. How parents interact with their children affects the child's development of cognitive and behavioral factors implicated in depression later on, as do interactions with peers in adolescence (e.g., Eisenberg, Spinrad, & Eggum, 2010). In fact, exemplifying the biopsychosocial approach to depression, a longitudinal study of adolescents found that genetic and neural predictors of depression at age 18 depend on parenting behaviors when the child is age 12 (Little et al., 2015). In adulthood, too, an individual's social relationships can influence how he or she copes with negative events. Having more close relationships (and, especially, high-quality relationships) can provide protection against maladaptive coping patterns and depressive symptoms (Marroquín & Nolen-Hoeksema, 2015).

Sociocultural Theories

Sociocultural theorists have focused on how differences in the social conditions of demographic groups lead to differences in vulnerability to depression. Three demographic factors are especially relevant to sociocultural theories of depression: cohort effects (meaning generational differences), gender, and ethnicity/race.

Cohort Effects A **cohort effect** exists when people's difference on some psychological variable depends not on their age per se, but instead on the era in which they were born and lived. Historical and cultural changes may have put more recent generations at higher risk for depression than previous generations (Kessler, 2003; Klerman & Weissman, 1989). For example, fewer than 20 percent of people born before 1915 appear to have experienced major depression, whereas over 40 percent of people born after 1955 appear to be at risk for major depression at some time in their lives. Some theorists suggest that more-recent generations are at higher risk for depression because of the rapid changes in social values beginning in the 1960s and the disintegration of the family unit (Klerman & Weissman, 1989). Additionally, younger adults are currently more comfortable disclosing their mental health. Studies show that many young people are undeterred by stigma, which allows them the freedom to discuss their psychological difficulties and seek professional help. Additionally, another important factor is the ease of sharing personal experiences in the digital information age. Unlike generations in the past who were more likely to suffer with mental health problems in solation, today a struggling younger person can readily find others with similar problems, either through social interaction or support groups (Keles, McCrae, & Grealish, 2020). Another possible explanation is that younger generations have unrealistically high expectations for themselves that older generations did not have, and thus more vulnerability to depression.

Gender Differences We noted earlier that women are about twice as likely as men to suffer from depression. Several explanations have been offered for this gender difference (Nolen-Hoeksema & Hilt, 2013). One is that men and women differ in how they respond to, or cope with, negative feelings. When faced with distress, men are more likely than women to turn to alcohol to cope and to deny that they are distressed, while women are more likely than men to ruminate about their feelings and problems (Nolen-Hoeksema & Hilt, 2013). Men therefore may be more likely to develop disorders such as alcohol abuse, while women's tendency to ruminate appears to make them more likely to develop depression. These different responses to stress may be due to social norms—it is more acceptable for men to turn to alcohol and for women to ruminate (Addis, 2008; Nolen-Hoeksema & Hilt, 2013).

Perhaps also due to gender socialization, women tend to be more interpersonally oriented than men (Feingold, 1994). On one hand, women's strong interpersonal networks may give them support in times of need. On the other hand, when bad things happen to others or when there is conflict in their relationships, women are more likely than men to experience depressive symptoms (Hammen, 2003; Rudolph, 2008). Women also appear more likely than men to base their self-worth on the health of their relationships (Jack, 1991). In addition, women in most societies have less status and power than do men, and as a result they experience more prejudice, discrimination, and violence (Nolen-Hoeksema & Hilt, 2013). Sexual abuse, particularly in childhood, occurs more often to girls and women, and contributes to depression throughout their lifetime (Widom, DuMont, & Czaja, 2007).

Earlier in this chapter, we noted biological explanations for women's greater vulnerability to depression compared to men. Biological and sociocultural factors likely interact to lead to the large gender difference in the incidence of depression (Nolen-Hoeksema & Hilt, 2013). For example, the increase in gender differences coincides with puberty, and social aspects of puberty—such as its timing relative to one's peers—play a role in depression (e.g., Alloy, Hamilton, Hamlat, & Abramson, 2016).

Ethnicity/Race Differences As society becomes increasingly diverse, ethnic and racial differences in the prevalence and patterns of depression support sociocultural theories. In the United States, compared to Caucasian Americans, Latinos show similar rates of depression overall (Kessler, 2003). However, rates vary widely depending on specific culture of origin, first versus second generation status, and acculturation (González, Tarraf, Whitfield, & Vega, 2010; Wassertheil-Smoller et al., 2014). Interestingly, Latinos born in the United States have higher rates of depression than those who immigrated from other countries. Relative to Caucasian Americans, Latinos show more chronic courses of depression and receive less adequate treatment (González et al., 2010; Wassertheil-Smoller et al., 2014).

Adult studies indicate that African Americans have lower rates of depression than Caucasian Americans (Anderson & Mayes, 2010; Kessler, 2003). This may seem puzzling given the disadvantaged status of African Americans in U.S. society. However, African Americans have high rates of anxiety disorders, suggesting that the stress of their social status may make them especially prone to anxiety disorders rather than to depression. Other studies have found extremely high rates of depression among Native Americans, especially the young (Saluja et al., 2004). Depression among Native American youth is tied to poverty, hopelessness, and alcoholism.

Asian Americans show lower rates of depression than other ethnic groups. Some findings indicate that, because of cultural differences, people of Asian descent may experience depression in a more somatic form—for example, reporting a headache rather than negative thinking (e.g., Ryder et al., 2008), although

evidence for this claim is mixed (Kim & Lopez, 2014). Ethnic/racial differences not only shed light on sociocultural factors in depression across demographics, but also help guide treatment and prevention efforts.

THEORIES OF BIPOLAR DISORDER

Most existing theories of bipolar disorder focus on biological causes. In recent years, however, there has been increasing interest in psychological and social contributors to new episodes in people with bipolar disorder.

Biological Theories of Bipolar Disorder

Theories of bipolar disorder center on the genetic factors, structural and functional brain abnormalities, and neurotransmitter factors.

Genetic Factors

The development of bipolar disorder is strongly and consistently linked to genetic factors, although the specific genetic abnormalities are still being explored through various studies. The GWAS have found significant biological support for many psychological disorders in addition to bipolar and depression, such as schizophrenia, substance use disorder, posttraumatic stress disorder (PTSD), anorexia, ADHD, and autism (Duncan, Ostacher, & Ballon, 2019). The GWAS have helped transform our understanding of mood disorders by producing evidence of specific genetic markers and illustrating the complex genetic architecture that overlaps with many psychiatric disorders, such as schizophrenia and major depressive disorder. The transdiagnostic nature of familial risk among individuals with mood disorders suggests that psychopathological, neurocognitive, neuroanatomical, and environmental factors are involved in the familial transmission of severe mental illness (Sandstrom, Sahiti, Pavlova, & Uher, 2019). Recent findings have established there is considerable overlap in the genetic variants for different psychiatric disorders, with approximately two-thirds of genetic influences shared across schizophrenia, bipolar disorder, and MDD. Studies suggest that family history remains the most powerful predictor for serious mental illnesses and offspring of parents with MDD, bipolar disorder, and schizophrenia are at high risk for disease onset (Gordovez & McMahon, 2020).

First-degree relatives (parents, children, and siblings) of people with bipolar disorder have 5 to 10 times higher rates of both bipolar disorder and depressive disorders than relatives of people without bipolar disorder (Craddock & Sklar, 2013). Also, the identical twins of individuals with bipolar disorder are 45 to 75 times more likely to develop the disorder than are people in the general population (McGuffin et al., 2003). Ongoing research seeks to identify the specific genes implicated in bipolar disorder, some of which likely contribute to other disorders like schizophrenia (Craddock & Sklar, 2013).

Structural and Functional Brain Abnormalities

Like the depressive disorders, bipolar disorder is associated with abnormalities in the structure and functioning of the amygdala, which is involved in the processing of emotions (Figure 5) and the prefrontal cortex, which is involved in cognitive control of emotion, planning, and judgment (Garrett et al., 2012; Phillips & Swartz, 2014). Some evidence also indicates alterations in the size or functioning of the hippocampus. Specifically, studies have found smaller hippocampal volumes have been reported in those with bipolar disorder as compared to healthy controls (Haukvik et al., 2020).

An area of the brain called the striatum, part of a structure called the basal ganglia, is involved in the processing of environmental cues of reward. For example, this brain structure becomes active when rewarding stimuli, such as tasty food or opportunities to earn money, are perceived by the individual. This area of the brain is activated abnormally in people with bipolar disorder but not consistently so in people with major depression, suggesting that people with bipolar disorder may be neurobiologically hypersensitive to rewarding cues in the environment (Nusslock et al., 2012). A circuit from the prefrontal cortex through the striatum to the amygdala is involved in adaptation to changing contingencies of reward (i.e., knowing when you should drop one strategy in favor of another in order to get a reward). Some researchers suggest that individuals with bipolar disorder have abnormalities in the functioning of this circuit that lead them to have inflexible responses to reward (Brotman et al., 2016; Philips & Swartz, 2014). When they are in a manic phase, they inflexibly and excessively seek reward; when they are in a depressive phase, they are highly insensitive to reward. Even between manic or depressive episodes, though, people with bipolar disorder respond to incentives and social rewards with more positive emotion, and this reactivity is linked with activity in the striatum (Dutra, Cunningham, Kober, & Gruber, 2015).

Some studies suggest that youth with bipolar disorder have abnormalities in the white matter of the brain, particularly in the prefrontal cortex (Frazier et al., 2007; Kafantaris et al., 2009). White matter is tissue that connects various structures in the brain and transmits messages between them. White-matter abnormalities are found in children at their first episodes of bipolar disorder, before they have been medicated (Adler et al., 2006), and in children at risk for bipolar disorder because of family history (Frazier et al., 2007). White-matter abnormalities could result in the brain's prefrontal area having difficulty communicating with and exerting control over other areas, such as the amygdala, leading to the disorganized emotions and extreme behavior characteristic of bipolar disorder (Brady et al., 2017; Garrett et al., 2012).

FIGURE 5

Amygdala Activation in Youth with Bipolar Disorder.
Youth with bipolar disorder showed significantly greater amygdala activation (yellow area) than did healthy youth when rating their fear of neutral faces.

Rich, B. A., Vinton, D. T., Roberson-Nay, R., Hommer, R. E., Berghorst, L. H., McClure, E. B., Leibenluft, E. (2006). Limbic hyperactivation during processing of neutral facial expressions in children with bipolar disorder. Proceedings of the National Academy of Science. Reprinted by permission.

Neurotransmitter Factors

The monoamine neurotransmitters have been implicated in bipolar disorder as well as in major depressive disorder. In particular, several studies have suggested that dysregulation in the dopamine system contributes to bipolar disorder (Brotman et al., 2016). High levels of dopamine are thought to be associated with high reward seeking, while low levels are associated with insensitivity to reward. Thus, dysregulation in the dopamine system may lead to excessive reward seeking during the manic phase and a lack of reward seeking in the depressed phase (Ashok et al., 2017).

Psychosocial Contributors to Bipolar Disorder

Although biological theories of bipolar disorder have received the most attention, psychosocial approaches have identified other important factors, including reward sensitivity, stress, and changes to bodily and social routines.

In line with biological evidence that dysregulation of reward systems plays a role in bipolar disorder, psychologists have examined relationships between bipolar disorder and behavioral indicators of sensitivity to reward. Reward sensitivity refers to the degree to which people experience emotional, behavioral, and biological responses to positive events they experience or anticipate. In some of these studies, individuals play games on the computer, such as gambling games, that assess their willingness to take risks in order to pursue possible rewards and their ability to detect what kinds of behaviors will be rewarded. These studies confirm that people with bipolar disorder, even when they are asymptomatic, show greater sensitivity to reward than do people without the disorder (Alloy et al., 2008; Johnson, Fulford, & Carver, 2012). In addition, a study that followed people with bipolar disorder for nearly 3 years found that those with greater sensitivity to reward relapsed into manic or hypomanic symptoms sooner than did those with lower sensitivity to reward (Alloy et al., 2008; Alloy, Olino, Freed, & Nusslock, 2016). Whereas a person without bipolar disorder might enjoy a fun evening out with friends and then go home to relax, a person with bipolar disorder might find the evening so rewarding that she stays up through the night. In contrast, individuals with high sensitivity to punishment relapse into depressive episodes sooner than those with lower sensitivity to punishment.

Another psychological factor that has been studied in people with bipolar disorder is stress. Experiencing stressful events and living with an unsupportive family where discord, criticism, and conflict are high may trigger new episodes of bipolar disorder. Increased evidence suggests that family psychoeducational treatments are effective in relapse prevention and symptom control when combined with standard drug treatment (Altman et al., 2006; Miklowitz & Chung, 2016). Even positive events can trigger new episodes of mania or hypomania, particularly if they involve striving for goals seen as highly rewarding. A study of college students found that among those with bipolar disorder, preparing for and completing exams tended to trigger hypomanic symptoms, particularly among students who were highly sensitive to rewards (Nusslock, Abramson, Harmon-Jones, Alloy, & Hogan, 2007). Thus, goal-striving situations may trigger high reward sensitivity, which in turn triggers manic or hypomanic symptoms in people with bipolar disorder.

Changes in bodily rhythms or usual routines also can trigger episodes in people with bipolar disorder. Dysregulation of the internal biological clock, known as circadian rhythms, has been hypothesized to be a central mechanism in bipolar disorders and recent studies have found considerable support. However, it is unclear whether circadian dysregulation provides vulnerability for the initial onset of bipolar disorders or if it is a causal factor in the course of these disorders. When individuals with bipolar disorders experience life events that disrupt their daily schedules or social rhythms, these schedule changes impact their circadian rhythms eventually culminating in bipolar mood episodes (Alloy et al., 2017). Irregular or inadequate sleep, in particular, appears to be a characteristic of many individuals with bipolar disorder that can lead to increased symptoms (Harvey, 2008b; Ng et al., 2015). Significant changes in daily routine can do the same, particularly if they are due to changes in the social climate, such as starting a new job. Some researchers believe that there is a close relationship between social and bodily rhythms and disruption in the neural and psychological systems underlying reward (Alloy, Nusslock, & Boland, 2015). Two psychosocial therapies we discuss later in this chapter, interpersonal and social rhythm therapy, help people with bipolar disorder keep their bodily and social rhythms regular.

TREATMENT OF MOOD DISORDERS

Many forms of treatment are now available for sufferers of mood disorders. In any given year, however, only about half the people who have bipolar disorder and about 60 percent of the people having an episode of major depression seek treatment in the United States, and many fewer seek treatment in developing nations (Kessler, 2003; Merikangas et al., 2011). Most often, those who eventually do seek treatment do so a number of years after the onset of their symptoms.

Biological Treatments for Mood Disorders

The most common first-line biological treatments for depression and bipolar disorder are medications. In addition to being treated with drugs, some people with mood disorders are treated with electroconvulsive therapy (ECT). Three new treatments for mood disorders—repetitive transcranial magnetic stimulation (rTMS), vagus nerve stimulation (VNS), and deep brain stimulation—hold out hope for many people. People with seasonal affective disorder (SAD) can benefit from a simple therapy: exposure to bright lights. It's important to note that there is no single treatment that is completely effective for everyone and these options are necessary for those whose symptoms are resistant to various methods of treatment.

Drug Treatments for Depression

The late twentieth century saw rapid growth in the number of drugs available for depression and in the number of people using them. Several classes of drugs are commonly used in treating depressive disorders and the depressive symptoms of bipolar disorder; these drugs include selective serotonin and/or norepinephrine reuptake inhibitors, tricyclic antidepressants, and monoamine oxidase inhibitors (MAOIs). Initially, they were thought to work by altering levels of the neurotransmitters serotonin, norepinephrine, or dopamine in synapses or by affecting the receptors for these neurotransmitters. However, these changes occur within hours or days of taking the drugs, whereas reductions in depressive symptoms typically don't appear for weeks. More recent theories suggest that these drugs have slow-emerging effects on intracellular processes in the neurotransmitter systems discussed in the section on genetic factors in depression (see Figure 1) and on the action of genes that regulate neurotransmission, the limbic system, and the stress response (Gitlin, 2015).

All of the different antidepressant drugs currently available reduce depression in about 50 to 60 percent of people who take them (Gitlin, 2015). These medications appear to work better for treating severe and persistent depression than for treating mild-to-moderate depression. A meta-analysis of 718 patients from 6 studies found that antidepressants were substantially better than a placebo in reducing symptoms only in very severely depressed patients; in patients with mild-to-moderate depression, the effects of the antidepressants were small to nonexistent (Fournier et al., 2010; Khan, Leventhal, Khan, & Brown, 2002; Kirsch et al., 2008). A large-scale meta-analysis also found support for the use of antidepressants in patients with MDD and these results show an approximate 58 to 67 percent response

rate (versus 39.9 percent for placebo). Although this research supports the efficacy of antidepressants in treatment for MDD, this therapy alone may not always be enough to treat depression (Ionescu & Papakostas, 2017). While research on the effectiveness of antidepressant medication is robust, it is important to note that half of those who receive and adequate dosage of antidepressants for an adequate duration of time still remain depressed (Kessler et al., 2018).

The choice of which drug to begin treatment with tends to be based on the experience of the physician and concerns about the patient's ability to tolerate side effects. It typically takes a few weeks to know whether a person will respond to a drug. Most people try more than one medication before they find the one that works for them. These days, antidepressant drugs are used to relieve the acute symptoms of depression. Then individuals usually are maintained on antidepressant drugs for at least 6 months after their symptoms have subsided, to prevent relapse. Discontinuing antidepressant use during the first 6 to 9 months after symptoms subside seems to double the risk of relapse in severe depression (Geddes, Burgess, Hawton, Jamison, & Goodwin, 2004). People with bipolar disorder often take antidepressants continually to prevent a relapse of depression.

Selective Serotonin Reuptake Inhibitors The **selective serotonin reuptake inhibitors,** or **SSRIs,** are widely used to treat depressive symptoms. SSRIs are not more effective in the treatment of depression than the other available antidepressants, but they have fewer difficult-to-tolerate side effects (Gitlin, 2015). In addition, they are much safer if taken in overdose than many of the older antidepressants, such as the tricyclic antidepressants and the MAOIs, described below. Finally, they have positive effects on a wide range of symptoms that co-occur with depression, including anxiety, eating disorders, and impulsiveness. Recent studies have shown that antidepressant medication was slightly more efficacious in improving overall depression severity than cognitive-behavioral therapy (CBT) (Boschloo et al., 2019).

The SSRIs do have side effects, however, and 5 to 10 percent of people have to discontinue their use because of these side effects (Gitlin, 2015). The most common side effects are gastrointestinal symptoms (e.g., nausea and diarrhea), tremor, nervousness, insomnia, daytime sleepiness, diminished sex drive, and difficulty achieving orgasm. When people first begin taking an SSRI, they sometimes report feeling "jittery" or having a feeling of "crawling out of one's skin." Some people who have bipolar disorder may develop manic symptoms when they take an SSRI. The agitation some people experience while taking an SSRI may contribute to an increase in suicidal thought and behavior, but this can also be due to increased motivation and energy as depression begins to lift. Some studies have suggested that SSRIs can increase suicidal behavior among children and adolescents, but overall, it seems SSRIs decrease such behavior in children and adults (Garland, Kutcher, Virani, & Elbe, 2016).

Selective Serotonin-Norepinephrine Reuptake Inhibitors The **selective serotonin-norepinephrine reuptake inhibitors (SNRIs)** were designed to affect levels of norepinephrine as well as serotonin. They act in the same way as SSRIs (that is, by influencing neurotransmission), but perhaps because these drugs influence both neurotransmitters, they show a slight advantage over the SSRIs in preventing a relapse of depression (Nemeroff et al., 2007). The dual action of these drugs also may account for their slightly broader array of side effects compared to the SSRIs.

Bupropion: A Norepinephrine-Dopamine Reuptake Inhibitor Bupropion affects the norepinephrine and dopamine systems and thus is known as a **norepinephrine-dopamine reuptake inhibitor.** These antidepressants increase the amount of active **norepinephrine** and **dopamine** neurotransmitters throughout the brain which provides similar therapeutic effects on emotional and reward processing to other antidepressants. Bupropion has been found to improve negative biases in emotional processing early in treatment but the beneficial effects on reward processing often occur later in treatment. It may be especially useful in treating people suffering from psychomotor retardation, anhedonia, hypersomnia, cognitive slowing, inattention, and craving—for example, bupropion can help people stop craving cigarettes. Recent studies have focused on the hypothesis that bupropion may be better suited to treat anhedonia; however research suggests that anhedonia may also initially worsen prior to clinical improvement before improving later in treatment (Walsh, Browning, Drevets, Furey, & Harmer et al., 2018). In addition, bupropion appears to overcome the sexual dysfunction side effects of the SSRIs and thus sometimes is used in conjunction with them. The effects of bupropion address the role of dopamine in pleasure, reward, and movement (see the chapter "Theories and Treatment of Abnormality" for reminders of how these various neurotransmitters work).

Tricyclic Antidepressants The **tricyclic antidepressants** were some of the first drugs shown to consistently relieve depression. However, they are used much less frequently these days than the other drugs reviewed in this section. The primary reason for this is that they have numerous side effects. Many of these are anticholinergic effects, so called because they are related to levels of the neurotransmitter acetylcholine.

The tricyclic antidepressants also can cause a drop in blood pressure and cardiac arrhythmia in people with heart problems. Further, the tricyclics can be fatal in overdose, and an overdose is only three to four times the average daily prescription for the drug. For this reason, physicians are wary of prescribing these drugs, particularly for people with depression who might be suicidal.

Monoamine Oxidase Inhibitors Another older class of drugs that is no longer used frequently to treat depression is the **monoamine oxidase inhibitors (MAOIs).** MAO is an enzyme that causes the breakdown of the monoamine neurotransmitters in the synapse. MAOIs decrease the action of MAO and thereby increase the levels of these neurotransmitters in the synapses.

The MAOIs are as effective as the tricyclic antidepressants, but their side effects are potentially quite dangerous. When people taking MAOIs ingest aged cheese, red wine, or beer, they can experience a potentially fatal rise in blood pressure. The MAOIs also can interact with several drugs, including antihypertension medications and over-the-counter drugs such as antihistamines. The MAOIs also can cause liver damage, weight gain, severe lowering of blood pressure, and several of the same side effects caused by the tricyclic antidepressants.

Mood Stabilizers

People with bipolar disorder may take antidepressants to relieve their depressive symptoms, but they also usually take a mood stabilizer (lithium or an anticonvulsant medication) to relieve or prevent symptoms of mania. Lithium can also have positive effects on depressive symptoms in people with depression. In addition, many people are prescribed atypical antipsychotic medications to control mood swings.

Lithium is successful in the prevention and treatment of mania and is regarded as the only substance that prevents both new depressive and new manic episodes, and reduces suicidal thoughts. Lithium is a naturally occurring salt that can be found in rocks and in the waters of many mineral springs. Although the exact mechanism of lithium is unknown, it alters the metabolism of neurotransmitters, specifically catecholamines and serotonin. Lithium may work by improving the functioning of the intracellular processes that appear to be abnormal in the mood disorders (Malhi, Tanious, Das, Coulston, & Berk, 2013). Most people with bipolar disorder take lithium even when they have no symptoms of mania or depression in order to prevent relapses. People maintained on adequate doses of lithium have significantly fewer relapses of mania and depression than people with bipolar disorder not maintained on lithium (Geddes et al., 2004; Ketter, Miller, Dell'Osso, & Wang, 2016).

Although lithium has literally been a lifesaver for many people with mood disorders, it poses some problems. Despite the positive effects of lithium, the rate of prescriptions has declined in recent past which could be, in part, due to the side effects and the fact that patients need close monitoring. There are many side effects to this medication that range from annoying to life threatening such as, nausea, vomiting and diarrhea, blurred vision, tremors, toxicity, and organ damage (Chokhawala, 2020; Won & Kim, 2017). One big problem with lithium is the difference between an effective dose and a toxic dose is small, leaving a narrow window of therapeutic effectiveness. People who take lithium must be monitored carefully by a physician, who can determine whether the dosage of lithium is adequate to relieve their symptoms but not so large as to induce toxic side effects. Lithium can cause diabetes, hypothyroidism, and kidney dysfunction and can contribute to birth defects if taken during the first trimester of pregnancy. Physicians and patients need to work together to ensure that the major benefits of lithium are balanced with these significant drawbacks.

Anticonvulsant and Atypical Antipsychotic Medications In the mid-1990s it was discovered that a medication that helps reduce seizures, valproate (trade name Depakote), also helped stabilize mood in people with bipolar disorder. Other anti-epileptic medications, carbamazepine (trade names Tegretol, Equetro) and lamotrigine (trade name Lamictal), have been approved for use in treating bipolar disorder. The side effects of these drugs include blurred vision, fatigue, vertigo, dizziness, rash, nausea, drowsiness, and liver disease. Valproate seems to induce fewer side effects and is used more often than carbamazepine. Lamotrigine is used especially for maintenance treatment and preventing episode recurrence. But the anti-epileptics can cause birth defects if women take them while pregnant, and they do not prevent suicide as effectively as lithium does. The anti-epileptics may work by restoring the balance between the neurotransmitter systems in the amygdala.

The atypical antipsychotic medications, which are described in more detail in the chapter "Schizophrenia Spectrum and Other Psychotic Disorders," are also used to quell the symptoms of severe mania. These drugs, which include olanzapine (Zyprexa), aripiprazole (Abilify), quetiapine (Seroquel), and risperidone (Risperdal), reduce functional levels of dopamine and seem to be especially useful in the treatment of psychotic manic symptoms (Ketter et al., 2016). The side effects of these drugs can include weight gain and problematic metabolic changes (e.g., increased risk of diabetes and increased insulin, glucose, and low-density lipoprotein cholesterol levels).

With the increased recognition of bipolar disorder and related syndromes in children, there has been an increase in the use of medications to treat children. These medications include mood stabilizers, atypical antipsychotics, and antidepressants. Existing studies show that these drugs can help stabilize children's moods, but the number of well-controlled, large group studies is small, and there are significant concerns about both the short-term and the long-term toxic effects of these drugs on children's developing brains and bodies (Liu et al., 2011).

Electroconvulsive Therapy

Although medications are the typical first line of treatment for people with depressive disorders, an alternative treatment option is **electroconvulsive therapy,** or **ECT.** This convulsive therapy was introduced in the early twentieth century and is now most commonly used for treating severe and persistent mood disorders. ECT was introduced in the early twentieth century, originally as a treatment for schizophrenia (see the chapter "Theories and Treatment of Abnormality") and although the practice of ECT has changed considerably over time, it remains one of the most controversial treatments for mood disorders. The early application of ECT in psychiatric hospitals and depiction of this practice in movies and media created a significant amount of stigma surrounding this treatment. The public viewed ECT as inhumane and torturous, and as a result, it fell out of favor in the 1960s and 1970s. It made a resurgence in the 1980s, however. Today, it is a widely accepted treatment for serious mental disorders and is administered at hospitals throughout the world. It is estimated that one million people annually receive ECT (Leiknes, Schweder, & Høie, 2012).

ECT consists of a series of treatments in which a seizure is induced by passing electrical current through the patient's brain. Anesthesia and muscle relaxants are administered at the start of the procedure to make this process more comfortable for the patient and reduce the risk of injury. Electrodes are applied to the head, and a current of 70 to 150 volts is passed through the brain for about ½ - to 1 second. Patients typically experience a seizure that lasts about 1 minute. The full series of treatments typically consists of 6 to 12 sessions.

Despite the tainted image, ECT is a very effective option for treatment-resistant depressive disorders, with approximately 50 to 80 percent of clients achieving remission, a higher response rate than response rates to antidepressant treatment. Clients who receive ECT are more likely to experience decreased symptoms than if they were taking an antidepressant medication (Kolar, 2017). Research has found that remission rates are highest when ECT is used as a first-line treatment for severe depression and most successful when used during a psychotic episode.

ECT has shown to be very effective when used to treat depression with suicidal features and is associated with substantial and rapid reduction in the expression of suicidal thoughts (Ferrier, 2019). Current ECT research suggests that this is one of the most effective treatments for major depressive disorder (Bewernick & Schlaepfer, 2015) and bipolar disorder (Perugi et al., 2017). Unfortunately, the negative perception of this therapy resulted in a decreased use of ECT in many countries and a reduction in consumer access to ECT, which many see as a violation of a right to access effective treatment (Gazdag & Ungvari, 2019).

While ECT is an effective treatment for depression, the mechanism of ECT is still unclear but may involve structural changes to the parts of the brain implicated in mood disorders. Recently, neuroimaging studies have reported that the prefrontal cortex, hippocampus, angular gyrus, insular and other brain regions are involved in the mechanism of ECT for depression. Growing literature suggests that ECT induces plasticity in specific brain regions, including the hippocampus, basal ganglia, anterior cingulate, and prefrontal cortex. Studies suggest that ECT does not affect only one brain region, but changes the structure and function of wide brain areas, which indicates that ECT may influence brain networks rather than one structure or area (Dukart et al., 2014; Leaver et al., 2018; Wei et al., 2018). Various theories suggest that ECT changes the function of neurotransmitters, such as serotonin and dopamine, reduces brain inflammation, and promotes restructuring of the brain. Recent studies also identify ECT as a strong stimulator of neurogenesis by promoting the proliferation of stem cells (Gazdag & Ungvari, 2019).

ECT can lead to memory loss and difficulty learning new information, particularly in the days following treatment (Kolar, 2017; Sackeim et al., 2007). When ECT was first developed, it was administered to both sides of the brain, and the effects on memory and learning sometimes were severe and permanent. These days, ECT usually is delivered to only one side of the brain—usually the right side, because this side is less involved in learning and memory. As a result, patients undergoing modern ECT are less likely to experience significant or long-term memory loss or learning difficulties, but people who have undergone ECT still experience a significant increase in memory problems (Sackeim et al., 2007). In addition, because this unilateral administration sometimes is not as effective as bilateral administration, some people are still given bilateral ECT.

Although ECT can be extremely effective in eliminating the symptoms of depression, the relapse rate among people who have undergone ECT can be as high as 85 percent, with over 30 percent of patients relapsing in the first 6 months after ECT (Fink, 2001; Jelovac, Kolshus, & McLoughlin, 2013). Continuing

Electroconvulsive therapy is an effective treatment for severe depression, but it is controversial, in part because of outdated depictions of it in the media. *JOEL SAGET/AFP/Getty Images*

ECT sessions after remission is a reasonable treatment option to prevent relapse for patients with depression who have responded well to ECT, especially for those individuals who did not experience cognitive impairment. Research has also shown that a gradual discontinuation of ECT may decrease the risk of early relapse. At this time however, there is a lot of controversy about continuation/ maintenance ECT, and no clear guidelines currently exist (Kolar, 2017).

Newer Methods of Brain Stimulation

In recent years, researchers have been investigating new methods of stimulating the brain without applying electric current. Each of these methods has been shown in randomized clinical trials to result in more improvement in depressive symptoms than a placebo in patients with depressive disorders or bipolar disorder whose depressive symptoms have not responded to other forms of treatment (Slotema, Blom, Hoek, & Sommer, 2010).

The procedure known as **repetitive transcranial magnetic stimulation (rTMS),** noninvasively exposes patients to repeated, high-intensity magnetic pulses focused on particular brain structures (Figure 6a). This procedure involves placing a machine around specific locations of the brain, and since it is noninvasive this procedure can can be done on an outpatient basis. In treating people with depression, researchers have targeted the left prefrontal cortex, which tends to show abnormally low metabolic activity in some people with depression. Clients who receive rTMS report few side effects—usually only minor headaches treatable by over-the-counter pain relievers. Patients can remain awake, rather than having to be anesthetized as in ECT, thereby avoiding possible complications of anesthesia. Studies suggest that this form of treatment is an effective and safe treatment for patients with treatment-resistant depression (Bewernick & Schlaepfer, 2015). There is a great deal of hope that these

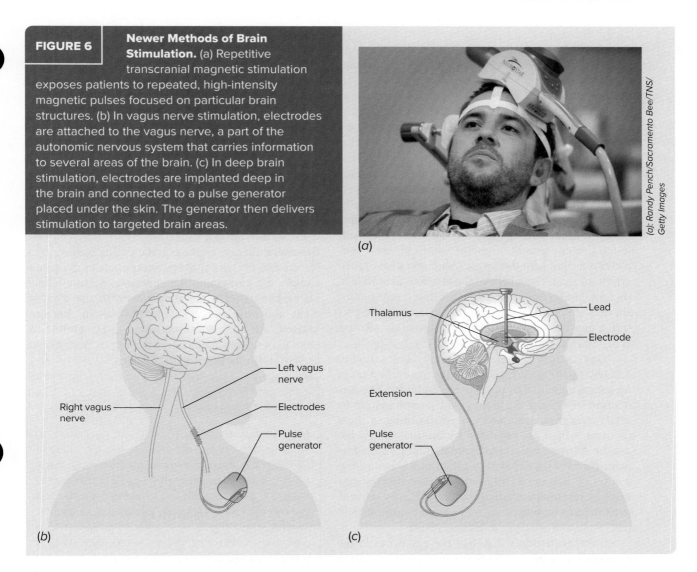

FIGURE 6 **Newer Methods of Brain Stimulation.** (a) Repetitive transcranial magnetic stimulation exposes patients to repeated, high-intensity magnetic pulses focused on particular brain structures. (b) In vagus nerve stimulation, electrodes are attached to the vagus nerve, a part of the autonomic nervous system that carries information to several areas of the brain. (c) In deep brain stimulation, electrodes are implanted deep in the brain and connected to a pulse generator placed under the skin. The generator then delivers stimulation to targeted brain areas.

(a): Randy Pench/Sacramento Bee/TNS/Getty Images

(a)

(b) Right vagus nerve · Left vagus nerve · Electrodes · Pulse generator

(c) Thalamus · Lead · Electrode · Extension · Pulse generator

techniques will be effective and safe alternative therapies, particularly for people who do not respond to drug therapies and may not be able to tolerate ECT. Researchers continue to explore how these treatments affect symptoms across a wide range of disorders, and when they are better or worse treatment options (Coles, Kozak, & George, 2018).

Vagus nerve stimulation (VNS; Figure 6b) is an invasive brain stimulation method where electrodes are surgically implanted at the vagus nerve, a part of the nervous system that carries information to several areas of the brain, including the hypothalamus and amygdala which are involved in depression. In VNS, the vagus nerve is stimulated by a small electronic device, much like a cardiac pacemaker, that is surgically implanted under the patient's skin in the left chest wall. These electrodes are connected to a pulse generator that delivers stimulation to the vagus nerve, which in turn travels to targeted areas of the brain. The results of a 5-year longitudinal study of clients treated with VNS resulted in superior outcomes in both effectiveness and mortality for patients with a chronic, severe, and treatment-resistant depression, but it is often difficult to receive this treatment since there is limited coverage from insurance providers which is a financial deterrent for many hospitals (Aaronson et. al., 2017; Bewernick & Schlaepfer, 2015).

The newest and least studied procedure to date is **deep brain stimulation.** In this procedure, electrodes are surgically implanted in specific areas of the brain (Figure 6c). The electrodes are connected to a pulse generator that is placed under the skin and stimulates these brain areas. Very small trials of deep brain stimulation have shown promise in relieving intractable depression (Mayberg et al., 2005). Understanding how these newer treatments for depression actually work is an important goal of researchers seeking to maximize effectiveness and minimize risks (e.g., Coles et al., 2018; De Raedt, Vanderhasselt, & Baeken, 2015).

Light Therapy

Recall that SAD is a specifier of major depressive disorder (MDD), mood disorder in which people become depressed during the winter months, when there are the fewest hours of daylight. Their moods improve in the summer months, when there are more hours of daylight each day. People with SAD may have deficient retinal sensitivity to light, meaning that their bodies react more strongly than most people's to changes in the amount of light each day (Rohan, Roecklein, Lacy, & Vacek, 2009). It turns out that exposing people with SAD to bright light for a few hours each day during the winter months, known as **light therapy,** can significantly reduce some people's symptoms. One study found that 57 percent of people with SAD who completed a trial of light therapy showed remission of their symptoms and 79 percent of those who had both light therapy and cognitive therapy (described below) showed remission, compared to 23 percent of a control group who did not receive intervention (Rohan et al., 2007; see also Rohan et al., 2015).

One theory is that light therapy helps reduce SAD by resetting circadian rhythms, natural cycles of biological activity that occur every 24 hours. The production of several hormones and neurotransmitters varies over the course of the day according to these rhythms, which are regulated by internal clocks but can be affected by environmental stimuli, including light. People with depression sometimes show dysregulation of their circadian rhythms. Light therapy may work by resetting circadian rhythms, thereby normalizing the production of hormones and neurotransmitters (Rohan, Roecklein, & Haaga, 2009).

Another theory is that light therapy works by decreasing levels of the hormone melatonin, which is secreted by the pineal gland (Rohan et al., 2009). Decreasing melatonin levels can increase the levels of norepinephrine and serotonin, reducing the symptoms of depression. Also, studies suggest that exposure to bright lights may directly increase serotonin levels, also decreasing depression.

Psychological Treatments for Mood Disorders

Each of the psychological theories has led to a treatment designed to overcome those factors the theory asserts cause and maintain mood disorders.

Behavioral Therapy

Behavioral therapy focuses on increasing positive reinforcers and decreasing aversive experiences in an individual's life by helping the depressed person change his or her patterns of interaction with the environment and with other people (Dimidjian, Barrera, Martell, Muñoz, & Lewinsohn, 2011; Hollon & Dimidjian, 2015). Behavioral therapy is designed to be short-term, lasting about 12 weeks.

People diagnosed with seasonal affective disorder (SAD) are often treated during darker winter months with a few hours each day of light. *Rocky89/iStock/Getty Images*

CASE STUDY

Mark worked constantly. When he was not actually at work, he was working at home. He had a position of considerable responsibility and was convinced that if he didn't stay focused on his job, he'd miss something that would result in his being fired or kicked off the career ladder. Mark had not taken a vacation in several years. Although he wanted to continue to get pay raises and promotions, as he has each year, he was also painfully aware that life was passing him by. He felt stressed, depressed, and hopeless about ever having a "normal" life.

Mark clearly felt rewarded for his one-dimensional life with praise, pay raises, promotions, and the absence of mistakes for which he might be punished. Mark's behavior was governed by his work focus. He engaged in no social activities, lived alone, and did not organize his time to include anything but his work. The behavior therapist suggested that if he wanted to improve his quality of life, and his outlook on life, he must learn some very specific new behaviors. Mark was encouraged to schedule time for social and recreational opportunities. He learned that he needed to actively and deliberately do things that are fun and pleasurable. He and the therapist practiced new ways to meet people and form social relationships (friendships, dating). The therapist also taught him relaxation skills to reduce his stress. Eventually, Mark felt a new sense of control over his life, and his depression lifted.

(Source: Adapted from Yapko, 1997.)

The first phase of behavioral therapy involves a functional analysis of the connections between specific circumstances and the depressed person's symptoms. When does the depressed person feel worst? Are there any situations in which he or she feels better? This analysis helps the therapist pinpoint the behaviors and interaction patterns that need to be the focus of therapy. It also helps the client understand the intimate connections between his or her symptoms and his or her daily activities or interactions.

Once the circumstances that precipitate the client's depressive symptoms are identified, therapists help the client change aspects of the environment that are contributing to the depression, such as isolation. They teach depressed clients skills for changing their negative circumstances, particularly negative social interactions. They also help clients learn new skills, such as relaxation techniques, for managing their moods in unpleasant situations. Several of these techniques are illustrated in the previous case study.

Cognitive-Behavioral Therapy

CBT represents a blending of cognitive and behavioral theories of depression (Beck, Weissman, Lester, & Trexler, 1974; Ellis & Harper, 1961; Lewinsohn, Muñoz, Youngren, & Zeiss, 1986; Rehm, 1977; see Hollon & Dimidjian, 2015). This therapy has two general goals. First, it aims to change the negative, hopeless patterns of thinking described by the cognitive models of depression. Second, it aims to help people with depression solve concrete problems in their lives and develop skills for being more effective in their world so they no longer have the deficits in reinforcers described by behavioral theories of depression.

CASE STUDY

Susan was a young, single, 24-year-old woman. Her goals for therapy were to learn how to overcome chronic feelings of depression and temptations to overeat. Susan was unemployed and living with her aunt and uncle in a rural area. She had no means of personal transportation. Hypersensitivity to the reactions of significant others and the belief that they could control her feelings seemed to be central to her negative self-concept and feelings of helplessness. Susan described her mother as knowing which "buttons to push." This metaphor was examined and challenged. She was questioned as to how her mother controlled her emotions: Where were these buttons? Once again, the principle was asserted that it is not the actions of others that cause emotions, but one's cognitions about them.

. . . During the last stage of therapy, Susan's mother visited. This provided a real test of the gains Susan had made, as it was her mother's criticism that she feared the most. At first, she reported feeling easily wounded by her mother's criticism. These examples were used as opportunities to identify and challenge self-defeating thoughts. Soon, Susan was able to see her mother's critical statements as her mother's problem, not her own. She also discovered that, as she became better at ignoring her mother's critical remarks and not taking them to heart, her mother began to be more relaxed and open around her and criticized her less.

(Source: Adapted from Thorpe & Olson, 1997, pp. 225–227.)

Like behavioral therapy, CBT is designed to be brief and time-limited. The therapist and client usually will agree on a set of goals they wish to accomplish in 6 to 12 weeks. These goals focus on specific problems that clients believe are connected to their depression, such as problems in their marriage or dissatisfaction with their job. From the beginning of therapy, the therapist urges clients to set their own goals and make their own decisions.

The first step in CBT is to help clients discover the negative automatic thoughts they habitually have and understand the link between those thoughts and their depression. Often, the therapist will assign clients the homework of keeping track of times when they feel sad or depressed and writing down on record sheets, such as the one in Figure 7, what is going through their mind at such times.

The second step in CBT is to help clients challenge their negative thoughts. People with depression often believe that there is only one way to interpret a situation—their negative way. Therapists use a series of questions to help clients consider alternative ways of thinking about a situation and the pros and cons of these alternatives, such as "What is the evidence that you are right in the way you are interpreting this situation?" "Are there other ways of looking at this situation?" and "What can you do if the worst-case scenario comes true?"

The third step in CBT is to help clients recognize the deeper, basic beliefs or assumptions they might hold that are fueling their depression. These might be beliefs such as "If I'm not loved by everyone, I'm a failure" or "If I'm not a complete success at everything, my life is worthless." The therapist will help clients question such beliefs and decide if they truly want to base their lives on them. The case of Susan illustrates some of the cognitive components of CBT.

Cognitive-behavioral therapists also use behavioral techniques to train clients in new skills they

FIGURE 7	**An Automatic Thoughts Record Used in Cognitive-Behavioral Therapy.** In cognitive-behavioral therapy, patients keep a record of the negative thoughts that arise when they feel negative emotions. This record is then used in therapy to challenge the patients' depressive thinking.

Date	Event	Emotion	Automatic thoughts
April 4	Boss seemed annoyed.	Sad, anxious, worried	Oh, what have I done now? If I keep making him mad, I'm going to get fired.
April 5	Husband didn't want to make love.	Sad	I'm so fat and ugly.
April 7	Boss yelled at another employee.	Anxious	I'm next.
April 9	Husband said he's taking a long business trip next month.	Sad, defeated	He's probably got a mistress somewhere. My marriage is falling apart.
April 10	Neighbor brought over some cookies.	A little happy, mostly sad	She probably thinks I can't cook. I look like such a mess all the time. And my house was a disaster when she came in!

TABLE 5   Interpersonal Therapy

Interpersonal therapists focus on four types of interpersonal problems as sources of depression.

Type of Problem	Therapeutic Approach
Grief, loss	Help the client accept feelings and evaluate a relationship with a lost person; help the client invest in new relationships
Interpersonal role disputes	Help the client make decisions about concessions willing to be made and learn better ways of communicating
Role transitions	Help the client develop more realistic perspectives toward roles that are lost and regard new roles in a more positive manner
Interpersonal skills deficits	Review the client's past relationships, helping the client understand these relationships and how they might be affecting current relationships; directly teach the client social skills, such as assertiveness

Source: Hollon et al., 2005.

might need to cope better. Often people with depression are unassertive in making requests of other people or in standing up for their rights and needs. This lack of assertiveness can be the result of their negative automatic thoughts. For example, a person who often thinks "I can't ask for what I need because the other person might get mad and that would be horrible" is not likely to make even reasonable requests of other people. The therapist first will help clients recognize the thoughts behind their actions (or lack of action). The therapist then may work with the clients to devise exercises or homework assignments in which they practice new skills, such as assertiveness, between therapy sessions.

Interpersonal Therapy

In interpersonal therapy (IPT), therapists look for four types of problems in depressed individuals (Table 5; Weissman & Verdeli, 2013). First, many depressed people are grieving the loss of a loved one, perhaps not from death but instead from the breakup of an important relationship. Interpersonal therapists help clients face such losses and explore their feelings about them. Therapists also help clients begin to invest in new relationships.

A second type of problem on which IPT focuses is interpersonal role disputes, which arise when people do not agree on their roles in a relationship. For example, a college student and a parent may disagree on the extent to which the student should follow the parent's wishes in choosing a career. Interpersonal therapists first help the client recognize the dispute and then guide them in making choices about what concessions might be made to the other person in the relationship. Therapists also may need to help clients modify and improve their patterns of communicating with others in relationships. For example, a student who resents his parents' intrusions into his private life may tend to withdraw and sulk rather than directly confront his parents about their intrusions. He would be helped to develop more effective ways of communicating his distress over his parents' intrusions.

The third type of problem addressed in IPT is role transitions, such as the transition from college to work or from work to full-time motherhood. People sometimes become depressed over the role they must leave behind. Therapists help clients develop more realistic perspectives toward roles that are lost and learn to regard new roles in a more positive manner. If a client feels unsure about their ability to perform a new role, the therapist helps the client develop a sense of mastery in the new role. Sometimes, clients need help developing new networks of social support to replace the support systems they have left behind in their old roles.

Fourth, people with depression also turn to IPT for help with problems caused by deficits in interpersonal skills. Such skill deficits can be the reason people with depression have inadequate social support networks. The therapist reviews with clients their past relationships, especially important childhood relationships, and helps them understand these relationships and how they might be affecting their current relationships. The therapist also might directly teach clients social skills, such as assertiveness.

Interpersonal and Social Rhythm Therapy and Family-Focused Therapy

Interpersonal and social rhythm therapy (ISRT) is an enhancement of IPT designed specifically for people with bipolar disorder (Frank et al., 2005). When people with bipolar disorder experience disruptions in either their daily routines or their social environment, they sometimes experience an upsurge in symptoms. ISRT combines IPT techniques with behavioral techniques to help patients maintain regular routines of eating, sleeping, and activity, as well as stability in their personal relationships. By having patients self-monitor their patterns over time, therapists help patients understand how changes in sleep patterns, circadian rhythms, and eating habits can provoke symptoms. Then therapists and patients work together to develop a plan to stabilize the patients' routines and activities. Similarly, patients learn how stressors in their family and work relationships affect their moods, and they develop better strategies for coping with these stressors. Studies show that patients who receive ISRT in conjunction with medication show fewer symptoms and relapses over time than patients who do not receive ISRT (Frank et al., 2005; Haynes, Gengler, & Kelly, 2016). Targeting the important role of sleep in bipolar disorder, related treatments increasingly address insomnia and other sleep problems directly. Preliminary evidence indicates that this emphasis may reduce relapses and improve functioning (Harvey et al., 2015).

Family-focused therapy (FFT) is also designed to reduce interpersonal stress in people with bipolar disorder, particularly within the context of families. Patients and their families are educated about bipolar disorder and trained in communication and problem-solving skills. Studies comparing FFT with standard therapy (medication with periodic individual checkups with a psychiatrist) have found that adults receiving FFT show lower relapse rates over time (Miklowitz & Chung, 2016). In addition, applications of FFT to adolescents with or at risk of developing bipolar disorder show promise in helping these youths and their families manage symptoms and reduce the impact of the disorder on the adolescents' functioning and development (Miklowitz et al., 2013). More generally, patients with bipolar disorder are strongly affected by their social environments (and vice versa). Including the family appears to be an overall positive addition to psychosocial treatment (Reinares et al., 2016).

Comparison of Treatments

Which of the many treatments for mood disorders is best? In the past few decades, several studies have compared behavioral, cognitive-behavioral, interpersonal, and drug therapies in the treatment of depressive disorders. Perhaps surprisingly, these therapies, despite their vast differences, appear to be about equally effective in treating most people with depression (Cuijpers, van Straten, van Oppen, & Andersson, 2008; DeRubeis, Gelfand, Tang, & Simons, 1999; Dimidjian et al., 2006; Hollon & Dimidjian, 2015; Weissman & Verdeli, 2013). For example, in one study, 240 people with major depression were randomly assigned to receive either the SSRI paroxetine (Paxil) or CBT for 16 weeks (DeRubeis et al., 2005).

At the end of treatment, about 60 percent in each group no longer experienced major depression. Another study compared the results of behavioral therapy, cognitive therapy (without behavioral interventions), and drug therapy (paroxetine) in 240 patients with major depressive disorder (Dimidjian et al., 2006). In this study, behavioral therapy led to improvement in the greatest number of patients, followed by cognitive therapy and then drug therapy. Various studies have demonstrated support for a combination of both psychotherapy and medication treatment for depressive disorders. Research has found that psychotherapy and pharmacotherapy alone are efficacious for improving function and quality of life, but psychotherapy and medication produce superior results when implemented together (Kamenov, Twomey, Cabello, Prina, & Ayuso-Mateos, 2017).

Relapse rates in depression are quite high, even among people whose depressions completely disappear with treatment. For this reason, many psychiatrists and psychologists argue that people with a history of recurrent depression should be kept on a maintenance level of therapy even after their depression is relieved (Gitlin, 2015). Usually, the maintenance therapy is a drug therapy, and many people remain on antidepressant drugs for years after their initial episodes of depression have passed. Studies of behavioral therapy, IPT, and CBT show that maintenance levels of these therapies—usually consisting of once-a-month meetings with therapists—also can substantially reduce relapse rates (Hollon & Dimidjian, 2015; Cuijpers, Donker, Weissman, Ravitz, & Cristea, 2016).

Even when maintenance doses of psychotherapy are not available, people who have had any of the empirically supported psychotherapies appear to be less likely to relapse than those who have had only drug therapy (Weissman & Cuijpers, 2017). For example, researchers followed the 240 patients in one of the studies described earlier for a year after they had recovered from acute depression. They found that those who had had CBT showed a lower rate of relapse than those who continued with the drug therapy (paroxetine) only and that both groups had much lower rates of relapse than those who were taking a placebo pill over those 12 months (Figure 8; Hollon et al., 2005). Interventions that specifically emphasize relapse prevention may be especially helpful for people at higher risk for depression relapse (Bockting, Hollon, Jarrett, Kuyken, & Dobson, 2015).

In the case of bipolar disorder, combining drug treatment with the psychological therapies may reduce the rate at which patients stop taking their medication and may lead more patients to achieve full remission of their symptoms, compared to lithium treatment alone (Miklowitz, 2010; Swartz & Frank, 2001). Psychotherapy can help people with bipolar

FIGURE 8   **Relapse Rates After Drug Versus Cognitive-Behavioral Therapy for Major Depression.**
Patients with major depression who had received CBT showed lower relapse rates in the next year than those who continued to take only an SSRI. Both groups showed lower rates of relapse than patients who received a placebo pill.

disorder understand and accept their need for lithium treatment as well as help them cope with the impact of the disorder on their lives.

In addition to treating mood disorders after their onset, another priority is preventing episodes before they emerge. Prevention programs can be effective in eliminating or delaying the onset of symptoms, especially if they are targeted at high-risk groups based on risk factors for depression (Muñoz, Beardslee, & Leykin, 2012). For example, programs aimed at women prior to childbirth appear somewhat effective in preventing postpartum depression (Sockol, Epperson, & Barber, 2013).

SUICIDE

According to the Centers for Disease Control and Prevention (CDC), more than 45,000 people in the United States die by suicide each year. Approximately 7 percent of U.S. citizens have experienced the death of a friend or family member due to suicide which makes this a public health concern (Hayes et al., 2020). Suicide is among the three leading causes of death worldwide among people ages 15 to 44 and it is currently the 10th leading cause of death in the United States (Ivey-Stephenson et al., 2017; World Health Organization [WHO], 2017). Around the world, more people die from suicide than from homicide. Suicide is associated with mood disorders, and thus we address it in the final section of this chapter. Note, however, that the risk of suicide is increased in people with any mental disorder.

Defining and Measuring Suicide

The CDC, one of the federal agencies in the United States that tracks suicide rates, defines **suicide** as "death from injury, poisoning, or suffocation where there is evidence (either explicit or implicit) that the injury was self-inflicted and that the decedent intended to kill themself." As clear as this definition seems, there is great variability in the form that suicide takes, and whether to call particular types of death suicide is open to debate. We may easily agree that a young man who is despondent and shoots himself in the head has committed suicide. It is harder to agree on whether an unhappy young man who goes on a drinking binge and crashes his car into a tree has committed suicide. Is an elderly person who refuses life support when dying from a painful disease committing suicide? Is a middle-aged person with severe heart disease who continues to smoke cigarettes, eat fatty foods, and drink excessive amounts of alcohol committing suicide? Clearly, suicide-like behaviors fall along the type of continuum we discuss throughout this book.

We can distinguish among *completed suicides,* which end in death; **suicide attempts,** which may or may not end in death; and **suicidal ideation** or thought. Many people with mental disorders think about committing suicide but never attempt to kill themselves. Also, actual suicide attempts are much more common than completed suicides, with some studies estimating that suicide attempts are 20 times as common as completed suicides (WHO, 2017).

Given the difficulty of defining suicide, it is not surprising that accurate suicide rates are difficult to obtain. Many deaths are ambiguous, particularly when no notes are left behind and no clues exist as to the victim's mental state before death. Recorded rates probably are low, because the stigma against suicide is a great incentive for labeling a death anything but a suicide. Accurate data on nonlethal suicide attempts are even harder to obtain.

Even so, the statistics indicate that suicide is more common than we would like to believe. More than 40,000 people kill themselves each year in the United States, an average of 113 people per day, or 1 every 13 minutes (CDC, 2015). In addition, as many as 3 percent of the population make a suicide attempt (with intent to die) sometime in their lives (Nock & Kessler, 2006), and more than 13 percent report having had suicidal thoughts at some time (Borges, Angst, Nock, Ruscio, & Kessler, 2008). Recent studies have found an increase in suicides among working-age adults aged 45 to 64 years. Regional and state differences in suicide rates are also documented in the United States and tend to be higher in the West than in the South, Midwest, and Northeast. And, specifically, suicide rates by sex, race/ethnicity, age group,

and mechanism of death for the general population are higher in rural communities than in urban areas (Ivey-Stephenson et al., 2017). Suicide is not just an American phenomenon, however. Internationally, an estimated 800,000 people die by suicide each year, or 1 person about every 40 seconds (WHO, 2017).

In the context of the tragic statistics just reviewed, *DSM-5* approaches suicide risk and behavior more deliberately than did *DSM-IV*. Throughout *DSM-5,* particular characteristics that make people more vulnerable to suicide are highlighted, and those mental disorders that are associated with an elevated risk for suicide are identified specifically (e.g., not just mood or personality disorders, but schizophrenia, anorexia, and posttraumatic stress disorder). By describing the suicidal patterns associated with a range of diagnoses, *DSM-5* encourages clinicians to attend to suicide risk early and often in treatment. In addition, *DSM-5* includes two new conditions for further research study in a special section toward the end of the manual. These include proposed criteria sets for suicidal behavior disorder and nonsuicidal self-injury, for which future research is encouraged, both of which represent major problems on college campuses. While the proposed criteria sets are *not* intended for clinical use (and are not yet officially recognized as disorders), their inclusion provides increased emphasis on suicide and self-harm as an important focus of future clinical research (American Psychiatric Association, 2013).

Gender Differences

While suicide significantly affects people worldwide each year, there are noted differences in the rates of suicide attempt and suicide completion between men and women. Research has found that women are more likely to attempt suicide whereas men have a higher rates of suicide completion, typically choosing more violent methods, such as firearms. It is worth noting that there are also significant differences in diagnostic rates of depression between men and women, with men less likely to receive a diagnosis and remain an undertreated population. The underdiagnosis of depression in males and suicide rates that are three times that of females highlight important patterns in mental health screening services that need to be appropriately addressed (Oliffe et al., 2019; Tsirigotis, Gruszczynski, & Tsirigotis, 2011).

Recent studies have shown changes in the rates of suicide completion and while men are still more likely to die by suicide, the gender differences have narrowed. Suicide rates among women, particularly young women, have increased disproportionately in the past four decades. From 2000 to 2016 research has found a 50 percent increase in suicides among women of all age groups. This increased risk of suicide among young women may be due, in part, to the

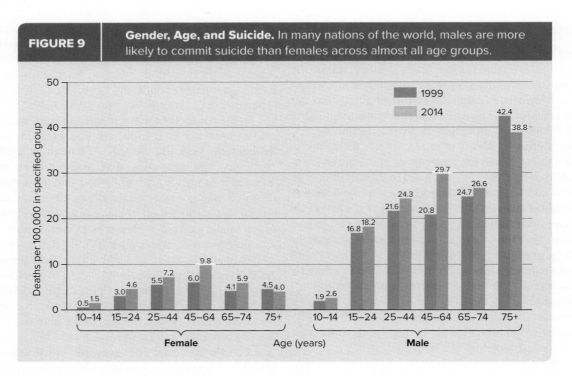

FIGURE 9 | **Gender, Age, and Suicide.** In many nations of the world, males are more likely to commit suicide than females across almost all age groups.

higher prevalence rates of depression and stress-related disorders like PTSD among this group which increases risk for suicidal behavior that may explain some variation across genders (Monaco, 2018; Polanco-Roman, Anglin, Miranda & Jeglic, 2019).

Research has found that the methods used for suicide vary by age group. Among girls ages 10 to 14, 70 percent of suicide deaths were due to suffocation, which includes hangings. This method was also the most common among women aged 15 to 24 which accounted for 44 percent of suicides, followed by firearm use (29 percent). For women 25 to 44 years of age, the most common method was firearms, accounting for 32 percent of suicides. However, poisoning was the most common method for women 45 years of age and older (40 percent), followed by use of firearms (32 percent). Research has shown that among boys aged 10 to 14, the use of firearms and suffocation was used equally (48 percent each) but firearm use was more common with increasing age (Monaco, 2018).

This gender difference is true across all age groups, as seen in Figure 9. Many people assume that suicide rates are highest among adolescents. Although rates are increasing in that age group (see below), in fact the most "typical" suicide in the United States involves a middle-aged, Caucasian man (CDC, 2015).

Ethnic and Cross-Cultural Differences

Within the United States, there are substantial differences in suicide rates among ethnic/racial groups (Figure 10; CDC, 2015; Oquendo et al., 2001; Polanco-Roman, Anglin, Miranda & Jeglic, 2019). Overall, the rates of suicide are higher for non-Hispanic white

(approximately 15 people per 100,000 population) and American Indian/Alaska Native (approximately 13 per 100,000) populations than for other racial/ethnic groups (CDC, 2015; Ivey-Stephenson et al., 2017). Suicide among Native Americans is tied to poverty, lack of education and hope, discrimination, substance abuse, limited access to care, and the easy availability of firearms (Wexler et al., 2015). Suicide rates among African American males have increased greatly in recent decades, but African Americans generally commit suicide at lower rates than other groups (about 6 per 100,000; CDC, 2015). Latino suicide rates are similar, but have increased markedly in recent years among young Latina females (CDC, 2015; Silva & Van Orden, 2018). Suicide risk among racial/ethnic minority populations is most pronounced among youth, as suicide deaths among Black and Latino/a adolescents have increased in the United States over the past two decades. Further, Black children ages 5 to 12 are about twice as likely to die by suicide than their white peers. In fact, among people of color, the age of highest risk for suicide deaths is under age 30, whereas middle-aged adults (ages 40 to 50) account for the highest proportion of suicide deaths among white populations (Polanco-Roman et al., 2019).

Racial/ethnic discrimination may be one factor associated with the increased suicidality among particularly among racial/ethnic minority emerging adults, who are most vulnerable to the harmful effects of discrimination. African Americans report a higher degree of racial discrimination than any other demographic group which (Arshanapally, Werner, Sartor & Bucholz, 2017). Recent studies have shown that these

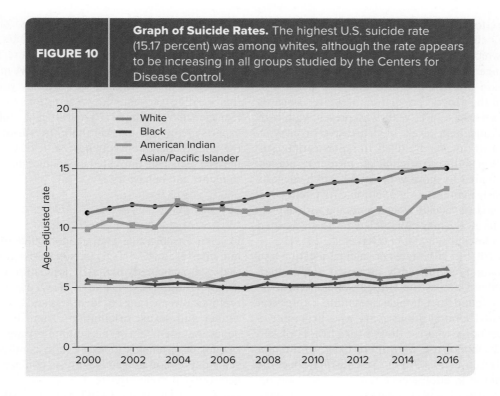

FIGURE 10 | **Graph of Suicide Rates.** The highest U.S. suicide rate (15.17 percent) was among whites, although the rate appears to be increasing in all groups studied by the Centers for Disease Control.

young and emerging adults are particularly sensitive to the detrimental effects of racial/ethnic discrimination. This group reports greater experiences of discrimination and poorer coping responses as compared to older minority adults. There is compelling evidence which suggests that racial/ethnic discrimination is linked to poor physical and mental health outcomes, namely depression, and suicidal thoughts and behavior which is independent of socioeconomic status (SES) and other sociodemographic factors. Unfortunately, racial/ethnic minority individuals remain underrepresented in suicide research. This lack of understanding emphasizes the need for more research that will shed light about cultural context of risk for suicidal thoughts and behavior among racial/ethnic minorities (Polanco-Roman et al., 2019).

There are also cross-national differences in suicide rates. Higher rates are found in much of Europe, the former Soviet Union and China, and lower rates in Latin America and South America (WHO, 2017). The suicide rates in Australia, the United States, Canada, and England fall between these two extremes. The differences may be due in part to cultural and religious norms. Followers of religions that expressly forbid suicide are less likely to attempt it (Gearing & Alonzo, 2018; L. O'Donnell, C. O'Donnell, Wardlaw, & Stueve, 2004).

Suicide in Children and Adolescents

Death by suicide is a serious public health issue for children in the United States and is now the second leading cause of death for youth ages 10 to 18 (Opara et al., 2020). Suicide among this age group is linked to risk factors such as mental health problems, family history of suicidal behavior, biological factors, family problems, and peer victimization and bullying. Research has shown that youth were commonly exposed to one or more problems that resulted in feeling burdensome to other and loneliness which likely fueled thoughts, and sometimes plans, for suicide attempts. Research also found that continued exposure to negative experiences and thoughts/plans about suicide resulted in an acquired capacity to self-harm and eventual suicide (Holland, Vivolo-Kantor, Logan, & Leemis, 2017). Studies have found a strong association between self-harm and risk of future suicide with approximately 50 percent of adolescents who die by suicide having previously self-harmed. Self-harm increases the risk of death by suicide approximately tenfold and the 6-month period, following an episode of self-harm has been identified as the period of time where the risk of is highest (Harris, Beese, & Moore, 2019). As is the case for adults, girls are much more likely to attempt suicide than boys, but boys are more likely to succeed (Jacobson & Gould, 2009). Males are up to six times more likely than females in this age range to commit suicide (CDC, 2015; Hawton, Saunders, & O'Connor, 2012).

Children with mood disturbance more frequently display irritability as a core symptom of depression than in adults. This feature typically manifests in the form of frequent temper outbursts typically occurring in response to frustration and can be verbal or behavioral. Irritability is reported by one-third of depressed children which makes this group more prone to increased anger. Chronic and severe irritability is the main feature of DMDD which affects 3 percent of children in the general population. Research suggests that children ages 6 to 12 years who present with high irritability and high levels of depressive or anxious mood are two times more likely to report serious suicidal ideation and/or to attempt suicide during adolescence compared to those without. Research suggests that this early manifestation of chronic irritability during childhood, especially when combined with depressive/anxious mood, may be associated with an elevated risk for adolescent suicidality (Orri et al., 2018).

From 2007 to 2017, rates of suicidal ideation and suicide planning significantly increased among high school students across the United States. Recent research has found that hopelessness and depression were elevated among adolescents who experienced suicidal ideations, whereas those with a history of self-injury and alcohol use were more likely to attempt suicide (Hayes et al., 2019). Suicide may become more common in adolescence than in childhood because the rates of several types of psychopathology tied to suicide, including depression, anxiety disorders, and substance abuse, increase in adolescence. Suicide rates also may rise during the teen years because adolescents are more sophisticated than children in their thinking and can contemplate suicide more clearly. Finally, adolescents simply may have readier access to the means to commit suicide (e.g., drugs and guns) than do children.

Among Black children under 12 years of age, there has been a statistically significant increase in death by suicide and suicidal ideation in recent years (Opara et al., 2020). Hispanic females have especially high rates of suicidal ideation and attempted suicides as compared to Hispanic adolescent male and those from other racial/ethnic groups (Jacobson & Gould, 2009; Silva & Van Orden, 2018). Luis Zayas and colleagues (Zayas, Lester, Cabassa, & Fortuna, 2005) suggest that these high rates are linked to clashes between Hispanic girls, who are highly acculturated to American values, and their parents, who may hold traditional cultural values of *familism* (centrality of family to one's life) and may reject their daughters' bids for independence.

Rates of suicide among children and teenagers more than doubled between the 1950s and the early 1990s, but they have steadily declined since 1994 (Hawton et al., 2012). The initial increase may have been linked to the increase in substance use by teenagers during that same period, coupled with an increased availability of firearms. The decrease in suicide rates since the mid-1990s is thought to be related to an increase in the use of antidepressants, particularly SSRIs, to treat depression in adolescents. Unfortunately, there has been a spike in adolescent suicide rates since 2004—the same year the FDA mandated a warning regarding the use of SSRIs by youth. Since that warning was required, prescriptions for SSRIs for teenagers have declined (Nemeroff et al., 2007). Some experts are concerned that the FDA warning has had the unintended consequence of leaving many depressed teenagers untreated and vulnerable to suicidal thoughts and behaviors.

Lesbian, Gay, Bisexual, Transgender, Queer, and Intersex (LGBTQI)

Lesbian, gay, bisexual, transgender, queer or questioning, intersexed (LGBTQI) persons are a group identified as a particularly high-risk population for suicidal ideations and behavior. The LGBTQI community represents a diverse range of identities and expressions of gender and sexual orientation. There is strong evidence that members of this community are at a higher risk for experiencing mental health conditions, especially depression and suicidality as compared to their heterosexual counterparts. Despite increased acceptance in recent years, LGBTQI people still face significant discrimination, prejudice, denial of civil and human rights, harassment and family rejection, which can lead to new or worsened psychological symptoms (National LGBT Health Education Center, 2018).

Research has found multiple factors associated with suicidal behavior among LGBTQ people, including isolation from family and peers, a history of mental health issues, substance use disorders, and victimization such as bullying and abuse. Even today, with increased awareness and social acceptance in the United States, many LGBTQ people find they must contend with harassment, discrimination, and bias enacted by peers, family, colleagues, workplaces, houses of worship, schools, places of public accommodation, and health care settings. Anti-LGBTQ attitudes can become internalized, leading to further stress and potential for suicidal thoughts (National LGBT Health Education Center, 2018). Given the prevalence of direct exposure to bias-based aggression like homophobia, it is no surprise that LGBTQ youth face an increased risk of developing mental health symptoms, such as anxiety, depression, and suicidality. Research suggests that depression is the strongest predictor of suicidal ideation. In one study, 85 percent patients with MDD experienced suicidal ideation. This is especially concerning since LGBTQ youth show increased levels of depression as compared to non-LGBTQ youth (Hayes et al., 2019). Research has shown that gay, lesbian, and bisexual adolescents attempt suicide at rates two to six times higher than those of heterosexual adolescents (Jacobson & Gould, 2009).

Research on LGBTQ young adults suggests that psychological distress and mental health problems are more prevalent among sexual and gender minorities than among their peers. This chronic stress is often associated with discrimination on the basis of one's sexual or gender identification (Woodford et al., 2018). For example, recent research has shown that LGBTQI students are often victimized in schools, with 85 percent of students reporting sexuality-based verbal harassment over the past year, with 40 percent reporting this experience at extremely high frequencies. Physical harassment is also reported among 27 percent of students from this sample reported being physically victimized at school because of their sexuality. These rates of LGBTQI victimization are also consistent across other forms of peer violence such as cyberbullying, relational aggression, and sexual harassment who report their sexual orientation is the most common focus of the attack (Hayes et al., 2019).

Likely an outcome of marginalization, research has shown that LGBTQ youth experience greater risks for mental health conditions and suicidality. Specifically, LGBTQ youth are more than twice as likely to report experiencing persistent feelings of sadness or hopelessness than their heterosexual peers. Transgender youth are twice as likely to experience depressive symptoms, suicide ideation, and attempt as compared to cisgender lesbian, gay, bisexual, queer and questioning youth. Suicide risk in LGBTQ people is at its highest during the teen years and early twenties. Research has found that depression, peer victimization, help-seeking beliefs, and intent to use drugs are predictors of both suicidal ideation and attempts. LGBTQ youth who report high levels of depression are significantly more likely to report suicidal ideation than LGBTQ youth with less depressive symptoms. LGBTQ youth with high levels of depression are three times more likely to attempt suicide as compared to LGBTQ youth with less depression (Hayes et al., 2019).

In 2015, more than 4.5 times as many LGB-identified high school students reported attempting suicide in the past 12 months compared to non-LGB students (29.4 vs. 6.4 percent). Of this sample, 43 percent expressed serious thoughts about completing suicide. Youth who are bisexual or questioning their sexual orientation and/or gender identity are even more likely to experience depression or suicidality than their LG-identified peers (National LGBT Health Education Center, 2018). Significantly higher rates of suicide attempt have been documented among sexual minorities in college with nearly 10 percent of transgendered students and 5 percent of cisgender LGBQ students reporting attempted suicide. Studies have found that psychological resilience had a significant effect on depression and moderate interpersonal microaggressions. The willingness to seek help has been shown as a powerful factor that can help protect individuals against the negative mental health outcomes for sexual minority youth in particular. Meaning, if a person feels positively about seeking help, they are more likely to access mental health services which result in more positive outcomes in the future. Research also suggests that strengthening psychological resilience among LGBTQ college students, campuses can help to promote positive mental health among students (Jacobson & Gould, 2009).

Negative mental health outcomes are not limited to LGBTQI youth and adults in the LGBTQI community are more than twice as likely as heterosexual adults to experience a mental health condition. Transgender individuals are nearly four times as likely as cisgender individuals (people whose gender identity corresponds with their birth sex) to experience a mental health condition (NAMI). Older LGBTQI adults (65 years and older) are an overlooked population in terms of suicide. Older adults in the general population account for approximately 17 percent of completed suicides even though they currently make up about 15 percent of the total U.S. population. Unfortunately, since older LGBTQ adults are an underresearched population, the percentage of completed suicides among this group is unknown. However, some studies have found higher suicide rates among LGB older adults as compared to their straight peers which could be expected as this group has likely endured a long life of stigmatization (National LGBT Health Education Center, 2018).

College Students

The transition to college can often bring heightened challenges that come with increased academic and social pressures. This often stressful period of time is associated with an increase risk of suicidality among young adults. Suicide is the second leading cause of death among traditionally aged college students in the United States, with a prevalence of approximately 14 deaths per 100,000 persons. Research suggests that, each year, 10 percent of college students seriously consider suicide and roughly 1.5 percent engage in suicide behavior these rates have increased slightly every year since 2010 (Hayes et al., 2020). Students who had contemplated or attempted suicide were more likely than those who had not to have experienced depression and hopelessness, loneliness, and problems with their parents. Regrettably, only 20 percent of the students who had contemplated suicide had sought any type of counseling. However, rates of suicidal thinking among college students are about the same as their same-age peers; rates of suicide attempts are somewhat lower (CDC, 2015). Studies have found that the development of effective coping skills are associated with decreased suicide risk and increased suicide protection (Yi et al., 2020).

College students are a group with high risk for suicide attempt who often do not seek out counseling services. *Galina Zhigalova / EyeEm/Getty Images*

Fortunately, effective programs designed to connect at-risk college students to campus counseling centers for psychological help have been developed for this population. In order for these programs to best serve students needs, college-based counseling centers recognize the importance of servicing high-risk students. As a result of these early intervention programs, students have attended more than a million sessions of psychotherapy on U.S. campuses during the 2016–2017 academic year. Studies show that those who seek psychotherapy are typically more depressed, hostile, and anxious than their peers. These students are also three times more likely than their classmates to report high levels of suicide ideation and five times more likely to have made a previous suicide attempt (Hayes et al., 2020).

Suicide in Older Adults

Although there has been a 50 percent decline in suicide rates among adults over age 65 in the past few decades, older people, particularly older men, still remain at relatively high risk for suicide. Among older adults, the highest risk is among European American men over age 85 (CDC, 2015). When they attempt suicide, older people are much more likely than younger people to be successful. It seems that most older people who attempt suicide fully intend to die (McIntosh, 1995).

Some older people commit suicide because they cannot tolerate the loss of their spouse or other loved ones. Suicide rates are highest in the first year after a loss but remain relatively high for several years (McIntosh, 1995). Other older people who commit suicide wish to escape the pain and suffering of debilitating illness. Escape from illness and disabilities may be a particularly strong motive for suicide among men, who are reluctant to become a burden to others (Conwell & Thompson, 2008). In one study of older people who committed suicide, 44 percent said they could not bear being placed in a nursing home and would rather be dead (J. P. Loebel, J. S. Loebel, Dager, Centerwall, & Reay, 1991).

Most older people who lose a spouse or become ill do not commit suicide. Those with a history of depression or other psychological problems are at greatest risk for responding to the challenges of old age with suicide (Harwood, Hawton, Hope, & Jacoby, 2000). Higher suicide rates among older adults may also reflect the impairments in cognitive abilities (such as problem solving and resisting impulses) that older adults sometimes experience during depressive episodes (Wang & Blazer, 2015).

Nonsuicidal Self-Injury

Some people—often adolescents—repeatedly cut, burn, puncture, or otherwise significantly injure their skin with no intent to die, a behavior known as **nonsuicidal self-injury,** or **NSSI** (Nock, 2010). NSSI seems to be relatively common, with lifetime prevalence of up to 18 percent internationally (Muehlenkamp, Claes, Havertape, & Plener, 2012). NSSI is especially prevalent among adolescents (17 percent) compared to young adults (13 percent) and adults (5.5 percent; Swannell, Martin, Page, Hasking, & St. John, 2014). Clinicians, teachers, and other health professionals report a dramatic increase in NSSI in recent years, but longitudinal data do not support this (Muehlenkamp et al., 2012; Swannell et al., 2014).

Individuals who engage in NSSI are at increased risk for suicide attempts (Klonsky, May, & Saffer, 2016; Nock, 2010). NSSI occurs at an elevated rate across most mood and anxiety disorders (Bentley, Cassiello-Robbins, Vittorio, Sauer-Zavala, & Barlow, 2015), as well as being a prominent feature of borderline personality disorder (see the chapter "Personality Disorders"). Theories of NSSI suggest that it functions as a way of regulating emotion and/or influencing the social environment (Fox, Toole, Franklin, & Hooley, 2017). People who engage in NSSI often report that the experience of feeling the pain and seeing the blood actually calms them and releases tension. There is some evidence that individuals who engage in NSSI do have more difficulty regulating their emotions, and use their behavior to regulate distress (Davis et al., 2014; Fox et al., 2017; Weinberg & Klonsky, 2012). Self-injury also draws support and sympathy from others or may punish others (Nock, 2008). Some risk factors for NSSI are similar to those for suicide, such as hopelessness (Fox et al., 2015), but much more research on what triggers self-injury is needed.

Understanding Suicide

Psychological Disorders and Suicide

More than 90 percent of people who commit suicide probably have been suffering from a diagnosable mental disorder (Borges et al., 2010; Jacobson & Gould, 2009; Joiner, Brown, & Wingate, 2005). Depression increases the odds of a suicide attempt by approximately six times, and bipolar disorder increases the odds of a suicide attempt by seven times (Nock et al., 2008). Internationally, one in every four people with bipolar I disorder, and one in every five people with bipolar II disorder, has a history of suicide attempts (Merikangas et al., 2011). The mood disorders are most closely associated with suicide, but borderline personality disorder, substance abuse, and, to a lesser extent, anxiety disorders are also predictors of suicidal behavior (Bentley et al., 2016; Klonsky et al., 2016).

By far the best predictor of future suicidal thoughts and behavior is past suicidal thoughts and behavior (Borges et al., 2008, 2010; O'Connor & Nock, 2014). Thus, it is critically important that suicidal thoughts and behaviors be assessed and that intervention be made, regardless of what other psychological problems they may be related to.

Stressful Life Events and Suicide

Studies across cultures have shown that the risk of suicide is increased by a variety of stressful life events, especially events related to abuse, interpersonal loss, perceived failure, economic hardship, and physical illness (Borges et al., 2010; O'Connor & Nock, 2014). A large cross-national study found that interpersonal violence, especially sexual abuse, is the traumatic event most strongly linked to suicidal thoughts and attempts (Stein et al., 2010). Such experiences not only are immediate triggers of suicidal thoughts and behavior but also are associated with increased risk over the victim's life span. For example, a nationwide study in the United States found that a history of child sexual abuse increased the odds of a suicide attempt by 2 to 4 times for women and by 4 to 11 times for men (Molnar, Berkman, & Buka, 2001), and risk increases with more instances of abuse (Bruffaerts et al., 2010).

Loss of a loved one through death, divorce, or separation is also consistently related to suicide attempts or completions (O'Connor & Nock, 2014). People feel they cannot go on without the lost relationship and wish to end their pain. Physical abuse by a partner is also a potent predictor of suicide attempts (McLaughlin, O'Carroll, & O'Connor, 2012).

Another stressful event consistently linked to increased vulnerability to suicide is economic hardship (Borges et al., 2010; Fanous, Prescott, & Kendler, 2004). Loss of a job, for example, can precipitate suicidal thoughts and attempts (Platt & Hawton, 2000).

Could media coverage of school shootings, such as the one at Santa Fe High School in Texas on May 18, 2018, and suicide inspire other students to commit similar acts? *Bob Levey/Getty Images*

Increases in the suicide rate among African American males may be tied to perceptions that their economic futures are uncertain as well as to comparisons of their economic status to that of the majority culture. Rates of suicide among African American males in the United States are highest in communities where the occupational and income inequalities are greatest (Joe & Kaplan, 2001).

Finally, a large international study found that physical illness, especially if it occurred early in life, was a risk factor for suicidal ideation, plans, and attempts even in people who did not have a mental disorder (Scott et al., 2010). The illness most strongly related to suicidal thoughts and behavior was epilepsy.

Suicide Contagion

The strong influence of both social media and traditional media outlets have been widely supported through research. We see this everyday, a video is trending on *TikTok,* it goes viral and before you know it, everyone is doing the same dance. Fashion, hairstyles, music, games, and even language have trends in which a particular style can become contagious. Can the same be said for harmful behavior, like suicide? Research has shown that certain types of media reports and portrayals of suicide can influence the attitudes, beliefs, and behaviors about suicide among young people. Suicide contagion often occurs when a suicide death that is widely publicized by the media results in increases in suicide rates (Ma-Kellams, Baek, & Ora-Keller, 2018). When two or more suicides or attempted suicides occur together in space or time professionals refer to them as a **suicide cluster** which primarily occurs among adolescents (Haw, Hawton, Niedzwiedz, & Platt, 2013; Poland, Lieberman, & Niznik, 2019). For example, a series of suicide attempts in the same high school or a series of completed suicides in response to the suicide of a celebrity is a contagion.

The dramatic increase in the number of digital platforms, like Netflix, has increased the exposure of adolescents and young adults to presentations of suicide that may negatively impact their mental health. For example, the controversial Netflix series *13 Reasons Why (13RW)* highlights concerns about the fictional portrayal of suicide in the media and its potential impact on youth. This suicide-revenge-fantasy chronicles the life and death of high school student, Hannah Baker, and depicts the events that lead to a graphic depiction of her suicide. Studies have shown that reports and portrayals of suicide in the media can trigger imitative suicidal behaviors in vulnerable individuals. Specifically, the repeated and glorified media coverage of suicide methods can lead to contagion effects, particularly in fictional stories where the rates of youth suicide and method used for suicide is already common in a society (McKenzie, Jenkin, Steers, Magill, & Collings, 2020).

Following the first season of *13RW*, mental health professionals expressed serious concerns about the adverse effects of this show on adolescent suicides. Additionally, the show's creators ignored internationally recognized best practices for the responsible portrayal of suicide in television and films. Research has shown that exposure to and identification with a role model who died by suicide can lead to increased suicides, particularly among similar demographic groups. Suicides are more likely to increase following the suicide death of someone with whom the individual can relate. Following the release of *13RW*, there was a significant increase in Internet searches for suicide-related terms, as as well as hospital admissions for suicidal behavior among adolescents. Overall increases in adolescent suicide rates were observed with slightly higher rates noted among females, as compared to the general U.S. population. Other studies confirm the negative impact of *13RW* on psychological health by reporting worsening moods among some adolescents, particularly those who were already experiencing poor mental health. Conversely, research has also found that some adolescents experienced beneficial effects from watching *13RW* that included increased discussions with parents and a better understanding of depression and suicide (McKenzie et al., 2020).

The manner in which the discussion of suicide is framed in the media also appears to have an effect on suicide rates. News stories containing sensationalized content may be more associated with increased suicide rates, whereas stories showing positive coping styles in response to adverse circumstances may be associated with decreased suicide rates. Evidence suggests that suicide contagion may be particularly pronounced when media coverage of a peer/celebrity suicide is detailed and uses dramatic language. These studies also suggest that at-risk individuals may further identify with the struggles experienced by the celebrity/peer as a result of such media coverage, potentially leading them conclude that suicide is an acceptable solution to ongoing struggles, or an act worthy of imitation. Interestingly, this theory is supported by several studies indicating that people who die by suicide after a celebrity/peer suicide are significantly more likely to use the same suicide methods (and sometimes the same location), the details of which may have been acquired through sensational and detailed media coverage (Carmichael & Whitley, 2019). Additional studies on suicide contagion confirms a growing concern among suicide prevention specialists that the prolonged media coverage of the details surrounding celebrity deaths may inadvertently exacerbate the suicide contagion effect. For example, in the 2 months following the suicide death of actor and comedian Robin Williams there was a 10 percent increase in suicides among men who completed suicide through the same method of suffocation (Ma-Kellams, Baek, & Ora-Keller, 2018).

In addition, the local and media attention given to a suicide can be attractive to some people who are feeling alienated and abandoned. After the murder-suicide rampage of two teenagers at Columbine High School in Littleton, Colorado, some teenagers said that receiving the same kind of media attention that was given to the shooters would be an attractive way to "go out." Such phenomena may become more prevalent with newer technologies that allow exposure to suicide or other negative peer influences via social media, although research in this area is only emerging (Twenge, Joiner, Rogers, & Martin, 2018). Given the dramatic increase of usage and wide-reach of social media platforms, recent studies are exploring the potential for contagion effects. Specifically, research examining the influence of Instagram on suicide contagion and self-harm has found that Instagram is frequently used for suicide-related communications. Additionally, research has also shown that self-harm is present in a majority of Instagram posts, and posts that mention suicide elicited higher engagement than

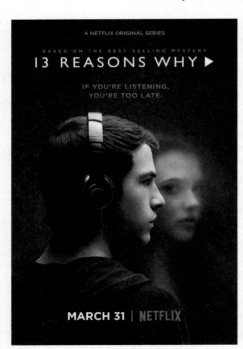

The controversial series, 13 Reasons Why (13RW), illustrated how a strong media presence can influence suicide contagion among adolescent viewers. PARAMOUNT TELEVISION/Album/Alamy Stock Photo

posts that did not. These studies found the relative absence of public health voices from the conversations about suicide on Instagram suggests that mental health professionals should consider increased involvement on this platform (Carlyle et al., 2018).

Research on suicide contagion through social networks suggests that the more exposure an individual has to suicidal behaviors, such as suicidal plans, attempts, or completions, the more acceptable and probable that behavior may become. Adolescents are a particularly vulnerable population since their self-image is still developing, they are particularly socially conscious, and more susceptible to others' influence. Research has found that exposure to suicidal behaviors is significantly associated with increased risk of suicide attempt, and it contributes to higher attempt risk among girls. As a result, suicidal behaviors spread through social networks and suicide contagion tends to amplify the existing gender differences (Poland, Lieberman, & Niznik, 2019; Yıldız, Orak, Walker, & Solakogluidiz, 2019).

Personality and Cognitive Factors in Suicide

One personality characteristic that seems to predict suicide is **impulsivity,** the general tendency to act on one's impulses rather than to inhibit them when it is appropriate to do so (Joiner, 2005). This trait has long been viewed as a risk factor for suicide, but the connection may not be as strong as once believed (Anestis, Soberay, Gutierrez, Hernández, & Joiner, 2014; Klonsky et al., 2016). Nevertheless, when impulsivity is overlaid on another psychological problem—such as depression, substance abuse, or living in a chronically stressful environment—it can be a contributor to suicidal thinking and behavior. One family history study showed that the children of parents with a mood disorder who also scored high on measures of impulsivity were at much greater risk of attempting suicide (Brent et al., 2002).

The cognitive variable that has most consistently predicted suicide is **hopelessness**—the feeling that the future is bleak and there is no way to make it more positive (Beck, Steer, Kovacs, & Garrison, 1985). Thomas Joiner (2005) suggested that hopeless feelings about being a burden on others and about never belonging with others are especially linked to suicide. This theory, known as the interpersonal theory of suicide, merges cognitive and social factors and has been supported by research (Chu et al., 2017). Hopelessness also may be one reason many people who are suicidal do not seek treatment. Other cognitive factors in suicide include cognitive rigidity, rumination, perfectionism, and poor problem solving (O'Connor & Nock, 2014).

Biological Factors in Suicide

As in the mood disorders, biological contributors to suicide include genetic predisposition and neurotransmitter dysfunction. Suicide runs in families. For example, one study found that the children of parents who had attempted suicide were 6 times more likely to also attempt suicide than were the children of parents who had a mood disorder but had not attempted suicide (Brent et al., 2002, 2003).

Although some of this clustering of suicide within families may be due to environmental factors, such as family members modeling each other or sharing common stressors, twin and adoption studies suggest that genetics is involved as well (Joiner, 2005). Twin studies estimate that the risk of suicide attempts increases by 5.6 times if a person's monozygotic twin has attempted suicide, and by 4.0 times if a person's dizygotic twin has attempted suicide (Glowinski et al., 2001; Joiner et al., 2005). Strong evidence of a genetic component to suicide remained when researchers controlled for histories of psychiatric problems in the twins and their families, for recent and past negative life events, for how close the twins were to each other socially, and for personality factors.

Many studies have found a link between suicide and low levels of the neurotransmitter serotonin (Mann, 2013). For example, postmortem studies of the brains of people who committed suicide find low levels of serotonin (Costanza et al., 2014). Also, people with a family history of suicide or who have attempted suicide are more likely to have abnormalities on genes that regulate serotonin (Antypa, Serretti, & Rujescu, 2013; Courtet et al., 2004; Joiner, 2005). People with low serotonin levels who attempt suicide are more likely to make another suicide attempt than are people with higher serotonin levels, and as in depression, the effects of genes and serotonin are stronger under conditions of negative life events (e.g., Ghasemi, Seifi, Baybordi, Danaei, & Rad, 2018). Differences in serotonin transmission are linked to suicidal tendencies even in people who are not depressed, suggesting that the connection between serotonin and suicide is not due entirely to a common connection to depression.

Treatment and Prevention

Some intervention and prevention programs appear to reduce the risk of suicide. Intervention programs target people immediately at risk of suicide. They include crisis intervention services (e.g., suicide hotlines) and dialectical behavior therapy. Prevention programs target the public in general, or people who have risk factors but are not immediately in crisis. Prevention programs have focused on educating people broadly about suicide risk and the steps to take if they are suicidal or know of someone who is suicidal. Because access to guns is associated with higher suicide rates, some prevention efforts focus on removing access to guns, which might reduce the chances of a person taking their own life impulsively.

Treatment of Suicidal Persons

A person who is gravely suicidal needs immediate care. Sometimes people require hospitalization to prevent an imminent suicide attempt. They may voluntarily agree to be hospitalized. If they do not agree, they can be hospitalized involuntarily for a short period of time (usually about 3 days). We will discuss the pros and cons of involuntary hospitalization in the chapter "Mental Health and the Law."

Community-based *crisis intervention programs* are available to help suicidal people deal in the short term with their feelings and then refer them to mental health specialists for longer-term care. Some crisis intervention is done over the phone, on suicide hotlines. Some communities have walk-in clinics or suicide prevention centers, which may be part of a more comprehensive mental health system.

Crisis intervention aims to reduce the risk of an imminent suicide attempt by providing suicidal persons someone to talk with who understands their feelings and problems. The counselor can help them mobilize support from family members and friends and can make a plan to deal with specific problem situations in the short term. The crisis intervention counselor may contract with the suicidal person that they will not attempt suicide, or at least will contact the counselor as soon as suicidal feelings return. The counselor will help the person identify other people they can turn to when feeling panicked or overwhelmed and make follow-up appointments with the suicidal person or refer them to another counselor for long-term treatment.

The SSRIs also may reduce the risk of suicide, because they reduce depressive symptoms and because they regulate levels of serotonin, which may have an independent effect on suicidal intentions (Gitlin, 2015; Mann, 2013). As we discussed earlier, however, there is some evidence that the SSRIs can increase the risk of suicide in some children and adolescents. Clinicians must weigh the potential benefits and risks and carefully monitor individuals for signs of increased suicidal thoughts when they begin taking an SSRI (Garland et al., 2016).

Psychological therapies designed to treat depression can be effective in treating suicidal individuals. *Dialectical behavior therapy (DBT)* was developed to treat people with borderline personality disorder, who frequently attempt suicide (see the chapter "Personality Disorders"; Linehan, 1999). This therapy focuses on managing negative emotions and controlling impulsive behaviors. It aims to increase problem-solving skills, interpersonal skills, and skill at managing negative emotions. Studies show that DBT and CBT can reduce suicidal thoughts and behaviors (Asarnow, Hughes, Babeva, & Sugar, 2017; Linehan et al., 2006; Ougrin, Tranah, Stahl, Moran, & Asarnow, 2015). Similar to

other clinical issues, clinicians and researchers are developing mobile technologies for addressing NSSI and suicide (Franklin et al., 2016).

What is clearest from the literature on the treatment of suicidal people is that they are woefully undertreated. Most people who are suicidal never seek treatment (Bruffaerts et al., 2011). Even when their families know they are suicidal, they might not be taken for treatment because of denial and a fear of being stigmatized. Recall that a suicide attempt is the strongest predictor of future suicide attempts and completed suicide. Suicide attempts tend to increase in intent and lethality after the first attempt (Goldston et al., 2015), so receiving professional attention early on is critical for suicidal individuals.

Suicide Prevention

Suicide hotlines and crisis intervention centers provide help to suicidal people in times of their greatest need, hoping to prevent a suicidal act until the suicidal feelings have passed. In addition, many prevention programs aim to educate entire communities about suicide. These programs often are based in schools or colleges. Students are given information about the rate of suicide in their age group, the risk factors for suicide, and actions to take if they or a friend is suicidal.

Some such programs have been shown to affect suicidal thinking and behavior (e.g., Schilling, Lawless, Buchanan, & Aseltine, 2014). Unfortunately, the evidence supporting broad-based prevention or education programs is mixed, and some may even do harm (Calear et al., 2016; Gould, Greenberg, Velting, & Shaffer, 2003). One major problem with these programs is that they often simultaneously target both the general population of students and those students at high risk for suicide. The programs may attempt to destigmatize suicide by making it appear quite common and by not mentioning that most suicidal people are suffering from a psychological disorder, in hopes that suicidal students will feel freer to seek help. But such messages can backfire with students who are not suicidal, making suicide seem like an understandable response to stress. In addition, studies of school-based suicide prevention programs have found that adolescents who had made prior suicide attempts generally reacted negatively to the programs, saying that they were less inclined to seek help after attending the program than before (Gould et al., 2003).

Researchers have tailored suicide prevention messages to specific populations—particularly high-risk populations—in hopes of getting the right kind of help to the neediest people. David Shaffer and his colleagues have designed a program that involves screening adolescents for risk of suicide, doing a diagnostic interview with high-risk adolescents, and then interviewing them to determine the most appropriate referral to a mental health specialist (Shaffer & Gould, 2000). This program has had some success in identifying high-risk youth and getting them into effective treatment. Similar programs have been developed for college students. In addition, clinicians and school administrators are increasingly aware of the prevalence of NSSI in adolescence and young adulthood, and of research showing that it presents a risk for suicidal behavior. Although interventions for NSSI are early in development, several appear promising and may affect suicide prevention as well (Glenn, Franklin, & Nock, 2015).

Parents and school officials often worry that asking teenagers about thoughts of suicide might "put the idea in their head." One study addressed this concern directly (Gould et al., 2005). The researchers randomly assigned more than 2,000 teenagers to complete questionnaires that either included or did not include questions about suicidal thoughts and behaviors. Two days later the researchers had all the teenagers fill out a measure of suicidal thought. Teenagers who had completed the suicide questionnaire did not report any more (or less) suicidal thought or distress than the teenagers who had not been asked about suicide. Thus, there was no evidence that answering questions about suicide induced teenagers to consider suicide or made them highly distressed.

Guns and Suicide

In the United States, the use of firearms accounts for more than half of fatal suicides. A significant proportion of suicide attempts are made impulsively, with the decision to act occurring within an hour of the attempt in 71 percent of cases, and within less than 5 minutes in 24 percent of cases. Various studies have established a consistent association between household firearm ownership and increased suicide rates. Since attempt survivors rarely die in subsequent attempts and most who complete suicide have no history of a past attempt, the access to highly lethal means has been recognized as one of the most important contributors to high rates of completed suicide (Nestadt et al., 2020). The majority of people who commit suicide by gun, however, use a gun that has been in their household for some time; the presence of a gun in the home increases the risk of suicide by 4 to 5 times (Houtsma, Butterworth, & Anestis, 2018; Miller & Hemenway, 2008). As mentioned, one explanation for higher rates of suicide deaths in men, despite higher rates of attempts in women, is that men use guns—a highly lethal method—more often than women.

The mere presence of a firearm in the home appears to be a risk factor for suicide when other risk factors are taken into account, especially when handguns are improperly secured or are kept loaded (Houtsma et al., 2018; Miller & Hemenway, 2008). These suicides do not occur only among people with mental disorders. This apparently counterintuitive finding is the result of the dramatic increase in impulsive suicides seen among residents of homes containing a loaded gun, even among people without a known risk factor such as psychopathology (Brent & Bridge, 2003; Westefeld, Gann, Lustgarden, & Yeates, 2016).

Can the number of such suicides be reduced by laws that restrict access to guns? Several studies have found that suicide rates are lower in cities, states, or countries with strict antigun legislation that limits people's access to guns (e.g., M. Anestis & J. Anestis, 2015). For example, one international study showed that the percentage of suicides by gun decreased proportionately

Restricting access to guns appears to lower suicide rates. *Cbenjasuwan/Shutterstock*

with the number of households owning guns; in addition, after countries enacted stricter gun control laws, the percentage of suicides involving guns decreased (Ajdacic-Gross et al., 2006). Similarly, in the United States, in states with unrestrictive firearm laws (e.g., Alaska, Kentucky, Montana) rates of suicide by firearm are much higher than in states with restrictive firearm laws (e.g., New York, Connecticut, Rhode Island) (M. Anestis & J. Anestis, 2015; Houtsma et al., 2018). Such patterns related to gun laws and suicide are found even after controlling for differences in socioeconomic status, race/ethnicity, and urbanization (M. Anestis & J. Anestis, 2015).

Although people who are intent on committing suicide can find other means to do so when guns are not available, restricting ready access to them appears to reduce impulsive suicides with guns. Suicides by means other than guns (e.g., by jumping off a building or inhaling carbon monoxide) show no increase when access to guns is restricted, suggesting that people do not consistently substitute different means of committing suicide when guns are not available (Miller & Hemenway, 2008; Westefeld et al., 2016). Instead, the unavailability of guns seems to give people a cooling off period during which their suicidal impulses can wane.

What to Do if a Friend Is Suicidal

What should you do if you suspect that a friend or family member is suicidal? The Depression and Bipolar Support Alliance (2008), a patient-run advocacy group, makes the following suggestions in *Suicide and Depressive Illness:*

1. Take the person seriously. Although most people who express suicidal thoughts do not go on to attempt suicide, most people who do commit suicide have communicated their suicidal intentions to friends or family members beforehand.

2. Get help. Call the person's therapist, a suicide hotline, 911, or any other source of professional mental health care.

3. Express concern. Tell the person concretely why you think he or she is suicidal.

4. Pay attention. Listen closely, maintain eye contact, and use body language to indicate that you are attending to everything the person says.

5. Ask direct questions about whether the person has a plan for suicide and, if so, what that plan is.

6. Acknowledge the person's feelings in a nonjudgmental way. For example, you might say something like "I know you are feeling really horrible right now, but I want to help you get through this" or "I can't begin to completely understand how you feel, but I want to help you."

7. Reassure the person that things can be better. Emphasize that suicide is a permanent solution to a temporary problem.

8. Don't promise confidentiality. You need the freedom to contact mental health professionals and tell them precisely what is going on.

9. Make sure guns, old medications, and other means of self-harm are not available.

10. If possible, don't leave the person alone until they are in the hands of professionals. Go with them to the emergency room if need be. Then, once they have been hospitalized or have received other treatment, follow up to show your care.

11. Take care of yourself. Interacting with a person who is suicidal can be extremely stressful and disturbing. Talk with someone you trust about it—perhaps a friend, family member, or counselor—particularly if you worry about how you handled the situation or that you will find yourself in that situation again.

Source: Depression and Bipolar Support Alliance, Suicide prevention: Responding to an emergency situation, 2008. http://www.ndma.org, accessed May 15, 2008. Copyright ©2008 by Depression and Bipolar Support Alliance. All rights reserved. Used with permission.

CHAPTER INTEGRATION

The mood disorders affect the whole person. Depression and mania involve changes in every aspect of functioning, including biology, cognitions, personality, social skills, and relationships. Some of these changes may be causes of the depression or mania, while others may be consequences.

The fact that the mood disorders are phenomena affecting the whole person illustrates the intricate connections among biology, cognitions, personality, and social interactions. These areas of functioning are so intertwined that major changes in any one area almost necessarily will provoke changes in other areas. Many recent models of the mood disorders suggest that most people who become depressed carry a vulnerability to depression for much of their lives. This may be a biological vulnerability, such as dysfunction in the neurotransmitter systems, or a psychological vulnerability, such as overdependence on others. Not until these vulnerabilities interact with certain stressors is a full-blown depression triggered, however (Figure 11).

Recent studies have established that depression is associated with altered gut microbiota composition which influences the brain. The gut microbiome is made up of the collection of bacteria, fungi, and viruses, harbored in the gastrointestinal tract which has a measurable impact on the brain. Studies have shown that the gut microbiome influences psychological factors like stress, anxiety, depressive symptoms, and

FIGURE 11 | **An Integrative Model of Depression.**

Genetic factors

Dysfunction in neurotransmitter and neuroendocrine systems

Personality characteristics that increase stress response and exposure to stressors (e.g., neuroticism)

Heightened vulnerability to stress

Encounters with new stressors

Depression

social behavior. This microbiome–gut–brain axis may be mediated by various mechanisms including neural, immune, and endocrine pathways that are relevant to psychiatric disorders.

Fortunately, the interconnections among these areas of functioning may mean that improving functioning in one area can improve functioning in other areas: Improving people's biological functioning can improve their cognitive and social functioning and their personalities, improving people's cognitive and social functioning can improve their biological functioning, and so on. Thus, although there may be many pathways into mood disorders (biological, psychological, and social), there also may be many pathways out.

SHADES OF GRAY   DISCUSSION

Carmen's symptoms—currently severe depressed mood in the context of long-standing unhappiness, excessive sleep every day (hypersomnia), difficulty concentrating to a degree that interfered with her ability to engage in her college classes, feelings of worthlessness, and significant weight loss (likely greater than 5 percent of her body weight) because she's skipping meals—are characteristic of a major depressive episode. We know she "spent days on end in her bedroom," but we are not entirely clear if her current symptoms meet the criterion of 2 consecutive weeks to receive a diagnosis of major depressive disorder. What we know more certainly is that she has experienced many years (> 2) struggling with moderately low mood, low self-esteem, pessimism, and chronic fatigue. Thus, she would clearly meet criteria for persistent depressive disorder, likely early onset (before age 21), severe, but we would need to get more information to add the specifier of "with intermittent major depressive episodes, with current episode." The addition of the specifier would indicate that full criteria for

a major depressive episode are currently met, but she has experienced periods of at least 2 months in the past 2 years with symptoms that fall below the threshold for a full major depressive episode.

Because Carmen's more severe symptoms began in the winter term, you may wonder if she is experiencing a major depressive disorder with seasonal pattern, or what used to be known as seasonal affective disorder (SAD). "With seasonal pattern" is a specifier that applies to recurrent major depressive disorder and highlights a temporal relationship between the onset of major depressive episodes and a particular time of year (e.g., in the fall or winter). The addition of this specifier is not currently warranted because (a) it requires evidence that Carmen has experienced seasonal changes in mood in the last 2 years, and we only have evidence that Carmen's depression has worsened in this year, and (b) the specifier requires that Carmen's depressive symptoms lift during the spring or summertime. Instead, Carmen's depressive symptoms seem to persist throughout the year.

CHAPTER SUMMARY

- People with depressive disorders experience only the symptoms of depression (sad mood, loss of interest, disruption in sleep and appetite, motor retardation or agitation, loss of energy, feelings of worthlessness and guilt, suicidal thoughts and behavior).

- People with bipolar disorder experience symptoms of both depression and hypomania or mania (elated or agitated mood, grandiosity, little need for sleep, racing thoughts and speech, increase in goals, and dangerous behavior). The presence of one or more hypomanic or manic episodes is the core feature of the bipolar disorders (see Table 4).

- Major depressive disorder is the classic condition among the depressive disorders. It is characterized by discrete episodes of depressed mood and/or loss of interest or pleasure and other symptoms that lasts at least 2 weeks. In addition, there are several

subtypes of major depressive disorder: with mixed features, with anxiety features, with melancholic features, with psychotic features, with catatonic features, with atypical features, with seasonal pattern, and with peripartum onset.

- Persistent depressive disorder (dysthymia) is a chronic form of depression that continues for at least 2 years in adults or 1 year in youth. It can be less severe than major depressive disorder (full criteria are not met in last 2 years) or it may represent intermittent or persistent major depressive episodes, and includes many of the same subtypes as major depressive disorder.

- Premenstrual dysphoric disorder is diagnosed in women who show increases in symptoms of distress in the week before the onset of menses, with relief of symptoms after menses begins.

- Cyclothymic disorder is a less severe but more chronic form of bipolar II disorder that does not include major depressive episodes.

- Depression is one of the most common disorders, but there are substantial age, gender, and cross-cultural differences in depression. Bipolar disorder is much less common than the depressive disorders and tends to be a lifelong problem. The length of individual episodes of bipolar disorder, as in depression, varies dramatically from one person to the next and over the life course.

- The neurotransmitters norepinephrine, serotonin, and dopamine have been implicated in the mood disorders. Disordered genes may lead to dysfunction in these neurotransmitter systems. In addition, neuroimaging studies show abnormal structure or activity in several areas of the brain, including the prefrontal cortex, hippocampus, anterior cingulate, and amygdala. There is evidence that people with depression have chronic hyperactivity in the HPA axis, which may make them more susceptible to stress.

- The gut microbiome influences psychological factors like stress, anxiety, depressive symptoms, and social behavior. This microbiome–gut–brain axis may be mediated by various mechanisms including neural, immune, and endocrine pathways that are relevant to psychiatric disorders.

- There is an association between the neurobiology of major depressive disorder and neuroinflammation. It is believed that inflammation of the nervous system moderates depressive symptoms and suicidal behavior. Inflammatory processes have been implicated in the pathophysiology of depression, but the specific mechanism still remains unclear.

- Behavioral theories of depression suggest that people with much stress in their lives may have too low a rate of reinforcement and too high a rate of punishment, leading to depression. Stressful events also can lead to learned helplessness—the belief that nothing you do can control your environment—which also is linked to depression.

- The cognitive theories argue that depressed people have negative views of themselves, the world, and the future and engage in biased thinking that promotes this negativity. People who ruminate in response to distress are more prone to depression.

- Interpersonal theories suggest that people prone to depression are highly sensitive to rejection and engage in excessive reassurance seeking. Levels of interpersonal stress and conflict are high in the lives of depressed people.

- Sociocultural theorists have tried to explain the differences in rates of depression among different demographic groups. The decreased risk of depression in older adults may be due to historical cohort effects. Women's greater risk for depression may be due to differences in the ways women and men respond to distress and to women's greater interpersonal orientation, lesser power and status, and higher rates of victimization. High rates of depression in Hispanic Americans may be due to low socioeconomic status.

- Bipolar disorder has an even greater connection to genetic factors than does depression. The areas of the brain most implicated in bipolar disorder are the amygdala, prefrontal cortex, and striatum. Adolescents with bipolar disorder show abnormalities in white-matter tissue. Dopamine is the neurotransmitter most implicated in bipolar disorder.

- People with bipolar disorder may have dysfunctional reward systems: They are hypersensitive to reward when in a manic state and insensitive to reward when in a depressed state.

- Four or more mood episodes that meet criteria for manic, hypomanic, or major depressive episode within 1 year lead to a diagnosis of rapid cycling bipolar disorder. Multiple studies have consistently found that evidence of poorer prognosis and greater disease burden in rapid cycling bipolar disorder

- Most of the biological therapies for mood disorders are drug therapies, including antidepressants and mood stabilizers. Electroconvulsive therapy is used to treat severe depression that does not respond to drugs. Newer methods of stimulating the brain, including repetitive transcranial magnetic stimulation, vagus nerve stimulation, and deep brain stimulation, hold promise for the treatment of mood disorders. Light therapy is helpful in treating major depressive disorder with seasonal pattern.

- Behavior therapies focus on increasing positive reinforcers and decreasing negative events by building social skills and teaching clients how to engage in pleasant activities and cope with their moods. Cognitive-behavioral therapies help people with depression develop more adaptive ways of thinking. Interpersonal therapy helps people with depression identify and change the patterns in their relationships.

- Interpersonal social rhythm therapy helps people with bipolar disorder manage their social relationships and daily rhythms to try to prevent relapse. Family-focused therapy may help people with bipolar disorder manage their disorder.

- Direct comparisons of various psychotherapies and drug therapies show that they tend to be equally effective in treating depression. Psychotherapies may be more effective than drug therapies in reducing relapse.

- Suicide is defined as death from injury, poisoning, or suffocation when there is evidence (either explicit or implicit) that the injury was self-inflicted and that the decedent intended to kill themself.

- Women are more likely than men to attempt suicide, but men are more likely than women to complete suicide. Cross-cultural differences in suicide rates may have to do with religious proscriptions, stressors, or cultural norms about suicide. Young people are less likely than adults to commit suicide, but suicide rates among youth have been fluctuating dramatically in recent decades. The elderly, particularly elderly men, are at high risk for suicide.

- Several mental disorders, including depression, bipolar disorder, substance abuse, schizophrenia, and anxiety disorders, increase the risk for suicide.

- Several negative life events or circumstances, including economic hardship, serious illness, loss, and abuse, increase the risk for suicide.

- Suicide clusters (also called suicide contagion) occur when two or more suicides or attempted suicides are nonrandomly bunched together in a place or time.

- Impulsivity and hopelessness predict suicidal behavior.

- Family history, twin, and adoption studies all suggest a genetic vulnerability to suicide. Many studies have found a link between low serotonin levels and suicide.

- Drug treatments for suicidal patients most often involve lithium or antidepressant medications. Psychotherapies for suicide are similar to those for depression. Dialectical behavior therapy addresses skill deficits and thinking patterns in people who are recurrently suicidal.

- Suicide hotlines and crisis intervention programs provide immediate help to people who are highly suicidal. Community prevention programs aim to educate the public about suicide and to encourage suicidal people to enter treatment.

- Guns are involved in the majority of suicides, and some research suggests that restricting access to guns can reduce the number of suicide attempts.

KEY TERMS

bipolar disorder

mania

depressive disorders

dysphoria

major depressive disorder (MMD)

seasonal affective disorder (SAD)

peripartum onset

persistent depressive disorder

premenstrual dysphoric disorder (PMDD)

black box warning

bipolar I disorder

bipolar II disorder

hypomania

cyclothymic disorder

rapid cycling bipolar disorder

disruptive mood dysregulation disorder

monoamines

norepinephrine

serotonin

dopamine

hypothalamic-pituitary-adrenal axis (HPA axis)

behavioral theories of depression

learned helplessness theory

negative cognitive triad

reformulated learned helplessness theory

rumination

interpersonal theories of depression

neuroinflammation

rejection sensitivity

cohort effect

selective serotonin reuptake inhibitors (SSRIs)

selective serotonin-norepinephrine reuptake inhibitors (SNRIs)

norepinephrine-dopamine reuptake inhibitor

tricyclic antidepressants

monoamine oxidase inhibitors (MAOIs)

lithium

electroconvulsive therapy, or ECT

repetitive transcranial magnetic stimulation (rTMS)

vagus nerve stimulation (VNS)

deep brain stimulation

light therapy

behavioral therapy

interpersonal and social rhythm therapy (ISRT)

family-focused therapy (FFT)

suicide

suicide attempts

suicidal ideation

nonsuicidal self-injury (NSSI)

suicide cluster

impulsivity

hopelessness

Chapter 8

riza azhari/Shutterstock

Schizophrenia Spectrum and Other Psychotic Disorders

CHAPTER OUTLINE

Schizophrenia Spectrum and Other Psychotic Disorders Along the Continuum

Normal thinking, communication, and social interactions

Deficits in attention and working memory *(may or may not lead to difficulties in communication, thought, or social interaction)*

Delusional disorder *(persistent beliefs that are unrealistic, but no other symptoms of schizophrenia)*

Schizophreniform disorder *(symptoms of schizophrenia for more than 1 month but less than 6 months)*

Schizoaffective disorder *(mixed symptoms of schizophrenia and a mood disorder)*

Functional

Dysfunctional

Schizotypal personality disorder *(paranoia, beliefs that random events are related to the individual, magical thinking, perceptual illusions, social isolation, restricted emotions)*

No longer distinguished in *DSM-5*

Brief psychotic disorder *(symptoms of schizophrenia for less than 1 month)*

Schizophrenia *(delusions, hallucinations, disorganized speech or behavior, and/or negative symptoms, and functional decline for 6 months)*

Schizophrenia is one of the most recognized psychological disorders and is often depicted in movies and on TV. When asked to describe this disorder, most students will be able to mention hallucinations and delusions as descriptors and, they are usually correct. People with schizophrenia see, hear, and feel things that aren't real (hallucinations) and may have false, unshakeable beliefs (delusions), for example, that there is a conspiracy to harm them that is being orchestrated by a government agency. Such experiences and beliefs that are out of touch with reality are called *psychotic symptoms,* but what many don't realize is these are only some of the symptoms experienced by people with schizophrenia spectrum disorders. Other symptoms include speaking incoherently, act in an unpredictable manner, have problems with communication and emotional expression, or unusual facial grimaces, tics or gait. The DSM identifies schizophrenia as the most severe psychotic disorder in this category, but as we shall see in this chapter there are others.

The continuum of disorders outlined in this section represents what the *DSM-5* has labeled the schizophrenia spectrum which includes a set of psychotic disorders that share similarities with schizophrenia but are not as severe or persistent. Schizophrenia is among the most extreme disorders that we will study. And, although psychotic disorders appear very different from normal experience, this category is still viewed on a continuum. The symptoms that make up schizophrenia can appear in mild to moderate form in many people who do not meet the full criteria for any disorder (Ahmed, Buckley, & Mabe, 2012; Linscott & van Os, 2010).

The *DSM-5* recognizes the continuum of psychotic experiences by listing schizophrenia and other psychotic disorders in order of severity. The first disorder along the continuum is *schizotypal personality disorder*, which involves moderate symptoms resembling those of schizophrenia but with a retained grasp on reality. People with this personality disorder often speak in odd and eccentric ways, have unusual beliefs or perceptions, and have difficulty relating to other people. Farther along the continuum are disorders in which people lose touch with reality. In *delusional disorder,* individuals have persistent beliefs that are contrary to reality, but they lack other symptoms of schizophrenia and often are not impaired in their functioning. Their delusions tend to be about things that are possible, but untrue. In *brief psychotic disorder,* individuals have symptoms of schizophrenia for 1 month or less. In *schizophreniform* disorder, individuals have symptoms of schizophrenia for 1 to 6 months but usually resume their normal lives. *Schizoaffective disorder* presents a mixed picture of schizophrenia and major depression or mania. Other psychotic disorders, including *substance-induced psychotic disorder* and *psychotic* (or *catatonic*) *disorder associated with another medical condition,* are psychoses specifically brought on by a substance or an illness. They may be short-term or longer lasting.

Extraordinary People

John Nash, *A Beautiful Mind*

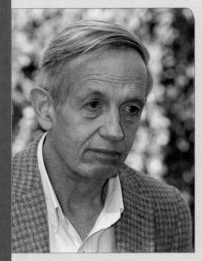

Bob Strong/AFP/Getty Images

In 1959, at age 30, John Nash was a widely recognized mathematician and professor at the Massachusetts Institute of Technology. While still a graduate student at Princeton, he had introduced the notion of equilibrium to game theory, which eventually would revolutionize the field of economics and win him the Nobel Prize.

As writer Sylvia Nasar details in her biography of John Nash, *A Beautiful Mind,* which was the basis for the Academy Award–winning film, Nash had always been eccentric and had few social skills. But in 1959 Nash began writing letters to the United Nations, the FBI, and other government agencies complaining of conspiracies to take over the world. He also began talking openly about his belief that powers from outer space, or perhaps from foreign governments, were communicating with him through the front page of the *New York Times*. Nash later described one of his delusions:

> I got the impression that other people at MIT were wearing red neckties so I would notice them. As I became more and more delusional, not only persons at MIT but people in Boston wearing red neckties [would seem significant to me] . . . [there was some relation to] a cryptocommunist plot. (Nasar, 1998, p. 242)

Nash's wife, Alicia, saw him become increasingly distant and cold toward her. His behavior grew more and more bizarre:

> Several times, Nash had cornered her with odd questions when they were alone, either at home or driving in the car. "Why don't you tell me about it?" he asked in an angry, agitated tone, apropos of nothing. "Tell me what you know," he demanded. (Nasar, 1998, p. 248)

In April 1959, after his threats to harm her became more severe and his behavior became increasingly unpredictable, Alicia had him committed to McLean Hospital. There Nash was diagnosed with paranoid schizophrenia and was given medication and daily psychoanalytic therapy. Nash learned to hide his delusions and hallucinations and to behave rationally, although his inner world remained unchanged. Upon his release, Nash resigned from MIT, furious that the institution had "conspired" in his commitment to McLean Hospital.

After traveling around Europe for 2 years, Nash walked the streets of Princeton with a fixed expression and a dead gaze, wearing Russian peasant garments and going into restaurants in his bare feet. He wrote endless letters and made many phone calls to friends and eminences around the world, talking of numerology and world affairs. Alicia was forced to have him committed again, this time in Trenton State Hospital. After 6 weeks, Nash was considered much improved and was moved to another ward of the hospital, where he began to work on a paper on fluid dynamics. After 6 months of hospitalization, a month after his 33rd birthday, he was discharged. Nash appeared to be well for some time, but then his thinking, speech, and behavior began to slip again. Eventually he ended up living with his mother in Roanoke, Virginia.

His daily rounds extended no farther than the library or the shops at the end of Grandin Road, but in his mind he traveled to the remotest reaches of the globe and lived in refugee camps, foreign embassies, prisons, and bomb shelters. At other times he felt that he was inhabiting an inferno, a purgatory, or a polluted heaven. His many identities included a Palestinian refugee, a Japanese shogun, and even, at times, a mouse (Nasar, 1998).

After his mother died, Nash returned to Princeton and lived with Alicia. During the 1970s and 1980s, his illness gradually subsided without treatment. Nash was awarded the Nobel Prize in economics for his contributions to game theory. He and Alicia lived in Princeton, where Nash worked on his mathematical theories and helped care for their son, Johnny, who obtained his PhD in mathematics and also developed paranoid schizophrenia. Although Johnny has received the newest treatments for schizophrenia, they help only a little, and he is hospitalized frequently. John Nash and his wife died in a traffic accident in 2015.

The biography of John Nash, and the subsequent motion picture of his life, illustrates the devastating brain disease, called schizophrenia. This disorder is one of the most debilitating psychological disorders that disrupts every area of personal function, often resulting in a decreased quality of life for the individual. Imagine what it must be like to not know what's real or who can be trusted. These episodes can be terrifying. Just as John Nash did during the acute phases of his illness, you might hear disturbing voices that no one else can hear, or voices that are not coming from other people but are only in your head, but you can't recognize this fact. You might believe that your thoughts and ideas are being broadcast over the radio or on television, and others already know what you are thinking. The inability to recognize the difference between reality and unreality is what defines **psychosis** and is the common feature that connects all psychotic disorders. Although schizophrenia tends to be the most commonly known psychotic disorder, there are other psychotic disorders with varying and similar symptoms that we will also discuss in this chapter. Recent research suggests that the prevalence of psychotic symptoms may be significantly higher than previously believed with a prevalence rate of 5 to 8 percent in the general population (Stevens, Prince, Prager, & Stern, 2014).

SYMPTOMS, DIAGNOSIS, AND COURSE

Schizophrenia is a complex neuropsychiatric disorder with psychosis as its core diagnostic symptom that affects perception, cognition, and emotion during acute episodes (Häfner, 2019). *DSM-5* refers to the **schizophrenia spectrum** to reflect the fact that there are five domains of symptoms that define psychotic disorders, and their number, severity, and duration distinguish psychotic disorders from each other. People with schizophrenia may show all or just some psychotic symptoms, and the disorder can look different across individuals. The five domains of psychotic symptoms include four kinds of *positive symptoms*—namely, delusions, hallucinations, disorganized thought (speech), and disorganized or abnormal motor behavior (including catatonia)—and *negative symptoms* (e.g., restricted emotional expression or affect). People with schizophrenia also often show numerous *cognitive deficits* that research has shown are linked to declines in functioning, although cognitive symptoms are not part of the diagnostic criteria (American Psychiatric Association, 2013). These symptoms of schizophrenia are not always present and, at times, people with schizophrenia think and communicate clearly, have an accurate view of reality, and function well in daily life. However, during the active phase of their illness, their thinking and speech are disorganized, they lose touch with reality, and they have difficulty caring for themselves.

Positive Symptoms

The **positive symptoms** of schizophrenia include delusions, hallucinations, and disorganized thought and speech. These are described as "positive" because they are in addition to behaviors that are expected. A common misconception is that positive symptoms are good or beneficial to the individual, but this is not true. Positive in this sense should be viewed in mathematical terms, meaning something has been added. In this case, the symptoms that have been added are overt, atypical, and disruptive.

Delusions

Delusions are false, unshakeable beliefs that are held with strong conviction despite contradictory evidence (Baker, Konova, Daw, & Horga 2019). These fixed beliefs are not amenable to change in light of conflicting evidence. Meaning, these strongly held false beliefs are not often subject to change even when presented with indisputable facts. Delusions are thoughts that are contrary to reality and often include ideas that are highly unlikely and often impossible to be true. The content of delusions may include a variety of themes (e.g., persecutory, referential, somatic, religious, grandiose) (Quinn, 2017). It is theorized that people with delusional thoughts ascribe inappropriately high amounts of meaning and attention to irrelevant events (Diaconescu, Hauke, & Borgwardt, 2019). Meaning, people with delusional thoughts over-focus on insignificant events and attribute great importance to things that are of no consequence.

Of course, most people occasionally hold beliefs that are likely to be wrong, such as the belief that they will win the lottery. These kinds of self-deceptions differ from delusions in at least three ways (Strauss, 1969). First, self-deceptions are at least possible, whereas delusions often are not. It is possible, if highly unlikely, that you are going to win the lottery, but it is not possible that your body is dissolving and floating into space. Second, people harboring self-deceptions may think about these beliefs occasionally, but people harboring delusions tend to be preoccupied with them. Delusional people look for evidence in support of their beliefs, attempt to convince others of these beliefs, and take actions based on them, such as filing lawsuits against the people they believe are trying to control their mind. Third, people holding self-deceptions typically acknowledge that their beliefs may be wrong, but people holding delusions often are highly resistant to arguments or compelling facts that

TABLE 1   Types of Delusions

These are some types of delusions that are often woven together in a complex and frightening system of beliefs.

Type of Delusion	Definition	Example
Persecutory delusion	False belief that oneself or one's loved ones are being persecuted, watched, or conspired against by others	Belief that the CIA, FBI, and local police are conspiring to catch you in a sting operation
Delusion of reference	Belief that everyday events, objects, or other people have an unusual personal significance	Belief that a newscaster is reporting on your movements, or that a random manhole cover was put there so you could see it
Grandiose delusion	False belief that one has great power, knowledge, or talent or that one is a famous and powerful person	Belief that you are Martin Luther King, Jr., reincarnated
Delusion of being controlled	Belief that one's thoughts, feelings, or behaviors are being imposed or controlled by an external force	Belief that an alien has taken over your body and is controlling your behavior
Thought broadcasting	Belief that one's thoughts are being broadcast from one's mind for others to hear	Belief that your thoughts are being transmitted via the Internet against your will
Thought insertion	Belief that another person or object is inserting thoughts into one's mind	Belief that your spouse is inserting blasphemous thoughts into your mind
Thought withdrawal	Belief that thoughts are being removed from one's mind by another person or by an object	Belief that your roommate is stealing all your thoughts while you sleep
Delusion of guilt or sin	False belief that one has committed a terrible act or is responsible for a terrible event	Belief that you have killed someone or that you are responsible for a disaster (e.g., flood)
Somatic delusion	False belief that one's appearance or part of one's body is diseased or altered	Belief that your intestines have been replaced by snakes

contradict their delusions. They may view the arguments others make against their beliefs as a conspiracy to silence them and as evidence of the truth of their beliefs. According to the *DSM 5*, the distinction between a delusion and a strongly held idea is sometimes difficult to make and depends in part on the degree of conviction with which the belief is held despite clear or reasonable contradictory evidence (American Psychiatric Association, 2013; Quinn, 2017). Table 1 lists some of the more common types of delusions. Delusions can also occur in other disorders such as severe forms of depression or bipolar disorder (see the chapter "Mood Disorders and Suicide"). For example, depressed individuals might believe they have committed some unforgivable sin, and those who are experiencing mania might believe they are a deity (Bentall et al., 2008).

Most commonly experienced by those with schizophrenia are **persecutory delusions,** often referred to as paranoid delusions, in which they believe others are plotting to harm them in some way (Bentall et al., 2008; Cannon & Kramer, 2012). People with persecutory delusions may believe they are being watched, harassed, conspired against, or tormented by people they know, such as their neighbors, professors, or by agencies or persons in authority with whom they have never had direct contact. For example, a person with a persecutory delusion may believe the the FBI, CIA, and members of the mafia are all involved in a conspiracy to assassinate them. This delusion may result in the belief that these groups are watching their every move with surveillance teams, following them in unmarked cars and have placed wiretaps throughout their home. Most importantly, this belief is so unshakeable that there is nothing anyone can typically do to convince them otherwise which results in high levels of psychological distress. While, some of these delusions sound very far-fetched and almost absurd, it's important to recognize that people suffering from these beliefs are terribly distressed, agitated, and fearful. Imagine that you couldn't trust anyone that you know and believe that everyone is part of a plot to harm you. Almost half of individuals with persecutory delusions have the lowest levels of psychological well-being of the general population.

These types of delusions are typically accompanied by anxiety, depression, and disturbed sleep. Paranoid delusions are more frequent in first episodes of psychosis and approximately 70 percent of individuals experience a persecutory delusion during their first psychotic break (Freeman & Garety, 2014). Recent research has found that the frequency of persecutory delusions may be positively correlated with age. Studies have found that paranoid delusions rose from near zero at young age to almost 30 percent for males and to over 40 percent for females by old age (Häfner, 2019). It is highly likely that the impetus for this type of paranoid thinking stems from worry, with rates similar to those with generalized anxiety disorder (GAD). Worry brings implausible ideas to mind, keeps them there, and increases the distress. A longitudinal national epidemiological survey showed that the presence of worry predicts new incidences of paranoid thoughts over time and predicts the persistence of existing non-clinical paranoia. Levels of rumination are also high in patients with persistent persecutory delusions. This suggests that worry may fuel these dysfunctional, inaccurate, and repetitive thoughts that cause very significant amounts of personal distress (Freeman & Garety, 2014).

PROFILES

Everyone is part of the plan!

Rashad knew things that no one else could understand, which meant there was no one he could trust, not even his closest friends and family. While he wasn't sure why they were after him, he knew that the CIA, FBI, and local police were working together with an organized street gang to assassinate him for things that he knew. Rashad saw conspiracies at every turn and knew that he had to stay one step ahead of the people who were working to harm him. Rashad was convinced that cars were following him everywhere that he went, his apartment had been bugged by the government who was listening to every word he said and that all people he encountered on a daily basis were all actors who were part of this plan to drug, kidnap, and kill him. Despite endless conversations with friends who attempted to reason with Rashad and convince him that there was no conspiracy and he was not in danger, his beliefs remained unchanged. These delusional thoughts worsened and as a result, Rashad spent long periods of time in his apartment alone, with the doors and windows locked and the curtains shut so no one could see him. He covered his windows and doors in aluminum foil to reduce the transmission of the wiretapping equipment, he installed additional locks and refused to let anyone into his home for weeks.

Grandiose delusions are unsupported beliefs that one has special powers, ability, wealth, mission, or identity that creates an inflated worth. Simply stated, it's the false belief that you are more important than you really are despite evidence to the contrary (Bortolon, Yazbek, Norton, Capdevielle, & Raffard, 2019). A person may believe they are a God or have divine powers, they are the reincarnated spirit of a celebrity, like Bruce Lee, or the most intelligent person on earth or they discovered the cure for a disease, like cancer. Grandiose delusions are commonly experienced and occur in about half of patients diagnosed with schizophrenia and two-thirds of patients with bipolar disorder. Both harm and distress can occur as a result of grandiose delusions for example, believing one is invincible and stepping into traffic. Research examining grandiose delusions found high rates of harmful or potentially harmful life effects that were direct consequences of grandiose beliefs. For example, physical harm may occur when trying to fly or walk on water, sexual harm may occur when going home with strangers they believed to be God, and social harm may be experienced when rejected or ridiculed by others for their delusional beliefs or behaviors. Some, especially the male participants, knowingly entered dangerous situations feeling themselves to be invulnerable. For example, Max described exaggerated self-confidence during an altercation at a nightclub because "I felt that people were looking out for me" because he believed that he was a trained member of the secret service (Isham et al., 2019).

Recent studies have found that grandiosity is not synonymous with arrogance, entitlement, or feelings of superiority despite the negative connotation. Power and self-efficacy, helping others, and making a valuable contribution to society were common themes found in a recent study on grandiose delusions. Participants in a recent study described their feelings during grandiose episodes in terms of social connectedness, often reporting they felt like they were "part of a team," respected by others, or involved in intimate relationships with the promise of comfort and protection. Since individuals experiencing grandiose delusions often report feelings of paranoia, depressed mood, self-loathing, and rejection these delusions may serve as a form of respite that helps compensate for negative self-beliefs in this population (Isham et al., 2019).

Another common type of delusion is the **delusion of reference,** in which people believe that random events or comments by others are directed at them. People with delusions of reference may believe that a news story they saw online was placed there specifically for them and may contain special codes or clues. It is theorized that this is the result of heightened attention to irrelevant cues and the incorrect assignment of significance or importance what are actually neutral stimuli (Pankow et al., 2016). For example, a person with a delusional reference may believe that a flickering streetlight across from their home is actually sending them important messages from God. John Nash believed that people in Boston were deliberately wearing red neckties so he would notice them as part of a "crypto-communist" plot. Another common type of delusion is **delusions of thought insertion,** or beliefs that one's thoughts are being controlled by outside forces. This type of delusion involves the inability of the individual to recognize their own thoughts and rather attribute these alien thoughts to someone else. For example, *"Thoughts are put into my mind like 'Kill God.' It's just like my mind working, but it isn't. They come from this chap, Chris. They are his thoughts"* (Ratcliffe & Wilkinson, 2015).

Delusional beliefs can be simple and transient, such as when a person with schizophrenia believes the pain he has just experienced in his stomach is the result of someone across the room shooting a laser beam at him. However, delusional beliefs often are complex and elaborate, with the person clinging to these beliefs for long periods. The following profile illustrates how several types of delusions—grandiose delusions, persecutory delusions, delusions of reference, and delusions of thought insertion—may work together in one person's belief system. Although the passage is written by a person with schizophrenia about his own experience, he speaks of himself in the third person.

David's grandiose delusions were that he had discovered the source of telepathy, that all the scientists thought highly of him, and that he might be the Messiah. These grandiose delusions were accompanied by persecutory delusions—that the scientists were criticizing him because they were jealous. David's delusions of reference were that all the scientists were talking about him, both directly and indirectly. David believed that he could read others' minds. Finally, he had delusions of thought control—that the scientists were determining his feelings with their facial expressions, gestures, and postures.

Hallucinations

Have you ever had a strange perceptual experience where your senses misled you? Perhaps you thought you saw someone when no one was there, maybe you thought you heard a voice say your name but no one did, or you felt as though someone reached out and touched you but there was no one around? Most of us have experienced this momentary confusion when our perceptual system creates a feeling of reality despite a lack of external stimuli. These transient moments can help us better understand and empathize with the hallucinations experienced by those with schizophrenia. Unlike delusions which are false beliefs, hallucinations are false perceptions. **Hallucinations** are false or inaccurate perceptions that affect the senses and cause people to hear, see, taste, touch, or smell what others do not. Meaning, people with schizophrenia may perceive a sound, like a voice, but there is no corresponding auditory stimulus detected by the sense organ, the ear. For the experiencer, hallucinations can have important personal meanings, and for clinicians they represent a significant diagnostic symptom that may impact daily functioning and prognosis (Waters & Fernyhough, 2017). Hallucinations are common and often stressful experiences, which can occur in all sensory modalities (e.g., auditory, visual, olfactory, tactile, and gustatory). Auditory verbal hallucinations (AVHs) are most commonly reported and often perceived as "voices" that are consistently reported in 70 to 80 percent of people with schizophrenia. The perception of these voices to those with schizophrenia can often be unpleasant and frightening (Castiajo & Pinheiro, 2017).

AVHs are core features of psychotic illness and are significant predictors of poor mental health outcome and risk (Upthegrove et al., 2016). These hallucinations may consist of a voice speaking the individual's thoughts aloud or carrying on a running commentary on the person's behavior, a collection of voices speaking about the individual in the third person, or voices issuing commands and instructions. The voices may seem to come either from inside the person's head or from somewhere outside. They often have a negative quality, criticizing or threatening the individuals or telling them to hurt themselves or others. People with schizophrenia may talk back to the voices even as they are trying to talk to people who are actually in the room with them. The content of auditory hallucinations, or what the voices actually say to the client, significantly varies among individuals. Individuals with AVHs often report that the voice(s) speak directly to them, they cannot control the voice(s), and the voice(s) are often evil. It has been hypothesized that the spontaneous fluctuation of the voices over time may reflect the underlying neuronal and neurochemical basis for auditory hallucinations (Hugdahl, 2017).

Neuroimaging literature has shown that AVHs are associated with a variety of alterations in brain structure and function that are concentrated in regions associated with auditory/verbal stimuli and executive control (Bohlken, Hugdahl, & Sommer, 2017). Various studies have also found spontaneous activation of speech production areas in the right hemisphere of the prefrontal cortex and the auditory cortex which might contribute to the single word or basic sentences that often characterize auditory hallucinations (Hugdahl, 2017)

In addition to this disorder, hearing voices occurs transdiagnostically and is found among individuals diagnosed with major depression, borderline personality disorder, bipolar disorder, dissociative disorders, and posttraumatic stress disorder (PTSD). Hearing voices is also found outside of psychiatric contexts occurring in the context of Alzheimer's and Parkinson's diseases and epilepsy, hearing loss, and eye disease. Studies also show that a low percentage (2 to 10 percent) of the general population reports voice-hearing experiences without meeting criteria for psychiatric diagnoses, evidencing that the experience may not be limited to dysfunction or impairment. Isolated experiences of voice-hearing may occur in the absence of any detectable illness in up to 50 percent of the general population, for example following the death of a loved one. The loudness of the voice heard, the external attribution and and the perceived location of the hallucinated voice are the main similarities shared by clinical and nonclinical individuals (Castiajo & Pinheiro, 2017; Corlett et al., 2019; McCarthy-Jones et al., 2015).

Visual hallucinations (VHs) are often accompanied by auditory hallucinations (or other sensory modalities), are the second most common type of hallucinations in psychotic patients (Dudley, Aynsworth, Cheetham, McCarthy-Jones, & Collerton, 2018). Research estimates the prevalence of VHs at approximately 24 to 72 percent, but these rates may be underestimated. For example, a woman may see a figure of a man standing at her bedside, telling her she is damned and must die. An individual's hallucinations may be consistent with her delusions—the person who sees Satan telling her she must die may think that she is related to Satan. VHs may also occur in a wide range of clinical conditions, such as ophthalmologic diseases, neurologic disorders, toxic and metabolic disorders (Castiajo & Pinheiro, 2017). *Tactile hallucinations* involve the perception that something is happening to the outside of the person's body—for example, that bugs are crawling up her back. *Somatic hallucinations* involve the perception that something is happening inside the person's body—for example, that worms are eating his intestines. These hallucinations often are very frightening (Torrey, 2013).

Hallucinations do not occur only in schizophrenia and other psychotic disorders. One study of individuals with VHs (Gauntlett-Gilbert & Kuipers, 2003) found that 60 percent were diagnosed with

schizophrenia or schizoaffective disorders (described below) but that 25 percent were diagnosed with depression and 15 percent with bipolar disorder (see the chapter "Mood Disorders and Suicide").

Disorganized Thought and Speech

The disorganized thinking of people with schizophrenia is often referred to as a **formal thought disorder.** One of the most common forms of disorganization in schizophrenia is a tendency to slip from one topic to a seemingly unrelated topic with little coherent transition, often referred to as *loose associations* or *derailment.* For example, one person with schizophrenia posted this "announcement":

> Things that relate, the town of Antelope, Oregon, Jonestown, Charlie Manson, the Hillside Strangler, the Zodiac Killer, Watergate, King's trial in L.A., and many more. In the last 7 years alone, over 23 Star wars scientists committed suicide for no apparent reason. The AIDS coverup, the conference in South America in 87 had over 1,000 doctors claim that insects can transmit it. To be able to read one's thoughts and place thoughts in one's mind without the person knowing it's being done. Realization is a reality of bioelectromagnetic control, which is thought transfer and emotional control, recording individual brain-wave frequencies of thought, sensation, and emotions.

The person who wrote this announcement saw clear connections among the events he listed in the first half of the paragraph and between these events and his concerns about mind reading and bioelectromagnetic control. However, it is difficult for us to see these connections.

A person with schizophrenia may answer questions with unrelated or barely related comments. For example, when asked why he is in the hospital, a man with schizophrenia might answer, "Spaghetti looks like worms. I really think it's worms. Gophers dig tunnels but rats build nests." At times the person's speech is so disorganized as to be totally *incoherent* to the listener, a form of speech known as "word salad." For example, "Much of abstraction has been left unsaid and undone in these products milk syrup, and others, due to economics, differentials, subsidies, bankruptcy, tools, buildings, bonds, national stocks, foundation craps, weather, trades, government in levels of breakages and fuses in electronics too all formerly states not necessarily factuated" (Maher, 1966, p. 395). The person may make up words that mean something only to them, known as *neologisms.* Or the person may make associations between words based on the sounds of the words rather than on the content, known as *clangs,* or may repeat the same word or statement over and over again.

Men with schizophrenia tend to show more severe deficits in language than do women with schizophrenia, possibly because language is controlled more bilaterally—that is, by both sides of the brain—in women than in men (see Mendrek & Mancini-Marie, 2016). Thus, the brain abnormalities associated with schizophrenia may not affect women's language and thought as much as they do men's because women can use both sides of their brain to compensate for deficits. In contrast, language is more localized in men, so when these areas of the brain are affected by schizophrenia, men may not be as able to compensate for the deficits.

Disorganized or Catatonic Behavior

The disorganized behavior of people with schizophrenia often frightens others. People with schizophrenia may display unpredictable and apparently untriggered agitation—suddenly shouting, swearing, or pacing rapidly. These behaviors may occur in response to hallucinations or delusions. For example, a man who believes he is being persecuted may hallucinate a frightening figure chasing him; in response, he screams and runs. Another man who believes a computer chip has been implanted under his skin to control him may pace agitatedly because no one will believe him and offer him the help he thinks he needs. People with schizophrenia often have trouble organizing their daily routines of bathing, dressing properly, and eating regularly. Because their attention and memory are impaired, it takes all their concentration to accomplish even one simple task, such as brushing their teeth. They may engage in socially unacceptable behavior, such as public masturbation. Many are disheveled and dirty, sometimes wearing few clothes on a cold day or heavy clothes on a very hot day.

Catatonia is disorganized behavior that reflects noticeable psychomotor dysfunction that may involve decreased or excessive and peculiar motor activity which can range from pronounced unresponsiveness to agitation (American Psychiatric Association, 2013). These disorganized behaviors can involve a lack of response to instructions (*negativism*), to showing a rigid, inappropriate, or bizarre posture, to a complete lack of verbal or motor responses (e.g., *mutism*). In *catatonic excitement*, the person shows purposeless and excessive motor activity for no apparent reason. The individual may articulate a number of delusions or hallucinations or may be incoherent (Mueser & Jeste, 2008).

Negative Symptoms

You might say to yourself that all the symptoms of schizophrenia seem negative. However, specific psychotic symptoms are explicitly labeled **negative symptoms** because they involve the loss of certain qualities of the person, rather than behaviors or thoughts that the person expresses overtly (Marder & Galderisi, 2017). The core negative symptoms in schizophrenia are restricted affect and avolition/asociality. Although the positive symptoms of schizophrenia may strike you as more severe and debilitating than the negative symptoms, the presence of strong negative symptoms is more associated with poor outcome than is the presence of strong positive symptoms, in part because the negative symptoms tend to be persistent and more difficult to treat (Galderisi et al., 2012; Patel, Cherian, Gohil, & Atkinson, 2014; Strauss, Harrow, Grossman, & Rosen, 2010). Negative symptoms are less prominent in other psychotic disorders.

Restricted Affect

Restricted affect refers to a severe reduction in or absence of emotional expression in people with schizophrenia. People with schizophrenia show fewer facial expressions of emotion, may avoid eye contact, and are less likely to use gestures to communicate emotional information than people without the disorder. Their tone of voice may be flat, with little change in emphasis, intonation (speech melody), rhythm, tempo, or loudness to indicate emotion or social engagement.

Do people with schizophrenia actually experience less affect than people without the disorder? Self-report questionnaires often find that people with schizophrenia report significant *anhedonia*, or a loss of the ability to experience pleasure (see Kring & Elis, 2013). Yet in laboratory studies in which individuals' responses to standardized positive stimuli (e.g., pleasant outdoor scenes or photos of food) are assessed, people with schizophrenia often report as much positive affect as people without the disorder (Minor & Cohen, 2010; Kring & Moran, 2008). Similarly, some studies have shown emotionally charged films to people with and without schizophrenia while recording their facial expressions and physiological arousal (Kring & Neale, 1996). The people with schizophrenia showed less facial responsiveness to the films than did the normal group, but they reported experiencing just as much emotion and showed even more physiological arousal. Thus, people with schizophrenia who show no emotion may be experiencing intense emotion that they cannot express. The self-reports of anhedonia by people with schizophrenia may reflect limitations in self-report questionnaires or secondary problems with depression, which is common in schizophrenia (Marder & Galderisi, 2017). Moreover, multiple studies show that even when emotion experience is intact, people with schizophrenia have trouble predicting future emotional experience, which can lead to problems in motivation and decision making (e.g., Moran & Kring, 2018).

Avolition/Asociality

Avolition is an inability to initiate or persist at common, goal-directed activities, including those at work, at school, and at home. The person is physically slowed down in his or her movements and seems unmotivated. He or she may sit around all day doing almost nothing. Personal hygiene and grooming are lacking. Avolition may be expressed as asociality, the lack of desire to interact with other people. Individuals with schizophrenia are often withdrawn and socially isolated. Some of this social isolation may be the result of the stigma of schizophrenia—many people with schizophrenia are shunned by their families and other people. Asociality should be diagnosed only when the individual has access to welcoming family and friends but shows no interest in socializing with them (Marder & Galderisi, 2017).

Cognitive Deficits

People with schizophrenia show deficits in basic cognitive processes, including attention, memory, and processing speed (Savla, Moore, & Palmer, 2008). Compared to people without schizophrenia, they have greater difficulty focusing and maintaining their attention at will—for example, in tracking a moving object with their eyes. In addition, people with schizophrenia show deficits in working memory, the ability to hold information in memory and manipulate it (Barch & Sheffield, 2017). These deficits in attention and working memory make it difficult for people with schizophrenia to pay attention to relevant information and to suppress unwanted or irrelevant information.

As a result, they find it difficult to distinguish the thoughts in their mind that are relevant to the situation at hand and to ignore stimuli in their environment that are not relevant to what they are doing. These deficits taken together may contribute to the hallucinations, delusions, disorganized thought and behavior, and avolition of people with schizophrenia (Barch & Sheffield, 2017). Information and stimulation constantly flood their consciousness, and they are unable to filter out what is irrelevant or to determine the source of the information. This makes it difficult for them to concentrate, maintain a coherent stream of thought or conversation, perform a basic task, or distinguish real from unreal. Social relationships and work performance are severely affected, and daily functioning is impaired (Bowie et al., 2008). Delusions and hallucinations may develop as individuals try to make sense of the thoughts and perceptions bombarding their consciousness (Beck & Rector, 2005; Garety & Freeman, 2013).

The immediate relatives of people with schizophrenia also show many of these cognitive deficits to a less severe degree, even if they do not show the symptoms of schizophrenia (Kemp, Bathery, Barrantes-Vidal, & Kwapil, 2020; Snitz, MacDonald, & Carter, 2006). In addition, longitudinal studies of people who develop schizophrenia suggest that many show these cognitive deficits before they develop acute symptoms of the disorder (Cannon et al., 2003; Keshavan, DeLisi, & Seidman, 2011) and cognitive deficits often do not improve over the course of the disorder or with treatment. Cognitive deficits may be an early marker of risk for schizophrenia and may contribute to the development of other symptoms (Gur et al., 2007) and strongly contribute to the disability of the illness (Kemp et al., 2020).

Diagnosis

Schizophrenia has been recognized as a psychological disorder since the early 1800s In 1883, German psychiatrist Emil Kraepelin labeled the disorder *dementia praecox* (precocious dementia) because he believed that the disorder results from premature deterioration of the brain. He viewed the disorder as progressive, irreversible, and chronic (Kendler, 2019).

Eugen Bleuler disagreed with Kraepelin's view that this disorder develops at an early age and always leads to severe deterioration of the brain (Bartley & Ross, 2020; Lavretsky, 2008). Bleuler introduced the label *schizophrenia* for this disorder, from the Greek words *schizein*, meaning "to split," and *phren*, meaning "mind." Bleuler believed that this disorder involves the splitting of usually integrated psychic functions of mental associations, thoughts, and emotions. (Bleuler did not view schizophrenia as the splitting of distinct

TABLE 2   *DSM-5* Diagnostic Criteria for Schizophrenia

A. Two (or more) of the following, each present for a significant portion of time during a 1-month period (or less if successfully treated). At least one of these must be 1, 2, or 3:

1. Delusions
2. Hallucinations
3. Disorganized speech (i.e., frequent derailment or incoherence)
4. Grossly disorganized or catatonic behavior
5. Negative symptoms (i.e., diminished emotional expression or avolition)

B. For a significant portion of the time since the onset of the disturbance, level of functioning in one or more major areas, such as work, interpersonal relations, or self-care, is markedly below the level achieved prior to the onset (or when the onset is in childhood or adolescence, there is failure to achieve expected level of interpersonal, academic, or occupational functioning).

C. Continuous signs of the disturbance persist for at least 6 months. This 6-month period must include at least 1 month of symptoms (or less if successfully treated) that meet Criterion A (i.e., active-phase symptoms) and may include periods of prodromal or residual symptoms. During these prodromal or residual periods, the signs of the disturbance may be manifested by only negative symptoms or by two or more symptoms listed in Criterion A present in an attenuated form (e.g., odd beliefs, unusual perceptual experiences).

D. Schizoaffective disorder and depressive or bipolar disorder with psychotic features have been ruled out because either (1) no major depressive or manic episodes have occurred concurrently with the active-phase symptoms, or (2) if mood episodes have occurred during active-phase symptoms, they have been present for a minority of the active and residual periods of the illness.

E. The disturbance is not attributable to the physiological effects of a substance (e.g., a drug of abuse, a medication) or another medical condition.

F. If there is a history of autism spectrum disorder or communication disorder of childhood onset, the additional diagnosis of schizophrenia is made only if prominent delusions or hallucinations in addition to the other required symptoms of schizophrenia are also present for at least 1 month (or less if successfully treated).

Specify if:

With catatonia

personalities, as in dissociative identity disorder, nor do modern psychiatrists and psychologists.)

Bleuler argued that the primary problem underlying the symptoms of schizophrenia is the "breaking of associative threads"—that is, a breaking of associations among thought, language, memory, and problem solving. He argued that the attentional problems seen in schizophrenia are due to a lack of the necessary links between aspects of the mind, and that the disorganized behavior is similarly due to an inability to maintain a train of thought (Lavretsky, 2008).

The *DSM-5* states that, in order to be diagnosed with schizophrenia, an individual must show two or more symptoms of psychosis, at least one of which should be delusions, hallucinations, or disorganized speech (see Table 2). These symptoms must be consistently and acutely present for at least 1 month, referred to as the *acute phase* of the disorder. In addition, the individual must have some symptoms of the disorder for at least 6 months to a degree that impairs

social or occupational functioning. These symptoms cannot be due to a medical disease, a mood disorder, or ingestion of a substance (see the chapter "Mood Disorders and Suicide"). When symptoms of catatonia are present, these symptoms are specified in the diagnosis (American Psychiatric Association, 2013).

During the 6 months before and after the active phase (meeting Criterion A in Table 2), the individual may show predominantly negative symptoms, with milder forms of the positive symptoms. These are often referred to as **prodromal symptoms** (before the acute phase) and **residual symptoms** (after the acute phase). When experiencing prodromal and residual symptoms, people with schizophrenia may be withdrawn and uninterested in others. They may express beliefs that are unusual but not delusional (Nelson & Yung, 2008). They may have strange perceptual experiences, such as sensing another person in the room, without reporting full-blown hallucinations. They may speak in a somewhat disorganized and tangential way but remain coherent. Their behavior may be peculiar—for example, collecting scraps of paper—but not grossly disorganized. During the prodromal phase, family members and friends may perceive the person with schizophrenia as "gradually slipping away" (Torrey, 2013). Left untreated, schizophrenia is both chronic and episodic; after the first onset of an acute episode, individuals may have chronic residual symptoms punctuated by relapses into acute episodes.

The odd behaviors and asociality seen in schizophrenia can resemble the symptoms of autism spectrum disorders (ASDs) (see the chapter "Neurodevelopmental and Neurocognitive Disorders"). Difficulties in social communication represent a transdiagnostic feature that overlaps between ASDs and schizophrenia. While there are some similarities between these disorders, each has distinct developmental patterns. Symptoms of ASD typically occur during early childhood, whereas most symptoms characteristic of schizophrenia do not appear before early adulthood. To distinguish the two disorders, the diagnostic criteria for schizophrenia specify that schizophrenia can be diagnosed only if delusions and/or hallucinations are clearly present (St Pourcain et al., 2018).

The impact of schizophrenia symptoms on people's lives is enormous. One review of 37 longitudinal studies that had followed individuals for an average of 3 years after their first episode of acute schizophrenia symptoms found that only about 40 percent were employed or in school and only about 37 percent had recovered a good level of functioning (Menezes, Arenovich, & Zipursky, 2006). Difficulties in functioning are tied to the negative symptoms of schizophrenia—the lack of motivation and appropriate emotional responding—as well as to the positive symptoms. People with schizophrenia who show many negative symptoms have lower levels of educational attainment and less success holding jobs, poorer performance on cognitive tasks, and a poorer prognosis than do those with predominantly positive symptoms (Andreasen, Flaum, Swayze, Tyrell, & Arndt, 1990; Marder & Galderisi, 2017). In addition, the negative symptoms are less responsive to medication than are the positive symptoms: With medication, a person with schizophrenia may be able to overcome the hallucinations, delusions, and thought disturbances but may not be able to overcome the restricted affect and avolition. Thus, the person may remain chronically unresponsive, unmotivated, and socially isolated even when not acutely psychotic (Marder & Galderisi, 2017).

You may have heard the media refer to people with schizophrenia as "paranoid schizophrenics." Prior versions of the DSM listed subtypes of schizophrenia, the best known of which was paranoid schizophrenia. People with this type of schizophrenia, such as John Nash, have delusions and hallucinations that involve themes of persecution and grandiosity. Their delusions often focus on being hunted, spied on, persecuted and conspired against by others, including government agencies, the media, family and friends, and complete strangers, perhaps because they have special knowledge or powers. They may believe that anyone who disagrees with their delusions is part of the conspiracy. They can become angry, suspicious, and even violent, as John Nash did. They often do not show grossly disorganized speech or behavior. They may be lucid and articulate, relating elaborate stories of plots against them.

Although paranoia is still recognized as a common symptom in schizophrenia, the DSM-5 dropped the DSM-IV subtypes of schizophrenia because evidence supporting their diagnostic stability, validity, and usefulness is not strong. Schizophrenia is currently viewed as part of the psychotic spectrum without differentiating subtypes. Additionally, research found that these subtypes had no meaningful impact on treatments outcomes for people with schizophrenia (Mattila et al., 2015; Linscott, Allardyce, & van Os, 2009).

Course

It is estimated that within the United States, 0.25 to 0.7 percent of the population will develop schizophrenia at some time in their lives, but recent studies suggest that this may be an overestimation. Research on the global prevalence of schizophrenia suggests the rates are approximately 0.33 to 0.75 percent, although this risk increases considerably when relatives with the disorder are present (Fosse, Joseph, & Jones, 2016). The psychotic features of schizophrenia typically emerge during the late teens through the mid-30s with prevalence peaking around 40 years before declining among older age groups. A recent study found that an overwhelming majority of cases (70.8 percent or 14.8 million) occurred in the 25 to 54 years age group (Charlson et al., 2018). Meaning, on average symptoms of schizophrenia are more likely to develop earlier in life than in late adulthood. The development of psychotic symptoms prior to adolescence is very uncommon but can be diagnosed. Early-onset schizophrenia (EOS) is diagnosed in childhood and adolescence prior to age 13 and is viewed on the same clinical and biological continuum as adults. Childhood-onset schizophrenia is rare, with an incidence lower than 1 in 10,000 children. These cases tend to have poor outcomes, prominent negative symptoms, and high rates of comorbidity with other psychological disorders. (Budisteanu et al., 2020; Stevens, Prince, Prager, & Stern, 2014).

Psychotic symptoms can develop rapidly (acute onset) but more likely the process will be slow and gradual. These symptoms and impairment are often seen in people with schizophrenia long before their first psychotic episode. Research has historically shown that the onset of overt psychosis is often preceded by a phase that is characterized by very mild (sometimes subclinical levels) positive and negative symptoms and generalized functional decline (Kemp et al., 2020; Keshavan et al., 2011). Most onsets of schizophrenia are marked by a **prodromal** stage extending over several years which produces the highest social consequences. Research on the age of onset shows culmination in males from 15 to 25 years, whereas females often a first peak at age 15 to 30 years and a second, flatter peak at 44 to 49 years around menopause (Häfner, 2019). Typically, an early age at onset is a predictor of poor prognosis with negative mental health outcomes. The course of this disorder is relatively chronic and individuals are more likely to experience more cognitive and functional impairment (Gatov, Rosella, Chiu, & Kurdyak, 2017). More recurrent episodes are likely during the first 10 to 15 years and chances of a full recovery are less likely than other psychological disorders with only about 13.5 percent of those with schizophrenia meeting full recovery criteria (Charlson et al., 2018).

When symptoms of schizophrenia no longer interfere with daily function, the disorder is considered to be in remission. Many sufferers will experience disorganized thinking and cognitive impairments even when other symptoms are in remission which contribute to the prolonged disability of the disease. Psychotic symptoms tend to diminish over the course of the lifespan it is theorized that age-related neurological changes, such as declines in dopamine activity, may account for the reduction in psychotic symptoms (American Psychiatric Association, 2013).

Studies have found that the prevalence of schizophrenia in less developed countries was significantly lower than in emerging and developed countries with some of the lowest prevalence rates found in the sub-Saharan Africa and North Africa/Middle East regions. Indian studies have suggested that the prevalence of schizophrenia is lower in India than in the West which could be a result of underreporting (Viswanath & Chaturvedi, 2012). Prevalence rates are consistent across countries but recent research has found higher prevalence estimates of schizophrenia in China more than any other country, worldwide. Despite these low prevalence rates, schizophrenia is globally ranked as one of the top 15 leading causes of disability (American Psychiatric Association, 2013; Charlson et al., 2018; Moreno-Küstner, Martín, & Pastor, 2018).

Schizophrenia causes significant impairments in psychosocial function which increases the chances that people with schizophrenia will be unemployed, homeless, living in poverty, having difficulties keeping up with household and self-care tasks, and relying on ongoing family support and mental health services. The largest burden from schizophrenia is in the 25- to 54-year age group, where individuals are most likely to be economically productive. This results in significant economic deficits due to losses in productivity by individuals and their families, out-of-pocket costs for treatment, and considerable burdens on health and welfare systems (Charlson et al., 2018). International studies show that nations spend up to 3 percent of their health care budgets treating people with psychotic disorders, and tens of billions of dollars more are lost in declines in productivity (Gustavsson et al., 2011; Jin & Mosweu, 2017).

Instead of pursuing their education, a career, or a family, people with schizophrenia may need continual services, including residential care, rehabilitative therapy, subsidized income, and the help of mental health professionals. Due to the chronic nature of this disorder, it is likely that they may need these services for the rest of their lives. Schizophrenia and other psychotic disorders exact a heavy toll, including high medical costs. Schizophrenia has also been linked to higher rates of comorbid illnesses and mortality rates which are often due to underlying physical illnesses, especially chronic diseases such as coronary heart disease, stroke, type II diabetes, respiratory diseases, and some cancers. Unnatural causes, including suicide, account for less than 15 percent of deaths (Charlson et al., 2018).

Prognosis

Schizophrenia is one of the most severe and debilitating mental disorders, and many people with the disorder suffer symptoms and impairment for many years, even with treatment (Harrow, Grossman, Jobe, & Herbener, 2005; Jobe & Harrow, 2010). Between 50 and 80 percent of people hospitalized for one episode of active-phase schizophrenia will be rehospitalized sometime in their lives (Eaton, Moortensenk, Herrman, & Freeman, 1992; Harrow et al., 2005). The life expectancy of people with schizophrenia is between 10 and 20 years shorter than that of people without schizophrenia (Laursen, Nordentoft, & Mortensen, 2014). People with schizophrenia suffer from infectious and circulatory diseases at a higher rate than do people without the disorder, due in part to underdiagnosis of physical illness, less access to care, higher rates of smoking, and being overweight due to diet, exercise, and side effects of medications (Laursen et al., 2014). Between 5 and 10 percent of people with schizophrenia commit suicide, with the highest rates among those recently diagnosed or experiencing a first psychotic episode (Laursen et al., 2014; Ventriglio et al., 2016). The following account of a woman's suicidal thoughts gives a sense of the psychological pain that many people with schizophrenia live with and wish to end through suicide.

PROFILES

I had major fantasies of suicide by decapitation and was reading up on the construction of guillotines. I had written several essays on the problem of the complete destruction of myself; I thought my inner being to be a deeply poisonous substance. The problem, as I saw it, was to kill myself, but then to get rid of my essence in such a way that it did not harm creation. (Anonymous, 1992, p. 334)

Despite the introduction of effective pharmacological treatments and psychosocial interventions, fewer than one in seven people fully recover from this disorder and the longitudinal and progressive course of schizophrenia may explain the poor outcomes observed over time. Advocates for early intervention have argued that early treatment has the potential to arrest a disease process that would otherwise result in severe mental deterioration. Studies have shown that 70 to 80 percent of individuals with a first episode of schizophrenia will experience a remission of psychotic symptoms within the first year of treatment. This percentage appears to remain stable when individuals are provided with ongoing comprehensive treatment. The relapse of psychotic symptoms following a remission from a first episode of schizophrenia occurs in over 80 percent of individuals. This relapse is mainly attributed to the discontinuation of antipsychotic medication rather than the effects of a continuous disease process. During the first year following the first psychotic episode, the risk of symptom recurrence following remission in persons receiving maintenance antipsychotic treatment is estimated to be in the range 0 to 5 percent as compared to 78 percent in the first year without medication and close to 100 percent after 3 years without medication (Zipursky & Agid, 2015).

Despite the dire statistics, many people with schizophrenia do not show a progressive deterioration in functioning across the life span but instead stabilize within 5 to 10 years of their first episode, showing few or no relapses and regaining a moderately good level of functioning (Menezes et al., 2006). Although cognitive deficits are clearly present at the time of the first psychotic episode, recent research has shown that these deficits significantly improve in the first year of treatment tend to remain stable or improve rather than decline over the longer term (Zipursky & Agid, 2015).

Gender and Age Factors

Clinical research has found differences between men and women with schizophrenia in terms of prevalence, age of onset, symptom presentation, disease severity, and responses to treatment. Men are more likely to present with an earlier age at onset, negative symptoms, lower social functioning, and comorbid substance abuse than women. Conversely, women display relatively late onset of the disease with more affective symptoms. While men and women have similar prevalence of Schizophrenia, most of studies demonstrate that female onset is typically 3 to 5 years later than males. The peak onset for the first psychotic episode is early-to-mid 20s for males and late 20s for females. Recent studies have found evidence that men have a single peak age of onset (21 to 25 years) and women have two peak ages of onset, one between 25 and 30 years old and another one is after 45 years old. The idea that women have two separate and delayed peak ages of symptom onset is evidenced by the fact that women make up about 66 to 87 percent of clients who develop symptoms after the age of 40 to 50 years (American Psychiatric Association, 2013; Li, Ma, Wang, Yang, & Wang, 2017).

There are also notable differences in the display of symptoms between men and women. For example, men with schizophrenia appear to have more negative symptoms such as social withdrawal, substance abuse, and blunted affect than female clients whereas women with schizophrenia often present with more mood disturbances and depressive symptoms. The age of onset is also associated with type of symptoms most experienced. For example, studies show that women with late onset of schizophrenia may have less severe negative symptoms and present with more positive symptoms, particularly sensory hallucinations and persecutory delusions (Li et al., 2017).

Women with schizophrenia tend to have a better prognosis than men with the disorder (Seeman, 2008). In a 20-year study of people with schizophrenia, 61 percent of the women had periods of recovery, compared to 41 percent of the men (Grossman, Harrow, Rosen, Faull, & Strauss, 2008). Women are hospitalized less often than men and for briefer periods of time, show milder negative symptoms between periods of active-phase symptoms, and have better social adjustment when they are not psychotic (Grossman et al., 2008). The reasons for these gender differences are not entirely clear. Women diagnosed with schizophrenia tend to have better prior histories than men: they are more likely to have graduated from high school or college, to have married and had children, and to have developed good social skills

(Seeman, 2008). This may be, in part, because the onset of schizophrenia in women tends to be in the late 20s or early 30s, whereas men more often develop schizophrenia in their late teens or early 20s. Women with schizophrenia also show fewer cognitive deficits than men with the disorder (Mendrek & Mancini-Marie, 2016). All these factors lead to expectations of a better prognosis for women but do not entirely explain it (Grossman et al., 2008).

Estrogen may affect the regulation of dopamine, a neurotransmitter implicated in schizophrenia, in ways that are protective for women (Mendrek & Mancini-Marie, 2016; Seeman, 2008). Some of the sex differences, particularly in cognitive deficits, may also be due to normal sex differences in the brain. The pace of prenatal brain development, which is hormonally regulated, is slower in males than in females and may place males at higher risk than females for abnormal brain development. Several studies suggest that males with schizophrenia show greater abnormalities in brain structure and functioning than do females with schizophrenia (Mendrek & Mancini-Marie, 2016).

In both men and women with schizophrenia, functioning seems to improve with age (Jablensky, 2000; Harrow et al., 2005). Why? Perhaps they find treatments that help them stabilize, or maybe they and their families learn to recognize the early symptoms of a relapse and seek treatment before the symptoms become acute (Torrey, 2013). Alternatively, the aging of the brain might somehow reduce the likelihood of new episodes of schizophrenia. Some think this might be related to a reduction in dopamine levels in the brain with age; as we will discuss, high dopamine levels have been implicated in schizophrenia.

Cultural Influences

Culture influences the epidemiology, phenomenology, outcome, and treatment of schizophrenia. Although the types of delusions we have discussed likely occur in all cultures, the specific content of delusions can differ across cultures since these themes often relate to the person's social background and cultural beliefs (Suhail & Cochrane, 2002; Viswanath, & Chaturvedi, 2012). Since the subjects of delusions relate to culture in which a person lives, it is common to see certain types of delusional content within particular cultures. For example, religious delusions are common in Christian societies and are more rare among Hindu, Muslim, or Buddhist societies. Magical religious delusions are more likely to be found in those living in rural societies, especially in women over the age of 30. Low rates of religious delusions, grandiose delusions, and delusions of guilt were found in Pakistan and conversely, religious grandiosity was more common in African countries. Studies have found that the cultural content of the delusions is likely to recurs in

future psychotic episodes (Viswanath, & Chaturvedi, 2012). For example, one study found that many of the delusions of British people with schizophrenia focused on being controlled by televisions, radios, and computers, but this focus was rare among Pakistani people with schizophrenia, whose delusions were more likely to involve being controlled by black magic (Suhail & Cochrane, 2002). Studies comparing Japanese people and Western Europeans with schizophrenia have found that, among the Japanese, delusions of being slandered by others and delusions that others know something terrible about them are relatively common, perhaps due to the emphasis in Japanese culture on being thought well of by others. In contrast, among Germans and Austrians with schizophrenia, religious delusions of having committed a sin (e.g., "Satan orders me to pray to him; I will be punished") are relatively common, perhaps due to the influence of Christianity in Western Europe (Tateyama et al., 1993). Even within a culture, delusional content differs across time based on sociocultural factors. For example, delusional content in the United States disproportionately focused on Germans during World War II, Communists during the Cold War, and technology in recent years (Cannon & Kramer, 2012).

Some theorists argue that odd or impossible beliefs that are part of a culture's shared belief system cannot be considered delusions (Fabrega, 1993). If the people of a particular culture believe that the spirits of dead relatives watch over the living, then individuals in that culture who hold that belief are not considered delusional. However, people who hold extreme manifestations of their culture's shared belief systems are considered delusional. For example, a person in the culture described who believed that their dead relatives were causing their heart to rot would be considered delusional. *DSM-5* also changed the definition of delusions to "fixed beliefs that are not amenable to change in light of conflicting evidence" from "erroneous beliefs" (as in *DSM-IV*) because it is often highly difficult to establish the fully false nature of a belief (Coltheart, Langdon, & McKay, 2011).

As with delusions, the types of hallucinations people experience in different cultures appear similar, but the content of the hallucinations can be culturally specific. For example, Asians with hallucinations might see the ghosts of ancestors haunting them, but not common among Europeans, who might hallucinate that they are being pursued by terrorists (Browne, 2001). It is important for clinicians to understand hallucinations in their cultural context (Larøi et al., 2014). Studies show that the characteristics of one's culture influences both the content and acceptance in society of hearing "voices." For example, "voices" are more emotionally negative in the United States than in developing countries. People from cultures that provide accepted explanations for the phenomenon such as hearing arch angels, or *Djinns* (genies) more often experience AVHs without necessarily causing consistent distress (Hugdahl & Sommer, 2018).

Other Psychotic Disorders

Most people assume that schizophrenia is the only psychotic disorder since it is commonly depicted in television and movies, but this is only one psychotic disorder on the continuum. The *DSM-5* recognizes other psychotic disorders that share features with schizophrenia and fall along a continuum in terms of severity. Schizophrenia has the worst long-term outcome of these disorders, followed by schizoaffective disorder, schizophreniform disorder, and the other psychotic disorders shown in the chapter-opening feature, "Schizophrenia Spectrum and Other Psychotic Disorders Along the Continuum."

Schizoaffective disorder is a mix of schizophrenia and a mood disorder (Table 3). People with schizoaffective disorder simultaneously experience psychotic symptoms (delusions, hallucinations, disorganized speech and behavior, and/or negative symptoms) and prominent mood symptoms meeting the criteria for a major depressive or manic episode (see the chapter "Mood Disorders and Suicide"). Mood symptoms must be present for the majority of the period of illness. Unlike mood disorders with psychotic features, a diagnosis of schizoaffective disorder requires at least 2 weeks of hallucinations or delusions without mood symptoms (American Psychiatric Association, 2013).

The diagnosis of **schizophreniform disorder** requires that individuals meet Criteria A, D, and E for schizophrenia but show symptoms that last only 1 to

A significant percentage of people with schizophrenia end up homeless and on the streets. *Christopher Kerrigan/McGraw Hill*

6 months (Table 4). The 1- to 6-month duration requirement is intermediate between that for brief psychotic disorder (discussed next) and schizophrenia. Although functional impairments may be present, they are not necessary for a diagnosis of schizophreniform disorder. Individuals with this disorder who have a good prognosis have a quick onset of symptoms, functioned well previously, and experience confusion but not blunted or flat affect. Individuals who do not show two or more of these features are said to be without good prognostic features. The majority (about two-thirds) of individuals with schizophreniform disorder will eventually receive a diagnosis of schizophrenia or schizoaffective disorder (American Psychiatric Association, 2013).

TABLE 3   *DSM-5* Diagnostic Criteria for Schizoaffective Disorder

A. An uninterrupted period of illness during which there is a major mood episode (major depressive or manic) current with Criterion A of schizophrenia. Note: The major depressive episode must include Criterion A1: Depressed mood.

B. Delusions or hallucinations for 2 or more weeks in the absence of a major mood episode (depressive or manic) during the lifetime duration of the illness.

C. Symptoms that meet criteria for a major mood episode are present for the majority of the total duration of the active and residual portions of the illness.

D. The disturbance is not attributable to the effects of a substance (e.g., a drug of abuse, a medication) or another medical condition.

Specify type:

Bipolar type: A manic episode is part of the presentation. Major depressive episodes may also occur.

Depressive type: If only major depressive episodes are part of the presentation.

Specify if:

With catatonia

TABLE 4   *DSM-5* Diagnostic Criteria for Schizophreniform Disorder

A. Criteria A, D, and E of Schizophrenia are met (see Table 2).

B. An episode of the disorder lasts at least 1 month but less than 6 months. When the diagnosis must be made without waiting for recovery, it should be qualified as "provisional."

Specify if:

With good prognostic features: as evidenced by two or more of the following:

   1. Onset of prominent psychotic symptoms within 4 weeks of the first noticeable change in usual behavior or functioning

   2. Confusion or perplexity

   3. Good premorbid social and occupational functioning

   4. Absence of blunted or flat affect

Without good prognostic features

With catatonia

TABLE 5   *DSM-5* Diagnostic Criteria for Brief Psychotic Disorder

A. Presence of one (or more) of the following symptoms. At least one of these must be (1), (2), or (3):

   1. Delusions

   2. Hallucinations

   3. Disorganized speech (e.g., frequent derailment or incoherence)

   4. Grossly disorganized or catatonic behavior

   Note: Do not include a symptom if it is a culturally sanctioned response.

B. Duration of an episode of the disturbance is at least 1 day but less than 1 month, with eventual full return to premorbid level of functioning.

C. The disturbance is not better explained by major depressive or bipolar disorder with psychotic features or another psychotic disorder such as schizophrenia or catatonia, and is not attributable to the physiological effects of a substance (e.g., substance of abuse, a medication) or another medical condition.

Specify if:

With marked stressor(s) (brief reactive psychosis): if symptoms occur in response to events that, singly or together, would be markedly stressful to almost anyone in similar circumstances in the individual's culture.

Without marked stressor(s): if symptoms do not occur in response to events that, singly or together, would be markedly stressful to almost anyone in similar circumstances in the individual's culture.

With postpartum onset: if onset is during pregnancy or within 4 weeks postpartum

With catatonia

Individuals with **brief psychotic disorder** show a sudden onset of delusions, hallucinations, disorganized speech, and/or disorganized behavior. However, the episode lasts only for 1 day to 1 month, after which the symptoms completely remit (Table 5). Symptoms sometimes emerge after a major stressor, such as being in an accident. At other times, no stressor is apparent. Approximately 1 in 10,000 women experience brief psychotic episodes shortly after giving birth (Steiner, Dunn, & Born, 2003; VanderKruik et al., 2017). Although risk of relapse is high, most people show an excellent outcome.

Individuals with **delusional disorder** (Table 6) have delusions lasting at least 1 month regarding

TABLE 6 *DSM-5* Diagnostic Criteria for Delusional Disorder

A. The presence of one (or more) delusions with a duration of 1 month or longer.

B. Criterion A of schizophrenia has never been met. Note: Hallucinations, if present, are not prominent and are related to the delusional theme (e.g., the sensation of being infested with insects associated with delusions of infestation).

C. Apart from the impact of the delusion(s) or its ramifications, functioning is not markedly impaired, and behavior is not obviously bizarre or odd.

D. If manic or major depressive episodes have occurred, these have been brief relative to the duration of the delusional periods.

E. The disturbance is not attributable to the physiological effects of a substance or another medical condition and is not better explained by another mental disorder, such as body dysmorphic disorder or obsessive-compulsive disorder.

Specify whether:

Erotomanic type: The central theme of the delusion is that another person is in love with the individual.

Grandiose type: The central theme of the delusion is the conviction of having some great (but unrecognized) talent or insight or having made some important discovery.

Jealous type: The central theme of the delusion is that one's spouse or lover is unfaithful.

Persecutory type: The central theme of the delusion is the belief that one is being conspired against, cheated, spied on, followed, poisoned or drugged, maliciously maligned, harassed, or obstructed in the pursuit of long-term goals.

Somatic type: The central theme of the delusion involves bodily functions or sensations.

Mixed type: No one delusional theme predominates.

Unspecified type: The dominant delusional belief cannot be clearly determined or is not described in the specific types (e.g., referential delusions without a prominent persecutory or grandiose theme).

Specify if:

With bizarre content: If delusions are clearly implausible, not understandable, and not derived from ordinary life experiences (e.g., delusional belief that one's internal organs have been removed by a stranger and replaced with someone else's organs without leaving any wounds or scars).

situations that occur in real life, such as being followed, being poisoned, being deceived by a spouse, or having a disease. Unlike schizophrenia, people with delusional disorder do not show any other psychotic symptoms. Other than the behaviors that are related to their delusions, they do not act oddly or have difficulty functioning. In the general population, delusional disorder is relatively rare, with an estimated lifetime prevalence range from 0.05 to 0.2 percent (American Psychiatric Association, 2013; Joseph & Siddiqui, 2020). The prevalence of delusional disorder is less common than other disorders like schizophrenia, bipolar disorder, and various mood disorders which may be due, in part, to underreporting. People with this disorder are less likely to seek out mental health services on their own and typically only receive therapeutic intervention when forced by family or friends. The mean age of onset is about 40 years, but the range is from 18 years to 90 years, which is considerable. The persecutory and jealous subtype of delusional disorder is more

common in males, while the erotomanic variety is more common in females.

Treatment can be difficult since these clients often have poor insight into their behaviors, but symptoms can improve with a combination of psychotherapy and antipsychotic medication. The prognosis of delusional disorder is better with treatment and medication compliance with almost 50 percent of clients making a full recovery, more than 20 percent of clients reporting decreased symptoms and less than 20 percent of clients reporting minimal to no change in symptoms. A good prognosis is also related to earlier onset of symptoms (prior to 30 years), higher social and occupational functioning, sudden onset of symptoms, and short duration. Women also have a better prognosis than men with delusional disorder (Joseph & Siddiqui, 2020).

Although included as part of the schizophrenia spectrum of disorders, **Schizotypal personality disorder** (Table 7) is the only disorder on the psychotic continuum that is not a psychotic disorder, but rather a

TABLE 7   Diagnostic Criteria for Schizotypal Personality Disorder

A. A pervasive pattern of social and interpersonal deficits marked by acute discomfort with, and reduced capacity for, close relationships as well as by cognitive or perceptual distortions and eccentricities of behavior, beginning by early adulthood and present in a variety of contexts, as indicated by five or more of the following:

1. Ideas of reference (excluding delusions of reference).

2. Odd beliefs or magical thinking that influences behavior and is inconsistent with subcultural norms (e.g., super-stitiousness, belief in clairvoyance, telepathy, or "sixth sense"; in children and adolescents, bizarre fantasies or preoccupations).

3. Unusual perceptual experiences, including bodily illusions.

4. Odd thinking and speech (e.g., vague, circumstantial, metaphorical, overelaborate, or stereotyped).

5. Suspiciousness or paranoid ideation.

6. Inappropriate or constricted affect.

7. Behavior or appearance that is odd, eccentric, or peculiar.

8. Lack of close friends or confidants other than first-degree relatives.

9. Excessive social anxiety that does not diminish with familiarity and tends to be associated with paranoid fears rather than negative judgments about self.

B. Does not occur exclusively during the course of schizophrenia, a bipolar disorder or depressive disorder with psy-chotic features, another psychotic disorder, or autism spectrum disorder. Note: If criteria are met prior to the onset of schizophrenia, add "premorbid," e.g., "schizotypal personality disorder (premorbid)."

personality disorder. Schizotypal personality disor-der falls below the threshold required for a diagnosis of a psychotic disorder, but the *DSM-5* recognizes it as part of the schizophrenia spectrum of disorders (Heckers et al., 2013). More information about schizotypal personality disorder is presented in the chapter "Personality Disorders." People with this dis-order have a lifelong pattern of peculiar behaviors that impact their personality and self-concept, their social and interpersonal function (empathy, inti-macy), and their thinking and behavior. The eccen-tric behaviors that characterize this disorder and disturbed thought and affect are similar to those seen in schizophrenia, however, the symptom develop-ment and course of this disorder resemble those of a personality disorder (PD).

Individuals with schizotypal personality disorder experience pathological personality traits that include psychoticism, eccentricity, cognitive and perceptual dysregulation, unusual beliefs, unusual beliefs, and re-stricted affect and emotional withdrawal character-ized by suspiciousness (Kirchner, Roeh, Nolden, & Hasan, 2018). They may have few close relationships and trouble understanding the behaviors of others. They tend to perceive other people as deceitful and hostile and may be socially anxious and isolated be-cause of their suspiciousness. People with schizotypal personality disorder think and behave in ways that are very odd, although they maintain their grasp on real-ity. People with this disorder may believe that random events or circumstances are related to them (*ideas of reference*). For example, they may think it highly sig-nificant that a fire occurred in a store in which they had shopped only yesterday. Their perceptions are also odd—for example, thinking they see people in the patterns of wallpaper. They may be easily distracted or fixate on an object for long periods of time, lost in thought or fantasy. The prevalence of schizotypal per-sonality disorder has been described as ranging from 0.6 percent in a Norwegian sample to 4.6 percent in an American sample, but appears to be less frequent in clinical settings (0 to 1.9 percent) (American Psychiatric Association, 2013).

On neuropsychological tests (see the chapter "Assessing and Diagnosing Abnormality"), people with schizotypal personality disorder show deficits in working memory, learning, and recall similar to, but less severe than, those shown by people with schizophrenia (Barch & Sheffield, 2017). They also share some of the same genetic traits and neurologi-cal abnormalities of people with schizophrenia (Cannon, van Erp, & Glahn, 2002). Some people diagnosed with schizotypal personality disorder have episodes symptomatic of brief psychotic disorder, and some eventually develop the full syndrome of schizophrenia.

Read the following case study (adapted from Andreasen, 1998).

Jeff, age 19, had been a normal but somewhat shy kid until about 2 years ago. On a high school trip to France, he had become acutely anxious and returned home early. After that, Jeff began to withdraw. He no longer wanted to be with friends, and he dropped off the football team. His grades plummeted from his usual A's and B's, but he was able to graduate. His parents commented that a gradual but dramatic personality change had taken place over the past 2 years, and he just seemed "empty." All their efforts to encourage him, to help him find new directions, or to reassess his goals seemed to have led nowhere.

Jeff had begun coursework in college but was unable to study and dropped out. He got a job delivering pizzas but couldn't even find his way around town—the town he had grown up in—to deliver the pizzas to the right addresses. His parents reported that he seemed suspicious much of the time and that he had no desire to be around friends or peers. Jeff didn't seem to care about anything. His grooming and hygiene had deteriorated. The apartment he rented was filthy and full of decaying food and dirty laundry. He had no history of drug abuse of any type.

When interviewed by a psychiatrist, Jeff said he did not feel sad or blue, just "empty." Jeff reported no experiences of hearing voices when no one was around, seeing things that other people can't see, or feeling like he'd lost control of his mind or body.

Does Jeff have schizophrenia or one of the disorders along the schizophrenia spectrum? (Discussion appears at the end of this chapter.)

BIOLOGICAL THEORIES

Given the similarity in the symptoms and prevalence of schizophrenia across cultures and time, biological factors have long been thought key to its development. There are several biological theories of schizophrenia. First, evidence indicates genetic transmission, although genetics does not fully explain who develops this disorder. Second, some people with schizophrenia show structural and functional abnormalities in specific areas of the brain, which may contribute to the disorder. Third, many people with schizophrenia have a history of birth complications or prenatal exposure to viruses, which may affect brain development. Fourth, neurotransmitter theories hold that excess levels of dopamine contribute to schizophrenia; newer research also focuses on the neurotransmitters serotonin, GABA, and glutamate.

Genetic Contributors to Schizophrenia

Genes are considered the strongest risk factor for development of schizophrenia. Family, twin, and adoption studies all indicate the presence of a genetic component in the transmission of schizophrenia which make genetics a critical risk factor. Studies conducted over the last few decades have found the genetic architecture of schizophrenia to be highly complex, heterogeneous, and polygenic, but much still remains unknown. Schizophrenia is a multifactorial disorder, which is largely influenced by the interplay of multiple susceptibility genes, epigenetic processes, and environmental factors (Tifu, Kohn, Vlasie, & Patrichi, 2020). Gene-environment interactions play a critical role in the neurodevelopmental model of schizophrenia. Research has demonstrated beyond doubt that genetics constitutes a strong risk factor for schizophrenia, but despite recent advances in molecular genetics, the cause and subsequent development of schizophrenia and the genotype-environment interactions remain largely unknown (Chou et al., 2017; Henriksen, Nordgaard, & Jansson, 2017). Various studies suggest the cause of schizophrenia is multifactorial and reflects an interaction between genetic vulnerabilities and environmental risk factors. Environmental contributors, such as pregnancy and birth complications, childhood trauma, urban birth, migration, social isolation, and substance abuse interact at various levels over time and influence the individual's likelihood to develop the disorder (Stilo & Murray, 2019). Research suggests that that multiple genes interact with environmental factors to increase the risk of schizophrenia (Schmidt-Kastner, Guloksuz, Kietzmann, Van Os, & Rutten, 2020). Meaning, it must be assumed that both genetics and environment experiences are strongly associated with the development of schizophrenia, but exactly how genetic vulnerabilities interact with environment risk factors to develop schizophrenia is still being explored.

Family Studies

A significant contribution of family, twin, and adoption studies is determining the proportional increase in risk for disease with the degree of genetic relationship to a person suffering from schizophrenia (Tifu, Kohn, Vlasie, & Patrichi, 2020). Meaning, how likely are you to develop schizophrenia if a member of your family has also developed this disorder? Psychologist Irving Gottesman compiled more than 40 studies to

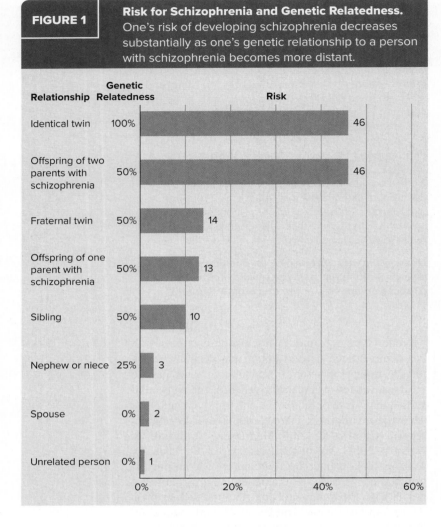

FIGURE 1 | **Risk for Schizophrenia and Genetic Relatedness.** One's risk of developing schizophrenia decreases substantially as one's genetic relationship to a person with schizophrenia becomes more distant.

research provides additional support for the heritability of schizophrenia finding that the prevalence of schizophrenia in individuals with an affected first-degree relative is six times higher than in the general population. Among individuals with an affected second-degree relative, the risk of developing schizophrenia increases by 2.4 percent (Chou et al., 2017).

The nature of heredity in schizophrenia goes beyond the simple genetic percentages of risk, and culminates in a complex landscape of different genetic levels of risk that are complex and variable. For example, recent studies have estimated a 27 percent risk of developing schizophrenia for children of two affected parents and 50 percent for MZ twins and an adopted child with a biological parent with schizophrenia, the risk for disease is 6 to 10 times higher than the general population (Tifu et al., 2020). Extensive research shows that the relationship between an individual's degree of genetic similarity to a relative with schizophrenia and the individual's own risk of developing schizophrenia play a role in the development of schizophrenia, but it's complicated.

Despite the growing evidence that schizophrenia is strongly genetically correlated, it is important to remember that biology is not destiny. Meaning, having a biological relative with schizophrenia may increase an individual's risk for the disorder, but it does guarantee that the disorder will develop. For example, of all children who have one parent with schizophrenia, 87 percent will not develop the disorder. Research has shown that a family history of schizophrenia is also associated with a higher degree of risk for developing schizophrenia, but also mood and delusional disorders. Offspring of parents with severe mental illness (SMI) are at increased risk for a range of psychiatric disorders and one-third of them may develop a mental illness by early adulthood. Interestingly, family members of people with schizophrenia are at elevated risk of having bipolar disorder—and vice versa—suggesting shared genetic factors (Lichtenstein et al., 2009). A nationwide study in Sweden found that a child of a parent with schizophrenia is five times more likely to develop bipolar disorder than the general population. Research also found that having an affected sibling increases the likelihood of developing bipolar disorder by more than three times.

Schizophrenia is regarded as a neurodevelopmental disorder in which defective genes and environmental factors interact to induce symptoms of the disorder. Additional research from the International Schizophrenia Consortium (ISC) found substantial shared genetic association between schizophrenia and bipolar disorder. Since heritability and environmental factors each account for half of the phenotypic variance, evidence suggests that both genetic and shared environmental factors contribute significantly to the development of this disorder. (Chou et al., 2017).

determine the lifetime risk of developing schizophrenia for people with various familial relationships to a person with schizophrenia (Gottesman & Shields, 1976). His conclusions are summarized in Figure 1. The children of two parents with schizophrenia and monozygotic (MZ, identical) twins of people with schizophrenia share the greatest number of genes with people with schizophrenia. As the top bars of the graph in Figure 1 show, these individuals also have the greatest risk of developing schizophrenia at some time in their lives.

As the genetic similarity to a person with schizophrenia decreases, an individual's risk of developing schizophrenia also decreases. Thus, a first-degree relative of a person with schizophrenia (e.g., a non-twin sibling), who shares about 50 percent of genes with the person with schizophrenia, has about a 10 percent chance of developing the disorder. In contrast, a niece or nephew of a person with schizophrenia, who shares about 25 percent of genes with the person with schizophrenia, has only a 3 percent chance of developing the disorder. The risk for developing schizophrenia is less than 1 percent in the general population. Recent

Adoption Studies

Even when the child of a person with schizophrenia develops the disorder, it may not be due to genetics. A home with a parent with schizophrenia is likely to be a stressful environment. When a parent is psychotic, the child may be exposed to illogical thought, mood swings, and chaotic behavior. Even when the parent is not actively psychotic, the residual negative symptoms of schizophrenia—restriction of affect, lack of motivation, and disorganization—may impair the parent's child-care skills.

Twin and adoption studies are the most frequently used study designs to examine heritability. For example, Seymour Kety and colleagues (1994) found that the biological relatives of adoptees with schizophrenia were 10 times more likely to have a diagnosis of schizophrenia than were the biological relatives of adoptees who did not have schizophrenia. In contrast, the adoptive relatives of adoptees with schizophrenia showed no increased risk for the disorder.

In one of the largest adoption studies, Pekka Tienari (Tienari et al., 2003; Tienari, Wahlberg, & Wynne, 2006) tracked 155 offspring of mothers with schizophrenia and 185 children of mothers without schizophrenia; all the children had been given up for adoption early in life. Approximately 10 percent of the children whose biological mother had schizophrenia developed schizophrenia or another psychotic disorder, compared to about 1 percent of the children whose biological mother did not have schizophrenia.

Twin Studies

If schizophrenia has strong genetic contributions, it makes sense to examine individuals who share the most DNA, like twins. In general, heritability estimates derived from twin studies are higher than those based on the general population often ranging between 41 and 87 percent. High rates of heritability have been shown among twins with schizophrenia in a meta-analysis that included 12 different European and North American studies. This research utilized a multi-group twin model and found heritability of up to 81 percent, as well as evidence for shared environmental influences on schizophrenia (Popovic et al., 2019; Tifu et al., 2020). Research conducted in Sweden found a slightly lower rate of heritability at 64.3 percent, while other studies in Taiwan found even lower rates at 47.3 percent in their population. Although these studies found lower rates of schizophrenia among twin sets, the heritability estimates are still substantial. Differences in these rates are most likely reflect variations in the research methods used (Chou et al., 2017). This research provides strong support for the genetic transmission of schizophrenia. Meaning the more genes shared with a person who is affected by schizophrenia the more likely the disorder will develop in that family member. Several adoption studies

The Genain quadruplets all later developed schizophrenia, but the specific forms of the disorder differed among the sisters. *AP Photo*

addressing the question of genes versus environment indicate that genetics plays an important role in schizophrenia. Figure 1 also shows the compiled results of several twin studies of schizophrenia. The results show a concordance rate for MZ (identical) twins of 46 percent, and a concordance rate for dizygotic (fraternal) twins of 14 percent.

Even when a person carries a genetic risk for schizophrenia, however, many other biological and environmental factors may influence whether and how he or she manifests the disorder. The classic illustration of this point is the story of the Genain quadruplets, who shared the same genes and family environment. All of them developed schizophrenia, but their specific symptoms, onset, course, and outcomes varied substantially (Mirsky et al., 2000).

Recently researchers have been investigating epigenetic factors that influence the expression of genes (Cromby, Chung, Papadopoulos, & Talbot, 2016). Recall from the chapter "Theories and Treatment of Abnormality" that DNA can be chemically modified by different environmental conditions, resulting in genes being turned on or off, thereby altering the development of cells, tissues, and organs. When MZ twins who were discordant for schizophrenia (i.e., one twin had schizophrenia, but the other twin did not) were compared with MZ twins who both had schizophrenia, researchers found that the MZ twins discordant for schizophrenia showed numerous differences in the molecular structure of their DNA, particularly on genes regulating dopamine systems. In contrast, the MZ twins concordant for schizophrenia showed many fewer molecular differences in their DNA (Petronis et al., 2003). The reasons for these epigenetic differences are unclear, but they likely involve effects of stress (Howes, McCutcheon, Owen, & Murray, 2017). A number of environmental events that could affect development in utero appear to increase the risk for schizophrenia. Some of these events might alter genes that guide brain development (Diwadkar, Bustamante, Rai, & Uddin, 2014).

The main justification for molecular genetics studies of enduring psychosis (schizophrenia) is high heritability estimates obtained from classical twin studies. The classical twin method rests upon the equal environment assumption (EEA), which holds that reared-together identical and fraternal twin pairs grow up experiencing equally similar environmental exposures. However, a review of prior twin studies shows that identical twins are more similar than fraternal twins on childhood exposures that are central to the etiology of psychosis. Such exposures include bullying, sexual abuse, physical maltreatment, emotional neglect and abuse, and general trauma. An additional assumption presented by twin researchers, that the differential intraclass correlation for child social adversities can be explained by evocative gene–environment covariation, is not consistent with the available evidence. Moreover, due to an array of methodological problems and questionable assumptions, adoption studies provide misleading indications in support of genetic effects. As a result, direct studies of DNA variations in schizophrenia must stand on their own ground. Possible minor findings

from such molecular genetics studies, when combined with the available evidence of environmental effects, support a stress-based sociopsychobiological model of schizophrenia etiology (Fosse Joseph & Jones, 2016).

Structural and Functional Brain Abnormalities

Clinicians and researchers have long believed that the brains of people with schizophrenia differ fundamentally from those of people without schizophrenia. With the development of technologies such as positron-emission tomography (PET scans), computerized axial tomography (CAT scans), and magnetic resonance imaging (MRI), scientists have been able to examine in detail the structure and functioning of the brain. These new technologies have shown major structural and functional deficits in the brains of some people with schizophrenia (Barch & Sheffield, 2017; Karlsgodt, Sun, & Cannon, 2010). Most theorists think of schizophrenia as a neurodevelopmental disorder, in which a variety of factors lead to abnormal development of the brain in the uterus and early in life.

The most consistent finding is a gross reduction in gray matter in the cortex of people with schizophrenia, particularly in the medial, temporal, superior temporal, and prefrontal areas (Figure 2; Karlsgodt et al., 2010). In addition, people who are at risk for schizophrenia because of a family history but have not yet developed the disorder show abnormal activity in the prefrontal cortex (Lawrie, McIntosh, Hall, Owens, & Johnstone, 2008). The prefrontal cortex is important in language, emotional expression, planning, and carrying out plans. The prefrontal cortex connects to all other cortical regions, as well as to the limbic system, which is involved in emotion and cognition, and to the basal ganglia, which is involved in motor movement. Thus, it seems logical that a person with an unusually small or inactive prefrontal cortex would show the deficits in cognition, emotion, and social interactions seen with schizophrenia, such as difficulty holding a conversation, responding appropriately to social situations, and carrying out tasks.

The prefrontal cortex undergoes major development in the years from adolescence to young adulthood (Galván & Tottenham, 2016). Aberrations in the normal development of the prefrontal cortex during mid- to late adolescence may help explain the emergence of the disorder during this period (Cannon et al., 2003). Neuroimaging studies of individuals who developed schizophrenia in adolescence show significant structural changes across the cortex, particularly in the prefrontal cortex, from before to after development of symptoms (Figure 2; Sun et al., 2009).

FIGURE 2 | **Enlarged Ventricles in People with Schizophrenia.** The left panel shows the brain of a healthy male. The right panel shows the brain of his identical twin, who has schizophrenia. Notice the larger ventricles (blue spaces midbrain) in the brain of the twin with schizophrenia.

Schizophrenia Patients (n=12)   Healthy volunteers (n=10)

Photo Researchers/Science History Images/Alamy Stock Photo

The hippocampus is another brain area that consistently differs from the norm in people with schizophrenia (Karlsgodt et al., 2010). The hippocampus plays a critical role in the formation of long-term memories. In some studies, people with schizophrenia show abnormal hippocampal activation when doing tasks that require them to encode information for storage in their memory or to retrieve information from memory (Barch, Csernansky, Conturo, & Snyder, 2002; Schacter, Chiao, & Mitchell, 2003). Other studies show that people with schizophrenia have abnormalities in the volume and shape of their hippocampus and at the cellular level (Knable, Barci, Webster, Meador-Woodruff, & Torrey, 2004; Lieberman et al., 2018). Similar abnormalities in the hippocampus are found in the first-degree relatives of people with schizophrenia (Seidman et al., 2002).

In addition to reductions in gray matter, the brains of people with schizophrenia show reductions and abnormalities in white matter (material that forms the connections between areas of the brain), particularly in areas associated with working memory (Karlsgodt et al., 2008). These white-matter abnormalities are present in individuals before they develop overt symptoms of schizophrenia, suggesting that they are early signs of the disorder rather than consequences of the disease process (Karlsgodt, Niendam, Bearden, & Cannon, 2009). White-matter abnormalities can impair the ability of various areas of the brain to work together, which could lead to the severe deficits seen in schizophrenia.

Along with these changes in the structure and activity of cortical and other brain areas, people with schizophrenia show enlargement of ventricles, fluid-filled spaces in the brain (Lawrie et al., 2008). Enlarged ventricles suggest atrophy, or deterioration, in other brain tissue. People with schizophrenia with enlarged ventricles tend to show social, emotional, and behavioral deficits long before they develop the core symptoms of schizophrenia. They also tend to have more severe symptoms than other people with schizophrenia and are less responsive to medication. These characteristics suggest gross alterations in the functioning of the brain, which are difficult to alleviate with treatment.

Damage to the Developing Brain

What causes the neuroanatomical abnormalities in schizophrenia? According to recent research, genetic and epigenetic factors seem to play a major role (Howes et al., 2017). In addition, these abnormalities may be tied to birth complications, traumatic brain injury, viral infections, nutritional deficiencies, and deficiencies in cognitive stimulation (Barch & Sheffield, 2017; Howes & Murray, 2014). A variety of birth complications are well-documented risk factors for

schizophrenia which includes emergency cesarean sections, bleeding during pregnancy, preeclampsia, gestational diabetes, and low birth weight. Additionally, the use of forceps and low birth weight typically predict earlier age of onset of psychosis (Patel, Cherian, Gohil, & Atkinson, 2014; Stilo & Murray, 2019).

Birth Complications Serious prenatal and birth difficulties are more frequent in the histories of people with schizophrenia than in those of people without schizophrenia and may play a role in the development of neurological difficulties (Cannon et al., 2003; Kotlicka-Antczak et al., 2017). While symptoms of schizophrenia typically manifest in young adulthood, the neurodevelopmental theory of schizophrenia suggests that a damage during neurodevelopment produces long-term detrimental effects on the brain. Studies have found evidence that perinatal factors including environment, parental influence on the fetus during pregnancy and obstetric complications contribute to the risk of developing schizophrenia. (Jenkins, 2013). Moreover, a longitudinal study of individuals at high risk for schizophrenia found that those with a history of obstetric difficulties were more likely to develop the full syndrome of schizophrenia than were those without such a history (Mittal et al., 2009).

One complication that may be especially important in neurological development is perinatal hypoxia which is a birth complication that occurs when a baby receives inadequate oxygen supply to the brain before, during, or after delivery. This lack of necessary oxygen can cause changes to brain function and anatomy that is associated with the subsequent development of schizophrenia. Research has shown brain abnormalities among people with schizophrenia who were exposed to perinatal hypoxia. It is posited that the lack of adequate oxygen to the developing brain impairs neuronal development.

Studies have shown that hypoxia seems to contribute to a reduction in the gray matter and an enlargement in the lateral ventricular zone. Interestingly, studies have also shown that a strong correlation between hypertension during pregnancy and women who became mothers to individuals with schizophrenia. Studies using rodents show that exposure to chronic hypoxia may lead to loss of tissue volume, decreased myelination, and increased ventricles, which are often brain abnormalities observed in people with schizophrenia (e Silva, Brito, Yuzawa, & Rosenstock, 2019). Immune system response and brain inflammation are significant prenatal risk factors for schizophrenia since inflammation produces similar outcomes to hypoxia (Schmidt-Kastner et al., 2020). Research has found that infants who suffered from perinatal hypoxia are twice as likely to develop schizophrenia later in later life. However, the exact

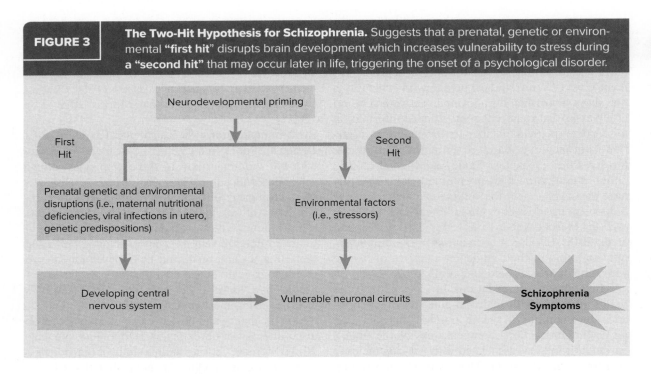

FIGURE 3   **The Two-Hit Hypothesis for Schizophrenia.** Suggests that a prenatal, genetic or environmental **"first hit"** disrupts brain development which increases vulnerability to stress during a **"second hit"** that may occur later in life, triggering the onset of a psychological disorder.

pathway from fetal exposure to the outbreak of the disease decades later are unknown. Research suggests that the effects of oxygen deprivation interact with a genetic vulnerability to schizophrenia, resulting in a person's developing the disorder. Most people experiencing oxygen deprivation prenatally or at birth do not develop schizophrenia, however (Hefter, Marti, Gass, & Inta, 2018). The two-hit model (Figure 3) suggests psychiatric conditions may be the result of a disturbance in brain developmental during the weeks before or after birth (*perinatal*). This disturbance disrupts the neuronal circuits and causes increased vulnerability to stress during periods of critical brain development. Psychosocial stressors that are experienced later in life may then trigger the onset of the disorder. Meaning, the first "hit" disrupts some aspect of brain development, and establishes increased vulnerability to a second "hit" that may occur later in life that riggers the onset of psychiatric symptoms (Popovic et al, 2019).

Maternal Illness and Prenatal Exposure Epidemiological studies have shown high rates of schizophrenia among persons whose mothers were exposed to infections and diseases such as influenza, rubella, toxoplasmosis, and herpes during pregnancy or delivery (Stilo & Murray, 2019). Research on this topic spans decades and has produced significant evidence of increased rates of schizophrenia in women who were pregnant during flu epidemics. These early studies were critical in identifying maternal risks of exposure to illness which clarified the boundaries of **pathogenic**

exposures and subsequently led contemporary studies to expand from viral to bacterial infections. Recent research on maternal bacterial infection during pregnancy was significantly associated with subsequent development of schizophrenia among offspring. A localized bacterial infection predicted a 1.6-fold increased risk of developing a psychotic disorder in adulthood, and system-wide bacterial infection predicted a nearly three-fold increase in the development of a psychotic disorder. Maternal bacterial infections during pregnancy are more strongly associated with the development of schizophrenia in male rather than female offspring for reasons that are not fully known (Kendler, 2020; Patel, Cherian, Gohil & Atkinson, 2014).

The idea that the development of schizophrenia could be traced to the fetal period was first hypothesized with correlational evidence of birth season and the incidence of this disorder (Kendler, 2020). Early studies found a relationship between flu season and the future development of schizophrenia in children whose mothers were infected with influenza. Interestingly, people with schizophrenia are somewhat more likely to be born in the spring months than at other times of the year (Ellman & Cannon, 2008). This suggests that pregnant women may be more likely to contract influenza and other viruses at critical phases of fetal development if they are pregnant during the fall and winter. Research has found an increased risk of developing schizophrenia after maternal exposure to viruses like influenza, measles, rubella, varicella-zoster, polio, and herpes, as well as bacterial and parasitic infections during pregnancy. It is posited that maternal and fetal inflammatory responses to infection may alter fetal neurodevelopment.

The COVID-19 pandemic began as a cluster of unknown viral pneumonias reported in Wuhan, China and now exceeds 17 million cases globally. Throughout the world, communities have experienced significant infection rates of COVID-19 which are expected to increase. Researches from previous viral pandemics and influenza epidemics have found increased incidences of psychiatric conditions such as anxiety, insomnia, depression, psychosis, and schizophrenia (Zimmer, Youngblood, Adnane, Miller, & Goldsmith, 2021). Coronaviruses may pose a significant risk for development of psychotic disorders, like schizophrenia, since they enter the brain through the olfactory pathway and have been found in human brain tissue after death (*post mortem*). Additionally, some studies suggest that COVID-19 may be transmitted from mother to fetus *in utero* which can directly impact fetal brain development. There is some evidence that viral infections like COVID-19 may be general risk factors for psychotic disorders and can have both acute and chronic effects on brain development. This suggests that viral infections prompt a mother's immune system to be more active, which can negatively impact the development of brain cells and dopamine systems in the fetus (see also Kneeland & Fatemi, 2013).

There is strong evidence that maternal immune activation (MIA) is linked to the development of psychiatric disorders such as autism spectrum disorder (ASD) and schizophrenia in offspring. C-reactive protein (CRP) is a biomarker of inflammation from both infectious and noninfectious exposures. A recent study of pregnant women infected with COVID-19 showed elevated concentrations of CRP which indicates the presence of severe inflammation. Due to the continued spread of COVID-19 around the world, the number of pregnant women exposed to this virus is expected to increase. This raises concerns among researchers who anticipate these increased rates of COVID-19 infection will likely increase the incidence of psychotic disorders worldwide (Cowan, 2020). Given the risk of MIA in neuropsychiatric disorders such as ASD and schizophrenia, follow-up investigations of pregnant women infected with COVID-19 are critical to better understand their impact on offspring.

Research studies have been conducted to assess the risks for schizophrenia using animals born to viral exposed mothers. Various studies have found similarities to human patients with schizophrenia, including structural abnormalities in brain changes in dopamine activation, increased markers of inflammation and impairments in attention and working memory. Additionally, some of these symptoms have been reversed with antipsychotic medications (Zimmer et al., 2021).

Studies suggest that an anti-inflammatory diet that includes leafy green vegetables like kale, cauliflower, broccoli, and brussels sprouts for pregnant women with COVID-19 infection and their children may reduce the risk of neuropsychiatric disorders such as ASD and schizophrenia (Hashimoto, 2020).

The second trimester of pregnancy is a crucial period for fetal brain development. It is hypothesized that disruption of brain development may cause the structural deficits found in the brains of some people with schizophrenia. Growing evidence suggests that maternal infections can lead to fetal brain injury, neurodevelopmental abnormalities, and an elevated lifetime risk for certain psychiatric disorders in the children. Additionally, research has found that maternal inflammation is also associated with changes in fetal serotonin production which may lead to atypical brain development. This effect on brain development and the subsequent development of psychiatric symptoms is likely dependent on the severity of infection and offspring sex. It is possible that an inflammatory fetal brain injury to an individual with genetic susceptibility creates an increased risk of developing future psychiatric conditions (Al-Haddad et al., 2019; Kendler, 2020). Individuals whose mothers had been exposed to the herpes simplex virus while pregnant were also more likely to have a psychotic disorder, most often schizophrenia (Buka, Cannon, Torrey, Yolken, & the Collaborative Study Group on the Perinatal Origins of Severe Psychotic Disorders 2008).

The Gut Microbiome Identifying the factors that are most associated with the development of psychological disorders is critical and currently there is no shortage of theories. There are countless studies that attempt to isolate the factors that predict the onset of psychiatric symptoms. One idea is the association of psychiatric illness with altered gut microbiota composition. As discussed in Chapter 7: Theories of Depression, the gut microbiome is made up of the collection of bacteria, fungi, and viruses, harbored in the gastrointestinal tract which significantly impacts brain function (Martinez, Leone, & Chang, 2017).

Neurotransmitters

The neurotransmitter dopamine has long been thought to play a critical role in schizophrenia (Howes, McCutcheon, & Stone, 2015). The original dopamine theory suggested that the symptoms of schizophrenia are caused by excess levels of dopamine in the brain, particularly in the prefrontal cortex and the limbic system, which are associated with positive symptoms, like hallucinations and delusions. The diathesis–stress model suggests that the hypothalamus-pituitary-adrenal (HPA) axis may trigger a cascade of events resulting in neural circuit dysfunction, including alterations in dopamine production (Stilo & Murray, 2019). Sensitivity to stress may increase an individual's vulnerability to developing schizophrenia since a stress-induced activation of the HPA axis contributes to dopamine release. These effects are important because increased amounts of this neurotransmitter are hypothesized as a critical factor in the pathophysiology of schizophrenia. This idea is further supported by the antipsychotic effects of dopamine receptor antagonists that block the action of dopamine (Popovic et al., 2019).

Medications used to reduce the symptoms of schizophrenia, such as **phenothiazines** or **neuroleptics,** block the reuptake of dopamine. Conversely, drugs that increase the levels of dopamine in the brain, such as amphetamines, tend to increase the incidence of the positive symptoms of schizophrenia (Davis, Kahn, Ko, & Davidson, 1991; Dela Peña, Gevorkiana, & Shi, 2015). The original dopamine theory of schizophrenia suggested that increased levels of this neurotransmitter contribute to symptomatology, but this theory proved too simple since many people do not respond to phenothiazines (Davis et al., 1991; Howes et al., 2015). Some people with schizophrenia who do respond to the phenothiazines tend to experience more relief from positive symptoms (hallucinations and delusions) than from negative symptoms. This suggests that simple dopamine depletion does not fully explain the negative symptoms. Furthermore, levels of dopamine change relatively soon after drug therapy begins, while changes in symptoms often require more time. This suggests that the level of dopamine in the brain is not the only determinant of symptoms (Hengartner & Moncrieff, 2018). Neuroimaging studies also suggest the presence of more dopamine receptors and higher levels of dopamine in some areas of the brain in people with schizophrenia than in people without the disorder.

Kenneth Davis and colleagues (1991) proposed a revised theory suggesting that different types of dopamine receptors and different levels of dopamine in various areas of the brain can account for the symptoms of schizophrenia. First, there may be excess dopamine activity in the **mesolimbic pathway,** a subcortical part of the brain involved in the processing of salience and reward (Figure 4). Abnormal functioning in this area of the brain may lead individuals to attribute importance to otherwise insignificant stimuli. This dysfunction may contribute to the development of symptoms such as hallucinations and delusions (Howes et al., 2015). Newer drugs in the treatment of schizophrenia, the *atypical antipsychotics,* may work to reduce the symptoms of schizophrenia by binding to a specific type of dopamine receptor common in the mesolimbic system, that blocks the action of dopamine.

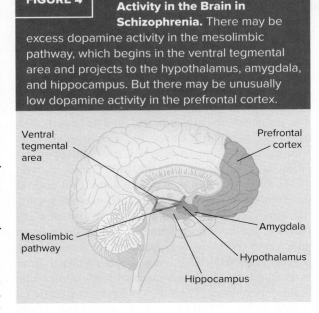

FIGURE 4   Areas of Abnormal Dopamine Activity in the Brain in Schizophrenia. There may be excess dopamine activity in the mesolimbic pathway, which begins in the ventral tegmental area and projects to the hypothalamus, amygdala, and hippocampus. But there may be unusually low dopamine activity in the prefrontal cortex.

Ventral tegmental area
Prefrontal cortex
Mesolimbic pathway
Amygdala
Hypothalamus
Hippocampus

Second, there may be unusually low dopamine activity in the prefrontal area of the brain, which is involved in attention, motivation, and the organization of behavior (Barch & Sheffield, 2017; Howes et al., 2015). Low dopamine activity here may lead to the negative symptoms of schizophrenia: lack of motivation, inability to care for oneself in daily functions, and the restriction of affect. This idea is consistent with the evidence associating structural and functional abnormalities in this part of the brain with the negative symptoms of schizophrenia. It also helps explain why the phenothiazines, which reduce dopamine activity, do not effectively alleviate the negative symptoms.

Although the revised version of the dopamine hypothesis was proposed over two decades ago, many of its components continue to be supported (see Howes et al., 2015). Dysregulation of dopamine systems seems to be involved in multiple forms of psychosis (and mood disorders), not just in schizophrenia.

Other neurotransmitters also play an important role in schizophrenia. Serotonin neurons regulate dopamine neurons in the mesolimbic system, and some of the newest drugs for treating schizophrenia bind to serotonin receptors (Howes et al., 2015). The interaction between serotonin and dopamine may be critical in schizophrenia. Still other research has found abnormal levels of the neurotransmitters glutamate and gamma-aminobutyric acid (GABA) in people with schizophrenia (Howes et al., 2015). Glutamate and GABA are widespread in the brain, and deficiencies could contribute to cognitive and emotional symptoms. Glutamate neurons are the major excitatory pathways linking the cortex, limbic system, and thalamus, regions of the brain shown to behave abnormally in people with schizophrenia. Drugs, such as PCP and ketamine, that block glutamate receptors cause hallucinations and delusions in otherwise healthy individuals.

PSYCHOSOCIAL PERSPECTIVES

Although schizophrenia is strongly linked to biological factors, social factors can influence its onset, course, and outcome.

Social Drift, Trauma, and Urban Living

People with schizophrenia are more likely than people without schizophrenia to experience chronically stressful circumstances, such as living in impoverished inner-city neighborhoods and having low-status occupations or being unemployed. The high correlation may be explained by **social drift** which is a theory that suggests that cumulative exposure to environmental risk factors in deprived and urban areas over time increases risk of psychological disorders, particularly for individuals with genetic predispositions. Risk factors such as, lack of social support, higher poverty and crime rates as well as reduced access to health care are associated with urban living (Dohrenwend, 2000., Lee et al., 2019; Patel, Cherian, Gohil, & Atkinson, 2014).

A classic study showing social drift tracked the socioeconomic status (SES)of men with schizophrenia and compared it to the status of their brothers and fathers (Goldberg & Morrison, 1963). The men with schizophrenia tended to end up in socioeconomic classes well below those of their fathers. In contrast, the healthy brothers of the men with schizophrenia tended to end up in socioeconomic classes equal to or higher than those of their fathers.

Since the symptoms of schizophrenia often interfere with a person's ability to complete an education and hold a job, it is theorized that people with schizophrenia tend to drift downward into lower SES or more deprived areas as compared to the class of their family of origin, but studies are inconclusive. For example, a recent longitudinal analysis showed that individuals with severe mental illnesses (SMIs) were more likely to move into areas with varying levels of deprivation and urban/rural indicators as compared to the general population after being diagnosed with a psychological disorder. Other studies have found only a slight downward social drift, measured by SES for communities in the USA, for individuals with schizophrenia during the course of 7-year hospitalization. Such drift was absent for individuals with other mental illnesses. Conversely, a recent Canadian study found evidence of social drift after migration from nonmetropolitan to metropolitan areas as well as from less socially to more socially deprived areas. Studies also show that younger individuals with schizophrenia move more frequently after illness onset which is typically related to the need for better access to mental health services. Frequent moves may also explain why individuals with schizophrenia experience more ongoing deprivation and unsupportive living arrangements when in cities before illness onset (Lee et al., 2019). While some recent data support the social drift theory, other research reaches the opposite conclusion: that social status and environments affect schizophrenia (Heinz, Deserno, & Reininghaus, 2013). Of course, both directions are possible or even likely (e.g., Lund & Cois, 2018), and the link may reflect other associated risk factors, such as genetics (Sariaslan et al., 2016).

Trauma and Social Adversity Various types of trauma and social adversities have been extensively examined as potential risk factors for schizophrenia across the lifespan. Childhood trauma is considered a severe form of stress that increases an individual's vulnerability to developing schizophrenia. Studies have found strong evidence that childhood adversity which includes sexual abuse, physical abuse, emotional/psychological abuse, neglect, parental death, and bullying, are associated with increased risk for psychosis in adulthood. Epidemiological studies show that childhood abuse and neglect increase the risk to later develop schizophrenia. Among persons with schizophrenia, the most frequent subtype of trauma was emotional neglect, but rates of physical abuse and physical neglect were also significantly higher (Popovic et al., 2019). Research has also found a robust relationship between childhood trauma and positive symptoms of schizophrenia in adulthood, particularly hallucinations and affective symptoms (Stilo & Murray, 2019).

People who grow up and/or live in an urban environment have an increased risk of developing schizophrenia or psychosis. Several studies also have shown that people with schizophrenia and other forms of psychosis are more likely to have been born in a large city than in a small town (Heinz et al., 2013; March et al., 2008; Stilo & Murray, 2019). For example, studies in the United States find that people with psychotic disorders are as much as five times more likely to have been born and raised in a large metropolitan area than in a rural area. Moving from a rural to an urban residence during childhood is also a risk factor that doubles the chances of developing schizophrenia, as does the amount of time a child spends in an urban area. As the number of years in an urban area increases, so does the risk of developing schizophrenia. There is significant evidence that higher rates of severe mental illness (SMI) are associated with urban neighborhoods characterized by higher levels of deprivation, poverty, and ethnic heterogeneity (Lee et al., 2020). Many explanations have been proposed such as greater exposure to maternal obstetrical complications, cannabis use, social deprivation, income inequality, and social fragmentation but none of them are conclusive (Stilo & Murray, 2019).

Many researchers argue that the link between urban living and psychosis is not limited to stressful conditions, but also to overcrowding which increases the risk that a pregnant woman or a newborn will be exposed to infectious agents. Many studies have shown that the rates of many infectious diseases—including influenza, tuberculosis, respiratory infections, herpes, and measles—are higher in crowded urban areas than in less crowded areas (Heinz et al., 2013). As noted earlier, there is a link between prenatal or perinatal exposure to infectious disease and schizophrenia. However, it is clear that social factors related to stress, including poverty, discrimination, and marginalization, also play a role (Heinz et al., 2013; Howes, McCutcheon, Owen, & Murray, 2017; March et al., 2008).

Various studies have shown that there is a strong relationship between psychotic experiences and exposure to cannabis use, childhood trauma, and living in cities. Studies suggest that cumulative exposure to these factors effectively predict persistent psychotic symptoms 3 years later in the general population. Research has also found that individuals who were exposed to four or more environmental risk factors had a significantly lower age of onset than those exposed to three factors. The amount of cumulative exposure to these environmental risk factors is likely to predict which individuals will display psychotic symptoms, and increased exposure is associated with early onset of symptoms (Stilo & Murray, 2019).

Stress and Relapse

Although stressful circumstances alone might not cause someone to develop schizophrenia, they might trigger new episodes in people with the disorder. Researchers have found higher levels of stress occurring shortly before the onset of a new episode compared to other times in the lives of people with schizophrenia (Norman & Malla, 1993). For example, in one study, researchers followed a group of people with schizophrenia for 1 year, interviewing them every 2 weeks to determine whether they had experienced any stressful events and/or any increase in their symptoms. Those

who experienced relapses of psychosis were more likely than those who did not to have experienced negative life events in the month before their relapse (Ventura, Neuchterlein, Lukoff, & Hardesty, 1989). Stressful events in adulthood may be especially important among people who experienced adverse events in childhood (Beards et al., 2013; Lataster, Myin-Germeys, Lieb, Wittchen, & van Os, 2011).

One major stressor linked to an increased risk for episodes in schizophrenia and other psychotic disorders is immigration (Alegría, Álvarez, & DiMarzio, 2017). Recent immigrants often have left behind extended networks of family and friends to move to a new country where they may know few people. They may face financial stress, particularly if the education they received in their native country isn't recognized in their new country. They may not know the language of their new country and may not be comfortable in the new culture. Studies in the United States and Britain have found that first- and second-generation immigrants have a higher incidence of acute symptoms of schizophrenia than individuals from their ethnic group who have been in the country longer or individuals native to the country. These findings have been consistently replicated in the United Kingdom, the Netherlands, Germany, Denmark, France, Italy, and to a lesser extent Canada with some evidence that the risk of schizophrenia and other psychotic disorders is especially high among refugees compared with nonrefugee migrants (Coid et al., 2008; Stilo & Murray, 2019)

It is clear that our life events, both positive and negative, impact our psychological health. Stressful life events such as the loss of loved one, financial hardship, or illness, are all examples of environmental factors that can contribute to the development of a psychological disorder. For those with schizophrenia and other psychotic disorders, research strongly supports the notion that stressful life events may exacerbate psychotic symptoms (Hussein, Jacoob, & Sharour, 2016). Relapse rates among individuals with psychotic disorders are particularly high and may be associated with stressful life events. Research has found a significant correlation between stressful life events like adult trauma, conflict, bereavement, and financial difficulties and the return of psychotic symptoms. Eighteen different studies found significant positive associations between adult stressful life events, occurring after the onset of psychosis, and psychotic relapse (N. Martland, R. Martland, Cullen, & Bhattacharyya, 2020; Mayo et al., 2017).

Volumes of research have consistently supported that negative life factors are likely to increase a person's vulnerability to developing schizophrenia. Conversely, there are also environmental factors that protect people from developing this disorder. Recent research suggests that exposure to household pets, specifically dogs, during infancy and early childhood may be associated with a significantly decreased risk of developing schizophrenia. Recent studies have found that exposure to a pet dog during pregnancy, infancy, or childhood has been associated with reduced inflammation and a decreased rate of immune-mediated disorders such as asthma and food allergies. It is theorized that exposure to a pet dog may alter immune activation and lower the risk of immune disorders and stress response, altering subsequent cortisol release. Research has also shown that exposure to a household pet dog can alter the intestinal microbiome of family members through contact with canine microflora, suggesting that exposure to pet dogs might affect intestinal inflammation and modulate the risk of schizophrenia through changes in the gut-brain axis. Recent studies have found lower rates of schizophrenia among those who had a pet dog present in the household at birth, which suggests in utero exposure during pregnancy, or during the first 3 years of life. Exposure during this period of time corresponds with immune activation which has been associated with altered neurodevelopment and an increased risk of psychiatric disorders (Yolken et al., 2019).

Schizophrenia and the Family

Historically, theorists blamed schizophrenia on mothers. Early psychodynamic theorists suggested that schizophrenia results when mothers are at the same time overprotective and rejecting of their children (Fromm-Reichmann, 1948). These schizophrenogenic (schizophrenia-causing) mothers dominated their children, not letting them develop an autonomous sense of self and simultaneously making the children feel worthless and unlovable. Similarly, Gregory Bateson and his colleagues (1956) argued that parents (particularly mothers) of children who develop schizophrenia put their children in a double bind by constantly communicating conflicting messages to them. Such a mother might physically comfort her child when he falls down and is hurt but, at the same time, be verbally hostile and critical to him. Children chronically exposed to such mixed messages supposedly cannot trust their feelings or their perceptions of the world and thus develop distorted views of themselves, of others, and of their environment that contribute to schizophrenia. These theories did not hold up to scientific scrutiny, but they heaped guilt on the family members of people with schizophrenia.

One factor in family interaction that research shows is associated with multiple episodes of schizophrenia is **expressed emotion.** Family members can positively support patients by providing care directly but, sometimes, can also negatively influence clinical

The role of family interaction in schizophrenia is an example of how biological, psychological, and social factors combine in mental illness. *Eric Risberg/AP Photo*

conditions by showing negative emotions toward patients (Wang, Chen, & Yang, 2017). Studies have shown that families high in expressed emotion are over involved with one another, are overprotective of the family member with schizophrenia, and voice self-sacrificing attitudes toward the family member while at the same time being critical, hostile, and resentful toward them (Hooley, 2007). Although these family members do not doubt their loved one's illness, they talk as if the ill family member can control his or her symptoms (Hooley & Campbell, 2002; Wang, Chen, & Yang, 2017). They often have ideas about how the family member can improve the symptoms or functioning. Expressed emotion has been assessed through lengthy interviews with people with schizophrenia and their families, through projective tests and direct observation of family interactions. A number of studies have shown that people with schizophrenia whose families are high in expressed emotion are more likely to suffer relapses of psychosis than are those whose families are low in expressed emotion (Ellapolla & Abayaweera, 2020; Hooley, 2007) and is consistently found as a reliable predictor of rehospitalization among people with schizophrenia. A longitudinal study of individuals at high risk for schizophrenia found that those living in a family characterized by low warmth and high criticism (components of high-expressed emotion) were more likely to develop the full syndrome of schizophrenia than were those living in a family with greater warmth and less criticism (Schlosser et al., 2010). Being in a family with high-expressed emotion may create stresses for persons with schizophrenia that overwhelm their ability to cope and thus trigger first or new episodes of psychosis. Additionally, the rehospitalization rate of individuals with schizophrenia with high emotional expression caregivers was higher than those with low emotional expression caregivers. Research has also found that higher levels of criticism was correlated with higher rates of rehospitalization (Wang, Chen, & Yang, 2017).

Expressed emotion is a reliable predictor of relapse in psychotic disorders worldwide, but cultural differences in the level and presentation of emotional expression have been reported. Emotional over-involvement (EOI) and critical comments/hostility have been strongly linked with higher levels of emotional expression (Cherry, Taylor, Brown, Rigby, & Sellwood, 2017). Recent studies have found that exposure to high emotional expression was associated with a 95 percent increased likelihood of relapse as compared to low emotional expression across the globe. Despite differences in cultural expression of emotion, this relationship appears to be universal. Studies have found cultural variations in both the degree and manifestation of emotional expression. It is noted that intrafamilial interactions vary across cultures and may influence the emotional responses of a family member toward a family member with schizophrenia.

How a family responds to an illness is variable and reflects their culture. For example, research has found that in relatively collectivist cultures, an absence of positive remarks could be more detrimental than the presence of criticism, given the strong emphasis of family bonds. Unlike Western countries, where personal independence is culturally emphasized, criticism may be particularly toxic. Among African American adult-caregiver relationships criticisms may be perceived as engagement, caring, and support. The link between high levels of family expressed emotion and higher relapse rates has been replicated in studies of several cultures, including those of Europe, the United States, Mexico, and India. The lower levels of expressed emotion in families in developing countries may help explain the lower relapse rates of people with schizophrenia in these countries. Although families often are forgiving of the positive symptoms of schizophrenia (e.g., hallucinations, delusions) because they view them as uncontrollable, they can be unforgiving of the negative symptoms (e.g., lack of social interest). This understanding may facilitate the development of culturally appropriate tools that could aid our cultural understandings and efforts to improve the effectiveness of family interventions in multicultural settings (Driscoll, Sener, Angmark, & Shaikh, 2019).

The link between high levels of family expressed emotion and higher relapse rates has been replicated in studies of several cultures, including those of Europe, the United States, Mexico, and India. The lower levels of expressed emotion in families in

developing countries may help explain the lower relapse rates of people with schizophrenia in these countries. Although families often are forgiving of the positive symptoms of schizophrenia (e.g., hallucinations, delusions) because they view them as uncontrollable, they can be unforgiving of the negative symptoms (e.g., lack of motivation, blunted affect), viewing them as controllable by the person with schizophrenia (Hooley & Campbell, 2002). People with more of the negative symptoms may elicit more expressed emotion from their families. They also may be especially prone to relapse, but for reasons other than exposure to expressed emotion.

High levels of emotional expression are not pathological but rather a robust predictor of prognosis. There is a strong association between emotional expression and EOI, and the mental health and well-being of carers is also widely noted. Family members who rate high on expressed emotion are also more likely to have some form of psychopathology (Cherry et al., 2017; Goldstein, Talovic, Nuechterlein, & Fogelson, 1992). Perhaps the best evidence that family expressed emotion does in fact influence relapse in people with schizophrenia is that interventions to reduce family expressed emotion tend to reduce the relapse rate in family members with schizophrenia (Hooley, 2007).

Cognitive Perspectives

Aaron Beck and Neil Rector (Beck & Rector, 2005) suggest that fundamental difficulties in attention, inhibition, and adherence to the rules of communication lead people with schizophrenia to try to conserve their limited cognitive resources. One way they do this is by using certain biases or thinking styles for understanding the overwhelming information streaming through their brain. Delusions arise as the person with schizophrenia tries to explain strange perceptual experiences, and "jumps to conclusions" based on limited evidence. Hallucinations result from a hypersensitivity to perceptual input, coupled with a tendency to attribute experiences to external sources. Rather than thinking "I'm hearing things," the person with schizophrenia will think "Someone is trying to talk to me." The negative symptoms of schizophrenia arise from expectations that social interactions will be aversive and from the need to withdraw and conserve scarce cognitive resources.

This cognitive conceptualization has received empirical support and has led to cognitive treatments for people with schizophrenia (Garety & Freeman, 2013). Researchers and clinicians increasingly recognize the role of cognition in combination with emotional, biological, and social factors in schizophrenia (Garety & Freeman, 2013; Howes &

CASE STUDY

Anik is a 29-year-old Javanese woman who was born in a rural area but has lived in the city of Yogyakarta for the past 4 years. She has been married 1½ years but is very unhappy in her marriage, feeling her husband is lacking in openness and compassion. Anik has been unable to care for her 8-month-old daughter for the past several months, so the daughter was living with Anik's aunt in Jakarta. When her illness began, Anik first became withdrawn and didn't sleep or eat. She developed hallucinations of accusatory voices criticizing her husband, his family, and their landlady. Anik also suffered from jealous delusions that her husband was having an affair. She was taken to the hospital by her brother, where her symptoms included *mondarmandir* ("wandering without purpose"), *ngamuk* ("being irritable"), being easily offended and suspicious, talking to herself, crying, insomnia, *malmun* ("daydreaming"), and quickly changing emotions. Her sister-in-law reported that she had been chronically fearful and irritable for some time and would frequently slam doors and yell. In Javanese culture, the control of emotions in social situations is of great importance, so Anik's outbursts were seen as clear signs of some sort of pathology.

Anik had several explanations for her behavior. First and foremost, she believed that she was in a bad marriage, and this stress was a contributing factor. Shortly before her symptoms began, her landlady said something harsh to her, and Anik believed that her startle reaction to this (*goncangan*) led to *sajithati,* literally "liver sickness." In addition, Anik's mother had a brief period during Anik's childhood when she "went crazy," becoming loud and violent, and Anik believes she may have inherited this tendency from her mother. Anik initially sought to overcome her symptoms by increasing the frequency with which she repeated Muslim prayers and asking to be taken to a Muslim boarding house. Once she was taken to the hospital, she agreed to take antipsychotic medications, which helped her symptoms somewhat. She was discharged from the hospital after a short time but was rehospitalized multiple times over the next year.

Murray, 2014). Cognitive therapies help patients identify and cope with stressful circumstances associated with the development and worsening of symptoms. They also teach patients to dispute their delusional beliefs or hallucinatory experiences. Negative symptoms are treated by helping patients develop the expectation that being more active and interacting more with other people will have positive benefits. This cognitive intervention has shown greater success in reducing symptoms than does simply providing patients with support (Beck & Rector, 2005; Garety & Freeman, 2013).

Cross-Cultural Perspectives

Different cultures vary greatly in how they explain schizophrenia (Hopper, 2008; Karno & Jenkins, 1993; Larøi et al., 2014). Most have a biological explanation for the disorder, including the general idea that it runs in families. Intermingled with biological explanations are theories that attribute the disorder to stress, lack of spiritual piety, and family dynamics. Kevin Browne (2001) offers a case study of a woman from Java, whose understanding of her schizophrenia symptoms included all these factors.

Anik's experience illustrates the interweaving in people with schizophrenia symptoms of traditional beliefs and practices and modern biological treatments. Although she agreed to take antipsychotic medications, the understanding she and her family had of her symptoms was not primarily a biological one but rather one rooted in concerns about stress and, to some extent, religion.

TREATMENT

Comprehensive treatment for people with schizophrenia involves many levels since this is such a complex disorder. Treatment typically includes medications to help reduce psychotic symptoms and prevent relapse, therapy to help people cope with the consequences of the disorder, and social services to provide support for community integration to ensure access to necessary resources that will allow individuals to participate in daily life.

Biological Treatments

Over the centuries, many treatments for schizophrenia have been developed, based on the scientific theories of the time. Physicians have performed brain surgery on people with schizophrenia in an attempt to "fix" or eliminate the part of the brain causing hallucinations or delusions. These patients sometimes were calmer after their surgeries, but they often also experienced significant cognitive and emotional deficits as a result of the surgery. *Insulin coma therapy* was used in the 1930s to treat schizophrenia. People with schizophrenia would be given massive doses of insulin—the drug used to treat diabetes—until they went into a coma. When they emerged from the coma, however, patients rarely were much better, and the procedure was very dangerous. *Electroconvulsive therapy*, or *ECT*, was also used to treat schizophrenia until it became clear that it had little effect (although it is effective in treating serious depression, including in people with schizophrenia, as discussed in the chapter "Mood Disorders and Suicide").

Mostly, however, people with schizophrenia were simply warehoused. In 1955, one out of every two people housed in psychiatric hospitals had been diagnosed with schizophrenia, although by today's standards of diagnosis some may actually have had different disorders (Rosenstein, Milazzo-Sayre, & Manderscheid, 1989). These patients received custodial care—they were bathed, fed, and prevented from hurting themselves, often with the use of physical restraints—but few received any treatment that actually reduced their symptoms and improved their functioning. Not until the 1950s was an effective drug treatment for schizophrenia—chlorpromazine—introduced. Since then, several other antipsychotic drugs (also called *neuroleptics*) have been added to the arsenal of treatments for schizophrenia. More recently, the atypical antipsychotics hold out the promise of relieving positive symptoms while inducing fewer intolerable side effects than the traditional or typical antipsychotics.

(First Generation) Typical Antipsychotic Drugs

In the early 1950s, French researchers Jean Delay and Pierre Deniker found that **chlorpromazine** (Thorazine), one of a class of antipsychotic drugs called the phenothiazines, calms agitation and reduces hallucinations and delusions in patients with schizophrenia. Other phenothiazines that became widely used include trifluoperazine (Stelazine), thioridazine (Mellaril), fluphenazine (Prolixin), and perphenazine (Trilafon). These drugs appear to block receptors for dopamine, thereby reducing its action in the brain. For the first time, many people with schizophrenia could control the positive symptoms of the disorder (hallucinations, delusions, thought disturbances) by taking these drugs even when they were asymptomatic. Unfortunately, while positive symptoms were reduced with these antipsychotic medications, they did not help and often had harmful effects on negative symptoms that involved, cognitive, affective, and/or motor domains (Solmi et al., 2017). Thanks to these drugs, by 1971 the number of people with schizophrenia who required

hospitalization had decreased to half of what would have been expected without the use of the drugs (Lavretsky, 2008). Other classes of antipsychotic drugs introduced after the phenothiazines include the *butyrophenones* (such as Haldol) and the *thioxanthenes* (such as Navane).

Among people who do respond, the typical antipsychotics are more effective in treating the positive symptoms of schizophrenia than in treating the negative symptoms (lack of motivation and interpersonal deficits). Many people with schizophrenia who take these drugs are not actively psychotic but still are unable to hold a job or build positive social relationships. People with schizophrenia typically must take an antipsychotic drug all the time in order to prevent new episodes of active symptoms. If the drug is discontinued, about 78 percent of people with schizophrenia relapse within 1 year and 98 percent relapse within 2 years, compared to about 30 percent of people who continue on their medications (Gitlin et al., 2001).

Unfortunately, however, these drugs have significant side effects that cause many people to want to discontinue their use (Adams, Awad, Rathbone, & Thornley, 2007; Patel, Cherian, Gohil, & Atkinson, 2014). The side effects include grogginess, dry mouth, blurred vision, drooling, sexual dysfunction, visual disturbances, weight gain or loss, constipation, menstrual irregularities in women, and depression. Another common side effect is *akinesia,* which includes slowed motor activity, monotonous speech, and an expressionless face. Patients taking the phenothiazines often show symptoms similar to those seen in Parkinson's disease, including muscle stiffness, freezing of the facial muscles, tremors and spasms in the extremities, and *akathesis,* an agitation that causes people to pace and be unable to sit still (Adams et al., 2007). The fact that Parkinson's disease is caused by a lack of dopamine in the brain suggests that these side effects occur because the drugs reduce the functional levels of dopamine (Patel et al., 2014).

One serious and permanent side effect is **tardive dyskinesia,** a neurological disorder that involves involuntary movements of the tongue, face, mouth, or jaw. People with this disorder may involuntarily smack their lips, make sucking sounds, stick out their tongue, puff their cheeks, or make other bizarre movements over and over again. Tardive dyskinesia often is irreversible and may occur in over 20 percent of persons with long-term use of the phenothiazines.

The side effects of the neuroleptics can be reduced by lowering dosages. For this reason, many clinicians prescribe for people with schizophrenia the lowest dosage possible that still keeps active symptoms at bay, known as a maintenance dose. Unfortunately, maintenance doses often do not restore an individual to full functioning. The negative symptoms of schizophrenia may still be strongly present, along with mild versions of the positive symptoms, making it hard for the individual to function in daily life. Some people with schizophrenia have frequent hospitalizations and ongoing difficulties outside the hospital.

(Second Generation) Atypical Antipsychotics

Fortunately, newer drugs, the **atypical antipsychotics,** seem to be more effective in treating schizophrenia than the neuroleptics, without the neurological side effects of the latter (Walker et al., 2009). One of the most common of these drugs, *clozapine* (sold in the United States as Clozaril), binds to the D4 dopamine receptor, but it also influences several other neurotransmitters, including serotonin (Sajatovic, Madhusoodanan, & Fuller, 2008). Studies have shown that clozapine is effective in treating schizophrenia spectrum disorders, particularly for individuals with treatment-resistant schizophrenia who did not respond to other drug therapies. This medication has been found as effective in reducing both the negative symptoms and positive symptoms associated with schizophrenia (Cho, et al., 2019; Okhuijsen-Pfeifer, 2018; Stroup, Gerhard, Crystal, Huang, & Olfson, 2016; Wimberley et al., 2017). The demonstrated efficacy of second-generation antipsychotics (SGAs) has increased their use for a wide range of psychiatric conditions besides schizophrenia spectrum disorders. These medications have become especially popular as add-on treatment for patients with MDD who show poor response to antidepressants and for behavioral symptoms associated with dementia (Solmi et al., 2017).

The introduction of antipsychotic medication had profound impacts on the treatment of schizophrenia and other psychotic disorders. However, for a considerable number of people with schizophrenia, these medications do not reduce their overall symptoms and the exact impact of this treatment remains unclear. The estimated percentage of patients that do not or only partially respond to treatment vary significantly. Various studies have estimated that 10 to 60 percent of patients have little or no response to drug therapy, with one recent study suggesting rates higher than 80 percent. The uncertainty about the effectiveness of drug therapy may be related to the various ways in which efficacy is defined. However, higher rates of nonresponse are associated with earlier onset of illness which has been consistently identified as a predictor of poor response to antipsychotic treatment, as well as those with lower symptoms severity (Pae, 2020; Samara, Nikolakopoulou, Salanti, & Leucht 2019). A large meta-analysis of the efficacy of anti-psychotic medications that included 6493 participants provided strong evidence that anti-psychotic drug therapy is a superior treatment. Research has found that antipsychotics reduced both the rates of relapse and rehospitalization to less than half (Stern, Linker, Vadodaria, Marchetto, & Gage, 2018).

Recent studies have identified clozapine as a superior treatment option that has high rates of efficacy for patients with treatment-resistant schizophrenia or those who have suicidal ideations and behavior. The question of long-term mortality risk is of particular clinical interest for those treated with clozapine. Like all medications, clozapine has side effects, including dizziness, nausea, sedation, seizures, hypersalivation, weight gain, and tachycardia. More concerning is the development of a condition called *agranulocytosis* that may occur while taking clozapine. This is a deficiency of granulocytes, substances produced by bone marrow, that fight infection. The condition can be fatal, so patients taking clozapine must be carefully monitored (Vermeulen et al., 2019). Recent studies have found that the enhanced clinical efficacy outweighs the potential long-term harmful side-effects of clozapine. Although this drug is associated with severe side effects, the reduction in psychiatric symptoms provides more long-term benefits as compared to those who are continuously treated with other antipsychotics. Researchers have speculated that the improved health among a group that typically is more sick than the average person may be due to the monitoring by health professionals. Monitoring of cardiac risk factors, such as hypertension or hyperglycemia or adverse lifestyle behaviors like smoking and drinking alcohol, may reduce mortality rates among patients treated with clozapine (Vermeulen et al., 2019). Clozapine has greater efficacy for treating this disorder than all the other antipsychotics and these recent studies are encouraging an increased use among prescribers (Haddad, & Correll, 2018).

There are a number of other second generation antipsychotics that have been introduced over the past two decades, including risperidone (trade name Risperdal), olanzapine (Zyprexa), quetiapine (Seroquel), and ziprasidone (Geodone, Zeldox). These drugs do not tend to induce agranulocytosis, but they can cause a number of side effects, including significant weight gain and increased risk for diabetes, as well as sexual dysfunction, sedation, low blood pressure, seizures, gastrointestinal problems, vision problems, and problems with concentration. A randomized clinical trial conducted by the National Institute of Mental Health in several sites across the United States compared the effectiveness of five of these drugs (quetiapine, perphenazine, risperidone, olanzapine, and ziprasidone) in over 1,000 patients with schizophrenia (Levine, Rabinowitz, Ascher-Svanum, Faries, & Lawson, 2011). The focus of the trial was how many patients would show remission of symptoms over an 18-month fol-low-up period. Unfortunately, only 44.5 percent of the patients experienced remission of any duration during this period, 21.0 percent showed remission for at least 3 months, and only 11.7 percent showed remission for at least 6 months. For the five medications, 6-month remission rates were highest (12.4 percent) for the olanzapine treatment group, followed by quetiapine (8.2 percent), perphenazine (6.8 percent), ziprasi-done (6.5 percent), and risperidone (6.3 percent).

Although the atypical antipsychotics are superior to older medications, more work is needed to deter-mine which of them are safest and most effective, and for which patients (Samara et al., 2016). The benefits of antipsychotics in terms of symptom reduction are greatest in those with the most severe symptoms. Multiple studies have found that antipsychotic use is associated with lower mortality than no antipsychotic use in people with schizophrenia, but more research is needed to better understand the mechanisms of the disorder to develop the most effective treatments (Haddad, & Correll, 2018). Most people with psy-chotic disorders will not be able to benefit from effec-tive rehabilitation programs without the use of antipsychotic drug therapies. It is critical that initia-tion of drug treatment occurs as soon as possible, par-ticularly within 5 years of the first acute psychotic episode, since this period reflects significant illness-related changes in the brain (Patel, Cherian, Gohil, & Atkinson, 2014).

Psychological and Social Treatments

Even when antipsychotic medications do help reduce the psychotic symptoms of schizophrenia, they often do not completely restore the life of a person with schizophrenia, as the following profile illustrates.

PROFILES

Medicine did not cause sanity; it only made it possi-ble. Sanity came through a minute-by-minute choice of outer reality, which was often without meaning, over inside reality, which was full of meaning. Sanity meant choosing reality that was not real and having faith that someday the choice would be worth the fear involved and that it would someday hold mean-ing. (Anonymous, 1992, p. 335)

Many individuals who are able to control the pos-itive symptoms of schizophrenia with drugs still expe-rience many of the negative symptoms, particularly problems in motivation and in social interactions.

Psychological interventions can help these individu-als increase their social skills and reduce their isola-tion and apathy. Such interventions also can help people with schizophrenia and their families reduce the stress and conflict in their lives, thereby reducing the risk of relapse into psychosis (Pharoah, Mari, Rathbone, & Wong, 2010; Turner, van der Gaag, Karyotaki, & Cuijpers, 2014). In addition, the lack of effectiveness of the antipsychotic drugs suggested by the studies reviewed in the preceding section is due in part to people discontinuing the drugs either because they do not think they need them or because they find the side effects intolerable (Barkhof, Meijer, de Sonneville, Linszen, & de Haan, 2012). Psychological interventions can help people with schizophrenia understand their disorder, appreciate the need to remain on their medications, and cope more effectively with the side effects of the medica-tions. Because of the severity of their disorder, many people with schizophrenia have trouble finding or holding a job, feeding and sheltering themselves, and obtaining necessary medical or psychiatric care. Psy-chologists, social workers, and other mental health professionals can assist people with schizophrenia in meeting these basic needs.

Behavioral, Cognitive, and Social Treatments

Most experts in the treatment of schizophrenia argue for a comprehensive approach that addresses the wide array of behavioral, cognitive, and social deficits in schizophrenia and is tailored to the specific deficits of each individual with the disorder (Liberman, 2008; Mueser, Deavers, Penn, & Cassisi, 2013). These treat-ments are given in addition to medication and can in-crease patients' level of everyday functioning and significantly reduce the risk of relapse (see review by Barkhof et al., 2012).

Cognitive impairments experienced by those with schizophrenia have been consistently identified as a critical target for treatments due to the severe impact on daily function. Research has suggested that these symptoms may be as important as positive symptoms in predicting recovery. With current drug therapies having a little impact on cognitive impair-ments, there is a clear need to develop effective treat-ments to tackle cognitive symptoms (Grant et al., 2017). Cognitive treatments include helping people with schizophrenia recognize and change demoraliz-ing attitudes they may have toward their illness so that they will seek help when needed and participate in society to the extent that they can (Beck & Rector, 2005; Garety & Freeman, 2013). Behavioral treat-ments, based on social learning theory (see the chap-ter "Theories and Treatment of Abnormality"), include the use of operant conditioning and mode-ling to teach persons with schizophrenia skills such as initiating and maintaining conversations with others, asking for help or information from physicians, and persisting in an activity, such as cooking or cleaning (Liberman, 2008). These interventions may be administered by the family. In that case, a therapist would teach a client's family members to ignore schizophrenia symptoms, such as bizarre comments, and instead reinforce socially appropriate behavior by giving it attention and positive emotional responses. In psychiatric hospitals and residential treatment centers, token economies sometimes are established, based on the principles of operant conditioning. Patients earn tokens that they can exchange for special privileges (such as additional outings beyond what is ordinarily provided) by completing daily self-care tasks (such as showering or changing clothing) or even by simply engaging in appropriate conversations with others.

Social interventions include increasing contact between people with schizophrenia and supportive others, often through self-help support groups (Liberman, 2008). These groups discuss the impact of the disorder on their lives, the frustration of trying to make people understand their disorder, their fear of relapse, their experiences with various medications, and other day-to-day concerns. Group members also can help one another learn social and problem-solving skills by giving feedback and providing a forum in which individual members can role-play new skills. People with schizophrenia also are often directly taught problem-solving skills applicable to common social situations. For example, they may practice generating and role-playing solutions for when a receptionist tells them no one is available at a company to interview them for a potential job.

Although behavioral, cognitive, and social treatments can improve functioning, studies show that the effects can be rather small, especially in the long term (Jauhar et al., 2014; Turner et al., 2014). Current research aims to understand how these treatments can be improved and tailored to individuals and their particular symptoms.

Family Therapy

Recall that high levels of expressed emotion within the family of a person with schizophrenia can substantially increase the risk and frequency of relapse. Many researchers have examined the effectiveness of family-oriented therapies for people with schizophrenia. Successful therapies combine basic education on schizophrenia with the training of family members in coping with their loved one's inappropriate behaviors and the disorder's impact on their lives (Pharaoh et al., 2010; Barkhof et al., 2012).

In the educational portion of these therapies, families are taught about the disorder's biological causes, its symptoms, and the medications and their side effects. The hope is that this information will reduce self-blame in family members, increase their tolerance for the uncontrollable symptoms of the disorder, and allow them to monitor their family members' use of medication and possible side effects. Family members also learn communication skills to reduce harsh, conflictual interactions, as well as problem-solving skills to help manage issues in the family such as lack of money, in order to reduce the overall level of stress in the family. They also learn specific behavioral techniques for encouraging appropriate behavior and discouraging inappropriate behavior on the part of their family member with schizophrenia.

These family-oriented interventions combined with drug therapy appear to be more effective at reducing relapse rate than treatment with antipsychotic medication alone. Better outcomes are demonstrated by a reduction in psychotic symptoms and relapse rates for the affected individual. Improvements that have been observed within the family include increased carer well-being, reduction in carer burden, and reduction in patient-directed negative expressed emotion, particularly criticism and hostility. This reduction in patient-directed criticism and conflict may reduce levels of stress and/or increases perceived levels of support (Carr, 2019; Morin & Franck, 2017).

Psychoeducation is a very effective therapeutic tool that has been consistently found to decrease relapse by 50 to 60 percent. These programs were initially developed to decrease high-expressed emotion to help prevent relapse, but later iterations focus on social and role functioning, as well as family well-being. Research has shown very promising results when psychoeducation therapy is applied in the first psychotic episode, combined with other evidence-based interventions. Research has shown a substantial return of functioning and avoidance of psychosis altogether (McFarlane, 2016).

Multifamily psychoeducational therapy, in which several families are treated together, may be especially effective because it provides families with a forum to increase mutual support, shared learning, and reduce feelings of isolation and stigmatization. Outcomes for family therapy for childhood onset psychosis are less favorable than for adolescents, possibly because this is a more severe and debilitating condition. Psychoeducational family therapy for psychotic disorders is designed to help families understand and manage the condition, antipsychotic medication, related stresses, and early warning signs of relapse. Psychoeducational family therapy also strives to reduce negative family processes associated with relapse, specifically high levels of expressed emotion, stigma, problems with communication, and life stressors with an emphasis on blame reduction (Morin & Franck, 2017). Psychoeducational family therapy also helps families develop skills to improve communication, problem-solving, coping, crisis management, and service access. Skills training commonly involves modeling, rehearsal, feedback, and discussion. Effective treatment typically lasts between 9 and 12 months. Typically there are more meetings at the beginning of treatment than toward the end (Carr, 2019).

Family-based therapies also can increase patients' adherence to taking antipsychotic medications. For example, Guo et al. (2010) randomly assigned 1,268 patients with early-stage schizophrenia to receive antipsychotic medication alone or medication plus family therapy, which included skills training and cognitive-behavioral interventions. The patients were followed for a year. In that time, those who had family therapy with medication were less likely to discontinue their medications than those without family therapy (33 percent vs. 47 percent). The patients receiving family-based intervention also experienced less relapse of symptoms and greater improvement in social functioning and quality of life than those who received medication alone.

For people with schizophrenia to be cared for by their family and to be deeply embedded in it is more likely in some cultures than in others. Family-oriented interventions may be even more critical for people in these cultures (Barrio & Yamada, 2010; Lopez, Kopelowicz, & Canive, 2002). The interventions must be culturally sensitive. One study found that behavior therapies to increase communication actually backfired in some Hispanic families, perhaps because these families already had low levels of expressed emotion and found the techniques suggested by the therapists to violate their cultural norms for how family members should interact (Telles et al., 1995). Some of the most traditional family members in this study expressed great discomfort during exercises that encouraged them to establish eye contact or express negative feelings to authority figures, because these actions were considered disrespectful. As with other disorders, therapists must take into account the culture of their clients in designing interventions.

Assertive Community Treatment Programs

People with schizophrenia require a significant amount of support and care for their diverse needs. Monitoring and adjustment of their medications, occupational training, assistance in receiving financial resources (such as Social Security and Medicaid), social skills training, emotional support, and sometimes basic housing make comprehensive community-based treatment programs a necessity.

Assertive Community Treatment (ACT) is regarded as a benchmark of best practice for treating persons living with severe and persistent mental illness, like schizophrenia. ACT is an evidence-based approach focused on intensive treatment, support, and rehabilitation This community-based framework has received extensive support and it has been shown to improve functional deficits and reduce hospitalizations (Guérin, Dupuis, Jacob & Prud'homme, 2019). ACT programs provide comprehensive services for people with schizophrenia, relying on the expertise of medical professionals, social workers, and psychologists to meet the variety of patients' needs 24 hours a day (Bustillo, Lauriello, Horan, & Keith, 2001). Outpatient care models like ACT have been developed for patients with severe mental illness (SMI) to best serve their complex treatment needs and have generally shown positive effects. Studies on the ACT treatment model have found that these community-based programs produced improvements in illness severity with low disengagement and hospitalization rates (Schöttle et al; 2018).

In the chapter "Looking at Abnormality" we discuss the community mental health movement, which was initiated by President Kennedy in the 1960s to transfer the care of people with serious mental disorders from primarily psychiatric hospitals to comprehensive community-based programs. The idea was that people with schizophrenia and other serious disorders would spend time in the hospital when severe symptoms required it but when discharged from the hospital would go to community-based programs to help them reintegrate into society, maintain their medications, gain needed skills, and function at their highest possible level. Hundreds of halfway houses, group homes, and therapeutic communities were established for people with serious mental disorders who needed a supportive place to live.

Other comprehensive treatment programs provide skills training, vocational rehabilitation, and social support to people with schizophrenia who live at home. Studies of these programs find that they reduce the amount of time spent in the hospital and, as a result, can be cost-effective. One classic example of such programs was The Lodge, a residential treatment center for people with schizophrenia established by George Fairweather and his colleagues (Fairweather, Sanders, Maynard, & Cressler, 1969). At The Lodge, mental health professionals were available for support and assistance, but residents ran the household and worked with other residents to establish healthy behaviors and discourage inappropriate behaviors. The residents also established their own employment agency to assist with finding jobs. Follow-up studies showed that Lodge residents fared much better than people with schizophrenia who were simply discharged from the hospital into the care of their families or into less intensive treatment programs (Fairweather et al., 1969). For example, Lodge residents were less likely to be rehospitalized and much more likely to hold a job than were those in a comparison group, even after The Lodge closed.

Although 38 states in the United States have adopted ACT to care for people with schizophrenia and other serious mental disorders, only 2 percent of individuals with these disorders are currently being served by such programs (Padgett & Henwood, 2011). Unfortunately, the *community mental health movement* was never funded at a level that could support its program goals. With the changes in medical insurance in recent years, funding for mental health care for the seriously mentally ill has been even tighter. Although billions of dollars are spent on mental health care each year in the United States, much of that money goes not to direct services to people with schizophrenia but instead to subsistence programs such as Social Security disability payments and to community services for people with less serious mental disorders (Torrey, 2013). Much of the financial burden of caring for people with schizophrenia falls to state and local governments, which lack the necessary resources, or to families, who too often are bankrupted by the cost of care.

As a result, 40 to 60 percent of people with schizophrenia receive little or no care in a given year. Those who do receive care often are hospitalized only when their symptoms are acute, and they remain in the hospital for an inadequate period of time to allow their symptoms to stabilize. They may be discharged with little or no follow-up. Some return to their families, but many end up in nursing homes, where they receive only custodial care, or in single-room-occupancy hotels or rooming houses, often in run-down inner-city neighborhoods. Many end up homeless or in prison (Torrey, 2013).

Stigma

Despite growing awareness and increased knowledge about mental health issues, people with serious and persistent mental illness, like schizophrenia, still face significant amounts of stigma. Studies have shown that people in the general population typically perceive individuals with psychological disorders as dangerous, unpredictable, and out of control. Various studies have provided strong support that the relationship between the majority of psychiatric disorders and violent behaviors does not exist, which suggests that negative attitudes toward people with mental illness (PWMI) are most likely related to prejudice and stereotypes. As a result of this biased perception, PWMI are often subjected to

People with mental illness often experience or anticipate discrimination and stigma due to negative public attitudes. *Monstar Studio/Shutterstock*

discriminative and stigmatizing behaviors in social situations, within their families and among friends. This constant exposure to stigmatizing attitudes has numerous negative effects, such as lower quality of life, decreased likelihood to seek professional help, discontinuing treatment, and higher treatment dropout rates (Mannarini & Rossi, 2019).

Mental illness stigma is as a major obstacle to well-being among PWMI. According to recent research on public attitudes toward mental illness in the United States, only 42 percent of Americans aged 18 to 24 believe PWMI can be successful at work, 26 percent believe that others have a caring attitude toward PWMI, and 25 percent believe that PWMI can recover from their illness. A robust body of evidence demonstrates that PWMI experience discrimination in nearly every domain of their lives, including employment, housing, and medical care. These stigmatizing experiences are associated with increased symptom severity, decreased treatment seeking, and treatment nonadherence. People with psychological disorders are aware of the negative stereotypes associated with mental illness and negative ways in which PWMI are treated. This knowledge may increase psychological distress and worry about people being afraid of/or avoiding them, being denied work or being perceived by others as weak or dangerous. People with SMI may anticipate this even if they have never personally experienced stigma (Fox, Earnshaw, Taverna, & Vogt, 2018).

Additionally, research has found that stigma toward PWMI is both a cross-diagnostic and cross-cultural phenomenon. Recent research conducted in Germany, Russia, and Mongolia examined stigma associated with major depression and schizophrenia finding comparable results regardless of strong differences in cultural backgrounds. Further, people were more likely to attribute depression to psychosocial causes and biological causes to schizophrenia. Meaning, among various countries and regardless of the culture, people were more likely to believe schizophrenia was caused by biological factors than was depression. Moreover, people who attributed biological causes to psychological disorders, were also more likely to report a stronger desire for social distance. People with SMI, like psychotic disorders, are more likely to experience isolation and stigma as a result of public perception. This increases the likelihood that they avoid seeking professional help from fear of disclosing a diagnosis that is associated with stigma (Mannarini & Rossi, 2019).

The stigmatization of mentally ill individuals is well documented in the scientific literature. In addition to the challenges of living with severe symptoms of mental illness, those affected individuals must also battle the burden of mental health stigma. Biased attitudes and behaviors like avoidance, negative stereotypes, adverse treatment interactions, and various forms of discrimination are still present and pose a significant social problem. Stigma for those with serious mental illness can be an impediment in everyday functions which impacts their quality of life. Studies examining the relationship between mental illness and stigmatizing attitudes toward

mentally ill people have been reported in many different countries. Schizophrenia still carries high rates of stigma and is of particular attention in this area (Fox et al., 2018).

CHAPTER INTEGRATION

There is probably more consensus among mental health professionals about the biological roots of schizophrenia than of any other psychopathology discussed in this book. The evidence that the fundamental vulnerability to schizophrenia is biological is compelling, yet there is growing consensus that psychosocial factors also contribute to the risk for schizophrenia among people who have a biological vulnerability. Theorists are increasingly developing models that integrate the biological and psychosocial contributors to schizophrenia in order to provide comprehensive explanations of the development of this disorder (Figure 5; Cannon, 2009; Howes et al., 2017).

Genetic factors clearly play a role in vulnerability to schizophrenia. Environmental factors early in a person's life, such as exposure to toxins or to viruses in utero or hypoxia during childbirth, can interact with a genetic liability stemming from epigenetic processes to increase the person's vulnerability to developing schizophrenia. If a person with this biological vulnerability to schizophrenia is raised in a supportive, low-expressed-emotion family and escapes

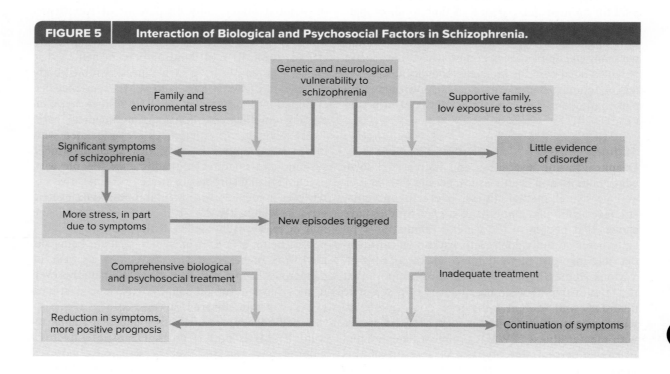

FIGURE 5 | **Interaction of Biological and Psychosocial Factors in Schizophrenia.**

exposure to major stressors, he or she may never develop the full syndrome of schizophrenia. The person still may have mild symptoms, however, because the biological underpinnings of this disorder play such an important role. Alternatively, a person who has a biological vulnerability and grows up in a stressful atmosphere is more likely to develop the full syndrome of schizophrenia.

The two-hit model suggests psychiatric conditions may be the result of a disturbance in brain developmental during the weeks before or after birth (*perinatal*). This disturbance disrupts the neuronal circuits and causes increased vulnerability to stress during periods of critical brain development. Psychosocial stress also clearly contributes to new episodes of psychosis in people with this disorder. Psychosocial stressors that are experienced later in life may then trigger the onset of the disorder. Meaning, the first "hit" disrupts some aspect of brain development, and establishes increased vulnerability to a second "hit"

that may occur later in life that riggers the onset of psychiatric symptoms.

Immune system response and brain inflammation are significant prenatal risk factors for schizophrenia. Recent research on maternal bacterial infection during pregnancy was significantly associated with subsequent development of schizophrenia among offspring. A localized bacterial infection predicted a 1.6-fold increased risk of developing a psychotic disorder in adulthood, and system-wide bacterial infection predicted a nearly threefold increase in the development of a psychotic disorder. Maternal bacterial infections during pregnancy are more strongly associated with the development of schizophrenia in male rather than female offspring for reasons that are not fully known.

There is widespread consensus among mental health professionals that the most effective therapies for schizophrenia are those that address both the biological and the psychosocial contributors to the disorder.

SHADES OF GRAY DISCUSSION

As you may have noticed, Jeff's symptoms do not fit neatly into any of the categories in the *DSM-5*. You might wonder if he is depressed, because he reports feelings of emptiness. But because he does not show most of the other symptoms of depression (see the chapter "Mood Disorders and Suicide"), this is not an appropriate diagnosis. His emptiness, social isolation, lack of motivation, and general deterioration in functioning all look like negative symptoms of schizophrenia. However, he does not appear to have the positive symptoms—delusions, hallucinations, or incoherence in speech or thought.

The psychiatrist treating Jeff believed that he was showing prodromal or early symptoms of schizophrenia, which often are predominantly negative. He was given antipsychotic medications and allowed to go

home with his parents. Remaining isolated and apathetic, he stopped taking the medications. Two months later, he said he was experiencing severe electrical sensations in his head that he believed were being transmitted through his father's mind. He also began to have "horrible thoughts" that were put there by his father. He became agitated and one night grabbed a knife, went into his parents' bedroom, and threatened to kill his father if he would not stop tormenting him. Fortunately, his father was able to talk him into dropping the knife and going to the emergency room.

Jeff was admitted to the hospital, given a diagnosis of schizophrenia, and placed on a higher dose of antipsychotic medications. His positive symptoms diminished, but his negative symptoms remained. (Adapted from Andreasen, 1998)

CHAPTER SUMMARY

- There are five domains of symptoms that define psychotic disorders. They include positive and negative symptoms.

- The positive symptoms of schizophrenia include delusions (fixed beliefs that are held strongly despite conflicting evidence), hallucinations (unreal perceptual experiences), thought disturbances (incoherent thought and speech), and grossly disorganized or catatonic behavior.

- The negative symptoms of schizophrenia include restricted affect and avolition (the inability to initiate and persist in goal-directed activities) or asociality. Separate prodromal and residual symptoms are mild versions of the positive and negative symptoms that occur before and after episodes of acute symptoms.

- Cognitive deficits in schizophrenia include problems in attention, working memory, processing speed,

- learning and memory, abstraction, and problem solving.

- Estimates of the prevalence of schizophrenia in various countries range from about 0.1 to 2.0 percent, but most estimates are between 0.5 and 1.0 percent. There are some slight ethnic differences in rates of schizophrenia, but these may be due to differences in socioeconomic status.

- The content of delusions and hallucinations varies somewhat across cultures, but the form of these symptoms remains similar, and many clinicians and researchers believe that schizophrenia can be diagnosed reliably across cultures.

- A number of other psychotic disorders are recognized by the *DSM-5*. Schizoaffective disorder is diagnosed when symptoms of schizophrenia occur with periods of major depression or mania. Individuals with schizophreniform disorder meet the criteria for schizophrenia but for a period of only 1 to 6 months. Those with brief psychotic disorder meet the criteria for schizophrenia but for a period of less than 1 month and sometimes in response to a major stressor. Delusional disorder is characterized by just one kind of psychotic symptoms, delusions. Schizotypal personality disorder is characterized by a life-long pattern of severe oddities in thought, behavior, and self-concept that fall short of psychosis.

- Biological theories of schizophrenia focus on genetics, structural and functional abnormalities in the brain, and neurotransmitters. There is clear evidence of a genetic transmission of schizophrenia. People with schizophrenia show abnormal functioning in the cortical areas of the brain, particularly prefrontal areas and the hippocampus, as well as enlarged ventricles. Many people with schizophrenia have a history of prenatal difficulties, such as exposure to the influenza virus during the second trimester of gestation, or birth complications, including perinatal hypoxia. Brain abnormalities and dysfunction in dopamine systems play a role in schizophrenia.

- Stressful events probably cannot cause schizophrenia in people who lack a vulnerability to the disorder, but they may trigger new episodes of psychosis in people with the disorder.

- Expressed emotion theorists argue that some families of people with schizophrenia are simultaneously overprotective and hostile and that this increases the risk of relapse.

- Cognitive theories suggest that some psychotic symptoms are attempts by the individual to understand and manage cognitive deficits.

- Drugs known as the phenothiazines, introduced in the 1950s, brought relief to many people with schizophrenia. The phenothiazines reduce the positive symptoms of schizophrenia but often are not effective in reducing the negative symptoms. Major side effects include tardive dyskinesia, an irreversible neurological disorder characterized by involuntary movements of the tongue, face, mouth, or jaw.

- Atypical antipsychotics, most of which were introduced in the past two decades, seem to induce fewer side effects than the phenothiazines and are effective in treating both the positive symptoms and the negative symptoms of schizophrenia for many people. Still, many people with schizophrenia do not respond or respond only partially to these drugs.

- Psychological and social treatments focus on helping people with schizophrenia reduce stress, improve family interactions, learn social skills, manage their illness, and cope with the impact of the disorder on their lives. Comprehensive treatment programs combining drug therapy with an array of psychological and social treatments have been shown to reduce relapse significantly.

KEY TERMS

psychosis

schizophrenia spectrum

positive symptoms

delusions

persecutory delusions

grandiose delusions

delusion of reference

delusions of thought insertion

hallucinations

formal thought disorder

catatonia

negative symptoms

restricted affect

avolition

prodromal symptoms

residual symptoms

prodromal

schizoaffective disorder

schizophreniform disorder

brief psychotic disorder

delusional disorder

schizotypal personality disorder

pathogenic

phenothiazines

neuroleptics

mesolimbic pathway

social drift

expressed emotion

chlorpromazine

tardive dyskinesia

atypical antipsychotics

assertive community treatment (ACT)

Chapter 9

Grigvovan/Shutterstock

Personality Disorders

CHAPTER OUTLINE

Personality Disorders Along the Continuum

Long-standing patterns of behavior, thought, and feeling that lead to positive social and occupational functioning

A student who is interested in classes, has good relationships with friends, can regulate his or her emotions, and reflects on him- or herself accurately

Potentially meets diagnostic criteria for a personality disorder:

Long-standing patterns of behavior, thought, and feeling that somewhat interfere with social and/or occupational functioning

A student who is often inappropriate with others or socially withdrawn, is having significant difficulties understanding him- or herself or others, and/or frequently overreacts emotionally or behaviorally

Functional ── Dysfunctional

Long-standing patterns of behavior, thought, and feeling that are unusual but do not interfere with social or occupational functioning

A student who is awkward or sometimes inappropriate with others; struggles with his or her sense of self, self-esteem, or life goals; and/or sometimes overreacts emotionally

Likely meets diagnostic criteria for a personality disorder:

Long-standing patterns of behavior, thought, and feeling that substantially interfere with social and/or occupational functioning

A student who is chronically inappropriate with others or socially withdrawn; has severe difficulties with identity, self-esteem, or self-direction; and/or becomes out of control emotionally in distressing situations

---

You'll love my friend, she has the *best* personality. Missy is so outgoing, everyone loves her; Dan is very quiet and serious; Ugh, Jill has no personality . . . at all! We hear descriptions of personality all the time, but what do they mean? Personality involves a unique combination of traits and characteristics that psychologically distinguish one person from another. Our personality includes the core elements that make us who we are and directly affect our daily life, social interactions, interpersonal relations, perception, and emotion.

A core aspect of your personality is your sense of self, or *identity.* On the functional end of the personality continuum are people who have a sense of self that is relatively stable and is distinct from others with the ability to appropriately adapt to social situations. Another core aspect of personality is the way we *relate to others* (Krueger & Markon, 2014). People with adaptive personalities empathize and cooperate with others, can appropriately express empathy, and appreciate the uniqueness of the different people in their lives. All of the individual traits and characteristics that make up their personality are relatively flexible and can adapt to new situations and events. No one personality characteristic encapsulates every moment of human behavior. In a healthy personality, these traits are not fixed or rigid and can ebb and flow based on the social context. For example, you may be a very outgoing and extroverted person who loves to chat with people, even strangers. While this is a characteristic of your personality, there must be flexibility in various social situations. Is it socially acceptable for someone to talk through a lecture a sermon in church? A healthy personality adapts to various social situations. Most people are able to draw upon their personality traits in a flexible manner, adjusting their responses to the needs of the situation. However, when personality traits become rigid and inflexible, they will typically cause a variety of social and personal dysfunctions and psychological distress.

People also vary greatly in their ability to form and maintain good interpersonal relationships. Some people find it difficult to care about others appropriately, being either too self-sacrificing or too self-absorbed to empathize with others. Some people have difficulty tolerating differing perspectives and differentiating their own needs and desires from those of others. Some may find interpersonal relationships too distressing or unrewarding and withdraw from other people altogether. When individuals have significant deficits in their identity and their capacity for interpersonal relationships, they may be diagnosed with a personality disorder (PD)

We've noted throughout this book that drawing a line between normal and abnormal, between functional and dysfunctional, is problematic for all the mental disorders. PDs have presented especially great challenges in defining where unhealthy functioning that constitutes a disorder begins. The *DSM-5* includes two models of PDs. Its current categorical model is nearly the same as *DSM-IV*. Its alternative dimensional model is based on ample evidence that PDs, for the most part, represent extreme versions of typical personality traits (Krueger & Markon, 2014; Morey, Benson, Busch, & Skodol, 2015; Widiger & Mullins-Sweatt, 2009).

Extraordinary People

Susanna Kaysen, *Girl, Interrupted*

Boston Globe/Getty Images

Susanna Kaysen was 18, depressed, drifting through life and endlessly oppositional toward her parents and teachers. She tried to commit suicide and eventually was hospitalized, remaining in the hospital for nearly 2 years. Later, Kaysen discovered that her diagnosis had been borderline personality disorder. In her autobiography, *Girl, Interrupted,* she raises many questions about this diagnosis.

After locating a copy of the *DSM*, she saw that many of her behaviors were characteristic of borderline personality disorder. "It's a fairly accurate picture of me at 18, minus a few quirks like reckless driving and eating binges," she has written.

Kaysen recognizes that sometimes symptoms of a disorder seem like normal developmental processes when she wryly likens the *DSM*'s description of the instability of self-image, interpersonal relationships, and mood characteristic of borderline personality disorder to the typical life of an adolescent.

She sees in the *DSM* other characteristics of her own, such as self-mutilating behavior and a chronic feeling of emptiness. "My chronic feelings of emptiness and boredom," she reports, "came from the fact that I was living a life based on my incapacities, which were numerous." She lists many aspects of school life that she simply couldn't manage.

At times Kaysen felt she was "crazy," asking herself and other people if something she did or said seemed disturbed. "I start a lot of sentences with 'Maybe I'm totally nuts,' or, 'Maybe I've gone round the bend.' If I do something out of the ordinary—take two baths in one day, for example—I say to myself, 'Are you crazy?'"

Was Susanna Kaysen just a mixed-up teenager whose parents expected too much of her and locked her away when she didn't comply? Or was she a deeply troubled young woman whose stay in the hospital prevented her complete psychological deterioration? Is the diagnosis of borderline personality disorder valid, or is it a label we attach to people who don't conform? Kaysen's *Girl, Interrupted* (which was made into a film starring Winona Ryder) brings life to the enduring debate about the validity and ethics of the diagnosis of borderline personality disorder.

Source: Adapted from Kaysen, 1993.

In your daily conversations, you likely refer to people's personalities all the time. **Personality** is enduring patterns of perceiving, feeling, thinking about, and relating to oneself and the environment. You might say that a person you just met is outgoing, or that you tend to be disorganized, or that a friend of yours is highly emotional. A **personality trait** is a prominent aspect of personality that is relatively consistent across time and across situations, such as being outgoing, caring and compassionate, exploitive or hostile, impulsive or unstable.

One of the leading theories of personality is the **five-factor model,** a dimensional perspective that posits that everyone's personality is organized along five broad personality traits, or factors. These factors are often referred to as the *Big 5:* negative emotionality, extraversion, openness to experience, agreeableness, and conscientiousness (McCrae & Costa, 1999, 2013). Each factor has a number of facets, or dimensions, as shown in Table 1. The table lists the facets that make up each of the five factors (in the leftmost

column), and descriptions of people who are high on that facet (in the second column) and descriptions of people low on that facet (in the third column). These descriptions give a sense of the two ends of each dimension. Basically, all people vary on each of these dimensions, and these dimensions cluster under the Big 5. Considerable research supports the five-factor model of personality. These traits seem to capture a great deal of the variation in people's personalities, and they have been replicated in cultures very different from that of the United States (Benet-Martinez & John, 1998; Yang et al., 2002; see Carlo, Knight, Roesch, Opal, & Davis, 2014). The personality traits, especially the facet dimensions, in the five-factor model appear to be strongly influenced by genetics (Briley & Tucker-Drob, 2012; Jang et al., 2006; Sanchez-Roige, Gray, MacKillop, Chen, & Palmer, 2018). You can probably find yourself among the traits and facets of the Big 5.

As mentioned earlier, the *DSM-5* includes two models of PDs. Similar to the *DSM-IV-TR,* the first

TABLE 1   The Big 5 Personality Factors

Each of the Big 5 personality factors is composed of different facets, or components.

FACTOR 1: NEGATIVE EMOTIONALITY VERSUS EMOTIONAL STABILITY

Facet	Individuals high on this facet are	Individuals low on this facet are
Anxiousness	fearful, apprehensive	relaxed, unconcerned, cool
Angry hostility	angry, bitter	even-tempered
Depressiveness	pessimistic, glum	optimistic
Self-consciousness	timid, embarrassed	self-assured, glib, shameless
Impulsivity	tempted, urgent	controlled, restrained
Vulnerability	helpless, fragile	clear-thinking, fearless, unflappable

FACTOR 2: EXTRAVERSION VERSUS INTROVERSION

Facet	Individuals high on this facet are	Individuals low on this facet are
Warmth	cordial, affectionate, attached	cold, aloof, indifferent
Gregariousness	sociable, outgoing	withdrawn, isolated
Assertiveness	dominant, forceful	unassuming, quiet, resigned
Activity	unassuming, quiet, resigned	passive, lethargic
Excitement seeking	reckless, daring	cautious, monotonous, dull
Positive emotions	high-spirited	placid, anhedonic

FACTOR 3: OPENNESS VERSUS CLOSEDNESS TO ONE'S OWN EXPERIENCE

Facet	Individuals high on this facet are	Individuals low on this facet are
Fantasy	dreamers, unrealistic, imaginative	practical, concrete
Aesthetics	aberrant interests, aesthetic	uninvolved, no aesthetic interests
Feelings	self-aware	constricted, unaware
Actions	unconventional, eccentric	routine, predictable, habitual, stubborn
Ideas	unusual, creative	pragmatic, rigid
Values	permissive, broad-minded	traditional, inflexible, dogmatic

FACTOR 4: AGREEABLENESS VERSUS ANTAGONISM

Facet	Individuals high on this facet are	Individuals low on this facet are
Trust	gullible, naïve, trusting	skeptical, cynical, suspicious, paranoid
Straightforwardness	confiding, honest	cunning, manipulative, deceptive
Altruism	sacrificial, giving	stingy, selfish, greedy, exploitative
Compliance	docile, cooperative	oppositional, combative, aggressive
Modesty	meek, self-effacing, humble	confident, boastful, arrogant
Tender-mindedness	soft, empathetic	tough, callous, ruthless

FACTOR 5: CONSCIENTIOUSNESS VERSUS UNDEPENDABILITY

Facet	Individuals high on this facet are	Individuals low on this facet are
Competence	perfectionistic, efficient	lax, negligent
Order	ordered, methodical, organized	haphazard, disorganized, sloppy
Dutifulness	rigid, reliable, dependable	casual, undependable, unethical
Achievement	workaholic, ambitious	aimless, desultory
Self-discipline	dogged, devoted	hedonistic, negligent
Deliberation	cautious, ruminative, reflective	hasty, careless, rash

Source: Widiger & Mullins-Sweatt, 2009.

model is categorical and defines 10 different PDs in terms of distinct criteria sets. The categorical model is intended for current clinical use. An alternative trait-specific, or dimensional, model was developed for *DSM-5* and is included in a different section of the manual designated for further study. It makes use of a continuum model of PDs such as that represented in the Big 5 model. The alternative model essentially assumes that normal and abnormal personality fall on an integrated continuum of personality, with PDs representing more extreme and maladaptive variants of personality traits, as described in this chapter's Along the Continuum feature. We will first describe the *DSM-5*'s current model before turning to a review of its limitations and the *DSM-5*'s alternative model of PDs.

GENERAL DEFINITION OF PERSONALITY DISORDER

The *DSM-5* carries forward the categorical perspective first established in *DSM-III* in 1980. It treats personality disorders (PDs) as if they were entirely different from "normal" personality traits. Unlike prior manuals, however, the *DSM-5* provides a general definition of **personality disorder (PD)** that applies to each of the 10 specific PDs (Table 2). The general criteria for a PD specify that an individual's personality pattern must *deviate markedly from the expectations of their culture* as shown in *styles of thinking about oneself, others, or events; emotional experience and expression; interpersonal functioning; and/or impulse control.* An individual's personality pattern must be *pervasive and inflexible* across situations, be *stable* over time, have an *onset in adolescence or early adulthood,* and lead to *significant distress or functional impairment.* An individual's long-term pattern of functioning also cannot be better explained as a manifestation or consequence of another mental, substance use, or medical disorder (American Psychiatric Association, 2013).

By definition, a PD is an enduring pattern of thinking, feeling, and behaving that is relatively stable over time, and the particular personality features must be evident by early adulthood. For a PD to be diagnosed in an individual younger than 18 years, the personality patterns must have been present for at least 1 year (with the exception of antisocial PD, which cannot be diagnosed before age 18). Most clinicians

will thus assess the stability of personality traits over time and across different situations, taking into account ethnic, cultural, and social background influences and taking care to distinguish the personality traits that define the PDs from characteristics that emerge in response to situational stressors or more transient mental states like mood, anxiety, or substance use disorders.

The *DSM-5* also moved away from a multiaxial system of diagnosis, first introduced in *DSM-III,* and collapsed Axes I and II into a common section (see the chapter "Assessing and Diagnosing Abnormality"). Until the *DSM-5,* the PDs were treated differently and placed on Axis II, because it was believed that PDs were especially pervasive and chronic, rather than occurring in more discrete or acute episodes, which characterize the clinical disorders coded on Axis I. Although most people diagnosed with a PD also experience another clinical disorder at some time in their life (Grant et al., 2004), the *DSM-5* had as one of its goals to reduce comorbidity and no longer regarded the Axis I and Axis II distinction as clinically useful (Links & Eynan, 2013; Morey et al., 2015).

The *DSM-5* groups 10 distinct PDs into three clusters based on their descriptive similarities (Table 3). Importantly, *DSM-5* explicitly recognizes that this clustering system is limited, has not been consistently validated, and fails to account for the fact that individuals often show co-occurring PDs from different clusters. *Cluster A* includes three disorders characterized by *odd or eccentric behaviors and thinking:* paranoid PD, schizoid PD, and schizotypal PD. Each of these has some of the features of schizophrenia, but people diagnosed with these PDs are not out of touch with reality. Their behaviors often appear odd, eccentric, and inappropriate. For example, they may be chronically suspicious of others or speak in odd ways that are difficult to understand.

Cluster B includes four disorders characterized by *dramatic, erratic, or emotional behavior and interpersonal relationships:* antisocial PD, histrionic PD, borderline PD, and narcissistic PD. People diagnosed with these disorders tend to be manipulative, volatile, and uncaring in social relationships and prone to impulsive behaviors. They may behave in exaggerated ways or even attempt suicide to try to gain attention.

Cluster C includes three disorders characterized by *anxious and fearful emotions and chronic self-doubt:*

TABLE 2   Personality Disorder

The general criteria for a personality disorder specify that an individual's personality pattern must deviate significantly from the expectations of their culture as shown in the styles of thinking about oneself, others, or events; emotional experience and expression; interpersonal functioning; and/or impulse control.

TABLE 3   Personality Disorder Clusters

The *DSM-5* groups personality disorders into three clusters based on descriptive similarities.

CLUSTER A: ODD-ECCENTRIC PERSONALITY DISORDERS

People with these disorders have symptoms similar to those of people with schizophrenia, including inappropriate or flat affect, odd thought and speech patterns, and paranoia. People with these disorders maintain their grasp on reality, however.

CLUSTER B: DRAMATIC-EMOTIONAL PERSONALITY DISORDERS

People with these disorders tend to be manipulative, volatile, and uncaring in social relationships. They are prone to impulsive, sometimes violent behaviors that show little regard for their own safety or the safety or needs of others.

CLUSTER C: ANXIOUS-FEARFUL PERSONALITY DISORDERS

People with these disorders are extremely concerned about being criticized or abandoned by others and thus have dysfunctional relationships with others.

---

dependent PD, avoidant PD, and obsessive-compulsive PD. People diagnosed with these disorders have little self-confidence and difficulty in relationships.

CLUSTER A: ODD-ECCENTRIC PERSONALITY DISORDERS

The behavior of people diagnosed with the odd-eccentric personality disorders (Table 4) is similar to that of people with schizophrenia, but these people retain their grasp on reality to a greater degree than do people who are psychotic. They may be paranoid, speak in odd and eccentric ways that make them difficult to understand, have difficulty relating to other people, and have unusual beliefs or perceptual experiences that fall short of delusions and hallucinations. Many researchers consider this group of personality disorders to be part of the *schizophrenia spectrum,*

particularly schizotypal personality disorder (Nelson, Seal, Pantelis, & Phillips, 2013), though they are below the threshold for the diagnosis of a psychotic disorder (see the chapter "Schizophrenia Spectrum and Other Psychotic Disorders"). That is, these disorders show some attenuated schizophrenia-like symptoms and, especially regarding schizotypal personality disorder, may be precursors to schizophrenia in a small proportion of people. These disorders also more often occur in people with first-degree relatives who have schizophrenia or persecutory type delusional disorder.

Paranoid Personality Disorder

The defining feature of **paranoid personality disorder (PPD)** is a pattern of pervasive distrust and suspiciousness of others such that their motives are interpreted as malevolent. People diagnosed with this disorder

---

TABLE 4   Cluster A: Odd-Eccentric Personality Disorders

People with an odd-eccentric personality disorder may exhibit mild signs of schizophrenia.

Label	Key Features	Relationship to Schizophrenia
Paranoid personality disorder	A pattern of distrust and suspiciousness such that others' motives are interpreted as malevolent	Weak relationship
Schizoid personality disorder	A pattern of detachment from social relationships and a restricted range of emotional expression	Unclear relationship
Schizotypal personality disorder	A pattern of acute discomfort in close relationships, cognitive or perceptual distortions, and eccentricities of behavior	Strong relationship—considered a mild version of schizophrenia

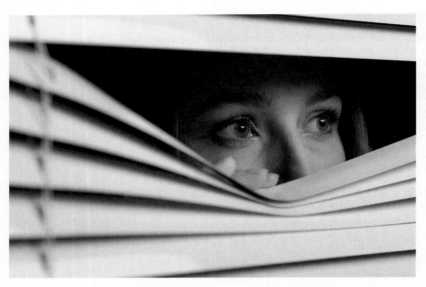

Individuals with paranoid personality disorder are suspicious and distrustful of others, often believing that unrelated events have personal significance to them. *D-Keine/Getty Images*

believe that other people are constantly trying to deceive or exploit them, and they are preoccupied with concerns about being victimized or mistreated. Convinced that others are plotting against them, they are hypervigilant (excessively on-edge) and constantly monitor their social environments looking for evidence to confirm their suspicions or for signs of danger. People with PDD are likely to attribute minor events that most people would dismiss as insignificant, as evidence that others are "out to get them." As a result, individuals with this disorder remain vigilant in scanning their environment for potential threats, feeling mistrustful of friendly gestures or any situation that may be ambiguous. People with PPD are more likely to notice a subtle grimace on the face of their boss or an apparently trivial slip of the tongue by a family member that would go unnoticed by others. People diagnosed with paranoid personality disorder consider these events to be highly meaningful and spend a great deal of time trying to decipher such clues to other people's true intentions. They are also very sensitive and angrily reactive to real or perceived criticism and tend to bear grudges. For example, watching co-workers engaged in a conversation across the room may be perceived to be talking about and plotting against the paranoid individual (Lewis & Ridenour, 2020).

This disorder directly impacts social relationships and people affected by PPD are more likely to have difficulty in social activities or settings, which results in more social withdrawal and isolating behaviors. Those individuals who are involved in romantic relationships often have trouble sustaining them without accusing the other person of being disloyal. People with paranoid personality disorder tend to misinterpret situations in line with their suspicions. For

example, a husband might interpret his wife's cheerfulness one evening as evidence that she is having an affair with someone at work. In contrast to paranoid thoughts occurring at the psychotic level, as seen in schizophrenia, the suspicious beliefs associate with paranoid personality disorder are typically somewhat plausible, and the individual diagnosed with paranoid personality disorder retains some degree of reality testing abilities (Lewis & Ridenour, 2020). These people are resistant to rational arguments against their suspicions and may consider the fact that another person is arguing with them as evidence that the person is part of the conspiracy against them. Some are secretive and withdraw from other people in an attempt to protect themselves, but others become hostile and argumentative, sure that their way of looking at the world is right and superior and that the best defense against the conspiring of others is a good offense. Felix, in the following case study, was diagnosed with paranoid personality disorder.

CASE STUDY

Felix is a 59-year-old construction worker who worries that his co-workers might hurt him. Last week, while he was using a table saw, Felix's hand slipped and his fingers came very close to being cut badly. Felix wonders if someone sabotaged the saw, so that somehow the piece of wood he was working with slipped and drew his hand into the saw blade. Since this incident, Felix has observed his co-workers looking at him and whispering to each other. He mentioned his suspicion that the saw had been tampered with to his boss, but the boss told him that was a crazy idea and that Felix obviously had just been careless.

Felix does not have any close friends. Even his brothers and sisters avoid him, because he frequently misinterprets things they say to be criticisms of him. Felix was married for a few years, but his wife left him when he began to demand that she should not see any of her friends or go out without him, because he suspected she was having affairs with other men. Felix lives in a middle-class neighborhood in a small town that has very little crime. Still, he owns three handguns and a shotgun, which are always loaded, in expectation of someone breaking into his house.

Recent research has found that among personality disorders, PPD is one of the least examined and there have been calls for its removal from the *DSM-5* from members of the psychiatric community (Poggi, Richetin, & Preti, 2019). What is well-known about

PPD is that this disorder is severe and difficult to treat since primary characteristics include suspicion, relentless, ruminative, and jealous which limit the chances of treatment initiation. Despite oddities that may resemble some aspects of psychotic disorders, symptoms of PPD do not include psychotic symptoms, such as paranoid delusions and hallucinations, commonly encountered in disorders like schizophrenia, schizoaffective, and psychotic states of bipolar disorder.

Epidemiological studies suggest that rates of PPD range from 1.21 to 4.4 percent of people in the general population throughout the world, but estimations within the clinical population are as high as 25 percent (Lee, 2017; Lewis & Ridenour, 2020). Not surprisingly, they are difficult to get along with, and their interpersonal relationships, including intimate relationships, tend to be unstable. Studies performed in the United States and Australia both indicate that PPD is a significant cause of disability. Additionally, global studies have found that persons with PPD, when not disabled, stop working earlier than nonpersonality disordered individuals. In clinical populations, this disorder is one of the strongest predictors of aggressive behavior. In the forensic realm, PPD is associated with violence and stalking and excessive litigation. People diagnosed with this disorder appear to be at increased risk for a number of clinical disorders, including major depression, anxiety disorders, substance abuse, and psychotic episodes (Grant, Stinson, et al., 2004; Trull, Jahng, Tomko, Wood, & Sher, 2010), as well as impaired vocational functioning (McGurk et al., 2013). Research has found that individuals with PPD are more likely to experience depressive disorders, social phobia and poor prognosis, despite intensive psychiatric treatment. The degree of suicide risk among this population is unclear due to limited data and more research is needed on this important clinical problem (Lee, 2017; Lewis & Ridenour, 2020).

Theories of Paranoid Personality Disorder

It has long been hypothesized that Cluster A personality disorders, like PPD, were related to schizophrenia. While there are some transdiagnostic patterns among these groups, currently there is insufficient research linking PPD with schizophrenia. Family studies have presented both sparse and mixed evidence on the increased familial risk for PPD among those families with schizophrenia. In one blind family study, researchers found that PPD was more common in relatives with unipolar depression than with schizophrenia-affected individuals. Other studies have found a stronger relationship between PPD and delusional disorder noting that 30 percent of family members of persons with delusional disorder sharing paranoid personality

disorder traits, as compared to only 3 percent of family members of healthy controls. In contrast, those with schizoid and schizotypal personality disorder are more commonly found in families with schizophrenia and less commonly found among families with delusional disorder. Additionally, the children of parents with schizophrenia have been found to be at higher risk for avoidant and schizotypal personality disorder, but not PPD. Overall, PPD remains an understudied disorder with many unanswered questions and some genetic relatedness between PPD and schizophrenia with more evidence of a relationship between PPD and delusional disorder (Lee, 2017).

Cognitive theorists view paranoid personality disorder as the result of an underlying belief that other people are malevolent and deceptive, combined with a lack of self-confidence about being able to defend oneself against others (Beck, Davis, & Freeman, 2015). Thus, the person must always be vigilant for signs of others' deceit or criticism and must be quick to act against others. A study of 17 patients diagnosed with paranoid personality disorder found that they endorsed beliefs as predicted by this cognitive theory more than did patients diagnosed with other personality disorders (Beck et al., 2001). Multiple studies have found that people experiencing paranoia tend to hastily "jump to conclusions" and require less information before drawing a conclusion than nonparanoid individuals. Additionally, studies have found the people with PPD are more likely to hold others responsible for their life circumstances rather than recognizing personal contributions to situations and outcomes. Research suggests that concentrating on signs of hostility and danger combined with an attribution style that erroneously externalizes and personalizes blame, may create the conditions in which the paranoid individual views themself as alone and unprotected in a dangerous world (Lewis & Ridenour, 2020).

As in many disorders, there are also social contributors to paranoid personality disorder. In the United States, African Americans report higher rates of paranoid personality disorder than whites. This disparity is likely due in part to increased exposure in this group to social and environmental risk factors that may lead individuals to be more mistrustful or suspicious. Differential exposure to discrimination, prejudice, childhood trauma, and especially socioeconomic status appear to contribute to this demographic disparity (Iacovino, Jackson, & Oltmanns, 2014).

Treatment of Paranoid Personality Disorder

Due to the inflexible distrust and suspicion of others, people diagnosed with paranoid personality disorder typically access mental health services only when they are in crisis. Meaning, it is rare to find an individual with PPD who voluntarily enters psychotherapy since their core symptoms make them more prone to be guarded and suspicious about treatment. This pervasive distrust also severely limits the amount of clinical trials and research that could provide useful information about best practices with no research studies focused on PPD and published clinical are primarily limited to individual case studies (Lewis & Ridenour, 2020). Currently, there are no FDA-approved medications for PPD and knowledge is limited about best therapeutic option for people with PPD. However, research on cognitive-behavioral therapy (CBT), psychoanalysis and transference-focused therapy, conditioned avoidant response (CAR) and dialectical behavioral therapy all show promise in helping people with PPD but there is not sufficient evidence to determine which therapy is most effective. Additionally, studies on mentalization-based treatment (MBT) find that this therapy which combines approaches from psychodynamic therapy, CBT, and interpersonal psychotherapy may also be effective option for those with PPD, especially if **borderline personality disorder (BPD)** is also present (Lee, 2017).

Cognitive therapy for people diagnosed with this disorder focuses on increasing their sense of self-efficacy in dealing with difficult situations, thus decreasing their fear and hostility toward others. Consider the following interchange below between a cognitive therapist and a woman, Ann, who believed that her co-workers were intentionally trying to annoy her and to turn her supervisor against her. They may seek treatment for severe symptoms of depression or anxiety, but they often do not feel a need for treatment of their paranoia. Their guarded and suspicious style will often undercut the development of a trusting, therapeutic relationship. In addition, therapists' attempts to challenge their paranoid thinking are likely to be misinterpreted in line with their paranoid belief system. For these reasons, treating paranoid personality disorder can be quite difficult (Millon, Grossman, Millon, Meagher, & Ramnath, 2004).

PROFILES

Therapist: You're reacting as though this is a very dangerous situation. What are the risks you see?

Ann: They'll keep dropping things and making noise to annoy me.

Therapist: Are you sure nothing worse is at risk?

Ann: Yeah.

Therapist: So you don't think there's much chance of them attacking you or anything?

Ann: Nah, they wouldn't do that.

Therapist: If they do keep dropping things and making noises, how bad will that be?

Ann: Like I told you, it's real aggravating. It really bugs me.

Therapist: So it would continue pretty much as it's been going for years now.

Ann: Yeah. It bugs me, but I can take it.

Therapist: And you know that if it keeps happening, at the very least you can keep handling it the way you have been—holding the aggravation in, then taking it out on your husband when you get home. Suppose we could come up with some ways to handle the aggravation even better or to have them get to you less. Is that something you'd be interested in?

Ann: Yeah, that sounds good.

Therapist: Another risk you mentioned earlier is that they might talk to your supervisor and turn her against you. As you see it, how long have they been trying to do this?

Ann: Ever since I've been there.

Therapist: How much luck have they had so far in doing that?

Ann: Not much.

Therapist: Do you see any indications that they're going to have any more success now than they have so far?

Ann: No, I don't guess so.

Therapist: So your gut reaction is as though the situation at work is really dangerous. But when you stop and think it through, you conclude that the worst they're going to do is to be really aggravating, and that even if we don't come up with anything new, you can handle it well enough to get by. Does that sound right?

Ann: [Smiling] Yeah, I guess so.

Therapist: And if we can come up with some ways to handle the stress better or handle them better, there will be even less they can do to you.

In this interchange, the therapist did not directly challenge Ann's beliefs about her co-workers' intentions but did try to reduce the sense of danger Ann felt about her workplace by helping her redefine the situation as aggravating rather than threatening. The therapist also enlisted Ann in an effort to develop new coping skills that might further reduce her aggravation and develop a sense of self-efficacy.

In order to gain the trust of a person diagnosed with a PPD, the therapist must be calm, respectful, and extremely straightforward. The therapist cannot directly confront the client's paranoid thinking but instead must rely on indirect means of raising questions in the client's mind about his or her typical way of interpreting situations. Although many therapists do not expect paranoid clients to achieve full insight into their problems, they hope that, by developing at least some degree of trust in the therapist, the client can learn to trust others a bit more and thus develop somewhat improved interpersonal relationships.

Similar to the longitudinal course of other personality disorder it is posited that symptoms of PPD diminish in severity over time. Some suggests that this disorder should be viewed as a variant of a psychotic-spectrum or delusional disorder, but there is still significant disagreement on this point. The degree to which paranoid personality disorder exists as a heritable condition, and its genetic relationship to other mental health conditions still remains unclear and additional studies are needed to develop a better overall understanding of this disorder (Lewis & Ridenour, 2020)

Schizoid Personality Disorder

You may have heard the term "schizoid" used to describe people who strongly prefer to turn their attention inward and away from the outside world, often engaging in solitary activities. People with SPD are often indifferent to opportunities to develop close relationships and derive little, if any, pleasure from family or social interactions (American Psychiatric Association, 2013). People diagnosed with **schizoid personality disorder (SPD)** show a pervasive pattern of detachment from social relationships and a restricted range of emotional expression in their interactions with others. This emotional coldness, detachment, and apathy may be related to the inability to process emotions among people with schizoid PD. Recent studies have shown higher rates of alexithymia among individuals with personality disorders a condition that is characterized by an impaired ability to recognize and express emotions. Alexithymia is associated with problems deciphering external emotions that may lead to emotional dysregulation, suicidal ideation, and comorbidity with other major psychiatric disorders.

Interestingly, the severity level of alexithymia was positively correlated with schizoid-affected individuals. Meaning, those with higher levels of alexithymia have less ability to correctly interpret emotional expresses. Perhaps as a result of this inability to interpret emotional expressions, people with schizoid PD have an elevated risk for major depression (Wang et al., 2020).

Symptoms of SPD are associated with higher levels of mental pain and recurrent depression which are acknowledged as risk factors for suicide. Limited studies have revealed an association between SPD and suicide behaviors. Clinical experience and research have shown that SPD is strongly associated with unbearable and inescapable loneliness and social withdrawal. SPD affected individuals are characterized by low interest in activities and significant affective indifference. It is theorized that these symptoms weaken the ability of the individual to effectively cope with mental pain which enhances the likelihood of lethal suicide attempt (Levi-Belz, Gvion, Levi, & Apter, 2019).

Studies in the United Kingdom and Greece have found a significant correlations between individuals with schizoid PD and the commitment of violent crimes, including homicides and violent behaviors. As compared with prisoners without personality disorders, the percentages of violent crimes and homicides/attempted homicides were significantly higher among those diagnosed with Cluster A personality disorder, particularly those with schizoid or schizotypal PD. Recent research has found high prevalence of paranoid and SPDs within the general prison population which suggests that Cluster A personality disorder diagnoses frequently co-exist within forensic samples. There is also a strong correlation between SPD and alcohol abuse (Apostolopoulos et al., 2018; Bennett & Johnson, 2017; Levi-Belz, Gvion, Levi, & Apter, 2019).

As with other personality disorders, SPD is a severe and highly treatment-resistant disorder that can lead to clinically significant distress or impairment in several important areas of functioning (Wang et al., 2020). Their experience and expression of positive emotions are very low, and their interest in having sexual experiences with another person is typically very limited. Other people describe them as emotionally aloof or cold, "loners," or "bland," uninteresting, and humorless. People diagnosed with this disorder are often indifferent to others' praise or criticism, and they take pleasure in few activities. While they tend to view relationships with others as unrewarding, messy, and intrusive, in those few situations in which they may temporarily feel comfortable talking about themselves, they may acknowledge having painful feelings, particularly related to social interactions. Recent research suggests that people with SPD may have a predisposition to fantasy and introspection which impacts the ability for individuals to express their feelings and experience pleasure (Căndel & Constantin, 2017). The case study of Roy described next shows several of these symptoms. Roy would be diagnosed with SPD because of his long-standing avoidance of relationships with other people and his lack of close relationships with family members.

CASE STUDY

Roy was a successful sanitation engineer involved in the planning and maintenance of water resources for a large city; his job called for considerable foresight and independent judgment but little supervisory responsibility. In general, he was appraised as an undistinguished but competent and reliable employee. There were few demands of an interpersonal nature made of him, and he was viewed by most of his colleagues as reticent and shy and by others as cold and aloof.

Difficulties centered around his relationship with his wife. At her urging they sought marital counseling, for, as she put it, "he is unwilling to join in family activities, he fails to take interest in the children, he lacks affection, and he is disinterested in sex."

The pattern of social indifference, flatness of affect, and personal isolation that characterized much of Roy's behavior was of little consequence to those with whom a deeper or more intimate relationship was not called for; with his immediate family; however, these traits took their toll. (Source: Millon, 1969, p. 224)

At this time, the amount of available literature on SPD is scarce which makes this disorder one of the most understudied disorders in the *DSM-5*. SPD is less common than other PDs with about 0.8 to 2.8 percent of adults manifesting the disorder at some time in their life, with some estimates as 5 percent of the general population. However, due to the social isolation experienced by people with this disorder, it may be possible that the actual prevalence is much higher than reported (Levi-Belz, Gvion, Levi, & Apter, 2019; Trull et al., 2010; Volkert, Gablonski, & Rabung, 2018). This disorder appears to occur somewhat more often in men than women (Trull et al., 2010; Zimmerman, Rothschild, & Chelminski, 2005). People with SPD can function in society, particularly in occupations that do not require frequent interpersonal interactions.

Theories of Schizoid Personality Disorder

There is a slightly increased rate of SPD in the relatives of persons with schizophrenia, but the link between the two disorders is not clear (Wang et al., 2020). Twin studies of the personality traits associated with SPD, such as low sociability and low warmth, strongly suggest that these personality traits may be partially inherited (Widiger & Costa, 2013). The evidence for the heritability of SPD is only indirect, however.

Treatment of Schizoid Personality Disorder

As you might expect, people with SPD may not be very motivated for treatment, and the interpersonal closeness of therapy may be experienced as stressful instead of supportive. Despite these treatment challenges, psychosocial treatments for SPD focus on increasing the person's awareness of their own feelings, as well as increasing their social skills and social contacts (Beck et al., 2015). The therapist may model the expression of feelings for the client and help the client identify and express their own feelings. Social skills training, done through role-playing with the therapist and homework assignments in which the client tries out new social skills with other people, is an important component of cognitive therapies. Some therapists recommend group therapy for people with SPD. In the context of group sessions, the group members can model interpersonal relationships, and each person with SPD can practice new social skills directly with other group members.

Schizotypal Personality Disorder

People affected with **schizotypal personality disorder (STPD)** have lifelong patterns of odd or peculiar behaviors and/or appearance that impact their interpersonal function, thinking, and behavior. This is the only PD that is included on the schizophrenia spectrum since people diagnosed with this disorder often display similar symptoms to those with schizophrenia. Although the eccentric behaviors, disturbance of thought and affect displayed in STPD are similar to those seen in schizophrenia, the symptom development and course of this disorder are not consistent with schizophrenia. Overall, this PD is understudied, often under-recognized or misdiagnosed, challenging to treat and associated with significant functional impairment (Rosell, Futterman, McMaster, & Siever, 2014). Like schizoid and paranoid personality disorders, people with STPD tend to be socially isolated, have a restricted range of emotions, and are uncomfortable with interpersonal interactions (Table 5). Symptoms of STPD often include odd and magical thinking and preoccupation with bizarre fantasies (See, Klimstra, Shiner, & Denissen,

TABLE 5   Schizotypal Personality Disorder*

A pervasive pattern of social and interpersonal deficits marked by acute discomfort with, and reduced capacity for, close relationships as well as by cognitive or perceptual distortions and eccentricities of behavior, beginning by early adulthood.

—Symptoms include:

- Restricted range of emotion

- Uncomfortable interpersonal interactions

- Odd and eccentric behavior

- Paranoia

—Prevalence rate is 3.9 percent of general population

—More commonly diagnosed in males than in females

*The information presented in this table is based solely on the author's interpretation of *DSM-5*. It does not reflect the exact language that appears in *DSM-5* and is not, therefore, formally endorsed by the American Psychological Association.

2020). This disruption of personality results in psychoticism, eccentricity, cognitive and perceptual dysregulation, unusual beliefs, restricted affect and emotional withdrawal, characterized by suspiciousness that disrupts daily function (Kirchner, Roeh, Nolden, & Hasan, 2018).

Problems with social interaction are common among those with STPD, who may have few close relationships and trouble understanding the behaviors of others. They tend to perceive other people as deceitful and hostile and may be socially anxious and isolated because of their suspiciousness. Although they maintain their grasp on reality, people with STPD think and behave in ways that are very odd. The distinguishing characteristics of STPD are the cognitive and perceptual distortions and odd and eccentric behaviors. For example, they may think they see people in the patterns of wallpaper or they may be easily distracted or fixate on an object for long periods of time, or lost in thought or fantasy (Beck et al., 2015). People with this disorder may have ideas of reference or they may believe that random events or circumstances are related to them. These misconceptions are associated with excessive social anxiety that tends to contribute to paranoid fears (Rosell, Futterman, McMaster, & Siever, 2014). For example, they may believe while out in a crowded public shopping area that everyone is staring at them or upon hearing someone laugh, they assume the laughter is directed at them.

In addition to demonstrating cognitive and perceptual distortions, people diagnosed with STPD tend to have speech that is tangential, circumstantial, vague, or overdetailed. In interactions with others, they may have inappropriate or odd emotional responses or no emotional response. They may be easily distracted or may fixate on an object for a long period of time, often lost in unusual thought or fantasy. Although these oddities of thought, speech, and behavior are similar in quality to those seen in schizophrenia, their severity is not as great as in schizophrenia, and people diagnosed with STPD retain basic contact with reality. The man in the following case study shows many of the oddities of STPD.

CASE STUDY

A 41-year-old man was referred to a community mental health center's activities program for help in improving his social skills. He had a lifelong pattern of social isolation, with no real friends, and spent long hours worrying that his angry thoughts about his older brother would cause his brother harm. He had previously worked as a clerk in civil service but had lost his job because of poor attendance and low productivity.

On interview the patient was distant and somewhat distrustful. He described in elaborate and often irrelevant detail his rather uneventful and routine daily life. For 2 days he had studied the washing instructions on a new pair of jeans: Did "Wash before wearing" mean that the jeans were to be washed before wearing the first time, or did they need, for some reason, to be washed each time before they were worn? He did not regard concerns such as these as senseless, though he acknowledged that the amount of time spent thinking about them might be excessive. He could recite from memory his most recent monthly bank statement, including the amount

(continued)

of every check and the running balance as each check was written. He knew his balance on any particular day, but he sometimes got anxious if he considered whether a certain check or deposit had actually cleared. (Reprinted with permission from the *DSM-IV Casebook: A Learning Companion to the Diagnostic and Statistical Manual of Mental Disorders*, 4th Edition. Copyright ©1994 by American Psychiatric Association. All Rights Reserved.)

The prevalence of STPD has been estimated as ranging from 0.6 percent in a Norwegian sample to 4.6 percent in an American sample, but appears to be less frequent in clinical settings (0 to 1.9 percent) (American Psychiatric Association, 2013). Men (4.2 percent) are slightly more affected with this disorder than women (3.7 percent). However, the likelihood of STPD was greater among Black woman, those with a low income, and people who were separated, divorced, or widowed. Conversely, research suggests that the odds of STPD were lowest among Asian men. Recent studies have found a significant relationship between STPD and bipolar I and II, PTSD, BPD, and narcissistic personality disorder (NPD) and schizophrenia (or isolated psychotic episodes). Common differential diagnoses are attention-deficit disorder, social anxiety disorder, autism-spectrum disorder, and dysthymia. Some people diagnosed with STPD have episodes symptomatic of brief psychotic disorder, and some eventually develop the full syndrome of schizophrenia. Concerns about the presence of additional disorders are significant, as these comorbidities can complicate understanding both the course of the disorder and treatment responses (Kirchner, Roeh, Nolden, & Hasan, 2018; Kwapil & Barrantes-Vidal, 2012; Rosell et al., 2014).

For a person to be given a diagnosis of STPD, their odd or eccentric thoughts cannot be part of cultural beliefs, such as a cultural belief in magic or specific superstitions. Still, some psychologists have argued that people of color are diagnosed more often with schizophrenia-like disorders, such as STPD, than are whites because white clinicians often misinterpret culturally bound beliefs as evidence of schizotypal thinking (Snowden & Cheung, 1990; see Schwartz & Blankenship, 2014). One large study of people in treatment found that African American patients were more likely than white or Hispanic patients to be diagnosed with STPD on both self-report and standardized diagnostic interviews (Chavira et al., 2003). This finding suggests that African Americans may be diagnosed with this disorder relatively frequently even when steps are taken to avoid clinician bias. It is possible that African Americans are more likely to be exposed to conditions that enhance a biological vulnerability to schizophrenia-like

disorders. These conditions include urban living and low socioeconomic status (see the chapter "Schizophrenia Spectrum and Other Psychotic Disorders" for a discussion of these conditions in schizophrenia).

Theories of Schizotypal Personality Disorder

STPD is the most well researched of the Cluster A personality disorders. Family history, adoption, and twin studies all suggest that STPD is transmitted genetically (Nelson et al., 2013). Indeed, a twin study found the heritability of STPD to be .81 (Coolidge, Thede, & Jang, 2004). In addition, STPD is much more common among first-degree relatives of people with schizophrenia than in the relatives of either psychiatric patients or healthy control groups (Kendler et al., 1993; Kwapil & Barrantes-Vidal, 2012). This supports the view that STPD is a mild form of schizophrenia that is transmitted through genes in ways similar to those in schizophrenia. A gene that regulates the NMDA receptor system has been associated with both schizophrenia and STPD (Ohi et al., 2012). Studies have also found that people with STPD share some of the same genetic traits and neurological abnormalities as people with schizophrenia (Cannon, van Erp, & Glahn, 2002). STPD is more frequently found in relatives of individuals with schizophrenia or a Cluster A personality disorder. Recent twin studies have showed highly stable genetic factors and intermittent environmental factors related to increased risk for the STPD. Additionally, genetic risk factors for schizophrenia may also be linked to development of STPD (Kirchner, Roeh, Nolden, & Hasan, 2018; Rosell et al., 2014).

On neuropsychological tests (see the chapter "Assessing and Diagnosing Abnormality"), people with STPD show deficits in working memory, learning, and recall similar to, but less severe than, those shown by people with schizophrenia (Barch & Sheffield, 2017). People with STPD show many of the same cognitive deficits as people with schizophrenia, including difficulties in verbal fluency, in inhibiting information when a task calls for it, and in memory (Barch & Sheffield, 2017; Cochrane, Petch, & Pickering, 2012; Mitropoulou et al., 2003). People with STPD, like those with schizophrenia, tend to show dysregulation of the neurotransmitter dopamine in the brain (Abi-Dargham et al., 2004). Thus, like people with schizophrenia, people with STPD may have abnormally high levels of dopamine in striatal and cortical regions of the brain that appears to play an important role in the development of these symptoms (Rosell et al., 2014).

Although people with STPD show abnormalities in the same areas of the brain as people with schizophrenia, these abnormalities tend to be less severe in STPD than in schizophrenia, perhaps reflecting the less severe symptoms (Barch & Sheffield, 2017; Kwapil & Barrantes-Vidal, 2012). For example, one study showed that people with both disorders show gray matter reductions in areas of the temporal lobe of the brain compared to controls, but the reductions were less in people with STPD than in people with schizophrenia (Rosell et al., 2014; Takahashi et al., 2011). Some research finds that people with STPD do not tend to show the abnormalities in the prefrontal areas of the brain shown by people with schizophrenia (e.g., Suzuki et al., 2005), perhaps reflecting the less severe symptoms in STPD.

As we have stated, STPD is likely a heritable condition. It is also influenced by such environmental factors as psychological trauma. Various studies suggest that childhood trauma increases vulnerability for schizophrenia-spectrum disorders, including STPD. A strong correlation between STPD and high frequencies of childhood adversity, have been found as compared to the general population. People with STPD are more likely to have experienced physical, emotional, and sexual abuse, and/or had a parent who was battered, abused substances, or spent time in jail. Research has found that all types of reported childhood trauma were significantly associated with the development of STPD and the severity of abuse was significantly linked to the disruption of interpersonal and cognitive function. It is posited that exposure to childhood trauma impacts long-term outcomes, especially paranoid ideation and suspiciousness, as well as complex social cognitive abilities (Quidé et al., 2018). STPD individuals who reported severe trauma were more likely to display diminished cognitive functioning in areas of working memory, visual learning, and verbal fluency. Severe sexual abuse was most associated with ideas of reference, odd belief, or magical thinking and severe emotional neglect was most associated with interpersonal dysfunction such as excessive social anxiety and constricted affect (Velikonja et al., 2019; Velikonja, Fisher, Mason, & Johnson, 2015).

Treatment of Schizotypal Personality Disorder

STPD is most often treated with the same drugs used to treat schizophrenia, including traditional neuroleptics such as haloperidol and thiothixene and atypical antipsychotics such as olanzapine, and typically at lower doses (Ripoll, Triebwasser, & Siever, 2011). As in schizophrenia, these drugs appear to relieve psychotic-like symptoms, which include distorted ideas of reference, magical thinking, and illusions. Antidepressants sometimes are used to help people with STPD who are experiencing significant distress.

Although there are few psychological theories of STPD, psychological therapies have been developed to help people with this disorder overcome some of their symptoms. In psychotherapy for STPD, it is especially important for the therapist to first establish a good relationship with the client, because these clients typically have few close relationships and tend to struggle with paranoid thoughts and excessive social anxiety (Beck et al., 2015). The next step in therapy is to help the client increase social contacts and learn socially appropriate behaviors through social skills training. Group therapy may be especially helpful in increasing clients' social skills.

The crucial component of cognitive therapy with clients diagnosed with STPD is teaching them to look for objective evidence in the environment to support their thoughts and to disregard bizarre thoughts. For example, a client who frequently thinks she is not real can be taught to identify that thought as bizarre and to discount the thought when it occurs, rather than taking it seriously and acting on it. This psychotherapy approach is similar to cognitive-behavioral approaches to psychotic disorders (see the chapter "Schizophrenia Spectrum and Other Psychotic Disorders"). Because symptoms are typically less severe than in schizophrenia, techniques like challenging perceptions and thoughts may be more readily accepted by the patient (Beck & Rector, 2005; Garety & Freeman, 2013).

CLUSTER B: DRAMATIC-EMOTIONAL PERSONALITY DISORDERS

Individuals affected by Cluster B personality disorder (PD) have difficulty regulating their emotions and behavior which results in what others consider to be dramatic, emotional, erratic, and impulsive behaviors. Cluster B disorders all share problems with impulsivity, inflated sense of self, a tendency to seek stimulation, and often a disregard for their own safety or the safety of others (American Psychiatric Association, 2013) (Table 6). People within this cluster have trouble regulating their emotions and impulses which seriously impacts their ability to maintain interpersonal relationships and daily function. For example, they may engage in suicidal behaviors or self-injury. They also may act in hostile, even violent, ways against others. There are four Cluster B PDs: borderline PD, histrionic PD, antisocial PD, and narcissistic PD. Borderline and antisocial PDs have been the focus of a great deal of research, whereas histrionic PD and narcissistic PD have received less attention in terms of study. As we will discuss, antisocial PD shares important symptom patterns that have a developmental continuity with conduct disorder, a separate disorder that is discussed in the chapter "Disruptive, Impulse-Control, and Conduct Disorders."

Borderline Personality Disorder

If there was one word that could best describe borderline personality disorder (BPD) it would be

TABLE 6   Cluster B Personality Disorders: Dramatic-Emotional

People with dramatic-emotional personality disorders tend to have unstable emotions and to engage in dramatic and impulsive behavior.

Label	Key Features	Similar Disorders
Antisocial personality disorder	A pattern of disregard for, and violation of, the rights of others; criminal, impulsive, deceitful, or callous behavior; lack of remorse	Conduct disorder (evidenced by age 15)
Borderline personality disorder	A pattern of instability in self-image, mood, and interpersonal relationships and marked impulsivity; transient dissociative states; highly reactive to real or imagined abandonment	Mood disorders
Histrionic personality disorder	A pattern of excessive emotionality and attention seeking; dramatic, seductive, or provocative behavior; suggestible; shallow emotional expression and relationships	Somatoform disorders, mood disorders
Narcissistic personality disorder	A pattern of grandiosity, need for admiration, and lack of empathy; entitled, arrogant, and exploitative attitudes and behavior	Manic symptoms

instability. This disorder is characterized by instability of emotions, interpersonal relationships and image that drastically impacts the ability to function. People with BPD have trouble regulating their emotion and often experience emotional extremes which are commonly displayed through intense bouts of anger, depression, and anxiety that may last only hours, or a few days (American Psychiatric Association, 2013). Someone with this marked instability may go from feeling on top of the world, to having thoughts of suicide or self-harm within hours. For example, Kurt was feeling great after hanging out with friends one night, but was quickly overwhelmed with thoughts of suicide when his girlfriend didn't answer his phone call. Kurt then started calling his friends threatening to drink bleach if they didn't come back and console him. The intense and volatile emotionality displayed by those BPD is associated with extreme sensitivity to perceived interpersonal slights. This feature combined with an unstable sense of self, intense and impulsive behaviors create behaviors that are often self-destructive (Gunderson, Herpertz, Skodol, Torgersen, & Zanarini, 2018).

Epidemiological studies suggest that symptoms of BPD emerge during early puberty and are likely to progressively impact a variety of areas of life. There is strong evidence that BPD will increasingly affect social relationships, which might lead to reduced social learning and opportunities to benefit from a healthy peer environment (Hutsebaut, Videler, Verheul, & Van Alphen, 2019). As a result, their interpersonal relationships are extremely unstable—they can switch from idealizing others to despising them without provocation. People with BPD often describe an emptiness that leads them to cling to new acquaintances or therapists in an attempt to fill their internal void. They worry about abandonment and misinterpret other people's everyday actions as desertion or rejection. For example, if a therapist has to cancel an appointment because of illness, a client with BPD might interpret this as rejection by the therapist and become very depressed or angry. Along with instability of self-concept and interpersonal relationships, the mood of people with BPD is unstable, with bouts of severe depression, anxiety, or anger seeming to arise frequently, often without cause. People with this disorder also show a strong tendency to engage in impulsive, self-damaging behaviors, including self-mutilating or suicidal behavior. Cindy's self-mutilating behavior was to cut and burn herself.

Susanna Kaysen, the author of *Girl Interrupted*, was featured in the **extraordinary people** profile on PDs which presented her experiences with BPD. In the following case study, a clinician describes her introduction to another woman who later was diagnosed with BPD.

CASE STUDY

At the initial meeting, Cindy was a 30-year-old, white, married woman with no children who was living in a middle-class suburban area with her husband. She had a college education and had successfully completed almost 2 years of medical school. Cindy was referred by her psychiatrist of 11 years, who was no longer willing to provide more than pharmacotherapy following a recent hospitalization for a near-lethal suicide attempt. In the 2 years prior to referral, Cindy had been hospitalized at least 10 times (one lasting 6 months) for psychiatric treatment of suicidal ideation; had engaged in numerous instances of parasuicidal behavior, including at least 10 instances of drinking Clorox bleach, multiple deep cuts, and burns; and had had three medically severe or nearly lethal suicide attempts, including cutting an artery in her neck.

Until age 27 Cindy was able to function well in work and school settings, and her marriage was reasonably satisfactory to both partners, although the husband complained of Cindy's excessive anger. When Cindy was in the second year of medical school, a classmate she knew only slightly committed suicide. Cindy stated that when she heard about the suicide, she immediately decided to kill herself also but had very little insight into what about the situation actually elicited the inclination to kill herself. Within weeks she left medical school and became severely depressed and actively suicidal. Although Cindy presented herself as a person with few psychological problems before the classmate's suicide, further questioning revealed a history of severe anorexia nervosa, bulimia nervosa, and alcohol and prescription medication abuse, originating at age 14.

Over the course of therapy, a consistent pattern associated with self-harm became apparent. The chain of events would often begin with an interpersonal encounter (almost always with her husband), which culminated in her feeling threatened, criticized, or unloved. These feelings would often be followed by urges either to self-mutilate or to kill herself, depending somewhat on her levels of hopelessness,

anger, and sadness. Decisions to self-mutilate and/or to attempt suicide were often accompanied by the thought "I'll show you." At other times, hopelessness and a desire to end the pain permanently seemed predominant. Following the conscious decision to self-mutilate or attempt suicide, Cindy would then immediately dissociate and at some later point cut or burn herself, usually while in a state of "automatic pilot." Consequently, Cindy often had difficulty remembering specifics of the actual acts. At one point, Cindy burned her leg so badly (and then injected it with dirt to convince the doctor that he should give her more attention) that reconstructive surgery was required. (Source: Linehan, M. M., Cochran, B. N., & Kehrer, K. C. Dialectical behavior therapy for borderline personality disorder. In D. H. Barlow (Ed.), *Clinical handbook of psychological disorders: A step-by-step treatment manual* (3rd ed., pp. 502–504). Copyright ©2001 by Guilford Press. Reprinted with permission. Permission conveyed through Copyright Clearance Center.)

Cindy's symptoms represent some of the core features of BPD: intense and out-of-control emotions that cannot be properly managed, a hypersensitivity to abandonment, a tendency to cling too tightly to other people, and a history of self-harm (see the *DSM-5* criteria in Table 7). The most commonly associated behaviors pattern among individuals with BPD are intentional, self-damaging acts, and suicide attempt. People with BPD often engage in parasuicidal gestures which involve nonlethal but intentional self-harm, as well as lethal suicide attempts. Research has shown that more than 70 to 75 percent of people with BPD have engaged in at least one deliberate act of

---

TABLE 7   Borderline Personality Disorder*

A pervasive pattern of instability of interpersonal relationships, self-image, and affect and marked impulsivity beginning by early adulthood.

—Symptoms include:
- Out-of-control emotions
- Unstable interpersonal relationships
- Concerns about abandonment
- Self-damaging behavior
- Impulsivity
- Frequently accompanied by depression, anxiety, or anger

—Prevalence rate is estimated between 1.6 and 5.9 percent of general population

—More commonly diagnosed in females than in males

*The information presented in this table is based solely on the author's interpretation of *DSM-5*. It does not reflect the exact language that appears in *DSM-5* and is not, therefore, formally endorsed by the American Psychological Association.

self-harm. These acts of self-harm can vary in terms of severity with some acts requiring little medical intervention such as cutting or scratching, cigarette burns and self-hitting or head banging to those requiring intensive medical interaction like overdoses, self-stabbing, or asphyxiation/suffocation. The greatest risk for suicide appears to be in the first year or two after diagnosis with the disorder, possibly because people often are not diagnosed until a crisis brings them to the attention of the mental health system. Suicide rates are estimated to be between 8 and 10 percent which is almost 50 times higher than the general population. BPD is the most common PD within clinical populations and is associated with intensive use of mental health services (Cristea et al., 2017; Linehan, 2018; Soloff & Chiapetta, 2012).

People with BPD are more likely to experience adverse long-term outcomes which include severe and persistent functional disability, physical illness, reduced quality of life, and reduced life expectancy from suicide and natural causes. In sum, even if the symptoms of BPD may be "waxing and waning" throughout the life course, the associated psychopathology and disability are often chronic and impact clients for many years (Hutsebaut et al., 2019; Pearce et al., 2018). The variety of symptoms in BPD and their shifting nature make it a complex disorder to diagnose and treat. This complexity is heightened by the fact that people with BPD frequently are also diagnosed with another mental disorder, such as depression, generalized anxiety disorder, specific phobia, agoraphobia, posttraumatic stress disorder (PTSD), panic disorder, substance abuse disorders, eating disorders, and psychotic disorders. Recent studies have found that anxiety disorders have the highest prevalence among individuals with BPD and eating disorders are among the lowest (Eaton et al., 2011; Hasin et al., 2011; Slotema, Blom, Niemantsverdriet, Deen, & Sommer, 2018).

The prevalence of BPD is estimated to be about 1.7 percent of the general population but significantly higher rates (15 to 28 percent) are found within psychiatric clinics or hospitals. In clinical settings, BPD is diagnosed much more often in women than in men, but the gender differences in a large nationwide study of adults in the community was small. BPD is often present in people in lower socioeconomic classes than in people in other classes (Chavira et al., 2003; De Genna & Feske, 2013). A large study of people in treatment for PDs found that Hispanics were more likely than whites or African Americans to be diagnosed with BPD. This could be because factors that contribute to the disorder, such as extreme stress, are more common among Hispanics. Or clinicians may over diagnose the disorder in Hispanic people because they do not take into account Hispanic cultural norms

that permit greater expression of strong emotions such as anger, aggressiveness, and sexual attraction (Chavira et al., 2003).

Although historically associated with white females, recent studies studies suggest that the rates of BPD are comparable among males and females, but are disproportionate among people of color. It is posited that issues with emotional regulation such as low awareness and understanding, unwillingness to accept emotions, the inability to control impulsive behaviors when distressed, and limited access to effective emotional regulation strategies may contribute to the development and maintenance of BPD. Research suggests that race may moderate the link between some difficulties with areas of emotional regulation and BPD. For example, the instability of emotions, limited ability to regulate emotions through effective coping strategies, and BPD identity disturbance were stronger among white individuals as compared to Black or East Asians with BPD (Haliczer et al., 2019).

BPD is associated with young adults and adolescents not only due to the high prevalence rates among these groups, but also because of the higher levels of distress experienced. Various studies have shown that symptoms of BPD generally decrease with age and spontaneous remission has been noted in 25 to 41 percent of patients with borderline, schizotypal, avoidant, and obsessive–compulsive PDs. Additionally, research has shown a further decline in the prevalence of BPD diagnoses from middle adulthood to old age which may be accounted for by different reasons. There may be less living people with BPD past middle adulthood since this population has a reduced life expectancy due to suicide and dysfunctional lifestyle. It is also possible that as people with BPD age, their symptoms change and shift toward more depressive, somatic, and passive-aggressive expressions that are less representative of borderline-type pathology. Although there is a noted stabilization of BPD with age, it is important to note that research has found some features of BPD to persist among older BPD patients, including emotional dysregulation and disturbed interpersonal relationships (Hutsebaut et al., 2019).

Although BPD has been viewed in the past as a chronic, intractable disorder by clinicians, recent studies have shown that over 85 percent of people diagnosed with this disorder show remission of symptoms within 10 to 15 years and that only a minority of those in remission have a relapse of the disorder (Gunderson et al., 2011; Zanarini, Frankenburg, et al., 2012). The ability of these individuals to hold a job significantly improved over the time period studied, but they continued to show difficulty in having stable, positive social relationships. Stressful life events and lack of social support are triggers for relapse in individuals whose symptoms have remitted (Gunderson et al., 2011). It is worth noting that despite renewed optimism influenced by the growing availability of evidence-based treatments, full social and professional recovery from BPD remains rather rare, and high levels of relapse following initial remission after treatment are typical, particularly in the areas of social and professional disability (Hutsebaut et al., 2019)

Most patients display a gradual remission of symptoms which can be accelerated by evidence-based psychosocial treatments. Studies have found that a majority of BPD symptoms improve over time, including self-harming behaviors and proneness to crisis. the natural course and otherwise effective treatments of BPD usually leave many patients with persistent and severe social disabilities related to depression or self-harming behaviors (Alvarez-Tomás et al., 2017; Gunderson et al., 2018). Like most psychological disorders, the impact of the illness impacts the caregivers and family members of those with BPD. Recent studies have shown that caregivers experience higher rates of psychological symptoms and distress than the general population. The reported levels of burden among families with a member with BPD are higher than those associated with other severe mental disorders. Qualitative studies have also highlighted the chronic and traumatic stress, burden, prolonged hopelessness, shrinking social support, and feelings of grief, guilt, and distress experienced by relatives of individuals with BPD (Pearce et al., 2018).

Theories of Borderline Personality Disorder

Given the emotional instability characteristic of BPD, it is not surprising that several theorists have argued that people with this disorder have fundamental deficits in regulating emotion (Baer, Peters, Eisenlohr-Moul, Geider, & Sauer, 2012; Carpenter & Trull, 2013; Selby, Anestis, Bender, & Joiner, 2009). People with BPD score higher than healthy subjects on measures of difficulty in regulating emotion and in laboratory tasks assessing unwillingness to tolerate emotional distress in order to reach a goal (Gratz, Moore, & Tull, 2016; Gratz, Rosenthal, Tull, Lejuez, & Gunderson, 2010). In one study, participants carried beepers that randomly cued them to provide ratings of their moods. People with BPD showed greater variability in their moods, particularly with regard to hostility, fear, and sadness, than people with no PD (Trull et al., 2008). A similar set of studies tracked the emotions of patients with BPD during their days and found that, compared to healthy individuals, patients experienced a more negative emotional baseline, more emotional variability, and somewhat slower return to their emotional baseline (Ebner-Priemer et al., 2015).

Cognitively, people with BPD are hyperattentive to negative emotional stimuli in the environment, their memories tend to be more negative, and they tend to make negatively biased interpretations of situations (Baer et al., 2012). While they frequently try to suppress their negative thoughts, their attempts usually are unsuccessful, and they end up ruminating about the negative thoughts or acting out impulsively or aggressively in response to them (Selby et al., 2009). The combination of emotional and cognitive dysfunction in BPD is also linked with the disruption in interpersonal behavior that can cause so much impairment. Laboratory and observational studies show that individuals with the disorder tend to hold more negative views of others and of relationships, sometimes struggle to empathize with others' perspectives, and engage in poor problem solving in social scenarios (Lazarus, Cheavens, Festa, & Rosenthal, 2014).

What do these difficulties in processing and regulating emotion stem from? Empirical studies have found that people with BPD are more likely than people without the disorder to report a childhood marked by instability, neglect, and parental psychopathology (Gunderson et al., 2011; Helgeland & Torgersen, 2004). They often have a history of physical and sexual abuse during childhood (Afifi et al., 2011; Martins, de Carvalho Tofoli, Von Werne Baes, & Juruena, 2011). This abuse, neglect, and instability could contribute to difficulties in regulating emotions and in attaining a positive, stable identity through several mechanisms.

Marsha Linehan (see Neacsiu & Linehan, 2014) suggests that a history of exposure to abuse, neglect, criticism, and emotional invalidation by significant others makes it difficult for people with BPD to learn appropriate emotion-regulation skills and to understand and accept their emotional reactions to events. People with this disorder come to rely on others to help them cope with difficult situations but do not have enough self-confidence to ask for this help in mature or effective ways. They become "manipulative" and indirect in their attempt to gain support from others (for example, by injuring themselves or creating crises), and their extreme emotional reactions to situations lead to impulsive actions.

Psychoanalytic theorists, particularly those in the object relations school (Kernberg, 1979; Klein, 1952), suggest that people with BPD never learned to fully differentiate their view of themselves from their view of others, making them extremely reactive to others' opinions of them and to the possibility of abandonment. When they perceive others as rejecting them, they reject themselves and may engage in self-punishment or self-mutilation. They also have never been able to integrate the positive and negative qualities of either their self-concept or their concept of others, because their early caregivers rewarded them when they remained dependent and compliant, but became hostile when they tried to separate from the caregivers. They tend to see themselves and other people as either all good or all bad and to vacillate between these two views, a process known as *splitting* (Flora, 2018). The instability in their emotions and interpersonal relationships is due to such splitting, reflecting their vacillation between the all-good and the all-bad self and the all-good and the all-bad other. For example, a person with BPD might view her partner as the sweetest, most caring person in the world when they are getting along, but when he does something frustrating, she might suddenly view him as totally unsupportive, unintelligent, and selfish, with no sense that he could have a mix of these positive and negative characteristics.

Neuroimaging studies show that the amygdala and hippocampus of people with BPD are smaller in volume than those of people without the disorder (Ruocco, Amirthavasagam, & Zakzanis, 2012). Recall that the amygdala is a part of the brain that is important in the processing of emotion and that the hippocampus is involved in the regulation of stress and in memory. In addition, people with BPD have greater activation of the amygdala in response to pictures of emotional faces, which may partly explain the difficulty they have in regulating their moods (Donegan et al., 2003; Mier et al., 2012). Neuroimaging studies also have found structural and metabolic abnormalities in the prefrontal cortex of patients with BPD (Soloff et al., 2012). This area of the brain is important in the regulation of emotional reactions and control of impulsive behavior. Impaired functioning in the amygdala and prefrontal cortex has been linked with the emotional lability and dysregulation found in people with BPD (Silvers et al., 2016).

The neurobiological differences between people with BPD and healthy individuals could be due to genetic factors. The disorder runs in families (Gunderson et al., 2011), and twin studies provide evidence that the symptoms of BPD are heritable (Distel et al., 2009). Early abuse and maltreatment also are associated with changes in the structure and organization of the brain, particularly the amygdala and hippocampus, which may explain in part why child abuse could contribute to the deficits seen in people with the disorder (Ruocco et al., 2012).

Treatment of Borderline Personality Disorder

One of the first psychotherapies shown to have positive effects in patients with BPD is **dialectical behavior therapy (DBT)** (Neacsiu & Linehan, 2014). Of all the available treatments of BPD, this form of therapy has assembled the most empirical support and is associated with a reduction in nonlethal self-injury, hospitalization, and anger. Additionally, research has also shown increased client retention and overall functioning (Sauer-Zavala et al., 2020). This therapy focuses

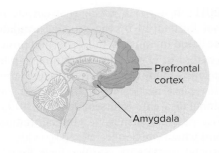

The amygdala and the prefrontal cortex have been implicated in borderline personality disorder.

on helping clients gain a more realistic and positive sense of self, learn adaptive skills for solving problems and regulating emotions, and correct dichotomous thinking. Therapists teach clients to monitor self-disparaging thoughts and black-or-white evaluations of people and situations and to challenge these thoughts and evaluations. Therapists also help clients learn appropriate assertiveness skills to use in close relationships so that they can express their needs and feelings in a mature manner. Clients may learn how to control their impulsive behaviors by monitoring situations most likely to lead to such behaviors and learning alternative ways to handle those situations. Controlled clinical trials comparing DBT to wait list controls have found that the therapy reduces depression, anxiety, and self-mutilating behavior while increasing interpersonal functioning (e.g., Bohus et al., 2004; Linehan et al., 2006; see Choi-Kain, Finch, Masland, Jenkins, & Unruh, 2017; Panos, Jackson, Hasan, & Panos, 2014).

Cognitive therapy treatments for BPD have also proven helpful. *Systems training for emotional predictability and problem solving* (STEPPS) is a group intervention for people with BPD that combines cognitive techniques challenging irrational and maladaptive cognitions and behavioral techniques addressing self-management and problem solving. A clinical trial of STEPPS compared to usual therapy (support plus medication) showed that clients receiving STEPPS showed greater improvement in negative affect, impulsivity, and functioning than clients receiving the usual therapy (Black, Blum, & Allen, 2018; Blum et al., 2008). Similarly, trials of CBT focusing on challenging patients' maladaptive core beliefs and teaching them more adaptive ways to function in daily life resulted in significant reductions in hospitalizations and suicide attempts, as well as greater improvements in mood, compared to patients receiving general support (Davidson et al., 2006; Giesen-Bloo et al., 2006; Sempértegui, Karreman, Arntz, & Bekker, 2013).

Recent studies suggest that psychodynamic approaches are effective for the treatment of borderline symptoms and related problems (Cristea et al., 2017). **Transference-focused therapy** uses the relationship between patient and therapist to help patients develop a more realistic and healthier understanding of themselves and their interpersonal relationships. Patients with BPD receiving this therapy showed reductions in suicidality, impulsivity, aggression, and anger (Clarkin, Levy, Lenzenweger, & Kernberg, 2007). **Mentalization-based treatment** is based on the theory that people with BPD have fundamental difficulty understanding the mental states of themselves and others because of traumatic experiences in childhood and poor attachment to their caregivers (Fonagy & Bateman, 2008; Sauer-Zavala et al., 2020). This psychodynamically oriented therapy provides patients with validation and support. Further, it attempts to help patients appreciate alternatives to their own subjective sense of self and others by using the relationship between the patient and the therapist, and the patient and others, to illustrate those alternatives. One long-term study found significant improvement in mood and functioning in patients receiving mentalization-based therapy compared to patients receiving typical community care. Also, over a 5-year follow-up, patients receiving mentalization-based therapy needed less medication, had fewer suicide attempts, and continued to function better on several dimensions than patients receiving the usual care (Bateman & Fonagy, 2008).

The first-line treatment for BPD is psychotherapy (Choi-Kain et al., 2017). Some medications may be useful in treatment, including the mood stabilizers aripiprazole and lamotrigine and the atypical antipsychotics, such as olanzapine and quetiapine (Black et al., 2014; Zanarini, Schulz, et al., 2012; Stoffers & Lieb, 2015). You might expect serotonin reuptake inhibitors to improve mood and reduce aggressiveness and impulsivity in people with BPD, but so far evidence of their effectiveness is lacking (Stoffers & Lieb, 2015). Overall, the results of drug treatment studies have been mixed. Adding a drug treatment to an effective psychotherapy such as DBT does not appear to improve recovery rates, and is recommended primarily for comorbid disorders (Choi-Kain et al., 2017; Neacsiu & Linehan, 2014; Simpson et al., 2004).

Histrionic Personality Disorder

Histrionic personality disorder (HPD) shares features with BPD, including rapidly shifting emotions and intense, unstable relationships, and is commonly described as dramatic, excitable, erratic, or volatile (French & Shrestha, 2018). However, people with BPD also show self-destructiveness, angry disruptions in close relationships, and chronic feelings of inner emptiness, while people with HPD behave in ways to draw attention to themselves across situations. HPD

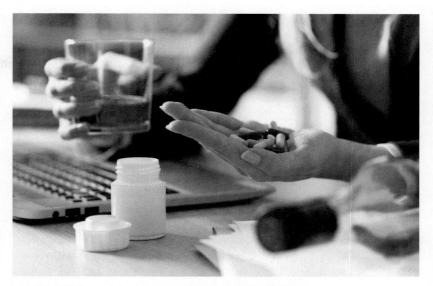

Suicidal behavior is common among people with borderline personality disorder. *Pheelings Media/Getty Images*

is characterized by excessive attention-seeking behavior and emotional display, impulsive and inappropriate or competitive sexual conduct. Those with HPD demand a significant amount of attention from those around them and research indicates that they often use excessive emotionality and provocative behavior to manipulate others (Hughes, Brewer, & Khan, 2020). A person with BPD may desperately cling to others as an expression of self-doubt and unstable identity, but a person with HPD simply wants flattering nurturance and preferential attention.

Individuals with HPD crave the spotlight and feel underappreciated or disregarded when they are not the center of attention. Often the life of the party, people with HPD tend to have a "larger than life" presence and are often enchanting, overly seductive, or inappropriately sexual with most of the people they meet, even if when they are not sexually attracted. Individuals with HPD pursue others' attention by being highly dramatic (e.g., gregarious, exaggerated emotional expression) and overtly seductive and by flamboyantly emphasizing the positive qualities of their physical appearance. Excessive emotion characterizes this disorder and it is not uncommon for those with HPD to display rapidly shifting and shallow emotions that others may perceive as insincere. Furthermore, their dramatic behaviors and desire to be the center of attention interfere with interpersonal relationships, sometimes causing embarrassment to friends and family with public displays of excessive emotions. Others often see them as self-centered and shallow, unable to delay gratification, demanding, and overly dependent, and they often end up alienating friends with the demands for constant attention. These individuals are also likely to be overly trusting of and easily influenced by others, particularly those in authority or people they admire. Additionally, they tend to consider relationships closer than they usually are in reality (French & Shrestha, 2018). Debbie, in the following case study, was diagnosed with HPD.

CASE STUDY

Debbie was a 26-year-old woman who worked as a salesclerk in a trendy clothing store and who sought therapy for panic disorder with agoraphobia. She dressed flamboyantly, with an elaborate and dramatic hairdo. Her appearance was especially striking, since she was quite short (under 5 feet tall) and at least 75 pounds overweight. She wore sunglasses indoors throughout the evaluation and constantly fiddled with them, taking them on and off nervously and waving them to emphasize a point. She cried loudly and dramatically at various points in the interview, going through large numbers of tissue. She continually asked for reassurance. ("Will I be OK?" "Can I get over this?") She talked nonstop throughout the evaluation. When gently interrupted by the evaluator, she was very apologetic, laughing and saying, "I know I talk too much," yet she continued to do so throughout the session. (Beck, A. T., & Freeman, A. M. *Cognitive therapy of personality disorders* (pp. 211–212). Copyright ©1990 by Guilford Press. Reprinted with permission. Permission conveyed through Copyright Clearance Center.)

HPD affects approximately 1 to 3 percent of general population and women are twice as likely to be diagnosed with this disorder than men (Hughes et al., 2020). People with this disorder are more likely to be separated or divorced than married (Disney, Weinstein, & Oltmanns, 2012). Like people with the somatoform disorders, they tend to exaggerate medical problems and make more medical visits than the average person, and this group has an increased rate of suicidal threats and behavior to coerce attentive caregiving (Kraus & Reynolds, 2001). People with this disorder have an increased risk of developing depression and substance use disorders such as cannabis use disorder and alcohol use disorder. They are also prone to having somatization disorder, panic attacks, and conversion disorders and their attention-seeking behavior may lead frequent suicidal threats and gestures (French & Shrestha, 2018).

Although discussions of histrionic personalities date back to the ancient Greek philosophers, the disorder is the focus of little research and currently there are no evidence-based interventions specifically designed to treat HPD. However, certain therapeutic approaches, such as CBT, can been utilized. Notably, there are numerous issues and disagreements related to the validity of HPD which includes the prevalence rate, empirical support, and potential gender biases. Furthermore, the future of HPD as a diagnosis remains unclear, as HPD has been proposed to be omitted from future revisions of the *DSM,* primarily due to the lack of active empirical research support (Blashfield, Reynolds, & Stennett, 2012; Lengel, 2020).

Family history studies indicate that HPD clusters in families, along with borderline and antisocial personality, as well as somatic symptom disorders. Whether this disorder is the result of genetic traits from experiences within the family or environment is unclear.

Treatment of Histrionic Personality Disorder

Psychodynamic psychotherapy is a successful approach to treat people with HPD (French & Shrestha, 2018). These treatments focus on uncovering repressed emotions and needs and helping people with the disorder to express them in more socially appropriate ways (for example, by reaching out calmly for support, and offering support to others as well). Cognitive therapy focuses on identifying clients' assumptions that they cannot function on their own and helping them formulate goals and plans for their life that do not rely on the approval of others (Beck et al., 2015). Therapists attempt to help clients tone down their dramatic evaluations of situations by challenging these evaluations and suggesting more adaptive ones. Several case-related studies of treatments that aim to promote appropriate behavior in daily life contexts have shown reductions in self-reported depression and interpersonal difficulties (Callaghan, Summers, & Weidman, 2003; Kellett, 2007). Group and family therapy are not typically recommended as the first-line option for treating HPD since people with this disorder often desire to be the center of attention, which may distract from the goals of therapy. Although psychotherapy is widely accepted as the gold-standard for treating HPD, there are medication options to be considered. Since individuals with HPD often experience mood swings, anger, anxiety, and depression the use of antidepressants, mood stabilizers, and antipsychotics are used, but there are currently no FDA-approved medications for HPD (French & Shrestha, 2018).

Narcissistic Personality Disorder

Most of us have encountered narcissists before—people who think they are better than everyone else and should get their way in all circumstances and who will walk all over others to accomplish their goals. The word *narcissist* comes from the Greek myth of Narcissus, who fell in love with the reflection of himself in a pool, was unable to leave it, and died as a result.

The characteristics of **narcissistic personality disorder (NPD)** are similar to those of HPD. In both disorders, individuals act in a dramatic manner, seek admiration from others, and are shallow in their emotional expressions and relationships with others. Unlike those with HPD who look to others for approval, people with NPD see themselves as superior and expect others to recognize this quality. As the name implies, grandiosity is a distinguishing feature, as they are preoccupied with thoughts of their self-importance and with fantasies of power and success. People with NPD believe that they are special or unique which enhances their self-esteem despite the fact that they often inflate their accomplishments and overestimate their abilities. They often refer to their actions or accomplishments with words like "perfect" or "the best" which further transfer to any individuals or institutions to which they are associated. People with this disorder lack empathy and often dwell on their belief that others should admire them. In interpersonal relationships, they make entitled demands on others to follow their wishes, ignore or devalue the needs and wants of others, exploit others to gain power, and are arrogant and condescending. In contrast to BPD, they do not experience the same abandonment concerns, despite needing the admiration of others (American Psychiatric Association, 2013). David, in the following case study, has been diagnosed with NPDr.

The word *narcissist* comes from the Greek myth of Narcissus, who fell in love with the reflection of himself in a pool, was unable to leave it, and died as a result. *Alinari Archives/Alinari/ Getty Images*

CASE STUDY

David was an attorney in his early forties when he sought treatment for depressed mood. He cited business and marital problems as the source of his distress and wondered if he was having a midlife crisis. David had grown up in a comfortable suburb of a large city, the oldest of three children and the only son of a successful businessman and a former secretary. David spoke of being an "ace" student and a "super" athlete but could not provide any details that would validate a superior performance in these areas. He also recollected that he had his pick of girlfriends, as most women were "thrilled" to have a date with him.

David went to college, fantasizing about being famous in a high-profile career. He majored in communications, planning to go on to law school and eventually into politics. He met his first wife during college, the year she was the university homecoming queen. They married shortly after their joint graduation. He then went on to law school, and she went to work to support the couple.

During law school, David became a workaholic, fueled by fantasies of brilliant work and international recognition. He spent minimal time with his wife and, after their son was born, even less time with either of them. At the same time, he continued a string of extramarital affairs, mostly brief sexual encounters. He spoke of his wife in an annoyed, devaluing way, complaining about how she just did not live up to his expectations. He waited until he felt reasonably secure in his first job so that he could let go of her financial support and then he sought a divorce. He continued to see his son occasionally, but he rarely paid his child support.

After his divorce, David decided that he was totally free to just please himself. He loved spending all his money on himself, and he lavishly decorated his condominium and bought an attention-getting wardrobe. He constantly sought the companionship of attractive women. He was very successful at making initial contacts and getting dates, but he rarely found anyone good enough to date more than once or twice.

At work, David believed that because he was "different" from other people, they had no right to criticize him. But he had every right to criticize others. He also believed that other people were weak and needed contact with someone like him in order to bring direction or pleasure into their lives. He saw no problem in taking advantage of other people if they were "stupid" enough to allow him to do so. (Beck, A. T., & Freeman, A. M. *Cognitive therapy of personality disorders* (pp. 211–212). Copyright ©1990 by Guilford Press. Reprinted with permission. Permission conveyed through Copyright Clearance Center.)

People with NPD can be successful in societies that reward self-confidence and assertiveness, such as the United States. Many high-functioning professionals with NPD may display these traits as workaholics who may make significant contributions to their field. However, they may also experience significant distress as their pursuit of perfection always falls short which can lead them to be controlling and overbearing (Crisp & Gabbard, 2020; Millon, Grossman, Millon, Meagher, & Ramnath, 2004). When they grossly overestimate their abilities, however, they can make poor choices in their careers and may experience many failures, and they annoy and often alienate the important people in their lives (Miller, Campbell, & Pilkonis, 2007). People with this disorder seek treatment most often for depression and for trouble adjusting to life stressors (Fabrega et al.,1991).

A nationwide study in the United States found an overall prevalence of 6.2 percent with higher likelihood of men presenting with NPD (7.7 percent) than women (4.8 percent) (Stinson et al., 2008; Yakeley, 2018). These data also suggest that NPD is more prevalent among younger adults, possibly supporting the impression that NPD is on the rise as a result of social and economic conditions that support more extreme versions of self-focused individualism (Bender, 2012; but see Wetzel et al., 2017). Studies have also found that NPD is more common in Black men and women and Hispanic women, younger adults and people who were separated, divorced, widowed, or never married. People diagnosed with the disorder have high rates of substance abuse and of mood and anxiety disorders. In addition, they have increased rates of physical and sexual aggression, impulsivity, homicidal thoughts, and suicidal behaviors (Pincus et al., 2009; Ronningstam, 2011a; Yakeley, 2018)).

Theories of Narcissistic Personality Disorder

Psychodynamically oriented theorists suggest that the symptoms of NPD are maladaptive strategies for managing emotions and self-views (Ronningstam, 2011b). People with this disorder did not develop a realistically positive view of themselves or adaptive strategies for handling stress and distress as children, so they rely on the praise and domination of others for their self-esteem (Kernberg, 1993; Kohut, 1977). Cognitive theorists have argued that some people with NPD develop unrealistically positive assumptions about their self-worth as the result of indulgence and overvaluation by significant others during childhood (Beck et al., 2015). Other people with this disorder develop the belief that they are unique or exceptional as a defense against rejection or unmet basic emotional needs by important people in their lives. One study found that people diagnosed with NPD were significantly more likely to endorse beliefs such as "I don't have to be bound by rules that apply to other people" than were people diagnosed with other disorders (Beck et al., 2001).

Researchers and clinicians often distinguish two different subtypes of narcissism: grandiose narcissism and vulnerable narcissism (Miller et al., 2017; Pincus & Lukowitzky, 2010). The grandiose narcissist copes with difficulties in self-esteem by viewing himself as superior and unique and by engaging in grandiose fantasies. Such people are arrogant, entitled, manipulative, exploitative, envious, and aggressive, particularly when distressed. They may engage in criminal or violent acts toward others. David, from the case study above, would be considered a grandiose narcissist. A vulnerable narcissist, by contrast, copes with difficulties in self-esteem by engaging in grandiose fantasies to quell intense shame. Such people are self-focused, hypersensitive to rejection and criticism, distrustful, and thus avoid others. For example, a vulnerable narcissist might feel extreme shame at being passed over for a job, and respond to this shame by claiming she was overqualified. There is evidence of these two subtypes of narcissism in the behaviors and thoughts endorsed by people who have NPD or who score high on measures of narcissism (Miller et al., 2017; Pincus & Lukowitzky, 2010; Ronningstam, 2011a; Stanton & Zimmerman, 2018). What the two subtypes share in common is the personality trait of interpersonal antagonism (Miller et al., 2017).

Like BPD, NPD is associated with a history of childhood adversity, including physical abuse and neglect, and with having a parent who was abused or who had a mental health problem (Afifi et al., 2011). Some evidence indicates that overly permissive or overly controlling parenting may give rise to grandiose and vulnerable narcissism, respectively, but more research is needed (Miller et al., 2017).

Treatment of Narcissistic Personality Disorder

People diagnosed with NPD lead troubled lives, often driving away those whose support they most need. Psychotherapy holds out hope for a group of suffering individuals who may have trouble finding human connection anywhere else in their lives. (Crisp & Gabbard, 2020).

People with NPD tend not to seek treatment except when they develop depression or are confronted with severe interpersonal problems (Ronningstam, 2011b). In general, they see any problems they encounter as due to the weakness and problems of others. Not surprisingly, narcissistic personality traits pose significant challenges to the development of a stable working alliance between a client and therapist. By emphasizing a collaborative therapeutic approach, a therapist using cognitive techniques can help these clients develop more realistic expectations of their abilities and more sensitivity to the needs of others by teaching them to challenge their initially self-aggrandizing ways of interpreting situations (Beck et al., 2015). Such self-understanding and changes in self-serving biases don't come easily for people with NPD, and often they do not remain in therapy once their acute symptoms or interpersonal problems lessen. Like HPD, however, no systematic psychotherapy or medication treatment studies have been published (Dhawan, Kunik, Oldham, & Coverdale, 2010; Stoffers et al., 2011).

CLUSTER C: ANXIOUS-FEARFUL PERSONALITY DISORDERS

The cluster C anxious-fearful personality disorders—avoidant personality disorder (AVPD), dependent personality disorder (DPD), and obsessive-compulsive personality disorder (OCPD)—are characterized by a chronic sense of anxiety or fearfulness and behaviors intended to ward off feared situations (Table 8). While people with each of these three personality disorders (PDs) fear something different, they all result in personal distress and dysfunction.

Avoidant Personality Disorder

AVPD is characterized by excessive avoidance of interpersonal interactions which are fueled by feelings of personal inadequacy and fears of criticism and rejection. Symptoms of this disorder have considerable overlap with social anxiety disorder (SAD), but it has received much less attention in terms of research (American Psychiatric Association, 2013; Lampe & Malhi, 2018). People with AVPD have low self-esteem, are prone to shame, and are extremely anxious about being criticized by others and thus avoid interactions in which there is any possibility of being criticized (see Table 9). They might choose occupations that are

TABLE 8   Cluster C: Anxious-Fearful Personality Disorders

People with the anxious-fearful personality disorders are often anxious or fearful.

Label	Key Features	Similar Disorders
Avoidant personality disorder	A pattern of social inhibition, feelings of inadequacy, and a fear of being criticized, which lead to the avoidance of social interactions and nervousness	Social phobia
Dependent personality disorder	A pattern of submissive and clinging behavior related to an excessive need to be taken care of, and leading to high levels of dependence on others	Separation anxiety disorder, persistent depressive disorder (dysthymia)
Obsessive-compulsive personality disorder	A pattern of preoccupation with orderliness, extreme perfectionism, and control, leading to emotional constriction, rigidity in one's activities and relationships, and anxiety about even minor disruptions in one's routines	Obsessive-compulsive disorder

TABLE 9   Avoidant Personality Disorder

People with avoidant personality disorder may choose professions that allow them to avoid other people.

—Symptoms include:

- Prone to shame
- Hypersensitive to criticism
- Restrained and detached
- Isolated from others
- Severe anxiety about social situations

—Prevalence rate is 2.4 percent of general population

—More commonly diagnosed in females than in males

—Frequently accompanied by depression and anxiety

more socially isolated or require less interaction with others, such as wilderness park rangers. The two pathological personality traits that characterize them are negative affectivity and detachment. When they must interact with others, people with AVPD are shy, inhibited, nervous, and hypersensitive to signs of being evaluated or criticized. They are terrified of saying something or doing something to embarrass themselves and assume that anything they do is wrong. People with avoidant PD view themselves as inferior and socially inept and as a result they often feel isolated and lonely. Although they often crave relationships with others, they feel unworthy of these relationships and isolate themselves, as the following case study illustrates (American Psychiatric Association, 2013).

CASE STUDY

Ruthann is a 32-year-old postal employee who petitioned her supervisors to assign her to a rural route where she wouldn't have to talk with anyone most of the day. Ruthann has always been terrified of interacting with others, believing that they would judge her. When she was forced to interact, she was sure other people found her stupid and ugly and caught the many "social mistakes" she felt she committed in these interactions. Ruthann lived alone and did not date because she was sure men would find her unattractive and silly and would reject her.

The prevalence estimates for AVPD range from between 1.5 and 2.5 percent with a slightly higher likelihood that women will develop this disorder, although this is not fully agreed upon by recent studies (Fariba & Sapra, 2020). AVPD is often comorbid with major depression and substance abuse which increases the risk of suicidal ideation and attempts. Recent studies suggest that AVPD is specifically likely to increase the risk of postpartum depression, possibly influenced by levels of depression and anxiety that are present right before childbirth. AVPD is also commonly comorbid with other PDs, especially within Cluster C (Lampe & Malhi, 2018). It is also hypothesized that AVPD may be a significant predictor of persistent depressive disorder, including bouts of major depression and severe anxiety (Grant et al., 2004; Sanislow, da Cruz, Gianoli, & Reagan, 2012).

There is overlap between the characteristics of AVPD and those of SAD (see the chapter "Trauma, Anxiety, Obsessive-Compulsive, and Related Disorders"), so much so that they may be alternate forms of the same disorder. In particular, people with either disorder are highly self-critical about their social

interactions (Cox, Turnbull, Robinson, Grant, & Stein, 2011). People with AVPD tend to have more severe and generalized anxiety about social situations than people with SAD and are more chronically impaired by their anxiety (Sanislow et al., 2012). Nonetheless, they also may desire acceptance and affection and sometimes fantasize about idealized relationships with others. Note that this is different from schizoid PD; although both disorders involve social isolation, in AVPD this is due to anxious avoidance, as opposed to the social detachment of schizoid PD.

Theories of Avoidant Personality Disorder

Twin studies show that genetics plays a role in AVPD and that some of the same genes likely are involved in AVPD and SAD (Torvik et al., 2016). Unlike other PDs, AVPD does not have a strong relationship to sexual or physical abuse in childhood, although people with this disorder do report higher rates of emotional neglect (Afifi et al., 2011).

Cognitive theorists suggest that people with AVPD develop dysfunctional beliefs about being worthless as a result of rejection by important others early in life (Beck, Davis & Freeman, 2015). Individuals with AVPD often describe their parents as less affectionate, more rejecting, guilt-engendering, and less encouraging of achievement than persons without this disorder. People with AVPD who experienced parental neglect or rejection often conclude, "If my parents don't like me, how could anyone?" Thus, they avoid interactions with others. Their thoughts are of this sort: "Once people get to know me, they see I'm really inferior." When they must interact with others, they are unassertive and nervous, thinking, "I must please this person in every way or she will criticize me." They also tend to discount any positive feedback they receive from others, believing that other people are simply being nice or do not see how incompetent they really are. Additionally, people with AVPD are more likely to report a history of neglect, abuse, overprotection, and lower standards of care. This suggests there may be a relationship between neglect and emotional abuse by early caregivers and later development of AVPD. However, given the hypersensitivity displayed by people with AVPD, it is also possible that recall bias may contribute or to these findings. Twin studies and negative experiences within the family do support the role of environmental factors in the development of these symptoms, at least to some degree (Lampe & Malhi, 2018).

Treatment of Avoidant Personality Disorder

AVPD is a chronic disorder that begins at early age and has a lifelong impact which makes effective treatment critical (Lampe & Malhi, 2018). Cognitive and behavioral therapies have proven helpful for people with

AVPD. These therapies have included graduated exposure to social settings, social skills training, and challenges to negative automatic thoughts about themselves and social situations. People receiving these therapies show increases in the frequency and range of social contacts, decreases in avoidance behaviors, and increases in comfort and satisfaction when engaging in social activities (Emmelkamp et al., 2006).

The serotonin reuptake inhibitors are sometimes used to reduce the social anxiety of people with AVPD, but little research on their effectiveness in treating AVPD separate from social anxiety has been done (Ripoll, Triebwasser, & Siever, 2011; Silk & Feurino, 2012).

Dependent Personality Disorder

The excessive and pathological need to be taken care of by others is the core feature of **DPD** which leads to clinging behaviors and fear of separation (American Psychiatric Association, 2013). The symptoms of this PD significantly disrupt their social interactions and cause psychological distress which occurs by denying their own thoughts and feelings. People with this disorder worry about displeasing others losing their approval and to avoid any possibility of disagreements. They frantically cling to others and are likely to submit to even the most unreasonable or unpleasant demands to avoid separation. People with this PD have difficulty making everyday decisions, instead heavily relying on others for advice and reassurance, and they do not initiate new activities except in an effort to please others (American Psychiatric Association, 2013). In contrast to people with AVPD, who avoid relationships unless certain of being liked, people with DPD can function only within a relationship and will overly accommodate others to obtain care and support. People with DPD often view themselves as helpless and incompetent and as a result they crave continuous emotional support and reassurance from others. This disorder is also characterized by a pathological attachment to a person of significance, separation anxiety, and insecurity. This excessive interpersonal dependency requires that others assume responsibility for their life and interferes with their ability to make basic decisions without excessive amounts of reassurance, like what shirt to wear, or where to get lunch. As a result, people with DPD fail to take initiative or start projects, and experience low self-confidence, fear of abandonment, and self-doubt that significantly impacts daily function (Kellett & Lees, 2020).

They deeply fear the loss of relationship supports and the prospect of having to assume independent responsibility, and they may allow themselves to be exploited and abused to maintain relationships, as in the following case of Francesca.

People with avoidant personality disorder may choose professions that allow them to avoid other people. *kali9/E+/Getty Images*

CASE STUDY

Francesco was in a panic because his husband Archie seemed to be getting increasingly annoyed with him. Last night, Archie became very angry when Francesco asked him to cancel an upcoming business trip because he was terrified of being left at home alone. In a rage, Archie shouted, "You can't ever be alone! You can't do anything by yourself! You can't even decide what to have for dinner by yourself! I'm sick of it. Grow up and act like an adult!"

It was true that Francesco had a very difficult time making decisions for himself. While he was in high school, he couldn't decide which courses to take and talked with his parents and friends for hours about what he should do, finally doing whatever his best friend or his father told him to do. When he graduated from high school, he didn't feel smart enough to go to college, even though he had gotten good grades in high school. He drifted into a job because his best friend had a job with the same company and he wanted to remain close to that friend. The friend eventually dumped Francesco, however, because he was tired of Francesco's incessant demands for reassurance. Francesco frequently bought gifts for the friend and offered to do the friend's laundry or cooking, in obvious attempts to win the friend's favor. But Francesco also kept the friend for hours in the evening, asking him whether he thought Francesco had made the right decision about some trivial issue, such as what to buy his mother for Christmas and how he thought Francesco was performing on the job.

(continued)

Soon after his friend dumped him, Francesco met his future husband, and when Archie showed some interest in him, he quickly tried to form a close relationship. He liked the fact that Archie seemed strong and confident, and when Archie asked him to marry him, Francesco thought that perhaps finally he would feel safe and secure. But especially since Archie has begun to get angry with him frequently, Francesco has been worrying constantly that Archie is going to leave him.

Studies have found that DPDs have a relatively low estimated lifetime prevalence of 0.78 percent (Volkert, Gablonski, & Rabung, 2018). Higher rates of the disorder are found with self-report methods than with structured clinical interviews, suggesting that many people feel they have this disorder when clinicians would not diagnose it in them. More women than men are diagnosed with this disorder (Trull, Jahng, Tomko, Wood, & Sher, 2010). Depressive and anxiety disorders commonly co-occur in people with DPD, often triggered by interpersonal conflict or relationship disruption (Bornstein, 2012; Grant, et al., 2004). DPD increases the risk for physical illness, partner and child abuse, suicidal behavior, and high levels of functional impairment and health care costs (Bornstein, 2012; Loas, Cormier, & Perez-Diaz, 2011). Research has consistently found a high degree of comorbidity and symptom overlap between PDs, particularly within clusters. Within cluster C, DPD and AVPD share the most commonalities (Lampe & Malhi, 2018).

Theories of Dependent Personality Disorder

DPD often runs in families, and results of one twin study estimate the heritability of this disorder to be .81 (Coolidge, Thede, & Jang., 2004). Children and adolescents with a history of separation anxiety disorder or chronic physical illness appear to be more prone to developing DPD.

Behavioral and cognitive models describe this pathological dependence as learned behaviors designed to elicit care and emotional rewards that occur during early interactions with caregivers which are later generalized adult relationships. This idea suggests that as children learn which behaviors are effective in eliciting the desired response they will adjust their care-seeking behaviors to maximize rewards (Simonelli & Parolin, 2017). Cognitive theories argue that people with DPD have exaggerated and inflexible beliefs related to their depending needs, such as "I am needy and weak," which in turn drive their dependent behaviors. A study of 38 patients with DPD found that they endorsed such beliefs more often than patients with other PDs (Beck et al., 2001).

DPD can also be explained by problems with the development of healthy attachment. This theory suggests that individuals with DPD tend to have an anxious-insecure attachment style which results in an anxious attachment. In adulthood, those with this attachment style tend to be self-critical and insecure. As a result, they seek constant approval and reassurance from others in an effort to validate their self-worth, but deep-seated expectations of rejection make them constantly distressed and unable to trust others. The five-factor model (Big Five Model) describes this degree of dependency as high levels of anxiety and insecurity and low levels of risk taking and perceived competence. Other theories combining cognitive, developmental, and psychodynamic concepts highlight the influence of overprotective and authoritarian parenting, the influence of gender role on self-concept in which individuals view themselves as weak and incompetent (especially for girls). This construct suggests that the combination of these factors have important consequences in their motivation to seek guidance and support from other people and their fears of rejection and abandonment (Simonelli & Parolin, 2017).

Treatment of Dependent Personality Disorder

Unlike people with many of the other PDs, persons with DPD frequently seek treatment (T. Millon, Grossman, C. Millon, Meagher, & Ramnath, 2004) and are likely to show greater insight and self-awareness. A critical goal in any psychotherapeutic intervention for DPDs is to increase the client's self-confidence and learn appropriate independence skills. A wide variety of therapeutic approaches have been found to be beneficial in the treatment of DPD such as short-term dynamic psychotherapy, supportive expressive psychotherapy, psychodynamic therapy, cognitive therapy, cognitive behavior therapy, and logotherapy. There is no evidence to support any one of these psychotherapies as most effective in the treatment of DPD (Kellett & Lees, 2020).

The desire of people with DPD to strengthen ties to caring authority figures likely facilitates early development of a positive working alliance with the therapist, although it also presents challenges (Bornstein, 2012; Paris, 1998). Although many psychosocial therapies are used in the treatment of this disorder, none have been systematically tested for their effectiveness. Psychodynamic treatment focuses on helping clients gain insight into the early experiences with caregivers that led to their dependent behaviors, often by examining their relationship style with the therapist and interpreting the transference process with the goal of increased independence. Nondirective and humanistic therapies may be helpful in fostering autonomy and self-confidence in persons with DPD (Millon et al., 2004).

SHADES OF GRAY

Ellen Farber, a single 35-year-old insurance company executive, came to a psychiatric emergency room of a university hospital with complaints of depression and the thought of driving her car off a cliff. . . . She reported a 6-month period of increasingly persistent dysphoria and lack of energy and pleasure. Feeling as if she were "made of lead," Ms. Farber had recently been spending 15 to 20 hours a day in her bed. She also reported daily episodes of binge-eating, when she would consume "anything I can find," including entire chocolate cakes or boxes of cookies. She reported problems with inter-mittent binge-eating since adolescence, but these epi-sodes had recently increased in frequency, resulting in a 20-pound weight gain over the past few months. . . .

She attributed her increasing symptoms to financial difficulties. Ms. Farber had been fired from her job 2 weeks before coming to the emergency room. She claimed it was because she "owed a small amount of money." When asked to be more specific, she reported owing $150,000 to her former employers and another $100,000 to various local banks due to spending sprees.

In addition to lifelong feelings of emptiness, Ms. Farber described chronic uncertainty about what she wanted to do in life and with whom she wanted to be friends. She had many brief, intense relationships with both men and women, but her quick temper led to frequent arguments and even physical fights. Although she had always thought of her childhood as happy and carefree, when she became depressed she began to recall episodes of abuse by her mother. Initially, she said she had dreamt that her mother had pushed her down the stairs when she was only 6, but then she began to report previously unrecognized memories of beatings or verbal assaults by her mother. (Reprinted with permission from the *DSM-IV Casebook: A Learning Companion to the Diagnostic and Statistical Manual of Mental Disorders,* Fourth Edition. Copyright ©1994 by American Psychiatric Association. All Rights Reserved.)

What diagnosis would you give Ms. Farber? (Discussion appears at the end of this chapter.)

Cognitive-behavioral therapy for DPD includes behavioral techniques designed to increase assertive be-haviors and decrease anxiety, as well as cognitive tech-niques designed to challenge clients' assumptions about the need to rely on others (Beck et al., 2015). Clients might be given graded exposure to anxiety-provoking situations, such as making everyday and then more im-portant decisions independently. For example, they and their therapists might develop a hierarchy of in-creasingly difficult independent actions that the clients gradually attempt on their own, beginning with decid-ing what to have for lunch and ending with deciding what job to take. After making each decision, clients are encouraged to recognize their competence and to challenge any negative thoughts they had about making the decision. They also may be taught relaxation skills to enable them to overcome their anxiety enough to engage in homework assignments. Regardless of the therapeutic approach, it is important for the therapist to consider the dependent person's social network. Sometimes marital or family therapy can help elucidate relationship patterns that foster dependency, reinforce feelings of helplessness and anxiety, and interfere with independent decision making (Bornstein, 2012).

Obsessive-Compulsive Personality Disorder

Self-control, attention to detail, perseverance, high productivity, and perfectionism are highly valued in many societies, including U.S. society (Chamberlain,

Redden, Stein, Lochner, & Grant, 2017). However, when these traits develop to an extreme they might result in an individual who is rigid, perfectionistic, dogmatic, ruminative, and emotionally blocked. This inflexibility and preoccupation with orderli-ness, perfection, and control are associated with **OCPD** and cause significant impairment and inter-personal difficulties for affected individuals. Just like those affected by AVPD, individuals with OCPD report significantly higher levels of interpersonal distress as compared to those without the disorder (Solomonov, Kuprian, Zilcha-Mano, Muran, & Barber, 2020). While OCPD is functionally impair-ing, some symptoms with mild presentation such as excessive commitment to work and productivity may prove to be potentially useful (Wheaton & Ward, 2020). Unlike almost all other PCDs, OCPD is not associated with higher occurrences of disabil-ity (Chamberlain et al.,2017). Some people with OCPD are actually quite productive and base their self-esteem on their productivity and on meeting unrea-sonably high goals. They are compulsive; preoccu-pied with rules, details, and order; and perfectionistic. They tend to persist in a task even when their ap-proach is failing, leading them to experience nega-tive affect. Interpersonally, they have difficulty appreciating others or tolerating their quirks and are rigidly bound to rules. They are often stubborn and may force others to follow strict standards of performance. Like all psychological disorders, the symptoms of OCPD impact daily function and cause a reduced quality of life, economic burden, and at least moderate impairments in psychosocial functioning (Lei et al., 2020).

While this disorder shares features with obsessive-compulsive disorder (OCD; see the chapter "Trauma, Anxiety, Obsessive-Compulsive, and Related Disorders") and has a small to moderate comorbidity with OCD, it should not be confused with OCD (Diedrich & Voderholzer, 2015; Lochner et al., 2011). OCPD involves a more general way of interacting with the world than does OCD, which often involves only specific obsessional thoughts and compulsive behaviors. While people with OCD will be focused on very specific thoughts, images, ideas, or behavior and may feel very anxious if they do not engage in these (e.g., becoming anxious if they cannot check whether they have turned off the stove), people with OCPD will be more generally prone to being perfectionistic, rigid, and concerned with order. Recall that people with OCD experience obsessions and compulsions as intrusive and unwanted; by contrast, people with OCPD typically view their concerns as part of their personalities.

OCPD is largely understudied despite the high community prevalence and subsequent societal burden (Wheaton & Ward, 2020). The lack of empirical data and the symptom overlap between OCD and OCPD can make differentiating OCD and OCPD difficult. And, while less common, it is possible for people to have both disorders simultaneously. Studies suggest that individuals with OCPD and comorbid OCD studies will have an earlier onset, more severe symptoms, and poor treatment outcomes. Some researchers suggest that OCPD may actually be a subtype of OCD but more research is needed to confirm this notion. There are notable differences between OCD and OCPD in terms of individual perception that are interesting. People with OCD are more likely to actively seek treatment because they consider their symptoms to be at odds with their self-image. In contrast, people with OCPD see their symptoms as part of their personality and consistent with their self-image which reduces the likelihood that they will seek out treatment (Luo et al., 2020).

People with OCPD often seem grim and strict, tensely in control of their emotions, and lacking in spontaneity (Millon et al., 2004). They are workaholics who see little need for leisure activities or friendships. Other people experience them as stubborn, stingy, possessive, moralistic, and officious (American Psychiatric Association, 2013). They tend to relate to others in terms of rank or status and are ingratiating and deferential to "superiors" but dismissive, demeaning, or authoritarian toward "inferiors." Although they are extremely concerned with efficiency, their perfectionism and obsession about following rules often interfere with completing tasks and getting along with others, as in the following case study.

CASE STUDY

Ronald Lewis is a 32-year-old accountant who is "having trouble holding on to a woman." He does not understand why, but the reasons become very clear as he tells his story. Mr. Lewis is a remarkably neat and well-organized man who tends to regard others as an interference to the otherwise mechanically perfect progression of his life. For many years he has maintained an almost inviolate schedule. On weekdays he arises at 6:47, has two eggs soft-boiled for 2 minutes, 45 seconds, and is at his desk at 8:15. Lunch is at 12:00, dinner at 6:00, bedtime at 11:00. He has separate Saturday and Sunday schedules, the latter characterized by a methodical and thorough trip through the *New York Times*. Any change in schedule causes him to feel varying degrees of anxiety, annoyance, and a sense that he is doing something wrong and wasting time.

Orderliness pervades Mr. Lewis's life. His apartment is immaculately clean and meticulously arranged. His extensive collections of books, records, and stamps are all carefully catalogued, and each item is reassuringly always in the right and familiar place. Mr. Lewis is highly valued at his work because his attention to detail has, at times, saved the company considerable embarrassment. . . . His perfectionism also presents something of a problem, however. He is the slowest worker in the office and probably the least productive. He gets the details right but may fail to put them in perspective. His relationships to co-workers are cordial but formal. He is on a "Mr. and Ms." basis with people he has known for years in an office that generally favors first names. Mr. Lewis's major problems are with women and follow the same repetitive pattern.

At first, things go well. Soon, however, he begins to resent the intrusion upon his schedule a woman inevitably causes. This is most strongly illustrated in the bedtime arrangements. Mr. Lewis is a light and nervous sleeper with a rather elaborate routine preceding his going to bed. He must spray his sinuses, take two aspirin, straighten up the apartment, do 35 sit-ups, and read two pages of the dictionary. The sheets must be of just the right crispness and temperature and the room must be noiseless. Obviously, a woman sleeping over interferes with his inner sanctum and, after sex, Mr. Lewis tries either to have the woman go home or sleep in the living room. No woman has put up with this for very long. (Adapted from Spitzer, R. L., Skodol, A. E., Gibbon, M., & Williams, J. B. W., *Psychopathology: A Case Book,* New York: McGraw Hill, 1983, pp. 63–64.)

OCPD is the most prevalent PD, with estimated lifetime prevalence ranging from 2 to 8 percent within the U.S. population. There are mixed findings on sex differences for prevalence rates of OCPD with some studies finding that men more than twice as likely as women to be affected by this disorder and others finding no differences between men and women. Similar inconsistent results exist for racial and ethnic differences as well with some studies noting no differences between groups and others suggesting lower rates among American Asians and Hispanic populations, as compared to Caucasian and African Americans (Luo et al., 2020; Solomonov et al., 2020). This disorder is typically diagnosed in adulthood and the diagnostic rates increase with age. OCPD is more likely to be found in individuals over the age of 30 than in younger individuals, but traits are thought to begin in childhood. The course of OCPD is believed to be chronic with fairly stable symptoms over the lifespan, but the evidence is mixed (Wheaton, Pinto, Fontenelle & Yücel, 2019).

People with this disorder are prone to depression, anxiety, and eating disorders, but not to the same extent as people with the other PDs already discussed (Grant et al., 2004). Interestingly, the majority of individuals with OCD do not also have OCPD but when they co-occur OCD and depression symptoms are more severe (Diedrich & Voderholzer, 2015; Gordon, Salkovskis, Oldfield, & Carter, 2013).

Theories of Obsessive-Compulsive Personality Disorder

Cognitive theories suggest that people with this disorder harbor beliefs such as "Flaws, defects, or mistakes are intolerable." One study found that people diagnosed with OCPD endorsed such beliefs significantly more often than people diagnosed with other PDs (Beck et al., 2001), but a more recent study found that they did not (Arntz, Weertman, & Salet, 2011).

OCPD appears to be related to genetic factors similar to those found in OCD (Lochner et al., 2011; Taylor, Asmundson, & Jang, 2011). People with OCPD have a slightly greater history of physical neglect than people with no disorder (Afifi et al., 2011). OCPD is more commonly found in the relatives of people with OCD than in those without OCD which suggests a familial and possibly genetic overlap with regards etiology (Chamberlain et al., 2017).

Despite the fact that OCPD is the second most common PD among the general and inpatient populations, the neurological research is scarce. However, some studies have found a reduced volume of gray matter in multiple brain regions, such as the prefrontal cortex, cingulate, and the insula, of OCPD individuals. Abnormalities in the prefrontal cortex have been found among people with OCD and OCPD which suggests a shared or similar neural mechanism that relates to decision-making, with better behavior performance found in those with OCPD (Luo et al., 2020). Additional research has also found that people with OCPD exhibit altered spontaneous neural activity as compared to healthy controls in multiple brain regions. This abnormal brain activity may account for various OCPD symptoms including cognitive inflexibility, excessive self-control, and lower levels of empathy (Lei et al., 2020).

Treatment of Obsessive-Compulsive Personality Disorder

Individuals with OCPD experience high levels of psychological distress and impairment in function that often results from the conflicting need for perfection and order and the failures of those around them to conform. As a result, those with OCPD frequently seek psychotherapy and medical treatment. However, no gold standard OCPD treatment exists for this substantially understudied affliction (Wheaton & Ward, 2020). There are no controlled psychological treatment studies focusing primarily on OCPD, and only one medication trial.

Supportive therapies may assist people with this disorder in overcoming the crises that bring them in for treatment, and behavioral therapies can decrease their compulsive behaviors (Beck et al., 2015; Millon et al., 2004). For example, a client may be given the assignment to alter his usual rigid schedule for the day, first by simply getting up 15 minutes later than usual and then by gradually changing additional elements of his schedule. The client may be taught to use relaxation techniques to overcome the anxiety created

People with obsessive-compulsive personality disorder are very concerned with orderliness, structure, and rules. *IPGGutenbergUKLtd/Getty Images*

by alterations in the schedule. He might also write down the automatic negative thoughts he has about changes in the schedule ("Getting up 15 minutes later is going to put my entire day off"). In the next therapy session, he and the therapist might discuss the evidence for and against these automatic thoughts, gradually replacing maladaptive thoughts and rigid expectations with more flexible beliefs and attitudes that include valuing close relationships, leisure and recreation, and feelings. Sometimes the selective serotonin reuptake inhibitor medications (e.g., Prozac) may be used to reduce obsessionality.

ALTERNATIVE *DSM-5* MODEL FOR PERSONALITY DISORDERS

The *DSM-5*'s definition of personality disorder (PD) and the criteria used for diagnosing the PDs reviewed in this chapter have not changed from those in the *DSM-IV-TR*. In fact, its categorical scheme for understanding PDs has remained in place for over 30 years since the publication of the *DSM-III* in 1980. However, the *DSM-5* includes an alternative model for diagnosing PDs that incorporates a *dimensional,* or continuum, perspective. It is presented in a separate section of the *DSM-5* designated for further study (Section III) and is not meant for current clinical use. It is reviewed here to provide a perspective on the evolution of the diagnosis of PDs, as well as one approach to responding to the problems with a categorical diagnostic system.

Over the years, many limitations of the *DSM*'s categorical approach to the diagnosis of PDs have been recognized by clinicians and researchers (see Krueger & Markon, 2014; Morey, Benson, Busch, & Skodol, 2015). Some of the most significant limitations include that the 10 separate PDs have a good deal of overlap in their diagnostic criteria (Grant, Stinson, Dawson, Chou, & Ruan, 2005; Zimmerman, Rothschild, & Chelminski, 2005). Indeed, it appears that although the different PDs are distinguished by their unique symptoms discussed above, there is also a more general personality pathology factor that is common across multiple PDs (Sharp et al., 2015). There was poor agreement among clinicians as to whether individuals met the criteria for these disorders (Morey et al., 2015; Zanarini et al., 2000). Although the PDs are conceptualized as stable characteristics of an individual, longitudinal studies found that people diagnosed with these disorders varied over time in how many symptoms they exhibited and in the severity of these symptoms, going into and out of the diagnosis (Shea et al., 2002). In particular, people often seemed as if they had a PD when they were

suffering from an acute disorder, such as major depressive disorder, but then their PD symptoms seemed to diminish when their depressive symptoms subsided. Finally, despite having 10 different PD diagnoses, the *DSM* criteria did not fit many people who seemingly had pathological personalities, nor did the criteria reflect the extensive literature on fundamental personality traits that are consistent across cultures (Verheul & Widiger, 2004).

The alternative *DSM-5* model characterizes PDs in terms of impairments in personality *functioning* and pathological personality *traits*. There are three steps in diagnosing a PD under this alternative model (see Waugh et al., 2017). The first step in diagnosing a PD is determining an individual's level of functioning in terms of their sense of self (or identity) or their relationships with others on a scale that goes from little or no impairment to extreme impairment. To diagnose a PD under this system, the person must have at least moderate impairment.

The second step in diagnosing a PD is determining whether the individual has any pathological personality traits. Although there is tremendous variability across people in the specific nature of their personalities, as noted at the beginning of this chapter regarding, for instance, the Big 5 model, there appears to be a relatively small set of personality traits or dimensions along which people's personalities vary (Krueger & Markon, 2014; McCrae & Terracciano, 2005). The pathological personality traits used in the alternative model have significant overlap with the Big 5 traits, but also some differences (Suzuki, Griffin, & Samuel, 2017).

There are five pathological traits assessed in the alternative model. One fundamental trait is the extent to which people tend to be even-tempered and calm, secure, and able to handle stress, versus being emotionally labile, insecure, and overreactive to stress, a dimension referred to in personality theories as *neuroticism* (McCrae & Costa, 1999) or in *DSM-5* alternative model terms as **negative affectivity.** A second core personality trait, **detachment,** involves the extent to which people are appropriately outgoing and trusting of others versus tending to be withdrawn, avoidant, and untrusting. The third dimension, **antagonism,** is anchored at the positive end by characteristics such as honesty, appropriate modesty, and concern for others and at the negative end by characteristics such as deceitfulness, grandiosity, and callousness. A fourth domain, called **disinhibition,** ranges from a tendency to be responsible, organized, and cautious to a tendency to be impulsive, risk-taking, and irresponsible. The fifth dimension, **psychoticism,** captures personality characteristics that are relatively rare in the general population but are important aspects of certain types of dysfunction (Krueger & Markon, 2014; Watson,

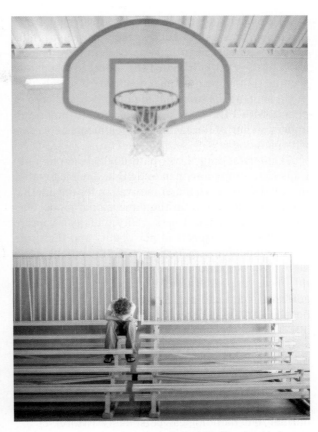

A core personality trait involves the extent to which people are appropriately outgoing and trusting of others (left) or tend to be withdrawn, avoidant, and untrusting (right). *(Left): JGI/Jamie Grill/Getty Images; (Right): L. Mouton/PhotoAlto*

Clark, & Chmielewski, 2008). People high on this dimension have highly unusual beliefs and perceptions and tend to be quite eccentric.

Taken together, the alternative *DSM-5* model specifies that, in order to diagnose an individual with a PD, he or she must show significant difficulties in identity and interpersonal functioning and significant pathological personality traits. In addition, these difficulties and traits must be unusual for the individual's developmental stage and sociocultural environment. For example, if an individual believed they could speak to dead relatives but this was a common belief in their culture, then they might not be rated high on the psychoticism trait domain. Finally, as in the official categorical model in the *DSM-5*, in the alternative model these difficulties and pathological traits cannot be due to ingesting a substance, such as hallucinatory perceptions while on a narcotic, or to a medical condition, such as a blow to the head, or better explained by another mental disorder.

Although the *DSM-5* explicitly incorporates a continuum approach into its general criteria in the alternative model for a PD, it also includes six specific PDs—*antisocial, avoidant, borderline, narcissistic, obsessive-compulsive,* and *schizotypal*—with which

individuals may be diagnosed based on their identified traits. Note that four PDs discussed in this chapter are not specifically recognized in the alternative model.

The third step in the diagnosis of PDs under this model is determining whether individuals meet the criteria for any of these six specific disorders. If an individual doesn't meet the criteria for any of these disorders but still has significant difficulties in his or her sense of self and relationships together with pathological personality traits, the diagnosis *PD–trait specified* is given. For example, a person who does not meet the definition for antisocial, avoidant, borderline, narcissistic, obsessive-compulsive, or schizotypal PD but is highly prone to being anxious about whether other people like him or her and also behaves irresponsibly in an attempt to get attention from others might be diagnosed as having PD–trait specified.

When clinicians diagnose someone with PD–trait specified, they then specify which pathological personality traits the person has. Thus, the *DSM-5* approach to PDs is a *hybrid model;* that is, it combines a dimensional or continuum approach with the categorical approach more typical of other types of disorders.

This hybrid dimensional-categorical model and its components aim to address the significant limitations of a purely categorical approach to PDs. The authors of the *DSM-5* included the model in a separate section of the manual to encourage research that might support the model in the diagnosis and care of people with PDs, as well as contribute to improved understanding of the causes and treatments of personality pathology.

Understanding how pathological personality traits factor into more than one PD and relate to other mental disorders is a major motivation for the alternative model. Research on the dimensional model suggests that pathological personality traits can capture the maladaptive aspects of personality and their role in poor functioning (Clark et al., 2015; Wright et al., 2015). More research is needed to determine whether this newer approach should replace the official categorical system, but studies suggest that it is useful in both research and clinical application (Waugh et al., 2017). The more dimensional perspective on PDs may also help researchers and clinicians better understand the complexities of mental disorders more broadly (Wright et al., 2012). Future research relating the alternative *DSM-5* model to general personality traits (e.g., the Big 5) might also facilitate integration of normal and pathological personality (Morey et al., 2015; Suzuki et al., 2017).

The approach to PDs in *DSM-5* is an excellent example of how the field of abnormal psychology continually faces the issues of defining abnormality and categorizing and diagnosing mental disorders discussed in this book's early chapters. This dimensional approach may also improve researchers' ability to understand how personality pathology develops in childhood and adolescence. This aspect is key not only to understanding pathology but also to prevention and intervention. As personality traits are viewed as more variable than they were in the past, and as diagnoses are less clearly categorical, studies of the biological predispositions and psychosocial factors in the development of personality pathology play an increasingly important role (De Fruyt & De Clercq, 2014).

CHAPTER INTEGRATION

Several of the personality disorders (PDs) discussed in this chapter, as well as antisocial PD (see the chapter "Disruptive, Impulse-Control, and Conduct Disorders"), are associated with a history of adversity in childhood, including abuse and neglect, and parental instability and psychopathology (Afifi et al., 2011). There are several possible explanations for this relationship (see Figure 1). It may be the result of genetic factors that create both parental

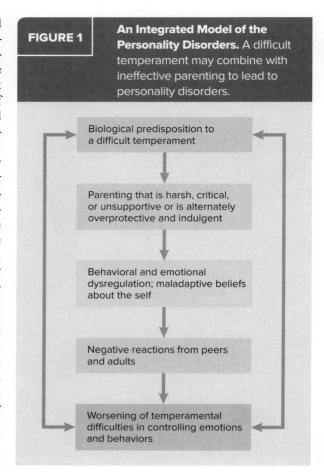

FIGURE 1   **An Integrated Model of the Personality Disorders.** A difficult temperament may combine with ineffective parenting to lead to personality disorders.

Biological predisposition to a difficult temperament

Parenting that is harsh, critical, or unsupportive or is alternately overprotective and indulgent

Behavioral and emotional dysregulation; maladaptive beliefs about the self

Negative reactions from peers and adults

Worsening of temperamental difficulties in controlling emotions and behaviors

psychopathology (which leads to neglectful and abusive parenting and an unstable household) and vulnerability to a PD in children. Abuse and neglect, along with a genetic predisposition, may produce permanent changes in the developing brain of some children that result in symptoms of certain PDs (Ruocco, Amirthavasagam, & Zakzanis, 2012). Abuse, neglect, and poor parenting resulting from parental psychopathology could also lead children to develop maladaptive ways of thinking about themselves and the world and poor regulation of their emotions (Beck, Davis, & Freeman, A. 2015; Millon, Grossman, Millon, Meagher, & Ramnath, 2004). Genetic factors may also contribute to the children developing maladaptive cognitions and emotion regulation strategies. Children who show early symptoms of PDs likely are more difficult to parent, which may lead to more hostile or neglectful behavior on the part of their parents. On the other hand, children born with a vulnerability to PD symptoms but have parents who validate their children's emotional experiences, are responsive to their needs, and help them develop an appropriate view of themselves and adaptive ways to cope with stress and relate to the world may never develop a full-blown PD.

SHADES OF GRAY   DISCUSSION

Ms. Farber shows signs of a mood disorder, with dysphoria, lack of energy or pleasure, and suicidal thoughts. Her sleeping and eating patterns have changed dramatically as well. This could suggest that she has a major depressive disorder, but other details of her story point to the possibility of a personality disorder. Ms. Farber's spending sprees, intense and even violent relationships with others, feelings of emptiness, and unstable sense of herself and her relationships suggest borderline personality disorder. This case illustrates a common problem clinicians face in making the diagnosis of a personality disorder: People with a personality disorder often come to the attention of mental health professionals when they are in a crisis, making it difficult to diagnose whether they have an acute disorder, such as depression, and/or a personality disorder.

CHAPTER SUMMARY

- Personality refers to a person's enduring patterns of perceiving, feeling, thinking about, and relating to oneself and the environment. A personality trait is a prominent aspect of personality that is relatively consistent across time and situations.

- The *DSM-5* defines personality disorder as an enduring pattern of inner experience and behavior (e.g., ways of perceiving and interpreting self, others, events; emotional responses; impulse control; interpersonal functioning) that deviates markedly from the expectations of an individual's culture. The personality pattern is pervasive and inflexible across time and situations, with onset in adolescence or early adulthood, and leads to clinically significant distress and/or functional impairment.

- Like *DSM-IV-TR,* the *DSM-5* takes a categorical approach toward classifying personality disorders and assumes that there is a dividing line between normal personality and pathological personality. However, the *DSM-5* no longer classifies personality disorders on a separate axis, as in *DSM-IV-TR.*

- It divides the personality disorders into three clusters based on their descriptive similarities: Cluster A includes the odd-eccentric disorders, cluster B includes the dramatic-emotional disorders, and cluster C consists of the anxious-fearful disorders.

- The cluster A odd-eccentric personality disorders include paranoid personality disorder (extreme mistrust of others), schizoid personality disorder (extreme social withdrawal and detachment), and schizotypal personality disorder (discomfort in close relationships, odd behavior, inappropriate social interactions, and cognitive-perceptual distortions). These disorders, particularly schizotypal personality disorder, may be genetically linked to schizophrenia and may represent mild versions of schizophrenia. People with these disorders tend to have poor social relationships and to be at increased risk for depression and schizophrenia.

- Psychotherapies for the odd-eccentric disorders have not been empirically tested for their efficacy.

They may be treated with traditional and atypical antipsychotics.

- The cluster B dramatic-emotional personality disorders include four disorders characterized by dramatic, erratic, and emotional behavior and interpersonal relationships: antisocial personality disorder (see the chapter "Disruptive, Impulse-Control, and Conduct Disorders"), borderline personality disorder, histrionic personality disorder, and narcissistic personality disorder. People with borderline personality disorder show profound instability in self-concept, emotional regulation, and interpersonal relationships, along with impulsive behavior. People with histrionic personality disorder show rapidly shifting moods, unstable relationships, a need for attention and approval, and dramatic, seductive behavior. People with narcissistic personality disorder show grandiosity, arrogance, and exploitation of others.

- Theories of borderline personality disorder argue that it is due to difficulties in self-concept and regulating emotions. These difficulties may be related to childhood adversity (especially abuse), which is commonly (though not always) reported by people with this disorder. The disorder is also associated with smaller volume in the hippocampus and amygdala, greater reactivity of the amygdala to emotional stimuli, and less activity in the prefrontal cortex, possibly leading to impulsive behavior and emotion regulation difficulties.

- Dialectical behavior therapy has been shown to be effective in treating people with borderline personality disorder. This therapy focuses on helping clients gain a more realistic and positive sense of self; learn adaptive skills for managing distress, regulating emotions, and solving problems; and correct dichotomous thinking. Cognitive and psychodynamic therapies (i.e., transference-focused and mentalization-based treatments) are also helpful. Mood stabilizers and atypical antipsychotics may be the most helpful medications.

- Treatments for histrionic and narcissistic personality disorders are less well developed, and people with these disorders tend not to seek therapy unless they develop significant distress (e.g., depression) or problems. Cognitive therapy may be helpful to them.

- The cluster C anxious-fearful personality disorders include three disorders characterized by anxious and fearful emotions and chronic self-doubt, leading to maladaptive behaviors: dependent personality disorder (extreme need to be cared for and fear of rejection), avoidant personality disorder (social anxiety and sense of inadequacy leading to social avoidance), and obsessive-compulsive personality disorder (rigidity in activities and interpersonal relationships).

- Genetic factors and childhood experiences of rejection by significant others are implicated in the development of avoidant personality disorder. Treatment involves cognitive-behavioral interventions to expose people to the interpersonal situations that make them anxious and to help them change the way they interpret criticism from others.

- People with obsessive-compulsive personality disorder often also have obsessive-compulsive disorder, and the disorders share some of the same genetic risk factors. Treatment with behavioral interventions to reduce compulsions and cognitive techniques to challenge rigid, perfectionistic beliefs can be helpful.

- In addition to the current categorical model for diagnosing personality disorders, the *DSM-5* includes an alternative dimensional trait model in a separate section of the manual designated for further study. The alternative model requires clinicians to diagnose a personality disorder based on particular difficulties in personality functioning and on specific patterns of pathological personality traits. The alternative model may represent how the diagnosis of personality disorders will evolve in the future and may facilitate integration of normal and pathological personality theories and research.

KEY TERMS

personality

personality trait

five-factor model

personality disorder (PD)

paranoid personality disorder (PPD)

schizoid personality disorder (SPD)

schizotypal personality disorder (STPD)

borderline personality disorder (BPD)

dialectical behavior therapy (DBT)

transference-focused therapy

mentalization-based treatment

histrionic personality disorder

narcissistic personality disorder (NPD)

avoidant personality disorder (AVPD)

dependent personality disorder

obsessive-compulsive personality disorder

negative affectivity

detachment

antagonism

disinhibition

psychoticism

Chapter 10

ferrantraite/Getty Images

Neurodevelopmental and Neurocognitive Disorders

CHAPTER OUTLINE

Neurodevelopmental and Neurocognitive Disorders Along the Continuum

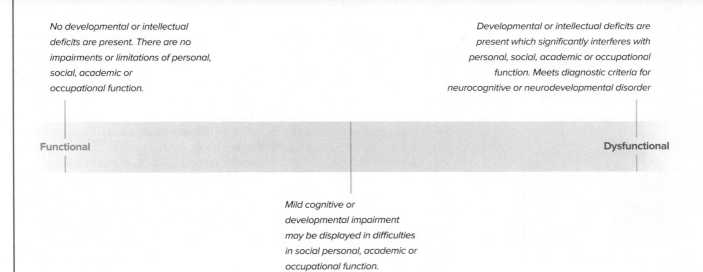

No developmental or intellectual deficits are present. There are no impairments or limitations of personal, social, academic or occupational function.

Developmental or intellectual deficits are present which significantly interferes with personal, social, academic or occupational function. Meets diagnostic criteria for neurocognitive or neurodevelopmental disorder

Functional

Dysfunctional

Mild cognitive or developmental impairment may be displayed in difficulties in social personal, academic or occupational function.

One of the most fascinating discoveries in the last few decades is how much the human brain changes across the life span. The pace of brain development is extraordinary in early life, with dramatic growth in its size and complexity in infancy and childhood, followed by further shaping and maturation into early adulthood (Casey, Tottenham, Liston, & Durston, 2005). The brain continues to change throughout adulthood in response to people's lifestyles, experiences, and health. Then, as people grow older, come gradual declines in the structural and functional integrity of the brain but adaptations in the ways the brain processes information that allow most people to retain a high level of functioning well into old age (Park & Reuter-Lorenz, 2009; Sowell et al., 2003).

Yet there is tremendous variability across people in the development and aging of the brain and in related cognitive, emotional, and behavioral functioning. Parents of young children often anxiously chart their child's progress on major milestones of development, such as talking, walking, and reading. Although some children reach these milestones later than others, most eventually gain the critical skills that allow them to function in everyday life. Some children, however, continue to have major problems with basic academic skills, such as reading, writing, and mathematics. Others have more global cognitive deficits that interfere with their ability to function in many domains of life. For others, the deficits are in their ability to regulate their emotions and behaviors and to understand social interactions. Although such difficulties may stem in part from adverse environmental experiences, such as trauma or poverty, they often have their roots in atypical brain development.

Similarly, as our brains age in middle age and older adulthood, they decrease in size and efficiency, leading most of us to experience gradual declines in how quickly we perceive and process information, in our ability to hold and manipulate information in working memory, and in long-term memory (see Figure 1). Most of us can use our accumulated knowledge and expertise to compensate for these declines in cognitive-processing ability.

However, for some people, deterioration in the brain is more severe and widespread than usual, leading to moderate or severe deficits in the processing of information and thus in their ability to function in daily life.

Brain dysfunction in either childhood or older age can be understood only in the context of what is typical or functional for individuals in those periods of life. Psychologists who focus on functional and dysfunctional development in children are referred to as *developmental psychopathologists*. Those concerned with functional and dysfunctional changes in older age are referred to as *geropsychologists*.

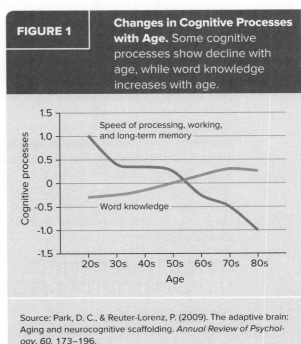

FIGURE 1 | **Changes in Cognitive Processes with Age.** Some cognitive processes show decline with age, while word knowledge increases with age.

Source: Park, D. C., & Reuter-Lorenz, P. (2009). The adaptive brain: Aging and neurocognitive scaffolding. *Annual Review of Psychology, 60,* 173–196.

Extraordinary People

Temple Grandin, *Thinking in Pictures*

MediaPunch/REX/Shutterstock

Dr. Temple Grandin, professor of animal sciences at Colorado State University, has designed one-third of the livestock-handling facilities in the United States. She has published dozens of scientific papers and gives lectures throughout the world. Some of her lectures describe her new equipment and procedures for safer and more humane animal handling. Others describe her life with autism.

Grandin showed the classic symptoms of autism (now called autism spectrum disorder) during childhood. As a baby, she had no desire to be held by her mother, though she was calm if left alone. As a young child, she seldom made eye contact with others and seemed to lack interest in people. She frequently threw wild tantrums. If left alone, she rocked back and forth or spun around repeatedly. She could sit for hours on the beach, watching sand dribble through her fingers, in a trance-like state. At age 2, she still had not begun talking and was labeled "brain-damaged" because doctors at that time did not know about autism spectrum disorder.

Fortunately, Grandin's mother was determined to find good teachers, learn ways to calm her daughter, and encourage her to speak and engage with others. Grandin did learn to speak by the time she entered elementary school, although most of her social interaction deficits remained. When she was 12, Grandin scored 137 on an IQ test (which falls in the very superior range) but still was thrown out of a regular school because she didn't fit in. She persisted, however, and eventually went to college, where she earned a degree in psychology, and then to graduate school, where she earned a PhD in animal sciences.

Grandin has been able to thrive in her career and personal life. Still, she finds it very difficult to understand emotions and social relationships. She does not "read" other people well and often finds herself offending others or being stared at because of her social awkwardness:

> I have always felt like someone who watches from the outside. I could not participate in the social interactions of high school life. . . . My peers spent hours standing around talking about jewelry or some other topic with no real substance. What did they get out of this? I just did not fit in. I never fit in with the crowd, but I had a few friends who were interested in the same things, such as skiing and riding horses. Friendship always revolved around what I did rather than who I was. (Grandin, 1995, p. 132)

Still, Grandin does not regret that she has autism. She says,

> If I could snap my fingers and be a nonautistic person, I would not. Autism is part of what I am. (p. 60)

All the disorders in this book are related to dysfunction in the brain to one degree or another. The disorders we discuss in this chapter are classified in the *DSM-5* specifically as neurological disorders. We consider a group of disorders that typically arise first in childhood, known as the **neurodevelopmental disorders:** attention-deficit/hyperactivity disorder; autism spectrum disorder; intellectual disability; and learning, communication, and motor disorders. Then we consider disorders that typically arise in older age. These are known as the **neurocognitive disorders:** various major and mild neurocognitive disorders, and delirium.

ATTENTION-DEFICIT/ HYPERACTIVITY DISORDER

"Pay attention! Slow down! You're so hyper today!" We've all heard parents say things like this from time to time, but what if these behaviors are always present? There are some children who can only concentrate on a task for a few minutes at a time whether the activity is doing homework, playing, or even watching television. These individuals may constantly fidget, blurt out whatever they are thinking, or display high levels of distractibility. As a result, theses behaviors may interfere with learning, friends, and social relationships. Socialization is a critical part of child development and helps children learn to pay attention, control their impulses, and organize their behaviors so that they can accomplish long-term goals. Unfortunately, due to problems with attention and hyperactivity, some children have tremendous trouble learning these skills and may be diagnosed with **attention-deficit/hyperactivity disorder (ADHD)** (see the *DSM-5* criteria in Table 1). Children with this disorder have persistent issues with attention and/or impulsivity-hyperactivity as shown in the case of Eddie, a young boy with ADHD.

TABLE 1 *DSM-5* Criteria for Attention-Deficit/Hyperactivity Disorder

A. A persistent pattern of inattention and/or hyperactivity that interferes with functioning or development, as characterized by (1) and/or (2):

1. *Inattention:* Six (or more) of the following symptoms have persisted for at least 6 months to a degree that is inconsistent with developmental level and that negatively impacts directly on social and academic/occupational activities: Note: The symptoms are not solely a manifestation of oppositional behavior, defiance, hostility, or failure to understand tasks or instructions. For older adolescents and adults (age 17 and older), at least five symptoms are required.

   a. Often fails to give close attention to details or makes careless mistakes in schoolwork, at work, or during other activities (e.g., overlooks or misses details, work is inaccurate)

   b. Often has difficulty sustaining attention in tasks or play activities (e.g., has difficulty remaining focused during lectures, conversations, or lengthy reading)

   c. Often does not seem to listen when spoken to directly (e.g., mind seems elsewhere, even in the absence of any obvious distraction)

   d. Often does not follow through on instructions and fails to finish schoolwork, chores, or duties in the workplace (e.g., starts tasks but quickly loses focus and is easily sidetracked)

   e. Often has difficulty organizing tasks and activities (e.g., difficulty managing sequential tasks; difficulty keeping materials and belongings in order; messy, disorganized work; poor time management; tends to fail to meet deadlines)

   f. Often avoids, dislikes, or is reluctant to engage in tasks that require sustained mental effort (e.g., schoolwork or homework; for older adolescents and adults, preparing reports, completing forms, or reviewing lengthy papers)

   g. Often loses things necessary for tasks or activities (e.g., school materials, pencils, books, tools, wallets, keys, paperwork, eyeglasses, mobile telephones)

   h. Is often easily distracted by extraneous stimuli (for older adolescents and adults, may include unrelated thoughts)

   i. Is often forgetful in daily activities (e.g., doing chores, running errands; for older adolescents and adults, returning calls, paying bills, keeping appointments)

2. *Hyperactivity and impulsivity:* Six (or more) of the following symptoms have persisted for at least 6 months to a degree that is inconsistent with developmental level and that negatively impacts directly on social and academic/occupational activities. Note: The symptoms are not solely a manifestation of oppositional behavior, defiance, hostility, or a failure to understand tasks or instructions. For older adolescents and adults (age 17 and older), at least five symptoms are required.

   a. Often fidgets with or taps hands or feet or squirms in seat

   b. Often leaves seat in situations when remaining seated is expected (e.g., leaves their place in the classroom, office or, other workplace, or other situations that require remaining in place)

   c. Often runs about or climbs in situations where it is inappropriate (Note: in adolescents or adults, may be limited to feeling restless)

   d. Often unable to play or engage in leisure activities quietly

   e. Is often "on the go," acting as if "driven by a motor" (e.g., is unable to be or uncomfortable being still for an extended time, as in restaurants, meetings; may be experienced by others as being restless and difficult to keep up with)

   f. Often talks excessively

   g. Often blurts out an answer before a question has been completed (e.g., completes people's sentences; cannot wait for turn in conversation)

   h. Often has difficulty waiting their turn (e.g., while waiting in line)

   i. Often interrupts or intrudes on others (e.g., butts into conversations, games, or activities; may start using other people's things without asking or receiving permission; for adolescents or adults, may intrude into or take over what others are doing)

B. Several inattentive or hyperactive-impulsive symptoms were present prior to age 12 years.

C. Several inattentive or hyperactive-impulsive symptoms are present in two or more settings (e.g., at home, school, or work; with friends or relatives; in other activities).

D. There is clear evidence that the symptoms interfere with, or reduce the quality of, social, academic, or occupational functioning.

E. The symptoms do not occur exclusively during the course of schizophrenia or another psychotic disorder and are not better explained by another mental disorder (e.g., mood disorder, anxiety disorder, dissociative disorder, personality disorder, substance intoxication, or withdrawal).

Specify Based on Current Presentation

Combined Presentation: If both Criterion A1 (Inattention) and Criterion A2 (Hyperactivity-Impulsivity) are met for the past 6 months.

Predominantly Inattentive Presentation: If Criterion A1 (Inattention) is met but Criterion A2 (Hyperactivity-Impulsivity) is not met for the past 6 months.

Predominantly Hyperactive/Impulsive Presentation: If Criterion A2 (Hyperactivity-Impulsivity) is met and Criterion A1 (Inattention) is not met for the past 6 months.

CASE STUDY

Nine-year-old Sean was referred to the child study team by his third grade teacher due to his disruptive classroom behaviors. Sean is often restless and unable to focus during class time, which is a significant distraction to his classmates. It is very common for Sean to be seen wandering around the classroom during a lesson talking to other children while they are working which has impacted their ability to concentrate. When seated, Sean often fidgets with any items on his desk like pencils, erasers, or his workbook or he constantly taps his feet and hands in a disruptive beat. Sean was recently suspended from school for climbing on top of the teacher's desk multiple times to see how far he could jump across the room. The teacher has found it impossible to focus her attention on other students who require instruction due to Sean's behavioral issues.

Sean's mother reports that his behavior has been difficult to manage since he was about 3-years-old when she noticed problems with hyperactivity and following directions. Sean has never been able to rest and often requires less sleep than one would expect for a child of his age. Sean's mother stated that when he was very young, he would often wake up before 5:00 am and go downstairs by himself where he would get "into everything in the house" and his parents would wake up to a mess everywhere. At the age of 4, Sean unlocked multiple latches on their front door and wandered out of the neighborhood because he wanted to get a "slushie." Sean was found and returned by a person passing him by on the street.

TV shows or games that require concentration and attention are of no interest to Sean. He prefers to play outdoors alone or with his dog and he has few friends since he is often overwhelming to children his age. Sean has many favorite games and toys, but they are often disorganized, broken or missing despite help from his mother to keep things in order.

Unlike Eddie, most elementary-school-age children of his age can sit still for a reasonable period of time and engage in games that require patience and concentration. They can inhibit their impulses to jump up in class or run across a busy street without looking. Children with ADHD, like Eddie, have driven and disorganized behaviors that interfere with daily function.

There are three subtypes or presentations of ADHD in the *DSM-5*. The *combined presentation* requires six or more symptoms of inattention and six or more symptoms of hyperactivity-impulsivity. The *predominantly inattentive presentation* is diagnosed if six or more symptoms of inattention but less than six symptoms of hyperactivity-impulsivity are present. The *predominantly hyperactive/impulsive presentation* is diagnosed if six or more symptoms of hyperactivity-impulsivity but less than six symptoms of inattention are present. Eddie appears to have this last presentation of ADHD.

ADHD is one of the most common neurodevelopmental disorders in childhood and research suggests that approximately 3.4 to 6 percent of all school-aged children across the world are diagnosed with this disorder, which is thought to be increasing (Hauck, Lau, Wing, Kurdyak, & Tu, 2017). ADHD begins in childhood and symptoms must be present prior to the age of 12 within multiple settings (e.g., home and school) to be diagnosed. It is also likely this range is an underestimate of the prevalence according to the new *DSM-5* criterion of onset by 12 years of age. One of the major changes in the diagnostic criteria for ADHD in the *DSM-5* is that the age limit for the onset of symptoms was raised from 7 years to 12 years, in response to research suggesting that the cutoff of 7 years failed to capture many children who eventually show ADHD but a cutoff of 12 years captured 95 percent of individuals who develop ADHD. Although this disorder focuses on childhood symptoms and diagnoses, the impairments associated with ADHD can persist into adulthood (American Psychiatric Association, 2013; Barkley, 2014; Jangmo et al., 2019; Pelsser, Frankena, Toorman, & Rodrigues Pereira, 2017; Voort, He, Jameson, & Merikangas, 2014).

There are long-established sex differences found within ADHD. Boys are a little more than two times more likely than girls to develop ADHD in childhood and early adolescence, although this difference narrows as they age into adulthood (Hinshaw, 2018). Girls with ADHD tend to present primarily with inattentive features and have less disruptive behavior than boys with ADHD, which may result in an underdiagnosis of this disorder. It is also speculated that these significant gender differences may be related to sex-specific stereotypes of ADHD. The stereotype of a "disruptive boy" may influence how male and female behaviors are perceived by individuals, like teachers and parents, who are often key to the referral and diagnostic process. Recent research found that parents underrated the hyperactive/impulsive symptoms in girls with ADHD and overrated those observed in boys. This suggests gender bias may be a factor that impacts the sex ratio and diagnostic rates of ADHD. Girls who do not display more gender-stereotypical symptoms or those who are less impaired may be overlooked for assessment (Mowlem, Agnew-Blais, Taylor, & Asherson, 2019). ADHD is found across most cultures and ethnic groups. Although the percentage of children with ADHD is similar across countries, children in the United States are diagnosed at somewhat higher rates (Hinshaw, 2018; Polanczyk, Willcutt, Salum, Kieling, & Rohde, 2014). Like Eddie, most children with ADHD are diagnosed in elementary school.

The symptoms associated with ADHD are strongly associated with poor school performance, both in childhood and later in life. Children with ADHD are at increased risk of lower scores on achievement tests, lower grade point average (GPA), grade repetition, and special education placement than those without ADHD. The same outcomes have been observed in adolescents with ADHD who often fail more grade levels and perform worse on academic achievement tests (Jangmo et al., 2019; Langberg et al., 2012). Children with ADHD have issues with concentration and attention that hinder their ability to learn the material and often perform below their intellectual capabilities. In addition to poor academic performance, peer relationships are often disrupted and children with ADHD are more likely to experience peer rejection and teasing as a result of hyperactivity and impulsivity. Peer neglect is often associated with symptoms related to elevated levels of inattention (American Psychiatric Association, 2013). Like Eddie, many children with ADHD have poor relationships with other children and are often rejected outright (Hoza et al., 2005). When interacting with their peers, children with ADHD may be intrusive, irritable, and demanding. They want to play by their own rules and sometimes show mood and temper problems. When things do not go their way, they may become aggressive. In addition to symptoms of ADHD interfering with their school performance, recent studies suggest that learning disorders (LDs) are commonly comorbid with this group. Specifically, Reading Disorder (RD), Disorder of Written Expression (DWE), and Developmental Coordination Disorder (DCD) are among the most common LDs that co-exist with ADHD (Parke, Thaler, Etcoff, & Allen, 2020). Research has found 20 to 25 percent of children with ADHD may have a specific learning disorder that makes it doubly hard for them to concentrate in school and to learn (Wilens, Biederman, & Spencer, 2002).

The behavior problems of some children with ADHD worsen over the course of development, and become severe enough to be diagnosed as a conduct disorder. This is particularly true for ADHD children with the combined presentation. Children with conduct disorders grossly violate the social and cultural norms for appropriate behavior toward others by acting in uncaring and even antisocial ways (see the chapter "Disruptive, Impulse-Control, and Conduct Disorders"). Between 45 and 60 percent of children

Children normally have high energy levels, but only a minority of children can be labeled hyperactive. *Dejan Dundjerski/Shutterstock*

with ADHD develop a conduct disorder, abuse drugs or alcohol, or violate the law (Ahmad & Hinshaw, 2016; Frick & Nigg, 2012). For some individuals, conduct problems persist into adulthood.

The long-term outcomes for children with ADHD vary considerably, but studies have found that impairing symptoms can persist into adulthood in 50 to 78 percent of cases (Hinshaw, 2018; Pelsser, Frankena, Toorman, & Rodrigues Pereira, 2017). Adults diagnosed with ADHD as children are at increased risk for antisocial personality disorder, substance abuse, mood and anxiety disorders, marital problems, traffic accidents, legal infractions, and frequent job changes (Fischer & Barkley, 2006; Wilens et al., 2002). Some adults who have had lifelong problems achieving success in school and at work and difficulties in social relationships might have had undiagnosed and untreated ADHD as children. An epidemiological study of the United States found that 4.4 percent of adults could be diagnosed with ADHD (Kessler, Adler, et al., 2006). They were more likely to be male, and they showed a wide range of difficulties at work and in their social lives. Most had not received treatment for ADHD specifically, although many had been treated for other disorders. Adults with ADHD are at higher risk for depression, anxiety disorders, substance abuse, and antisocial personality disorder (Asherson, Buitelaar, Faraone, & Rohde, 2016; Klassen et al., 2010). ADHD significantly impacts quality of life of the child, parents and siblings and contributes to a long term burden on the family and society. Additionally, ADHD may more than double the risk of premature death from unnatural causes, like accidents (Pelsser, Frankena, Toorman & Rodrigues Pereira, 2017).

Biological Factors

The difficulties in attention, planning and carrying through with activities, and impulse control seen in ADHD appear to be tied to fundamental abnormalities in the brain (Cubillo, Halari, Smith, Taylor, &

The prefrontal cortex is smaller and shows abnormal activity in children with ADHD.

Rubia, 2012; Hoogman et al., 2017). Abnormal activity has been seen in several areas, including the prefrontal cortex, which is key to the control of cognition, motivation, and behavior; the striatum, which is involved in working memory and planning; and the cerebellum, which is involved in motor behaviors. The cerebral cortex is smaller in volume in children, and there is less connectivity between frontal areas of the cortex and areas of the brain that influence motor behavior, memory and attention, and emotional reactions. Because the cortex continues to develop well into adolescence, one hypothesis is that children with ADHD are neurologically immature—that is, their brains are slower to develop than the brains of unaffected children—leaving them unable to maintain attention and control their behavior at an age-appropriate level. This immaturity hypothesis helps explain why in some children the symptoms of ADHD, especially hyperactivity symptoms, decline with age (Cubillo et al., 2012; Hoogman et al., 2017).

The catecholamine neurotransmitters, particularly dopamine and norepinephrine, appear to function abnormally in individuals with ADHD (del Campo, Chamberlain, Sahakian, & Robbins, 2011). We have previously discussed the role of these neurotransmitters in mood, but they also play important roles in sustained attention, inhibition of impulses, and processing of errors. Drugs that affect levels of these neurotransmitters are useful in treating ADHD.

ADHD is a highly heritable childhood disorder with a chronic course that is strongly tied to genetic factors (Larsson, Chang, D'Onofrio, & Lichtenstein, 2014). Siblings of children with ADHD are three to four times more likely to develop it than siblings of children without the disorder (Todd, Lobos, Sun, & Neuman, 2003). Several other disorders also tend to run in the families of children with ADHD, including antisocial personality disorder, alcoholism, and depression. Autism spectrum disorders (ASD) and ADHD frequently co-occur and studies suggest a genetic link between these disorders that is supported by twin studies. However, the genetic architecture and overlap between ASD and ADHD remains largely unclear. (Ahmad & Hinshaw, 2016; Ghirardi et al., 2018) Twin studies and adoption studies suggest that genetic factors play a role in vulnerability to ADHD (Pingault et al., 2015). Attentional and hyperactivity symptoms of ADHD both seem to have a genetic basis (Nikolas & Burt, 2010). Molecular genetics studies suggest that genes that influence dopamine, noradrenaline, and serotonin may be abnormal in individuals with ADHD (Li, Chang, Zhang, Gao, & Wang, 2014).

Many children with ADHD have a history of prenatal and birth complications. ADHD is associated with low birth weight, premature delivery, and difficult delivery leading to oxygen deprivation (see Sciberras, Mulraney, Silva, & Coghill, 2017). Some investigators suspect that moderate to severe drinking or heavy use of nicotine or barbiturates by mothers during pregnancy can lead to the kinds of behavioral inhibition deficits seen in children with ADHD. Others regard these associations as a result of shared genetic risk among ADHD and drinking and smoking habits. Some studies have found small to moderate risk associated with exposure to lead during childhood, including through ingesting lead-based paint (Goodlad, Marcus, & Fulton, 2013).

The links between diet and symptoms of ADHD are inconsistent. An unhealthy "Western" diet full of fat, sodium, sugar, and food additives is associated with greater symptoms of hyperactivity both in healthy children and in children with ADHD, but it is not clear that this diet causes ADHD or other forms of psychopathology (Howard et al., 2011). A small number of children with ADHD show improvement in their symptoms when synthetic food colorings are removed from their diet (Nigg, Lewis, Edinger, & Falk, 2012). The International Society for Nutritional Psychiatry Research, recently stated that there is 'emerging and compelling evidence for nutrition as a crucial factor' in mental disorders. At this time however, the mechanism of nutrition on the development of ADHD is unclear but future research should focus on the gut-brain axis. Studies have shown that the gut microbiota responds rapidly to a change of diet and produces neurochemicals comparable to those in the brain which may help usbetter understand the development of this and other psychiatric disorders (Pelsser et al., 2017).

Psychological and Social Factors

Children with ADHD are more likely than children without a psychological disorder to belong to families that experience frequent disruptions and in which the parents are prone to aggressive and hostile behavior and substance abuse (Ahmad & Hinshaw, 2016; Harold et al., 2013). Some of these associations may be due to shared genetic effects on impulsivity and cognitive problems, which lead to both the parental behaviors and the children's ADHD symptoms. However, it appears that genetic factors in ADHD prompt disruptive behavior in children and, in turn, hostile parenting, even in adoptive (i.e., genetically unrelated) parents (Harold et al., 2013). Family interaction patterns, especially in early childhood, influence the course and severity of ADHD, including the development of conduct problems (Musser, Karalunas, Dieckmann, Peris, & Nigg, 2016).

Treatments for ADHD

Most children with ADHD are treated with stimulant drugs, such as Ritalin, Dexedrine, and Adderall (Barkley, 2014). It may seem odd to give a stimulant to a hyperactive child, but 70 to 85 percent of ADHD children respond to these drugs with decreases in demanding, disruptive, and noncompliant behavior (Chan, Fogler, & Hammerness, 2016; Swanson et al., 2008). The children also show increases in positive mood, in the ability to be goal-directed, and in the quality of their interactions with others. The stimulants may work by increasing levels of dopamine in the synapses of the brain, enhancing release, and inhibiting reuptake of this neurotransmitter (Swanson et al. 2011).

The side effects of stimulants include reduced appetite, insomnia, edginess, and gastrointestinal upset. Stimulants also can increase the frequency of tics in children with ADHD. There has been concern that stimulants may stunt growth, and some evidence exists that children with ADHD who begin taking stimulants show a decrease in their growth rate (Swanson et al., 2017). Stimulants also carry a risk of abuse by people looking for a high, to make money by resale, or hoping to gain an edge in high school, college, or the workplace (see the chapter "Substance Use and Gambling Disorders").

Nationwide, the number of children prescribed stimulant medications in the United States increased by 200 to 300 percent in the 1980s and 1990s, and then increased more slowly after 2000 (Zuvekas & Vitiello, 2012). However, rates of prescriptions continue to increase, especially among adolescents and adults (Safer, 2016). Some researchers argue that this increase reflects greater recognition of children and adults with ADHD and of their need for treatment. Others say that it represents an inappropriate overuse of the drugs, particularly for children who are difficult to control (Angold, Erkanli, Egger, & Costello, 2000). There is scant empirical evidence on which to judge these competing claims.

Other drugs that treat ADHD include atomoxetine, clonidine, and guanfacine, which are not stimulants but affect norepinephrine levels. These drugs can help reduce tics, common in children with ADHD, and increase cognitive performance (del Campo et al., 2011; Kratochvil et al., 2007). Side effects of these drugs include dry mouth, fatigue, dizziness, constipation, and sedation.

Antidepressant medications are often prescribed to children and adolescents with ADHD since anxiety and depressive disorders are very common in this population (Hauck e al., 2017). These drugs have some

SHADES OF GRAY

Read the following description of Jake, a college student.

Jake had just earned a 2.4 GPA in his freshman year at the University of Washington when his parents took him to see a psychologist about his academic performance. At the meeting with the psychologist, his parents described their middle son as lazy, unmotivated, stubborn, and disorganized. His brothers were successful at school, as his parents had been. Growing up, Jake had seemed smart, but he often sabotaged his grades by forgetting to do his homework, quitting in the middle of assignments, and not finishing tests. When he completed a project, he would often leave it behind or lose it. He could be engrossed in TV or a video game, but when it came to his homework, he lacked focus. His parents also noted that he was constantly late and didn't seem to care about making everyone else wait for him.

When the psychologist spoke with Jake alone, Jake seemed like a nice, polite teenager. Jake felt discouraged and confused about school. He agreed that he didn't get the good grades his brothers did and knew his parents expected more of him. When he was younger he did well in school, and in elementary school he thought of himself as smart. But his grades had slipped when he transitioned into middle school, then again when he entered high school, and now again in college. He thought he understood what was going on in class but was always forgetting or losing things, and his mind would often wander. Outside of the classroom, he had a small but supportive group of friends, and he was involved in a wide variety of sports and activities. He denied any involvement with drugs or illegal activity. (Source: Adapted from Vitkus, J., *Casebook in abnormal psychology*. New York: McGraw-Hill, 2004, pp. 193–199)

What might be causing Jake's problems? What additional information would you want before making a diagnosis? (Discussion appears at the end of this chapter.)

positive effects on cognitive performance but are not as effective for ADHD as the stimulants (Wilens et al., 2002). Bupropion, an antidepressant with particularly strong effects on dopamine levels, appears to be more effective for ADHD than some other antidepressants. Unfortunately, the gains made by ADHD children treated with medications alone are short-term. As soon as medication is stopped, symptoms often return.

Behavioral therapies for ADHD focus on reinforcing attentive, goal-directed, and prosocial behaviors and extinguishing impulsive and hyperactive behaviors (Barkley, 2014; Evans, Owens, Wymbs, & Ray, 2018). These therapies typically engage parents and teachers in changing rewards and punishments in many aspects of the child's life. A child and his or her parents might agree that he or she will earn a chip every time he or she obeys a request to wash hands or put away the toys. At the end of each week, they can exchange their chips for fun activities. Each time the child refuses to comply, they lose a chip. Such techniques can help parents break the cycle of engaging in arguments with their children that escalate problem behaviors, which in turn lead to more arguments and perhaps physical violence. The children learn to anticipate the consequences of their behaviors and to make less impulsive choices. They are taught to interact more appropriately with others, including waiting their turn in games, finding nonaggressive ways to express frustration, and listening when others speak. Meta-analyses of hundreds of studies have found strong and consistent evidence that behavioral therapy is highly effective in reducing symptoms of ADHD in children (Catala-Lopez et al., 2017; Fabiano et al., 2009). For adults with ADHD, cognitive-behavioral treatments that incorporate organizational, planning, and time management skills appear to be effective as well (Knouse, Teller, & Brooks, 2017).

Some studies suggest that the combination of stimulant therapy and psychosocial therapy is more likely to produce short-term improvements than either therapy alone. In one multi-site study, 579 children with ADHD were randomly assigned to receive the combination of Ritalin and behavior therapy, one therapy alone, or routine community care (Jensen et al., 2001). After 14 months, 68 percent of the combined-treatment group had reduced or discontinued their ADHD behaviors, such as aggression and lack of concentration. In the medication-alone group, 56 percent showed reduced or discontinued symptoms. Behavior therapy alone reduced symptoms in only 34 percent of group members, and only 25 percent of those given routine community care showed reductions in their symptoms. In follow-ups 3, 6, and 8 years later, all three treatment groups continued to have fewer ADHD symptoms than they had had before treatment, but there were no differences between

In behavioral therapies for ADHD, a child and her parents might agree that she will earn a chip every time she obeys a request to wash her hands. At the end of each week, she can exchange her chips for fun activities such as eating an ice cream cone or extra screen time. *Adam Gault/Getty Images*

treatment groups in outcome (Jensen et al., 2007; Molina et al., 2009). In addition, 6 and 8 months after treatment ended, all three groups still had more symptoms than classmates who had not been diagnosed with ADHD (Molina et al., 2009).

AUTISM SPECTRUM DISORDER

Autism spectrum disorder (ASD) involves impairment in two fundamental behavior domains—deficits in social interactions and communications and restricted, repetitive patterns of behaviors, interests, and activities (see Table 2). Richard, a child with ASD, shows a range of deficits characteristic of this disorder.

CASE STUDY

It was clear by the age of 3 that Robyn lacked social skills and interest in others, appearing almost standoffish. Her parents felt like they had done something wrong when the child would not show any emotional response towards them. Robyn never seemed excited to see her parents or connected to them on an emotional level. When left with a baby-sitter, it was common for Robyn to scream for long periods of time, despite knowing the babysitter very well. Robyn would often ignore her older brother and other children preferring to play alone. As an infant, her patterns of babbling had no conversational intonation and only recently could Robyn understand simple instructions. It appeared that she was developing appropriate language until her parents noticed that her speech only consisted of echoing certain words and phrases she heard in the past. When practicing the ABCs with her

TABLE 2 *DSM-5* Diagnostic Criteria for Autism Spectrum Disorder

A. Persistent deficits in social communication and social interaction across multiple contexts, as manifested by the following, currently or by history (examples are illustrative, not exhaustive; see text [of the *DSM-5*]):

1. Deficits in social-emotional reciprocity; ranging from abnormal social approach and failure of normal back-and-forth conversation, to reduced sharing of interests, emotions, or affect or failure to initiate or respond to social interactions.

2. Deficits in nonverbal communicative behaviors used for social interaction, ranging, for example, from poorly integrated verbal and nonverbal communication, to abnormalities in eye contact and body language, to deficits in understanding and use of gestures, or to a total lack of facial expression or nonverbal communication.

3. Deficits in developing, maintaining, and understanding relationships, ranging, for example, from difficulties adjusting behavior to suit various social contexts, to difficulties in sharing imaginative play or in making friends, or to an absence of interest in peers.

B. Restricted, repetitive patterns of behavior, interests, or activities as manifested by at least two of the following, currently or by history (examples are illustrative, not exhaustive; see text [of the *DSM-5*]):

1. Stereotyped or repetitive motor movements, use of objects, or speech (e.g., simple motor stereotypies, lining up toys or flipping objects, echolalia, idiosyncratic phrases).

2. Insistence on sameness, inflexible adherence to routines, or ritualized patterns of verbal or nonverbal behavior (such as extreme distress at small changes, difficulties with transitions, rigid thinking patterns, greeting rituals, need to take same route, or eat same food each day).

3. Highly restricted, fixated interests that are abnormal in intensity or focus (such as strong attachment to or preoccupation with unusual objects, excessively circumscribed or perseverative interests).

4. Hyper- or hyporeactivity to sensory input or unusual interest in sensory aspects of environment (such as apparent indifference to pain/temperature, adverse response to specific sounds or textures, excessive smelling or touching of objects, fascination with lights or movement).

C. Symptoms must be present in the early developmental period (but may not become fully manifest until social demands exceed limited capacities, or may be masked by learned strategies in later life).

D. Symptoms cause clinically significant impairment in social, occupational, or other important areas of current functioning.

E. These disturbances are not better explained by intellectual disability or global developmental delay. Intellectual disability and autism spectrum disorder frequently co-occur; to make comorbid diagnoses of autism spectrum disorder and intellectual disability, social communication (Criteria A) must be below that expected for general developmental level.

Reprinted with permission from the *Diagnostic and Statistical Manual of Mental Disorders,* Fifth Edition. Copyright ©2013 by American Psychiatric Association. All Rights Reserved.

mother, it became obvious that Robyn was simply repeating the letters and sentence of her mother . . . "Let's say our ABCs, ok?" Robyn could use some simple phrases to communicate her needs, but her parents noticed some differences in how she would ask for things as compared to their other child. For example, when asking for a drink, Robyn would say "Do you want a drink?" to indicate that she was thirsty. Additionally, Robyn did not utilize eye contact, facial expressions or gestures to communicate with others.

Robyn loved to play with toy cars and blocks and would spend hours lining them up all over the house. It was common to see Robyn flapping her hands or rocking back and forth as she played alone. Robyn had a strong attachment to a small flashlight that she always carried in her hand, even though she did not use it at any time for practical or play purposes. This flashlight was always with her, otherwise Robyn would become distraught. Robyn would become very difficult to manage if there were any changes to her typical routine, schedule, or placement of her favorite objects. Once, by accident, a friend of the family "cleaned up" her line of blocks and cars that ran throughout the house. Robyn exploded into screams of terror and began hitting herself with an open hand. The fastest way to stop these episodes was to return her items to their designated place. Robyn's family was very conscious of this as a trigger for her outbursts and they made every effort not to upset her routine.

The deficits in social interactions and communications of **autism** may first show up in infants' and toddlers' interactions with their parents, which are usually characterized by reciprocal adoration (Harbison et al., 2018). Compared to normally developing children, infants with ASD may not smile and coo in response to their caregivers or initiate play with their caregivers. They may not want to cuddle with their parents, even when they are frightened. They may hardly ever make eye contact relative to cultural norms or show joint attention (i.e., failure to follow a caregiver's pointing or eye gaze). Other early symptoms often include delayed language development. When they are a bit older, children with ASD may not be interested in playing with other children, preferring solitary play. They also do not seem to react to other people's emotions (American Psychiatric Association, 2013). In the chapter opener, Temple Grandin describes how she had to work hard to overcome her lack of understanding of social interactions.

Approximately 25 to 30 percent of individuals with ASD do not develop useful speech by school age and those who do develop language may not use it as expected for their age. Children with ASD typically use a small number of single words or fixed phrases to request items (Chenausky, Brignell, Morgan, & Tager-Flusberg, 2019). In the case study about Richard, he showed several of the communication problems characteristic of children with ASD. Rather than generating his own words, he simply echoed what he had just heard, a behavior called **echolalia.** He reversed pronouns, using *you* when he meant *I.* When he did try to generate his own words or sentences, his language was one-sided and lacked social reciprocity and he did not modulate his voice for expressiveness, instead sounding almost like a monotone voice-generating machine.

The second group of deficits concerns the activities and interests of children with ASD. Rather than engaging in symbolic play with toys, they are preoccupied with one feature of a toy or an object. Richard was preoccupied with his miniature car, carrying it everywhere without playing with it, and Temple Grandin was interested only in watching sand dribble through her fingers. They may engage in bizarre, repetitive behaviors with toys. Rather than using two dolls to play "house," a child with ASD might take the arm off one doll and simply pass it back and forth between her two hands. Routines and rituals often are extremely important to children with ASD. When any aspect of their daily routine is changed—for example, if their mother stops at the bank on the way to school—they may become excessively frightened and highly distressed. Some children perform stereotyped and repetitive behaviors using some part of their body, such as incessantly flapping their hands or banging their head against a wall. These behaviors sometimes are

In the movie *Rain Man,* Dustin Hoffman plays a man with autism who had some extraordinary abilities. Most people with autism do not fall into this category of "savants" portrayed in the film.
United Artists/courtesy of Everett Collection

referred to as *self-stimulatory behaviors,* under the assumption that these children engage in such behaviors for self-stimulation. It is not clear, however, that this is their true purpose.

Children with ASD often do poorly on measures of intellectual ability, such as IQ tests, with approximately 50 percent of autistic children showing at least moderate intellectual disability (Mattila et al., 2011; Sigman, Spence, & Wang, 2006). The deficits of some children with ASD are confined to skills that require language and understanding others' points of view, and they may score in the average range on tests that do not require language skills. Temple Grandin is clearly of above average intelligence despite her ASD. Language skills are critical as they significantly contribute to school placements and academic performance, as well as, the ability to engage in social interaction. Overall, professionals agree that verbal skills are critical in predicting long-term outcomes for children with ASD in terms of psycho-social adjustment and well-being (Brignell et al., 2018). Much has been made in the popular press about the special talents of some children with ASD, such as the ability to play music without having been taught or to draw extremely well, or exceptional memory and mathematical calculation abilities as depicted in the movie *Rain Man*. These persons sometimes are referred to as *savants*. Such cases are quite rare, however (Bölte & Poustka, 2004).

For the diagnosis of ASD, symptoms must have their onset in early childhood and are typically observed by age 2 (American Psychiatric Association, 2013). It is important to note that there is wide variation in the severity and outcome of this disorder. By far the best predictor of the outcome of ASD is a child's IQ and the amount of language development before age 6 (Anderson, Liang, & Lord, 2014; Howlin, Goode, Hutton, & Rutter, 2004). Children who have an IQ above 50 and communicative speech before age 6 have a much better prognosis than do others. People diagnosed with ASD who had an IQ of 70 or above were especially likely to achieve a "good" or "very good" outcome (Howlin et al., 2004). Childhood IQ and early language ability have been found to be the strongest predictors of adult outcomes (Brignell et al., 2018).

In the *DSM-5*, there is only one ASD, as defined in Table 2 which is a change from previous editions. These changes were made due to evidence that different pervasive developmental disorders (PDDs), especially autism and Asperger's disorder, share common etiologies and it was reliably distinguishing these was unreliable (Lord & Bishop, 2015; Swedo et al., 2012). Moreover, because the disorder presents differently depending on symptom severity, developmental level (e.g., IQ), and age, *DSM-5* uses the term "spectrum" to capture the range of related but varied presentations. The impact of the changes in the treatment of ASDs in the *DSM-5* is a matter of some debate and concern. Several initial studies that reanalyzed data on children diagnosed under the *DSM-IV-TR* criteria found that the *DSM-5* criteria for ASD captured only about 50 to 60 percent of children who previously would have been diagnosed with autism, Asperger's disorder, or PDD-NOS (Mattila et al., 2011; McPartland, Reichow, & Volkmar, 2012). These studies indicated that the children most likely not to fit the *DSM-5* criteria for ASD are those who have higher IQs and who lack deficits in verbal communications. Only about one-quarter of individuals previously diagnosed with Asperger's syndrome or PDD-NOS meet the criteria for ASD based on the *DSM-5* criteria. These findings raised concerns about the effects of these changes on access to services for individuals who have previously been diagnosed with autistic disorders other than classic, low-functioning autism (McPartland et al., 2012). The most recent and largest study of this kind, however, found that *DSM-5* criteria identified 91 percent of children with established *DSM-IV* PDD diagnoses (Huerta, Bishop, Duncan, Hus, & Lord, 2012), suggesting that most children would remain eligible for the diagnosis and related services. Future studies will likely further clarify the impact of these changes to the diagnostic criteria.

Contributors to Autism Spectrum Disorder

Over the years, a wide variety of theories of autism have been proposed. The psychiatrist who first described autism, Leo Kanner (1943), thought that autism was caused by a combination of biological factors and poor parenting. He and later psychoanalytic theorists (Bettelheim, 1967) described the parents of children with autism as cold, distant, and uncaring. The child's symptoms were seen as a retreat inward to a secret world of fantasies in response to unavailable parents. However, research over the decades has shown clearly that unresponsive parenting plays little or no role in the development of autism.

Several biological factors have been implicated in the development of ASD. Family and twin studies strongly suggest that genetics plays a role in the development of the disorder. The siblings of children with ASD are 50 times more likely to have the disorder than are the siblings of children without ASD (Sigman et al., 2006). Twin studies show concordance rates for ASD to be about 60 percent for monozygotic (MZ) twins and 0 to 30 percent for dizygotic (DZ) twins (Chen, Peñagarikano, Belgard, Swarup, & Geschwind, 2015; Hallmayer et al., 2011). In addition, about 90 percent of the MZ twins of children with ASD have a significant cognitive impairment, compared to 10 percent of DZ twins. Also, children with ASD have a higher-than-average rate of other genetic disorders associated with cognitive impairment, including fragile X syndrome and PKU (Chen et al., 2015; Volkmar, State, & Klin, 2009). These data suggest that a general vulnerability to several types of cognitive impairment, only one of which is manifested as ASD, runs in families. No single gene seems to cause ASD; instead, abnormalities in several genes have been associated with ASD (Chen et al., 2015).

Neurological factors probably play a role in ASD. The array of deficits seen in ASD suggests disruption in the normal development and organization of the

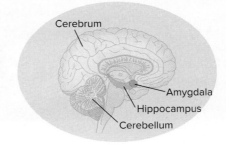

These areas of the brain have been implicated in autism.

brain (Chen et al., 2015). In addition, approximately 30 percent of children with ASD develop seizure disorders by adolescence, suggesting a severe neurological dysfunction (Fombonne, 1999). A consistent finding is greater head and brain size in children with the disorder than in children without it (Lotspeich et al., 2004; Via, Radua, Cardoner, Happé, & Mataix-Cols, 2011).

Neuroimaging studies have suggested a variety of structural abnormalities in the brains of individuals with ASD, including in the cerebellum, the cerebrum, the amygdala, and possibly the hippocampus (Chen et al., 2015; Via et al., 2011). When children with ASD are doing tasks that require perception of facial expressions, joint attention with another person, empathy, or thinking about social situations, they show abnormal functioning in areas of the brain that are recruited for such tasks. For example, when shown photos of faces, children with ASD show less activation than do typically developing children in an area of the brain involved in facial perception called the fusiform gyrus (Figure 2; Schultz, 2005). Another study showed that adults with ASD show atypical patterns of brain activation when hearing their own name (Nijhof, Dhar, Goris, Brass, & Wiersema, 2018). Difficulty in perceiving and understanding facial expressions and verbal communications could contribute to these children's deficits in social interactions.

ASD is one of the most heritable neuropsychiatric disorders. However, no specific gene for ASD has been identified and single gene mutations explain less than 1 percent of all ASD cases, which implicates environmental factors and complex gene interactions in the development of this disorder (Doenyas, 2018). Alternatively, children with autism have a higher-than-average rate of prenatal and birth complications, and these complications might create the neurological abnormality (Chen et al., 2015). Furthermore, studies have found differences between children with and without ASD in levels of the neurotransmitters serotonin and dopamine; more research is needed to understand how these neurotransmitters factor into the disorder (Muller, Anacker, & Veenstra-VanderWeele, 2016).

The profound influence of the prenatal environment on fetal brain development and long-term developmental outcomes is well established. It is widely acknowledged that the mother's health impacts the developing person, but new areas of interest may shed light on the development of various psychological disorders, like ASD. Imbalance (*dysbiosis*) of the maternal gut microbiome in response to events such as infection, altered diet, and stress during pregnancy is associated with abnormalities in brain function and behavior of the offspring. The brain is especially vulnerable to insults during such critical periods of development as *in utero,* infancy and early childhood; and insults that occur during these critical periods have the potential to cause long-term damage. Maternal immune activation (MIA) and inflammation have been linked with several neurodevelopmental disorders like ASD, schizophrenia, cerebral palsy, epilepsy, and depression. MIA is the activation of the immune system in response to events such as infection, stress, asthma, allergies, or inflammation. This theory suggests that MIA acts as a disease primer or first "hit" to the developing nervous system which makes these individuals vulnerable for further cumulative exposures or "hits" later in life increasing the likelihood of psychopathology. An individual's response to inflammatory events results from various interactions between their underlying genetic disposition and the various environmental factors to which they are exposed. Studies have found inflammatory markers, such as C-reactive protein, among mothers who have children with ASD (Jiang, Cowan, Moonah, & Petri, 2018)

In recent years, the microbiota-gut-brain axis has become a considerable focus of investigation for its role in the development of ASD behaviors. Children with ASD experience more gastrointestinal (GI) symptoms than children without ASD and these GI symptoms strongly correlate with their symptom severity. A recent review of four decades of literature on the physiological abnormalities in ASD found that 95 percent of studies identified an association between ASD and immune dysregulation and inflammation (Doenyas, 2018). Excessive

| FIGURE 2 | Scans such as these help researchers to understand the brain activity of autism spectrum disorder. |

EVAN VUCCI/AP Images

gut inflammation (*enteropathy*) has been linked to poor health outcomes and can trigger widespread systemic inflammation and the release of cytokines. Cytokytines are small secreted proteins produced by almost every cell that are crucial for healthy immune system function. However, too many cytokines can have a negative effect and overwhelm the body (Kany, Vollrath, & Relja, 2019). Cytokine imbalances during the early periods of neurodevelopment may have profound long-term impacts on a variety of diseases, including ASD, schizophrenia, and cerebral palsy (Jiang et al., 2018).

A mechanism by which the gut may influence neurodevelopment is through intestinal inflammation which is linked to poor neurodevelopmental outcomes among those growing up with childhood adversity. It is well-known that adverse environments which may include exposure to poverty, stress, war, or neglect can have lasting effects on child development. The impact of adversity on inflammation is likely multifactorial, including exposure to infectious disease, malnutrition, psychosocial stress, and poor caregiver interactions. The release of cytokines may act as a mediator across these risk factors, but the cumulative effect of cytokine elevation is inflammation (Jiang et al., 2018).

Treatments for Autism Spectrum Disorder

A number of drugs have been shown to improve some of the symptoms of ASD, including overactivity, stereotyped behaviors (e.g., head banging and hand flapping), sleep disturbances, and tension. However, although medications are often prescribed, the evidence for their effectiveness is quite mixed (Madden et al., 2017; Stepanova, Dowling, Phelps, & Findling, 2017). The selective serotonin reuptake inhibitors appear to reduce repetitive behaviors and aggression and improve social interactions in some, but not all, people with ASD. The atypical antipsychotic medications have shown more reliable effectiveness; they are used to reduce obsessive and repetitive behaviors and to improve self-control. Finally, stimulants are used to improve attention. Although these drugs do not alter the core features of ASD, they sometimes make it easier for people with ASD to participate in school and in behavioral treatments.

Psychosocial therapies for ASD combine behavioral techniques and structured educational services (Reichow, Barton, Boyd, & Hume, 2012; Vismara & Rogers, 2010; Wong et al., 2015). Operant conditioning strategies are used to reduce excessive behaviors, such as repetitive or ritualistic behaviors, tantrums, and aggression, and to alleviate deficits or delays, such as deficits in communication and in interactions

with others. These techniques may be implemented in highly structured schools designed especially for children with ASD or in regular classrooms if children are mainstreamed. The specific deficits a child has in cognitive, motor, or communication skills are targeted, and materials that reduce possible distractions (such as books that do not have words printed in bright colors) are used. Parents may be taught to implement the techniques consistently when the children are at home. Several other studies have shown strong improvements in cognitive skills and behavioral control in children with ASD who were treated with a comprehensive behavior therapy administered both by their parents and in their school setting from an early age (see meta-analysis by Eldevik et al., 2009).

Many well-established treatments for ASD include behavioral treatment models that are based on the principles of applied behavior analysis. These models attempt to reinforce socially acceptable behaviors and decrease or eliminate undesirable ones. Early intensive behavioral intervention for children with ASD is strongly recommended and have shown to dramatically affect developmental outcomes. These programs can reduce or remove problematic behaviors and improve core symptoms common to children with ASD, such as daily living skills, social skills, and communication. There are many options for the treatment of ASD and no one universal treatment for all individuals with ASD has been endorsed because developmental levels and symptoms vary substantially in children with ASD (Xu et al., 2019).

INTELLECTUAL DISABILITY

Intellectual disability (ID) (or intellectual developmental disorder), formerly referred to as mental retardation, involves significant deficits in intellectual abilities and life functioning. The first *DSM-5* criterion for ID requires significant deficits in intellectual functioning, such as abstract thinking, reasoning, learning, problem solving, and planning (Table 3, American Psychiatric Association, 2013). The *DSM* requires that these deficits be confirmed by clinical assessment and formal assessments such as IQ tests.

The second criterion for the diagnosis involves deficits in functioning in three broad domains of daily living, such that the person cannot live reasonably independently without some support (American Psychiatric Association, 2013). First, in the conceptual domain, individuals show deficits in skills such as language, reading, writing, math, reasoning, knowledge, memory, and problem solving. Second, in the social domain, individuals have difficulty in being aware of and understanding others' experiences, in interpersonal communication skills, in the ability to make and keep friends, in social judgment, and in

TABLE 3   *DSM-5* Criteria for Intellectual Disability (ID)

Intellectual disability (intellectual developmental disorder) is a disorder with an onset during the developmental period that includes both intellectual and adaptive functioning deficits in conceptual, social, and practical domains. The following three criteria must be met:

A. Deficits in intellectual functions, such as reasoning, problem solving, planning, abstract thinking, judgment, academic learning, and learning from experience, confirmed by both clinical assessment and individualized, standardized intelligence testing.

B. Deficits in adaptive functioning that result in failure to meet developmental and sociocultural standards for personal independence and social responsibility. Without ongoing support, the adaptive deficits limit functioning in one or more activities of daily life, such as communication, social participation, and independent living, across multiple environments, such as home, school, work, and community.

C. Onset of intellectual and adaptive deficits during the developmental period.

The severity of intellectual disability can be classified as mild, moderate, severe, or profound, on the basis of adaptive function (and not IQ alone) and the level of supports required.

regulating their own reactions in social interactions. Third, in the practical domain, individuals show deficits in managing personal care (such as maintaining hygiene, grocery shopping, cooking), managing their own finances, recreation, transportation, and organizing themselves to hold a job or attend school. People with ID also often have problems with motor skills, such as eye–hand coordination and balance. These deficits have to be significant compared to other people who are the same age and have a similar sociodemographic background and culture.

The *DSM-5* classifies ID into four levels of severity: mild, moderate, severe, and profound. Children and adults with a *mild level of ID* generally have some limitations in their ability to acquire typical academic or job-related skills, may seem immature in social interactions and overly concrete in their communications with others, show limited social judgment and understanding of risk, and may be able to care for themselves reasonably well except in complex situations such as making legal or health decisions. Adults with mild ID often hold competitive jobs that don't emphasize conceptual skills.

Children with a *moderate level* of *ID* typically have significant delays in language development, such as using only 4 to 10 words by age 3. They may be physically clumsy and have some trouble dressing and feeding themselves. They typically do not achieve beyond the second-grade level in academic skills but, with special education, can acquire simple vocational skills. As adults, they may be able to hold a job requiring only an elementary-school level of conceptual skills, but they likely will require considerable assistance. With extensive training, they can learn to care for their personal needs (eating, personal hygiene). Their social interactions may be impaired by communication difficulties, and they may show poor social judgment.

Individuals with *severe* ID have a very limited vocabulary and may speak in two- or three-word sentences. As children they may have significant deficits in motor development and may play with toys inappropriately (e.g., banging two dolls together). As adults, they can feed themselves with a spoon and dress themselves if the clothing is not complicated (with many buttons or zippers). They cannot travel alone for any distance and cannot shop or cook for themselves. Some individuals may be able to learn some unskilled manual labor, but many are unable to do so. In the social domain, they generally lack awareness of risk, and may easily be led by others due to naiveté in social situations. They require support for all aspects of daily living.

At the *profound level* of ID, individuals often don't develop conceptual skills beyond simple matching of concrete physical features of objects. Co-occurring sensory and motor impairments may prevent functional use of objects and limit participation in everyday activities to watching. In the social domain, the individual may only be able to understand simple concrete instructions and gestures. Even in adulthood, the individual is fully dependent on others for all aspects of daily living, including physical care, health, and safety. Maladaptive behavior is present in a significant minority of individuals with profound ID.

Individually administered intelligence tests are used to assess the level of intellectual functioning of a person suspected of having ID. Intelligence tests measure verbal comprehension, working memory, perceptual reasoning, quantitative reasoning, abstract thought, and processing speed. Individuals with ID generally have scores of two standard deviations below the mean IQ score of the general population of 100; in other words, an IQ score of 70 ($\pm$ 5, or 65–75) or lower. However, *DSM-5* de-emphasizes intelligence test scores in the diagnostic criteria to determine level of severity, and rather focuses clinicians' attention on the individual's level of adaptive functioning across the conceptual, social, and practical domains, in part because IQ scores can be misleading or misused. It is estimated that 1 to 3 percent of the population has intellectual development disorder (Humeau, Gambino, Chelly, & Vitale, 2009).

Biological Causes of Intellectual Disability

Many biological factors can cause ID, including chromosomal and gestational disorders, exposure to toxins prenatally or in early childhood, infections, brain injury or malformations, metabolism and nutrition problems, and some kinds of seizure disorders (e.g., infantile spasms). We examine these factors first and then turn to sociocultural factors.

Genetic Factors

Nearly 300 genes affecting brain development and functioning have been implicated in the development of ID (Ellison, Rosenfeld, & Shaffer, 2013). These genes do not lead to the disorder as such but rather to one or more of the types of deficits people with ID show. It is not surprising, then, that families of children with ID tend to have high incidences of a variety of intellectual problems, including the different levels

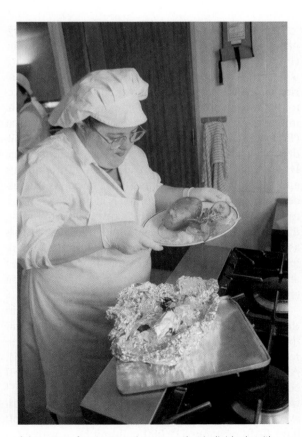

Advocates of mainstreaming argue that individuals with intellectual disabilities should be integrated into everyday life. *John Birdsall/Shutterstock*

of ID and autism spectrum disorder (Ellison et al., 2013; Humeau et al., 2009).

Two metabolic disorders that are genetically transmitted and that cause ID are phenylketonuria (PKU) and Tay-Sachs disease. PKU is carried by a recessive gene and occurs in about 1 in 20,000 births. Children with PKU are unable to metabolize phenylalanine, an amino acid. As a result, phenylalanine and its derivative, phenylpyruvic acid, build up in the body and cause brain damage. Fortunately, children who from an early age receive a special diet free of phenylalanine can attain an average level of intelligence. Most states mandate testing for PKU in newborns. If left untreated, children with PKU typically have an IQ below 50 and severe or profound ID.

Tay-Sachs disease also is carried by a recessive gene and occurs primarily in Jewish populations. When an affected child is 3 to 6 months old, a progressive degeneration of the nervous system begins, leading to mental and physical deterioration. These children usually die before age 6, and there is no effective treatment.

Several types of chromosomal disorders can lead to ID (Williams, 2010). Normally children are born with 23 pairs of chromosomes. Twenty-two of these pairs are known as autosomes, and the twenty-third pair contains the sex chromosomes. One of the best known causes of ID is Down syndrome, which occurs when chromosome 21 is present in triplicate rather than in duplicate. (For this reason, Down syndrome is also referred to as trisomy 21.) Down syndrome occurs in about 1 in every 800 children born in the United States.

From childhood, almost all people with Down syndrome have ID, although the severity level varies from mild to profound. Their ability to care for themselves, live somewhat independently, and hold a job depends on their level of intellectual deficit and the training and support they receive. Children with Down syndrome have a round, flat face and almond-shaped eyes; a small nose; slightly protruding lip and tongue; and short, square hands. They tend to be short in stature and somewhat obese. Many have congenital heart defects and gastrointestinal difficulties. As adults, they seem to age more rapidly than normal, and their life expectancy is shorter than average. People with Down syndrome have abnormalities in the neurons in their brains that resemble those found in Alzheimer's disease. Nearly all individuals with Down syndrome past age 40 develop the thinking and memory deficits characteristic of a neurocognitive disorder due to Alzheimer's disease and lose the ability to care for themselves (Visser et al., 1997). Individuals with Down syndrome represent the largest group of individuals under 65 years of age with early onset Alzheimer's disease making it the leading genetic risk factor (Gomez, Morales, Maracaja-Coutinho, Parra, & Nassif, 2020) (see the section later in this chapter, "Neurocognitive Disorder Due to Alzheimer's Disease").

Fragile X syndrome, another common cause of ID, is caused when a tip of the X chromosome breaks off (Turk, 2011). This syndrome affects primarily males because they do not have a second, normal X chromosome to balance the mutation. The syndrome is characterized by severe to profound ID, speech defects, and severe deficits in interpersonal interaction. Males with fragile X syndrome have large ears, a long face, and enlarged testes. Females with the syndrome tend to have a less severe level of ID (Koukoui & Chaudhuri, 2007). Two other chromosomal abnormalities that cause severe ID and shortened life expectancy are trisomy 13 (chromosome 13 is present in triplicate) and trisomy 18 (chromosome 18 is present in triplicate).

The risk of having a child with Down syndrome or any other chromosomal abnormality increases with the age of the parents. This may be because the older a parent is, the more likely chromosomes are to have degenerated or to have been damaged by toxins.

Brain Damage During Gestation and Early Life

Intellectual development can be profoundly affected by the fetus's prenatal environment (King, Hodapp, & Dykens, 2005). When a pregnant woman contracts the rubella (German measles) virus, the herpes virus, or syphilis, there is a risk of damage to the fetus that can cause ID. Chronic maternal disorders, such as high blood pressure and diabetes, can interfere with fetal nutrition and brain development and thereby affect the intellectual capacities of the fetus. If these maternal disorders are treated effectively throughout the pregnancy, the risk of damage to the fetus is low.

CASE STUDY

Abel Dorris was adopted when he was 3 years old by Michael Dorris. Abel's mother had been a heavy drinker throughout the pregnancy and after Abel was born. She had subsequently died at age 35 of alcohol poisoning. Abel had been born almost 7 weeks premature, with low birth weight. He had been abused and malnourished before being removed to a foster home. At age 3, Abel was small for his age, was not yet toilet-trained, and could only speak about 20 words. He was diagnosed with a mild intellectual disability. His adoptive father hoped that, in a positive environment, Abel could catch up.

Yet, at age 4, Abel was still in diapers and weighed only 27 pounds. He had trouble remembering the names of other children, and his activity level was unusually high. When alone, he would rock back and forth rhythmically. At age 4, he suffered the first of several severe seizures, which caused him to lose consciousness for days. No drug treatments seemed to help.

When he entered school, Abel had trouble learning to count, to identify colors, and to tie his shoes. He had a short attention span and difficulty following simple instructions. Despite devoted teachers, when he finished elementary school, Abel still could not add, subtract, or identify his place of residence. His IQ was in the mid-60s.

Eventually, at age 20, Abel entered a vocational training program and moved into a supervised home. His main preoccupations were his collections of stuffed animals, paper dolls, newspaper cartoons, family photographs, and old birthday cards. At age 23, he was hit by a car and killed. (Source: Adapted from Dorris, M., *The unbroken cord.* New York: Harper & Row, 1989; Lyman, R., "Michael Dorris dies at 52: Wrote of his son's suffering," *New York Times*, April 15, 1997, 24.)

Children whose mothers abuse alcohol during pregnancy are at increased risk for **fetal alcohol syndrome** (FAS; see Mukherjee, Hollins, & Turk, 2006). Alcohol is a teratogen that can pass through the placental barrier, which is why it has been established as a risk factor for adverse pregnancy outcomes including stillbirth, miscarriage, premature birth, and low birthweight (Popova, Lange, Probst, Gmel, & Rehm, 2017). Children with fetal alcohol syndrome have a below average IQ of 68, have poor judgment, increased distractibility, and difficulty understanding social cues. As adolescents, their academic functioning is at only the second-to fourth-grade level, and they have trouble following directions. These neurodevelopmental impairments associated with FAS can lead to significant secondary impairments such as academic failure, substance abuse, inability to live independently, and maintain employment which have lifelong implications.

It is estimated that 2 to 15 children per 10,000 in the United States have fetal alcohol syndrome, and three times that number are born with lesser alcohol-related neurological and birth defects (CDC, 2018d). Approximately, 10% of women around the world consume alcohol during pregnancy and one in 67 women delivered a child with FAS. This suggests an average of 15 of every 10,000 births worldwide will have FAS, or about 119,000 children born with FAS globally every year. There are notable differences in prevalence rates around the globe with the highest

Children whose mothers abuse alcohol during pregnancy are at increased risk for *fetal alcohol syndrome. Realistic Reflections*

being in the European Region (Russia, UK, Denmark, Belarus, and Ireland) where the FAS prevalence is 2·6 times higher than the global average. Countries in the Eastern Mediterranean Region and South-East Asia Region (Oman, United Arab Emirates, Saudi Arabia, Qatar, and Kuwait) report low levels of alcohol use during pregnancy and the lowest FAS rates in the world (Popova et al., 2017). Abel Dorris, in the case study above, was born with fetal alcohol syndrome.

Even low to moderate levels of drinking during pregnancy can lead to negative outcomes, such as higher rates of miscarriage, delivery before full gestation, lower birth weight, congenital abnormalities, and impaired social and cognitive development (S. Jacobson & L. Jacobson, 2000). For example, longitudinal studies of children exposed prenatally to alcohol show negative effects on growth at age 6 and on learning and memory skills at age 10, even if the children do not evidence the full syndrome of FAS (Cornelius, Goldschmidt, Day, & Larkby, 2002). One study found that a mother's consumption of even one to three drinks per week during pregnancy was associated with significant deficits in young children's social engagement and interaction skills (Brown, Olson, & Croninger, 2010).

Severe head traumas that damage children's brains also can lead to ID. Shaken baby syndrome results when a baby is shaken, leading to intracranial injury and retinal hemorrhage (see Mian et al., 2015). Babies' heads are relatively large and heavy compared to the rest of their body, and their neck muscles are too weak to control their head when they are shaken. The rapid movement of their head when shaken can lead to their brains being banged against the inside of the skull and bruised. Bleeding in and around the brain or behind the eyes can lead to seizures, partial or total blindness, paralysis, ID, or death. Although the shaking of a baby may be part of a pattern of chronic abuse, shaken baby syndrome can occur when an otherwise nonabusive parent becomes frustrated and shakes the baby only once.

Young children face a number of other hazards that can cause brain damage. Exposure to toxic substances—such as lead, arsenic, and mercury—during early childhood can lead to ID by damaging areas of the brain. Children also can incur traumatic brain injury leading to ID through accidents, including motor vehicle accidents in which they are not properly restrained.

Sociocultural Factors

Children with ID are more likely to come from low socioeconomic backgrounds (Emerson, Shahtahmasebi, Lancaster, & Berridge, 2010). It may be that their parents also have ID and have not been able to acquire well-paying jobs. The social disadvantages of being poor also may contribute to lower-than-average intellectual development. Poor mothers are less likely to receive good prenatal care, increasing the risk of premature birth. Children living in lower socioeconomic areas are at increased risk for exposure to lead, because many older buildings have lead paint, which chips off and can be ingested. Poor children are concentrated in poorly funded schools, where those with lower IQs receive less favorable attention from teachers and fewer learning opportunities, especially if they are also members of a minority group. Poor children also are less likely to have parents who read to them and are involved in their schooling. These factors may directly affect a child's intellectual development and exacerbate the biological conditions that impede a child's cognitive development (Zigler, Gilliam, & Jones, 2006).

Treatments for Intellectual Disability

Interventions for children and adults with ID must be comprehensive, intensive, and long-term to show benefits (Singh, 2016; Zigler et al., 2006; Zigler & Styfco, 2004, 2008).

Drug Therapy

Medications are used to reduce seizures, which are common in people with ID; to control aggressive or self-injurious behavior; and to improve mood (Matson & Neal, 2009). Neuroleptic medications (see the chapter "Schizophrenia Spectrum and Other Psychotic Disorders") can reduce aggressive, destructive, and antisocial behavior; however, the potential for neurological side effects has made these medications controversial. The atypical antipsychotics, such as risperidone, have been shown to reduce aggression and self-injurious behavior in adults with ID without having serious neurological side effects (Unwin & Deb, 2011). Antidepressant medications can reduce depressive symptoms, improve sleep patterns, and help control self-injurious behavior in individuals with ID.

Behavioral Strategies

A child's parents or caregivers and teachers can work together using behavioral strategies to enhance the child's positive behaviors and reduce negative behaviors. These strategies help children and adults learn new skills, from identifying colors correctly to applying vocational skills. Social and communication skills also may be taught. Individuals may learn to initiate conversations by asking questions and to articulate what they want to say more clearly. The desired behavior may be modeled in incremental steps and rewards given to the individual as he or she comes closer to mastering the skill. Behavioral strategies also can help reduce self-injurious and other maladaptive behaviors. Typically, behavioral methods do not simply focus on isolated skills but rather are integrated into a comprehensive program designed to maximize the individual's ability to function in the community (Feldman, 2004). Various treatment models are linked to evidence-based interventions that focus on parent skill training and mindfulness interventions designed to reduce parental stress and improve children's behavioral skills. There is significant evidence to support the effectiveness of parent training to reduce disruptive behavior in young children and a range of behavioral parent training models. These treatments have been shown to reduce challenging behavior in children and adolescents with ID (Crnic, Neece, McIntyre, Blacher, & Baker, 2017).

Social Programs

Social programs have focused on integration of the child into the mainstream where possible, on placement in group homes that provide comprehensive care, and on institutionalization when necessary. The earlier these interventions begin, the greater the chance that the child will develop to full potential.

Early Intervention Programs Many experts recommend beginning comprehensive interventions with children at risk for intellectual development disorder from the first days of life. These measures include intensive one-on-one interventions to enhance their development of basic skills; efforts to reduce the social conditions that might interfere with the children's development, such as child abuse, malnutrition, or exposure to toxins; and adequate medical care (Perry, Koudys, & Blacklock, 2016; Zigler & Styfco, 2004).

One such program was the Infant Health and Development Program (Gross, Brooks-Gunn, & Spiker, 1992), which focused on children with a birth weight of 2,500 grams (5½ pounds) or less and a gestational age of 37 completed weeks or less. This program had three components. First, specially trained counselors visited each child's home during the first 3 years of the child's life, providing support to the mother and fostering parent–child activities that would enhance the child's development. The mothers were given training in good parenting practices and in ways to facilitate their children's cognitive development. For example, they were taught ways to calm their babies (who tended to be irritable), provide appropriate levels of stimulation as well as opportunities for exploration, and reduce stress in the family's environment. Second, the children went daily to a child development center with specially trained teachers, who worked to overcome the children's intellectual and physical deficits. Third, parent support groups were started to help the parents cope with the stresses of parenting.

At 36 months of age, the children in the intervention group were significantly less likely to have IQ scores in the low range than were those in the control group, who received only medical care (Infant Health and Development Program, 1990). The children who received the program intervention also showed fewer behavioral and emotional problems at age 36 months than did the children in the control group.

What accounted for the positive effects of the intervention? Several factors were noted. The home environments of the children in the intervention group improved significantly (Berlin, Brooks-Gunn, McCartoon, & McCormick, 1998; McCormick, McCarton, Brooks-Gunn, Belt, & Gross, 1998). More learning materials were available, and their mothers more actively stimulated the children's learning. The mothers of the children in the intervention program were better able to assist their children in problem solving, remaining more responsive and persistent with their children. In turn, these children showed more enthusiasm for and involvement in learning tasks. In addition, the mothers in the intervention program reported better mental health than the mothers in the control group and also were less likely to use harsh discipline with their children. All these psychosocial factors are associated with better outcomes for ID children who receive intervention. The complex developmental factors which include social and contextual influences have been found to influence competencies both directly and indirectly of ID children which suggests that early intervention programs have important developmental benefits (Crnic et al., 2017).

Mainstreaming Providing more opportunities for inclusion for students with ID and special education needs (SEN) has influenced education systems around the world. This agenda has resulted in improved access to mainstream education for students with special educational needs, such as those with ID. The rights of people with ID to receive mainstream education in schools together with their peers provide equal opportunities to participate in society. Many children today spend some time in special education, where they receive intensive training to overcome skills deficits, and some time in regular classrooms over the course of the week. Comparative studies have consistently shown that students placed in mainstream educational settings perform as well as or better than students in self-contained special educational settings. It is possible that the higher expectations and focus on academic achievement in mainstream school settings may explain these differences. In terms of social outcomes, studies have found both positive and negative results and no definitive conclusions can be drawn at this time. Some studies have found higher rates of stigma reported by students with ID in mainstream schools but others report a positive psychosocial situation with regard to peer relations and motivation to study. While it is agreed upon that the overall academic performance of those with ID is comparable or better to those in special education settings, studies on the social benefits of mainstreaming students need further attention (Klang, 2020).

Group Homes Many adults with ID live in group homes, where they receive assistance in performing daily tasks (e.g., cooking, cleaning) and training in vocational and social skills. They may work in sheltered workshops during the day, performing unskilled or semiskilled labor. Increasingly, they are being mainstreamed into the general workforce, often in service-related jobs (e.g., in fast-food restaurants or as baggers in grocery stores). Some community-based programs for adults with ID have been shown to be effective in enhancing their social and vocational skills (Chilvers, Macdonald, & Hayes, 2006; Toogood, Totsika, Jones, & Lowe, 2016).

LEARNING, COMMUNICATION, AND MOTOR DISORDERS

Rather than having deficits in a broad array of skills, as in intellectual disability, children with learning, communication, or motor disorders have deficits or abnormalities in specific skills or behaviors. These disorders are not due to intellectual disability, global developmental delay, neurological disorders, or general external factors like economic disadvantage. The severity of these disorders can range from mild to severe.

Specific Learning Disorder

Individuals with **specific learning disorder** have deficits in one or more academic skills: reading, written expression, and/or mathematics (see Table 4). The *DSM-5* diagnosis is given only when the individual's performance in one or more of these domains is significantly below than expected for their age, schooling, and overall level of intelligence (American Psychiatric Association, 2013). Although the threshold for diagnosis of a specific learning disorder is somewhat arbitrary, unexpected low performance on individually administered, culturally and linguistically appropriate, standardized academic achievement tests is a generally used criterion for school-age individuals (e.g., ≤ 1 or 1.5 standard deviations below the age-based population mean).

Difficulties in reading, often referred to as *dyslexia,* are usually apparent by the fourth grade and represent the most common specific learning disorder. Reading impairments include poor word reading accuracy, slow reading rate, and reading comprehension weaknesses. They are seen in about 7 percent of children, more commonly boys (Peterson & Pennington, 2015; Rutter et al., 2004). Difficulties in mathematics may include problems in understanding mathematical terms, recognizing numerical symbols, clustering objects into groups, counting, mastering math facts, and understanding mathematical principles. Although many people feel that they are not great at math, deficits in math skills severe enough to warrant this diagnosis occur in only about 1 percent of children (Tannock, 2005). Difficulties in written expression involve significant weaknesses in spelling, constructing a sentence or paragraph, or grammar and punctuation.

Children with learning disorders often struggle with low academic performance or have to put forth extraordinarily high levels of effort to achieve average grades. They can become demoralized or disruptive in class. If left untreated, they are at high risk for dropping out of school, with as many as 40 percent never

TABLE 4   *DSM-5* Criteria for Specific Learning Disorder

A. Difficulties learning and using academic skills, as indicated by the presence of at least one of the following symptoms that have persisted for at least 6 months, despite the provision of interventions that target those difficulties:

1. Inaccurate or slow and effortful word reading (e.g., reads single words aloud incorrectly or slowly and hesitantly, frequently guesses words, has difficulty sounding out words).

2. Difficulty understanding the meaning of what is read (e.g., may read text accurately but not understand the sequence, relationships, inferences, or deeper meanings of what is read).

3. Difficulties with spelling (e.g., may add, omit, or substitute vowels or consonants).

4. Difficulties with written expression (e.g., makes multiple grammatical or punctuation errors within sentences; employs poor paragraph organization; written expression of ideas lacks clarity).

5. Difficulties mastering number sense, number facts, or calculation (e.g., has poor understanding of numbers, their magnitude, and relationships; counts on fingers to add single-digit numbers instead of recalling the math fact that peers do; gets lost in the midst of arithmetic computation and may switch procedures).

6. Difficulties with mathematical reasoning (e.g., has severe difficulty applying mathematical concepts, facts, or procedures to solve quantitative problems).

B. The affected academic skills are substantially and quantifiably below those expected for the individual's chronological age, and cause significant interference with academic and occupational performance, or with activities of daily living. Skill impairments are confirmed by individually administered standardized achievement measures and comprehensive clinical assessment. For individuals ≥17 years, a documented history of impairing learning difficulties may be substituted for the standardized assessment.

C. The learning difficulties begin during school-age years and may not become fully manifest until the demands for those affected academic skills exceed the individual's limited capacities (e.g., as in timed tests, reading, or writing lengthy complex reports for a tight deadline, excessively heavy academic loads).

D. The learning difficulties are not better accounted for by intellectual disabilities, uncorrected visual or auditory acuity, other mental or neurological disorders, psychosocial adversity, lack of proficiency in the language of academic instruction, or inadequate educational instruction.

Specify all academic domains and subskills that are impaired. When more than one domain is impaired, each one should be coded according to the following specifiers:

With impairment in reading:
   Word reading accuracy
   Reading rate or fluency
   Reading comprehension

With impairment in written expression:
   Spelling accuracy
   Grammar and punctuation accuracy
   Clarity or organization of written expression

With impairment in mathematics:
   Number sense
   Memorization of arithmetic facts
   Accurate or fluent calculation
   Accurate math reasoning

finishing high school. As adults, they may have problems getting and keeping a good job, and often avoid leisure or work activities that require reading, arithmetic, and/or writing. The emotional side effects of their learning disorder may also affect their social relationships (Fletcher, Lyon, Fuchs, & Barnes, 2018).

Communication Disorders

The **communication disorders** involve persistent difficulties in the acquisition and use of language and other means of communication (see Table 5). Children with **language disorder** have difficulties with

Learning disorders can lead to frustration and low self-esteem.
Corbis/VCG/Getty Images

a high prevalence condition in preschool children which has resulted in the development of numerous interventions which vary in the method used to achieve change in a child's speech (Wren, Harding, Goldbart, & Roulstone, 2018). Most children with this disorder respond well to treatment and issues with speech may improve over time, shortening the duration of the disorder (American Psychiatric Association, 2013).

A third *DSM-5* communication disorder is **childhood-onset fluency disorder** or stuttering. Children who stutter have significant problems with speaking evenly and fluently, often voicing frequent repetitions of sounds or syllables (such as "I-I-I-I see him"). Some children also repeat whole words or short phrases, for example, "Kids tease me about my, about my s-s-s-stutter." The severity of their speech problems varies by the situation but usually is worse when they are under pressure to speak well, as when giving an oral report (American Psychiatric Association, 2013). Stuttering often begins gradually and almost always starts before age 10. Estimates of the prevalence of stuttering range from 0.3 percent to 5 percent, with roughly twice as many boys as girls diagnosed (Howell, 2007; D. McKinnon, S. McLeod, & Reilly, 2008; Proctor, Yairi, Duff, & Zhang, 2008). As many as 80 percent of children who stutter recover on their own by age 16 (Drayna & Kang, 2011). Others, however, continue to stutter as adults. Stuttering can lower children's self-esteem and cause them to limit their goals and activities.

spoken language, written language, and other language modalities (e.g., sign language). Their symptoms may include problems with vocabulary, grammar, narrative (i.e., knowing how to describe something or put together a story), and other pragmatic language abilities. Children with **speech sound disorder** have persistent difficulties in producing speech. They may not use speech sounds appropriate for their age or dialect, or they may substitute one sound for another (e.g., use a *t* for a *k* sound) or omit certain sounds (such as final consonants on words). Their words come out sounding like baby talk. They might say *wabbit* for *rabbit,* or *bu* for *blue* (Kartheiser, Ursano, & Barnhill, 2007). Speech sound disorder is

TABLE 5   Diagnostic Features of Communication Disorders

Disorder	Description
Language Disorder	Persistent difficulties in the acquisition and use of language in speech, written, or sign language due to deficits in the comprehension or production of vocabulary, sentence structure, or discourse.
Speech Sound Disorder	Persistent difficulty with speech sound production that interferes with speech intelligibility or prevents verbal communication of messages. Includes deficits in the phonological knowledge of speech sounds and/or difficulty coordinating movements of the jaw, tongue, or lips for clear speech with breathing and vocalizing for speech.
Childhood-Onset Fluency Disorder (Stuttering)	A disturbance in the normal fluency and time patterning of speech (e.g., sound syllable repetitions, sound prolongations of consonants and vowels, pauses within words).
Social (Pragmatic) Communication Disorder	Persistent difficulties with pragmatics or the social use of language and nonverbal communication in naturalistic contexts, which affects the development of social relationships and social participation. Symptoms are not better explained by autism spectrum disorder, intellectual disability, or low abilities in the domains of word structure and grammar or general cognitive ability.

Source: *Diagnostic and Statistical Manual of Mental Disorders,* Fifth Edition. American Psychiatric Association, 2013.

U.S President Joe Biden's public acknowledgment of his life-time battle with stuttering may help reduce stigma for those affected with this condition. *YASAMIN JAFARI TEHRANI/Shutterstock*

Finally, children with **social communication disorder** have deficits in using verbal and nonverbal communication for social purposes, such as greeting and sharing information, in a manner that is appropriate for the social context. Because children with social communication disorder have difficulty changing their communication to match the needs of the listener or following rules for conversation and storytelling, their social participation and social relationships are often impaired. Note that children with autism spectrum disorder (ASD) have difficulties in social communication. The *DSM-5* specifies that the diagnosis of social communication disorder can be given only if the child's communication difficulties are not better explained by ASD, and thus the child cannot currently or by history also show evidence of restricted/repetitive patterns of behavior, interests, or activities (American Psychiatric Association, 2013).

Causes and Treatment of Learning and Communication Disorders

Genetic factors are implicated in all the learning and communication disorders (Carrion-Castillo, Franke, & Fisher, 2013; Davis, Haworth, & Plomin, 2009; Drayna & Kang, 2011). While there may not be specific genes responsible for specific disorders in most cases, certain genetic abnormalities may account for a number of different learning disorders (Davis et al., 2009; Peterson & Pennington, 2015).

Abnormalities in brain structure and functioning have long been thought to cause learning disorders. Studies of people with difficulties in reading have identified three areas of the brain involved in three separate but interrelated skills (Shaywitz & Shaywitz, 2008). An area of the inferior frontal gyrus called *Broca's area* is involved in the ability to articulate and analyze words. An area in the parietotemporal region is involved in the ability to map the visual perception of the printed word onto the basic structures of language. Another area, in the occipitotemporal region, is involved in the rapid, automatic, fluent identification of words (S. Shaywitz & B. Shaywitz, 2008). In individuals with dyslexia, a condition in which the individual has difficulty with accurate and fluent word recognition, neuroimaging studies show unusually low activity in the parietotemporal and occipitotemporal regions (Shaywitz, 2003).

Environmental factors linked to the learning disorders include lead poisoning, birth defects, sensory deprivation, and low socioeconomic status (Fletcher et al., 2018). These conditions may create the risk of damage to critical brain areas. Children whose environments offer fewer opportunities to develop language skills are less likely to overcome biological contributors to learning problems (Peterson & Pennington, 2015; S. Shaywitz & B. Shaywitz, 2008).

The treatment of these disorders usually involves therapies designed to build the missing skills (Fletcher et al., 2018). Under the provisions of the Individuals with Disabilities Education Act, these interventions are bundled in a child's comprehensive Individualized Education Plan (IEP). The IEP describes the child's specific skills deficits as determined by formal tests and observations by parents and teachers. The plan also involves parents and teachers in strategies to help the child overcome these deficits. A child with dyslexia might receive systematic instruction in word recognition while in school, supplemented with practice at home, possibly using computerized exercises. Such programs appear to significantly improve skills in children with learning disorders (Scammacca et al., 2016).

Studies suggest that specialized instruction to overcome skills deficits actually can change brain functioning. In one study, children with dyslexia received daily individual tutoring. Before, immediately after, and 1 year after the intervention, the children underwent neuroimaging. Children who received this intervention not only improved their reading but also demonstrated increased activation in the parietotemporal and occipitotemporal regions (Shaywitz et al., 2004). Other researchers also have seen neural effects of specialized training to overcome learning problems (Gabrieli, 2009; Temple et al., 2003).

Motor Disorders

The *DSM-5* specifies four neurodevelopmental **motor disorders** (see Table 6). Two of these are tic disorders, **Tourette's disorder** and **persistent motor or vocal tic disorder (PMVTD)**. These disorders involve motor tics and/or vocal tics that consistently and are present for at least 12 months. They are relatively common, with prevalence rates of 1 percent and 3 to 4 percent, respectively (Roessner, Hoekstra, & Rothenberger, 2011).

TABLE 6 Criteria for Motor Disorders

Disorder	Description
Tourette's Disorder	Both multiple motor *and* one or more vocal tics that have been present at some time during the illness, although not necessarily concurrently
Persistent Motor or Vocal Tic Disorder	Single motor *or* vocal tics, persistent for at least 1 year, and with onset before age 18
Stereotypic Movement Disorder	Repetitive, seemingly driven, and apparently purposeless motor behavior (e.g., hand shaking or waving, body rocking, head banging, self-biting) causing clinically significant distress or functional impairment
Developmental Coordination Disorder	Motor performance that is substantially below expected levels, given the person's chronologic age and previous opportunities for skill acquisition (e.g., poor balance, clumsiness, dropping or bumping into things; marked delays in acquiring basic motor skills such as walking, crawling, sitting, catching, throwing, cutting, coloring, or printing)

Note: For tic disorders that do not meet the criteria for Tourette's Disorder or Persistent Motor or Vocal Tic Disorder, the *DSM-5* provides diagnoses of Other Specified or Unspecified Tic Disorder.

Tics are sudden, rapid, recurrent, nonrhythmic motor movements or vocalizations. Examples of motor tics include jerking of the head, arm, or leg; eye blinking; facial grimacing; and neck stretching. Vocal tics can be almost any sound or noise, but common ones include throat clearing, sniffing, and grunting (Singer, 2005). People with Tourette's disorder have multiple motor tics and at least one or more vocal tics that have persisted for more than a year since the first tic onset. About 10 percent of people with Tourette's have a complex form of vocal tic that involves uttering or shouting obscenities or other socially objectionable words or phrases (Singer, 2005). People with PMVTD have *only* motor *or* vocal tics, not both.

People with these disorders often feel a premonition that a tic is imminent and an urge just before the tic occurs; the urge to tic is temporarily reduced by the tic behavior (Flessner, 2011). The frequency of tics in both disorders increases when people are under stress or do not have alternative activities to occupy them. Tourette's disorder and PMVTD are often comorbid with other psychological disorders, such as obsessive-compulsive disorder (OCD), attention deficit hyperactivity disorder (ADHD), ASD, anxiety disorders, and affective disorders. Several studies have shown that quality of life for those with these disorders is significantly impacted (Rizzo, Pellico, Silvestri, Chiarotti, & Cardona, 2018).

The distinctions between Tourette's disorder and PMVTD may seem minor, and studies show that similar genetic and other biological factors may underlie both tic disorders (e.g., Harris & Singer, 2006). Tourette's disorder, especially with the presence of complex vocal tics, is more debilitating and more often comorbid with other disorders than is PMVTD such as ADHD or OCD, so the authors of the *DSM-5* chose to keep them as separate diagnoses (Walkup, Ferraõ, Leckman, Stein, & Singer, 2010).

People with **stereotypic movement disorder** engage in repetitive, seemingly driven, and apparently purposeless motor behavior, such as hand shaking or waving, hair twirling, body rocking, head banging, and self-biting. These behaviors differ from tics in that the individual may continue to engage in them for an extended period of time (Stein, Grant et al., 2010). They are often seen in individuals with other disorders, particularly ASD, intellectual disability, and attention-deficit/hyperactivity disorder (Stein, Grant, et al., 2010).

All three of these motor disorders typically begin in childhood and increase in adolescence and then decline in adulthood (Roessner et al., 2011; Walkup et al., 2010). All three are highly comorbid with OCD and likely share common causes with OCD (Walkup et al., 2010). Specifically, these three motor disorders and OCD co-occur in families and may be due to similar genetic factors. Further, these disorders are associated with dysfunctions in dopamine systems in areas of the brain involved in control of motor behavior, such as the cerebrum, basal ganglia, and frontal cortex, as is the case in OCD (see reviews in Roessner et al., 2011; Stein, Grant, et al., 2010; Walkup et al., 2010). Tourette's syndrome and PMVTD both respond to drugs that alter dopamine systems, such as atypical antipsychotic medications (Roessner et al., 2013; Walkup et al., 2010).

All three motor disorders also can be treated with a behavioral therapy called *habit reversal therapy* (Azrin & Nunn, 1973), in which the triggers for and signs of impending tics or stereotypic behaviors are identified and clients are taught to engage in competing behaviors (e.g., squeezing their hands when they feel a vocal tic coming on, crossing their arms when they feel they are about to engage in hand flapping). Habit reversal therapy and related behavioral treatments have shown positive results in randomized controlled trials. Tic awareness training, relaxation training, contingency management, and generalization training are also included in this behavioral therapy. These behavioral therapies are very successful in reducing tic severity and are recommended as a first-line intervention (McGuire et al., 2014; Rizzo et al., 2018).

Developmental coordination disorder is another motor disorder involving fundamental deficits or significant delays in the development of basic motor skills, such as sitting, crawling, walking, running, simple athletic skills (throwing or catching a ball), and motor skills involved in writing, cutting, or coloring. These deficits cannot be due to a medical condition such as muscular dystrophy. Significant deficits such as these are fairly common, with a prevalence of 5 to 6 percent in children (affecting more boys than girls), and can cause moderate to severe distress and dysfunction in a child's life (Blank, Smits-Engelsman, Polatajko, & Wilson, 2012). These deficits are frequently comorbid with other disorders, especially ADHD (Sigurdsson, van Os, & Fombonne, 2002). The causes of developmental coordination disorder are not known, and may be highly heterogeneous (Blank et al., 2012). The disorder is most often treated with physical or occupational therapy.

TABLE 7   *DSM-5* Criteria for Major Neurocognitive Disorder (NCD)

A. Evidence of significant cognitive decline from a previous level of performance in one or more cognitive domains (complex attention, executive function, learning and memory, language, perceptual-motor, or social cognition) based on:

1. Concern of the individual, a knowledgeable informant, or the clinician that there has been a significant decline in cognitive function; *and*

2. A substantial impairment in cognitive performance, preferably documented by standardized neuropsychological testing or, in its absence, another quantified clinical assessment.

B. The cognitive deficits interfere with independence in everyday activities (i.e., at a minimum, requiring assistance with complex instrumental activities of daily living such as paying bills or managing medications).

C. The cognitive deficits do not occur exclusively in the context of delirium.

D. The cognitive deficits are not better explained by another mental disorder (e.g., major depressive disorder, schizophrenia).

Note: NCDs are specified by their etiological subtypes, such as whether, for example, they are due to Alzheimer's disease, frontotemporal lobar degeneration, Lewy body disease, traumatic brain injury, or substance/medication use.

Reprinted with permission from the *Diagnostic and Statistical Manual of Mental Disorders,* Fifth Edition. Copyright ©2013 by American Psychiatric Association. All Rights Reserved.

MAJOR AND MILD NEUROCOGNITIVE DISORDERS

In the remainder of the chapter, we discuss disorders that most often arise later in life, namely the neurocognitive disorders (NCDs), which include major and mild NCD and delirium. These disorders result from medical conditions that cause impairment in cognition or from substance intoxication or withdrawal. Cognitive problems include memory deficits, language disturbances, perceptual disturbances, impairment in the capacity to plan and organize, and failure to recognize or identify objects. We begin our discussion with major and mild NCD.

Major NCD is more commonly known as **dementia** when referring to older adults with degenerative disorders like Alzheimer's disease (AD) (see the *DSM-5* criteria in Table 7). People with this disorder cannot remember the most fundamental facts of their lives, express themselves through language, or carry out basic everyday tasks. Milder versions of this disorder

that involve modest cognitive decline from a previous level of performance, but do not yet result in significant impairment in functioning, can be diagnosed as **mild NCD.**

Major NCD typically occurs in late life. The estimated prevalence of the most common type of major NCD—that due to AD—is 5 to 10 percent of people over age 65 (Alzheimer's Association, 2018; Hebert, Weuve, Scherr, & Evans, 2013). The prevalence of most types of major NCD increases with age, and experts estimate that 30 percent of individuals age 85 and older are living with major NCD (Ferri et al., 2005).

Symptoms of Major Neurocognitive Disorder

Major NCD is characterized by a decline in cognitive functioning severe enough to interfere with daily living (see Table 7). Memory deficits are prominent (American Psychiatric Association, 2013). In the early stages of major NCD, the memory lapses may be similar to those we all experience from time to time—forgetting the name of someone we know casually, our phone number, or what we went into the next room to get. Most of us eventually remember what we temporarily forgot, either spontaneously or by using tricks that jog our memory. The difference in major NCD is that memory does not return spontaneously and may not respond to reminders or other cues.

People in the early stages of major NCD, or who have mild NCD, may repeat questions because they do not remember asking them moments ago or do not remember getting an answer. They frequently misplace items, such as keys or wallets. They may try to compensate for their memory loss. For example, they may carefully write down their appointments or things they need to do. Eventually, however, they forget to look at their calendars or lists. As memory problems become more significant, they may become angry when asked questions or may make up answers in an attempt to hide their memory loss. As the disorder progresses, they may become lost in familiar surroundings and be unable to find their way when not accompanied by someone.

Eventually, long-term memory also becomes impaired. People with major NCD will forget the order of major events in their life, such as graduation from college, marriage, and the birth of their children. After a time, they will be unable to recall the events at all and may not even know their own name.

Another cognitive deficit of major NCD is **aphasia,** a deterioration of language. People with major NCD will have tremendous difficulty producing the names of objects or people and often may use terms such as *thing* or vague references to the objects or people to hide their inability to produce concrete names. If asked to identify a cup, for example, they may say that it is a thing for drinking but be unable to name it as a cup. They also may be unable to understand what another person is saying or to follow simple requests such as "Turn on the lights and shut the door." In advanced stages of major NCD, people may exhibit echolalia, simply repeating what they hear, or **palilalia,** repeating sounds or words over and over.

Another common cognitive deficit is **apraxia,** impairment of the ability to execute common actions such as waving good-bye or putting on a shirt. This deficit is not caused by problems in motor functioning (e.g., moving the arm), in sensory functioning, or in comprehending what action is required. People with major NCD simply are unable to carry out actions that are requested of them or that they wish to carry out.

Agnosia is the failure to recognize objects or people. People with major NCD may not be able to identify common objects, such as chairs or tables. At first, they fail to recognize casual friends or distant

Former President Ronald Reagan, who died in 2004 at age 93, was diagnosed with Alzheimer's disease. *National Archives and Records Administration (NLS-WHPO-A-C584(12))*

family members. With time, they may not recognize their spouse or children or even their own reflection in a mirror.

Most people with major NCD eventually lose **executive functions,** those brain functions that involve the ability to plan, initiate, monitor, and stop complex behaviors. Cooking Thanksgiving dinner, for example, requires executive functioning. Each menu item (the turkey, the stuffing, the pumpkin pie) requires different ingredients and preparation. The cooking of various menu items must be coordinated so that all the items are ready at the same time. People with mild NCD may attempt to cook Thanksgiving dinner but forget important components (such as the turkey) or fail to coordinate the dinner, burning certain items and undercooking others. People with major NCD are unable even to initiate such a complex task.

Deficits in executive functioning also involve difficulty in the kind of abstract thinking required to evaluate new situations and respond appropriately to these situations. For example, if a man with major NCD is presented with the proverb "People who live in glass houses shouldn't throw stones," he might be unable to interpret the abstract meaning of the proverb and instead interpret it concretely to mean "People don't want their windows broken."

In addition to these cognitive deficits, people with major NCD often show changes in emotional functioning and personality. Shoplifting and exhibitionism are common manifestations of a decline in judgment and an inability to control impulses. People with NCDs may become depressed when they recognize their cognitive deterioration. Often, however, they do not recognize or admit to their cognitive deficits. This can lead them to engage in unrealistic or dangerous actions, such as driving a car when they are too impaired to do so safely. They may become paranoid and angry with family members and friends, whom they see as thwarting their desires and freedom. They may accuse others of stealing belongings they have misplaced. They may believe that others are conspiring against them—the only conclusion left to them when they simply do not remember conversations in which they agreed to some action (e.g., starting a new medication or moving into a treatment facility for people with major NCD). Violent outbursts and combative behavior sometimes occur, particularly in moderate to severe stages of major NCDs.

Types of Major and Mild Neurocognitive Disorder

There are several types of NCD based on their causes. *DSM-5* recommends that the type of major or mild NCD be specified based on its medical or substance/medication-induced cause(s). The most common NCD worldwide is AD which accounts for up to two-thirds of all cases of NCDs. The prevalence of AD are increasing due, in part, to the higher aging world population. In the United States, AD-related deaths have increased by 89 percent between 2000 and 2014 (Gatz, 2007; Weller & Budson, 2018). These disorders also can be caused by vascular disease (blockage or leakage of blood to the brain, commonly referred to

as a stroke); by traumatic brain injury (TBI); by progressive diseases, such as Parkinson's disease and HIV disease; and by chronic substance abuse.

Neurocognitive Disorder Due to Alzheimer's Disease

People with NCD due to **AD** meet the criteria for major or mild NCD, and show clear evidence of decline in learning and memory. Individuals with AD experience progressive cognitive decline which typically begins with an inability to form recent memories, but ultimately affects all intellectual functions creating a loss of independence and premature death (Dindelegan, Faur, Purza, Bumbu, & Sabau, 2020). AD is a chronic and incurable disease that affects an estimated 5.4 million people in the United States (Efthymiou & Goate, 2017). The disease typically begins with mild memory loss, but as the disease progresses the memory loss and disorientation quickly become profound. About two-thirds of Alzheimer's patients show psychiatric symptoms, including agitation, irritability, apathy, and dysphoria. Often these emotional and behavioral symptoms are as difficult for caregivers of people with AD to deal with as the cognitive symptoms. As the disease worsens, sufferers may become violent and may experience hallucinations and delusions. The disease usually begins after age 65, but there is an early-onset type of AD that tends to progress more quickly than the late-onset type (Gatz, 2007; Scheltens et al., 2016). On average, people with this disease die within 8 to 10 years of its diagnosis, usually as a result of physical decline or independent diseases common in old age, such as heart disease.

Brain Abnormalities in AD What we now call AD was first described in 1906 by Alois Alzheimer. He observed severe memory loss and disorientation in a 51-year-old female patient. Following her death at age 55, an autopsy revealed that filaments within nerve cells in her brain were twisted and tangled. These **neurofibrillary tangles** are common in the brains of Alzheimer's patients but rare in people without an NCD (Figure 3). The tangles, which are made up of a protein called tau, impede nutrients, and other essential supplies from moving through cells to the extent that cells eventually die. Another brain abnormality seen in AD *is* plaques (see Figure 3). **Plaques** are deposits of a class of protein, called **beta-amyloid,** that are neurotoxic and accumulate in the spaces between the cells of the cerebral cortex, hippocampus, amygdala, and other brain structures critical to memory and cognition (Villemagne, Doré, Burnham, Masters, & Rowe, 2018).

There is extensive cell death in the cortex of Alzheimer's patients, resulting in shrinking of the cortex and enlargement of the ventricles of the brain (Figure 4). The remaining cells lose many of their

| FIGURE 3 | **Neurofibrillary Tangles and Beta-Amyloid Plaques in Alzheimer's Disease.** Protein deposits build up and cause neurofibrillary tangles and beta-amyloid plaques in neurons in the brains of people with Alzheimer's disease. |

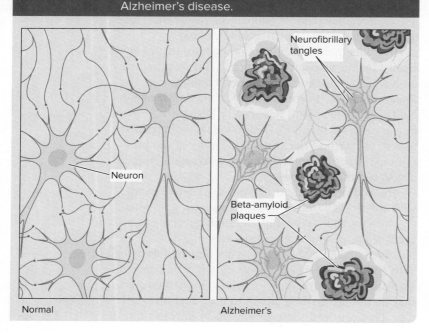

Normal   Alzheimer's

FIGURE 4	Cortical Regions in Alzheimer's Disease. Cell death causes shrinkage of cortical regions in the brains of people with advanced Alzheimer's disease (left; compare to healthy brain on right).

Science History Images / Alamy Stock Photo

FIGURE 5	Cell Damage in Alzheimer's Disease. Cells lose their dendrites, which connect cells to one another, in the brains of people with Alzheimer's disease.

Healthy cells   Alzheimer's cells

dendrites—the branches that link one cell to other cells (Figure 5). The result of all these brain abnormalities is profound memory loss and an inability to coordinate self-care and other daily activities.

Causes of AD Genetic factors appear to predispose some people to the brain changes seen in AD. Studies have found that AD is a highly heritable and complex disease with very limited effective prevention and treatment methods (Efthymiou & Goate, 2017). Family history studies suggest that 24 to 49 percent of first-degree relatives of patients with AD eventually develop the disease (Gatz, 2007). The lifetime risk of developing AD is 1.8 to 4 times higher for people with a family history of the disorder than for those without such a history. Twin studies confirm an important role of genetics in the risk for AD, as well as for other types of NCD. Concordance rates for all types of NCD in monozygotic twins are 44 percent for men and 58 percent for women; concordance rates for dizygotic twins are 25 percent for men and 45 percent for women (Gatz, Reynolds et al., 2006).

Several genes have been linked to AD. The gene most consistently associated with the disease is the apolipoprotein E gene (ApoE), which is on chromosome 19. This gene regulates the ApoE protein, which is involved in the transport of cholesterol through the blood. ApoE also binds to beta-amyloid protein and may play a role in its regulation. The ApoE gene has three alleles, or versions: e2, e3, and e4. People who inherit an e4 allele from one parent have a 2 to 4 times greater risk of developing AD than people who do not inherit an e4 allele, and people who

Plaques accumulate between cells in these and other areas of the brain in Alzheimer's disease.

inherit e4 alleles from both parents have an 8 to 12 times greater risk of developing the disorder (Coon et al., 2007; Naj, Schellenberg, & Alzheimer's Disease Genetics Consortium, 2017).

Neuroimaging studies show that people with the e4 version of the ApoE gene have reduced cortex and hippocampus volume compared to people without the e4 version of the ApoE gene, even as children or adolescents (Jack et al., 2007; Shaw et al., 2007; Thompson et al., 2004). As adults, people with the e4 version of the ApoE gene show greater cognitive deficits and earlier onset of Alzheimer's disorder (Perneczky, Alexopoulos, Wagenpfeil, & Kurz, 2012).

Other genes are implicated in the development of less common forms of AD, which begin in middle age and are more strongly familial. One of these genes is on chromosome 21 (Naj et al., 2017; Webb & Murphy, 2012). The first clue that a defective gene on chromosome 21 might be linked with AD came from the fact that people with Down syndrome are more likely than people in the general population to develop AD in late life. Researchers hypothesized that the gene responsible for some forms of AD may be on chromosome 21 and that people with Down syndrome are more prone to AD because they have an extra chromosome 21.

This hypothesis has been supported by studies of families with high rates of AD. These studies have found links between the presence of the disease and the presence of an abnormal gene on chromosome 21 (Webb & Murphy, 2012). Also, this abnormal gene on chromosome 21 is near the gene responsible for producing a precursor of the amyloid protein known as the amyloid precursor protein gene, or APP gene. It may be that defects along this section of chromosome 21 cause an abnormal production and buildup of amyloid proteins in the brain, resulting in AD. A number of other genes have been implicated in AD, though somewhat inconsistently (Gatz, 2007; Naj et al., 2017). Even taken altogether, however, the genes shown to be associated with AlD account for only about 50 percent of cases.

People with AD also show deficits in a number of neurotransmitters, including acetylcholine, norepinephrine, serotonin, somatostatin (a corticotropin-releasing factor), and peptide Y (Micheau & Marighetto, 2011). The deficits in acetylcholine are particularly noteworthy because this neurotransmitter is thought to be critical in memory function. The degree of cognitive decline seen in patients with Alzheimer's is significantly correlated with the degree of deficit in acetylcholine (Micheau & Marighetto, 2011). Drugs that enhance levels of acetylcholine can slow the rate of cognitive decline in some Alzheimer's sufferers.

We will likely know much more about the causes of AD in the next few years (see Scheltens et al., 2016). The technologies for studying the genetic and neurological processes of the disease are advancing rapidly, and many researchers are investigating this disorder. Five and a half million people in the United States and 18 million people worldwide are estimated to have AD, and this number is expected to increase by at least 300 percent by 2050 (Alzheimer's Association, 2018; Hebert et al., 2013). The annual cost of caring for people with NCD in the United States is expected to be $400 billion by 2050 (Lyketsos, Miller, & Neuropsychiatric Syndromes Professional Interest Area of the International Society to Advance Alzheimer's Research and Treatment, 2012). We can hope that by then we will understand the disorder well enough to treat it effectively.

Vascular Neurocognitive Disorder

Another common type of NCD is **vascular neurocognitive disorder.** People with this disorder meet the criteria for major or mild NCD, depending on the severity of cognitive symptoms and functional decline. The most prominent cognitive symptoms are significant declines in processing speed, in the ability to pay attention, and in the executive functions described earlier. In addition, there must be evidence of a recent vascular event or cerebrovascular disease. **Cerebrovascular disease** occurs when the blood supply to areas of the brain is blocked, causing tissue damage in the brain. Neuroimaging techniques, such as PET and MRI, can detect areas of tissue damage and reduced blood flow in the brain, confirming cerebrovascular disease.

Sudden damage to an area of the brain due to the blockage of blood flow or to hemorrhaging (bleeding) is called a **stroke.** Vascular NCD can occur after one large stroke or after an accumulation of small strokes. Cerebrovascular disease can be caused by high blood pressure and the accumulation of fatty deposits in the arteries, which block blood flow to the brain. It also can be a complication of diseases that inflame the brain and of traumatic brain injuries.

About 25 percent of stroke patients develop cognitive deficits severe enough to qualify for a diagnosis of NCD (Burhan, Moradizadeh, & Marlatt, 2018; Stephens et al., 2004). A greater risk of developing vascular NCD is seen in stroke patients who are older (over age 80), who have less education, who have a history of strokes, or who have diabetes.

Even stroke patients who do not immediately develop NCD are at increased risk of cognitive decline compared to people of the same age who do not suffer a stroke (Burhan et al., 2018; Hachinski, 2008). The patients most likely to eventually develop NCD tend to have additional strokes over time, some of which were obvious and others that were "silent" (or without obvious symptoms) and detected only later. In addition, patients who have medical events or conditions that cause widespread oxygen or blood deficiency—such as seizures, cardiac arrhythmias, congestive heart failure, and pneumonia—are more likely to develop vascular NCDs.

Neurocognitive Disorders Associated with Other Medical Condition

A variety of other serious medical conditions can produce NCDs, including Lewy body disease, Parkinson's disease, the human immunodeficiency virus (HIV), and Huntington's disease. Parkinson's disease is a degenerative brain disorder that affects about 0.3 percent of people in the general population and 2 percent of people over age 65 (Poewe et al., 2017). Muhammed Ali, who died in 2016, and Michael J. Fox are two well-known people with Parkinson's disease. Its primary symptoms are tremors, muscle rigidity, and the inability to initiate movement. The symptoms result from the death of brain cells that produce the neurotransmitter dopamine. Approximately 75 percent of people with Parkinson's disease develop NCD (Aarsland & Kurz, 2009).

Michael J. Fox is a well-known person suffering from Parkinson's disease. Despite his symptoms, he continues his acting career and is an active advocate. *Mike Coppola/MJF2015/Getty Images*

NCD due to Lewy body disease is a leading cause of non-Alzheimer disease-related NCDs. This disorder is associated with progressive cognitive impairment but also a combination of motor and sleep dysfunction, as well as, neurocognitive and neuropsychiatric symptoms, such as recurrent visual hallucinations, delusions, and depressive symptoms (American Psychiatric Association, 2013; How, Lo, Xiong, 2018). Characteristic symptoms include changes in attention and alertness, visual hallucinations, and the symptoms of Parkinson's disease. There is a significant overlap in cognitive symptoms between Lewy body disease and Parkinson's disease dementia which includes progressive impairment of executive functions, visual-spatial abnormalities, and memory problems (Jellinger & Korczyn, 2018).

The HIV, the virus that causes AIDS, affects an estimated 38 million people and can cause a mild or major NCD. Approximately 50 percent of HIV patients display neurocognitive dysfunction termed HIV-Associated Neurocognitive Disorder (HAND). HAND results from chronic low-level neuroinflammation due to HIV presence in the brain. HAND is widely associated with systemic inflammation driven, in part, by HIV but is also due to persistent disruption of microorganisms across the GI tract which compromise the gut microbiome. This neurocognitive disruption causes impairment of memory and concentration. HAND creates multiple types of cognitive impairments, predominantly with attention, memory, processing speed, and executive function. Difficulties with emotion, such as depression and apathy, and some motor deficits also occur (Olivier, Cacabelos, & Naidoo, 2018; Rizzo et al., 2020). As their mental processes slow—people with this condition may have difficulty following conversations or may take much longer to organize their thoughts and to complete simple, familiar tasks. They may withdraw socially and lose their spontaneity. Weakness in the legs or hands, clumsiness, loss of balance, and lack of coordination are also common. If the NCD progresses, the deficits worsen. Speech becomes increasingly impaired, as does the understanding of language. People become confined to bed, often indifferent to their surroundings.

HIV-associated major NCD is diagnosed when the deficits and symptoms become severe and global, with significant disruption of daily activities and functioning. As antiretroviral therapies have become widely used in treating people with HIV, new onsets of HIV-related NCD have decreased, as has its severity. On the other hand, as more patients with HIV survive into older age due to these drugs, the number of people with HIV-related NCD is increasing, particularly among people who abused drugs or also had a hepatitis C infection (Nath et al., 2008).

Huntington's disease is a rare genetic disorder that afflicts people early in life, usually between ages 25 and 55. People with this disorder eventually develop a major NCD and chorea—irregular jerks, grimaces, and twitches. Huntington's disease is transmitted by a single dominant gene on chromosome 4 (Ross et al., 2014). If one parent has the gene, their children have a 50 percent chance of inheriting the gene and developing the disorder. Huntington's disease affects many neurotransmitters in the brain, but which of these changes causes chorea and NCD remains unclear.

Mild and major NCD can also be caused by a rare disorder called prion disease (also known as Creutzfeld–Jacob's disease); by brain tumors; by endocrine conditions, such as hypothyroidism; by nutritional conditions, such as deficiencies of thiamine, niacin, and vitamin B12; by infections, such as syphilis; and by other neurological diseases, such as multiple sclerosis. In addition, the chronic heavy use of alcohol, inhalants, and sedatives, especially in combination with nutritional deficiencies, can cause brain damage and NCD. As many as 10 percent of chronic alcohol abusers may develop NCD (Ridley, Draper, & Withall, 2013). Alcohol-related NCD usually has a slow, insidious onset. While it can be slowed with nutritional supplements, it often is persistent, particularly when use was prolonged and as age increases.

NCD due to TBI often results from penetrating injuries, such as those caused by gunshots, or closed head injuries, typically caused by impact to the head and/or concussive forces such as caused by motor vehicle accident, explosion, or sports injury. This TBI is accompanied by cognitive decline and impairments of memory, moral judgment and social cognition (Hwang, Jang, Soh, H. Lee, & S. Lee, 2019). Individuals with NCD as a result of TBI may also experience disruption in emotional functioning such as, irritability and personality changes, and neurological symptoms such as speech and gait abnormalities. Depression is an often comorbid with this disorder which can worsen day-to-day function and compound difficulties with independent living and self-care (Rose, 2019). In the United States, falls account for 28 percent of traumatic brain injuries, motor vehicle accidents for 20 percent, being struck by an object for 19 percent, violence for 11 percent, and bicycle accidents for 3 percent (Langlois, Rutland-Brown, & Wald, 2006). Leland, in the case study below, developed a major NCD after a motor vehicle accident.

CASE STUDY

A 41-year-old factory worker named Leland was returning home along a rural road one night after work. A drunk driver ran a stop sign and collided at a high rate of speed with the driver's side of Leland's car. Leland was not wearing a seat belt. The collision sent Leland through the windshield and onto the pavement. He lived but sustained a substantial brain injury, as well as many broken bones and cuts. Leland was unconscious for more than 2 weeks and then spent another 2 months in the hospital, recovering from his injuries.

When he returned home to his family, Leland was not himself. Before the accident, he was a quiet man who doted on his family and frequently displayed a wry sense of humor. After the accident, Leland was sullen and chronically irritable. He screamed at his wife or children for the slightest annoyance. He even slapped his wife once when she confronted him about his verbal abuse of the children.

Leland did not fare much better at work. He found he now had great trouble concentrating on his job, and he could not follow his boss's instructions. When his boss approached Leland about his inability to perform his job, Leland could not express much about the trouble he was having. He became angry at his boss and accused him of wanting to fire him. Leland had always been much liked by his co-workers, and they welcomed him back after the accident with sincere joy, but soon he began to lash out at them, as he was lashing out at his wife and children. He accused a close friend of stealing from him. These symptoms continued acutely for about 3 months. Gradually, they declined. Finally, about 18 months after the accident, Leland's emotional and personality functioning appeared to be back to normal. His cognitive functioning also improved greatly, but he still found it more difficult to pay attention and to complete tasks than he did before the accident.

Leland's symptoms are characteristic of people with a severe **traumatic brain injury(TBI).** He showed changes both in his cognitive abilities and in his usual emotional and personality functioning. Fortunately, Leland's symptoms subsided after several months.

Many victims of moderate to severe brain injury never fully recover.

NCDs that follow single closed head injuries are typically mild and more likely to dissipate with time than are NCDs that follow repeated closed head injuries, such as those experienced by boxers, some soldiers, or people in multiple motor vehicle accidents. Between 2001 and 2012, over 3 million traumatic brain injuries in the United States were the result of sports and recreation activities; boys and young men are most likely to suffer NCD due to brain injury because they take more risks associated with brain injuries than do other groups (Coronado et al., 2015).

Soldiers who have served in Iraq and Afghanistan have had high rates of TBI due to blasts from roadside bombs and other explosive devices. A recent study on Iraq and Afghanistan war veterans accessing services through the veteran's administration (VA) found that 9.6 percent had been diagnosed with a TBI. Traumatic injuries are classified from mild to severe, with 75 to 80 percent of TBI cases among both Veterans and civilians classified as mild (Wyse, Pogoda, Mastarone, Gilbert, & Carlson, 2020). For veterans, such events may result from blast exposure, motor vehicle crashes, falls, or other head trauma and frequently co-occur with mental health diagnoses such as posttraumatic stress disorder (PTSD). Soldiers with traumatic brain injuries show declines in neurocognitive function similar to those seen in NCD, as well as depression, aggressive behavior, long-term unemployment, and problems in their social relationships.

The Impact of Gender, Culture, and Education on Neurocognitive Disorder

AD affects an estimated 30 million people worldwide with 4.6 million new cases annually. Among this population, women are more likely than men to develop AD and experience greater cognitive impairment. These sex differences increase with advanced age resulting in increased impairment (Laws, Irvine, & Gale, 2016). This may be simply because women tend to live longer than men and thus live long enough to develop an age-related NCD. Among people with the same degree of the brain changes due to Alzheimer's, women tend to show greater cognitive impairment than men (Barnes et al., 2005; Perneczky, Drzezga, Diehl-Schmid, Li, & Kurz, 2007). The reasons for these gender differences are not known.

In general, African Americans and Caribbean Hispanics show higher incidence of dementia than European Americans (Chin, Negash, & Hamilton, 2011; Mehta & Yeo, 2017). African Americans have higher rates of hypertension and cardiovascular

Soldiers who have served in Iraq and Afghanistan have had high rates of traumatic brain injury.
PETER PARKS/AFP/Getty Images

disease, both of which contribute to vascular NCD. However, the genetic factors leading to NCD may be more prevalent in European Americans than in African Americans.

Differences in people's level of education also may contribute to differences in rates of NCD. Neuroimaging studies of people with NCD find that those with less education show more of the brain deterioration associated with NCD than do those with more education. It may be that people with more education have a higher socioeconomic status, which in turn provides them with better nutrition and health care that protect them against the conditions contributing to AD. Education and, more generally, cognitive activity throughout one's life actually may increase brain resources in ways that forestall the development of NCD in people prone to the disorder (Gatz, Prescott, & Pedersen, 2006; Scheltens et al., 2016).

The likelihood that a person with NCD will be institutionalized rather than cared for in the family is greater among European Americans than among Asians or Hispanics and Latinos (Chin et al., 2011; Mausbach et al., 2004; Torti, Gwyther, Reed, Friedman, & Schulman, 2004). One reason may be that European Americans are more likely to have the substantial financial resources it takes to treat family members with NCD (Chin et al., 2011). In addition, Asian and Latino cultures may have a more positive view of caring for sick and elderly family members than European American culture. Asian and Latino cultures also exert greater societal pressure to care for ill family members in the home.

Treatments for and Prevention of Neurocognitive Disorder

Two classes of drugs are approved for treatment of the cognitive symptoms of NCD (Martorana, Esposito, & Koch, 2010). The first class is cholinesterase inhibitors, such as donepezil (Aricept), rivastigmine (Exelon), and galantamine (Reminyl). These drugs help prevent the breakdown of the neurotransmitter acetylcholine, and randomized trials show that they have a modest positive effect on NCD symptoms (Martorana et al., 2010). The side effects of these drugs include nausea, diarrhea, and anorexia. The second class is drugs that regulate the activity of the neurotransmitter glutamate, which plays an essential role in learning and memory; memantine (Namenda) is one such drug. Developing new drugs is an international priority due to projected increases in the number of people with NCD (Cummings et al., 2016).

Many other drugs used to treat people with NCD affect the secondary symptoms of the disorder rather than the primary cognitive symptoms. Antidepressants and antianxiety drugs may be used to help control emotional symptoms. Antipsychotic drugs may help control hallucinations, delusions, and agitation (Scheltens et al., 2016; Sultzer et al., 2008).

Behavior therapies can be helpful in controlling patients' angry outbursts and emotional instability (Fitzsimmons & Buettner, 2002; Teri et al., 2003). Often, family members are given training in behavioral techniques to help them manage patients at home.

The School Sisters of Notre Dame have participated in a fascinating study of the effects of early intellectual activity on mental and physical health in old age. *Scott Takushi/Newscom*

These techniques not only reduce stress and emotional distress in family caregivers but also may result in fewer behavior problems in the family member with NCD (Teri et al., 2003). Many people are interested in behavioral means of reducing their risk for NCD. Aerobic exercise and mental activity may have some protective value (Deeny et al., 2008; Valenzuela, 2008). Reducing the risk factors for stroke—for example, avoiding smoking, obesity, and hypertension—may reduce the risk for vascular NCD (Gatz, 2007; Scheltens et al., 2016).

Although some memory decline is typical of aging, research shows that some people who notice a significant decline are in fact in the early stages of dementia (Rabin, Smart, & Amariglio, 2017). Early identification of memory problems and treatment with cognitive training may help slow the progression into major NCD (Smart et al., 2017).

One of the most fascinating studies to show a link between intellectual activity beginning early in life and a reduced risk of AD is the Nun Study, a longitudinal study of several hundred elderly nuns in the School Sisters of Notre Dame. Nuns who entered old age with greater intellectual strengths were less likely to develop severe NCD, even when their brain showed evidence of significant neurofibrillary tangles and senile plaques (Snowdon, 1997). For example, the level of linguistic skill the nuns showed in journal writings when they were in their twenties significantly predicted their risk of developing NCD in later life (Snowdon et al., 1996). The best example was Sister Mary, who had high cognitive test scores right up until her death at age 101. An evaluation of Sister Mary's brain revealed that AD had spread widely through her brain, even though her cognitive test scores slipped only from the "superior" range to the "very good" range as she aged. Other results from this study showed that tiny strokes may lead a mildly deteriorating brain to develop a major NCD (Snowdon et al., 1997).

DELIRIUM

Delirium is characterized by disorientation, recent memory loss, and a clouding of attention (Table 8). A delirious person has difficulty focusing, sustaining, or shifting attention. These signs arise suddenly, within several hours or days. They fluctuate over the course of a day and often become worse at night, a condition known as *sundowning*. The duration of these signs is short—rarely longer than a month. Delirious patients often are agitated or frightened. They also may experience disrupted sleep-wake cycles, incoherent speech, delusions, and hallucinations (American Psychiatric Association, 2013). Delirium increases with age and it is present in 11 to 42 percent of patients admitted to the hospital who are 65 years or older (Helgesen et al., 2020).

The symptoms of delirium usually follow a common progression (Inouye, Westendorp, & Saczynski, 2014). In the early phase, patients report mild symptoms such as fatigue, decreased concentration, irritability, restlessness, or depression. They may experience mild cognitive impairments or perceptual disturbances, or even visual hallucinations. As the delirium worsens, the person's orientation becomes disrupted. A patient may think their childhood home instead of in the hospital. If undetected, the delirium progresses, and the person's orientation to familiar people

TABLE 8   *DSM-5* Criteria for Delirium
A. A disturbance in attention (i.e., reduced ability to direct, focus, sustain, and shift attention) and orientation to the environment and awareness (reduced orientation to the environment).
B. The disturbance develops over a short period of time (usually hours to a few days), and represents a change from baseline attention and awareness, and tends to fluctuate in severity during the course of a day.
C. An additional disturbance in cognition (e.g., memory deficit, disorientation, language, visuospatial ability, or perception).
D. The disturbances in Criteria A and C are not better explained by another pre-existing, established, or evolving neurocognitive disorder and do not occur in the context of a severely reduced level of arousal, such as coma.
E. There is evidence from the history, physical examination, or laboratory findings that the disturbance is a direct physiological consequence of another medical condition, substance intoxication or withdrawal, or exposure to a toxin, or due to multiple etiologies.

becomes distorted. For example, a delirious person may misidentify his wife or fail to recognize his child. Immediate memory is the first to be affected, followed by intermediate memory (memories of events occurring in the past 10 minutes) and finally by remote, or distant, memory. When intervals of these symptoms alternate with intervals of lucid functioning and the symptoms become worse at night, a diagnosis of delirium is likely. If the person is not disoriented (to time, place, or person) or if recent memory loss is absent, then a diagnosis of delirium is unlikely.

The onset of delirium may be dramatic, as when a normally quiet person suddenly becomes loud, verbally abusive, and combative or when a compliant hospital patient tries to pull out his intravenous tube. Sometimes, though, the onset of delirium manifests as an exaggerated form of an individual's normal personality traits. For example, a generally cranky person recovering from surgery may complain loudly and harshly about the "inadequate" care she is receiving from the attending nurses. It would be easy for attending staff to regard her irritability as consistent with her personality style: "She must be feeling better; she's beginning to complain." In this type of case, the delirium may go unrecognized until more severe symptoms emerge.

Sometimes, delirious individuals simply appear confused. People who know the person well might say, "He just doesn't seem like himself." These delirious individuals may call an acquaintance by the wrong name or forget how to get to a familiar location, such as their room. In such cases, the first indication of delirium often comes from the observations of family or medical staff. They notice that the person seems calm during the day but becomes agitated at night. It is important to monitor such a person around the clock. Detecting delirium also may require the frequent testing of the person's orientation (by asking their name, the date and time, and the location). Close monitoring is also important because, with delirium, accidents such as falling out of bed or stepping into traffic are common.

Delirium typically signals a serious medical condition. When it is detected and the underlying medical condition is treated, delirium is temporary and reversible (Cole, Ciampi, Belzile, & Zhong, 2009). The longer delirium continues, however, the more likely the person is to suffer permanent brain damage, because the causes of delirium, if left untreated, can induce permanent changes in the functioning of the brain (Fong, Vasunilashorn, Libermann, Marcantonio, & Inouye, S. K., 2019).

Causes of Delirium

Neurocognitive disorder is the strongest predictor of delirium, increasing the risk fivefold (Inouye et al.,

2014). A wide range of medical disorders, including stroke, congestive heart failure, infectious diseases, a high fever, and HIV infection, is associated with a risk for delirium. Intoxication with illicit drugs and withdrawal from these drugs or from prescription medications also can lead to delirium. Other possible causes include fluid and electrolyte imbalances, medication side effects, and toxic substances.

Delirium may be caused when a medical condition, a drug, or a toxic substance affects the level of acetylcholine in the brain. Abnormalities in a number of other neurotransmitters, including dopamine, serotonin, and GABA, are seen in people who are delirious.

Delirium is probably the most common psychiatric syndrome found in general hospitals, particularly in older people. About 18 to 35 percent of older people are delirious on admission to the hospital for a serious illness, and another 11 to 14 percent develop delirium while in the hospital (Inouye et al., 2014). Older people often experience delirium following surgery. The delirium may be the result of the person's medical disorder or the effect of medications. It also may result from sensory isolation. A syndrome known as ICU/CCU psychosis—a type of delirium—occurs in intensive care and cardiac care units (Brown, 2014). Patients who are kept in unfamiliar surroundings that are monotonous may hear noises from machines as human voices, see the walls quiver, or hallucinate that someone is tapping them on the shoulder. Among the elderly, a high mortality rate is associated with delirium (Inouye et al., 2014). The typical reason is that the underlying condition or the cause of the delirium is very serious. Delirium also has negative effects on health, functioning, and survival well after the episode itself, and can increase risk for dementia as well (Inouye et al., 2014).

Delirium is a common problem in older adult hospital patients. *Fuse/Getty Images*

Some people are at increased risk for delirium. Risk factors include age (the older the person, the higher the risk), gender (males are at greater risk than females), and pre-existing brain damage or neurocognitive disorder. African Americans have higher rates of delirium than European Americans, possibly because African Americans are less likely to have health insurance and thus do not receive early intervention for a serious illness. As a result, their illness may be more likely to become severe enough to cause delirium.

Treatments for Delirium

It is extremely important that delirium be recognized and treated quickly. If a delirious person is not already hospitalized, immediate referral to a physician should be made. If another medical condition is associated with the delirium (e.g., stroke or congestive heart failure), the first priority is to treat that condition. Drugs that may contribute to the delirium must be discontinued. Antipsychotic medications sometimes are used to treat the person's confusion and agitation, although they do not seem to affect prognosis of delirium (Inouye et al., 2014). It also may be necessary to prevent people with delirium from harming themselves accidentally. Often, nursing care is required to monitor people's state and prevent them from wandering off, tripping, or ripping out intravenous tubes and to manage their behavior if they should become noncompliant or agitated and combative. In some instances, restraints are necessary. Providing a reassuring atmosphere filled with familiar personal belongings, such as family photographs and the person's own clothing, can help patients prone to delirium be less agitated and feel more secure and in control. Psychosocial treatments that improve sleep, address sensory issues, and encourage mobility and therapeutic activity have shown some promise but require further research (Inouye et al., 2014).

CHAPTER INTEGRATION

As noted in the Along the Continuum feature at the beginning of this chapter, both developmental psychopathologists and geropsychologists emphasize the importance of understanding the neurodevelopmental and neurocognitive disorders in the context of normal development and aging. Development and aging are not simply biological processes but rather involve the interaction of biological, environmental, and psychosocial processes, as depicted in Figure 6.

All the disorders in this chapter are related to genetic abnormalities, but the environment can affect

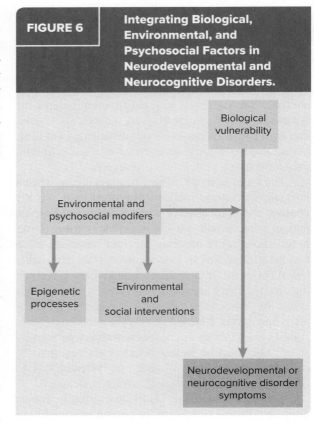

FIGURE 6 Integrating Biological, Environmental, and Psychosocial Factors in Neurodevelopmental and Neurocognitive Disorders.

the expression of genes through epigenetic processes (see the chapter "Theories and Treatment of Abnormality"). For example, there is evidence that the risk of autism spectrum disorder is higher among children whose biological fathers are older (e.g., over 40) at the time of conception (Hultman, Sandin, Levine, Lichtenstein, & Reichenberg, 2011). This may be because sperm deteriorates due to aging, or it may be that accumulated exposure to toxins over the lifespan causes DNA damage that results in a higher risk for autism spectrum disorder in their children.

In addition, the impact of biological vulnerabilities to neurodevelopmental or neurocognitive disorders on functioning can be significantly influenced by the environment and people's behavior. Children with autism spectrum disorder who receive early, intense behavioral intervention may eventually function very similarly to a child without the disorder, whereas children with autism spectrum disorder who receive no intervention are much less likely to develop typical functioning. As another example, the likelihood of developing many diseases in old age is substantially influenced by a person's behavior as a younger adult—people who keep mentally active into middle and old age may be less likely to develop Alzheimer's disease or develop less severe versions of NCDs.

Similarly, the social and emotional environment can affect the severity of deficits among people with neurodevelopmental and neurocognitive disorders. A child with ADHD whose parents are overwhelmed by his behavior and withdraw or become aggressive in response is less likely to develop the ability to regulate his behavior than is a child whose parents respond more effectively. If an older adult who is easily confused or forgetful is further stressed by family members who frequently become annoyed with her or expect too much of her, then her cognitive deficits can become even more severe. Thus, even though the neurodevelopmental or neurocognitive disorders are rooted in brain malfunction, psychosocial factors can influence the severity and manifestation of these disorders.

SHADES OF GRAY   DISCUSSION

Before giving Jake a diagnosis, there are several possibilities worth considering. First, you might consider whether Jake has a learning disability that is hurting his academic performance. You might administer testing to see if this is the case. Second, you may note that people with the inattentive type of ADHD are not hyperactive and often may seem absent-minded. Jake's tendencies to forget things, to leave projects incomplete, to have his mind wander, and to be late all fit the symptoms of a predominantly inattentive presentation of ADHD. However, they also could be caused by depression. Jake's parents often were critical of him and felt that he wasn't living up to their expectations, and difficulty with concentration, memory, and work completion are common features of depression. Also, the fact that Jake's grades tended to drop at times of transition could suggest trouble coping with change. You would need to thoroughly investigate these possibilities before making a diagnosis. More than just the presence of symptoms, an accurate diagnosis of ADHD requires that symptoms have a childhood onset, be developmentally inappropriate and persistent, be present in multiple settings, cause significant functional problems, and not be due to any other psychiatric disorder.

CHAPTER SUMMARY

- Attention-deficit/hyperactivity disorder (ADHD) is characterized by inattentiveness and hyperactivity. Children with ADHD often do poorly in school and in peer relationships and are at increased risk for developing behavior problems. ADHD is more common in boys than in girls.

- Biological factors that have been implicated in the development of ADHD include genetics, exposure to toxins prenatally and early in childhood, and abnormalities in neurological functioning.

- Treatments for ADHD usually involve stimulant drugs and behavior therapy designed to decrease children's impulsivity and hyperactivity and help them increase attention.

- Autism spectrum disorder is characterized by significant impairment in social interaction, communication with others, and everyday behaviors, interests, and activities. Many children with autism spectrum disorder score in the intellectual disability range on IQ tests. Outcomes of autism spectrum disorder vary widely, although the majority of people must receive continual care, even as adults. The best predictors of a good outcome in autism spectrum disorder are an IQ above 50 and language development before age 6.

- Possible biological causes of autism spectrum disorder include a genetic predisposition to cognitive impairment, central nervous system damage, prenatal complications, and neurotransmitter imbalances.

- Drugs reduce some symptoms in autism spectrum disorder but do not eliminate the core of the disorder. Behavior therapy is used to reduce inappropriate and self-injurious behaviors and encourage prosocial behaviors.

- Intellectual disability is defined as significant deficits in conceptual, social, and practical skills that affect everyday functioning with onset during the developmental period. It is not diagnosed by low IQ alone, and its level of severity is determined by adaptive functioning deficits.

- A number of biological factors are implicated in intellectual disability, including metabolic disorders (PKU, Tay-Sachs disease); chromosomal disorders (Down syndrome, fragile X, trisomy 13, trisomy 18); prenatal exposure to rubella, herpes, syphilis, or drugs (especially alcohol, as in fetal alcohol syndrome); premature delivery; and traumatic brain injury (such as that arising from being shaken as an infant).

- There is some evidence that intensive and comprehensive educational interventions, administered very early in a child's life, can help decrease the level of intellectual disability.

- Specific learning disorder affects skills in reading, mathematics, or written expression.

- The communication disorders involve persistent difficulties in the acquisition and use of language and other means of communication.

- Children with language disorder have difficulties with spoken language, written language, and other language modalities (e.g., sign language). Their symptoms may include problems with vocabulary, grammar, narrative (i.e., knowing how to describe something or put together a story), and other pragmatic language abilities.

- Children with speech disorder have persistent difficulties in producing speech.

- Children with social communication disorder have difficulties in the acquisition and use of spoken or written language or other, nonverbal forms of communication for social communication in naturalistic settings that interfere with their social relationships.

- Some of the learning and communication disorders may have genetic roots. Abnormalities in brain structure and functioning have been implicated in these disorders. Environmental factors, including lead poisoning, birth defects, sensory deprivation, and low socioeconomic status, may contribute to brain dysfunction.

- Treatment of the learning and communication disorders usually focuses on building skills in problem areas through specialized training, as well as computerized exercises.

- Tourette's disorder and chronic motor or vocal tic disorder are motor disorders involving the presence of persistent tics. Stereotypic movement disorder is a motor disorder characterized by repetitive, seemingly driven, and apparently purposeless motor behavior. These disorders are highly comorbid with obsessive-compulsive disorder and may be related to similar biological factors.

- Developmental coordination disorder involves deficits in fundamental motor skills.

- Neurocognitive disorders involve deterioration in cognitive functioning, often accompanied by emotional and behavioral changes. Cognitive impairments in neurocognitive disorder include memory impairment, aphasia, apraxia, agnosia, and loss of executive functioning.

- The most common type of neurocognitive disorder is that due to Alzheimer's disease. The brain of an Alzheimer's patient shows neurofibrillary tangles, plaques made up of beta-amyloid protein, and cortical atrophy. Recent theories of Alzheimer's disease focus on genes that might contribute to the buildup of beta-amyloid protein in the brain of Alzheimer's patients, particularly the ApoE gene.

- Neurocognitive disorder also can be caused by cerebrovascular disease, traumatic brain injury, and progressive disorders such as Parkinson's disease, Lewy body disease, HIV infection, Huntington's disease, and prion disease (Creutzfeldt–Jakob disease). Chronic substance abuse and the nutritional deficiencies that often accompany it also can lead to neurocognitive disorder.

- Drugs may help reduce the cognitive symptoms of neurocognitive disorder and the accompanying depression, anxiety, and psychotic symptoms in some patients.

- Delirium is characterized by disorientation, recent memory loss, and a global attention disturbance. Delirium typically is a signal of a serious medical condition, such as a stroke, congestive heart failure, an infectious disease, a high fever, or drug or medication intoxication or withdrawal. It is a common syndrome in hospitals, particularly among elderly surgical patients.

- Treating delirium involves treating the underlying condition leading to the delirium and keeping the patient safe until the symptoms subside.

KEY TERMS

neurodevelopmental disorders	language disorder
neurocognitive disorders	speech sound disorder
attention-deficit/hyperactivity disorder (ADHD)	childhood-onset fluency disorder
autism spectrum disorder (ASD)	social communication disorder
autism	motor disorders
echolalia	Tourette's disorder
intellectual disability (ID)	persistent motor or vocal tic disorder (PMVTD)
fetal alcohol syndrome (FAS)	stereotypic movement disorder
specific learning disorder	developmental coordination disorder
communication disorders	major neurocognitive disorder

dementia

mild neurocognitive disorder

aphasia

palilalia

apraxia

agnosia

executive functions

Alzheimer's disease (AD)

neurofibrillary tangles

plaques

beta-amyloid

vascular neurocognitive disorder

cerebrovascular disease

stroke

traumatic brain injury (TBI)

delirium

Chapter 11

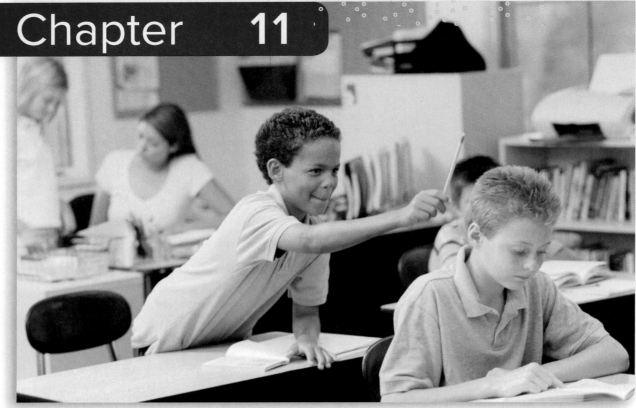

Bananastock/age fotostock

Disruptive, Impulse-Control, and Conduct Disorders

CHAPTER OUTLINE

Disorders of Conduct and Impulse Control Along the Continuum

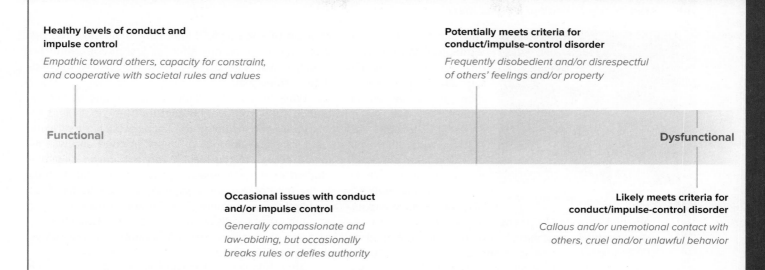

Healthy levels of conduct and impulse control

Empathic toward others, capacity for constraint, and cooperative with societal rules and values

Potentially meets criteria for conduct/impulse-control disorder

Frequently disobedient and/or disrespectful of others' feelings and/or property

Functional

Dysfunctional

Occasional issues with conduct and/or impulse control

Generally compassionate and law-abiding, but occasionally breaks rules or defies authority

Likely meets criteria for conduct/impulse-control disorder

Callous and/or unemotional contact with others, cruel and/or unlawful behavior

The disorders discussed in this chapter all involve disruptive, impulsive, and antisocial behavior that violates major social norms. You've no doubt observed that people vary in how cooperative they are with social norms and in how empathetic and caring they are toward other people. On one end of the continuum are people who exemplify a strong social and moral code and who deeply care for others, even sacrificing their own well-being on behalf of others (think Mother Teresa). Most of us are a little farther along the continuum: Although we generally are law-abiding and try to be compassionate toward others, we break a few rules now and then (e.g., driving too fast) and are sometimes unkind to others, especially when we are stressed or in a bad mood. Yet farther along the continuum are people who think some social norms don't apply to them and who can be downright cruel toward others, particularly when it helps them accomplish their goals, such as Kevin Spacey's character Francis Underwood in the television program *House of Cards* or Prince Joffrey in *Game of Thrones*.

The individuals who receive the diagnoses discussed in this chapter persistently break basic social rules regulating behavior and often treat others very badly, even being aggressive or violent toward others. Two of the disorders we discuss apply only to children. Children diagnosed with *oppositional defiant disorder* are chronically angry and irritable; are argumentative and defiant, refusing to comply with adult requests; and are

vindictive toward others, often blaming others for their own mistakes and bad behavior. Children diagnosed with *conduct disorder* act in even more antisocial ways, repeatedly being aggressive and cruel toward animals and people, vandalizing and destroying others' property, stealing and lying, and violating basic family and school rules. The other two disorders are diagnosed only in individuals age 18 and older. *Intermittent explosive disorder* is characterized by repeated outbursts of verbal or physical aggression toward others that is far out of proportion to any provocation. *Antisocial personality disorder* is characterized by a chronic pattern of disregard for the basic rights of others. People with this disorder are selfish, manipulative, deceitful, cruel, and often aggressive toward others in order to get what they want.

Throughout this chapter, we discuss biological and psychosocial factors that appear to contribute to the development of these disorders. These factors may also help account for bad behavior that falls short of meeting any of the diagnoses—the everyday bad behavior we see in people with whom we interact or people in the media. Fundamentally, all behavior, good and bad, moral and immoral, is tied to biological and psychosocial factors. This raises the following question: What are the implications of identifying causes of bad behavior for how society should deal with people who violate major social norms and hurt others?

Extraordinary People

Ted Bundy, *Portrait of a Serial Killer*

Bettmann/Contributor/Getty Images

Ted Bundy was born in Burlington, Vermont. He did well in school and typically earned A's in most of his classes, although he was sometimes in trouble for fighting with other children. He later attributed much of his scholastic success to his mother's diligent efforts to encourage him. Despite his fondness for his mother, they never discussed personal matters, and he stated that their relationship was not an open one. Bundy reported that he found it difficult to socialize and often chose to be alone or engage in solitary hobbies when in high school. Although he was described as charming, intelligent, and attractive, he had limited social contacts because he did not enjoy drinking and preferred the role of a scholar. He also had relatively few experiences with girls in high school and only went on one date.

After graduation, Bundy became involved with politics and worked on several successful campaigns, where he was described as being responsible, dedicated, and hardworking. Through this experience he was able to establish a wide social network. Bundy used his charm and quick wit to establish himself as an up-and-coming politician and even was referred to as a "young JFK" for his political savvy.

At age 27, Bundy began abducting, raping, and murdering young women. He often lured these women into his car by deception, such as by impersonating a police detective. The brutal murders included bludgeoning, mutilation, and rape. The murders attracted media and police attention, yet Bundy continued to abduct women and evade detection. He planned and executed the kidnappings with great care, in order to avoid discovery. His colleagues found him charming and endearing, and they could not imagine that he was capable of such acts. Bundy was finally arrested approximately 15 months after his first murder. After his arrest, he was linked to several murders and was scheduled to stand trial.

While in custody, his charm, good looks, and cooperation soon won over his captors. They gave him special treatment, including the least restrictive restraints. He insisted on defending himself in court and was allowed access to the local library, where he diligently studied legal documents. He proved to be a quick study in the field of law and was able to delay his hearings and trial for quite some time. During this delay he lost enough weight to fit his body through a 12-inch aperture and escaped by crawling through openings above the jail cells and offices.

After escaping custody he settled near Florida State University. Not long after, he was once again raping, beating, and killing women. During this time, he lived under a false name and supported himself by using stolen credit cards. He was eventually arrested after bludgeoning to death many members of a sorority house as they slept. He was subsequently found guilty and twice sentenced to death. However, his legal acumen was so high during the trial that, after sentencing him, the judge stated that Bundy "should have been a lawyer." These legal skills continued to serve him while in prison as he delayed his execution for 10 years. Others, however, suggested that his arrogant self-confidence contributed to a failure to obtain competent legal counsel and that his effort to serve as his own lawyer ultimately was harmful to his defense.

While in prison, Bundy granted numerous interview requests and revealed that he committed the murders as a way to gain full possession of the women. He claimed that the rapes were not brutal and that he had attempted to make the murders as painless as possible for the victims. Bundy never expressed any explicit or compelling feelings of remorse for the murders. In fact he withheld the identities of many of his victims as a way to delay his execution. (Adapted from T. A. Widiger, personal communication, 2009)

Ted Bundy was one of the most extreme examples of what many people call a *psychopath* or *sociopath*. He could be charming, charismatic, cunning, and hideously sadistic, deriving great pleasure from inflicting pain on others. He never accepted responsibility for his actions, blaming his unlawful behavior on the bad influence of the violent pornography he was attracted to as a youth.

The disorders we consider in this chapter all reflect the tendency to engage in behavior that violates the basic rights of others or major social norms. In most cases these antisocial behaviors are nowhere near as extreme as Ted Bundy's, but they can still exact a heavy toll on the targets of the behavior. We start with conduct disorder and oppositional defiant disorder, which by definition begin during childhood. Then we discuss intermittent explosive disorder, which, as the name implies, is characterized by intermittent but recurrent aggressive outbursts. Finally, we cover antisocial personality disorder, which is diagnosed only in adults and could be applied to Ted Bundy.

CONDUCT DISORDER AND OPPOSITIONAL DEFIANT DISORDER

Have you ever lied, stolen something, or hit someone? Most of us would have to answer yes to at least one of these. However, relatively few would answer yes to the following questions:

- Have you ever pulled a knife or a gun on another person?
- Have you ever forced someone into sexual activity at knifepoint?
- Have you ever deliberately set a fire with the hope of damaging someone's property?
- Have you ever broken into someone else's car or house with the intention of stealing?

Many young people who have **conduct disorder** answer yes to these questions and engage in other serious transgressions of societal norms for behavior (see the *DSM-5* criteria in Table 1). These children have a chronic pattern of unconcern for the basic rights of others. Consider Phillip, in the following case study.

CASE STUDY

Phillip, age 12, was suspended from a small-town Iowa school and referred for psychiatric treatment by his principal, who sent the following note:

This child has been a continual problem since coming to our school. He does not get along on the playground because he is mean to other children. He disobeys school rules, teases the patrol children, steals from the other children, and defies all authority. Phillip keeps getting into fights with other children on the bus.

The truth is not in Phillip. When caught in actual misdeeds, he denies everything and takes upon himself an air of injured innocence. He believes we are picking on him. His attitude is sullen when he is refused anything. He pouts, and when asked why he does these things, he points to his head and says, Because I'm not right up here. This boy needs help badly. He does not seem to have any friends. His aggressive behavior prevents the children from liking him. Our school psychologist tested Phillip, and the

results indicated average intelligence, but his school achievement is only at the third- and low fourth-grade level. (Source: Jenkins, R. L., *Behavior disorders of childhood and adolescence.* Springfield, IL: Charles C Thomas, 1973, 60–64.)

Conduct disorder is defined as a repetitive and persistent pattern of aggressive, defiant, cruel, deceitful, and destructive antisocial behaviors that violate the basic rights of others or rules of society. The behaviors of children with conduct disorder fall into four categories: (1) aggression to people and animals, (2) destruction of property, (3) deceitfulness or theft, and (4) serious violations of rules. Conduct disorder is one of the most challenging and unmanageable mental health problems in children and adolescents. When it persists, it is one of the strongest predictors for the development of antisocial personality disorder, substance abuse, and criminal behavior, especially violent and severe crimes (Kerekes et al., 2020; Moore, Silberg, Roberson-Nay, & Mezuk, 2017).

Conduct disorder typically develops in childhood or adolescence with behaviors rarely, if ever, emerging in adulthood. In addition to the heightened risk for legal problems and contact with police, individuals with this disorder are also more likely to experience poor physical health, comorbid psychiatric conditions, and earlier death. Conduct disorder can have its onset before 10 years of age and children with early-onset conduct disorder are at an increased risk for persistent difficulties. The prevalence of conduct disorder ranges from 2 to 5 percent in children (5 to 12 years) and 5 to 9 percent in adolescents (13 to 18 years). The lifetime prevalence of conduct disorder is approximately 12 percent in males and 7 percent in females (Kerekes et al., 2020; Patel, Amaravadi, Bhullar, Lekireddy, & Win, 2018).

Boys are more likely to present with symptoms of conduct disorder than girls, but this gender difference may vary across the lifespan. During adolescence this changes and both genders show increased rates of conduct disorder, but boys are still two to three times more likely to be diagnosed than girls. The prevalence of conduct disorder is fairly consistent across countries that differ in race and ethnicity, but factors such as socioeconomic status (SES), neighborhood, and parenting practices may play a role in the development of this disorder. The lifetime prevalence of conduct disorder is 6.9 percent among Hispanics, 4.9 percent in Blacks, and 5.0 percent in whites. Caucasian children are more likely to be diagnosed with oppositional defiant disorder (ODD), whereas African American children are more likely to be diagnosed with conduct disorder (Patel et al., 2018).

TABLE 1   *DSM-5* Criteria for Conduct Disorder

A. A repetitive and persistent pattern of behavior in which the basic rights of others or major age-appropriate societal norms or rules are violated, as manifested by the presence of at least three of the following 15 criteria in the past 12 months from any of the categories below, with at least one criterion present in the past 6 months:

Aggression to People and Animals

1. Often bullies, threatens, or intimidates others
2. Often initiates physical fights
3. Has used a weapon that can cause serious physical harm to others (e.g., a bat, brick, broken bottle, knife, gun)
4. Has been physically cruel to people
5. Has been physically cruel to animals
6. Has stolen while confronting a victim (e.g., mugging, purse snatching, extortion, armed robbery)
7. Has forced someone into sexual activity

Destruction of Property

8. Has deliberately engaged in fire setting with the intention of causing serious damage
9. Has deliberately destroyed others' property (other than by fire setting)

Deceitfulness or Theft

10. Has broken into someone else's house, building, or car
11. Often lies to obtain goods or favors or to avoid obligations (e.g., "cons" others)
12. Has stolen items of nontrivial value without confronting a victim (e.g., shoplifting, but without breaking and entering; forgery)

Serious Violations of Rules

13. Often stays out at night despite parental prohibitions, beginning before age 13 years
14. Has run away from home overnight at least twice while living in the parental or parental surrogate home, or once without returning for a lengthy period
15. Is often truant from school, beginning before age 13 years

B. The disturbance in behavior causes clinically significant impairment in social, academic, or occupational functioning.

C. If the individual is age 18 years or older, criteria are not met for antisocial personality disorder.

An important distinction is made between conduct disorder that begins in childhood and conduct disorder that begins in adolescence (Frick & Nigg, 2012; Moffitt, 2006), and the *DSM-5* requires that conduct disorder be specified based on its age at onset. Children with **childhood-onset conduct disorder** (beginning before age 10) often show behavioral problems in preschool or early elementary school, and their problems tend to worsen as they grow older. They are more likely than individuals with **adolescent-onset conduct disorder** (beginning at age 10 or later) to continue to engage in antisocial behavior into adolescence and adulthood, a pattern called **life-course-persistent antisocial behavior** (American Psychiatric Association, 2013; Moffitt, Caspi, Harrington, & Milne, 2002; Odgers et al., 2008). For example, as adolescents, about 50 percent of those diagnosed with childhood-onset conduct disorder engage in criminal behavior and drug abuse. As adults, about 75 to 85 percent are chronically unemployed, have a history of unstable personal relationships, frequently engage in impulsive physical aggression, or abuse their spouse (Moffitt et al., 2008). Between 35 and 40 percent are diagnosed with antisocial personality disorder as adults. Those with early-onset conduct disorder are more likely to experience lower quality of life in adulthood due to their persistent antisocial behavior, which includes poorer mental health, substance use problems, unemployment, and family relationship issues (Moore et al., 2017).

The *DSM-5* allows another specifier for the diagnosis—*"with limited prosocial emotions"*—which can be applied to children who meet the full criteria for conduct disorder and show at least two of the following characteristics in multiple relationships and settings: (a) lack of remorse or guilt for their actions, (b) lack of empathy for others (callousness), (c) lack of concern about performance at school, at work, or in other important activities, and (d) shallow or deficient emotions (e.g., insincerity in emotions, using emotions to manipulate others). Children with this callous, unemotional presentation are less reactive to signs of fear and distress in others and less sensitive to punishment (Frick, 2012, 2016). They tend to be fearless and thrill-seeking. These traits characterize **psychopathy,** a more severe, aggressive, and difficult-to-treat pattern predictive of more long-term problems into adulthood (Cleckley, 1941/1982; Hare & Neumann, 2008; Kimonis , 2015). Because psychopathy has been studied more in adults than in children, we will discuss it below in relation to antisocial personality disorder.

African American males under the age of 11 are at the highest risk of inpatient hospitalization for conduct disorder. Children from low-income families with conduct disorder are 1.5 times more likely to require inpatient admission as compared to higher-income families. Additionally, these children are eleven times more likely to have comorbid psychosis and seven times more likely to have depression. This very significant chance that additional psychiatric disorders will be present in children with conduct disorder may exacerbate the illness and require inpatient care which makes this disorder debilitating for both the children and families (Patel et al., 2018).

The *DSM-5* also recognizes a less severe pattern of chronic misbehavior, **oppositional defiant disorder (ODD)** (see Table 2). Note that the symptoms are grouped into three types, reflecting both emotional and behavioral symptom categories. Unlike children

---

TABLE 2   *DSM-5* Criteria for Oppositional Defiant Disorder

A. A pattern of angry/irritable mood, argumentative/defiant behavior, or vindictiveness lasting at least 6 months as evidenced by at least four symptoms from any of the following categories, and exhibited during interaction with at least one individual who is not a sibling.

Angry/Irritable Mood

1. Often loses temper
2. Is often touchy or easily annoyed
3. Is often angry and resentful

Argumentative/Defiant Behavior

4. Often argues with authority figures, or for children and adolescents, with adults
5. Often actively defies or refuses to comply with requests from authority figures or with rules
6. Often deliberately annoys others
7. Often blames others for his or her mistakes or misbehavior

Vindictiveness

8. Has been spiteful or vindictive at least twice within the past 6 months

Note: The persistence and frequency of these behaviors should be used to distinguish a behavior that is within normal limits from a behavior that is symptomatic. For children under 5 years of age, the behavior should occur on most days for a period of at least 6 months unless otherwise noted (Criterion A8). For individuals 5 years or older, the behavior should occur at least once per week for at least 6 months, unless otherwise noted (Criterion A8). While these frequency criteria provide guidance on a minimal level of frequency to define symptoms, other factors should also be considered, such as whether the frequency and intensity of the behaviors are outside a range that is normative for the individual's developmental level, gender, and culture.

B. The disturbance in behavior is associated with distress in the individual or others in his or her immediate social context (e.g., family, peer group, work colleagues), or it impacts negatively on social, educational, occupational, or other important areas of functioning.

C. The behaviors do not occur exclusively during the course of a psychotic, substance use, depressive, or bipolar disorder. Also, the criteria are not met for disruptive mood dysregulation disorder.

with conduct disorder, children with ODD are not aggressive toward people or animals, do not destroy property, and do not show a pattern of theft and deceit. They are, however, chronically negativistic, defiant, disobedient, and hostile which can be limited to only one setting, like home for example. Children with ODD experience impaired social function even if the setting in which they display these symptoms is limited (American Psychiatric Association, 2013; Frick & Nigg, 2012). We see several symptoms of ODD in 9-year-old Jeremy in the following case study.

CASE STUDY

12-year-old Dylan was recently referred to the school-based therapist for his problematic classroom behaviors. Dylan has displayed behaviors that concern his teachers and parents since kindergarten, and they appear to be worsening. Dylan is often in trouble at school for harassing other children which is commonly displayed in teasing, name calling and physically aggressive behaviors. Dylan tends to pick fights with his classmates and is described by others as angry, difficult and mean. There are moments, despite his behavior, where Dylan appears to enjoy school, but these are short-lived when he cannot control the situation. Teachers have consistently reported that it appears as if Dylan enjoys antagonizing other children and he is almost always the one who starts a fight. Dylan denies that this is the case, but he is frequently involved in physical or verbal altercations with various classmates.

Dylan also has trouble with adult interactions. When asked to follow the rules at school or home, Dylan often becomes angry and combative, sometimes screaming or throwing items in response. Class work is particularly difficult for Dylan who does not believe he should have to complete assignments or listen to the teachers. For example, at the end of gym class, Dylan refused to stop playing basketball and wanted more time rather than returning to class. When approached by the gym teacher, Dylan became enraged and repeatedly threw basketballs at the teacher, striking him multiple times. Dylan's parents are also frustrated with this behaviors at home. While Dylan will sometimes follow directions and listen to his parents, more likely than not, he is defiant and disrespectful. Dylan will often lie about things that he has done and takes no responsibility for his actions, particularly those that cause others pain.

Often thought to be a more mild precursor to conduct disorder, symptoms of ODD often begin during the toddler and preschool years. Being defiant and obstinate are common characteristics of "the terrible twos," and concerns have been raised that the diagnosis of ODD pathologizes a behavior that is typical in young children. Indeed, some children who meet the criteria for ODD seem to outgrow these behaviors by late childhood or early adolescence. Children diagnosed with ODD, however, are significantly more likely than children who do not meet the criteria for the diagnosis to subsequently develop conduct disorder, substance use disorders, and mood and anxiety disorders (Erskine et al., 2016; Loeber, Burke, & Pardini, 2009b).

Across cultures, boys are about three times more likely than girls to be diagnosed with conduct disorder or ODD; this discrepancy is less stark in adolescence than in childhood (Canino, Polanczyk, Bauermeister, Rohde, Frick, 2010; Frick & Nigg, 2012). Males are 10 to 15 times more likely than females to have life-course-persistent antisocial behavior (Moffitt, 2006). The biological and psychosocial causes of these disorders may be present more often in boys than in girls. Also, boys with conduct disorder tend to be more physically aggressive than girls with conduct disorder and thus more likely to draw attention (Maughan, Pickles, Rowe, Costello, & Angold, 2000; Tiet, Wasserman, Loeber, McReynolds, & Miller, 2001).

Some researchers have suggested that antisocial behavior is not rarer in girls than in boys but just looks different (Crick, Ostrov, & Kawabata, 2007). Girls' aggression is more likely to be indirect and verbal

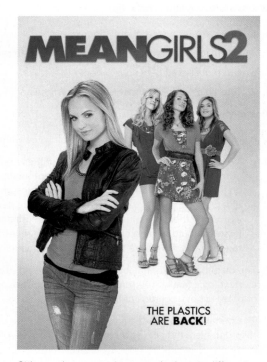

Girls may be aggressive toward others in different ways than boys. *AF archive/Alamy Stock Photo*

rather than physical. Girls appear to engage in relational aggression, such as excluding their peers, gossiping about them, and colluding with others to damage the social status of their targets (Crick et al., 2007).

However, girls and boys with conduct disorder are equally likely to engage in stealing, lying, and substance abuse (Tiet et al., 2001). Long-term studies of girls diagnosed with conduct disorder find that, as adolescents and adults, they also show high rates of depression and anxiety disorders, severe marital problems, criminal activity, and early, unplanned pregnancies (Loeber & Burke, 2011; Moffitt, Caspi, Rutter, & Silva, 2001).

Contributors to Conduct Disorder and Oppositional Defiant Disorder

The risk factors for conduct disorder and ODD are largely the same, so we discuss them together, referring primarily to conduct disorder because the majority of the research has focused on this disorder.

Biological Factors

Children with conduct disorder are more likely than children without the disorder to have parents with a history of antisocial behavior (Salvatore & Dick, 2016). Twin and adoption studies indicate that this aggregation of antisocial behaviors in families is due to both genetic and environmental factors (Polderman et al., 2015; Silberg, Maes, & Eaves, 2012). Genetics appears to play a particularly strong role in childhood-onset conduct disorder. Several specific genes have been associated with an increased risk of conduct disorder and ODD primarily genes involved in the regulation of the neurotransmitters dopamine, serotonin, and norepinephrine (Moffitt et al., 2008; Salvatore & Dick, 2016). One of these genes is the monoamine oxidase A (MAOA) gene, which encodes an enzyme that metabolizes serotonin, dopamine, and norepinephrine (see meta-analyses by Ficks & Waldman, 2014; Taylor & Kim-Cohen, 2007). Several studies have found that children who have both an abnormal variant of the MAOA gene and a history of childhood maltreatment (including physical and sexual abuse as well as neglect) are especially likely to develop aggressive traits in general, and conduct disorder in particular (e.g., Caspi et al., 2002). This is another example of interactions between genes and environment contributing to psychopathology. As in other disorders, however, more recent findings on such interactions in conduct disorder and ODD are more mixed (Dick et al., 2015; Salvatore & Dick, 2016).

The exact mechanisms by which genetic and environmental vulnerabilities create conduct disorder are still being mapped (Dodge, 2009; Frick, 2016). Children with conduct disorder may have neurological deficits in those brain systems responsible for planning and controlling behavior and processing reward and punishment (Matthys, Vanderschuren, & Schutter, 2013). They have high rates of comorbid attention-deficit/hyperactivity disorder (ADHD; see the chapter "Neurodevelopmental and Neurocognitive Disorders"; Beauchaine, Hinshaw, & Pang, 2010), a fundamentally neurological disorder characterized by difficulties in attention, impulsivity, and hyperactivity.

Neuroimaging studies show abnormalities in the functional areas of the prefrontal cortex involved in responding to emotional stimuli, including the anterior cingulate (Stadler et al., 2007; Sterzer, Stadler, Krebs, Kleinschmidt, & Poustka, 2005). They also show less amygdala activity in response to emotional stimuli (Sterzer et al., 2005), possibly suggesting that children with conduct disorder do not process emotional cues as do healthy children (see Matthys et al., 2013). Individuals with ODD and conduct disorder display deficits in multiple neurocognitive processes. Disruptive behavior has been linked to impaired facial emotion recognition and cognitive functioning that may lead to decreased self-regulation. There is also a hypersensitivity to negative emotions, such as anger, which may facilitate "hot-tempered" aggressive responses which are characteristic of ODD. Conversely, there is a noted decreased sensitivity to signs of distress of others, such as sad or frightened facial expressions, which suggest an impairment in empathy, a common issue found within the antisocial populations. Among those with conduct disorder, impaired emotion recognition has most often been found for fear and sadness, but recent research also finds problems with other basic emotions like disgust, anger, and surprise. The ability to recognize emotions is a complex process that requires attention and working memory. Individuals with conduct disorder and ODD may have problems with executive function and visual working memory which may contribute to difficulties recognizing various emotions in others (Kleine Deters et al., 2020). Indeed, children with conduct disorder show deficits on tasks that measure planning and organizing ability and the processing of emotional cues (Forslund, Brocki, Bohlin, Granqvist, & Eninger, 2016; Hobson, Scott, & Rubia, 2011).

In addition to genetics, another source of the neurological deficits these children have may be exposure to neurotoxins and drugs prenatally or during the preschool years. Boys whose mothers smoke during pregnancy are 2.6 times more likely to demonstrate oppositional behavior in early childhood, followed by increasingly more aggressive and severe antisocial behavior as they grow older (Wakschlag, Pickett, Kasza, & Loeber, 2006).

Serotonin has been widely known for its influence on emotions, but recent studies find this

SHADES OF GRAY

Consider the description below of Jake.

Jake has been larger than most kids from the day he was born. Now, at age 10, he towers over all the other boys and is 15 pounds heavier than most, with most of the extra weight being muscle. Over the last couple of years, Jake's parents encouraged him to channel his size and energies into sports, but he wasn't very coordinated and was teased by other kids, who called him "the gorilla." When this happened, Jake would sometimes lash out at the child who teased him, punching or kicking him. Given Jake's size advantage, this behavior usually resulted in moderate to severe injury for the other child. In the last 6 months Jake has been ambushing children who have been mean to him in the past on their way home from school and beating them up fairly severely. This has accomplished Jake's goals—the retribution against the other children feels good, and he doesn't get teased much anymore. Lately he's taken to ambushing children who have never teased him, just to send a message to others to stay clear of him and treat him with respect.

Could Jake be diagnosed with a conduct disorder based on the information in the description? (Discussion appears at the end of this chapter.)

neurotransmitter is also significantly correlated with the regulation of violence and aggression (Hantoosh, Ameen, & Amin, 2021; Schechter et al., 2017). Recent research has found a relationship between disrupted serotonin production and aggressive and impulsive behavior which may help clarify potential genetic influences of antisocial behavior. (Cherepkova, Maksimov & Aftanas, 2018). One study of a large community-based sample found that young men with high blood serotonin levels relative to the levels of other men their age were much more likely to have committed a violent crime (Moffitt et al., 1998). Several other studies, but not all, have found an association between measures of serotonin activity and antisocial behavior in children (Matthys et al., 2013).

Several studies have shown that children with conduct disorder have a slower heart rate than children without the disorder, both while resting and especially when confronted with a stressor (Fanti, 2018; Ortiz & Raine, 2004). They also show abnormal cortisol levels both at rest and in response to a stressor (Matthys et al., 2013). Because they become less physiologically aroused than other children when confronted by stressors, children with conduct disorder may be more willing to take risks and may have more difficulty learning from being punished for their behavior. However, children with conduct disorder who also experience anxiety symptoms and emotion dysregulation may show more, rather than less, physiological reactivity (Fanti, 2018).

People often link aggressive behavior to the hormone testosterone. A meta-analysis of of studies on testosterone and aggression in humans found a small but statistically significant correlation of .14 (Book, Starzyk, & Quinsey, 2001). The association between testosterone and aggression depends on the social context of the participants. In a study of 9- to 15-year-old boys, higher testosterone levels were associated with more conduct disorder symptoms in boys whose peers engaged in socially deviant behaviors (Rowe, Maughan, Worthman, Costello, & Angold, 2004). In boys whose peers did not engage in such behaviors, testosterone was associated with leadership rather than with conduct disorder symptoms.

Social Factors

Conduct disorder and ODD are found more frequently in children in lower socioeconomic classes and in urban areas than in children in higher socioeconomic classes and in rural areas (Shaw & Shelleby, 2014; Yoshikawa, Aber, & Beardslee, 2012). An "experiment of nature" provided evidence that poverty may play a causal role in antisocial behavior. For several years, researchers had been following 1,420 children in rural North Carolina, about one-quarter of whom were Native American (Costello, Compton, Keeler, & Angold, 2003). During the study, a casino operated by Native Americans opened, providing a sudden and substantial increase in income for the families of some of these children. The rates of conduct and ODD decreased in those Native American children whose families benefited from the casino money.

The quality of parenting that children receive, particularly children with vulnerability to conduct disturbances, is strongly related to whether they develop the full syndrome of conduct disorder (Kim-Cohen, Caspi, Rutter, Polo Tomas, & Moffitt, 2006; Loeber, Burke, & Pardini, 2009a; Shaw & Shelleby, 2014). Children who develop conduct disorder symptoms tend to have been difficult babies, toddlers, and younger children, at least as reported by their parents (Forbes, Rapee, Camberis, & McMahon, 2017). They are described as having been irritable, demanding, disobedient, and impulsive. They seemed to lack self-control and responded to frustration with aggression. Some theorists argue that such children are born with a biologically based difficult temperament that interacts with parenting and environmental factors to produce behavioral problems (Caspi et al., 2003).

Children who are physically abused or severely neglected by their parents are more likely to develop disruptive and delinquent behavior (Stouthamer-Loeber, Loeber, Homish, & Wei, 2001). Children whose parents are not involved in their everyday life—for example, whose parents do not know who their children's friends are or what their children are doing in school—are more likely to develop conduct disturbances. When parents do interact with their children with conduct disturbances, the interactions often are characterized by hostility, physical violence, and ridicule. Such parents frequently ignore their children or are absent from home, but when the children transgress, the parents lash out violently (Kim-Cohen et al., 2006; Shaw & Shelleby, 2014; Smith & Farrington, 2004). These parents are likely to physically punish boys more severely than girls, which may account partially for the higher rate of conduct disturbances in boys than in girls.

Malnutrition is increasingly recognized as a childhood risk factor for externalizing behaviors, such as aggression, hyperactivity, delinquency, conduct disorder, and antisocial personality disorder. Malnutrition can interfere with brain development by reducing neuronal growth, altering neurotransmitter performance, and impairing cognitive functions. Poor nutrition adversely impacts neuropsychological functioning which can significantly decrease self-control and elevate the risk of misconduct. Protein deficiency impacts brain development and significantly contributes to the development of antisocial behavior. Since proteins are synthesized primarily from amino acids, it is important to acknowledge that diet poor in amino acid tryptophan may lead to high rates of aggressive and antisocial behavior (Hantoosh et al., 2021).

Young people living in such families may turn to their peers to receive validation and escape their parents. Unfortunately, their peer group may consist of others with similar conduct disturbances who tend to

Children are more likely to exhibit disruptive and delinquent behavior if they have been physically abused. *Piotr Wawzyniuk/ Shutterstock*

encourage delinquent acts and even provide opportunities for those acts. For example, they may dare a new group member to commit a robbery to "show he is a man" and even provide him with a weapon and a getaway car. Children who become part of a deviant peer group are especially likely to begin abusing alcohol and illicit drugs, which in turn leads to further deviant acts (Loeber et al., 2009a).

Individuals with antisocial tendencies also tend to choose mates with similar tendencies (Smith & Farrington, 2004). Conversely, those who form close relationships with others who do not have a conduct disturbance are much more likely to outgrow their behaviors. Delinquent young men who marry young women with no history of conduct problems tend to cease their delinquent acts permanently (Sampson & Laub, 1992).

Cognitive Factors

Children with conduct disorder tend to process information about social interactions in ways that promote aggressive reactions (Forslund et al., 2016). They assume that others will be aggressive toward them, and they use these assumptions—rather than cues from specific situations—to interpret the actions of their peers (Helseth, Waschbusch, King, & Willoughby, 2015). For example, when accidentally bumped into by another child, a child with conduct disorder will assume that the bump was intentional and meant to provoke a fight. Children with conduct disorder tend to consider a narrow range of responses to perceived provocation by a peer, usually including aggression (see Fontaine & Dodge, 2006). When pressed to consider other responses, they generate ineffective or vague ideas and often judge anything besides aggression as a useless or unattractive response (Helseth et al., 2015).

Children who think about social interactions this way are likely to act aggressively toward others. Others then may retaliate—other children will hit back, parents and teachers will punish them, and people will perceive them negatively. These reactions feed the children's assumption that the world is against them, causing them to misinterpret future actions by others. A cycle of interactions can be built that maintains and encourages aggressive, antisocial behaviors.

Again, the best evidence that thinking patterns are causes, rather than simply correlates, of antisocial behavior in children comes from studies showing that changing children's aggressive thinking patterns can reduce their aggressive behavior. We will look to these and other interventions as they are used with children with conduct disorder.

An Integrative Model

Biological, social, and cognitive factors contributing to conduct disorder often may coincide and interact,

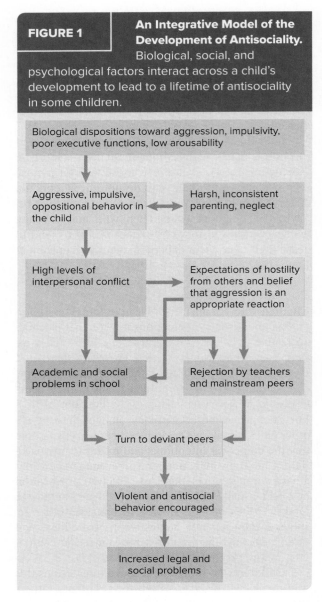

FIGURE 1

An Integrative Model of the Development of Antisociality. Biological, social, and psychological factors interact across a child's development to lead to a lifetime of antisociality in some children.

Biological dispositions toward aggression, impulsivity, poor executive functions, low arousability

Aggressive, impulsive, oppositional behavior in the child

Harsh, inconsistent parenting, neglect

High levels of interpersonal conflict

Expectations of hostility from others and belief that aggression is an appropriate reaction

Academic and social problems in school

Rejection by teachers and mainstream peers

Turn to deviant peers

Violent and antisocial behavior encouraged

Increased legal and social problems

in children with conduct disorder are more irritable, impulsive, awkward, overreactive, inattentive, and slow to learn than their peers. This makes them difficult to care for and puts them at increased risk for maltreatment and neglect. Early symptoms of aggression and oppositional behavior in a child lead to and interact with harsh discipline and a lack of warmth from parents and conflicts with aggressive peers. These children are at risk for academic and social problems in school, which can motivate them to turn to deviant peer groups that encourage antisocial behavior. Along the way, such children learn that the world is hostile and that they must defend themselves rapidly and aggressively. They are prone to impulsive behaviors or rash reactions to others. These children enter adulthood with a long history of negative interactions with others, violent and impulsive outbursts, and alienation from mainstream society. All these factors feed on one another, perpetuating the cycle of antisocial behavior into adulthood.

In a longitudinal study following children from age 3 into adulthood, Terri Moffitt, Avshalom Caspi, and colleagues (Moffitt & Caspi, 2001; Moffitt et al., 2001) found that the combination of a biological disposition toward cognitive deficits and a difficult temperament plus growing up in a risky environment characterized by inadequate parenting and disrupted family bonds tended to lead to conduct disorder that developed in childhood and persisted into adulthood. In contrast, youth who were antisocial only in adolescence were much less likely to have this combination of biological and environmental risk factors. Another study found impulsivity in boys to be linked to a greater risk for late-adolescent delinquency only among those who grew up in poor and violent neighborhoods (Lynam et al., 2000).

Treatments for Conduct Disorder and Oppositional Defiant Disorder

Psychological and social treatments can reduce violent and disruptive behavior in children with these disorders. Some children are also given medications to decrease their emotional dysregulation and difficult behaviors.

Psychological and Social Therapies

Most psychotherapies for conduct disorder are cognitive-behavioral in focus and aim to change children's ways of interpreting interpersonal interactions by teaching them to take and respect the perspectives of others, to use *self-talk* to control impulsive behaviors, and to use more adaptive ways of solving conflicts than aggression (Kazdin, 2015; Powell, Lochman, Boxmeyer, Barry, & Pardini, 2017). Many

sending a child on a trajectory toward antisocial behaviors that is difficult to stop (Figure 1) (Frick, 2016; Loeber et al., 2009a). Antisocial parents appear both to confer on their children a genetic vulnerability to conduct disturbances and to parent them in ways that engender antisocial behaviors—for example, exhibiting violence and hostility, neglect, and a lack of warmth (Frick, 2016; Loeber et al., 2009a; Silberg et al., 2012). These children also may be exposed to maternal drug use, poor prenatal nutrition, pre- and postnatal exposure to toxic agents, child abuse, poverty, and the stress of growing up in a violent neighborhood (Jennings, Perez, & Reingle Gonzalez, 2018; Loeber et al., 2009a; Silberg et al., 2003). Infants and toddlers with the neuropsychological problems seen therapies try to involve parents in order to change family interaction patterns that are helping maintain the children's antisocial behaviors (Webster-Stratton & Reid, 2017).

The first step in cognitive-behavioral therapy is to teach children to recognize situations that trigger anger or aggressive and impulsive behaviors. Therapists observe children in their natural settings and then point out situations in which they misbehave or seem angry. They then discuss hypothetical situations and how the children would react to them, asking older children to keep a diary of their feelings and behaviors. The children also learn to analyze their thoughts in these situations and to consider alternative ways to interpret them. The children's assumptions that others intentionally act meanly toward them are challenged, and they learn to adopt other people's perspectives on situations. Children may be taught to use self-talk, repeating phrases to help them avoid reacting negatively to situations.

Therapists teach adaptive problem-solving skills by discussing real and hypothetical problem situations with children and helping them generate positive solutions. For example, if a therapist and a child are discussing how to respond to another child who has cut in line in the lunchroom, the therapist initially might model an assertive (rather than aggressive) response, such as saying "I would like you to move to the back of the line" to the child cutting in. Then the child in therapy might practice the assertive response, perhaps also pretending to be the child cutting in line in order to gain some perspective on the other child's behavior.

Some psychosocial therapies for children with conduct disorder include parents, particularly if the family dynamics support the children's behavior (Kazdin, 2017, 2018). Parents learn to reinforce positive behaviors in their children and to discourage aggressive or antisocial behaviors. They also are given nonviolent discipline techniques and strategies for controlling their own angry outbursts. These behavioral techniques are especially important in treating younger children, who may not be able to analyze and challenge their thinking and problem-solving processes.

Unfortunately, it can be difficult to get those parents who need the most improvement in parenting skills to participate in therapy (Kazdin, 2017). Therapists also need to be sensitive to cultural differences in behavioral norms for children and parents. For example, in families of color it often is useful to engage the extended family (grandparents, aunts, uncles) in family therapy as well as the parents, depending on cultural values and norms (Chu & Leino, 2017).

All these cognitive-behavioral therapies—particularly interventions made in the home, in the classroom, and in peer groups—reduce aggressive and impulsive behaviors in children (Kazdin, 2015;

Webster-Stratton & Reid, 2017). Unfortunately, many children relapse, particularly if their parents have poor parenting skills, a history of alcoholism or drug abuse, or some other psychopathology. Interventions are most likely to have long-term positive effects if they begin early in a child's life, and booster sessions after a course of initial therapy can help a child avoid relapse (Kazdin, 2017; Shaw & Shelleby, 2014).

One ambitious program attempted to delay or prevent the onset of conduct disorder in children who showed a number of risk factors, such as a parental history of antisocial behavior. This program, called Fast Track, provided intensive cognitive-behavioral therapy to children and behavioral training to parents as described above, as well as academic tutoring from kindergarten through grade 10. After the first 3 years, the children in the intervention group showed better social interaction skills and peer relations and less aggressive behavior in the classroom than children in the control group, who received no intervention (Conduct Problems Prevention Research Group, 2002). After 5 years, 22 percent of the intervention group had conduct disorder compared to 29 percent of the control group (Conduct Problems Prevention Research Group, 2007). As adolescents, those in the intervention group reported less antisocial behavior and were less likely to seek outpatient care for mental health problems (Jones et al., 2010). At age 25, those in the intervention group reported fewer internalizing, externalizing, and substance abuse symptoms (59 percent) than those in the control group (69 percent), as well as fewer crime convictions, less risky sexual behavior, and higher well-being (Conduct Problems Prevention Research Group, 2015).

Drug Therapies

Nonpharmacological treatment is considered the "first-line" treatment for conduct disorder and oppositional defiant disorder, but many children who exhibit severely aggressive behavior have been prescribed a variety of drugs. Stimulants are the most widely prescribed drugs for conduct disorder in the United States, Canada, and many other countries, in part because conduct disorder often is comorbid with ADHD. A meta-analysis of clinical trials found that stimulants are highly effective in relieving ADHD symptoms in children with conduct disorder, and moderately effective in reducing aggression in these children (Balia, Carucci, Coghill, & Zuddas, 2018; Pappadopulos et al., 2006). Antidepressants, particularly the selective serotonin reuptake inhibitors and the serotonin-norepinephrine reuptake inhibitors, may help reduce episodes of irritable and agitated behavior in children (Balia et al., 2018; Savill et al.,

2015). Children with conduct disorder and ODD sometimes are prescribed atypical antipsychotics, which seem to suppress aggressive behavior (Balia et al., 2018). Whether they affect other symptoms of conduct disorder, such as lying and stealing, is unclear. Traditional antipsychotic medications, such as Haldol and Mellaril, also have been used to treat children with conduct disorder, with some success (Balia et al., 2018; Pappadopulos et al., 2006). However, the neurological side effects of these drugs (for additional information on these issues with conduct disorder, see the chapter "Schizophrenia Spectrum and Other Psychotic Disorders") have discouraged many physicians from prescribing them. Some controlled studies suggest that mood stabilizers, including lithium and anticonvulsants (see the chapter "Mood Disorders and Suicide"), may effectively treat children with aggressive conduct disorder (Balia et al., 2018).

ANTISOCIAL PERSONALITY DISORDER

In the Extraordinary People feature at the beginning of this chapter, you read the chilling account of Ted Bundy, the serial rapist and killer. People like Bundy who exhibit chronic antisocial behaviors are diagnosed as having **antisocial personality disorder (ASPD; Table 3)**. ASPD diagnostic criteria are presented in the "Personality Disorders" chapter in the *DSM-5,* but

ASPD is also dual-coded as a conduct disorder in *DSM-5*. ASPD is reviewed in this chapter because it is very closely connected to the spectrum of disruptive, impulse-control, and conduct disorders, including in its developmental origins, while still sharing the key features of a personality disorder (see the chapter "Personality Disorders").

The key features of ASPD, as defined by the *DSM-5,* are an impairment in the ability to form positive relationships with others, a tendency to engage in behaviors that violate basic rights of others and major social norms and values, and a focus on doing whatever it takes to gratify one's personal desires. People with this disorder are deceitful, repeatedly lying or conning others for personal profit or pleasure (American Psychiatric Association, 2013). Due to the problems with conduct, violence, and criminal activity, ASPD is considered the most socially destructive personality disorder since it produces extraordinary consequences to society. ASPD is highly prevalent among the most serious and antisocial criminal offenders (DeLisi, Drury, & Elbert, 2019). Like Ted Bundy, they may commit violent criminal offenses against others—including assault, murder, and rape—in order to gain pleasure or get what they want. When caught, they tend to have little remorse and seem indifferent to the pain and suffering they have caused others.

A prominent characteristic of antisocial personality disorder is poor impulse control. People with this disorder have low frustration tolerance and

---

TABLE 3   *DSM-5* Diagnostic Criteria for Antisocial Personality Disorder

A. A pervasive pattern of disregard for and violation of the rights of others, occurring since age 15 years, as indicated by three (or more) of the following:

  1. Failure to conform to social norms with respect to lawful behaviors, as indicated by repeatedly performing acts that are grounds for arrest.

  2. Deceitfulness, as indicated by repeated lying, use of aliases, or conning others for personal profit or pleasure.

  3. Impulsivity or failure to plan ahead.

  4. Irritability and aggressiveness, as indicated by repeated physical fights or assaults.

  5. Reckless disregard for safety of self or others.

  6. Consistent irresponsibility, as indicated by repeated failure to sustain consistent work behavior or honor financial obligations.

  7. Lack of remorse, as indicated by being indifferent to or rationalizing having hurt, mistreated, or stolen from another.

B. The individual is at least age 18 years.

C. There is evidence of conduct disorder with onset before age 15 years.

D. The occurrence of antisocial behavior is not exclusively during the course of schizophrenia or bipolar disorder.

often act impetuously, with no apparent concern for the consequences of their behavior. They often take chances and seek thrills, with no concern for danger. They are easily bored and restless, unable to endure the tedium of routine or to persist at the day-to-day responsibilities of marriage or a job (DeLisi et al., 2019; T. Millon, Grossman, C. Millon, Meagher, & Ramnath, 2004). As a result, they tend to drift from one relationship to another and often have lower-status jobs. They may impulsively engage in criminal activity—50 to 80 percent of men and about 20 percent of women in prison may be diagnosable with **ASPD** (Cale & Lilienfeld, 2002; Fazel & Danesh, 2002; Warren et al., 2002).

We noted earlier that Ted Bundy would be called a *psychopath* by some theorists. The definition of *psychopathy* by pioneers in the field such as Hervey Cleckley (1941/1982) and Robert Hare (Hare & Neumann, 2008) extends the *DSM-5* criteria for **ASPD**, emphasizing certain broad personality traits. The *DSM-5* criteria for **ASPD** and definitions of psychopathy overlap, but are not entirely the same. Psychopaths are characterized by a superficial charm, a grandiose sense of self-worth, a tendency toward boredom and a need for stimulation, a history of pathological lying, cunning and manipulativeness, and a lack of remorse. People with psychopathy are cold and callous, gaining pleasure by competing with and humiliating everyone and anyone. They can be cruel and malicious. They often insist on being seen as faultless and are dogmatic in their opinions. However, when they need to, people with psychopathy can be gracious and cheerful—until they get what they want. Then they may revert to being brash and arrogant. Cleckley (1941/1982) noted that although psychopaths often end up in prison or dead, many become successful business people and professionals. He suggested that the difference between successful psychopaths and those who end up in prison is that the successful ones are better able to maintain an outward appearance of normality. They may be able to do this because they have superior intelligence and can put on a "mask of sanity" and superficial social charm in order to achieve their goals.

ASPD is one of the most common personality disorders in the general population. The estimated lifetime prevalence of ASPD is 1 to 4 percent with males three to five times (6 percent) more likely to be diagnosed with ASPD than females (2 percent). However, within the prison population, ASPD prevalence rates may be as high as 50 percent (Azevedo, Vieira-Coelho, Castelo-Branco, Coelho, & Figueiredo-Braga. 2020). Epidemiological studies have not found ethnic or racial differences in rates of diagnosis (Fisher & Hany, 2020; Werner, Few, & Bucholz, 2015). Education and intelligence are negatively correlated with a higher prevalence of ASPD among those with lower IQs and reading levels. Research has shown reductions in the prevalence rate with increasing age in criminal populations suggesting that age-related changes in personality and increased mortality due to antisocial behaviors may best explain these changes.

Additionally, individuals with ASPD are significantly more likely to have substance abuse disorders which is a strong predictor of poor prognosis. Research has found that the comorbidity of ASPD positively correlates with the severity of the substance abuse disorder. The more severe the symptoms of ASPD, the more severe the substance abuse (Fisher & Hany, 2020; Parmar & Kaloiya, 2018; Williams et al., 2020). As many as 80 percent of people with ASPD abuse substances such as alcohol and illicit drugs (Trull, Jahng, Tomko, Wood, & Sher, 2010). Substance use, such as binge drinking, may be just one form of impulsive behavior that is part of ASPD. Substance use probably feeds impulsive and antisocial behavior in people with this personality disorder. Alcohol and other substances may reduce any inhibitions they do have, making them more likely to lash out violently at others. People with this disorder also are at somewhat increased risk for suicide attempts (particularly females) and violent death (Cale & Lilienfeld, 2002).

Adults with ASPD typically have shown a disregard for societal norms and a tendency toward antisocial behavior since childhood, and most would have been diagnosed with conduct disorder by mid-adolescence (see Table 3, Criterion C). Conduct disorder is considered a precursor to ASPD and studies show that approximately 80 to 90 percent of

In part because antisocial personality disorder is defined in terms of behaviors that involve rule-breaking, a large proportion of prisoners meet criteria for this disorder. *Nagel Photography/ Shutterstock*

individuals with ASPD also exhibited symptoms of conduct disorder earlier in life (DeLisi et al., 2019). For some people with this disorder, however, there is a tendency for their antisocial behavior to diminish as they age. This is particularly true of people who were not antisocial as children but became antisocial as adolescents or young adults This tendency may be due to psychological or biological maturation or to the possibility that many people with this disorder have been jailed or otherwise constrained by society from acting out their antisocial tendencies (Fisher & Hany, 2020; Moffitt, 1993).

Contributors to Antisocial Personality Disorder

Because most adults diagnosed with ASPD have exhibited antisocial tendencies since childhood, the biological and psychosocial factors associated with this disorder are similar to those associated with conduct disorder. Here we summarize those factors, focusing on studies that have been done with adults with antisocial tendencies. Many of these studies have used samples of individuals (mostly men) exhibiting criminal behaviors, rather than those specifically with ASPD.

The precise etiology of ASPD remains unknown, but it is most likely that the development of this disorder is multifactorial with both biological and environmental influences. There is substantial evidence of a genetic influence on antisocial behaviors, particularly criminal behaviors. Heritability estimates for ASPD range from 38 to 69 percent which suggests that genetics likely play a significant role in the development of this disorder (DeLisi et al., 2019; Rosenström et al., 2017). Twin studies find that the concordance rate for such behaviors is nearly 50 percent in monozygotic twins, compared to 20 percent or lower in dizygotic twins (Larsson et al., 2007; Rosenström et al., 2017). Adoption studies find that the criminal records of adopted sons are more similar to the criminal record of their biological father than to that of their adoptive father (Cloninger & Gottesman, 1987; Mednick, Reznick, Hocevar, & Baker, 1987).

Those genes most frequently implicated in adult antisociality are genes associated with functioning in the serotonin system, which is involved in impulsivity and aggression (Ficks & Waldman, 2014). Although not all studies support the role of these specific genes (Vassos, Collier, & Fazel, 2014), there may be complex interactions between these genes and others in the production of ASPD (e.g., Arias et al., 2011). As in studies of children, studies of adults find that those who have a genotype that influences serotonin functioning and who grow up in socioeconomically deprived circumstances are at particularly increased risk for developing symptoms of ASPD (Lyons-Ruth et al., 2007). Some newer epigenetic research suggests that early environmental factors might affect gene expression, including genes involved in serotonin and oxytocin, in ways that affect antisocial behavior (Checknita et al., 2015; Raine, 2018).

People with antisocial personalities tend to show deficits in verbal skills and in the executive functions of the brain: the ability to sustain concentration, abstract reasoning, concept and goal formation, the ability to anticipate and plan, the capacity to program and initiate purposive sequences of behavior, self-monitoring and self-awareness, and the ability to shift from maladaptive patterns of behavior to more adaptive ones (Raine, 2018). In turn, studies have found differences between antisocial adults and the general population in the structure or functioning of specific areas of the prefrontal cortex of the brain. These areas are involved in a wide range of advanced cognitive processes, such as decision making, planning, impulse control, regulation of emotions, learning from punishments and rewards, and feeling empathy for others (Ogilvie, Stewart, Chan, & Shum, 2011; Siever, 2008). For example, Adrian Raine and colleagues (2000) observed an 11 percent reduction in the volume of gray matter in the prefrontal cortex of males with ASPD compared to males without the disorder. In another study, Raine and colleagues (2011) observed reductions in the volume of the prefrontal cortex of both males and females with symptoms of ASPD compared to individuals with no symptoms. In addition, across the sample as a whole, males had less volume in the prefrontal cortex than females, and the differences between males and females in prefrontal cortex volume accounted for the differences in the number of antisocial symptoms they had. Thus, Raine and colleagues suggest that a tendency toward less gray matter in specific areas of the prefrontal cortex in males compared to females helps explain the gender differences in rates of ASPD. In addition to decreased volume in the prefrontal cortex, studies have found decreased volume and activity in the amygdala, which processes emotion and threat, and increased volume and activity in the striatum, which is involved in reward processing (Raine, 2018).

These deficits in structure and brain functioning could be tied to the genetic abnormalities that have been seen in people with ASPD. They may also be caused by medical illnesses or exposure to toxins during infancy and childhood, both of which are more common among people who develop antisocial and criminal behavior than among those who do not. Whatever their causes, the deficits in executive functions, empathy for others, and learning from punishment might contribute to stimulation seeking, poor impulse control, and difficulty in anticipating the consequences of one's actions.

The risk taking, fearlessness, and difficulty in learning from punishment seen in people with ASPD have also been tied to low levels of arousability as measured by a relatively low resting heart rate, low skin conductance activity, or excessive slow-wave electroencephalogram readings (Latvala, Kuja-Halkola, Almqvist, Larsson, & Lichtenstein, 2015; Sylvers, Brubaker, Alden, Brennan, & Lilienfeld, 2008). One interpretation of these data is that low levels of arousal indicate low levels of fear in response to threatening situations (Raine, 2018). Fearlessness can be put to good use—bomb disposal experts and British paratroopers also show low levels of arousal (McMillan & Rachman, 1987; O'Connor, Hallam, & Rachman, 1985). However, fearlessness also may predispose some people to antisocial and violent behaviors that require fearlessness to execute, such as fighting and robbery. In addition, low-arousal individuals may not fear punishment and thus may not be deterred from antisocial behavior by the threat of punishment.

Chronically low arousal also may be an uncomfortable state and may lead to stimulation seeking (Eysenck, 1994). If an individual seeks stimulation through prosocial or neutral acts, such as skydiving, this trait may not lead to antisocial behavior. Some individuals, however, may seek stimulation through antisocial acts that are dangerous or impulsive, such as fighting. The direction stimulation seeking takes—toward antisocial activities or toward more neutral activities—may depend on the reinforcement individuals receive for their behaviors. Those who are rewarded for antisocial behaviors by family and peers may develop antisocial personalities, whereas those who are consistently punished for such behaviors and are given alternative, more neutral options for behavior may not.

Like the other personality disorders, ASPD is linked to a history of childhood adversity and maltreatment. Several studies have found that criminal offenders experience greater amounts of childhood abuse and neglect, as compared to the general population. Among various forms of abuse and neglect, research has found that physical abuse and sexual abuse by a caregiver were most associated with the development of ASPD. It is believed that these adverse experiences in childhood contribute to the development of the most serious and violent acts of criminal behavior, typically displayed by those with ASPD (DeLisi et al., 2019). A study of a nationally representative sample found that adults diagnosed with ASPD had elevated rates of having been battered by a caregiver and of having a parent who had a substance use problem, who went to jail, and/or who attempted suicide (Afifi et al., 2011). They also had over twice the rates of physical, emotional, and sexual abuse as individuals without the disorder.

As in children with conduct disorder, the genetic, neurobiological, and social factors associated with ASPD probably interact (see Figure 1 in the section "An Integrative Model") to create a cycle of violence in the lives of people with the disorder. They then perpetuate that violence in their own relationships and families.

Treatments for Antisocial Personality Disorder

There is little to no evidence of effective treatment methods for those with ASPD. This population is often excluded from mental heath services which may be one explanation for this lack of evidence (Azevedo et al., 2020; Van den Bosch, Rijckmans, Decoene, & Chapman, 2018). Conversely, people with ASPD tend to believe they do not need treatment. They may submit to therapy when forced to because of marital discord, work conflicts, or incarceration, but they are prone to blaming others for their current situation rather than accepting responsibility for their actions. As a result, many clinicians do not hold much hope for effectively treating persons with this disorder through psychotherapy (Kraus & Reynolds, 2001; Millon et al., 2004).

There are no medications currently approved by the US Food and Drug Administration for treatment of ASPD. The use of medications may be effective in treating comorbid disorders (e.g., panic disorder, major depression), or to target symptoms of aggression and impulsivity. Lithium and the atypical antipsychotics have been used successfully to control impulsive and aggressive behaviors in people with ASPD (Black, 2017; Ripoll, Triebwasser, & Siever, 2011). Antiseizure drugs also have been used to reduce impulsiveness and aggressiveness (Ripoll et al., 2011). Cognitive-behavioral therapy (CBT) has been found effective for milder cases of ASPD (Black, 2017). When clinicians do attempt psychotherapy, they tend to focus on helping the person with ASPD gain control over his or her anger and impulsive behaviors by recognizing triggers and developing alternative coping strategies (Kraus & Reynolds, 2001). Some clinicians also try to increase the individual's understanding of the effects of his or her behaviors on others (Hare & Hart, 1993).

TABLE 4   *DSM-5* Criteria for Intermittent Explosive Disorder

A. Recurrent behavioral outbursts representing a failure to control aggressive impulses as manifested by either of the following:

    1. Verbal aggression (e.g., temper tantrums, tirades, verbal arguments, or fights) or physical aggression toward property, animals, or other individuals, occurring twice weekly, on average, for a period of 3 months. The physical aggression does not result in damage or destruction of property and does not result in physical injury to animals or other individuals.

    2. Three behavioral outbursts involving damage or destruction of property and/or physical assault involving physical injury against animals or other individuals occurring within a 13-month period.

B. The magnitude of aggressiveness expressed during the recurrent outbursts is grossly out of proportion to the provocation or to any precipitating psychosocial stressors.

C. The recurrent aggressive outbursts are not premeditated (i.e., are impulsive and/or anger-based) and are not committed to achieve some tangible objective (e.g., money, power, intimidation).

D. The recurrent aggressive outbursts cause either marked distress in the individual or impairment in occupational or interpersonal functioning, or are associated with financial or legal consequences.

E. Chronological age is at least 6 years (or equivalent developmental level).

F. The recurring aggressive outbursts are not better explained by another mental disorder (e.g., major depressive disorder, bipolar disorder, disruptive mood dysregulation disorder, a psychotic disorder, antisocial personality disorder, borderline personality disorder) and are not attributable to another medical condition (e.g., head trauma, Alzheimer's disease) or to the physiological effects of a substance (e.g., a drug of abuse, a medication). For children 6 to 18 years, aggressive behavior that occurs as part of an adjustment disorder should not be considered for this diagnosis.

Note: This diagnosis can be made in addition to attention-deficit/hyperactivity disorder, conduct disorder, oppositional defiant disorder, or autism spectrum disorder when recurrent impulsive aggressive outbursts are in excess of those usually seen in these disorders and warrant independent clinical attention.

INTERMITTENT EXPLOSIVE DISORDER

Children with conduct disorder and adults with antisocial personality disorder often engage in aggressive acts, which may be impulsive outbursts or premeditated behavior that unfolds over a longer period of time. The diagnosis of **intermittent explosive disorder** is given to individuals age 6 and older who engage in relatively frequent impulsive acts of aggression (see Table 4). The aggression may be verbal or physical (though noninjurious), and must be grossly out of proportion to the situation (e.g., angrily throwing a water bottle at a salesperson who won't give you a discount). The outbursts can't be the kind that are calculated to gain some advantage, such as a baseball player yelling at an umpire who has called a strike on him. Instead, they must be "out of control" as the result of anger, and represent an inability to inhibit the impulse to be aggressive in the immediate context of frustration or a perceived stress that would not typically result in an aggressive outburst. Epidemiological studies suggest that between 3.5 and

7 percent of the population could be diagnosed with intermittent explosive disorder (Coccaro, Fanning, & Lee, 2017; Kessler, et al., 2006). It typically begins in late childhood or adolescence and rarely onsets after age 40. This chronic disorder can lead to legal difficulties and to failed relationships and loss of employment (McCloskey, Noblett, Deffenbacher, Gollan, & Coccaro, 2008).

One theory of intermittent explosive disorder is that the impulsive aggressive behavior is caused by an imbalance in serotonin levels, although only a small amount of research has been conducted (Coccaro, Lee, & Kavoussi, 2010; Fanning, Coleman, Lee, & Coccaro, 2019). While not yet fully understood, brain imaging studies show diminished activity in the orbitofrontal cortex (OFC) and hyperactivity of the amygdala. Individuals with IED also display abnormal OFC-amygdala function when viewing threatening (angry) faces. These recent advancements are contributing significantly to a better understanding of the neurobiological basis of aggressive behavior (Fanning et al., 2019). The disorder runs in families, but it is not known whether this is due to genetic factors or to environmental and parenting factors (Coccaro, 2012).

Cognitive-behavioral treatments for intermittent explosive disorder help individuals identify and avoid triggers for explosive outbursts and appraise situations in ways that do not provoke aggression on their part. Multiple studies have found that both individual and group cognitive-behavioral therapy were very effective in reducing anger, aggression, hostile thinking, and depressive symptoms while improving anger control in individuals with intermittent explosive disorder, as compared to those placed on a waitlist (Hewage et al., 2018; McCloskey et al., 2008). Serotonin and norepinephrine reuptake inhibitors and mood stabilizers (e.g., lithium) have been shown to reduce aggression in individuals with this disorder in small, uncontrolled studies (Myrseth & Pallesen, 2010).

FIGURE 2 Reciprocal Effects Between Biological and Psychosocial Factors in the Disruptive, Impulse-Control, and Conduct Disorders

CHAPTER INTEGRATION

We noted earlier that integrative models of the disruptive, impulse-control, and conduct disorders view them as the result of interactions between biological and psychosocial factors. The reciprocal effects of these factors on each other in these disorders are striking (see Figure 2). Parents who are antisocial pass on their genes to their children, and parent them in ways that promote uncontrolled, aggressive, rule-breaking behavior. In addition, families whose members engage in antisocial behavior may experience *downward social drift:* The adults in these families cannot keep good jobs, and the families' socioeconomic status tends to decline, leading to the children growing up in poor surroundings, where they are exposed to toxins that can damage their developing brains.

These children tend to be irritable and difficult and thus draw hostility from their parents, teachers, and peers. The negative reactions of others feed these children's own hostile tendencies, convincing them that the world is against them. They join deviant peer groups, whose members reinforce their bad behavior. Their lack of achievement in school, inability to get along with others, and criminal behavior cause them to live in poverty. Then, when they have children of their own, the cycle begins again.

SHADES OF GRAY   DISCUSSION

The criteria for conduct disorder require three symptoms over a 12-month period, one of which is present in the past 6 months. Jake's current behavior of ambushing other children would likely meet the criteria if it continues—he's initiating fights, being physically cruel, and intimidating others intentionally. Prior to his beginning to ambush other kids, the fights he got into were provoked by teasing, so it's not clear that they would count toward a diagnosis of conduct disorder.

Jake seems to have turned into a bully, repeatedly harassing and victimizing innocent and often helpless others (Olweus, 2011). A study of American students found that 11 percent have been victims of bullying, 13 percent have been bullies, and 6 percent have been both (Tanner, 2001). Adults can be bullies, too, as in Michael Douglas's portrayal of Gordon Gekko in the movie *Wall Street.* Bullying is associated with a broad array of antisocial behaviors in children and adults, including physical fights, school and work attendance problems, cruelty to animals, stealing, and harassment (Vaughn et al., 2010). Bullies are significantly more likely than non-bullies to be diagnosed with conduct disorders as children and to have a history of parental antisocial behavior. As adults, they are more likely to commit crimes and to be diagnosed with antisocial personality disorder and substance use disorders (Ttofi, Farrington, & Lösel, 2012; Vaughn et al., 2010).

CHAPTER SUMMARY

- Conduct disorder is characterized by a persistent pattern of (a) aggression toward people and animals, (b) destruction of property, (c) deceitfulness or theft, and (d) serious violations of rules and social norms.

- Conduct disorder is more common in boys than in girls and is highly stable across childhood and adolescence. Childhood-onset conduct disorder is more persistent than adolescent-onset conduct disorder.

- A diagnosis of conduct disorder with limited prosocial emotions is given to children who meet the full criteria for conduct disorder and have at least two of the following characteristics: (a) lack of remorse or guilt for their actions, (b) lack of empathy for others, (c) lack of concern about performance in important life domains, and (d) shallow or deficient emotions (e.g., insincerity in emotions, using emotions to manipulate others).

- Children with oppositional defiant disorder are chronically negativistic, defiant, disobedient, and hostile. Unlike children with conduct disorder, they do not tend to be aggressive toward other people or animals, to steal, or to destroy property.

- Conduct and oppositional defiant disorders have been linked to genes involved in the regulation of the neurotransmitters dopamine, serotonin, and norepinephrine. The combination of certain genes and a history of maltreatment is especially strongly linked to conduct disorder.

- Children with conduct disorder show a range of neurological deficits in brain systems responsible for controlling behavior and impulses. These deficits may be caused by genetic factors and/or exposure to toxins.

- Abnormal serotonin levels, low physiological arousal, and high testosterone levels may also be linked to conduct disorder.

- Poverty, maltreatment, parenting characterized by harsh discipline with a lack of warmth, and deviant peer groups are social factors associated with conduct disorder.

- Children with conduct disorder tend to process information about social interactions in hostile ways and to see aggression as the only way to respond.

- The treatment for conduct disorder is most often cognitive-behavioral therapy, focusing on changing children's ways of interpreting interpersonal situations and helping them control their angry impulses. Parents are taught methods to control their children's behavior with appropriate punishments and reinforcements. Antipsychotic drugs, antidepressants, and stimulant drugs also are sometimes used to treat conduct disorder.

- Antisocial personality disorder is characterized by an impairment in the ability to form positive relationships with others, a tendency to engage in behaviors that violate basic rights of others and social norms and values, deceit and manipulativeness, and a focus on doing whatever it takes to gratify one's personal desires.

- Psychopathy is not recognized in *DSM-5* but overlaps with antisocial personality disorder. Psychopathy extends the criteria for antisocial personality disorder beyond persistent violations of others' rights and social norms to include traits like egocentricity, shallow emotions, manipulativeness, and lack of empathy, guilt, and remorse.

- Genetic factors, particularly those that affect serotonin and dopamine systems, may play a role in antisocial personality disorder. As in conduct disorder, the interaction between certain genes and growing up in deprived circumstances is associated with antisocial behavior.

- People with antisocial personalities tend to show deficits in areas of the brain associated with verbal skills, planning, and control of behavior.

- Low levels of arousability may contribute to the risk taking, fearlessness, and difficulty in learning from experience in people with antisocial personality disorder.

- Psychotherapy is not considered to be very effective for people with antisocial personality disorder. Lithium, antipsychotic drugs, and antiseizure drugs may help control their impulsive behaviors.

- Intermittent explosive disorder is characterized by persistent intermittent anger-based outbursts of noninjurious and nondestructive physical or verbal aggression greatly out of proportion to the circumstances (e.g., in response to a minor stress).

- Intermittent explosive disorder may be related to imbalances in serotonin systems or to genetic factors, but little research into its causes has been done.

- Cognitive-behavioral treatments for intermittent explosive disorder help individuals identify and avoid triggers for explosive outbursts and appraise situations in ways that do not provoke aggression on their part. Serotonin and norepinephrine reuptake inhibitors and mood stabilizers (e.g., lithium) have been shown to reduce aggression in individuals with this disorder.

KEY TERMS

conduct disorder

childhood-onset conduct disorder

adolescent-onset conduct disorder

life-course-persistent antisocial behavior

psychopathy

oppositional defiant disorder (ODD)

antisocial personality disorder (ASPD)

intermittent explosive disorder

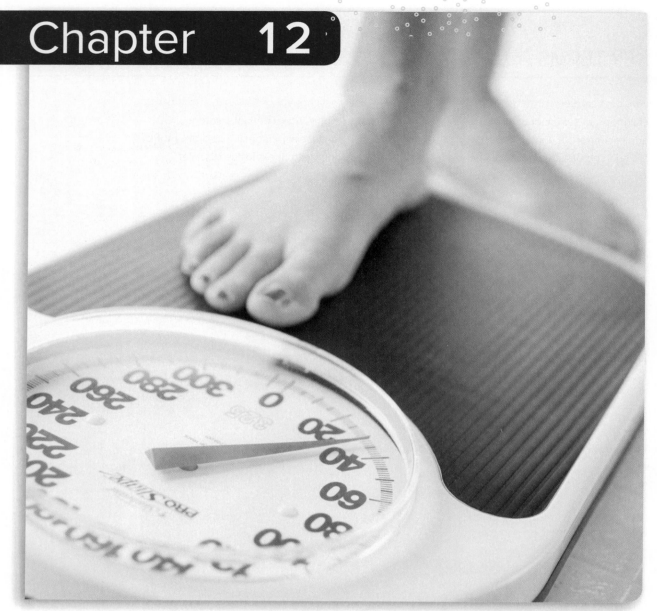

Chapter 12

Photodisc/Getty Images

Eating Disorders

CHAPTER OUTLINE

Eating Disorders Along the Continuum

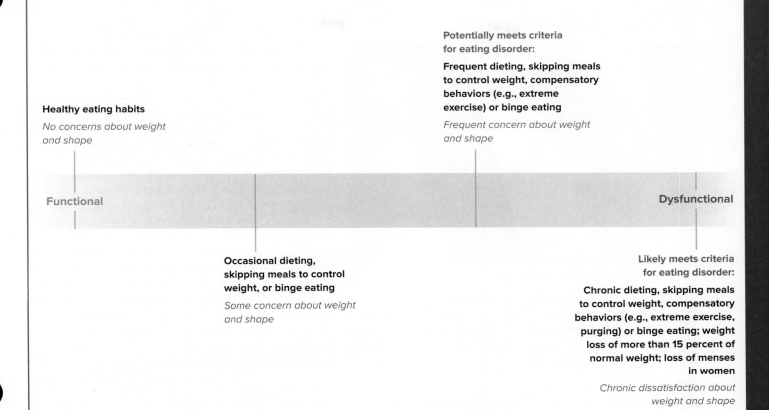

Healthy eating habits

No concerns about weight and shape

Potentially meets criteria for eating disorder:

Frequent dieting, skipping meals to control weight, compensatory behaviors (e.g., extreme exercise) or binge eating

Frequent concern about weight and shape

Functional

Dysfunctional

Occasional dieting, skipping meals to control weight, or binge eating

Some concern about weight and shape

Likely meets criteria for eating disorder:

Chronic dieting, skipping meals to control weight, compensatory behaviors (e.g., extreme exercise, purging) or binge eating; weight loss of more than 15 percent of normal weight; loss of menses in women

Chronic dissatisfaction about weight and shape

A "normative discontent"—that's how researchers 30 years ago labeled the dissatisfaction with weight and shape that is rampant among women, particularly young women, in developed countries (Rodin, Silberstein, & Striegel-Moore, 1984). Sadly, this discontent has only gotten worse in the last 30 years, and it has spread worldwide through mass media (Becker et al., 2011). A study in Iceland found that 64 percent of women who were of normal weight felt they needed to lose weight (Matthiasdottir, Jonsson, & Kristjansson, 2012). In the United States, 69 to 84 percent of women exhibit body dissatisfaction and prefer a smaller figure than their own. It is this desire for an often unattainable, incredibly thin body shape can contribute to body dissatisfaction and unhealthy eating behaviors (Allen, Robson, & Laborde, 2020; Runfola et al., 2013). Although men are less likely to be concerned with their weight, in recent years men have become increasingly concerned with attaining the lean lower body and strong, toned upper body celebrated in pop culture, and the media. Nearly half of men and 90 percent of adolescent boys want to be leaner and more muscular than they are (Murray et al., 2017; Neighbors & Sobal, 2007; Tiggemann, Martins, & Kirkbride, 2007).

Recent studies on body preference have found that children as young as age 3 reliably demonstrate a preference for thinness. This is seen through children assigning more positive and desirable characteristics to thinner figures and displaying negative attitudes toward larger figures which suggests that attitudes about body size and weight may develop very early in life. Various studies also show that this *weight bias* increases with age as children transition into adolescence and young adulthood. Children with strong weight bias are also more likely to experience higher levels of depression, anxiety, low self-esteem, body dissatisfaction, and disordered eating (Harriger, Schaefer, Thompson, & Cao, 2019).

At the far end of the continuum are people whose concerns about weight significantly impact their daily function and indicate the presence of an eating disorder. As you will see in this chapter, while relatively few people meet the full criteria for these eating disorders, many more people have some symptoms, what researchers call *partial-syndrome eating disorders* (Allen et al., 2020; Lewinsohn, Striegel-Moore, & Seeley, 2000).

In this chapter, we discuss the diagnosis and epidemiology of eating disorders; the causes of eating disorders, including the psychological and biological factors that may lead some people to develop the disorders; and effective treatments for eating disorders.

Extraordinary People

Fashion Models, *Dying to Be Thin*

Thierry Lopez/ZUMAPRESS/Newscom

They glide down runways, extraordinary examples of beauty, sophistication, and superiority. They represent the ultimate look, not just in the clothes they display but in the shape of their bodies. Lean to the point of being emaciated, perfect. But fashion models are literally dying in their attempt to attain and maintain the extreme thinness demanded by the industry. When French model and actress Isabele Caro was photographed in an Italian advertising campaign about the fashion industry's insistence that models be ultrathin, she weighed 60 pounds (she was 5 feet 4 inches tall). She survived on just one chocolate square and a cup of tea per day. She had lost her hair and several teeth. More than once she had lapsed into a coma. But the notoriety that her anorexic photos gained her landed her a spot as a judge on the French version of "America's Next Top Model." A couple of years later she was dead at the age of 28. Before Caro's death, Brazilian model Ana Carolina Reston died at the age of 21, weighing only 88 pounds. Model Luisel Ramos of Uruguay died from heart failure resulting from self-starvation just after stepping off a fashion show runway. In 2010, male model Jeremy Gillitzer died from complications of anorexia nervosa at age 38. When he had spoken to reporters a couple of years earlier, he had weighed only 88 pounds.

The deaths of models from complications of self-starvation have prompted European cities such as Madrid to set minimum weight standards for fashion models. In March 2012 the Israeli government passed a law requiring a minimum weight for any models working in that country. The fashion industry in the United States says it is instituting measures to reduce self-starvation in models.

But we all know that the shape and weight these models represent is unattainable by most people, so no one really believes they should look like them, right? Studies show that adolescent and adult females' attitudes toward themselves *are* affected by the thin ideal promoted by models and in articles about weight and shape in fashion magazines (see Grabe, Ward, & Hyde, 2008; Groesz, Levine, & Murnen, 2002). For example, Eric Stice and Heather Shaw (1994) showed college-age women, for just 3 minutes, either images of models from fashion magazines or images that didn't portray thin models. Those women who saw the fashion magazine images experienced increases in depression, shame, guilt, stress, insecurity, and body dissatisfaction compared to those women who were exposed to the other images. Other studies show that teenage girls given subscriptions to fashion magazines become more depressed and more dissatisfied with their body, diet more, and show more bulimic symptoms over time compared to teenage girls given subscriptions to nonfashion magazines, especially if the girls already expressed dissatisfaction with their body and had little social support (Stice, Spangler, & Agras, 2001). Similar results have been found in studies that expose adolescent or adult males to media depictions of idealized male bodies (Blond, 2008).

Obviously, not everyone who reads fashion magazines or sees fashion models on television becomes obsessed with their weight and shape or develops symptoms of an eating disorder. Later in this chapter, we discuss factors that enhance vulnerability to these pressures. But there is good reason to think that the extraordinary standards set by fashion models and media stars do affect how women and men view and treat their own bodies.

Jeremy Gillitzer *Nick Vlcek/Barcroft Media Ltd.*

Does the following profile, excerpted from a college student's diary, sound like someone you know?

PROFILES

This morning I had a half of a grapefruit for breakfast, and some coffee—no sugar or cream. For lunch, I had an apple and a diet soda. For dinner, I had some plain white rice and a salad with just some lemon squeezed over it. So I was feeling really good about myself, really virtuous. That is, until Jackie came over, and completely messed up my day. She brought over a movie to watch, which was fine. But then she insisted on ordering a pizza. I told her I didn't want any, that I wasn't hungry (which was a lie, because I was starving). But she ordered it anyway. The pizza arrived, and I thought I could be good and not have any. But it was just sitting there on the table, and I couldn't think of anything except having some. I couldn't concentrate on the movie. I kept smelling the pizza and feeling the emptiness in my stomach. Like a weakling, I reached out and got one piece, a small piece. It was ice cold by then, and kind of greasy, but I didn't care. I ate that piece in about 5 seconds flat. Then I had another piece. And another. I stopped after four pieces. But I still couldn't pay attention to the movie. All I could think about was what a pig I was for eating that pizza, and how I'll never lose 10 pounds so I can fit into size 2 jeans. Jackie's gone now, and I still keep thinking about how ugly and fat I am, and how I have no willpower. I didn't deserve to have that pizza tonight, because I haven't lost enough weight this month. I'm going to have to skip breakfast and lunch tomorrow, and exercise for a couple of hours, to make up for being a complete pig tonight.

Being overweight can have many negative consequences, such as high blood pressure, heart disease, and diabetes, as we discuss later in this chapter. But most people care about their weight because what a person weighs is equated with a person's self-worth in our society. Eating has become more than a source of nourishment, and exercise more than a means of improving health. What people eat and how much they exercise have become linked to feelings of worth, merit, guilt, sin, rebelliousness, and defiance, in turn affecting people's self-esteem.

In this chapter we focus on people whose concern with weight and shape, and whose eating behaviors, are severe enough not only to interfere with their functioning in daily life but also to threaten their lives. As discussed in Eating Disorders Along the Continuum, however, people's attitudes and behaviors toward food and their bodies cover a wide range of problems.

CHARACTERISTICS OF EATING DISORDERS

Many professionals and researchers argue that body image dissatisfaction is one of the most significant factors in the development of eating disorders, such as anorexia and bulimia nervosa (Soares Filho et al., 2020). Although we discuss anorexia nervosa, bulimia nervosa, and binge-eating disorder separately, most individuals who initially meet the criteria for one of these disorders "migrate" between them, meeting the criteria for two or more of the disorders at different times (Hilbert et al., 2014; Keel, Brown, Holland, & Bodell, 2012). Moreover, many individuals show behaviors and concerns characteristic of one or more of the eating disorders without meeting the full criteria for one of these diagnoses. Such individuals may be given the diagnosis *other specified feeding or eating disorder.*

Anorexia Nervosa

People with **anorexia nervosa (AN)** starve themselves, subsisting on little or no food for very long periods of time resulting in abnormally low body weight. Despite this weight loss, it is common for those individuals to remain convinced that they need to lose more weight (Duncan et al., 2017). As a result, their body weight is significantly below what is minimally normal for their age and height (see the *DSM-5* criteria in Table 1). The spectrum of individuals who develop AN is wide, ranging from adolescents who try to eat healthier or exercise more to be more competitive in sports, to individuals who have experienced trauma, to those who have lifelong body image issues. Regardless of the presentation and the path that led them to develop AN, they all have in common a discrepancy between their conscious motivation for how much they restrict food intake versus the body's need to stay at a healthy body weight. For example, Isabele Caro, described in the Extraordinary People feature, was 5 feet 4 inches tall and weighed only 60 pounds.

Eating disorders are among those psychological disorders with the highest mortality rate with most deaths occurring between the ages of 16 and 29 year and is approaching 6 percent mortality rate per decade. More than one-quarter of these deaths are suicide-related, but greater than 50 percent of AN deaths are the result of medical complications (Frank, DeGuzman, & Shott, 2019; Gibson, Workman, & Mehler, 2019). AN is ranked as the third leading cause of chronic illness in adolescents and is responsible for multi-system organ damage, including cardiac abnormalities, structural and functional brain impairment, and early-onset bone disease (Murray, Quintana, Loeb, Griffiths, & Le Grange, 2019).

Self-starvation and drastic weight loss are also associated with serious medical consequences, including bradycardia (extreme slowing of heart rate), arrhythmia

TABLE 1   *DSM-5* Criteria for Anorexia Nervosa

A. Restriction of energy intake relative to requirements, leading to a significantly low body weight in the context of age, sex, developmental trajectory, and physical health. Significantly low weight is defined as a weight that is less than minimally normal or, for children and adolescents, less than that minimally expected.

B. Intense fear of gaining weight or of becoming fat, or of persistent behavior that interferes with weight gain, even though at a significantly low weight.

C. Disturbance in the way in which one's body weight or shape is experienced, undue influence of body weight or shape on self-evaluation, or persistent lack of recognition of the seriousness of the current low body weight.

Specify current subtype:

Restricting type: During the last 3 months, the individual has not engaged in recurrent episodes of binge eating or purging behavior (i.e., self-induced vomiting or the misuse of laxatives, diuretics, or enemas). Weight loss is accomplished primarily through dieting, fasting, and/or excessive exercise.

Binge-Eating/Purging type: During the last 3 months, the individual has engaged in recurrent episodes of binge eating or purging behavior (i.e., self-induced vomiting or the misuse of laxatives, diuretics, or enemas).

(irregular heart beat), heart failure, hypotension, electrolyte disturbances, gastrointestinal issues, liver problems, low bone density, and increased risk of fracture (Gibson, Workman, & Mehler, 2019; Hanachi et al.,2020). Another potentially serious complication of anorexia is acute expansion of the stomach, to the point of rupturing. Kidney damage has been seen in some people with anorexia, and impaired immune system functioning may make people with anorexia more vulnerable to medical illnesses. Extreme weight loss often causes women and girls who have begun menstruating to stop having menstrual periods, a condition known as **amenorrhea.** However, some women who meet the other *DSM-5* criteria for anorexia nervosa still report some menstrual activity which is one reason the *DSM-5* eliminated the previous requirement for amenorrhea from its diagnostic criteria (Attia & Roberto, 2009). Bone strength is an issue for women who have amenorrhea, presumably because low estrogen levels reduce bone strength.

Despite being underweight, people with anorexia nervosa have a distorted image of their body, often believing that they are disgustingly fat and need to lose more weight. They struggle with an intense fear of gaining weight or of becoming fat, yet despite low weight they routinely engage in behavior that interferes with any weight gain. They feel good and worthwhile only when they have complete control over their eating and when they are losing weight. Their weight loss causes people with anorexia to be chronically fatigued, yet they drive themselves to exercise excessively and to keep up a grueling schedule at work or school (American Psychiatric Association, 2013).

People with anorexia nervosa often develop elaborate rituals around food, as writer Marya Hornbacher describes in her autobiography, *Wasted.*

PROFILES

I would spread my paper out in front of me, set the yogurt aside, check my watch. I'd read the same sentence over and over, to prove that I could sit in front of food . . . to prove it was no big deal. When five minutes had passed, I would start to skim my yogurt . . . take your spoon and run it over the top of the yogurt, being careful to get only the melted part. Lick it— wait, be careful, . . . only lick a teeny bit at a time . . . Then set the yogurt aside again. Read a full page, but don't look at the yogurt . . . Do not take a mouthful . . . Do not fantasize about toppings, crumbled Oreos, or chocolate sauce. Do not fantasize about a sandwich. A sandwich would be so complicated (Hornbacher, 1998, pp. 254–255).

Hornbacher describes one of the two types of anorexia nervosa—the restricting type (Table 2). People with the **restricting type of anorexia nervosa** often use dieting, fasting and/or excessive exercise as a way of preventing weight gain which results in dramatic weight loss (American Psychiatric Association, 2013; Maïmoun et al., 2018). Some people attempt to go for days without eating anything; most eat very small amounts of food each day, in part simply to stay alive and in part in response to pressure from others to eat. Hornbacher survived for months on one cup of yogurt and one fat-free muffin per day. Daphne, in the following case study, also has the restricting type of anorexia nervosa, one that includes excessive exercise as part of her weight-loss behavior pattern.

TABLE 2   Comparison of Eating Disorders

The eating disorders vary on several characteristics.

Characteristic	Anorexia Nervosa Restricting Type	Anorexia Nervosa Binge/Purge Type	Bulimia Nervosa	Binge-Eating disorder
Body weight	Significantly underweight	Significantly underweight	Often normal weight or overweight	Often significantly overweight
Body image	Severely disturbed	Severely disturbed	Overconcerned with weight and shape	Often very distressed with overweight
Bingeing	No	Yes	Yes	Yes
Purging or other compensatory behaviors	No	Yes	Yes	No
Sense of lack of control over eating	No	During binges	Yes	Yes

CASE STUDY

Olivia has never felt comfortable in her own skin and for as long as she could remember always felt "big" in comparison to other girls. These feelings became stronger after a growth spurt in eighth grade that made her much taller than her peers. At 5'10, Olivia felt awkward and huge next to her classmates which motivated her to begin dieting. Olivia began running everyday and eliminated sugar and carbs from her diet which made her feel less "fat". Olivia continued this routine for two years and dropped to a lean 130lbs. However, Olivia was disturbed that she wasn't losing more weight, so she increased her exercise and only ate 1,000 calories per day. Still discouraged by her lack of weight loss, Olivia began fully restricting her food and would not allow herself to eat anything until she had run at least 10 miles and only then she she eat a small serving of vegetables and one ounce of cheese. Now weighing 115lbs, Olivia stopped menstruating, her hair was falling out and her gaunt appearance worried her mother.

Olivia was initially excited to go away to college, but upon graduation she had become very worried. In high school, Olivia was an honor roll student and at the top of her class but now she was concerned she wouldn't be able to maintain a high college GPA. Olivia felt like a failure her first semester both academically and socially after her girlfriend ended their relationship over concerns about her weight loss. In an effort to regain control over her life, Olivia reduced her total daily food intake to two apples and a half ounce of cheese and ran at least 15 miles each day. By the end of fall semester, Olivia was down to 100 lbs. but she was unable to attend classes most days as she was chronically tired, had trouble con-

centrating, and occasionally fainted. Despite her skeletal appearance, Olivia only saw herself as a fat and unattractive woman who needed to lose more weight. Olivia was referred to the university counseling center by a concerned professor for assessment.

The other type of anorexia (AN) is the **binge/ purge type of anorexia nervosa,** in which people periodically engage in binge eating or purging behaviors (e.g., self-induced vomiting or the misuse of laxatives or diuretics). This disorder is different from bulimia nervosa in that people with the binge/purge type of anorexia nervosa continue to be substantially below a healthy body weight, whereas people with bulimia nervosa typically are at normal weight or somewhat overweight. Often, a person with the binge/purge type of anorexia nervosa does not engage in binges in which large amounts of food are eaten. If even a small amount of food is eaten, the person feels as if she has binged and will purge this food (Stoving et al., 2012). A number of studies have found that people with restrictive type of AN have different clinical presentation than those with the purging type. Specifically, there are noted differences in impulsivity, neurocognitive functioning, emotion regulation and self-regulatory behaviors and brain activity between these groups (Maïmoun et al., 2018).

Individuals with anorexia nervosa are required by Criterion A (see Table 1) to be at a significantly low body weight. *DSM-5,* however, provides guidance regarding how to determine whether an individual is at a significantly low weight and severity specifiers. For example, *DSM-5* suggests using a body mass index (BMI) of 18.5 kg/m^2 as the lower limit of normal body weight, a benchmark employed by the Centers for Disease Control and Prevention (CDC) and the World

Health Organization (WHO). The level of severity of anorexia nervosa would be mild if BMI ≥ 17 kg/m^2, moderate if BMI $= 16-16.99$ kg/m^2, severe if BMI $= 15-5.99$ kg/m^2, and extreme if BMI < 15 kg/m^2. However, the level of severity is not based only on BMI, but can be adjusted based on clinical symptoms, the degree of functional disability, or the need for supervision (American Psychiatric Association, 2013).

Anorexia nervosa (AN) has a lifetime prevalence of approximately 1 percent and disproportionately affects females. Its prevalence in young females is approximately 0.4 percent per year (Maïmoun et al., 2018). The rate among males was 0.3 percent in the U.S. studies (Hudson et al., 2007; Swanson, Crow, et al., 2011). Newer studies using the *DSM-5* criteria have found higher prevalence rates. One study followed girls for 8 years from adolescence to early adulthood and found that 0.8 percent had diagnosable anorexia nervosa by age 20 (Stice, Marti, & Rohde, 2013). Some estimate lifetime prevalence among adult women to be up to 4 percent (Smink, van Hoeken, & Hoek, 2013). Although AN tends to impact women at higher rates than men, new research has found an increasing prevalence of male body dissatisfaction and eating disorders which may fuel a diverse array of disordered eating practices. Men have historically been understudied in terms of AN and which has resulted in disproportionately sparse amounts of clinical information and a decreased recognition of eating disorders in males. Despite increasing prevalence among males in both community and clinical samples, less than 1 percent of empirical research relating to AN has focused on men. Due to the subjective nature of body dissatisfaction boys generally report more concerns with muscularity than thinness and engage in behaviors designed to enhance their muscle mass. While the presentation is different, it is possible that this type of disordered eating and behavioral practices to increase muscle mass (Murray, Quintana, Loeb, Griffiths, & Le Grange, 2019; Nagata et al., 2017).

In the United States, Caucasians are more likely than African Americans and Hispanic Americans to develop the disorder (Perez, Ohrt, & Hoek, 2016; Striegel-Moore & Franko, 2008; Swanson, Crow, et al., 2011). This may be because Caucasians are more likely to accept the thin ideal promoted in the media (Smolak & Striegel-Moore, 2001). Similarly, there is some evidence that cultures that do not value thinness in females have lower rates of anorexia nervosa than those in the United States and Europe (Hoek et al., 2005).

The incidence of AN has increased substantially since the early part of the twentieth century (Gordon, 2017). For example, a study of over 30,000 Swedish twins found significantly higher rates of anorexia nervosa among those born after 1945 than among those born before 1945 (Bulik et al., 2006). The motivations

for self-starvation also seem to vary across culture and time. In centuries past, and outside the United States and Europe, the stated motivations for excessive fasting have had less to do with weight concerns than with stomach discomfort or religious considerations (Keel & Klump, 2003). Patients with AN in Asian countries do not have the distorted body image characteristic of anorexia in the United States and Europe and readily admit to being very thin. Nonetheless, they stubbornly refuse to eat, as illustrated by the following case study of one Chinese woman.

CASE STUDY

Miss Y, age 31, was 5 foot 3 inches. She had formerly weighed 110 pounds but now weighed 48 pounds. Her anorexia began 4 years previously, when she was suddenly deserted by her boyfriend. . . . Miss Y started to complain of abdominal discomfort and reduced her food intake. She became socially withdrawn and unemployed. At her psychiatric examination, she wore long hair and was shockingly emaciated—virtually a skeleton. She had sunken eyes, hollow cheeks, and pale, cold skin. She recognized her striking wasting readily but claimed a complete lack of hunger and blamed the weight loss on an unidentifiable abdominal problem. . . . When asked whether she consciously tried to restrict the amount she ate, she said, "No." When questioned why she had gone for periods of 8 or more waking hours without eating anything, she said it was because she had no hunger and felt distended, pointing to the lower left side of her abdomen. . . . Miss Y . . . resisted all attempts to discuss this loss in detail and all other psychological and medical treatments. Miss Y later died of cardiac arrest. Postmortem examination revealed no specific pathology other than multiple organ atrophy due to starvation. (Adapted from Sing, 1995, pp. 27–29)

One question that can be raised is whether self-starvation in the absence of expressed weight concerns can be called AN, given that weight concerns are a defining feature of the disorder in the *DSM-5* (see Table 1, Criterion B). Alternatively, it is possible that the more culturally sanctioned rationale for dietary restriction involving gastrointestinal discomfort was put forth by Miss Y, substituting for the expression of weight concerns. *DSM-5* Criterion B was expanded to include not only overtly expressed fear of weight gain but also persistent behavior that interferes with weight gain; Miss Y clearly shows the latter. While the *DSM-5* itself is a culture-bound document, representing views of mental disorders in "Western" cultures, its text often addresses culture-related diagnostic issues in understanding and describing illness experiences.

Anorexia nervosa usually begins in adolescence or young adulthood (Nagata et al., 2017; Stice et al., 2013). The course of the disorder varies greatly from person to person. Long-term studies suggest that the median number of years from onset to remission of the disorder is 7 years for women and 3 years for men, even among patients in treatment (Stoving, Andries, Brixen, Bilenberg, & Horder, 2011). Multiple long-term studies around the world found that more than 20 years after onset of the diagnosis, about 51 to 76 percent of patients no longer qualify for a diagnosis, but many continue to have eating-related problems or other psychopathology, particularly depression (Dobrescu et al., 2020). Individuals with the binge/purge type of anorexia nervosa tend to have more comorbid psychopathology than people with the restricting type, particularly impulsive, suicidal, and self-harming behaviors (Peat, Mitchell, Hoek, & Wonderlich, 2009), and a more chronic course of the disorder (Stoving et al., 2012).

Bulimia Nervosa

The core characteristic of **bulimia nervosa** is uncontrolled eating, or **bingeing,** followed by inappropriate compensatory behaviors used to prevent weight gain from the binges (see the *DSM-5* criteria in Table 3), such as self-induced vomiting, misuse of laxatives, fasting, or excessive exercise (Hail & Le Grange, 2018). Mild presentations of bulimia include an average of 1 to 3 episodes of inappropriate compensatory behavior per week, while more extreme forms involve an average of 14 or more episodes per week. The *DSM-5* defines a binge as occurring over a discrete period of time, such as 1 or 2 hours, and involving an amount of food definitely larger than most people would eat during a similar period of time and in similar circumstances (American Psychiatric Association, 2013; Donnelly et al., 2018). People with eating disorders show tremendous variation in the size of their binges, however. Some people consume 3,000 to 4,000 calories in one sitting, focusing on food high in fat and carbohydrates; in other cases, the binge is between 1,200 and 2,000 calories (Hilbert, Wilfley, Dohm, & Striegel-Moore, 2011; Wolfe, Baker, Smith, & Kelly-Weeder, 2009). What makes these lesser amounts binges is people's sense that they are violating some dietary rule they have set for themselves and that they have no control over their eating but feel compelled to eat even though they are not hungry (Goldschmidt et al., 2016; Wolfe et al., 2009). Recognizing this aspect of binges, the *DSM-5* criteria for a binge include a sense of lack of control over eating (Criterion A2).

The behaviors people with bulimia use to control their weight include self-induced vomiting; the abuse of laxatives, diuretics, or other purging medications; fasting; and excessive exercise. Like people with anorexia nervosa, people with bulimia nervosa have self-evaluations that are heavily influenced by their body shape and weight. When they are thin, they feel like a "good person." However, people with bulimia nervosa, unlike people with anorexia nervosa, do not tend to show gross distortions in their body images (Hail & Le Grange, 2018). Whereas a woman with anorexia nervosa who is absolutely emaciated looks in the mirror and sees herself as obese, a woman with bulimia nervosa has a more realistic perception of her actual body shape and weight. Still, people with bulimia nervosa are constantly dissatisfied with their shape and weight and concerned about losing weight.

Self-induced vomiting is the behavior people most often associate with bulimia. Bulimia is often discovered by family members, roommates, and friends when

TABLE 3 *DSM-5* Criteria for Bulimia Nervosa
A. Recurrent episodes of binge eating. An episode of binge eating is characterized by both of the following:
1. Eating, in a discrete period of time (e.g., within any 2-hour period), an amount of food that is definitely larger than most people would eat during a similar period of time under similar circumstances.
2. A sense of lack of control over eating during the episode (e.g., a feeling that one cannot stop eating or control what or how much one is eating).
B. Recurrent inappropriate compensatory behaviors in order to prevent weight gain, such as self-induced vomiting; misuse of laxatives, diuretics, or other medications; fasting; or excessive exercise.
C. The binge eating and inappropriate compensatory behaviors both occur, on average, at least once per week for 3 months.
D. Self-evaluation is unduly influenced by body shape and weight.
E. The disturbance does not occur exclusively during episodes of anorexia nervosa.

people with the disorder are caught vomiting or leave messes after they vomit. Dentists also recognize people with bulimia because frequent vomiting can rot teeth due to exposure to stomach acid. The cycle of bingeing and then purging or using other compensatory behaviors to control weight becomes a way of life.

Other people use excessive exercise or fasting to control their weight. The man in the following profile fasted for a day or longer after a binge to control his weight. As the pressures of his job and a failed marriage increased, his bulimic pattern of bingeing and then fasting grew more serious.

Men with bulimia nervosa are more likely than women with bulimia nervosa to use excessive exercising to control their weight. *Pierre Charriau/age fotostock*

PROFILES

I would sigh with relief when Sunday evening came, since I had no responsibilities until the next morning. . . . I would carefully shop for cheese, meats, snacks and sweets . . . buy paperback novels and settle down for a 3-hour session of reading and slow eating until I could barely keep my eyes open. My binges took the place of Sunday dinner, averaging approximately 6,000 calories. I would typically schedule the following day as a heavy working day with evening meetings to distract myself from increasing hunger as I fasted. I began running . . . and walked to work as a further weight control measure . . . As time went on, I increased the frequency of these binges . . . I was physically exhausted most of the time, and my hands, feet, and abdomen were frequently puffy, which I interpreted as body fat . . . which contributed to my obsession . . . I weighed myself several times per day . . . as though my life depended on them. (Source: Wilps, 1990)

The lifetime prevalence of bulimia nervosa is estimated to be 1 to 1.5 percent in adults and 0.1 to 2 percent in adolescent youth. However, when studies evaluate disordered eating behavior rather than applying strict *DSM* criteria significantly higher prevalence (14 to 22 percent) was found for both adults and adolescents (Hail & Le Grange, 2018; Yao et al., 2021). It is much more common in females than in males. As with anorexia nervosa, the criteria for the diagnosis of bulimia nervosa were loosened somewhat in the *DSM-5* (by reducing the minimum average number of times per week binge/purge behaviors must occur from two to one). Partly due to this change, studies using *DSM-5* criteria find higher lifetime prevalence of up to 2.6 percent among women (Smink et al., 2013; Stice et al., 2013). Men with bulimia nervosa are more likely than women with the disorder to exercise excessively to control their weight and to be focused on developing a lean, muscular look rather than on being excessively thin (Murray et al., 2017).

There is clear evidence of cultural, racial/ethnic, and historical differences in the prevalence of bulimia nervosa. In the United States, it is more common in Caucasians and Hispanic Americans than in African Americans (Perez et al., 2016; Striegel-Moore & Franko, 2008; Swanson, Crow, et al., 2011), and a meta-analysis found that bulimia nervosa is considerably more common in Westernized cultures than in non-Westernized cultures (Keel & Klump, 2003). In addition, the prevalence of bulimia nervosa increased significantly in the second half of the twentieth century. Some studies indicate that rates in the United States, Europe, and Australia reached a peak in the 1990s, remaining stable or decreasing somewhat in the 2000s (Crowther, Armey, Luce, Dalton, & Leahey, 2008; Smink et al., 2016).

The onset of bulimia nervosa most often occurs in adolescence (Hail & Le Grange, 2018). Although the death rate among people with bulimia is not as high as among people with anorexia, bulimia also has serious medical complications and a death rate nearly double that in the general population (Arcelus, Mitchell, Wales, & Nielson, 2011). One of the most serious complications is an electrolyte imbalance, which results from fluid loss following excessive and chronic vomiting, laxative abuse, and diuretic abuse. Imbalances in electrolytes can lead to heart failure. US adults with lifetime eating disorders have significantly elevated risk of suicide attempt. Those with a lifetime history of eating disorders have roughly five- to-sixfold risk of suicide attempt. Prevalence estimates of suicide attempts for those with bulimia are approximately 31 percent which is significantly higher than found in the general population (Donnelly et al., 2018; Udo, T., Bitley, S., & Grilo, 2019). Adolescents with bulimia report suicidality at higher rates than adults with bulimia and at higher rates than their peers with any other eating disorder. Multiple studies have found approximately more than half of adolescents with bulimia (53 percent) report suicidal ideation, more than 25 percent report having a plan and more than 33 percent report a prior suicide attempt, with 17 percent reporting multiple past suicide attempts (Hail & Le Grange, 2018).

Bulimia nervosa tends to be a chronic condition. A long-term study of people seeking treatment found that 15 years after the disorder about 50 percent showed remission of their symptoms but the other 50 percent still had symptoms qualifying for a diagnosis The frequent use of purging is a predictor of a poorer outcome (Stoving et al., 2011; Stoving et al., 2012).

Binge-Eating Disorder

Binge-eating disorder (BED) was included in *DSM-IV* as a proposed condition in need of further study. As a result of extensive research supporting its clinical usefulness and validity over the past 20 years, it is included in *DSM-5* as a mental disorder. **Binge-eating disorder (BED)** resembles bulimia nervosa, except that a person with binge-eating disorder consumes an unusually large quantity of food while experiencing a lack of control and then does not regularly engage in purging, fasting, or excessive exercise to compensate for binges (Table 4). This type of eating results in excessive weight gain and obesity. During these binge-eating episodes, the affected individual typically reports behaviors such as eating faster than usual or eating until uncomfortably full. As a result of these binge eating episodes, people with BED experience clinically significant distress or impairment

(Tanofsky-Kraff, Schvey, & Grilo, 2020). People with BED may eat continuously throughout the day, with no planned mealtimes (Masheb, Grilo, & White, 2011). Others engage in discrete binges of large amounts of food, often in response to stress and to feelings of anxiety or depression (Munsch, Meyer, Quartier, & Wilhelm, 2012; Wonderlich, Gordon, Mitchell, Crosby, & Engel, 2009). They may eat very rapidly and appear almost in a daze as they eat, as the man in the following case study describes.

CASE STUDY

"The day after New Year's . . . I kept reminding myself about my resolution about dieting. . . . but all of my good intentions just seemed to fade away. . . . I just said, 'What the hell,' and started eating . . ."

Starting in a grocery store he bought a cake, several pieces of pie, and boxes of cookies. He drove through traffic with one hand, pulling food out of the bag and eating as fast as he could. After consuming all of his groceries, he went to restaurants, staying only a short time in each and eating only small amounts. . . . in constant dread of discovery, he had no idea what "sin" he felt he was committing. He knew only that it was not pleasurable. "I didn't enjoy it at all. It just happened. It's like a part of me just blacked out." Finally he went into a deli, bought another $20 worth of food and drove home, eating all the way, "until my gut ached" (Stunkard, 2003).

TABLE 4   *DSM-5* Criteria for Binge-Eating Disorder

A. Recurrent episodes of binge eating. An episode of binge eating is characterized by both of the following:

   1. Eating, in a discrete period of time (e.g., within any 2-hour period), an amount of food that is definitely larger than most people would eat in a similar period of time under similar circumstances.

   2. A sense of lack of control over eating during the episode (e.g., a feeling that one cannot stop eating or control what or how much one is eating).

B. The binge-eating episodes are associated with three (or more) of the following:

   1. Eating much more rapidly than normal.

   2. Eating until feeling uncomfortably full.

   3. Eating large amounts of food when not feeling physically hungry.

   4. Eating alone because of feeling embarrassed by how much one is eating.

   5. Feeling disgusted with oneself, depressed, or very guilty afterward.

C. Marked distress regarding binge eating is present.

D. The binge eating occurs, on average, at least once a week for 3 months.

E. The binge eating is not associated with the recurrent use of inappropriate compensatory behavior and does not occur exclusively during the course of bulimia nervosa or anorexia nervosa.

People with BED often are significantly overweight and say they are disgusted with their body and ashamed of their bingeing (Stunkard, 2011; Tanofsky-Kraff et al., 2020). In fact, as many as 30 percent of people currently in weight-loss programs may have BED (Stunkard, 2011). In the United States the rate in the general population is 2 to 3.5 percent; in other countries the rates are somewhat lower (Kessler et al., 2013; Smink et al., 2013). Individuals with a lifetime diagnosis of BED are four times more likely to have severe obesity (Tanofsky-Kraff et al., 2020).

Developing most often in early adulthood, BED is estimated to impact approximately 1 to 2.6 percent of the general population, with higher rates observed among adults with overweight/obesity. Among adolescents with BED, prevalence rates range from 0.7 to 2.3 percent, with approximately 2 percent of girls and under 1 percent of boys reporting the disorder. It has been reported that approximately 7 percent of adolescents with high body weight meet subthreshold rates. The core feature of BED is the loss of control during eating episodes that may provide researchers more insight into the development of the disorder. Children as young as 8 years report loss of control (LOC) eating episodes which increase the risk of BED in adulthood (Tanofsky-Kraff et al., 2020).

There are two peaks of onset in this disorder. The first immediately after puberty (mean age of 14 years), and the second in late adolescence between 18 and 20 years. In the general population, international research has reported that 26 percent of female and 13 percent of male adolescents have experienced an episode of binge eating at least once in the last 12 months. These subclinical symptoms of BED are often associated with an increased risk of developing BED and adverse outcomes, such as, low self-esteem and higher body dissatisfaction. In comparison to adults with BED, adolescents may experience less frequent episodes of binge eating than is required to make a diagnosis of BED according to the *DSM-5*. For this reason, it is important for clinicians to consider subthreshold binge-eating disorder (SBED) in adolescents. There are noted differences in the clinical presentation of BED with female adolescents frequently reporting less overeating than male adolescents, but more severe loss of control and distress during binge-eating episodes (Marzilli, Cerniglia, & Cimino, 2018).

BED disorder is associated with various adverse consequences among adults such as higher distress and concerns about body shape and weight, social impairment, and psychological dysfunction often manifested in symptoms of anxiety and depression. BED in adolescence was predictive of a broad spectrum of negative outcomes, including obesity, school, work and social impairment, symptoms of depression and anxiety, as well as emotional distress, substance use, self-harm, and suicidality (Marzilli, Cerniglia, & Cimino, 2018).

BED is somewhat more common in women than in men, both in the general community and among people in weight-loss programs, although the gender difference is not significant in some studies (Hudson, Hiripi, Pope, & Kessler, 2007; see Ágh et al., 2015). In the United States, there do not appear to be racial or ethnic differences in rates of BED (Perez et al., 2016; Striegel-Moore & Franko, 2008). Some studies suggest that sexual and gender minority youths may be at greater risk for disinhibited eating behaviors but more research is needed in this area. It is possible that a family history of obesity may interact with various psychosocial risk factors that may exacerbate an individual's predisposition to LOC eating. Additionally, weight-based teasing has been reported by approximately 60 percent of youth with high body weight which has been identified as a predictive factor for binge eating (Tanofsky-Kraff et al., 2020).

People with this disorder also have high rates of depression and anxiety and possibly a higher incidence of alcohol abuse and personality disorders (Marzilli et al., 2018; Tanofsky-Kraff et al., 2020; Striegel-Moore & Franko, 2008). BED tends to be chronic; one retrospective study found the mean duration of the disorder to be 8 years (Hudson et al., 2007), and another study found a mean duration of 14.4 years (Pope et al., 2006).

Other Specified Feeding or Eating Disorder

As noted in Eating Disorders Along the Continuum, subclinical symptoms of eating disorders are quite common, particularly among adolescent and adult populations. *Partial-syndrome eating disorders* are used to identify those who meet some, but not the full criteria for AN or bulimia nervosa. For example, adolescents with partial-syndrome eating disorders may binge a couple of times a month but not every week. They may be underweight but not severely so. They tend to be highly concerned with their weight and judge themselves on the basis of their weight, but their symptoms don't add up to a full-blown eating disorder. There is a recent increase in reported incidences of pre- and early-adolescents experiencing partial-syndrome and full-syndrome eating disorders. As a result, there is an urgent need to develop prevention programs that focus on the age prior to when adolescents begin to show dangerous weight control behaviors, like restrictive eating and purging behaviors (Buerger et al., 2019).

The *DSM-5* created a new diagnostic category called **other specified feeding or eating disorder** to capture presentations of an eating disorder that cause clinically significant distress or impairment but do not meet the full diagnostic criteria for any of the eating disorders previously discussed. The partial-syndrome eating disorders would fit into this new category. This issue was addressed in *DSM-5* through the addition of other specified feeding or eating disorder, the broadening of the criteria for anorexia nervosa and bulimia nervosa, and the addition of BED (Smink et al., 2013).

The *DSM-5* other specified feeding or eating disorder category includes disorders like **atypical anorexia nervosa** wherein all the criteria for anorexia nervosa are met, except that despite significant weight loss, the individual's weight is within or above the normal range. Another example is *bulimia nervosa of low frequency and/or limited duration,* which involves meeting all of the criteria for bulimia nervosa, except that the binge eating and inappropriate compensatory behaviors occur, on average, less than once a week and/or for less than 3 months. One last example is **night eating disorder,** a new disorder introduced in *DSM-5.* People with this disorder regularly eat excessive amounts of food after dinner and into the night (Allison, 2017). The eating behavior is not part of cultural or social norms—this is not the typical ordering of pizza with friends after a party or the occasional bout of the late-night munchies. People with night eating disorder feel an overwhelming desire to eat at night most nights of the week and are highly distressed that they cannot control their eating behavior. They experience frequent insomnia and may believe they need to eat in order to fall asleep. They typically are not hungry in the morning and skip breakfast. Night eating disorder most often begins in early adulthood and tends to be long-lasting. People with this disorder often are overweight and suffer from depression. Night eating disorder differs from *sleep-eating,* which can occur in some sleep disorders (see the chapter "Health Psychology"), in that people with night eating disorder are awake and aware when they are eating while people who sleep-eat are not.

Obesity

Although obesity is not included in *DSM-5* as a mental disorder, it is common among people with BED and is one of the greatest public health concerns internationally (Brownell & Walsh, 2017; Gearhardt et al., 2012). It is included here because obesity is highly associated with numerous mental disorders, is a risk factor for the development of some mental disorders (e.g., depressive disorders), and is the result of psychotropic medication side effects (e.g., atypical antipsychotics; see the chapter "Schizophrenia Spectrum and Other Psychotic Disorders").

Obesity (excess body fat) is defined as a body mass index (BMI) of 30 or over. BMI is based on kg/m^2; using the Imperial system of measurement, it is calculated as your weight in pounds multiplied by

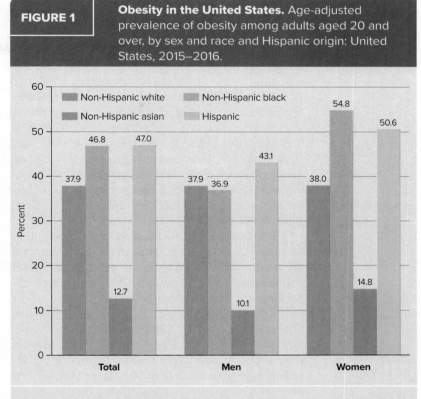

FIGURE 1

Obesity in the United States. Age-adjusted prevalence of obesity among adults aged 20 and over, by sex and race and Hispanic origin: United States, 2015–2016.

Prevalence of Obesity Among Adults and Youth: United States, 2015–2016, NCHS Data Brief No. 288, October 2017, Centers for Disease Control and Prevention

703, then divided by the square of your height in inches (Centers for Disease Control & Prevention [CDC], 2018b). Between 1980 and 2002, the prevalence of obesity in the United States doubled in adults and tripled in children and adolescents (Flegal, Carroll, Ogden, & Johnson, 2002; Hedley et al., 2004; Ogden, Flegal, Carroll, & Johnson, 2002). Rates have continued to climb, and currently it is estimated that nearly 40 percent of American adults and 19 percent of American children are obese (CDC, 2018b; Ogden, Carroll, Kit, & Flegel, 2012). African Americans and Hispanic Americans have the highest obesity rate, followed by non-Hispanic whites and Asian Americans (CDC, 2018b; Figure 1). Rates of obesity also are climbing around the world, particularly in countries where the standard of living and access to American fast foods are increasing (Novak & Brownell, 2011; World Health Organization, 2018c).

Obesity is associated with an increased risk of coronary heart disease, hypertension and stroke, type 2 diabetes, and some kinds of cancer (Novak & Brownell, 2011). In the United States, 5 to 7 percent of all health care costs are due to the effects of obesity. People with obesity suffer not only more physical illnesses but also a lower quality of life and more emotional problems, due in part to the stigmatization of obese people (Gearhardt et al., 2012; Pearl, 2018). For example, experimental studies have shown that employers are less likely to hire or promote individuals described in vignettes as overweight than they are to hire or promote individuals with identical credentials not described as overweight (Roehling, Pichler, & Bruce, 2013). Children and adolescents who are obese report frequent teasing and bullying and report that they skip school as a result (Van Geel, Vedder, & Tanilon, 2014). Although many laypeople think such stigmatization could serve as motivation for obese people to lose weight, experimental studies show that exposure to stigmatizing media portrayals leads obese people to eat more rather than less (Pearl, 2018; Pearl, Puhl, & Brownell, 2012).

The dramatic historical increases in obesity point to environmental causes. Researcher Kelly Brownell argues that we live in a toxic environment of high-fat, high-calorie, inexpensive food and advertisers who promote the consumption of large quantities of this food (Brownell & Horgen, 2004; Brownell & Walsh, 2017; Gearhardt et al., 2012). Added to this "Super-Size Me" culture is a significant reduction over the past several decades in the amount of physical activity people engage in. More than 60 percent of Americans do not get 30 minutes of physical exercise per day, and 25 percent get no exercise at all (Godfrey & Brownell, 2008). In the United States, only 2 percent of high schools, 8 percent of middle schools, and 4 percent of elementary schools require daily physical education (Story, Nanney, & Schwartz, 2009). A typical day for many Americans involves driving to work or school, passing through the drive-through at a fast-food restaurant to get a fat- and cholesterol-laden breakfast sandwich, sitting at work or school all day, getting up only to go to another fast-food restaurant for a lunch that may have thousands of calories, and then driving home to spend the evening sitting in front of the television. Eating like this is a prescription for obesity.

In addition, there is increasing evidence that the ultraprocessed foods sold by fast-food restaurants can create addictions similar to those created by drugs of abuse (Gearhardt et al., 2012; Schulte, Grilo, & Gearhardt, 2016). Food companies have manipulated the fat, sugar, salt, food additives, flavor enhancers, and caffeine in processed food in ways that increase flavor and result in quicker absorption of ingredients such as sugar into the bloodstream, increasing the foods' addictive properties (Gearhardt, Davis, Kuschner, & Brownell, 2011). Rats fed this type of food are more likely than rats fed regular rat food to endure repeated electric shocks in order to get more high-fat, high-sugar foods, and they show changes in the brain similar to those seen in people addicted to substances like cocaine (Johnson & Kenny, 2010). In humans, obese people, who tend to eat more ultraprocessed foods, show more

activity in reward areas of the brain associated with drug abuse when exposed to photos of such foods than do lean people (Rothemund et al., 2007; Stoeckel et al., 2008). Obese people show less activity in certain reward areas of the brain than do lean people when they actually consume such food, however, suggesting that changes in the brain similar to those seen in drug addicts occur after chronic exposure to ultraprocessed foods (Stice, Spoor, Bohon, Veldhuizen, & Small, 2008; Stice, Spoor, Ng, & Zald, 2009). Finally, people who show behavioral signs of food addiction, such as craving, tolerance, and withdrawal from high-fat, high-sugar ultraprocessed foods, have brain activity in response to viewing food photos and consuming processed foods similar to that of obese people (and drug addicts) (Gearhardt, Yokum, et al., 2011; Schulte et al., 2016). Cravings may be especially cued by food stimuli in the environment (Joyner, Kim, & Gearhardt, 2017). Thus, the environments and ultraprocessed foods that are the staple of American and, increasingly, international diets may be causing addictions to these foods that make them hard to resist.

Not everyone living in a toxic food environment becomes overweight or obese. Genes appear to account for a substantial percentage of the variability in obesity (Albuquerque, Stice, Rodríguez-López, Manco, & Nóbrega, 2015). Genes affect the number of fat cells and the likelihood of fat storage, the tendency to overeat, and the activity level in the brain in response to food. These genetic factors interact with the toxic environment to contribute to obesity. For example, Eric Stice and colleagues (Stice, Spoor, et al., 2008; Stice, Yokum, Bohon, Marti, & Smolen, 2010) found that individuals who showed atypical activity in reward areas of the brain in response to tasty food were at risk for future weight gain only if they had a certain variant of a gene associated with reward processing.

Millions of people try to lose weight on their own, with the aid of self-help books; millions of others participate in commercial weight-loss programs such as Weight Watchers. Evaluations of popular weight-loss programs suggest that they can result in modest weight loss (Gearhardt et al., 2012). For example, Christopher Gardner and colleagues (2007) randomly assigned women with a BMI of 27 to 40 to follow the Atkins (carbohydrate-restricted), the Ornish (fat-restricted), the Zone (macronutrients balance), or the LEARN (exercise and changes in eating patterns) program. At the end of 1 year, the women on the Atkins program had lost an average of about 10 pounds, significantly more weight loss than that of women on the Zone program (3.5 pounds) but not significantly different from that of women on the Ornish program (4.8 pounds) or the LEARN program (5.7 pounds). Another study that included both men and women found that the Atkins, Ornish, Zone, and Weight

TV weatherman Al Roker underwent bariatric surgery to lose weight. *(Left): Nick Elgar/Getty Images;* *(Right): Jason LaVeris/FilmMagic/Getty Images*

Watchers programs all resulted in similar weight loss (Dansinger, Gleason, Griffith, Selker, & Schaefer, 2005). Weight Watchers led to an average loss of 4 to 7 pounds, but only 50 to 65 percent of people stuck to the diet for 1 year. Even for those who do stick to these programs, the modest weight loss is discouraging, especially given the advertisements suggesting that these programs can result in much greater weight loss for obese people. Yet even a modest weight loss of 5 to 10 percent of body weight can result in significant health improvements for obese people.

Weight-loss drugs, such as orlistat (Xenical), lorcaserin (Belviq), liraglutide (Saxenda), and phentermine/topirimate (Qsymia) can suppress appetite and can help people lose weight. Randomized controlled trials have shown that these drugs can lead to weight loss of 3 to 9 percent over a year (S. Yanovski & J. Yanovski, 2014). However, all these medications have side effects, including gastrointestinal upset (orlistat), nausea, and increased heart rate (liraglutide), and risk of birth defects among pregnant women (phentermine/topiramate). Lifestyle changes are currently recommended first.

For obese people with a BMI between 30 and 39, low-calorie diets (900 to 1,200 calories per day), often using prepackaged, portion-controlled servings (such as meal replacement shakes), are recommended (Wadden, Neiberg, et al., 2011). Individuals also are encouraged to increase their level of physical activity. Such a program results in significantly more weight loss than when individuals consume a self-selected diet of conventional food (Berkowitz et al., 2011). For extremely obese people with a BMI of 40 or over who

have at least one severe health problem (e.g., diabetes), bariatric surgery is an option. A small pouch is created at the base of the esophagus, severely limiting food intake, and the stomach may be stapled, banded, or bypassed. Such surgery can result in a substantial weight loss, on average 60 percent of excess weight (Chang et al., 2014). One person who underwent bariatric surgery is TV weatherman Al Roker.

It is difficult for overweight and obese people to lose weight, and even more difficult to keep it off. To combat the discouragement many people feel about losing weight, researchers are encouraging obese people to adopt reasonably modest goals for weight loss and to focus on increasing their physical activity, both of which can lead to substantial improvements in cardiac functioning and diabetes risk (Wadden, Wilson, Stunkard, & Berkowitz, 2011). In general, the proven methods for preventing weight gain and reducing weight are these:

- Eat more nutrient-dense foods and fewer foods with empty calories.
- Aim for a minimum of 30 minutes of physical activity daily.
- Structure your environment so that healthy choices are easier to make; for example, keep low-fat foods readily available in your house and purge your cabinets of junk food.
- Be more active throughout the day: Use the stairs rather than the elevator, park in the farthest spot from the building rather than the closest, and seek other opportunities that encourage movement over standing or sitting (Godfrey & Brownell, 2008).

UNDERSTANDING EATING DISORDERS

A number of biological, sociocultural, and psychological factors have been implicated in the development of the eating disorders. As we have discussed, people frequently "migrate" between the eating disorder diagnoses and symptoms, so as you might expect, some of the risk factors are shared among the disorders. These disorders are often chronic with frequent relapse and burden experienced by those affected and their loved-ones is high (Frank, DeGuzman, & Shott, 2019; Hilbert et al., 2014). As we discuss at the end of this chapter, it is likely that it takes an accumulation of several of these factors for any individual to develop an eating disorder. In this section, however, we consider each factor separately.

Biological Factors

Like most psychological disorders, AN, BN, and BED tend to run in families (Frank et al., 2019; Trace, Baker, Peñas-Lledó, & Bulik, 2013). Twin studies consistently support a genetic basis for AN, with heritability estimates ranging 48 to 74 percent (Duncan et al., 2017). A twin study of BED found a heritability of 41 percent (Bulik, Sullivan, & Kendler, 2003). Genes appear to carry a general risk for eating disorders rather than a specific risk for one type of eating disorder (Bulik et al., 2010; Culbert, Racine, & Klump, 2015). A genetic risk for developing eating disorders appears to interact with the biological changes of puberty to contribute to the onset of eating disorders in girls, but not in boys (Klump et al., 2012). That is, in girls changes in hormones at puberty may activate a genetic risk for the eating disorders. The biological changes of puberty are accompanied by changes in girls' social worlds that likely contribute to their risk for eating disorders, as we discuss below.

The hypothalamus plays a central role in regulating eating and is implicated in the disordered eating behaviors characteristic of bulimia nervosa and anorexia nervosa.

Much of the current research on the biological causes of the eating disorders focuses on those bodily systems that regulate appetite, hunger, satiety, initiation of eating, and cessation of eating (Stice & Shaw, 2017; Trace et al., 2013). The hypothalamus plays a central role in regulating eating (Berthoud & Morrison, 2008). It receives messages about the body's recent food consumption and nutrient level and sends messages to cease eating when the body's nutritional needs are met. These messages are carried by a variety of neurotransmitters, including norepinephrine, serotonin, and dopamine, and by a number of hormones, including cortisol and insulin. Disordered eating behavior might be caused by imbalances in or dysregulation of any of the neurochemicals involved in this system or by structural or functional problems in the hypothalamus (Culbert et al., 2015). For example, disruptions of this system could cause the individual to have trouble detecting hunger accurately or to stop eating when full, both of which are characteristics of people with eating disorders.

People with AN show lowered functioning of the hypothalamus and abnormalities in the levels of several hormones important to its functioning, including serotonin and dopamine (Culbert et al., 2015; Stice & Shaw, 2017). Whether these disruptions are causes or

SHADES OF GRAY

Read the following case study.

Rachel, a 19-year-old college freshman, received a psychiatric evaluation at her parent's request over concerns about her recent weight loss. Rachel explained that she began running several mornings each week and "cut out junk food" to protect herself from gaining "that freshman 15." Once school began, Rachel increased her running, often skipped breakfast . . . and her lunch and dinner was limited to salad.

When Rachel returned home for winter break her family noticed that she looked thin and tired. Despite encouragement to rest, she awoke early each morning to run. She returned to school in January and thought she might be depressed. Courses seemed less interesting, and she wondered whether the college was right for her . . . When Rachel returned home for spring break, her parents asked her to step on the bathroom scale . . . her weight had fallen to 104 pounds, and she agreed to a visit to her physician who recommended a psychiatric consultation. (Source: Adapted from Attia & Walsh, 2007, p. 164.)

Does Rachel have an eating disorder? What criteria does she meet? Are there any criteria that she doesn't meet? (Discussion appears at the end of this chapter.)

consequences of the self-starvation of anorexia is unclear. Some studies have found that people with anorexia continue to show abnormalities in hypothalamic and hormonal functioning and neurotransmitter levels after they gain some weight, whereas other studies have found that these abnormalities disappear with weight gain (Polivy & Herman, 2002).

Dopamine helps regulate motor activity, feeding behaviors, and reinforcement and reward learning. An increasing number of functional brain imaging studies have found altered activation in reward-processing brain regions in those with AN. It is posited that such abnormalities together with anxious traits could contribute to AN-specific brain dysfunction and drive extreme food restriction by altering dopamine function. This research suggests that food restriction sensitizes various dopamine receptors and may be an underlying mechanism for enhanced dopamine activation that occurs in response to weight loss (Frank et al., 2019).

Many people with bulimia show abnormalities in the systems regulating the neurotransmitter serotonin (Culbert et al., 2015; Keel, Brown, Holland, & Bodell, 2012). Deficiencies in serotonin might lead the body to crave carbohydrates, and people with bulimia often binge on high-carbohydrate foods. These people may then engage in self-induced vomiting or some other type of purge in order to avoid gaining weight from carbohydrates. Thus, a number of biological abnormalities have been found to be associated with AN and BN. These abnormalities could contribute to disordered eating behavior by causing the body to crave certain foods or by making it difficult for a person to read the body's signals regarding hunger and fullness. Exactly why people with eating disorders also develop a distorted body image and the other cognitive and emotional problems seen in the eating disorders is not clear.

Finally, it is worth mentioning that recent research has found a direct influence of gut microbiota on eating disorders. Increased levels of bacterial induced autoantibodies have been reported in individuals with AN, bulimia, and BED. Among animal studies, the induction of these autoantibodies in mice influenced food intake and anxiety (Sanz & Aidy, 2019). Neurocognitive deficits may contribute to the etiology and/or maintenance of eating disorders. Executive functioning (aka, cognitive control) involves complex processes that are inherent components of self-regulation and are essential for adaptive emotional, social, and physical functioning (Donnelly et al., 2018).

Sociocultural and Psychological Factors

Societal pressures to be thin and attractive probably play a role in the eating disorders, although, as noted earlier, many people who are exposed to these pressures do not develop an eating disorder. Certain psychological factors may also need to come into play for an eating disorder to develop.

Social Pressures and Cultural Norms

Psychologists have linked the historical and cross-cultural differences in the prevalence of the eating disorders to differences in the standards of beauty for women at different historical times and in different cultures (Garner & Garfinkel, 1980; Keel & Klump, 2003; McCarthy, 1990; Sobal & Stunkard, 1989). Society is exposed to images and information that represents the cultural standards of beauty through the media. This outlet cultivates beauty ideals that influence psychological constructs like body image, disordered eating, and self esteem in both in males and females. These psychological factors are acknowledged as important predictors in the development of eating disorders.

Social Media Online media has rapidly evolved in recent years and social networking sites like Twitter, Instagram, and Facebook, are quickly becoming the primary media source used by young adults. Research has historically shown that exposure to traditional media (TV, movies and magazines) is associated with core features of eating disorders, such as body dissatisfaction. The increased use of online social networks is associated with decreased self esteem, happiness, life satisfaction, and increased depression and loneliness reported among young adult users. Image-centered digital media, such as Instagram, YouTube, Snapchat, and Tik Tok often increase appearance concerns among users which may promote self-consciousness about body image. Additionally concerning is the fact that social media exposure is subject to "social filtering," which is an algorithmic process in which an individual's social media behavior is used to predict interests which results in customized social media content designed to appeal to that individual. Therefore, individuals searching for or engaging with body-idealizing social media content will increase the delivery of body-related content to that individual in the future (Griffiths et al., 2018).

The easy and constant access to cameras and photo editing software via smartphones has led to the development of "selfie" culture. Individuals experiment with multiple photos using the most flattering angles, poses, filters, selfie sticks, and photo editing to create a flawless image for posting. This focus on perfection increases attention to ideal body image, which includes pressure to conform to the young, thin ideal that is highly valued in our society. For those who are more psychologically vulnerable, this may increase body dissatisfaction, desire for thinness, and the development of disordered eating. Research has found a correlation between social network usage and body image concerns, low self-esteem, dieting and disordered eating among adolescents and young adults. Participation in specific social media activities may predict issues with body image and the amount of time spent online may influence eating disorder symptoms and related concerns, but the research remains mixed on this topic since it is possible that social media does not solely influence the thin ideal, but rather the photos and videos reflect what the current society and individuals already idealize (Derenne & Beresin, 2018; Santarossa & Woodruff, 2017).

As online social media networks rapidly evolve there has been a dramatic increase adolescent users. According to the Pew Research Center, 71 percent of 13- to 17-year-olds reported using Facebook, with most confirming use of a "portfolio" of several additional social networking sites each day. Research suggests that individuals who are vulnerable to overly restrictive eating and exercise habits may be adversely influenced by social media posts that relate to various meal plans and daily workouts. They may also be triggered by fitness and *thinspiration* photos that glorify unrealistically lean, muscled, or emaciated bodies and are extremely popular online. Estimates obtained from popular search engines suggest that thinspiration images can be counted in the millions. Newer internet trends have increased the desire for previously unrecognized characteristics such as a "thigh gap" which suggests that the inner thighs should not touch, or "bikini bridge" where the hip bones protrude such that the material from a swimwear bottom stretches over them creating a gap underneath. Research has found that individuals affected by eating disorders who report frequent use of image-centric social media are more likely to make physical appearance comparisons and experience increased symptom severity (Griffiths et al., 2018). Additionally, many are triggered by online research, viewing documentaries, or being given assignments to calculate their body mass index, or increase their daily activity for a health, biology, or gym class. Additional pressures are imposed by online monitors, such as Fitbit, and apps that monitor caloric intake, steps, and miles run daily (Derenne & Beresin, 2018).

The Thin Ideal and Body Dissatisfaction The ideal shape for women in many developed nations has become thinner and thinner since the mid-twentieth century (Keel & Klump, 2003). Models in fashion magazines, winners of the Miss America and Miss Universe pageants, and Barbie dolls—icons of beauty for women—all have been getting thinner for years, something that is only recently beginning to change. Also, as discussed in the Extraordinary People feature, the average model in a fashion magazine these days is pencil-thin, with a figure that is physically unattainable by most adult women. Several studies show that women who internalize the thin ideal promoted in the media are at risk for eating disorders (see Hausenblas et al., 2013; Keel & Forney, 2013).

Both AN and BN are much more common in females than in males, perhaps because thinness is more valued and more strongly encouraged in females than in males. For example, studies of popular women's and men's magazines find 10 times more diet articles in women's magazines than in men's magazines (Andersen & DiDomenico, 1992; Grieve & Bonneau-Kaya, 2007). As discussed in the Extraordinary People feature, the more exposure young females have to media pressure to be thin, the more dissatisfied they become with their bodies (Grabe et al., 2008; Groesz et al., 2002; Hausenblas et al., 2013). Body dissatisfaction fed by pressures to be thin is one of the strongest predictors of risk for the development of eating disorders in young women. In one longitudinal study of high school girls, 24 percent of those with the greatest body dissatisfaction developed a diagnosable eating disorder, compared to 6 percent of those with less body dissatisfaction (Stice, Marti, & Durant, 2011). Media portrayals of male beauty emphasize muscularity over thinness, and have done so increasingly in recent years. Coinciding with this increase, boys' and men's body dissatisfaction and disordered eating has increased (Murray et al., 2017).

People can avoid some pressures to conform to the ideal of thinness by avoiding fashion magazines and other media depictions. People can't completely avoid their friends, however, and sometimes peers are

Boys and men are increasingly experiencing dissatisfaction with their bodies just as women have, especially when they compare themselves to celebrities such as Zac Efron. *Frederick M. Brown/Getty Images Entertainment/Getty Images*

the most effective carriers of appearance-related messages. Stice and colleagues had women college students talk to another college woman they thought was simply another student but actually was an accomplice in the study (Stice, Maxfield, & Wells, 2003). This accomplice was a thin, attractive 19-year-old woman. In the pressure condition, the accomplice complained about how dissatisfied she was with her weight and discussed her extreme exercise routine and restrictive diet. In the neutral condition, the accomplice talked about classes she was currently taking and her plans for the weekend. The target women in the pressure condition became significantly more dissatisfied with their bodies after talking with the thin accomplice about her weight concerns. In contrast, the women in the neutral condition did not become more dissatisfied with their bodies after talking with the same woman about matters unrelated to weight or dieting.

A study of adolescent girls in Fiji demonstrated the dual influences of peers and the media on eating behavior (Becker et al., 2011). In Fiji's indigenous population, access to popular media (television and the Internet) varies greatly from one region to another. Girls who had more direct media exposure had more eating disorder symptoms, but the strongest predictor of symptoms was the amount of media exposure the girls' friends had. Those girls whose friends watched the most television and had the most Internet access had the highest scores on a measure of eating pathology. When a girl is barraged by messages promoting the thin ideal in the media and these messages are reinforced in her peer network, her risk of developing an eating disorder increases significantly.

The thin ideal remains a strong sociocultural factor in eating disorders, but evidence suggests that its power may be decreasing. A meta-analysis of studies of body dissatisfaction found that thinness-oriented body dissatisfaction among girls and women has decreased over time (Karazsia, Murnen, & Tylka, 2017). It may be that increases in body-accepting messages in the media, visibility of fuller-sized models and celebrities, and ethnic diversity have begun to have psychological effects. Notably, the study showed no comparable decrease in muscularity-oriented body dissatisfaction among men.

Athletes and Eating Disorders One group with additional pressure to maintain a specific weight and body shape is athletes, especially those participating in sports in which weight is considered an important factor in competitiveness, such as gymnastics, ice skating, dancing, horse racing, wrestling, and bodybuilding (Joy, Kussman, & Nattiv, 2016; Smolak, Murnen, & Ruble, 2000). Researchers in Norway assessed all 522 elite female athletes between ages 12 and 35 for the presence of eating disorders. They found that those participating in sports classified as "aesthetic"

TABLE 5 Rates of Eating Disorders in Elite Women Athletes

Sports that emphasize weight are especially likely to encourage eating disorders.

Sport	Percentage with an Eating Disorder (%)
Aesthetic sports (e.g., figure skating, gymnastics)	35
Weight-dependent sports (e.g., judo, wrestling)	29
Endurance sports (e.g., cycling, running, swimming)	20
Technical sports (e.g., golf, high jumping)	14
Ball game sports (e.g., volleyball, soccer)	12

Source: Data from Sundgot-Borgen, 1994.

or "weight-dependent," including diving, figure skating, gymnastics, dance, judo, karate, and wrestling, were most likely to have AN or BN (Table 5; Sundgot-Borgen, 1994; see also Krentz & Warschburger, 2011). Many of the women athletes with eating disorders reported feeling that the physical changes of puberty had decreased their competitive edge. They had

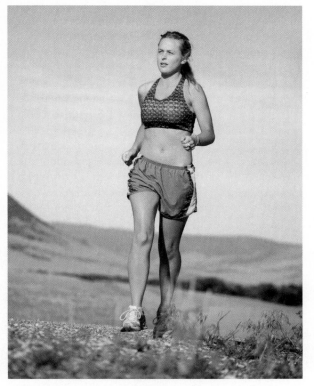

Some people with eating disorders may control their weight through excessive exercise. *Thinkstock Images/Getty Images*

started dieting severely to try to maintain their prepubescent figure. The case of Heidi, described by her therapist, illustrates several of these triggers.

Among men, bodybuilding is an increasingly popular sport, but bodybuilders routinely have substantial weight fluctuations as they shape their bodies for competition and then binge in the off-season. Male bodybuilders tend to have a pattern of eating and exercising as obsessive as that of men with eating disorders, but with a focus on gaining muscle rather than on losing fat (Murray et al., 2017). There is mixed evidence as to whether amateur athletics contributes to eating-disorder behaviors. One study of women college students found that varsity athletes showed the highest rates of eating-disorder behaviors, but club athletes and independent exercisers still had higher rates of some eating-disorder behaviors than did women who did not exercise (Holm-Denoma, Scaringi, Gordon, van Orden, & Joiner, 2009). However, a meta-analysis of studies concluded that, although elite athletes do show increased rates of eating disorders, nonelite athletes—particularly those participating in sports in which thinness is not emphasized—showed lower rates of eating problems than nonathletes (Smolak et al., 2000).

CASE STUDY

Heidi , a 16-year-old gymnast, trains with the university team . . . 4 hours a day, 6 days a week. . . . and anticipates a scholarship to a Big Ten school. Heidi glowed when she talked about gymnastics, but her eyes were red and her voice was hoarse. "I've had this problem for 2 years, but lately it's affecting my gymnastics. I am too weak, particularly on the vault . . . I blame my training for my eating disorder . . . Our coach has weekly weigh-ins where we count each other's ribs. If they are hard to count we're in trouble."

. . . Coach took her and the team to a steak house . . . After she ate, she obsessed about the weigh-in the next day, and decided . . . to get rid of her meal. . . . "It was harder than you would think . . . I thought, 'I'll never do that again,' . . . At first it was weekly . . . Now it's almost every day. (Source: Adapted from Pipher, 1994, pp. 165–168)

Cognitive Factors

When the body dissatisfaction that comes from social pressures to achieve a certain shape or weight is combined with low self-esteem and perfectionism, the result is a toxic mix of cognitive factors that strongly predict the development of an eating disorder (Boone, Soenens, & Luyten, 2014; Culbert et al., 2015; Fairburn, Cooper, Shafra, Bohn, & Hawker, 2008; Vohs et al., 2001).

Women who feel they need a perfect body, are dissatisfied with their body, and have low self-esteem will engage in maladaptive strategies to control their weight, including excessive dieting and purging.

In addition, people with eating disorders tend to be more concerned with the opinions of others and are more conforming to others' wishes, perhaps making them more susceptible to social pressures to be thin (Fairburn et al., 2008; Wade et al., 2008). People with eating disorders tend to have a dichotomous thinking style, judging things as either all good or all bad. For example, if they eat one cookie, they may think that they have blown their diet and might as well eat the whole box of cookies. They will say that they cannot break their rigid eating routines or they will completely lose control over their eating. They obsess over their eating routines and plan their days around these routines, down to the smallest detail (Abramson, Bardone-Cone, Vohs, Joiner, & Heatherton, 2006).

Women with eating disorders may be concerned with body size at an unconscious level (see Keel et al., 2012). Women with and without symptoms of bulimia were shown photos of women who varied in terms of both their body size and the emotions shown on their faces. The participants were not told that these were the critical dimensions along which the photos varied. Women with bulimic symptoms were more likely than the other women in the study to attend to information about body size rather than to information about facial emotion and to classify the photos on the basis of body size rather than facial emotion (Viken, Treat, Nosofsky, McFall, & Palmeri, 2002). Thus, women who show bulimic symptoms unconsciously organize their perceptions of the world around body size more so than do women who do not show significant bulimic symptoms.

Not everyone who diets, or exercises more, develops an eating disorder which suggests that specific underlying factors are involved. Feelings of control (cognitive-emotional dynamics) often drive food restriction in AN, but to what extent this need for control influences the development of the illness is unclear. It is believed that anxious temperaments and perfectionistic traits may facilitate the development and maintenance of core AN behaviors. Research suggests that these type of traits which motivate a desire to do things correctly are strong motivators of eating disorder behaviors. It is also theorized that using weight loss as an indicator of success makes it a a conditioned reward and cognitive reinforcer which increases the likelihood that recurrent weight loss will occur (Frank et al., 2019).

Emotion Regulation Difficulties

Eating-disorder behaviors may sometimes serve as maladaptive strategies for dealing with painful emotions (Kober & Boswell, 2018; Oldershaw, Lavender, Sallis, Stahl, & Schmidt, 2015). Individuals suffering depressive symptoms or, more generally, negative affect are at risk for the development of anorexic, bulimic, and BED symptoms (Leehr et al., 2015; Stice, 2016). Stice and colleagues (2002) followed a group of adolescent girls over a period of 2 years and found that girls who engaged in emotional eating—eating when they felt distressed in an attempt to feel better—were significantly more likely to develop chronic binge eating over those 2 years.

Stice and colleagues have identified two subtypes of disordered eating patterns involving binge eating (Stice, 2002; Stice, Bohon, Marti, & Fischer, 2008). One subtype is connected to excessive attempts to lose weight. Women with this *dieting subtype* are greatly concerned about their body shape and size and try their best to maintain a strict low-calorie diet, but they frequently abandon their regimen and engage in binge eating. They then often use vomiting or exercise to try to purge themselves of the food or of the weight it puts on their bodies. The other subtype is the *depressive subtype*. Women with this subtype also are concerned about their weight and body size, but they are plagued by feelings of depression and low self-esteem and often eat to quell these feelings.

Women with the depressive subtype of disordered eating patterns suffer greater social and psychological consequences over time than do women with the dieting subtype (Stice, 2002; Stice, Bohon, et al., 2008). They face more difficulties in their relationships with family and friends; are more likely to suffer significant psychiatric disorders, such as anxiety disorders; and are less likely to respond well to treatment. Longitudinal studies find that women with the depressive subtype are more likely to be diagnosed with major depression or an anxiety disorder over time and also are more likely to continue to engage in severe binge eating, compared to women with the dieting subtype (Stice & Fairburn, 2003; Stice, Bohon, et al., 2008). Over an 8-year follow-up, 80 percent of the women with the depressive subtype developed major depression. Among those women who suffered both elevated depressive symptoms and body dissatisfaction, 43 percent developed a diagnosable eating disorder (Stice et al., 2011).

Family Dynamics

Many factors may contribute to the development of eating disturbances such as genetics, body dissatisfaction, or fear of weight gain. Also included are cultural and family factors. Family has been identified as a social agent that helps cultivate attitudes and behaviors that relate to healthy and unhealthy eating practices. Parents can both directly and indirectly contribute to body dissatisfaction and the development of eating disorders in children. The quality of family relationships, levels of family conflict and dysfunction, poor communication and inappropriate boundaries have been linked to the development of eating disorders, particularly among adolescents with anorexia (Ioannou, Argyrides, & Mousoulidou, 2020; Leys, Kotsou, Goemanne, & Fossion, 2017). Disordered eating attitudes and behaviors may be related to various family dynamics that include negative experiences with food, weight-related teasing, perceived pressure from parents to be thin and low emotional expression. Families that emphasize thinness and appearance are at higher risk of having children practicing unhealthy eating patterns. For example, research has found that college women who come from families where appearance is highly valued were at higher risk in the family were at higher risk of developing disturbed eating patterns. Additionally, rigid, demanding and controlling (authoritarian) parenting styles are also associated with problematic eating patterns (Leys et al., 2017). It was previously believed that eating disorders and negative body image were problems of "Western" cultures, but recent research suggests that these issues can be found in a variety of cultures that significantly affects girls and women in non-Western countries including India, Singapore, China, United Arab Emirates, Iran, and Cyprus (Ioannou et al., 2020).

Hilde Bruch (1973, 1982), a pioneer in the study of eating disorders, argued that AN often occurs in girls who have been unusually "good girls"—high achievers, dutiful and compliant daughters who are always trying to please their parents and others by being "perfect." These girls tend to have parents who are overinvested in their daughters' compliance and achievements, are overcontrolling, and will not allow the expression of feelings, especially negative feelings (see also Minuchin, Rosman, & Baker, 1978). As a result, the daughters do not learn to identify and accept their own feelings and desires. Instead, they learn to monitor closely the needs and desires of others and to comply with others' demands, as can be seen in the case of Renee and her family.

CASE STUDY

Renee is a 16-year-old trans-girl with anorexia nervosa. Her parents are highly educated and very successful, having spent most of their careers in the diplomatic corps. Renee, her two brothers, and her parents are "very close, as are many families in the diplomatic corps, because we move so much," although the daily care of the children has always been left to nannies. The children had to follow strict rules for appropriate conduct, both in and outside the home. These rules were driven partly by the requirements of the families of diplomats to "be on

(continued)

their best behavior" in their host country and partly by Renee's parents' very conservative religious beliefs. Renee, as the only daughter in the family, always had to behave as "a proper lady" to counteract the stereotype of American girls as brash and sexually promiscuous. All the children were required to act mature beyond their years, controlling any emotional outbursts, accepting defeats and disappointments without complaint, and happily picking up and moving every couple of years when their parents were reassigned to another country.

Renee's anorexic behaviors began when her parents announced they were leaving the diplomatic corps to return to the United States. Renee had grown very fond of their last post in Europe, because she had finally found a group of friends that she liked and of whom her parents approved and she liked her school. She had always done well in school but often had hated the harshly strict teachers. In her present school, she felt accepted by her teachers as well as challenged by the work. When Renee told her parents she would like to finish her last year of high school in this school rather than go to the United States with them, they flatly refused to even consider it. Renee tried to talk with her parents, suggesting she would stay with the family of one of her friends, who was willing to have her, but her parents cut her off and told her they would not discuss the idea further. Renee became sullen and withdrawn and stopped eating shortly after the family arrived in the United States.

One important task of adolescence is separation and individuation from one's family. Bruch argues that girls from overcontrolling families deeply fear separation because they have not developed the ability to act and think independently of their family. They also fear involvement with peers, especially sexual involvement, because they neither understand their feelings nor trust their judgment. Yet at some level they recognize their need to separate from their family. They harbor rage against their parents for their overcontrol and become angry, defiant, and distrustful. They also discover that controlling their food intake both gives them a sense of control over their life and elicits concern from their parents. Their rigid control of their body provides a sense of power over the self and the family that they have never had before. It also provides a way of avoiding peer relationships by presenting herself as sickly, distant, untouchable, and superior in her self-control.

Research has confirmed that the families of girls with eating disorders have high levels of conflict, discourage the expression of negative emotions, and

emphasize control and perfectionism (Holtom-Viesel & Allan, 2014; Wade, Gillespie, & Martin, 2007; see Treasure & Cardi, 2017). Several of these negative characteristics are also prevalent in the families of children with depression, anxiety disorders, and several other forms of psychopathology. What may distinguish families in which AN or BN develops is that the mothers in these families believe their daughters should lose more weight, criticize their daughters' weight, and are themselves more likely to show disordered eating patterns (Arroyo, Segrin, & Andersen, 2017; Hill & Franklin, 1998). One longitudinal study showed that eating and weight-related concerns in 10-year-old children were predicted by the amount of conflict over eating habits and issues of control during mealtimes when the children were 5 years old (Stein et al., 2006). In addition, a lack of awareness of their bodily sensations may allow some girls in these families to ignore even the most severe hunger pangs (Leon, Fulkerson, Perry, & Early-Zald, 1995). Girls from these troubled families who cannot completely ignore their hunger may fall into the binge/purge type of AN or into BN.

Studies of adult women with BED suggest that the combination of low parental warmth and high parental demands or control seems to distinguish girls and women who develop BED from those who develop other forms of psychopathology (Striegel-Moore et al., 2005; Wilfley, Pike, & Striegel-Moore, 1997). Another family characteristic that distinguishes people with BED from individuals with other mental disorders is a history of binge eating among other family members (Striegel-Moore et al., 2005). Thus, individuals who develop the tendency to binge may come from families that modeled and reinforced bingeing behavior (e.g., Braden et al., 2014).

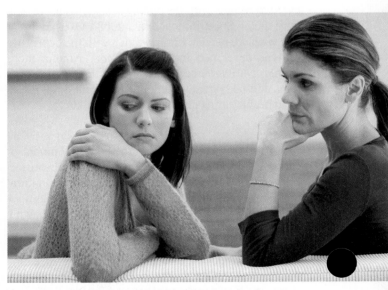

One theory of eating disorders emphasizes the role of overcontrolling families. *STOCK4B/Getty Images*

Unfortunately, the majority of studies of the families and personality characteristics associated with eating disorders have compared people who already have an eating disorder with those who do not. As a result, we do not know to what extent these family and personality characteristics actually are causes of eating disorders. The controlling nature of parents' behaviors toward their child may be a consequence as well as a cause of the disorder, with parents exerting control in order to try to save their child's life.

TREATMENTS FOR EATING DISORDERS

In this section, we discuss psychotherapies and drug treatments for people with eating disorders. There are many more studies of treatments for BN and BED than for AN in part due to prevalence rate among these disorders. Current behavioral and pharmaceutical treatments for eating disorders are presented within this section, but options and efficacy are limited (Frank et al. 2019).

Psychotherapy for Anorexia Nervosa

AN is among the most lethal of all psychiatric conditions and can persist for 20 years or longer among more than half of those affected which makes effective treatment crucial (Murray, Quintana, Loeb, Griffiths, & Le Grange, 2019). Unfortunately, there is limited evidence of effective pharmacological or psychological treatments for AN despite high morbidity and mortality (Duncan et al., 2017). It can be difficult to engage people with AN in psychotherapy. Because they so highly value the thinness they have achieved and believe they must maintain absolute control over their behaviors, people with AN can be resistant to therapy in general, and to therapists' attempts to change their behaviors or attitudes in particular. Regardless of the type of psychotherapy a therapist uses with a client with anorexia, he or she must do much work to win the client's trust and encourage participation in the therapy and to maintain this trust and participation as the client begins to regain the dreaded weight (Wade & Watson, 2012).

Winning the trust of someone with anorexia can be especially difficult if the therapist is forced to hospitalize the client because she has lost so much weight that her life is in danger. However, hospitalization and forced refeeding sometimes are necessary (Olmsted et al., 2010). Because people with AN typically do not seek treatment themselves, often they do not come to the attention of a therapist until they are so malnourished that they have a medical crisis, such as a cardiac problem, or until their families fear for their life. During hospitalization, the therapist will try to engage the client in facing and solving the psychological issues causing her to starve herself.

Psychotherapy can help many people with anorexia, particularly adolescents, but it typically is a long process, often marked by many setbacks (Wade & Watson, 2012). Along the way, many people with anorexia who have an initial period of recovery—with restoration of normal weight and healthy eating patterns—relapse into bulimic or anorexic behaviors (Carter et al., 2012). They often continue to have self-esteem issues, family problems, and periods of depression and anxiety.

CBTs are the most researched treatment for AN (Linardon, Wade, de la Piedad Garcia, & Brennan, 2017). The client's overvaluation of thinness is confronted, and rewards are made contingent on the person's gaining weight. If the client is hospitalized, certain privileges in the hospital are used as rewards, such as going outside the hospital for a shopping trip or receiving family visits (assuming all parties agree to this plan). The client also may be taught relaxation techniques to use as she becomes extremely anxious about ingesting food. Randomized clinical trials find that CBT can lead to weight gains and reductions in symptoms, although a substantial percentage of patients drop out of therapy or return to anorexic behaviors over time (Linardon et al., 2017; Wade & Watson, 2012). So far, comparisons of cognitive-behavioral treatments with other active treatments (e.g., supportive and family treatments) have shown them to be similar in efficacy (Byrne et al., 2017; Linardon et al., 2017).

In family therapy, the person with anorexia and her family are treated as a unit. The best-studied family therapy is the Maudsley model (Lock & le Grange, 2013). The intervention involves 10 to 20 sessions over 6 to 12 months. Parents are initially coached to take control of their child's eating and weight as the child's weight increases to a stable level. As the therapy progresses, the child gains greater autonomy over her eating, in collaboration with her family and therapist. There is evidence that family therapy can be successful in treating girls with AN (Lock, Agras, Bryson, & Kraemer, 2005; Rienecke, 2017).

Psychotherapy for Bulimia Nervosa and Binge-Eating Disorder

CBT has received substantial support as the leading treatment approach for bulimia, with relatively good outcomes for most (Fairburn, 2005; Hail & LaGrange, 2018; Linardon et al., 2017). CBT for BN is based on the view that the extreme concerns about shape and weight are the central features of the disorder (Fairburn et al., 2008). The therapist teaches the client to monitor the cognitions that accompany her eating, particularly the binge episodes and purging episodes. Then the therapist helps the client confront these cognitions and develop more adaptive attitudes toward weight and body shape. An interchange between a therapist and a client might go like this:

Therapist: What were you thinking just before you began to binge?

Client: I was thinking that I felt really upset and sad about having no social life. I wanted to eat just to feel better.

Therapist: And as you were eating, what were you thinking?

Client: I was thinking that the ice cream tasted really good, that it was making me feel good. But I was also thinking that I shouldn't be eating this, that I'm bingeing again. But then I thought that my life is such a wreck that I deserve to eat what I want to make me feel better.

Therapist: And what were you thinking after you finished the binge?

Client: That I was a failure, a blimp, that I have no control, that this therapy isn't working.

Therapist: Okay, let's go back to the beginning. You said you wanted to eat because you thought it would make you feel better. Did it?

Client: Well, as I said, the ice cream tasted good and it felt good to indulge myself.

Therapist: But in the long run, did bingeing make you feel better?

Client: Of course not. I felt terrible afterward.

Therapist: Can you think of anything you might say to yourself the next time you get into such a state, when you want to eat in order to make yourself feel better?

Client: I could remind myself that I'll feel better only for a little while, but then I'll feel terrible.

Therapist: How likely do you think it is that you'll remember to say this to yourself?

Client: Not very likely.

Therapist: Is there any way to increase the likelihood?

Client: Well, I guess I could write it on a card or something and put the card near my refrigerator.

Therapist: That's a pretty good idea. What else could you do to prevent yourself from eating when you feel upset? What other things could you do to relieve your upset, other than eat?

Client: I could call my friend Keisha and talk about how I feel. Or I could go for a walk—someplace away from food—like up in the hills, where it's so pretty. Walking up there always makes me feel better.

Therapist: Those are really good ideas. It's important to have a variety of things you can do, other than eat, to relieve bad moods.

The behavioral components of this therapy involve introducing forbidden foods (such as bread) back into the client's diet and helping the client confront her irrational thoughts about these foods, such as "If I have just one doughnut, I'm inevitably going to binge." Similarly, the client is taught to eat three healthy meals a day and to challenge the thoughts she has about these meals and about the possibility of gaining weight. CBT for bulimia usually lasts about 3 to 6 months and involves 10 to 20 sessions. In addition to CBT, there is evidence to support other approaches, such as interpersonal therapy (IPT) and integrative cognitive-affective therapy (Hail & LaGrange, 2018).

Controlled studies of the efficacy of CBT for bulimia find that about half the clients completely stop the binge/purge cycle (Fairburn, 2005; Shapiro et al., 2007). Clients undergoing this therapy also show a decrease in depression and anxiety, an increase in social functioning, and a lessening of concern about dieting and weight. CBT is more effective than drug therapies in producing complete cessation of binge eating and purging and in preventing relapse over the long term (Fairburn, 2005; Linardon et al., 2017). Expanded CBTs that also address emotion-regulation difficulties are especially effective in people with a combination of eating disorders and depression (Fairburn et al., 2009).

Other studies of the treatment of bulimia have compared CBT with three other types of psychotherapy: IPT, supportive-expressive psychodynamic therapy, and behavioral therapy without a focus on cognitions (Wilson, Fairburn, Agras, Walsh, & Kraemer, 2002; Linardon et al., 2017). In IPT, the client and the therapist discuss interpersonal problems related to the client's eating disorder, and the therapist works actively with the client to develop strategies to solve these problems. In supportive-expressive psychodynamic therapy, the therapist also encourages the client to talk about problems related to the eating disorder—especially interpersonal problems—but in a highly nondirective manner. In behavioral therapy, the client is taught how to monitor her food intake, is reinforced for introducing avoided foods into her diet, and is taught coping techniques for avoiding bingeing. In the studies, all the therapies resulted in significant improvement in the clients' eating behaviors and emotional well-being, but the CBT and IPT clients showed the greatest and most enduring improvements (Linardon et al., 2017). Comparisons of CBT and IPT suggest that CBT is significantly more effective than IPT in treating bulimia and works more quickly, with substantial improvement being shown by 3 to 6 weeks into treatment with CBT (Agras, Walsh, Fairburn, Wilson, & Kraemer, 2000; Fairburn et al., 2015). CBT and IPT appear to be comparably effective in preventing relapse in 1- and 6-year follow-ups (Agras et al., 2000; Linardon et al., 2017).

For BED, CBT has been shown to be more effective than other psychotherapies or antidepressant medications (Brownley et al., 2016; Linardon et al, 2017). CBT reduces binges as well as overconcern with weight, shape, and eating in people with BED.

Despite the efficacy of psychotherapy for eating disorders, and CBT in particular, good treatment can be hard to access (Kazdin, Fitzsimmons-Craft, & Wilfley, 2017). Efforts to improve treatment access include modifying treatment for delivery online and through mobile apps (Agras, Fitzsimmons-Craft, & Wilfley, 2017). In addition, especially because eating disorders tend to develop in adolescence and early adulthood, researchers have developed promising prevention programs that target risk factors such as media exposure and internalization of the thinness ideal (Becker & Stice, 2017; Le, Barendregt, Hay, & Mihalopoulos, 2017).

Biological Therapies

Currently, the only approved medication options for eating disorders are limited to selective serotonin reuptake inhibitors (SSRIs), like fluoxetine (Prozac) for BN and in some countries lisdexamfetamine (Vyvanse) for BED (Lutter, 2017). Vyvanse is a stimulant, often used in the treatment of attention-deficit/hyperactivity disorder, was approved by the FDA in 2015 for the treatment of moderate to severe BED in adults. Although Vyvanse reduces the frequency of binge-eating episodes it is not prescribed for weight loss. As commonly found with the use of stimulants, there is a potential for abuse and dependence as well as serious cardiovascular reactions (Hornberger & Lane, 2021). The use of SSRIs like, fluoxetine (Prozac), have been the focus of much research on biological treatments for BN. These drugs appear to reduce binge-eating and purging behaviors, but often they fail to restore the individual to normal eating habits. Unfortunately, there are no approved treatments for AN, but studies on the use of olanzapine and dronabinol are promising (Flament, Bissada, & Spettigue, 2012; Himmerich, Kan, Au, & Treasure, 2020; Linardon et al., 2017). Adding CBT to antidepressant treatment increases rates of recovery (Fairburn, 2005). Olanzapine, an atypical antipsychotic (see the chapter "Schizophrenia Spectrum and Other Psychotic Disorders"), leads to increases in weight in people with AN (see Flament et al., 2012). Meta-analyses of medications for binge eating found that a number of drugs, including the SSRIs, antiepileptic medications (such as topiramate), and obesity medications (such as orlistat), all are better than a placebo in reducing binge eating but do not tend to reduce concerns about body shape or weight (Brownley et al., 2016; Flament et al., 2012; Reas & Grilo, 2008).

CHAPTER INTEGRATION

Experts generally have suggested that biological, psychological, and social factors interact to cause the eating disorders (see Brownell & Walsh, 2017; Culbert et al., 2015). Any one factor alone may not be enough to lead someone to develop AN or BN, but combined they may do so (Figure 2).

Societal pressures for thinness clearly provide a potent influence on the development of unhealthy attitudes toward eating, especially for women. If these pressures were simply toward achieving a healthy weight and maintaining fitness, they would not be so dangerous. However, the ideal weight for women promoted by beauty symbols in developed countries is much lower than that considered healthy and normal for the average woman, and thus women may develop a negative body image. This leads them to engage in excessive dieting. Unfortunately, excessive dieting sets up conditions for impulsive binge eating, which leads to negative emotions and even lower self-esteem.

The increased use of online social networks is associated with decreased self esteem, happiness, life satisfaction, and increased depression and loneliness reported among young adult users. Image-centered digital media, such as *Instagram, YouTube, Snapchat,* and *Tik Tok* often increase appearance concerns among users which may promote self-consciousness about body image. Participation in specific social media activities may predict issues with body image and the amount of time spent online may influence eating-disorder symptoms and related concerns, but the research remains mixed on this topic since it is possible that social media does not solely influence the thin ideal, but rather the photos and videos reflect what the current society and individuals already idealize.

Biological factors may interact with these societal pressures to make some people more likely than others to develop an eating disorder. People who develop eating disorders may have a genetic predisposition to these disorders or to dysregulation of the hormone or neurotransmitter system. Exactly how the genetic vulnerabilities lead to the symptoms of eating disorders is unclear, but they may contribute to an ability to diet excessively. Another biological factor that may predispose some people to acquiesce to the pressures to diet and to be thin is a tendency toward anxiety or mild depression. Many people with eating disorders, especially people with bulimia nervosa, are often depressed and eat impulsively in response to their moods. Although problems in mood in people with an eating disorder may be the result of environmental circumstances or of the stresses of the disorder, they also may have a biological origin in some people.

Personality factors may interact with societal pressures to be thin and/or with the biological predispositions described to lead some people to develop an eating

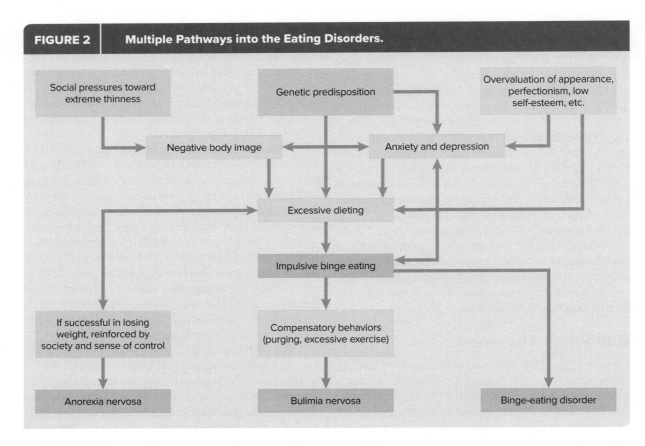

FIGURE 2   Multiple Pathways into the Eating Disorders.

disorder. Perfectionism, all-or-nothing thinking, and low self-esteem may make people more likely to engage in extreme measures to control their weight in pursuit of an ideal of attractiveness. These personality characteristics are more likely to develop in children whose parents are lacking in affection and nurturance and who at the same time are controlling and demanding of perfection.

Whatever pathway an individual takes into the eating disorders, these behaviors tend to be maintained once they begin. The excessive concern over weight among people with AN or BN is constantly reinforced by societal images, and any weight loss they do achieve is reinforced by peers and family. People with anorexia

also may be reinforced by the sense of control they gain over their lives by highly restrictive dieting. People with BN and BED may greatly desire control but are unable to maintain it, so they fall into binge eating to escape negative emotions. The compensatory behaviors of bulimia nervosa help the individual regain some sense of control, however fragile, and thereby are reinforced.

Thus, it may take a mixture of these factors, rather than any single factor, to lead someone to develop a diagnosable eating disorder. Once the disorder sets in, however, it tends to be reinforced and perpetuated. Note also that many of the same factors contribute to each different eating disorder.

SHADES OF GRAY   DISCUSSION

Rachel's eating and exercise behaviors are common for college women and, to some extent, are in line with recommendations to cut out junk food, eat more fruits and vegetables, and get more exercise. Yet Rachel's weight has dropped to a level that is well below what is considered healthy for her height. She also has become obsessive about her exercise routine, her mood is chronically low, and she is losing interest in school.

Prior to the *DSM-5,* Rachel would not have been diagnosed with anorexia nervosa because there is no evidence that her menstrual periods have stopped. Rachel might have received a *DSM-IV* diagnosis of

eating disorder not otherwise specified because she has significant symptoms that nonetheless do not meet the criteria for anorexia nervosa, bulimia nervosa, or binge-eating disorder. The *DSM-5* does not require cessation of menses for the diagnosis of anorexia nervosa, so Rachel's symptoms now would probably qualify for the diagnosis. Rachel's case illustrates questions that have been debated over the last few decades about whether the diagnostic criteria for the eating disorders are too strict or whether it would be better to avoid applying a psychiatric diagnosis to such common behavior.

CHAPTER SUMMARY

- The eating disorders include anorexia nervosa, bulimia nervosa, and binge-eating disorder.

- Anorexia nervosa is characterized by self-starvation, a distorted body image, intense fears of becoming fat, and often amenorrhea. People with the restricting type of anorexia nervosa refuse to eat and/or engage in excessive exercise in order to prevent weight gain. People with the binge/purge type periodically engage in bingeing and then purge to prevent weight gain.

- The lifetime prevalence of anorexia is under 1 percent, with 90 to 95 percent of cases seen in females. Anorexia nervosa usually begins in adolescence, and the course is variable from one person to another. It is a very dangerous disorder with a relatively high death rate from complications of self-starvation and suicide.

- Bulimia nervosa is characterized by uncontrolled bingeing followed by inappropriate compensatory behaviors designed to prevent weight gain from the binges (e.g., self-induced vomiting, misuse of laxatives or diuretics, excessive exercise).

- Bulimia nervosa is more common in females than in males. The onset of bulimia nervosa most often is in adolescence. Although people with bulimia do not tend to be underweight, bulimia nervosa has several dangerous medical complications.

- People with binge-eating disorder engage in bingeing, but not in purging or in behaviors designed to compensate for the binges. People with the disorder tend to be significantly overweight.

- The *DSM-5* diagnosis other specified feeding or eating disorder replaced the *DSM-IV* eating disorder not otherwise specified. It may be given to individuals who show severe symptoms of an eating disorder but do not meet the full criteria for one of the eating disorders (e.g., atypical anorexia nervosa, bulimia nervosa of low frequency and/or limited duration). People with night eating disorder, who ingest much of their caloric intake at night, may be given this diagnosis.

- Obesity is defined as a body mass index of 30 or more. Obesity rates have skyrocketed in recent years, largely due to increases in the intake of high-fat, low-nutrient food and decreases in physical activity. Treatments for obesity include commercial weight-loss programs, medications, low-calorie diets, and bariatric surgery.

- The biological factors implicated in the development of the eating disorders include genetics, the dysregulation of hormone and neurotransmitter systems, and generally lower functioning in the hypothalamus.

- Sociocultural theorists have attributed the eating disorders to pressures to be thin, especially in developed nations.

- Social media has been identified as a significant factor in the development of eating disorders. Image-centered digital media, such as Instagram, YouTube, Snapchat, and Tik Tok often increase appearance concerns among users which may promote self-consciousness about body image. Those individuals who are vulnerable to overly restrictive eating and exercise habits may be adversely influenced by social media posts that relate to various meal plans and daily workouts.

- Eating disorders may develop in some people as maladaptive strategies for coping with negative emotions. Also, certain cognitive factors, including overvaluation of appearance, perfectionism, low self-esteem, excessive concern about others' opinions, and a rigid, dichotomous thinking style, may contribute to the development of the eating disorders.

- The families of girls with eating disorders may be overcontrolling, overprotective, and hostile and may not allow the expression of feelings, especially negative feelings. In adolescence, these girls may develop eating disorders as a way of exerting control.

- Cognitive-behavioral therapy and family therapy have been shown to be effective in the treatment of anorexia nervosa.

- Cognitive-behavioral therapy has proven to be the most effective therapy for reducing the symptoms of bulimia and binge-eating disorder and preventing relapse. Interpersonal therapy, supportive-expressive psychodynamic therapy, and behavioral therapy also appear to be effective in treating bulimia nervosa.

- Antidepressants can reduce symptoms in anorexia nervosa, bulimia nervosa, and binge-eating disorder. The atypical antipsychotic olanzapine can help restore weight in people with anorexia nervosa.

KEY TERMS

anorexia nervosa (AN)

amenorrhea

restricting type of anorexia nervosa

binge/purge type of anorexia nervosa

bulimia nervosa

bingeing

binge-eating disorder (BED)

other specified feeding or eating disorder

atypical anorexia nervosa

night eating disorder

obesity

Chapter 13

Sam Wordley/Shutterstock

Sexual Disorders and Gender Diversity

CHAPTER OUTLINE

Sexuality and Gender Along the Continuum

Sexual functioning, sexual practices, and gender identity that bring the individual positive well-being and relationships

Potentially meets diagnostic criteria for a sexual disorder:

- **Difficulties in sexual functioning that cause moderate distress or difficulties in relationships** *(frequent difficulty reaching orgasm)*
- **Atypical sexual practices that cause distress or difficulties in social functioning** *(one's partner disapproves of the objects used in sexual practice)*
- **Uncertainty about gender identity**

Functional ———————————————————————— **Dysfunctional**

- **Occasional difficulties in sexual functioning that do not cause distress or relationships difficulties** *(occasional difficulty reaching orgasm)*
- **Atypical sexual practices that do not cause distress or difficulties in social functioning** *(use of objects as part of sex play with a consenting partner)*
- **Questions about gender identity that eventually are resolved**

Likely meets diagnostic criteria for a sexual disorder:

- **Chronic difficulties in sexual functioning that cause significant distress or difficulties in relationships** *(complete lack of sexual desire)*
- **Atypical sexual practices that cause significant distress or difficulties in social functioning** *(inappropriate objects become the sole focus of sexual activities, arrests for illegal sexual behavior)*
- **Significant distress regarding gender identity, desire to change genders**

Before the work of researchers William Masters and Virginia Johnson in the 1950s and 1960s, we knew little about typical or atypical **sexual functioning**—that is, what happens in the body during sexual activity. Occasional problems with sexual functioning, such as difficulty reaching orgasm or lack of sexual desire, are extremely common. When people have difficulties in sexual functioning that are persistent and that cause significant distress or interpersonal difficulty, they may be diagnosed with *a sexual dysfunction* (Balon, Segraves, & Clayton, 2007; Wincze & Weinberg, 2015). Studies around the world suggest that 40 to 45 percent of women and 20 to 30 percent of men frequently experience sexual dysfunctions (Lewis et al., 2010).

The activities and objects that people find arousing vary tremendously. When people focus their sexual activity on something considered inappropriate by society—for example, nonliving objects, prepubescent children, nonconsenting adults, or suffering or humiliation—they may be diagnosed with a *paraphilic disorder*. Many people have occasional paraphilic fantasies which fall within the spectrum of normal sexual behavior. Fantasies involving spanking or being spanked, domination and submission, as well as incest, bestiality, transsexuals, and "grannies" were also identified as common themes. A recent study found that more than half (58.6 percent) of participants reported at least one "paraphilic" sexual fantasy, including voyeurism (34.9 percent), fetishism (30 percent), and sadism (21.8 percent) (Joyal, Cossette, & Lapierre, 2015). For example, rape fantasies are relatively common among men and women and are considered part of the normal sexual experience. While various themes may fuel a sexual encounter many who report these fantasies also note their disinterest in acting out that fantasy. In a recent analysis of internet-based search content, erotic themes of incest and violence which are typically considered taboo are also common themes found in sexual fantasy (Seehuus, Stanton, & Handy, 2019). Unlike fantasy which is considered a healthy dimension of sexual behavior, people diagnosed with a paraphilic disorder often feel compelled to engage in their paraphilias, even though their behaviors cause them distress or create social, occupational, or legal problems.

Finally, individuals also vary in their **gender identity**—their perception of themselves as male, female, another gender, or without gender. Gender identity differs from *gender roles,* which are society's expectations for how males and females should act. Many females engage in behaviors considered part of the traditional masculine gender role, such as playing aggressive sports or pursuing competitive careers, but still have a fundamental sense of themselves as female. Similarly, many males engage in behaviors considered part of the traditional feminine gender role, such as caring for children, cooking, or sewing, but still have a fundamental sense of themselves as male. When an individual believes they were born with the body of the wrong gender and experiences significant distress, the *DSM-5* defines this as *gender dysphoria* (formerly called gender identity disorder).

Extraordinary People

David Reimer, *The Boy Who Was Raised as a Girl*

In April 1966, 8-month-old Bruce Reimer underwent a routine circumcision to alleviate a painful medical condition on his penis. The operation went terribly wrong, however, and Bruce's penis was accidentally severed. None of the doctors whom Bruce's anguished parents consulted could offer any hope of restoring the penis and suggested that he would never be able to function as a normal male. But Dr. John Money offered them a solution: Raise Bruce as a girl and have him undergo sex reassignment therapy. Dr. Money firmly believed that male or female identity depends on the environment in which a child is raised, not on genes or the genitals with which he or she is born. Bruce's condition presented Dr. Money with the perfect opportunity to prove his theory. Not only had Bruce been born male, but he had an identical twin brother as well. If surgically reassigning Bruce's sex and raising him as a girl resulted in Bruce fully accepting himself as a girl, when his twin brother identified himself as a boy, Money's theories of gender identity would be soundly supported.

Bruce's parents renamed him Brenda Lee and began dressing him in feminine clothes. The child underwent a bilateral orchidectomy—removal of both testicles—at the age of 22 months. Brenda's parents then furnished her with dolls and tried to reinforce her identity as a girl. Brenda, however, resisted. As brother Brian recalled, "When I say there was nothing feminine about Brenda . . . I mean there was nothing feminine. She walked like a guy. Sat with her legs apart. We both wanted to play with guys, build forts and have snowball fights and play army. She'd get a skipping rope for a gift, and the only thing we'd use that for was to tie people up, whip people with it" (Colapinto, 2000, p. 57).

As Brenda grew up, she refused surgery to create a vagina for her and insisted on urinating standing up. Beginning at age 12, Brenda was given estrogen, and as a result she began to develop breasts. However, her voice began to crack, just like her brother's. Finally, when Brenda was 14, her father told her the truth about the botched circumcision and her parents' decision to raise her as a girl. Brenda said, "I was relieved. . . . Suddenly it all made sense why I felt the way I did. I wasn't some sort of weirdo. I wasn't crazy" (Colapinto, 2000, p. 180).

Brenda immediately decided to revert to her biological sex. She renamed herself David, after the biblical king and giant-slayer. David began to take injections of testosterone and in 1980 underwent a double mastectomy to remove the breasts he had grown. Then, a month before his sixteenth birthday, he had surgery to create a rudimentary penis. Still, David's reentry into life as a boy was difficult. He still looked and talked differently from other boys and, as a result, was teased and shunned. The artificial genitals that had been fashioned for him frequently became blocked, and he went through several additional surgeries and treatments. Over the next few years, David attempted suicide and secluded himself in a mountain cabin for months at a time.

Finally, after his 22nd birthday, David had a new kind of surgery to create a more acceptable and functional penis. In 1990, David married a young woman named Jane, and things went well for a while. But after losing his job, experiencing financial difficulties, and separating from his wife, David committed suicide in 2004. According to his mother, he had also been grieving the death of his brother, which had occurred 2 years before the suicide. In a news story after David's death, John Colapinto, his biographer, noted, "David's blighted childhood was never far from his mind. Just before he died, he talked to his wife about his sexual 'inadequacy,' his inability to be a true husband. Jane tried to reassure him. But David was already heading for the door" (Colapinto, 2004).

David Reimer's story raises many questions about the biological and social contributors to our self-concept as male or female, our sexual preferences, and the role of sexuality and gender in our psychological well-being. In this chapter, we consider how biology interacts with social norms and psychological factors to produce both sexual health and sexual disorders.

As noted in Sexuality and Gender Along the Continuum, much of what we know about what happens in the human body during sexual activity is rooted in Masters and Johnson's (1970) groundbreaking work. They observed people engaging in a variety of sexual practices in a laboratory setting and recorded the physiological changes that occurred, concluding that the human sexual response cycle consists of five phases of physical and emotional change: desire, arousal or excitement, plateau, orgasm, and resolution (Figure 1). **Sexual desire** is the urge to engage in any type of sexual activity, even imaginal, such as fantasy. The **arousal phase,** or excitement phase, combines a psychological experience of pleasure and the physiological changes known as *vasocongestion* and *myotonia.* Vasocongestion, or *engorgement,* occurs when blood vessels and tissues fill with blood. In males, erection of the penis is caused by an increase in the flow of blood into the arteries of the penis, accompanied by a decrease in the outflow of blood from the penis through the veins. In females, vasocongestion causes the clitoris to enlarge, the labia to swell, and the vagina to become moist. Myotonia is muscular tension. During the arousal phase, many muscles in the body become tenser, culminating in the muscular contractions known as orgasm.

After arousal is the **plateau phase,** when excitement remains at a high but stable level. This period is pleasurable in itself, and some people try to extend the plateau phase as long as possible before reaching **orgasm,** the discharge of the neuromuscular tension built up during the excitement and plateau phases. In males, orgasm involves rhythmic contractions of the prostate and the entire length of the penis and urethra, accompanied by the ejaculation of semen. After ejaculation, a *refractory* period, lasting from a few minutes to a few hours, occurs in which the male cannot achieve full erection and another orgasm, regardless of the type or intensity of sexual stimulation. In females, orgasm generally involves rhythmic contractions of the vagina and more irregular contractions of the uterus, which are not always felt. Because females do not have a refractory period, they are capable of experiencing additional orgasms immediately following one. However, not all women find multiple orgasms easy to achieve or desirable. Following orgasm, the entire musculature of the body relaxes, and men and women tend to experience a state of deep relaxation, the stage known as **resolution.**

If you are sexually active, you may or may not have recognized all these phases in your sexual response cycle. People vary greatly in the length and distinctiveness of each phase. Although the work of Masters and Johnson was critical to our understanding of sexual functioning, it soon became clear that people vary tremendously in the extent to which they consciously experience each of these phases anytime they engage in sexual activity. For example, Masters and Johnson's depiction of the sexual response cycle may be more characteristic of men than of women, as women's responses tend to be more variable than men's (Basson et al., 2001; Giraldi, Kristensen, & Sand, 2015). Sometimes, the excitement phase is short for a female, and she reaches a discernible orgasm quickly. At other times, the excitement phase is longer, and she may or may not experience a full orgasm.

Occasional difficulties at one or more of the phases of the sexual response cycle are common (Michael, Gagnon, Laumann, & Kolata, 1994). As we discuss later, these difficulties may be tied to stresses in individuals' lives, medications they are taking, illness, or problems in their relationships. Individuals

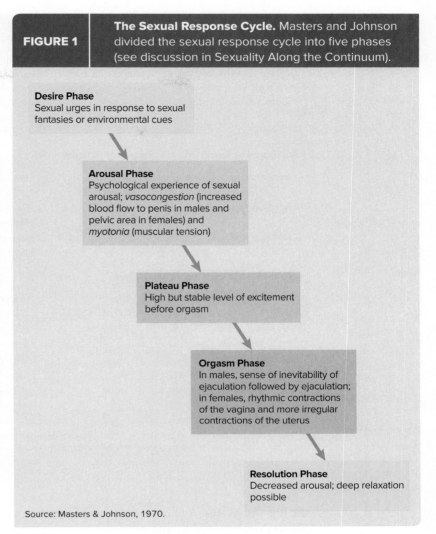

FIGURE 1

The Sexual Response Cycle. Masters and Johnson divided the sexual response cycle into five phases (see discussion in Sexuality Along the Continuum).

Desire Phase
Sexual urges in response to sexual fantasies or environmental cues

Arousal Phase
Psychological experience of sexual arousal; *vasocongestion* (increased blood flow to penis in males and pelvic area in females) and *myotonia* (muscular tension)

Plateau Phase
High but stable level of excitement before orgasm

Orgasm Phase
In males, sense of inevitability of ejaculation followed by ejaculation; in females, rhythmic contractions of the vagina and more irregular contractions of the uterus

Resolution Phase
Decreased arousal; deep relaxation possible

Source: Masters & Johnson, 1970.

who have persistent difficulties that cause them distress or interfere with their social or occupational functioning may be diagnosed with a sexual dysfunction.

SEXUAL DYSFUNCTIONS

The **sexual dysfunctions** are a set of disorders in which people have difficulty responding sexually or experiencing sexual pleasure (Table 1). To qualify for a diagnosis of a sexual dysfunction, the difficulty must be more than occasional or transient, and must cause significant distress or interpersonal difficulty. The distress and impairment criteria are especially important when considering a diagnosis of sexual dysfunction, because there is a great deal of variability in what is considered a normal human sexual experience. The *DSM-5* recognizes seven distinct sexual dysfunction disorders, which can roughly be divided into disorders of desire and arousal and disorders of orgasm and sexual pain (see Table 1). To be diagnosed with any of these disorders, the dysfunction must occur most of

TABLE 1   *DSM-5* Sexual Dysfunctions*

The sexual dysfunction disorders can be roughly divided into disorders of sexual desire and arousal and disorders of orgasm and sexual pain. If a sexual dysfunction is caused by a substance (e.g., alcohol) or medication, it is given the diagnosis substance/medication-induced sexual dysfunction. All sexual dysfunctions (except substance/medication-induced sexual dysfunction) require a minimum duration of approximately 6 months.

Disorder	Description
Disorders of Sexual Interest/Desire or Arousal	
Female sexual interest/arousal disorder	Persistent lack of, or significantly reduced, interest in sexual activity and/or lack of arousal in response to sexual activity
Male hypoactive desire disorder	Persistently absent or deficient sexual/erotic thoughts or fantasies, or desire for sexual activity
Erectile disorder	Recurrent inability to attain or maintain an erection or a marked decrease in erectile rigidity
Disorders of Orgasm or Sexual Pain	
Female orgasmic disorder	Reduced intensity, or recurrent delay or absence of orgasm during sexual activity
Early ejaculation	Recurrent ejaculation within 1 minute of initiation of partnered sexual activity when not desired
Delayed ejaculation	Marked delay, infrequency, or absence of ejaculation during sexual encounters
Genito-pelvic pain/penetration disorder	Marked difficulties having vaginal penetration; pain or tightening of pelvic floor muscles during penetration

*The information presented in this table is based solely on the author's interpretation of DSM-5. It does not reflect the exact language that appears in DSM-5 and is not, therefore, formally endorsed by the APA.

Source: *Diagnostic and Statistical Manual of Mental Disorders,* 5th Edition. American Psychiatric Association, 2013.

the time for at least 6 months, must cause significant distress or impairment, and must not be due to another, nonsexual psychiatric problem (e.g., depression); a substance or medication; a general medical condition; or stressors. If individuals do have a sexual dysfunction caused by a substance (such as chronic alcohol abuse) or a medication (such as an antidepressant), they may be diagnosed with *substance/medication-induced sexual dysfunction.* In reality, these dysfunctions overlap significantly, and many people who seek treatment for a sexual problem have more than one nonsexual dysfunction (American Psychiatric Association, 2013).

When considering whether or not someone suffers from a sexual dysfunction, clinicians should assess for several factors that may contribute to the symptoms, in order to fully understand the patient and as a tool in formulating interventions. These factors include partner factors such as health issues and sexual problems; relationship factors, including conflict and communication issues; individual vulnerability factors such as a history of abuse; cultural or religious beliefs; and relevant medical conditions (American Psychiatric Association, 2013, p. 423).

Disorders of Sexual Interest/ Desire and Arousal

Sexual desire can be manifested in a person's sexual thoughts and fantasies, a person's interest in initiating or participating in sexual activities, and a person's awareness of sexual cues from others (Krakowsky & Grober, 2016; Sand & Fisher, 2007). People vary tremendously in their levels of sexual desire or interest, and an individual's level of sexual desire or interest can vary greatly across time (Michael et al., 1994). Low sexual desire or arousal is among the most common problems for which people seek treatment (Leiblum, 2010; Wincze, Bach, & Barlow, 2008).

Male Hypoactive Sexual Desire Disorder

Men with **male hypoactive sexual desire disorder** have little desire for sex and have deficient or absent sexual thoughts or fantasies—they do not fantasize about sex or initiate sexual activity and may be unresponsive when a partner initiates sex (American Psychiatric Association, 2013). This lack of sexual desire causes them marked distress or interpersonal difficulty. In some rare cases, men report never having had much interest in sex, either with other people or privately (e.g., viewing of erotic films, masturbation, or fantasy). These men are diagnosed with *lifelong male hypoactive sexual desire disorder,* as the disturbance has always been present. In most cases, the man used to enjoy sex but has lost interest in it, a condition diagnosed as *acquired male hypoactive sexual desire disorder*. Inhibited desire can be either generalized to all partners and situations or specific to certain partners or types of stimulation. Obviously, the judgment about when a man's sexual desire has been too low for too long is subjective. The *DSM-5* specifies that the clinician should make this determination with consideration of other aspects of the person's life, including age. Between 15 and 20 percent of men report frequent problems involving hypoactive sexual desire, with higher rates among older men than among younger men (Krakowsky & Grober, 2016; McCabe et al., 2016).

Female Sexual Interest/Arousal Disorder

The nature of sexual desire or interest may be different for men and women. For men, the *DSM-5* defines desire as the presence of sexual fantasies and yearning to have sex, but many women say they seldom engage in sexual fantasies or yearning for sex yet do desire and enjoy sex (Sand & Fisher, 2007). In addition, sexual interest or desire and sexual arousal seem to be more intimately connected with each other in women than in men. In some women, sexual interest precedes arousal, while in others it follows it. As a result of these differences between women and men, and because for women problems with arousal and desire frequently coexist, the *DSM-5* combines difficulties in sexual interest or arousal into one diagnosis for women, **female sexual interest/arousal disorder.** In order to receive this diagnosis, a woman must, for at least 6 months, report at least three of the following symptoms: absent or significantly reduced interest in sexual activity, in sexual or erotic thoughts or fantasies, in initiation of sex or receptiveness to sex, in excitement or pleasure in most sexual encounters, in sexual responsiveness to erotic cues, or in genital or nongenital responses to sexual activity. As in male hypoactive sexual disorder, female sexual interest/arousal disorder can be either lifelong or acquired. It is important to note that female sexual interest/arousal disorder should not be diagnosed simply when there is a difference of interest between sexual partners, and that "most" in the criteria refers to having absent or significantly reduced excitement or pleasure in approximately 75 to 100 percent of sexual encounters (American Psychiatric Association, 2013).

The data we have on these problems in women come mostly from the *DSM-IV* diagnostic scheme, which separated sexual desire problems and sexual arousal problems in women. More than 30 percent of women report an occasional lack of desire for sex (McCabe et al., 2016). In a study of over 31,000 women, unusually low sexual desire was diagnosed in 9.5 percent of them (Clayton, 2007). Rates of low sexual desire increase to 26 percent in postmenopausal women (Leiblum, Koochaki, Rodenberg, Barton, & Rosen, 2006). For diagnosable levels of low desire, researchers estimate prevalence of 8.9 percent of women between 18 and 44, 12.3 percent between 45 and 64, and 7.4 percent age 65 or older (Parish & Hahn, 2016). Women with low sexual desire are more likely than men to report anxiety, depression, and life stress. About 20 percent of women report difficulties with lubrication or arousal during sexual activity (Lewis et al., 2010; McCabe et al., 2016). The study of over 31,000 women found that 5.4 percent could be diagnosed with a *DSM-IV* sexual arousal disorder (Clayton, 2007). Some discrepancy in prevalence rates has been reported depending on whether or not "distress" accompanies reported symptoms. Some women who experience problems with arousal and desire are not distressed by this (American Psychiatric Association, 2013).

Erectile Disorder

Erectile disorder (ED) in men (sometimes referred to as *impotence*) involves the recurrent inability to attain or maintain an erection until the completion of sexual activity or a marked decrease in erectile rigidity. Men with the lifelong form of erectile disorder have never been able to sustain an erection for a desired period of time. Men with the acquired form of the disorder were able to sustain an erection in the past but no longer can. This dysfunction can be identified as generalized or situational (American Psychiatric Association, 2013). Occasional problems in achieving or sustaining an erection are common, with as many as 30 million men in the United States having erectile problems at some time in their life. Erectile dysfunction is strongly associated with age and more likely to affect older men than younger men. Approximately 40 percent of men aged 40 and 70 percent of men aged 70 have some form of ED (Retzler, 2019). One U.S. study found a fourfold increase in the prevalence of ED among men in their seventies as compared with men in their twenties. While advanced age and poor cardiovascular function is most associated with ED, there is evidence of increasing incidence of ED in men younger than 40 years. It is posited that the prevalence rates among younger men may be underestimated due to underreporting (Nguyen, Gabrielson, & Hellstrom, 2017).

Epidemiological studies estimate that ED affects 8 percent men (20–29 years) and 11 percent among those aged 30 to 39 years. Most of the studies involving young men under the age of 40 years have been performed in Europe where the prevalence of ED ranges

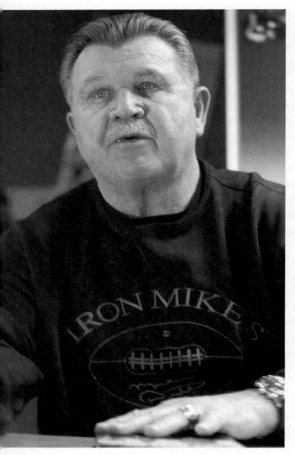

Thanks in part to endorsements by celebrities such as baseball player Rafael Palmeiro, former Senator Bob Dole, and former Chicago Bears coach Mike Ditka (pictured), sales of medications to treat erectile disorder have skyrocketed.
Shutterstock

between 1 and 10 percent (Rastrelli & Maggi, 2017). ED is an increasing health concern around the world that significantly impacts the quality of life of men and their sexual partners each year. It is estimated that 322 million men worldwide will be affected by ED by 2025, which is a significant increase from 152 million men in 1995 (Kessler, Sollie, Challacombe, Briggs, & Van Hemelrijck, 2019).

Such problems do not constitute a disorder until they become persistent and significantly interfere with a man's interpersonal relationships or cause distress. The criteria for erectile disorder specify that a man must fail to achieve or maintain an erection until completion of sexual activity on all or almost all (75 to 100 percent) occasions over a period of approximately 6 months (American Psychiatric Association, 2013).

ED affects approximately 15.5 to 69.2 percent of men worldwide, but various definitions and assessment methods impact the range of ED prevalence (Kessler et al., 2019). One nationwide study (Saigal et al., 2006) found that one in five men over age 20 could be diagnosed with erectile dysfunction; similar or slightly lower rates have been found internationally (McCabe et al., 2016). The prevalence of erectile dysfunction increases dramatically with age, with over 77 percent of men over age 75 affected by it (Lewis et al., 2010; McCabe et al., 2016; Saigal et al., 2006). The *DSM-5* reports that many clinicians have noted that lifelong dysfunction is associated with psychological contributors that are often amenable to treatment, whereas acquired cases are more often associated with biological causes. Problems with erectile functioning can be both the result and the cause of other difficulties in a couple's relationship.

Disorders of Orgasm or Sexual Pain

Individuals can desire to have sex, become aroused during sexual activity, but not experience an orgasm. In addition, women can experience significant pain or tightening of the pelvic muscles upon penetration.

Female Orgasmic Disorder

Women with **female orgasmic disorder,** or *anorgasmia*, experience markedly reduced intensity of orgasms, or delay or absence of orgasm, after having reached the excitement phase of the sexual response cycle in at least 75 percent of sexual encounters. Female orgasmic disorder can be either lifelong or acquired.

About one in four women reports occasional difficulty reaching orgasm (Laumann, Paik, & Rosen, 1999; McCabe et al., 2016), and 4.7 percent can be diagnosed with orgasmic disorder (Clayton, 2007). The problem is greater among postmenopausal women, with about one in three reporting some problem reaching orgasm during sexual stimulation (Clayton, 2007). As has been found with female sexual interest/arousal disorder, some women who have symptoms of female orgasmic disorder are not distressed by this and therefore would not warrant a diagnosis.

Early Ejaculation and Delayed Ejaculation

The most common form of orgasmic disorder in males is **early or premature ejaculation.** Men with this disorder persistently ejaculate with minimal sexual stimulation before they wish to ejaculate. Again, it is a judgment call as to when early ejaculation becomes a sexual dysfunction. The *DSM-5* specifies that, in order to receive this diagnosis, a man must ejaculate within 1 minute of penetration in partnered sexual activity and before the man wishes it on 75 percent of occasions over a period of at least 6 months. It can be either lifelong or acquired. The *DSM-5* also notes that early ejaculation may be applied to nonpenetrative sexual activities, but specific duration criteria are not known.

Edward Laumann and colleagues (1999) found that 21 percent of men reported problems with early ejaculation; others report rates as high as 40 percent (Williams & Johnson, 2016). Some men seeking treatment for this problem simply cannot prevent ejaculation before their partner reaches orgasm. Others ejaculate after very little stimulation, long before their partner is fully aroused. A community-based study found that 13 percent of men could be diagnosed with premature ejaculation by the *DSM-IV-TR* criteria, which were less specific than the *DSM-5* criteria in defining early ejaculation or requiring that it occur at least 75 percent of the time (Patrick et al., 2005). When the 1-minute criterion is applied, the prevalence of men who meet the criteria for the disorder falls to 1 to 3 percent (American Psychiatric Association, 2013, p. 444).

Men try to manage problems with early ejaculation by applying desensitizing cream to the penis before sex, wearing multiple condoms, distracting themselves with other thoughts while having sex, not allowing their partner to touch them, and masturbating multiple times shortly before having sex (Althof, 1995). These tactics generally are unsuccessful and

CASE STUDY

Bill and Margaret were a couple in their late twenties who had been married for 2 years. They had had a tumultuous dating relationship before marriage. A therapist helped Bill and Margaret deal with issues in their relationship. However, the therapist made an incorrect assumption that with increased intimacy and the commitment of marriage, Bill's ejaculatory control problem would disappear. . . .

Margaret saw the early ejaculation as a symbol of lack of love and caring on Bill's part. As the problem continued over the next 2 years, Margaret became increasingly frustrated and withdrawn. She demonstrated her displeasure by resisting his sexual advances, and their intercourse frequency decreased from three or four times per week to once every 10 days. A sexual and marital crisis was precipitated by Margaret's belief that Bill was acting more isolated and distant when they did have intercourse. When they talked about their sexual relationship, it was usually in bed after intercourse, and the communication quickly broke down into tears, anger, and accusations. Bill was on the defensive and handled the sexual issue by avoiding talking to Margaret, which frustrated her even more.

Unbeknownst to Margaret, Bill had attempted a do-it-yourself technique to gain better control. He had bought a desensitizing cream he'd read about in a men's magazine and applied it to the glans of his penis (the caplike structure at the end of the penis) 20 minutes before initiating sex. During intercourse he tried to keep his leg muscles tense and think about sports as a way of keeping his arousal in check. Bill was unaware that Margaret felt emotionally shut out during sex. Bill was becoming more sensitized to his arousal cycle and was worrying about erection. He was not achieving better ejaculatory control, and he was enjoying sex less. The sexual relationship was heading downhill, and miscommunication and frustration were growing. (McCarthy, B. W. [1989]. Cognitive-behavioral strategies and techniques in the treatment of early ejaculation. In S. R. Leiblum, & R. C. Rosen [Eds.], *Principles and practice of sex therapy: Update for the 1990s* [pp. 151–152]. New York: Guilford Press. Used with permission. Permission conveyed through Copyright Clearance Center.)

can make the man's partner feel shut out of the sexual encounter, as in the following case study.

Men with **delayed ejaculation** experience a marked delay in or the absence of orgasm following the excitement phase of the sexual response cycle in at least 75 percent of sexual encounters. Unlike early ejaculation, the definition of "delay" is not precisely defined and research does not yet suggest a clear definition. In most cases of this disorder, a man cannot ejaculate during intercourse but can ejaculate with manual or oral stimulation. Eight percent of men report problems reaching orgasm (Laumann et al., 1999; see also McCabe et al., 2016); it is estimated that less than 3 percent of men could be diagnosed with delayed ejaculation (Perelman & Rowland, 2008).

Genito-Pelvic Pain/Penetration Disorder

In community surveys, 12 to 39 percent of women report frequent pain during intercourse (Farmer, Kukkonen, & Binik, 2008; McCabe et al., 2016). The pain may be shallow during intromission (insertion of the penis into the vagina) or deep during penile thrusting. Some women also experience pain when inserting tampons, having a gynecological exam, riding a bike, or even walking (Farmer, Kao, & Binik, 2009). The pain can be the result of dryness of the vagina caused by antihistamines or other drugs, infection of the clitoris or vulvar area, injury or irritation to the vagina, or tumors of the internal reproductive organs. Pain during intercourse is rare in men, but when it does occur, it involves painful erections or pain during thrusting (Farmer et al., 2009).

In addition, some women experience involuntary contraction of the muscles surrounding the outer third of the vagina when penetration with a penis, finger, tampon, or speculum is attempted. These contractions are often called vaginismus. These women may experience sexual arousal and have an orgasm when their clitoris is stimulated. In other women, even the anticipation of vaginal insertion may result in this muscle spasm. It is estimated that 1 to 9 percent of women experience such muscle tightening (Perez, Brown, & Binik, 2016).

Women who for approximately 6 months recurrently experience either pain or muscle tightening during sex, or who have marked fear or anxiety about experiencing such pain, can be diagnosed with **genito-pelvic pain/penetration disorder.**

Causes of Sexual Dysfunctions

Most sexual dysfunctions probably have multiple causes, including both biological and psychosocial causes.

Biological Causes

The *DSM-5* specifies that to receive a diagnosis of any sexual dysfunction, the dysfunction cannot be caused exclusively by a medical condition. Still, many medical illnesses can cause problems in sexual functioning in both men and women. One of the most common contributors to sexual dysfunction is diabetes, which can lower sexual drive, arousal, enjoyment, and satisfaction, especially in men (Maiorino, Bellastella,

& Esposito, 2014). Diabetes often goes undiagnosed, leading people to believe that psychological factors are causing their sexual dysfunction when the cause actually is undiagnosed diabetes. Other diseases that are common causes of sexual dysfunction, particularly in men, are cardiovascular disease, hypertension, chronic kidney disease, multiple sclerosis, kidney failure, vascular disease, spinal cord injury, and injury to the autonomic nervous system due to surgery or radiation (Chen et al., 2019; Lewis et al., 2010).

As many as 40 percent of cases of erectile disorder are caused by one of these medical conditions (Lewis, Yuan, & Wangt, 2008). In men with cardiovascular disease, sexual dysfunction can be caused directly by the disease, which can reduce blood flow to the penis, or it may be a psychological response to the presence of the disease. For example, a man who recently has had a heart attack may fear he will have another one if he engages in sex.

In men, abnormally low levels of the androgen hormones, especially testosterone, or high levels of the hormones estrogen and prolactin can cause sexual dysfunction (Isidori et al., 2014). In women, levels of both androgens and estrogens may play a role in sexual dysfunction, although less consistently so than in men (Meston & Bradford, 2007). Estrogen problems in women may result in low arousal due to reduced vaginal lubrication. Levels of estrogen drop greatly at menopause; thus, postmenopausal women often complain of lowered sexual desire and arousal. Similarly, women who have had a radical hysterectomy—which removes the main source of estrogen, the ovaries—can experience reductions in both sexual desire and arousal. Androgens seem to play a role in the maintenance of sexual desire and mood and also may enhance the function of vaginal tissue.

Although many people drink alcohol to decrease their sexual inhibitions, alcohol also can impair sexual performance. *Blend Images - DreamPictures/Getty Images*

Vaginal dryness or irritation, which causes pain during sex and therefore lowers sexual desire and arousal, can be caused by antihistamines, douches, tampons, vaginal contraceptives, radiation therapy, endometriosis, and infections such as vaginitis or pelvic inflammatory disease (Meston & Bradford, 2007). Injuries during childbirth that have healed poorly, such as a poorly repaired episiotomy, can cause sexual pain in women (Salvatore, Redaelli, Baini, & Candiani, 2016). Women who have had gynecological cancers sometimes report pain, changes in the vaginal anatomy, and problems with their body image or sexual self-concept (Sears, Robinson, & Walker, 2018).

Several prescription drugs can diminish sexual drive and arousal and interfere with orgasm (Clayton, 2007; A. Montejo, L. Montejo, & F. Navarro-Cremades, 2015). These include antihypertensive drugs taken by people with high blood pressure, antipsychotic drugs, antidepressants, lithium, and tranquilizers. Indeed, sexual dysfunction is one of the most common side effects of the widely used selective serotonin reuptake inhibitors (Meston & Bradford, 2007; Montejo et al., 2015).

Many recreational drugs, including marijuana, cocaine, amphetamines, and nicotine, can impair sexual functioning (Lewis et al., 2010). Although people often drink alcohol to make them feel sexier and less inhibited, even small amounts of alcohol can significantly impair sexual functioning. Chronic alcohol abusers and alcohol dependents often have diagnosable sexual dysfunctions (Lewis et al., 2008). As noted previously, when a sexual dysfunction is caused by substance use, it is given the diagnosis **substance-induced sexual dysfunction.**

To determine whether a man is capable of attaining an erection, clinicians can do a psychophysiological assessment with devices that directly measure men's erections. In a laboratory, strain gauges can be attached to the base and glans of a man's penis to record the magnitude, duration, and pattern of arousal while he watches erotic films or listens to erotic audio recordings (Lewis et al., 2008). For women, the physical ability to become aroused can be measured with a vaginal photoplethysmography, a tampon-shaped device inserted into a woman's vagina that records the changes accompanying vasocongestion, the rush of blood to the vagina during arousal.

Psychological Causes
People's emotional well-being and beliefs and attitudes about sex greatly influence their sexuality.

Mental Disorders Again, the *DSM-5* criteria for the diagnosis of sexual dysfunction exclude that caused by other (nonsexual) mental disorders, but a number of mental disorders can cause sexual dysfunction (Waldinger, 2015). A person with depression may have no desire for sex or may experience any of the problems in sexual arousal and functioning discussed in this chapter. Unfortunately, the medications used to treat depression often lead to problems in sexual functioning. Similarly, people with an anxiety disorder, such as generalized anxiety disorder, panic disorder, or obsessive-compulsive disorder, may find their sexual desire and functioning waning. Loss of sexual desire and functioning also is common in people with schizophrenia (Waldinger, 2015).

Attitudes and Cognitions People who have been taught that sex is dirty, disgusting, or sinful or is a "necessary evil" understandably may lack the desire to have sex. They also may know so little about their own body and sexual responses that they do not know how to make sex pleasurable.

Although such negative attitudes toward sex may be less common among younger people these days, many younger and older women still report a fear of "letting go," which interferes with orgasm (Nobre & Pinto-Gouveia, 2006; Peixoto & Nobre, 2014). They

say they fear losing control or acting in some way that will embarrass them. This fear of loss of control may result from a distrust of one's partner, a sense of shame about sex, a poor body image, or a host of other factors. Cognitions among men that can contribute to dysfunction include all-or-nothing beliefs about erection quality, satisfying one's partner, and viewing foreplay as a waste of time (Peixoto & Nobre, 2014).

Another set of attitudes that interfere with sexual functioning is often referred to as performance concerns or **performance anxiety** (Masters & Johnson, 1970). People worry so much about whether they are going to be aroused and have an orgasm that this worry interferes with their sexual functioning: "What if I can't get an erection? I'll die of embarrassment!" "I've got to have an orgasm, or he'll think I don't love him!" These worry thoughts are so distracting that people experiencing them cannot focus on the pleasure that sexual stimulation is giving them and thus do not become as aroused as they want to or need to in order to reach orgasm (Figure 2; Barlow, Sakheim, & Beck, 1983; Perelman & Watter, 2016). Significant

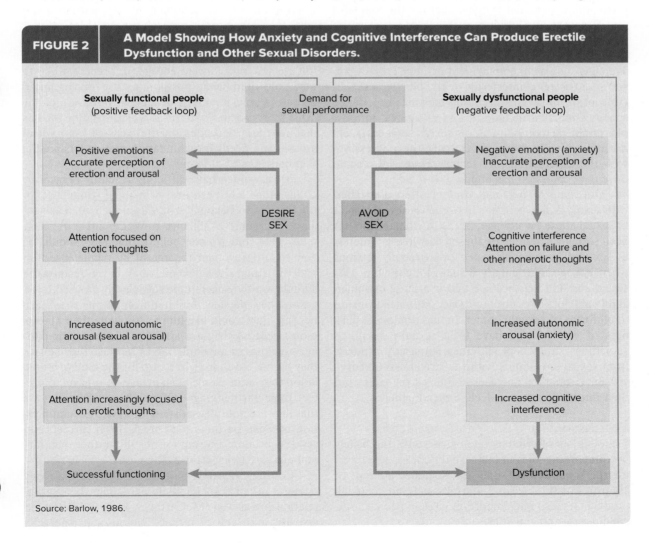

FIGURE 2 A Model Showing How Anxiety and Cognitive Interference Can Produce Erectile Dysfunction and Other Sexual Disorders.

Source: Barlow, 1986.

stress, challenges within a relationship and psychological disorders such as depression, anxiety, and posttraumatic stress disorder can also contribute to sexual dysfunctions like erectile disorder (Retzler, 2019).

In addition, many people engage in *spectatoring:* They anxiously attend to reactions and performance during sex as if they were spectators rather than participants (Masters & Johnson, 1970). Spectatoring distracts from sexual pleasure and interferes with sexual functioning. For example, men with concerns about the appearance of their penis are more likely to engage in higher levels of spectatoring which predicts greater erectile and orgasmic dysfunction (Wyatt, de Jong, & Holden, 2019). Unfortunately, people who have had some problems in sexual functioning only develop more performance concerns, which then further interfere with their functioning. By the time they seek treatment for sexual dysfunction, they may be so anxious about "performing" sexually that they avoid all sexual activity.

Trauma Reductions in sexual desire and functioning often follow personal trauma, such as the loss of a loved one, the loss of a job, or the diagnosis of severe illness in one's child. Unemployment may contribute to declines in sexual desire and functioning in men. Traumas such as unemployment can challenge a person's self-esteem, interfering with their sexual self-concept. Trauma can also cause a person to experience a depression that includes a loss of interest in most pleasurable activities, including sex. In such cases, clinicians typically focus on treating the depression, with the expectation that sexual desire will resume once the depression has lifted.

One type of personal trauma often associated with sexual desire disorders in women is sexual assault or sexual abuse (Waldinger, 2015). A woman who has been sexually assaulted or abused may lose all interest in sex and become disgusted or extremely anxious when anyone, particularly a man, touches her. Her sexual aversion may become tied to a sense of vulnerability and loss of control or to a conditioned aversion to all forms of sexual contact. In addition, male partners of women who have been sexually assaulted sometimes cannot cope with the trauma and withdraw from sexual encounters with the sexual assault survivor. Survivors then may feel victimized yet again, and their interest in sex may decline even further.

Interpersonal and Sociocultural Factors

Although our internal psychological states and beliefs play important roles in our sexuality, sex is largely an interpersonal activity—one that societies attempt to control. For this reason, interpersonal and sociocultural factors also play important roles in people's sexual interests and activities.

Interpersonal Factors Problems in intimate relationships are extremely common in people with sexual dysfunctions. Sometimes these problems are the consequences of sexual dysfunctions, as when a couple cannot communicate about the sexual dysfunction of one partner and the two grow distant from each other. Relationship problems also can be the direct cause of sexual dysfunctions (McCarthy & Ross, 2017).

Conflicts between partners may be about the couple's sexual activities. One partner may want to engage in a type of sexual activity that the other partner is uncomfortable with, or one partner may want to engage in sexual activity much more often than the other partner. People with inhibited desire, arousal, or orgasm often have sexual partners who do not know how to arouse their partner or are not concerned with their partner's arousal, focusing only on themselves. Couples often do not communicate with each other about what is arousing, so even if each partner intends to please the other, neither knows what the other desires.

Anorgasmia (lack of orgasm) characteristic of female orgasmic disorder may be tied to lack of communication between a woman and her partner about what the woman needs to reach orgasm (McCarthy & Ross, 2017). In sexual encounters between men and women, men still are more likely to decide when to initiate sex, how long to engage in foreplay, when to penetrate, and what position to use during intercourse. A man's pattern of arousal often is not the same as a woman's pattern of arousal, and he may be making these decisions on the basis of his level of arousal and needs for stimulation, not understanding that hers may be different.

Most women have difficulty reaching orgasm by coitus alone and need oral or manual stimulation of the clitoris to become aroused enough to reach orgasm (Carpenter, Williams, & Worly, 2017). Because many men and women believe that men should be able to bring women to orgasm by penile insertion and thrusting alone, women may never receive the stimulation they need to be sufficiently aroused to orgasm. They may feel inhibited from telling their partner that they would like him to stimulate their clitoris more, because they are afraid of hurting their partner's feelings or angering him or because they believe they do not have the right to ask for the kind of stimulation they want. Some women fake an orgasm to protect their partner's ego. Often, their partner knows that they are not fully satisfied, however. Communication between partners may break down further, and sex may become a forum for hostility rather than mutual pleasure (McCarthy & Ross, 2017).

Conflicts between partners that are not directly related to their sexual activity can affect their sexual relationship as well (McCarthy & Ross, 2017). Anger, distrust, and lack of respect for one's partner can greatly interfere with sexual desire and functioning. When one partner suspects that the other partner has been unfaithful or is losing interest in the relationship, all sexual interest may disappear. Often, there is an imbalance of power in a relationship, and one partner feels exploited, subjugated, and underappreciated by the other partner, leading to problems in their sexual relationship.

Among people seeking treatment for sexual problems, women are more likely than men to report problems in their marital relationship, other stressful events in their life, and higher levels of psychological distress (Meston & Bradford, 2007). Men seeking treatment are more likely than women to be experiencing other types of sexual dysfunction in addition to low sexual desire, such as erectile dysfunction.

Cultural Factors Other cultures recognize types of sexual dysfunction not described in the *DSM-5* (see Hall, 2016; Hall & Graham, 2013). For example, both the traditional Chinese medical system and the Ayurvedic medical system, which is native to India, teach that loss of semen is detrimental to a man's health (Dewaraja & Sasaki, 1991). Masturbation is strongly discouraged because it results in semen loss without the possibility of conception. A study of 1,000 consecutive patients seeking treatment in a sexual clinic in India found that 77 percent of the male patients reported difficulties with premature ejaculation and 71 percent were concerned about nocturnal emissions associated with erotic dreams (Verma, Khaitan, & Singh, 1998).

A depersonalization syndrome known as *Koro,* thought to result from semen loss, has been reported among Malaysians, Southeast Asians, and southern Chinese. This syndrome involves an acute anxiety state, characterized by a feeling of panic and impending death, and a delusion that the penis is shrinking into the body and disappearing (American Psychiatric Association, 2013). To stop the penis from disappearing into the body, the patient or his relatives may grab and hold the penis until the attack of Koro is ended.

Sexual function is more than just propagating the human species and has both recreational and psychological value. Sexuality is a socially constructed and culturally sensitive topic that is rooted in many complicated psychosocial factors. When sexual dysfunction occurs it can affect the quality of life, emotional bonding, and relationship harmony among couples. Despite less attention, sexual dysfunction is more common in women (43 percent) than in men (31 percent) and includes psychological factors such as dissatisfaction, emotional frustration, and mental impairment (Santana et al., 2019; Vaishnav, Saha, Mukherji, & Vaishnav, 2020). Epidemiological data show the estimated global prevalence of sexual dysfunction among women may be 30 to 63 percent with variation among countries and within regions. Research performed in the United States and Europe report female sexual dysfunction at about 19 to 50 percent, whereas studies on Middle Eastern and Japanese women estimate the prevalence of sexual disorders at about 30 percent (Lou et al., 2017).

Sexual dysfunction among women is common but due to culture and social customs, these affected women and their clinicians often avoid discussing the topic. Additionally, when making diagnoses, providers tend not to investigate the causes of female sexual dysfunction (Santana et al., 2019). For example, among women with sexual dysfunction in Beijing, China 30 percent never sought help, 29 percent considered looking for information on the Internet or in books, and only 23 percent had visited a doctor. A partner's sexual ability, the level of sexual satisfaction or dissatisfaction, and marital affection are factors associated with female sexual dysfunction. A study of Iranian women found that an overwhelming majority of women attributed their sexual dysfunction with their spouse's erectile dysfunction (82 percent) and poor marital affection (72 percent). Sexual difficulties of the spouse or romantic partner are potential risk factors for female sexual dysfunction. Recent studies have found that dissatisfaction with the spouse's sexual ability increased the risk of female sexual dysfunction by approximately seven times. A national survey of Swedish women found that erectile dysfunction or abnormal ejaculation also increased the incidence of female sexual dysfunction. Research in Taiwan, China also found that erectile dysfunction was directly linked to female arousal dysfunction, orgasmic dysfunction, and sexual dissatisfaction. Culture influences how sexual dysfunction is perceived by those affected women which impacts treatment. For example, in traditional Chinese culture, it is more likely that Chinese women will point out sexual dysfunctions and dissatisfaction in themselves rather than acknowledge the sexual problems of their spouse, such as erectile dysfunction. Interestingly, various studies have found that physiological issues such as reproductive organ inflammation, fibroids of the uterus, cervical lesions, urinary incontinence, and other medical dysfunctions are rarely the cause of female sexual dysfunction (Lou et al., 2017).

In addition to cultures' recognition of unique disorders, aspects of culture such as gender roles and religion affect the expression of disorders recognized in the *DSM-5* (Hall & Graham, 2013). For example, in cultures in which women's desire for sex is not expected, female sexual interest/arousal disorder is less prevalent and is likely experienced differently. For men, premature ejaculation is a primary complaint across cultures. By contrast, Western women seek treatment for sexual desire problems most often, whereas women in non-Western and more male-centric cultures seek treatment for vaginismus and genito-pelvic pain/penetration disorder (Hall, 2016).

In surveys in the United States, less educated and poorer men and women tend to experience more sexual dysfunctions. Problems include having pain during sex, not finding sex pleasurable, being unable to reach orgasm, lacking interest in sex, climaxing too early, and, for men, having trouble maintaining an erection (Laumann, Gagnon, Michael, & Michaels, 1994; Lewis et al., 2010). People in lower educational and income groups may have more sexual dysfunctions because they are under more psychological stress, because their physical health is worse, or because they have not had the benefit of educational programs that teach people about their bodies and about healthy social relationships. In addition, people from cultural backgrounds that teach negative attitudes toward sex are more likely to develop sexual dysfunctions resulting from these attitudes (Hall & Graham, 2013).

Trends Across the Life Span

Our culture conveys the message that young adults, particularly men, can't get enough sex but that sexual activity declines steadily with age. Supposedly, older adults (i.e., over about age 65) hardly ever have sex. Although younger adults tend to engage in more sexual activity than older adults, many adults remain sexually active well into old age (Lindau et al., 2007; Hillman, 2017).

Age-related biological changes can affect sexual functioning (Hillman, 2017). Both men and women need adequate levels of testosterone to maintain sexual desire. Testosterone levels begin to decline in a person's fifties and continue to decrease steadily throughout the rest of the person's life. Lower testosterone levels and age-related decreases in blood flow are associated with increased difficulty in achieving and maintaining an erection, increased time to ejaculation, and less intense orgasms (Hillman, 2017; Hockenberry & Masson, 2016). Diminished estrogen levels in postmenopausal women can lead to vaginal dryness and lack of lubrication and thus to a reduction in sexual responsivity (Hillman, 2017). In many cases of sexual dysfunction in older adults, the cause is not age itself but instead medical conditions, which are more common in older age.

For both older men and older women, the loss of a lifelong spouse, losses of other family members and friends, health concerns, and discomfort with one's own aging can contribute to sexual problems. Conflicts and dissatisfactions in a couple's relationship can worsen as the couple spends more time together following retirement and/or their children's moving out of the house. Older couples may need to learn to be more flexible and patient with each other as their bodies change and to try new techniques for stimulating each other. A number of biological and psychosocial treatments are available for sexual dysfunctions in both older and younger people.

Treatments for Sexual Dysfunctions

Because most sexual dysfunctions have multiple causes, treatment may involve a combination of approaches, often including biological interventions, psychosocial therapy focusing on problems in a relationship or on the concerns of an individual client, and sex therapies to help clients learn new skills for increasing their sexual arousal and pleasure.

Biological Therapies

If a sexual dysfunction is the direct result of another medical condition, such as diabetes, treating the medical condition often will reduce the sexual dysfunction (Maiorino et al., 2014). Similarly, if medications are contributing to a sexual dysfunction, adjusting the dosage or switching to a different type of medication can relieve sexual difficulties. Also, getting a person to stop using recreational drugs such as marijuana can often cure sexual dysfunction.

A number of biological treatments are available for men with erectile disorder (Bennett, 2016). The drug that has received the most media attention in recent years is sildenafil (trade name Viagra). This drug has proven effective both in men whose erectile dysfunction has no known organic cause and in men whose erectile dysfunction is caused by a medical condition, such as hypertension, diabetes, or spinal cord

Many older adults remain sexually active and experience little decline in sexual functioning. *Ronnie Kaufman/Blend Images*

injury. Three other drugs, Cialis, Levitra, and Stenix, have similar positive effects. These drugs do have side effects, though, including headaches, flushing, and stomach irritation, and they do not work for about a third of men (Chen et al., 2015).

Some antidepressants, particularly the selective serotonin reuptake inhibitors (SSRIs), can cause sexual dysfunctions (Montejo et al., 2015). Other drugs can be used in conjunction with these antidepressants to reduce their sexual side effects. One drug that has proven helpful in this regard is bupropion, which goes by the trade names Wellbutrin and Zyban. Bupropion appears to reduce the sexual side effects of the SSRIs and can itself be effective as an antidepressant. Sildenafil also may help men whose erectile dysfunction is caused by taking antidepressants, allowing them to continue taking the antidepressants without losing sexual functioning.

In men with erectile disorder, certain drugs can be injected directly into the penis to induce an erection. Although this method is effective, it has the obvious drawback of requiring injections (Bednarchik, Kottwitz, & Geiger, 2016). Mechanical interventions are also available for men with erectile dysfunction (Köhler & McVary, 2016). One device includes a cylinder that fits over the penis and connects to a manual or battery-powered vacuum pump, which induces engorgement of the penis with blood. Alternatively, prosthetic devices can be surgically implanted into the penis to make it erect. One prosthesis consists of a pair of rods inserted into the penis. The rods create a permanent erection, which can be bent either up or down against the body. Another type is a hydraulic inflatable device, which allows a man to create an erection by pumping saline into rods inserted in the penis and then to relieve the erection by pumping out the saline. Erections achieved with these devices technically are full erections but frequently do not evoke bodily or mental feelings of sexual arousal.

For men suffering from premature ejaculation, some antidepressants can be helpful, including fluoxetine (Prozac), clomipramine (Anafranil), and sertraline (Zoloft). Several studies suggest that these drugs significantly reduce the frequency of premature ejaculation (Rowland & Cooper, 2017).

Several studies have examined the effects of hormone therapy, specifically the use of testosterone, to increase sexual desire in men and women with hypoactive sexual desire disorder. Hormone replacement therapy can be very effective for men whose low levels of sexual desire or arousal are linked to low levels of testosterone; they are not effective for men whose low sexual desire or arousal is not linked to low levels of testosterone (Hockenberry & Masson, 2016; Isidori et al., 2014). In multiple randomized controlled trials, testosterone also appears to be effective in women with low levels of desire or arousal, particularly postmenopausal women (Achilli et al., 2017). Side effects can include increased hair growth in a minority of cases. Bupropion has proven helpful in treating some women with hypoactive sexual desire (Parish & Hahn, 2016).

Large controlled studies investigating the effects of sildenafil for women with sexual dysfunctions report mixed results (see Brotto, 2017). The drug does increase vasocongestion and lubrication in women, but these physiological changes do not consistently lead to greater subjective arousal, and sildenafil has been largely discarded as a pharmacological treatment for women. A newer medication, flibanserin (Addyi), was approved in the United States in 2015 and dubbed by some as the "female Viagra." Flibanserin acts on multiple neurotransmitters and has shown very modest effects on sexual desire (Brotto, 2017). It is taken daily and the woman cannot use alcohol while taking it, due to risk of developing severe low blood pressure. Because the drawbacks often outweigh the benefits, this drug is not widely prescribed.

Psychotherapy and Sex Therapy

The introduction of drugs, such as sildenafil, that can overcome sexual dysfunctions, at least in men, has dramatically changed the nature of treatments for these disorders. Given the financial and time constraints imposed by managed care, many people seeking treatment for a sexual dysfunction are offered only a medication and not psychotherapy (McCarthy & Ross, 2017). Also, many people want only a medication and do not want to engage in psychotherapy to address possible psychological and interpersonal contributors to their sexual problems.

A variety of psychotherapeutic techniques have been developed, however, and have been shown to help people with sexual dysfunctions (see Frühauf, Gerger, Schmidt, Munder, & Barth, 2013; McCarthy & Ross, 2017; Peterson, 2017). One option is individual psychotherapy in which individuals explore the thoughts and previous experiences that impede them from enjoying a positive sexual life. Couples therapy often helps couples develop more satisfying sexual relationships. As part of both individual and couples therapy, behavioral techniques are used to teach people skills to enhance their sexual experiences and to improve communication and interactions with their sexual partners.

Individual and Couples Therapy A therapist begins treatment by assessing the attitudes, beliefs, and personal history of an individual client or of both members of a couple in order to discover experiences, thoughts, and feelings that might be contributing to sexual problems. Cognitive-behavioral interventions

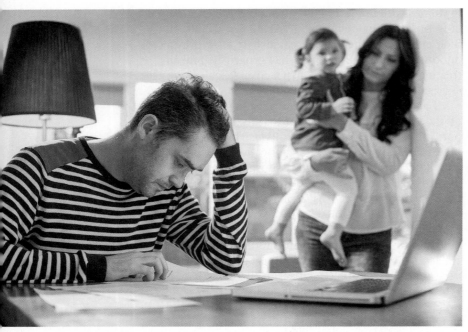

Many busy couples do not take time for activities that can maintain their sexual interest in each other. *sturti/Getty Images*

often are used to address attitudes and beliefs that interfere with sexual functioning (McCarthy & Ross, 2017; Wincze & Weinberg, 2015). For example, a man who fears that he will embarrass himself by not sustaining an erection in a sexual encounter may be challenged to examine the evidence of this having happened to him in the past. If this has been a common occurrence for the man, his therapist would explore the thought patterns surrounding the experience and then help the man challenge these cognitions and practice more positive ones. Similarly, a woman who has low sexual desire because she was taught by her parents that sex is dirty would learn to challenge this belief and to adopt a more accepting attitude toward sex.

When one member of a couple has a sexual dysfunction, it may be the result of problems in the couple's relationship, or, conversely, it may be contributing to problems in the relationship. For this reason, many therapists prefer to treat sexual dysfunctions in the context of the couple's relationship, if possible, rather than focusing only on the individual with the sexual dysfunction. The therapist may use role playing during therapy sessions to observe how the couple discusses sex and how the partners perceive each other's role in their sexual encounters (McCarthy & Ross, 2018).

Some couples in long-term relationships have abandoned the seduction rituals—those activities that arouse sexual interest in both partners—they followed when they were first together (McCarthy & Ross,

2018). Couples in which both partners work may be particularly prone to try squeezing in sexual encounters late at night, when both partners are tired and not really interested in sex. These encounters may be rushed or not fully satisfying and can lead to a gradual decline in interest in any sexual intimacy. A therapist may encourage a couple to set aside enough time to engage in seduction rituals and satisfying sexual encounters. For example, partners may decide to hire a babysitter for their children, have a romantic dinner out, and then go to a hotel, where they can have sex without rushing or being interrupted by their children.

Partners often differ in their scripts for sexual encounters—their expectations about what will take place during a sexual encounter and about what each partner's responsibilities are. Resolving these differences in scripts may be a useful goal in therapy. For example, if a woman lacks desire for sex because she feels her partner is too rough during sex, a therapist may encourage the partner to slow down and show the woman the kind of gentle intimacy she needs to enjoy sex. In general, therapists help partners understand what each wants and needs from sexual interactions and helps them negotiate mutually acceptable and satisfying repertoires of sexual exchange.

When the conflicts between partners involve matters other than their sexual practices, the therapist will focus primarily on these conflicts and only secondarily on the sexual dysfunction. Such conflicts may involve an imbalance of power in the relationship, distrust or hostility, or disagreement over important values or decisions. Cognitive-behavioral, psychodynamic, and family systems therapies are all applied to couple problems, including those affecting sexual dysfunction. Cognitive-behavioral therapies have been researched more than other types of couple therapy and have been shown to be effective for several types of sexual dysfunction (see Benson & Christensen, 2016; Johnson, Simakhodskaya, & Moran, 2018; Wincze & Weinberg, 2015).

Sex Therapy Whether a therapist uses a cognitive-behavioral or some other therapeutic approach to address the psychological issues involved in a sexual dysfunction, direct sex therapy using behavioral techniques may be a part of the therapy. When a sexual dysfunction seems to be due, at least in part, to inadequate sexual skill on the part of the client and their partner, sex therapy that focuses on practicing skills can be useful (Frühauf et al., 2013). Some people have never learned what gives them or their partner pleasure or have fallen out of the habit of engaging in some practices. Sex therapy both teaches skills and helps partners develop a regular pattern of engaging in satisfying sexual encounters.

Sex therapy often includes teaching or encouraging clients to masturbate (Vaishnav, Saha, Mukherji, & Vaishnav, 2020). The goals of masturbation are for people to explore their bodies to discover what is arousing and to become less inhibited about their sexuality. Then individuals are taught to communicate their newly discovered desires to their partners. This technique can be especially helpful for anorgasmic women, many of whom have never masturbated and have little knowledge of what they need in order to become aroused (Meston & Bradford, 2007). Studies show that more than 80 percent of anorgasmic women are able to have an orgasm when they learn to masturbate and that 20 to 60 percent are able to have an orgasm with their partner after learning to masturbate (Heiman, 2000). These women also report increased enjoyment and satisfaction from sex, a more relaxed attitude toward sex and life, and increased acceptance of their body.

The client's cognitions while engaging in new sexual skills can be evaluated and used as a focus of therapy sessions (McCarthy & Ross, 2017). For example, a woman who is learning how to masturbate for the first time may realize that while she is masturbating, she has thoughts such as "I'm going to get caught, and I'll be so embarrassed"; "I shouldn't be doing this—this is sinful"; and "Only pathetic people do this." A cognitive-behavioral therapist can then help the woman address the accuracy of these thoughts and decide whether she wants to maintain this attitude toward masturbation. If the woman is in psychodynamic therapy, the therapist might explore the origins of the woman's attitudes about masturbation in her early relationships. Thus, the behavioral techniques of sex therapy not only directly teach the client new sexual skills but also provide material for discussion in therapy sessions.

Sensate Focus Therapy One of the mainstays of sex therapy is **sensate focus therapy** (Masters & Johnson, 1970; Vaishnavet al., 2020; Weiner & Avery-Clark, 2017). In the early phases of this therapy, partners are instructed not to be concerned about or even to attempt intercourse. Rather, they are told to focus intently on the pleasure created by the exercises. These instructions are meant to reduce performance anxiety and any concern about achieving orgasm.

In the first phase of sensate focus therapy, partners spend time gently touching each other, but not around the genitals. They are instructed to focus on the sensations and to communicate with each other about what does and does not feel good. The goal is to have the partners spend intimate time together communicating, without pressure for intercourse. This first phase may continue for several weeks, until the partners feel comfortable with the exercises and have learned what gives each of them pleasure.

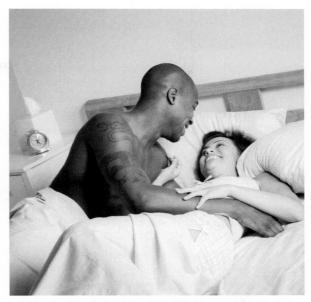

In sensate focus therapy, couples are encouraged to spend time exploring what sexually arouses each of them without feeling pressured to reach orgasm. *Andersen Ross/Getty Images*

In the second phase of sensate focus therapy, the partners spend time directly stimulating each other's breasts and genitals, but still without attempting intercourse. If the problem is a female sexual interest/arousal disorder, the woman guides her partner to stimulate her in arousing ways. It is acceptable for a woman to be aroused to orgasm during these exercises, but the partners are instructed not to attempt intercourse until she regularly becomes fully aroused by her partner during the sensate focus exercises. If the problem is a male erectile disorder, the man guides his partner in touching him in ways that feel arousing. If he has an erection, he is to let it come and go naturally. Intercourse is forbidden until he is able to have erections easily and frequently during the sensate focus exercises.

Throughout these exercises, the partner with the problem is instructed to be selfish and to focus only on the arousing sensations and on communicating with their partner about what feels good. The touching should proceed in a relaxed and nondemanding atmosphere. Once the partner with the problem regularly experiences arousal with genital stimulation, the partners may begin having intercourse, but the focus remains on enhancing and sustaining pleasure rather than on orgasm or performance.

Sensate focus therapy has been shown to be effective for disorders of desire, arousal, and orgasm, often in combination with other therapies (Linschoten, Weiner, & Avery-Clark, 2016). The following case study indicates how the behavioral techniques of sensate focus therapy can help couples recognize and confront the complex personal and interpersonal issues that may be interfering with their enjoyment of sex.

CASE STUDY

Murray, a 53-year-old successful insurance agent, and his wife, a 50-year-old nutritional counselor, had been married for 28 years. With the exception of time spent on vacation, Murray had a 7-year history of erectile dysfunction. The frequency of their lovemaking had gradually declined to its current level of once every 4 months. Murray reported considerable performance anxiety, enhanced by his competitive personality style. He summed up his dilemma: "When you have a life full of successes, you don't get much practice at how to deal with inadequacy."

During the first hour of therapy, sensate focus exercises were suggested and instructions given to engage in sensual nongenital touching. They returned in a week, noting how difficult it had been to find time to pleasure one another. Their mutual avoidance was discussed and understood as a means of warding off feelings of inadequacy. Working through the resistance allowed the couple to engage in the exercises three times over the course of the next week. With the pleasuring, Murray began to achieve good, long-lasting erections.

Therapy then progressed to include genital touching. After the first week, they talked about their problem of "silliness." They realized that humor had been used to cope with the dysfunction. Now, however, joking in bed seemed to inhibit sexual closeness. Murray's good erections were maintained, although he was having trouble concentrating on his sensations. Further exploration revealed that he was focusing his attention in a driven, intense manner. To counter this, the therapist redirected him to maintain a relaxed awareness akin to meditation. Murray found this analogy helpful, and the couple felt ready to proceed with vaginal containment. During the following week, they "disobeyed" and moved on to have mutually satisfying intercourse. They feared the recurrence of the old problem, but it did not return, and the remaining two sessions were spent talking about their sexual life. Despite otherwise good communication, they had never been able before to broach this topic with one another. (Althof, S. E. "Erectile dysfunction: Psychotherapy with men and couples. In S. R. Leiblum, & R. C. Rosen (Eds.), *Principles and practice of sex therapy* (3rd ed, p. 270.). New York: Guilford Press. Copyright ©2000 by Guilford Press. Reprinted by permission. Permission conveyed through Copyright Clearance Center.)

Techniques for Treating Early Ejaculation   Two techniques are useful in helping a man with early ejaculation gain control over his ejaculations: the stop-start technique (Semans, 1956) and the squeeze technique (Masters & Johnson, 1970; Vaishnav et al., 2020). The **stop-start technique** can be carried out either through masturbation or with a partner. In the first phase, the man is told to stop stimulating himself or to tell his partner to stop stimulating him just before he is about to ejaculate. He then relaxes and concentrates on the sensations in his body until his level of arousal declines. At that point, he or his partner can resume stimulation, again stopping before the point of ejaculatory inevitability. If stimulation stops too late and the man ejaculates, he is encouraged not to feel angry or disappointed but to enjoy the ejaculation and reflect on what he has learned about his body and then resume the exercise. If a man is engaging in this exercise with a partner, they are instructed not to engage in intercourse until he has sufficient control over his ejaculations during his partner's manual stimulation of him.

In the second phase of this process the man lies on his back with his partner on top of him who inserts his penis and remains quiet. Most men with premature ejaculation have intercourse only in the on-top position, with quick and short thrusting during intercourse, which makes it very difficult for them to exert control over their ejaculations. The goal is for the man to enjoy the sensation of penetration without ejaculating. During the exercise, he is encouraged to touch or massage his partner and for each to communicate about what they are experiencing. If he feels he is reaching ejaculatory inevitability, he can request that his partner dismount and lie next to him until his arousal subsides. Partners are encouraged to engage in this exercise for at least 10 to 15 minutes, even if they must interrupt it several times to prevent the man from ejaculating (Vaishnav et al., 2020).

In the third phase of the stop-start technique, the man's partner creates some thrusting motion while still on top of him but uses slow, long strokes. The partners typically reach orgasm and experience the entire encounter as highly intimate and pleasurable. Female partners of men with premature ejaculation often have trouble reaching orgasm during intercourse themselves, because the men lose their erection after ejaculating, long before the women are highly aroused, and tension is high between the partners during sex. The stop-start technique can create encounters in which men's partners receive the stimulation they need to reach orgasm as well.

The **squeeze technique** is used somewhat less often because it is harder to teach to partners (McCarthy, 2001). The man's partner stimulates him to an erection, and then, when he signals that ejaculation is imminent, his partner applies a firm but gentle squeeze to his penis, either at the head or at the base, for 3 or 4 seconds. This results in a partial loss of erection. The partner then can stimulate him again to the point of ejaculation and use the squeeze technique to stop the ejaculation. The goal of this technique, as with the stop-start technique, is for the man with a premature ejaculation disorder to learn to identify the point of ejaculatory inevitability and control his arousal level at that point.

Techniques for Treating Pelvic Muscle Tightening
Pelvic muscle tightening is often treated by deconditioning the woman's automatic tightening of her vaginal muscles (Stein, 2016). She is taught about the muscular tension at the opening of her vagina and the need to learn to relax those muscles. In a safe setting, she is instructed to insert her fingers into her vagina. She examines her vagina in a mirror and practices relaxation exercises. She may also use silicon or metal vaginal dilators made for this exercise. Gradually, she inserts larger and larger dilators as she practices relaxation exercises and becomes accustomed to the feel of the dilator in her vagina. If she has a partner, his or her fingers may be used instead of the dilator. If the woman has a male partner, eventually she guides his penis into her vagina while remaining in control.

Some physical therapists specifically treat sexual dysfunctions by focusing on weakness of the pelvic floor muscles, problems with blood flow in the penis, joint dysfunction, and pain associated with intercourse. They utilize techniques of muscle reeducation, nerve and joint mobilization, and massage.

Considerations for Gay, Lesbian, Bisexual, and Transgendered People

Gay, lesbian, bisexual and transgendered people experience sexual dysfunctions for the same reasons as heterosexual people, such as medical disorders, medications, aging, or conflicts with partners, and do so at similar rates (Cohen & Savin-Williams, 2017; Kerckhof et al., 2019). LGBTQI people face additional stressors related to their sexuality due to continuing stigma and discrimination against them, which can affect sex and health (Gilman et al., 2001; Plöderl & Tremblay, 2015).

Individuals with gender dysphoria (GD) experience psychological distress due to the incongruence between their biological sex and their gender identity and are commonly referred to as "transgender." Historically, the sexual experiences of transgender individuals received little research attention. However, it is now recognized that achieving a healthy sexual life is a vital component to psychological well-being and often a challenge for transgender individuals. The psychological distress caused by GD often interferes with the development of their sexual health. Transgender individuals are also at a high risk of experiencing sexual violence and transphobia which are negatively

associated with sexual satisfaction. Transgender individuals frequently report sexual dysfunctions that include difficulties initiating and seeking sexual contact and difficulties achieving an orgasm (Kerckhof et al., 2019). Hypoactive sexual desire disorder (HSDD) represents a common condition among transgender women (Cocchetti et al., 2021).

Therapists treating gay, lesbian, or bisexual clients must be sensitive to the psychological stresses these clients face as a result of society's rejection of their sexual orientation, as well as to the contributions of these stresses to their sexual functioning. Compared to heterosexual people, these clients may be influenced by unique developmental influences on identity and sexuality (such as coming out processes or cultural expectations) that affect the various domains of sexual function (Cohen & Savin-Williams, 2017). Most of the sex therapy treatments can readily be adapted for gay, lesbian, or bisexual couples.

Gay, lesbian, and bisexual people are discussed here to emphasize unique characteristics relevant to this population's experience of the sexual disorders. Researchers and clinicians do not consider minority sexual orientation itself as pathological. The attitude of clinical psychology as a profession toward homosexuality changed several decades ago. Early versions of the *DSM* listed homosexuality, particularly *ego-dystonic homosexuality* (which meant that the person did not want to be homosexual), as a mental disorder. Gay men, lesbians, and bisexual people argue that their sexual orientation is a natural part of themselves. Apart from society's homophobia, their orientation causes them no discomfort. Ample psychological research supports this idea; moreover, there is little evidence that psychotherapy can lead a homosexual person to become heterosexual, and substantial evidence that it can do harm. In 1973 the American Psychiatric Association removed homosexuality from its list of recognized psychological disorders (Spitzer, 1981). All of the major American mental health organizations explicitly reject the classification of minority sexual orientation as a disorder, as well as the use of so-called "conversion" therapies as these practices are considered harmful and ineffective (e.g., American Psychological Association, 2009; Flores, Mallory, & Conron, 2020).

PARAPHILIC DISORDERS

Sexual experiences and preferences are a typical and important aspect of human behavior but are often shrouded in secrecy. People vary greatly in the sexual activities they find arousing and sexual attitudes change over time (see Table 2). Understanding the diversity of sexual expression can help people to feel "seen" or better represented in terms of their sexualities.

TABLE 2   The Kinds of Sexual Practices People Find Appealing

A national survey of 2,201 adults (ages 18 to 70+) found that many different sexual practices appeal to people, with men finding more activities appealing than do women.

Practice	Percent Saying "Very Appealing" (%)	
	Men	Women
Vaginal intercourse	73	70
Watching partner undress	46	29
Receiving oral sex	61	43
Giving oral sex	41	21
Having sex in other parts of the house	38	33
Watching your partner masturbate in front of you	29	14
Watching sexually erotic videos (Porn)	25	11
Dirty talk	21	20
Watching a romantic movie	19	42
Anal sex	15	3
Watching others do sexual things	16	8.5
Flirting over text/SnapChat	13	16
Using dildos/vibrators	12	23
Taking or sharing nude photos with a partner	12.5	9
Wearing sexy underwear or lingerie	12	41
Having your anus stimulated by your partner's fingers	10	8
Having sex with a stranger	10	2
Tying up your partner or being tied up as part of sex	8	9
Group sex	7	2
Spanking or being spanked as part of sex	7	11
Having sex over FaceTime or Skype	5	2

Source: Herbenick et al., 2017

The society in which we live and various cultural events can influence sexual behavior which was seen, for example, after the release of the book *Fifty Shades of Grey*. The popularity of this book series prompted researchers to examine sexual activities like bondage, domination, submission, sadism, and masochism (BDSM) also referred to as "kink" behaviors. This moment in pop-culture led scholars to explore whether reading the book influenced sexual behavior within the general population. Interestingly, there were noted increases in rope sales in hardware stores, sex toy sales, as well as BDSM sex toy-related injuries following the release of the book series and 2015 film. While it is impossible to fully assess whether sexual practices changed as a result of *Fifty Shades of Grey*, it does show how sexual attitudes, preferences, and activities can be influenced by culture. There have been a number of societal level changes relevant to Americans' sexual practices such as greater acceptance of same-sex partnerships and marriage, as well as increased

representations in mainstream media of open relationships and marriages. Innovations in technology have provided greater access to sexually explicit material and greater ease of taking and sharing sexually explicit photographs and videos (Herbenick et al., 2017).

While there is great variability within typical sexual activities and function, there are behaviors that fall outside the normal spectrum. Atypical sexual preferences have been called *paraphilias* which comes from the Greek prefix "*para*," meaning around or beside and "*philia*" an ancient Greek word for love (Thibaut, 2020). Paraphilias are sometimes divided into those that involve the consent of others (e.g., some sadomasochistic practices) and those that involve nonconsenting others (e.g., voyeurism). They also can be divided into those that involve contact with others (e.g., pedophilia) and those that do not necessarily involve contact with others (e.g., some fetishes). A **paraphilic disorder** involves atypical sexual activity that causes the individual significant distress or

TABLE 3 Paraphilic Disorders

The paraphilic disorders involve atypical, recurrent, intense sexually arousing fantasies, sexual urges, or behaviors that cause the individual significant distress or impairment, or entail harm to others or the risk of harm.

Diagnosis	Object of Fantasies, Urges, or Behaviors
Fetishistic disorder	Nonliving objects (e.g., female undergarments) or nongenital body part(s)
Transvestic disorder	Cross-dressing
Sexual sadism disorder	Acts (real, not simulated) involving the physical or psychological suffering (including humiliation) of another person
Sexual masochism disorder	Acts (real, not simulated) of being humiliated, beaten, bound, or otherwise made to suffer
Voyeuristic disorder	Act of observing an unsuspecting person who is naked, in the process of undressing, or engaged in sexual activity
Exhibitionistic disorder	Exposure of one's genitals to an unsuspecting stranger
Frotteuristic disorder	Touching and rubbing against a nonconsenting person
Pedophilic disorder	Sexual activity with a prepubescent child or children

impairment, or entails personal harm or risk of harm to others. Individuals with paraphilic disorders have recurrent, intense sexually arousing fantasies, sexual urges, or behaviors involving one of the following: (1) nonhuman objects, (2) nonconsenting adults, (3) the suffering or humiliation of oneself or one's partner, or (4) children. Table 3 lists the paraphilic disorders recognized by the *DSM-5* (Thibaut, 2020).

The definitions of the paraphilias and paraphilic disorders are highly controversial. The *DSM-5* attempted to tighten the definition of a paraphilic disorder by specifying that the presence of a paraphilia does not constitute a disorder and that a diagnosis can be given only when the behaviors cause the person distress or impairment or cause others harm. However, questions remain as to why some variations in sexual behavior are considered mental disorders while others are not (Beech, Miner, & Thornton, 2016). On the other hand, labeling sexual behaviors that involve victims, such as pedophilia, as mental disorders runs the risk of providing an "excuse" for behaviors that society wishes to forbid and punish.

Some researchers wanted to include a disorder called paraphilic coercive disorder in the *DSM-5*; this diagnosis would apply to individuals who derive sexual pleasure from coercing others into nonconsensual sex (i.e., rape). Not surprisingly, this proposal raised a firestorm of concern (Frances & First, 2011; Knight, 2010; Wollert & Cramer, 2011), and the authors of the *DSM-5* decided to reject the proposal, once again confirming that rape is not a mental disorder but a criminal act (Beech et al., 2016). Another diagnosis proposed but rejected for inclusion in *DSM-5* is hypersexual disorder, which is characterized by excessive preoccupation with sexual fantasies, urges, and activities (sometimes referred to as sexual addiction) and lasts at least 6 months. Again, initial proposals to include this diagnosis in the *DSM-5* (Kafka, 2010) met with sharp criticism that there was insufficient evidence for its validity as a psychiatric disorder (Halpern, 2011; Moser, 2011; see Beech et al., 2016), though a later study suggested high reliability and validity when applied in a clinical setting (Reid et al., 2012). The problem of sexual addiction awaits further study, while those individuals with such behavior (such as excessive pornography use) and associated distress or impairment will seek treatment for a problem that is not yet defined as a mental disorder.

Drag queens such as RuPaul perform in exaggerated female dress and behavior, often as a form of performance art. Most identify as gay men, and do not dress as women for sexual arousal or as an expression of transgender identity. *Mark Boster/Los Angeles Times/ Getty Images*

These controversies are difficult to resolve because they involve moral judgments and powerful social norms. In addition, the research literature on most paraphilic disorders is limited and inconsistent, providing little information on which to base judgments about how pathological these behaviors are (Beech et al., 2016).

Fetishistic Disorder and Transvestic Disorder

The word "fetish" describes an inanimate object which can arouse sexual desire (Ventriglio, Bhat, Torales, & Bhugra, 2019). **Fetishistic disorder** involves repetitive and intense sexual arousal or gratification from nonliving objects or a highly specific focus on nongenital body parts. Commonly eroticized body parts include feet, toes, and hair. The sexual arousal is also achieved by touching, smelling or licking fabrics, materials, such as clothing, rubber, leather, footwear. A classic study performed by Chalkley et al. found more than half of their participants had a fetish for clothes and nearly a quarter for leather. The focus on multiple targets was also found in this study with more than 65 percent reporting two or more fetishes. Soft fetishes are objects that are soft, furry, or lacy, such as frilly lingerie, stockings, and garters. Hard fetishes are objects that are smooth, harsh, or black, such as spike-heeled shoes, black gloves, and garments made of leather or rubber (Darcangelo, Hollings, & Paladino, 2008; Eusei & Delcea, 2019).

These soft and hard objects are somewhat arousing to many people and, indeed, are promoted as such by their manufacturers. For most people, however, the objects simply add to the sexiness of the people wearing them, and their desire is for sex with those people. For the person with a fetish, the desire is for the object, not a human partner, and is needed for sexual gratification. For example, a man may prefer that his sexual partner wear a stiletto high heel during sex which enhances his arousal. A man with a fetish is aroused by the stiletto high heel and masturbates with this object in place of a human partner. The affected individual requires the object for sexual arousal and gratification, whereas other people just have a preference (Darcangelo et al., 2008; Eusei & Delcea, 2019).

While fetishism is not considered to be rare, it is not often seen in clinical settings and affected individuals are more likely forced to seek clinical treatment due to problems in their relationship or under court-ordered conditions that relate to criminal activity. For example, in 2015 a man in the United Kingdom was arrested for having sex with 450 tractors and more than 5,000 tractor images were found on his laptop. While his fetish for green John Deere tractors and the axle grease used in these machines is a psychological disorder, this behavior also violated state laws. As a result of this illegal behavior, his fetish was identified, he was placed on a sexual offenders' registry and ordered into treatment. Due to these frequent conditions, the motivation for seeking treatment will vary which influences engagement in the process and treatment outcomes . These behaviors tend to develop in childhood or early adolescence and may become more fully defined as the individual enters adulthood, as fetishism is more focused than paraphilias (Ventriglio, Bhat, Torales, & Bhugra, 2019). Due to the secrecy associated with these disorders, the prevalence of fetishistic disorder is not fully known, but it is almost exclusively reported in males in clinical samples. Although many men may engage in fetishistic behavior, perhaps less than 1 percent would be diagnosed with a disorder, because their behavior does not cause significant distress or impairment (American Psychiatric Association, 2013; Darcangelo, 2008; Eusei & Delcea, 2019; Ventriglio et al., 2019).

One variation on fetishism is **transvestic disorder,** which is applied to individuals who fantasize about dressing in the clothes specific to the opposite sex which results in sexual arousal and subsequent emotional distress and significant dysfunction. This can be manifested in the form of fantasies, sexual impulses, or specific behaviors that are present for a minimum of 6 months (Lescai, 2020). Transvestic disorder can be distinguished from transvestism, which is cross-dressing behavior that may or may not be for the purposes of sexual arousal or gratification (Wheeler, Newring, & Draper, 2008). The prevalence is not fully known but it is believed to be rare in men (less than 3 percent) and extremely rare in women. The majority of men with this disorder identify as heterosexual, although some individuals have occasional sexual interactions with other males when they are cross-dressed (American Psychiatric Association, 2013; Lescai, 2020). One community-based study found that 2.8 percent of men and 0.4 percent of women reported engaging in cross-dressing for sexual arousal (Langstrom & Zucker, 2005).

For many men who engage in cross-dressing, it is not the women's clothes themselves that are sexually arousing but instead the activity of dressing in women's clothes. They may surreptitiously wear only one women's garment, such as a pair of women's underpants. Or they may dress fully in women's garments, complete with makeup and a wig. Some men engage in cross-dressing alone. Others participate in transvestite subcultures, in which groups of men gather for drinks, meals, and dancing while dressed as women. Sexual arousal may also occurs as a result of a man fantasizing about himself in female form or other aspects of this feminine representation (Lescai, 2020; Wheeler et al., 2008). Some men with transvestic disorder are sexually aroused by thoughts of being a woman—having a woman's physical traits or functions (for example, breasts or menstruation) or engaging in traditionally feminine tasks, such as sewing. This accompanying arousal is called autogynephilia and is distinct from both gender dysphoria and transgender identity which is discussed below (Lescai, 2020).

Most adults who engage in cross-dressing report that the behavior began secretly prior to or during puberty (Wheeler et al., 2008). During childhood, the disorder is often manifested as a preoccupation with either a specific item of women's clothing or with women's clothing in general. Puberty is often the period of development in which interest in clothes of the opposite sex becomes associated with sexual arousal and may lead to ejaculation. The fullest intensity of sexual interest and manifestations are reached during young adulthood but may diminish with older age as affected individuals get only a state of well-being associated with the interest in the clothes of the opposite sex (Lescai, 2020). The function of the cross-dressing at young ages may not be explicitly sexual but instead may be more generally pleasurable or exciting or may alleviate negative psychological states associated with male gender roles. With puberty, cross-dressing activities increasingly are paired with sexual behavior. Most men who engage in cross-dressing are married and have children (Langstrom & Zucker, 2005).

Many individuals who display these behaviors or fantasies often do not meet the *DSM-5* diagnostic criteria. About half of men who engage in cross-dressing for sexual gratification find the behavior acceptable and thus might not meet the *DSM-5* criteria for the disorder (Langstrom & Zucker, 2005). Transvestic disorder is a paraphilia reported almost exclusively in men. Sexual arousal in young men in drag often leads to masturbation following the removal of the women's clothes. Men with female partners sometimes end the transvestite episode by having sex with their partners, but may experience difficulty maintain an erection to complete intercourse in the absence of women's clothing or without related fantasies. However, elderly men learn to avoid masturbation because avoiding ejaculation allows them to prolong the time dedicated to transvestism (Lescai, 2020). With age, the sexual function of cross-dressing may diminish even as men continue to cross-dress as a self-soothing behavior to achieve feelings of comfort or well-being (Newring, Wheeler, & Draper, 2008).

Sexual Sadism and Sexual Masochism Disorders

Sexual sadism disorder and **sexual masochism disorder** are two separate diagnoses, although sadistic and masochistic sexual practices often are considered together as a pattern referred to as **sadomasochism.** In sexual sadism disorder, a person's sexual fantasies, urges, or behaviors involve inflicting pain and humiliation on their sex partner. These acts of cruelty and bodily punishment produce sexual arousal or pleasure, including orgasm. Further, for the diagnosis to be given, the urges must cause the person significant distress or impairment in functioning or the person must have acted on these urges with a nonconsenting person. The diagnosis of sexual sadism is fraught with challenges such as low reliability and validity, as well as poor consistency across assessments and studies (Longpré, Guay, Knight, & Benbouriche, 2018). These definitional and diagnostic issues have led to disagreement among professionals when assessing sexual sadism. It is widely accepted that people with sexual sadism disorder feel pleasure from the suffering they cause to their victims and are more likely to behave antisocially. These individuals get pleasure from being cruel to others and are more likely to behave this way both online and in-person. However, new research suggests that dominance and feelings of power may precipitate sadistic sexual behaviors and sadism is not exclusively about pleasure (Foulkes, 2019; Marchis, 2019).

Sexual sadism is largely associated with criminal offenders with prevalence estimates ranging up to 10 percent of those convicted of rape. Among perpetrators of sexual homicide, the prevalence of sexual sadism disorder has been reported at approximately 36 percent in German and 29 percent in United States samples. The exact prevalence in this population is still unclear but sexual sadism is believed to be a primary force behind committing sexual offenses (Stefanska, Nitschke, Carter, & Mokros, 2019). The majority of research on sexual sadism was previously limited to criminal offenders with an estimated prevalence of 2 to 30 percent among this group. However, more recently, this phenomenon that is recognized among the noncriminal population. Sadistic traits are consistently found in both community and forensic samples and these behaviors range from the enjoyment of embarrassing others to the enjoyment of committing torture and murder (Foulkes, 2019). For example, in a sample of individuals aged 40 to 79, approximately 22 percent reported sadistic sexual fantasies. It is posited that most people in the noncriminal population under-report such sadistic fantasies due to legal and social concerns. Sexual sadism is predominant found among men and strongly associated with antisocial behaviors (Marchis, 2019).

In sexual masochism disorder, a person's sexual fantasies, urges, or behaviors involve suffering pain or humiliation during sex, and they must cause the person significant distress or impairment in functioning. In both disorders, distress may manifest as guilt, shame, loneliness, or intense sexual frustration. It is

Sexual sadism and sexual masochism exist along a continuum. More moderate forms that occur between consenting adults, such as those portrayed in the blockbuster romance *Fifty Shades of Grey,* by E. L. James, would likely not qualify for a *DSM-5* diagnosis. *Chuck Zlotnick/Focus/Universal/Kobal/Shutterstock*

uncommon for those with these types of sexual behaviors to seek treatment (American Psychiatric Association, 2013; Mirica, 2020). Some people occasionally engage in mild or moderately sadistic or masochistic behaviors during sex or simulate such behaviors without actually carrying through with the infliction of pain or suffering (Hucker, 2008). These people probably would not be given a diagnosis, especially if their behaviors occur in the context of a trusting relationship in which boundaries have been set and safety measures are in place (e.g., having a "safe word" that, when uttered by either partner, stops the behavior). This is a good example of sexuality along the continuum, as well as the challenges in defining abnormality in the sexual disorders (Beech et al., 2016). People diagnosed with sexual sadism disorder or sexual masochism disorder typically engage in sadistic and masochistic behaviors as their preferred or exclusive form of sexual gratification.

The sexual rituals in sadism and masochism disorders are of four types: physical restriction, which involves the use of bondage, chains, or handcuffs as part of sex; the administration of pain, in which one partner inflicts pain or harm on the other with beatings, whippings, electrical shock, burning, cutting, stabbing, strangulation, torture, mutilation, or even death; hypermasculinity practices, including the aggressive use of enemas, fists, and dildos in the sexual act; and humiliation, in which one partner verbally and physically humiliates the other during sex

(Sandnabba, Santtila, Alison, & Nordling, 2002). The partner who is the victim in such encounters may be either a masochist and a willing "victim" or a nonconsenting victim. A variety of props may be used in these encounters, including black leather garments, chains, shackles, whips, harnesses, and ropes. Men are much more likely than women to enjoy sadomasochistic sex, in the roles of both sadist and masochist (Sandnabba et al., 2002). Some women find such activities exciting, but many consent to them only to please their partners or because they are paid to do so, and some are nonconsenting victims of sadistic men.

Although sadomasochistic sex between consenting adults typically does not result in physical injury, the activities can get out of control or go too far. A particularly dangerous activity is hypoxyphilia, which involves sexual arousal by means of oxygen deprivation, obtained by placing a rope around the neck, putting a plastic bag or mask over the head, or exerting severe chest compression (Hucker, 2008). Accidents involving hypoxyphilia can result in permanent injury or death. Unsurprisingly given the role of lack of consent in the diagnosis, sexual sadism disorder is found at higher rates among forensic populations of sexually motivated murderers and sex offenders (Beech et al., 2016).

Voyeuristic, Exhibitionistic, and Frotteuristic Disorders

Voyeurism, as a form of sexual arousal, involves watching an unsuspecting person who is naked, undressing, engaging in sexual activities, or activities that are considered private in nature. Voyeurism is probably the most common illegal paraphilia (Baruch, 2020; Beech et al., 2016; Langstrom, 2009). A survey of 2,450 randomly selected adults from the general population of Sweden found that 12 percent of the men and 4 percent of the women reported at least one incident of being sexually aroused by spying on others having sex (Langstrom & Seto, 2006). A study of 60 male college students in the United States suggested that 42 percent had secretly watched others in sexual situations (Templeman & Stinnet, 1991).

For a diagnosis of **voyeuristic disorder** to be made, the voyeuristic behavior must be repeated over 6 months and must be compulsive. Further, for a diagnosis to be given, the urges must cause the person significant distress or impairment in functioning or the voyeur must have acted on these urges with a nonconsenting person. Most people who engage in voyeurism are men who watch women (Lavin, 2008). They may masturbate during or immediately after the act of watching. This disorder typically develops in adolescence before the age of 15. As with other paraphilias, prevalence rates are difficult to determine but voyeuristic disorder is estimated to affect 12 percent of men and 4 percent of women in the general population over the lifespan (Mirica, 2020). One study in Sweden found that individuals (18 to 60 years) reported sexual arousal by exhibitionism (3 percent) or voyeurism (8 percent) in the general population with more men reporting they had engaged in exhibitionism and voyeurism, as compared to women (Thibaut et al., 2020).

The person who engages in *exhibitionism* obtains sexual gratification by exposing their genitals to involuntary observers, who usually are strangers. The survey in Sweden cited above found that 4.1 percent of men and 2.1 percent of women reported having experienced sexual arousal from exposing their genitals to a stranger at least once in their life (Baruch, 2020; Langstrom & Seto, 2006). In order to obtain the diagnosis of **exhibitionistic disorder,** individuals must have acted on their urges to engage in the behavior, or the behavior must cause significant distress or impairment. Most exhibitionists are men, and their targets tend to be women, children, or adolescents (Murphy & Page, 2008). Clinically, it is important to know that exhibitionists who target children may also have a co-occurring pedophilic disorder. The exhibitionist typically confronts his victim in a public place, such as at a park or on a bus. His arousal comes from observing the victim's surprise, fear, or disgust or from a fantasy that his victim is becoming sexually aroused. His behavior often is compulsive and impulsive—he feels a sense of excitement, fear, restlessness, and sexual arousal and then feels compelled to find relief by exhibiting himself (Murphy & Page, 2008). Some people who engage in exhibitionism masturbate while exhibiting themselves. Others draw on memories or fantasies of exposing themselves to arouse themselves while masturbating.

People who engage in exhibitionism are more likely than most sex offenders to get caught, in part because of the public nature of their behavior. In addition, some of them repeatedly return to places where they have already exhibited themselves. The danger of being caught heightens their arousal. People who engage in exhibitionism are also likely to continue their behavior after having been caught (Murphy & Page, 2008). Castellini et al. (2018), in a sample of Italian university students (243 men and 532 women), reported that 50 percent of the men and 42 percent of women reported at least one paraphilic behavior. Within this sample, there was a higher prevalence of voyeurism, and exhibitionism among men (Thibaut et al., 2020).

Frotteurism is a paraphilia that often co-occurs with voyeurism and exhibitionism. The person who engages in frotteurism gains sexual gratification from rubbing against and fondling parts of the body of a nonconsenting person. Often, this happens in crowded

Digital Vision./Getty Images

places, such as a subway train or an elevator, and the target may not recognize the contact as sexual. During the act, the affected individual usually fantasizes that he is in an affectionate and sensual relationship with the victim. Part of the excitement experienced by those with frotteurism comes from the risk of being caught, which heightens the sexual response. The majority of these cases involve males inappropriately touching females, but there have been incidences of females touching males, females touching females, males touching males, and adults touching children (Baruch, 2020; Stan, 2020). In order to receive the diagnosis of **frotteuristic disorder,** individuals must experience recurrent and intense sexual arousal from nonconsensual rubbing or touching for more than 6 months that is manifested in thoughts, urges, or behaviors. These fantasies and urges cause significant distress or dysfunction in personal relationships and daily activities of the perpetrator or those around him (Stan, 2020).

Most people who engage in frotteurism are males, and the onset of the disorder most often is in adolescence or early adulthood (Beech et al., 2016; Lussier & Pichê, 2008). Most frotteuristic acts occur between the ages of 15 to 25 years, after which there is a gradual decline in frequency. The prevalence of frotteurism is estimated between 7.9 and 9.7 percent in the general population. Like most paraphilic disorders, little is known about the etiology or course of frotteurism. Individuals with frotteurism are frequently involved in antisocial activities and this disorder may result from various social issues or an inability to control one's sex drive. There are many theories on causation but ultimately no definitive conclusions. The course of frotteurism is likely to vary with time and sexual preferences and behaviors may decline with older age, as is common with other paraphilic disorders (Thibaut et al., 2020).

Frotteurism has been documented in cultures all over the world. In 2005, Japan and India, frotteurism became such a widespread problem that special women-only train cars and buses were created. This was developed after studies revealed more than 66 percent of female passengers in their twenties and thirties had experienced frotteuristic acts (rubbing, touching, groping) on public trains in Tokyo. In Japan this is called "chikan" which describes public sexual harassment or molestation. It is common that women in various cultures rarely report incidents of sexual harassment or assault on public transportation. As a result, female-only public transportation and taxi services have been introduced in at least 15 countries, including Brazil, Egypt, India, and Indonesia, in an effort to protect women. Embarrassment, concerns about whether it is a crime, and general acceptance of these behaviors are often factors that contribute to a lack of reporting which impact definitive frotteurism statistics (Stan, 2020).

Pedophilic Disorder

People with **pedophilic disorder** are adults (16 years +) who have recurrent, intense and uncontrollable sexual fantasies, urges, and behaviors focused on sexually immature children, generally 13 years and younger. To be diagnosed with pedophilic disorder, the individual must have acted on the urges involving children or child sexual exploitation materials, or experience distress because of these urges (American Psychiatric Association, 2013; Jahnke, 2018; Thibaut et al., 2020). Studies have found that not all men with this disorder act on their impulses and commit a sexual offense. However, those who commit a sexual crime often report struggling with their sexual urges for 10 years prior to the act. Most researchers emphasize the difference between pedophilic interests and sexual offending against children. Not all individuals with pedophilic interests sexually approach children, and not all child molesters have "recurrent and intense" pedophilic interests. Research has found that about half of the cases of child sexual abuse are committed by nonpedophilic offenders (Landgren, Malki, Bottai, Arver, & Rahm, 2020; Münch, Walter, & Müller, 2020). *DSM-5* recognizes that pedophilic disorder can be exclusive (i.e., attracted only to children) or nonexclusive. Additional specifiers indicate whether an individual is sexually attracted to males, females, or both, and whether the pedophilic behavior is limited to incest.

Not all individuals with pedophilic fantasies engage in sexual contact with children; instead, many use child pornography to become sexually aroused (Münch et al., 2020; Seto, 2009). Still, most of what we know about pedophilia is based on studies conducted with individuals who have committed sexual offenses with children. Sexual encounters between people with pedophilic disorder and their child victims often are brief, although they may recur frequently. People with pedophilic disorder may threaten children with harm, physically restrain them, or tell them that they will punish them or their loved ones if the children do not comply. Other people with pedophilic disorder are loving, caring, and gentle to the child, using emotional closeness to gain sexual access. This is especially true in incestuous relationships, in which people with pedophilic disorder may see themselves as simply being good, loving parents. They believe that what they do to the child is not sexual but loving (Seto, 2009).

CASE STUDY

Michael Robbins, a 45-year-old, single Caucasian cis-male, was recently found guilty of sexual assault after inappropriately touching multiple girls who were all under the age of 12. Friends and neighbors were shocked, appalled and irate when these incidents were reported since Michael had been a very active member of the community with a good reputation for helping others.

Michael had his first sexual experience at 7 years old when a female neighbor performed various sexual acts on him over the course of summer break. As he grew older, he noticed that he remained sexually attracted to young girls and he frequently had intense and repetitive sexual thoughts and urges for girls under the age of 12. Young girls were always his source of sexual arousal and he would frequently masturbate while fantasizing about a girl in that age range. Michael strategically developed opportunities to spend time with young girls, whether it was dating a single mother or volunteering to coach the local softball team. On more than one occasion, Michael developed strong emotional feelings for a much younger girl and professed his love to her. Sometimes, he described this affection to the girls as fatherly love, but he knew it was sexual.

Michael knew that these sexual fantasies and urges for young girls would never be approved by others, so he made every effort to hide these desires. While he understood that others would not approve of these thoughts, Michael felt that these relationships would be beneficial to the girls who he was teaching sexual pleasure. Despite this belief, Michael often experienced conflicting emotions and guilt surrounding his urges and prayed for help. So many times Michael successfully resisted acting upon these urges, but ultimately he could not.

The impact on the child victims of people with pedophilic disorder can be great. The most frequent symptoms shown by sexually abused children are fearfulness, shame, depression, complex posttraumatic stress disorder, conduct disorder and hyperactivity, sexualized behaviors (promiscuity and sexual behavior inappropriate for their age), and poor self-esteem (Alix et al., 2017; Murray, Nguyen, & Cohen, 2014). More severe symptoms are experienced by children who endure frequent abuse over a long period, who are penetrated by the perpetrator, who are abused by a family member (typically, a father or stepfather), and whose mother does not provide support on learning of the abuse. About two-thirds of victimized children show significant recovery from their symptoms within 12 to 18 months following cessation of the abuse, but significant numbers of abused children continue to experience psychological problems even into adulthood (Nelson, Baldwin, & Taylor, 2012; Vonderlin et al., 2018).

Causes of Paraphilias

Behavioral theories of the paraphilias explain them as being due to an initial classical pairing of intense early sexual arousal with a particular stimulus (Figure 3). For example, a child may become aroused when spying on the babysitter's lovemaking with her boyfriend or while being held down and tickled erotically. This may be followed by intensive operant conditioning in which the stimulus is present during masturbation.

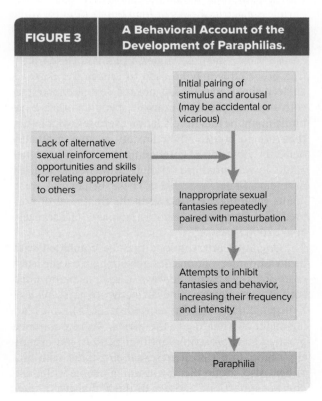

| FIGURE 3 | A Behavioral Account of the Development of Paraphilias. |

Initial pairing of stimulus and arousal (may be accidental or vicarious)

Lack of alternative sexual reinforcement opportunities and skills for relating appropriately to others

Inappropriate sexual fantasies repeatedly paired with masturbation

Attempts to inhibit fantasies and behavior, increasing their frequency and intensity

Paraphilia

For example, the individual may repeatedly fantasize about a particular scenario, such as watching the babysitter have sex, while masturbating. This reinforces the association between the stimulus and sexual arousal. The individual may try to suppress the undesired arousal or behaviors, but these attempts at inhibition increase the frequency and intensity of the fantasies. Eventually, the sexual arousal may generalize to other stimuli similar to the initial fantasy, such as actually watching other people's lovemaking, leading to paraphilic behavior (e.g., voyeurism). Some people with paraphilia appear to have a strong sex drive and masturbate often, providing many opportunities for the pairing of their fantasies with sexual gratification (Kafka & Hennen, 2003). Often, the person with a paraphilia also has few opportunities for other types of sexual reinforcement and has difficulty relating appropriately to other adults.

These classic behavioral theories have been supplemented with principles of social learning theory (see the chapter "Theories and Treatment of Abnormality"), which suggest that the larger environment of a child's home and culture influences their tendency to develop deviant sexual behavior. Children whose parents frequently use corporal punishment and engage in aggressive contact with each other are more likely to engage in impulsive, aggressive, and perhaps sexualized acts toward others as they grow older. Many people with pedophilia have poor interpersonal skills and feel intimidated when interacting sexually with adults (Seto, 2008).

A study of 64 convicted sex offenders with various types of paraphilia found that they had higher rates of childhood abuse and family dysfunction than did offenders who had committed property crimes and did not have a paraphilia (Lee, Jackson, Pattison, & Ward, 2002). Childhood sexual abuse among boys is associated with an increased risk for developing pedophilic disorder. Similarly, studies of juvenile sex offenders, most of whom assaulted a younger child, find that many likely suffered sexual abuse (Berlin, 2019; Gerardin & Thibaut, 2004).

Cognitive theorists have also identified a number of distortions and assumptions that people with a paraphilia have about their behaviors and the behaviors of their victims (Gerardin & Thibaut, 2004; Maletzky, 1998). These distortions may have been learned from parents' deviant messages about sexual behavior. They are used to justify the person's victimization of others when that is part of the behavior.

In the development of pedophilic disorder, there is evidence which suggests both nature and nurture are influential. In addition to previously mentioned psychosocial and environmental factors alterations in the development of the brain and hormonal systems may also contribute to pedophilia (Berlin, 2019; Seto, 2008).

Men with pedophilia are more likely to have had a head injury before age 13, to have cognitive and memory deficits, to have lower intelligence, and to have differences in brain structure volume (Fonteille et al., 2019). In addition, some small studies suggest that men with pedophilia have dysfunctions in the frontal areas of the brain involved in regulating impulsive and aggressive behavior and in testosterone levels (Jordan, Fromberger, Stolpmann, & Müller, 2011). How these factors specifically contribute to pedophilia is not yet clear.

Treatments for the Paraphilic Disorders

Most people with a paraphilia or a paraphilic disorder do not seek treatment for their behaviors (Darcangelo, 2008). Treatment is often forced on those who are arrested after engaging in illegal acts including voyeurism, exhibitionism, frotteurism, or pedophilia. Simple incarceration does little to change these behaviors, and convicted sex offenders are likely to become repeat offenders (Seto, 2008). Research has documented very strong punitive attitudes in relation to people with a pedophilic disorder and high stigmatizing attitudes that may hinder access to treatment. Some argue that stigmatization may indirectly increase the risk of sexual offending through deficits in social and emotional functioning, such as an inability to cope with stress, a stronger belief that adult-child sex is morally permissible, and reduced willingness to seek professional help. In a recent prevalence survey, only 12 percent of men with sexual interest in children considered seeking professional help. However, the rate increased to 50 percent among those whose sexual attraction to children surpassed their attraction to adults (Jahnke, 2018). Studies have found that access to effective treatment could reduce psychosocial stress for the affected individual and prevent child sexual abuse (Landgren et al., 2020). Unfortunately, individuals with pedophilia report strong fears of others finding out about their sexual interests and attempt to keep their pedophilic interests a secret. This fear of being discovered was significantly associated with more psychological and physical problems, fear of negative evaluation, loneliness, and emotional coping (as a dysfunctional coping style often found among sexual (Jahnke, 2018).

Biological interventions generally are aimed at reducing the sex drive in order to reduce paraphilic behavior. Surgical castration, which removes the testes and thereby almost completely eliminates the production of androgens, lowers repeat offense rates among sex offenders (Maletzky & Field, 2003; Seto, 2009). Castration has been performed on hundreds of convicted sex offenders in the Netherlands, Germany, and the United States, although it is rarely used today (Seto, 2009).

Sex offenders can also be treated by chemical castration, in which they are given antiandrogen drugs that suppress the production of testosterone and thereby reduce the sex drive. These drugs typically are used in conjunction with psychotherapy and can be useful for hypersexual men who are motivated to change their behavior (Holoyda & Kellaher, 2016). Follow-up studies have shown that people with a paraphilia treated with antiandrogen drugs show reductions in their paraphilic behavior (Garcia, Delavenne, Assumpção, & Thibaut, 2013; Holoyda & Kellaher, 2016). These drugs have a number of side effects, however, including fatigue, sleepiness, depression, weight gain, leg cramps, breast formation, hair loss, and osteoporosis. Seven U.S. states have laws that require some sex offenders who want to be paroled to take antiandrogen drugs or undergo surgical castration.

The SSRIs have been used to reduce sexual drive and paraphilic behavior (Holoyda & Kellaher, 2016). Some studies find that these drugs have positive effects on sexual drive and impulse control, although the effects are not totally consistent across studies.

Behavior modification therapies commonly are used to treat paraphilia and can be successful if people with a paraphilia are willing to change their behavior. **Aversion therapy** is used to extinguish sexual responses to objects or situations a person with a paraphilia finds arousing. During such therapy, a person with a paraphilia might be exposed to painful but harmless electric shocks or loud bursts of noise while viewing photographs of what arouses them, such as children, or while actually touching objects that arouse them, such as women's panties. Desensitization procedures may be used to reduce the person's anxiety about engaging in normal sexual encounters with other adults. For example, people with a paraphilia might be taught relaxation exercises, which they then use to control their anxiety as they gradually build up fantasies of interacting sexually with other adults in ways that are fulfilling to them and to their partners (Maletzky, 1998). These behavioral treatments generally are effective in the treatment of nonpredatory paraphilias such as fetishism (Darcangelo et al., 2008).

Cognitive interventions may be combined with behavioral interventions designed to help people learn more socially acceptable ways to approach and interact with people they find attractive (e.g., Kaplan & Krueger, 2012; Wong Sarver & Gros, 2014). Role playing might be used to give the person with a paraphilia practice in approaching another person and eventually negotiating a positive sexual encounter with him or her. Also, group therapy in which people with paraphilias support one another through changes in their behavior can be helpful. Multiple studies find that these combined cognitive-behavioral treatments can effectively treat nonpredatory paraphilias in individuals motivated to change (Darcangelo et al., 2008; Kaplan & Krueger, 2012).

Cognitive-behavioral therapy also has been used to help people with a predatory paraphilia (e.g., pedophilia, exhibitionism, voyeurism) identify and challenge thoughts and situations that trigger their behaviors and serve as justifications for the behaviors (Kaplan & Krueger, 2012). Some clinical trials of cognitive-behavioral therapy for sex offenders have found a significantly lower recidivism rate in men who received the therapy compared to those who did not (W. Marshall & L. Marshall, 2015). However, the evidence base is small and somewhat mixed (Kaplan & Krueger, 2012; Marques, Wiederanders, Day, Nelson, & van Ommeren, 2005).

Due to the nature of this disorder, opinions on best practices are often passionate. Current interventions with empirical support include psychotherapy and antidepressants as well as testosterone-suppressing medications for high-risk individuals. Chemical castration is used as a compulsory legal sentence for child sexual offenders in some jurisdictions in the United States, Asia, and Europe. Other countries prohibit this practice due to uncertain efficacy and ethical concerns. Studies have found that paraphilic disorder often co-occurs with depressive and anxiety disorders, symptoms of ADHD and antisocial personality disorder (ASD), and slightly lower IQ within the normal range. These comorbid psychological conditions create additional challenges to treating this underserved population (Landgren et al., 2020).

GENDER DYSPHORIA

Gender dysphoria is a new *DSM-5* diagnostic category that replaces *DSM-IV*'s *gender identity disorder*. While gender identity disorder emphasized cross-gender identification, *DSM-5*'s gender dysphoria is diagnosed when there is a discrepancy between individuals' gender identity (i.e., sense of themselves as male or female) and their biological sex (Table 4). Stephanie, in the following case study, would be diagnosed with gender dysphoria.

DSM-5 acknowledges the wide variation of gender-incongruent conditions and provides separate criteria sets for gender dysphoria in children and in adolescents and adults, the latter of which are more detailed (see Table 4; Zucker, Lawrence, & Kreukels, 2016). Importantly, the diagnosis of gender dysphoria requires significant distress or impairment associated with the gender incongruence; the incongruence is not in itself viewed as a disorder. As with adults, children with gender dysphoria experience incongruence between their assigned gender and the way they experience themselves as male or female. *Gender dysphoria in children* is a rare condition in which a child persistently rejects their anatomic sex and strongly desires to be or insists they are a member of the other sex. Girls with this disorder seek masculine-type activities and male peer groups to a degree far beyond that of a tomboy. Sometimes these girls express the belief that they will eventually grow a penis. Boys with the disorder seek feminine-type activities and female peer groups and tend to begin cross-dressing in girls' clothes at a very early age (Zucker & Wood, 2011). They express disgust with their penis and wish it

---

TABLE 4   *DSM-5* Criteria for Gender Dysphoria in Adolescents or Adults

A. A marked incongruence between one's experienced/expressed gender and assigned gender, of at least 6 months duration, as manifested by at least two of the following:

1. A marked incongruence between one's experienced/expressed gender and primary and/or secondary sex characteristics (or, in young adolescents, the anticipated secondary sex characteristics)
2. A strong desire to be rid of one's primary and/or secondary sex characteristics because of a marked incongruence with one's experienced/expressed gender (or, in young adolescents, a desire to prevent the development of the anticipated secondary sex characteristics)
3. A strong desire for the primary and/or secondary sex characteristics of the other gender
4. A strong desire to be of the other gender (or some alternative gender different from one's assigned gender)
5. A strong desire to be treated as the other gender (or some alternative gender different from one's assigned gender)
6. A strong conviction that one has the typical feelings and reactions of the other gender (or some alternative gender different from one's assigned gender)

B. The condition is associated with clinically significant distress or impairment in social, occupational, or other important areas of functioning.

would disappear. The onset of these behaviors typically is in the preschool years. Boys are referred more often than girls for concerns regarding gender dysphoria. This may reflect a greater prevalence of gender dysphoria in males than in females, or it may reflect a greater concern on the part of parents with violations of gender roles in boys than in girls (Zucker & Cohen-Kettenis, 2008).

CASE STUDY

Stephanie was 30 when she first attended our clinic. She gave a history of conviction that she was, in fact, male and wished to rid herself of identifiably female attributes and acquire male traits and features. She said she had been cross-living and employed as a male for about 1 year, following the breakdown of a 10-year marriage. She was taking testosterone prescribed by her family physician. She presented at our clinic with a request for removal of her uterus and ovaries.

She did not give a childhood history of tomboy attitudes, thoughts, or behavior. She said social interaction with other children, boys or girls, was minimal. Desperate for a friend, she fantasized "an articulate and strong" boy, exactly her age, named Ronan. They were always together and they talked over everything: thoughts and feelings and the events of her life. Cross-dressing in her father's clothing also began during childhood. There was no history of sexual arousal associated with or erotic fantasy involving cross-dressing.

Puberty at age 12 and the accompanying bodily changes apparently did not overly distress Stephanie. Sexual and romantic feelings focused on "slender, feminine-appearing men." . . .

At 19, she met a slender, good-looking man. They were compatible and married soon after. The marriage was a success. Stephanie's preferred position for intercourse was with both kneeling, she behind her husband, rubbing her pubic area against him while masturbating him. She would imagine she had a penis and was penetrating him. . . . She decided to live full-time in the male role as Jacob. While on the West Coast, she started treatment with male hormones. She moved back east and presented at our clinic for assessment. She saw herself as a male, primarily attracted to gay or gay-appearing males. (Dickey & Stephens, 1995, pp. 442–443)

Adults with gender dysphoria might cross-dress or dress in gender-nonconforming ways, either occasionally or regularly. Unlike people with transvestic disorder, these people are not sexually aroused by this practice;

they simply believe they are putting on the clothes of the gender to which they really belong. The sexual preferences of individuals with gender dysphoria vary. Some individuals are asexual, having little interest in either sex; some are heterosexual; and some are homosexual (Lawrence, 2008). People with gender dysphoria who can afford it may seek a sex-change operation.

Gender dysphoria is rare. Studies of prevalence vary, but a meta-analysis estimated prevalence of 6.8 in 100,000 natal (born) males and 2.6 in 100,000 natal females (Arcelus et al., 2015). Some people with gender dysphoria are so disturbed by their misassignment of gender and its social consequences that they develop mood and anxiety disorders, and to a lesser degree, alcohol and other substance abuse problems (Yarbrough, 2018; Zucker et al., 2016). Rates of suicide, suicide attempts, and nonsuicidal self-injury are also elevated in this group. Low self-esteem and psychological distress also result from their rejection by others. High rates of HIV infection among people with gender dysphoria have been reported in some studies, especially among individuals who also face poverty, racism, and employment discrimination (American Psychological Association, 2015; Wiewel, Torian, Merchant, Braunstein, & Shepard, 2016). HIV may be contracted through risky sexual behaviors or through the sharing of needles during drug use or hormone injections. Many people with gender dysphoria avoid seeking medical attention because of negative interactions with physicians. Indeed, some physicians refuse to treat people with gender dysphoria.

The diagnosis of gender dysphoria represents one piece—and a quite controversial piece—of gender diversity more broadly (Zucker & Duschinsky, 2016; Zucker et al., 2016). A number of terms are used by and for people whose gender identity or expression does not correspond with binary, biologically based male/female categories, and who would not necessarily be diagnosed with gender dysphoria. These terms include "transgender," "gender variant," "genderqueer," "gender nonconforming," "nonbinary," and "transsexual," among others. The term **transgender** (or "trans") is currently the most widely used, and refers to the broad spectrum of individuals who transiently or persistently identify with a gender different from their natal sex. This may include nontraditional gender identity that is recognized as neither male nor female. The term "transsexual," more widely used in the past, refers primarily to people who have chosen to undergo sexual reassignment surgery or hormonal treatment to align their biology with their gender identity (American Psychological Association, 2015). It is a more medically based term than the broader, socially based "transgender" umbrella term, and is considered offensive by some. The term "cisgender" applies to people whose gender identity aligns with their natal sex.

In recent years the experiences of transgender individuals have become more visible in the culture, including the coming out of Caitlyn Jenner (previously Bruce Jenner), an Olympic athlete and reality TV star. *(Left): Focus on Sport/Getty Images; (Right): Joe Seer/Shutterstock*

People who identify as transgender may or may not be diagnosed with gender dysphoria, depending on whether their gender incongruence causes distress or impairment. This was a major concern in the development of the *DSM-5* criteria (Zucker et al., 2016). Some transgender groups advocated for removing gender identity disorder altogether, just as homosexuality was removed in 1973. However, it was retained in order to maintain access to care for people distressed by their gender incongruence, and was reformulated to emphasize this incongruence rather than cross-sex identification (Zucker et al., 2016). Notably, whereas gender dysphoria is quite rare, population-based studies in the United States estimate that 0.6 percent identify as transgender (Flores, Herman, Gates, & Brown, 2016). Like the sexual disorders, the gender dysphoria diagnosis is a good example of the continuum approach, and of how defining and classifying abnormality are inherently affected by social, historical, and cultural contexts (see the chapters "Looking at Abnormality" and "Assessing and Diagnosing Abnormality").

Contributors to Gender Dysphoria

Biological theories of gender dysphoria have focused on the effects of prenatal hormones on brain development (Zucker et al., 2016; Zucker & Wood, 2011). Although several specific mechanisms have been implicated, most theories suggest that people who develop gender dysphoria have been exposed to unusual levels of hormones, which influence later gender identity and sexual orientation by influencing the development of brain structures involved in sexuality. In genetic females, female-to-male gender dysphoria has been associated with hormonal disorders resulting in prenatal exposure to high levels of androgens (Baba et al., 2007), whereas in genetic males, male-to-female gender dysphoria has been associated with prenatal exposure to very low levels of androgens (Hines, Ahmed, & Hughes, 2003; Swaab & Garcia-Filgueras, 2009).

Awareness of issues of gender dysphoria and transgender identity has increased in recent years, due in part to increased depiction in film and television, as in the 2017 film *A Fantastic Woman*. *Moviestore Collection Ltd/Alamy Stock Photo*

Researchers have identified multiple differences in brain anatomy and function among people with gender dysphoria (Kreukels & Guillamon, 2016; Zucker et al., 2016). In multiple studies, a cluster of cells in the hypothalamus called the bed nucleus of the stria terminalis, which plays a role in sexual behavior, has been implicated in gender dysphoria (Chung, De Vries, & Swaab, 2002; Garcia-Filgueras & Swaab, 2008; see Kreukels & Guillamon, 2016). Typically this cluster of cells is smaller in women's brains than in men's. Studies have found that this cluster of cells is half as large in men with gender dysphoria as in men without the disorder and close to the size usually found in women's brains. Other differences include gray matter volume, white matter structure, and cortical thickness. People with gender dysphoria, compared to people who do not experience gender incongruence, show patterns in these brain areas that are more like those in people of the other biological sex. However, these findings require further investigation. They apply more to natal men with gender dysphoria than to natal women, and also differ depending on sexual orientation (Kreukels & Guillamon, 2016; Zucker et al., 2016).

Hormonal factors and neural factors are closely related; they affect one another. Moreover, both may be tied to genetic factors. Family and twin studies suggest that gender dysphoria may have genetic causes (Coolidge, Thede, & Young, 2002; Heylens et al., 2012), although the specific genetic factors involved are not yet known (Ujike et al., 2009; Zucker et al., 2016).

In general, the evidence in support of psychological contributors to gender dysphoria has been weak (Zucker et al., 2016; Zucker & Wood, 2011). Most psychosocial theories of gender dysphoria focus on the role parents play in shaping their children's gender identity. Parents encourage children to identify with one sex or the other by reinforcing "gender-appropriate" behavior and punishing "gender-inappropriate" behavior. From early infancy, they buy male or female clothes for their children and sex-stereotyped toys (dolls or trucks). They encourage or discourage playing rough-and-tumble games or playing with dolls.

A long-term study of a large sample of boys with gender dysphoria found that their parents were less likely than the parents of boys without gender dysphoria to discourage cross-gender behaviors (Green, 1987). That is, these boys were not punished, either subtly or overtly, for engaging in feminine behavior such as playing with dolls or wearing dresses as much as were boys who did not have gender dysphoria. Further, boys who were highly feminine (although not necessarily with gender dysphoria) tended to have mothers who had wanted a girl rather than a boy, saw their baby sons as girls, and dressed their baby sons as girls. When the boys were older, their mothers tended to prohibit rough-and-tumble play, and the boys had few opportunities to have male playmates. About one-third of these boys had no father in the home, and those who did have a father in the home tended to be very close to their mother. However, conclusions about the role of parenting and psychosocial factors are limited by the design of most studies in this area (see Zucker et al., 2016).

Gender identity tends to be quite stable from childhood into adulthood. However, this stability is less clear among children with gender dysphoria. Many such children grow up to identify with their natal sex. One 24-year longitudinal study found that gender dysphoria in childhood is a better predictor of adult homosexual orientation than of adult gender dysphoria (e.g., Steensma, Van der Ende, Verhulst, & Cohen–Ketteni, 2013). Persistence of gender dysphoria from childhood into adolescence is higher among natal girls, children who express more intense dysphoria, and children who have begun taking on a cross-sex social role (Steensma, McGuire, Kreukels, Beekman, & Cohen-Kettenis, 2013). Importantly, research in this area is new, ongoing, and hotly debated, with major social and treatment implications for children (Olson, 2016; Temple Newhook et al., 2018; Zucker, 2018).

Treatments for Gender Dysphoria

Therapists who work with people with gender dysphoria help these individuals clarify their gender identity or experienced gender and their desire for treatment. In addition to psychotherapy, there are three principal treatments for gender dysphoria: (1) cross-sex hormone therapy, (2) social transition to full-time real-life experience in the desired gender role, and (3) gender-affirming surgery (GAS), which provides the genitalia and secondary sex characteristics (e.g., breasts) of the gender with which the individual identifies (Bizic et al., 2018; Byne et al., 2012). Treatment of gender dysphoria has historically raised numerous ethical concerns. Identifying the best treatment is fraught with challenges since there are existing concerns about the most appropriate way to define gender dysphoria (mental/medical illness, social construct, and variation of sex) and a lack of agreement on etiology. The most prominent topics and ethical questions associated with gender dysphoria treatment relate underage individuals, compromised fertility and possibility of regret following GAS (Bizic et al., 2018).

Cross-sex hormone therapy stimulates the development of secondary sex characteristics of the preferred sex and suppresses secondary sex characteristics of the birth sex. Estrogens are used in feminizing hormone therapy for male-to-female individuals with gender dysphoria. These hormones cause fatty deposits to develop in the breasts and hips, soften the skin, and inhibit the growth of a beard. Testosterone is used to induce masculinization in female-to-male individuals with gender dysphoria. This hormone causes the voice to deepen, hair to become distributed in a male pattern, fatty tissue in the breast to recede, and muscles to enlarge; the clitoris also may grow larger (Bizic et al., 2018; Byne et al., 2012). Hormone therapy may be given to individuals regardless of whether they wish to undergo sex reassignment surgery.

The social transition includes using a different name, pronouns, transformation of physical appearance, use of suitable bathrooms, and taking social roles of the affirmed gender (Bizic et al., 2018). Before undergoing sex reassignment surgery, individuals spend up to a year or more living full-time in the gender role they seek. Some choose to live full-time in their desired gender role even if they do not undertake sex reassignment surgery or hormone therapy (Byne et al., 2012).

Mental health professionals, endocrinologists, and surgeons are often part of the medical treatment team of experienced experts. GAS requires a series of surgeries and hormone treatments which often occurs over 2 years. Individuals who select GAS are required to provide two letters of recommendation from certified psychiatrists and another from a gender specialist. Additionally, an endocrinologist must confirm that they received hormonal therapy for a minimum period of 1 year. GAS is an inclusive concept that refers to all surgical procedures that a patient selects to become as similar as possible to the desired gender. In male-to-female surgery, the penis and testicles are removed, and tissue from the penis is used to create an artificial vagina. The construction of male genitals for a female-to-male reassignment is technically more difficult (Bizic et al., 2018; Byne et al., 2012). First, the internal sex organs (ovaries, fallopian tubes, uterus) and any fatty tissue remaining in the breasts are removed. Then the urethra is rerouted through the enlarged clitoris, or an artificial penis and scrotum are constructed from tissue taken from other parts of the body. This penis allows urination while standing but cannot achieve a natural erection. Other procedures, such as artificial implants, may be used to create an erection.

GAS surgery is controversial for a variety of reasons, most notably because it is irreversible. Other than suicide, postoperative regret is considered one of the worst complications. Research has found that the most common reasons for GAS regret were related to inadequate psychiatric assessment, a lack of social transition that limited "real-life experience," improperly administered cross-sex hormonal therapy, and recommendations made by inexperienced psychiatrists (Bizic et al., 2018). Follow-up studies suggest that the outcomes tend to be positive when patients are carefully selected for gender reassignment procedures based on their motivation for change and their overall psychological health and are given psychological counseling to help them through the change (Byne et al., 2012; Gorin-Lazard et al., 2013). Reviews of outcome studies have found adequate levels of sexual functioning and high sexual satisfaction following sex reassignment surgery (Klein & Gorzalka, 2009; Murad et al., 2010).

Perhaps the most controversial topic in this area is the treatment of children and adolescents. Treatment primarily focuses on psychotherapy to help children clarify their gender identity and deal with interpersonal and psychological issues created by that identity. Most clinicians consider cross-sex hormone therapies and surgeries unacceptable for children and adolescents because of their long-term consequences and children's inability to give fully informed consent for such procedures (Byne et al., 2012). However, current biological treatment options include medications known as gonadotropin-releasing hormone analogues, which delay the progression of puberty. These medications slow the progression of secondary sex characteristics, reducing gender dysphoria and giving children, parents, and clinicians more time to assess gender identity and appropriate treatment for dysphoria (Chew, Anderson, Williams, May, & Pang, 2018; Nahata, Chelvakumar, & Leibowitz, 2017). These drugs have potential side effects, including low bone density.

CHAPTER INTEGRATION

Nowhere is the interplay of biological, psychological, and social forces more apparent than in matters of sexuality (Figure 4). Biological factors influence gender identity, sexual orientation, and sexual functioning.

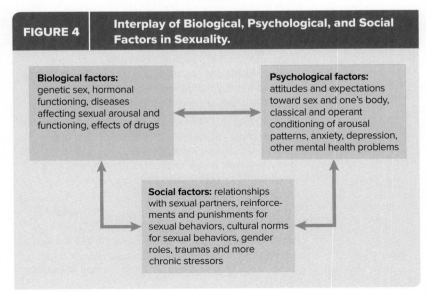

FIGURE 4 | Interplay of Biological, Psychological, and Social Factors in Sexuality.

Biological factors: genetic sex, hormonal functioning, diseases affecting sexual arousal and functioning, effects of drugs

Psychological factors: attitudes and expectations toward sex and one's body, classical and operant conditioning of arousal patterns, anxiety, depression, other mental health problems

Social factors: relationships with sexual partners, reinforcements and punishments for sexual behaviors, cultural norms for sexual behaviors, gender roles, traumas and more chronic stressors

These biological factors can be greatly moderated, however, by psychological and social factors. The meaning people assign to a sexual dysfunction, an unusual sexual practice, or an atypical gender identity is heavily influenced by their attitude toward their sexuality and gender, and by the reactions of people around them. In addition, as we saw with sexual dysfunctions, purely psychological and social conditions can cause a person's body to stop functioning as it normally would.

CHAPTER SUMMARY

- The sexual response cycle can be divided into the desire, arousal, plateau, orgasm, and resolution phases.

- Disorders of sexual desire/interest and arousal (male hypoactive sexual desire disorder, female sexual interest/arousal disorder, and erectile disorder) are among the most common sexual dysfunctions. People with these disorders experience a chronically lowered or absent desire for sex or deficiencies in sexual arousal.

- Women with female orgasmic disorder experience a persistent or recurrent delay in or the complete absence of orgasm, after having reached the excitement phase of the sexual response cycle.

- Men with early ejaculation persistently experience ejaculation (after minimal sexual stimulation) before, on, or shortly after penetration and before they wish it. Men with delayed ejaculation experience a persistent or recurrent delay in or the absence of ejaculation following the excitement phase of the sexual response cycle.

- Genito-pelvic pain/penetration disorder involves genital pain associated with intercourse or, in women, involuntary contraction of the muscles surrounding the outer third of the vagina when the vagina is penetrated.

- A variety of biological factors, including medical illnesses, the side effects of drugs, nervous system injury, and hormonal deficiencies, can cause sexual dysfunction. The psychological and sociocultural factors leading to sexual dysfunction most commonly involve negative attitudes toward sex, traumatic or stressful experiences, or conflicts with sexual partners.

- Fortunately, most sexual dysfunctions can be treated successfully. Biological treatments include drugs that increase sexual functioning, such as Viagra, and the alleviation of medical conditions that might be contributing to sexual dysfunction.

- Psychological treatments combine (1) psychotherapy focused on the personal concerns of the individual with the dysfunction and on the conflicts between the individual and their partner and (2) sex therapy designed to decrease inhibitions about sex and teach new techniques for achieving optimal sexual enjoyment.

- One set of techniques in sex therapy is sensate focus exercises. The exercises lead partners through three stages, from gentle nongenital touching to direct genital stimulation and finally to intercourse focused on enhancing and sustaining pleasure, rather than on orgasm and performance.

- Men experiencing premature ejaculation can be helped with the stop-start technique or the squeeze technique.

- The paraphilic disorders involve recurrent atypical sexual fantasies, urges, and behaviors that cause the individual distress or impairment, or cause harm or risk of harm to others.

- Fetishistic disorder is a paraphilic disorder that involves sexual fantasies, urges, or behaviors focused on nonliving objects or nongenital body parts. A particular form of fetish is transvestism, in which individuals cross-dress in order to become sexually aroused.

- Sexual sadism disorder involves sexual fantasies, urges, or behaviors focused on inflicting pain and humiliation on a sex partner. Sexual masochism disorder involves sexual fantasies, urges, or behaviors focused on experiencing pain or humiliation during sex.

- Voyeuristic disorder involves sexual fantasies, urges, or behaviors focused on secretly watching another person undressing, doing things in the nude, or engaging in sex. Almost all people who engage in voyeurism are men who watch women.

- Exhibitionistic disorder involves sexual fantasies, urges, or behaviors focused on exposing the genitals to involuntary observers, usually strangers.

- Frotteuristic disorder often co-occurs with voyeurism and exhibitionism. The person who engages in frotteurism has sexual fantasies, urges, or behaviors focused on rubbing against and fondling parts of the body of a nonconsenting person. Usually this occurs in a crowded public space.

- People with pedophilic disorder have sexual fantasies, urges, or behaviors focused on prepubescent children.

- Some neurodevelopmental differences are found between people with pedophilic disorder and people without the disorder.

- Behavioral theories suggest that the sexual behaviors of people with paraphilic disorder result from classical and operant conditioning.

- Treatments for the paraphilic disorders include biological interventions to reduce sexual drive, behavioral interventions to decondition arousal due to paraphilic objects, and cognitive-behavioral interventions to combat cognitions supporting paraphilic behavior and increase coping skills.

- Gender dysphoria is diagnosed when an individual believes that they were born with the wrong genitals and is fundamentally a person of the other sex. People with this disorder experience a chronic discomfort and sense of inappropriateness with their gender and genitals, wish to be rid of them, and want to live as members of the other sex.

- Gender dysphoria of childhood is a rare condition in which a child persistently rejects their anatomic sex, desires to be or insists they are a member of the other sex, and shows a strong preference for cross-gender roles and activities.

- Biological theories suggest that gender dysphoria is due to prenatal exposure to hormones that affect development of the hypothalamus and other brain structures involved in gender and sexuality. Socialization theories suggest that the parents of children (primarily boys) with gender dysphoria do not strictly encourage gender-appropriate behaviors.

- Treatment for gender dysphoria includes cross-sex hormone therapy, real-life experience as a member of the desired sex, and sex reassignment surgery.

KEY TERMS

sexual functioning

gender identity

sexual desire

arousal phase

plateau phase

orgasm

resolution

sexual dysfunctions

male hypoactive sexual desire disorder

female sexual interest/arousal disorder

erectile disorder (ED)

female orgasmic disorder

early or premature ejaculation

delayed ejaculation

genito-pelvic pain/penetration disorder

substance-induced sexual dysfunction

performance anxiety

sensate focus therapy

stop-start technique

squeeze technique

paraphilic disorder

fetishistic disorder

transvestic disorder

sexual sadism disorder

sexual masochism disorder

sadomasochism

voyeuristic disorder

exhibitionist disorder

frotteuristic disorder

pedophilic disorder

aversion therapy

gender dysphoria

transgender

antoniodiaz/Shutterstock

Substance Use and Gambling Disorders

CHAPTER OUTLINE

Substance Use Along the Continuum

Abstinence

Light social drinking

No significant social, occupational, or physical consequences

Potentially meets criteria for a mild alcohol use disorder:

Heavy drinking with some social, occupational, legal, or physical consequences

(DUI, misbehavior while intoxicated that affects job, frequent under-performance at work or school, increased blood pressure, damage to liver, etc.)

Likely meets diagnostic criteria for a severe alcohol use disorder:

- Clear evidence of significant social, occupational, legal, and/or physical consequences
- May have tolerance and withdrawal
- Unsuccessful attempts to control or cut down on consumption
- Life becomes taken over by obtaining, using, and recovering from the substance

Functional

Dysfunctional

Moderate drinking, mostly in social situations

Usually no social, occupational, or physical consequences, but accidents may occur *(driving while "buzzed"),* performance may be impaired the next day, and physical consequences may occur in vulnerable people *(increases in blood pressure in people with cardiac problems)*

Likely meets diagnostic criteria for a moderate alcohol use disorder:

- Clear evidence of significant social, occupational, legal, and/or physical consequences
- Continued use despite these consequences

As a student, you likely know more people along the continuum of substance use than any other continuum. TV shows and movies often show substance use as a rite of passage into adulthood—think of the college drinking scenes in movies like *21 & Over* or *Neighbors.* Illegal drug use is highest among young adults (Figure 1; Substance Abuse and Mental Health Services Administration [SAMHSA], 2017), with about 23 percent of college students reporting current use. At one end of the continuum are people who abstain completely from drugs or alcohol, for various reasons. Further along the continuum are people who use drugs and alcohol "recreationally." Nearly half the U.S. population admit to having tried an illegal substance at some time in their life (SAMHSA, 2017). Although movies and TV often make substance use seem cool, the consequences are staggeringly serious. There are more deaths from traffic accidents involving substance-impaired drivers than from all other types of accidents. About 20 percent of emergency room visits in the United States are related to the misuse of alcohol or of illegal or prescription drugs (SAMHSA, 2013). At the other end of the continuum are individuals who live their lives around substances. Their excessive substance use impairs their everyday functioning—they may avoid job and family responsibilities, act impulsively or bizarrely, or endanger their own and others' lives. These people have a substance use disorder.

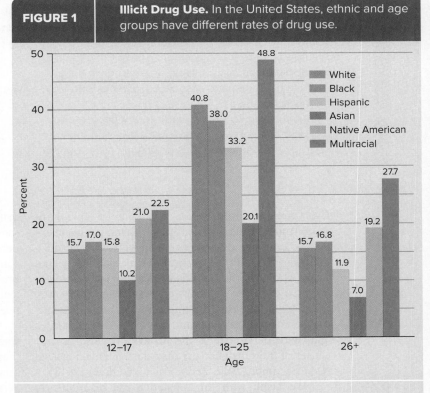

FIGURE 1

Illicit Drug Use. In the United States, ethnic and age groups have different rates of drug use.

Legend: White, Black, Hispanic, Asian, Native American, Multiracial

Percent (y-axis), Age (x-axis)

12–17: 15.7, 17.0, 15.8, 10.2, 21.0, 22.5
18–25: 40.8, 38.0, 33.2, 20.1, 48.8
26+: 15.7, 16.8, 11.9, 7.0, 19.2, 27.7

Source: SAMHSA, 2017, Table 1.30B, 226.
https://www.samhsa.gov/data/sites/default/files/NSDUH-DetTabs-2016/NSDUH-DetTabs-2016.pdf

Note: Illicit drugs include marijuana, cocaine, heroin, hallucinogens, inhalants, or prescription drugs used nonmedically. No estimate is given for Native Americans 12–17 years old because of a low response rate.

Extraordinary People

Celebrity Drug Abusers

Whitney Houston died of a drug overdose in 2012. *Patrick Seeger/ Epa/Shutterstock*

Whitney Houston was one of the most successful music artists of all time, selling over 170 million albums, singles, and music videos and winning more awards for her music than any other female artist. Her single "I Will Always Love You" from the movie *The Bodyguard,* which she also starred in, became the best-selling single in history by a female artist. She rode the top of the pop charts through the 1980s and 1990s, but then the hits stopped coming and her album sales plummeted as stories emerged about drug use leading to bizarre behavior and the loss of her once extraordinary voice. In a 2002 interview on *ABC News,* she admitted to abusing cocaine, marijuana, and pills. She attempted comebacks, but her voice was often frayed and shaky in public appearances. Then, in February 2012, Whitney Houston, age 48, was found drowned in the bathtub of a Beverly Hills hotel room. A coroner's report ruled the death an accident due to the effects of cocaine, marijuana, and multiple other drugs in her system and to heart damage associated with her long-term drug abuse.

Whitney Houston is only one in a long line of celebrity drug abusers who have died early as a result of their drug use. Heath Ledger's portrayal of the Joker in *The Dark Knight* won him an Oscar in 2009. However, the actor was not present to accept his award because on January 22, 2008, he had died of an overdose of prescription drugs, including oxycodone, hydrocodone, Valium, Restoril, Xanax, and doxylamine (a sleep aid). Ledger was 28 and on the brink of a promising career. Many other celebrities have had public problems with drugs and alcohol, including Kate Moss, Britney Spears, Lindsey Lohan, Robert Downey Jr., Drew Barrymore, and Courtney Love. Celebrities who have died from drug-related causes include Michael Jackson, D.J. AM, Chris Farley, Philip Seymour Hoffman, Prince, Russell Jones (Ol' Dirty Bastard), Amy Winehouse, and Rick James. As guitarist Keith Richards of the Rolling Stones said, "I used to know a few guys that did drugs all the time, but they're not alive anymore. . . . And you get the message after you've been to a few funerals."

Are celebrities more vulnerable to drug addiction than regular folks? Probably not. As we discuss in this chapter, alcohol and drug use disorders are among the most common mental health problems in the United States and around the world. Celebrities have more money to buy illicit drugs, and drugs and alcohol are a big part of the social scene in the entertainment industry. Some celebrities can't handle the pressure to stay on top of their field and may turn to drugs to cope. Also, when celebrities do abuse drugs or alcohol, the media broadcast their missteps widely. But much celebrity drug abuse probably is due to the same biological and psychosocial factors that contribute to drug and alcohol use disorders in noncelebrities.

Everyone has temptations, and some people have more trouble resisting them than others. In this chapter, we consider disorders that involve chronic difficulties in resisting the desire to drink alcohol or take drugs, known in the *DSM-5* as **substance use disorders.** We also consider **gambling disorder,** which involves the inability to resist the impulse to gamble, because the behavioral patterns and causes of this disorder appear to be similar to the behavioral patterns and causes of the substance use disorders (Denis, Fatséas, & Auriacombe, 2012; Petry, Zajac, & Ginley, 2018).

We begin with the substance use disorders. A **substance** is any natural or synthesized product that has psychoactive effects—it changes perceptions, thoughts, emotions, and behaviors. Some of the substances we discuss in this chapter are popularly referred to as drugs (e.g., cocaine and heroin). People who abuse these drugs are often referred to as *drug addicts.* Yet a person need not be physically dependent on a substance, as the term *addict* implies, in order to have a problem with it. For example, some who are not physically addicted to Ecstasy or Molly still may think they need the drug to have a good time.

Societies differ in their attitudes toward substances with psychoactive effects, with some seeing their use as a matter of individual choice and others seeing it as a grave public health and security concern. Within the United States, attitudes have varied greatly over time and across subgroups, depending upon the drug (Keyes et al., 2011). Many substances have been used for medicinal purposes for centuries. As long ago as 1500 BCE, people in the Andes highlands chewed coca leaves to increase their endurance (Cocores, Pottash, & Gold, 1991). Coca leaves can be manufactured into cocaine, which was used legally throughout Europe and the United States into the twentieth century to relieve fatigue. It was an ingredient in the original Coca-Cola drink and in more than 50 other widely available beverages and elixirs. Psychoactive substances also have traditionally appeared in religious ceremonies. When chewed, peyote causes visual hallucinations of colored lights or of geometric forms, animals, or people. Native groups in North America have used it in religious rituals for hundreds of years. Regardless of its purpose, the societal perception of psychoactive substances will likely continue to change throughout time as do most behaviors within various cultures.

DEFINING SUBSTANCE USE DISORDERS

There are four conditions that have historically been seen as important in defining individuals' use of substances: intoxication, withdrawal, abuse, and dependence. We first define these conditions.

Substance intoxication is a set of behavioral and psychological changes that occur as a result of the physiological effects of a substance on the central nervous system. People become intoxicated soon after they ingest a substance, and the more they ingest, the more intoxicated they become. Intoxication declines as the amount of the substance in blood or tissue declines, but symptoms may last for hours or days after the substance no longer is detectable in the body (Procyshyn, Bezchlibnyk-Butler, & Jeffries, 2017).

The specific symptoms of intoxication depend on what substance is taken, how much of it is taken and when, the user's tolerance, and the context. For example, you may have observed that alcohol makes some people aggressive and others withdrawn. Short-term, or acute, intoxication can produce symptoms different from those of chronic intoxication. The first time people take a moderate dose of cocaine, they may be outgoing and upbeat. With chronic use over days or weeks, they may begin to withdraw socially (Procyshyn et al., 2017). People's expectations about a substance's effects also can influence the types of symptoms they show. People who expect marijuana to make them relaxed may experience relaxation, whereas people who are frightened of disinhibition may experience anxiety (Ruiz & Strain, 2014).

The setting also can influence the types of intoxication symptoms people develop. People who consume a few alcoholic drinks at a party may become uninhibited and loud, but when they consume the same amount at home alone they may become tired

The setting in which a person becomes intoxicated can influence the type of symptoms people develop. People who consume a few alcoholic drinks at a party may become uninhibited and loud, but when they consume the same amount at home alone they may become tired and depressed. *John Rensten/Getty Images*

and depressed (Brick, 2008). The environment can also influence the extent to which intoxication is maladaptive. People who drink alcohol only at home may be less likely to cause harm to themselves or others than are people who drink at bars and drive home under the influence of alcohol. The diagnosis of intoxication with a substance is given only when the behavioral and psychological changes the person experiences are significantly maladaptive, that is, when they substantially disrupt the person's social and family relationships, cause occupational or financial problems, or place the individual at significant risk for adverse effects, such as a traffic accident, severe medical complications, or legal problems. For example, getting into a fist fight while clearly under the influence of a substance would merit a diagnosis of intoxication. Substance intoxication is common among individuals with a substance use disorder, but also occurs among those without a substance use disorder.

People who are dependent on a substance often show **tolerance**—they experience diminished effects from the same dose of a substance and need more and more of it to achieve intoxication. People who have smoked cigarettes for years often smoke more than 20 cigarettes a day, an amount that would have made them violently ill when they first began smoking. A person highly tolerant of a substance may have a very high blood level of it without being aware of its effects.

The risk for tolerance varies greatly among substances. Alcohol, opioids, stimulants, and nicotine have high risks for tolerance, whereas cannabis and PCP appear to have lower risks (Brick, 2008). People who are physiologically dependent on a substance often show severe withdrawal symptoms when they stop using it. Sometimes the substance must be withdrawn gradually to prevent these symptoms.

Substance withdrawal is a set of physiological and behavioral symptoms that result when people who have been using substances heavily for prolonged periods of time stop or greatly reduce their use. Symptoms typically are the opposite of those of intoxication. The diagnosis of withdrawal from a substance requires significant distress or impairment in a person's everyday functioning. Affected individuals may continue using the substance to relieve or avoid symptoms of withdrawal (Brick, 2008; Famitafreshi & Karimian, 2020).

The *DSM-5* combined substance abuse and dependence into one diagnosis, substance use disorder, because of difficulties in distinguishing between abuse and dependence in clinical and research settings and because of the low reliability of the diagnosis of substance abuse (Hasin, Fenton, Beseler, Park, & Wall, 2012). Substance use disorder is a cluster of cognitive,

behavioral, and physiological symptoms that suggests an individual continues using a substance despite significant problems that result in their life. The *DSM-5* diagnostic criteria for substance use disorder include impaired control, the continued use of substances despite negative social, occupational, and health consequences, risky use, as well as evidence of tolerance or withdrawal (see Table 1). Users must show two or more of the symptoms associated with substance use disorder over the course of a year to receive the diagnosis. Craving was added as a criterion in *DSM 5* because it is a common and diagnostically important symptom among people with substance use issues. Clinicians also rate the severity of the substance use disorder as mild (two or three of the criteria are met), moderate (four or five criteria are met), or severe (six or more criteria are met) (American Psychiatric Association; 2013; Hasin et al., 2012; Jemberie et al., 2020).

Substance abuse disorders most closely resemble what the lay person refers to as *drug addiction,* but it is important to note that this language is not included in the *DSM 5*, in part to reduce the stigma associated with addiction. People with substance use disorder have significant dysfunction in their daily lives as a

---

TABLE 1   Criteria for Substance Use Disorder

Impaired control

1. The substance is taken in increasingly larger amounts or over a longer period of time than originally intended.
2. The substance user craves the substance.
3. The substance user feels an ongoing desire to cut down or control substance abuse, or has made unsuccessful attempts to do so.
4. Much time is spent in obtaining, using, or recovering from the substance.

Social impairment

5. The ongoing use of the substance often results in an inability to meet responsibilities at home, work, or school.
6. Important social, work-related, or recreational activities are abandoned or cut back because of substance use.
7. Ongoing substance use despite recurring social or relationship difficulties caused or made worse by the effects of the substance.

Risky use

8. Ongoing substance use in physically dangerous situations such as driving a car or operating machinery.
9. Substance use continues despite the awareness of ongoing physical or psychological problems that have likely arisen or been made worse by the substance.

Pharmacological

10. Tolerance: the need for increased amounts of the substance to achieve the desired effect or by a diminished experience of intoxication over time with the same amount of the substance.
11. Withdrawal: the substance user experiences the characteristic withdrawal syndrome of the substance and/or takes the same or similar substance to relieve withdrawal symptoms.

Source: *Diagnostic and Statistical Manual of Mental Disorders*, Fifth Edition. American Psychiatric Association, 2013.

Note: Two or more of the above 11 criteria are required to make a diagnosis of substance abuse disorder. Symptoms are organized here by categories for clarity; these categories are not themselves in the *DSM-5*.

result. The affected individual may be unable to fulfill important obligations at work, school, or home. They may fail to show up at work or for classes, may be unable to concentrate and therefore perform poorly, or may even consume the substance at work or school. The use of substances may occur in certain situations in which it is physically hazardous, such as while driving. As a result of such behaviors, it is not uncommon for an individual to experience problems with the law, such as arrests for drunk driving or for the possession of illegal substances. Substance use disorder impacts daily function and is also associated with health problems and increased risk of mortality (Jemberie et al., 2020).

One study reanalyzed data from a large, nationally representative sample of the United States to determine the effects of changes from the *DSM-IV* to the *DSM-5* criteria for the diagnosis of alcohol-related disorders and found that the 12-month prevalence of alcohol use disorder based on the *DSM-5* criteria (10.8 percent) was quite similar to the combined 12-month prevalence of *DSM-IV* diagnoses of alcohol abuse or alcohol dependence (9.7 percent) (Agrawal, Heath, & Lynskey, 2011). This suggests that the combined prevalences of abuse and dependence diagnoses for each substance based on the *DSM-IV* criteria can be used to estimate the prevalence of substance use disorders for each substance discussed in this chapter.

DSM-5 recognizes 10 substance classes around which substance use disorders emerge. This chapter organizes these substance use disorders into five categories: (1) central nervous system depressants, including alcohol, barbiturates, benzodiazepines, and inhalants; (2) central nervous system stimulants, including cocaine, amphetamines, nicotine, and caffeine; (3) opioids, including heroin and morphine; (4) hallucinogens and phencyclidine (PCP); and (5) cannabis. We consider the characteristics of the problems people experience from using substances in each category and then discuss certain other drugs commonly misused.

DEPRESSANTS

Depressants slow the central nervous system. In moderate doses, they make people relaxed and somewhat sleepy, reduce concentration, and impair thinking, judgment, and motor skills. In heavy doses, they can induce stupor or even death (see Table 2).

Alcohol

Alcohol's effects on the brain occur in two distinct phases (Brick, 2008). In low doses, alcohol causes many people to feel more self-confident, more relaxed, and perhaps slightly euphoric. They may be less inhibited, and this disinhibitory effect may be what many people find attractive. At increasing doses, however, alcohol induces many of the symptoms of depression, including fatigue and lethargy, decreased motivation, sleep disturbances, depressed mood, and confusion. Also, although many people take alcohol to feel sexier (mainly by reducing their sexual inhibitions), even low doses can impair sexual functioning.

People intoxicated by alcohol slur their words, walk unsteadily, have trouble paying attention or remembering things, and are slow and awkward in their physical reactions. They may act inappropriately, becoming aggressive or belligerent, or saying rude things. Their moods may swing from exuberance to despair. With extreme intoxication, people may fall into a stupor or a coma. Often they do not recognize that they are intoxicated or may flatly deny it. Once sober, they may have amnesia, known as a *blackout*,

TABLE 2   Intoxication with and Withdrawal from Depressants

The depressant drugs depress activity in the central nervous system.

Drug	Intoxication Symptoms	Withdrawal Symptoms
Alcohol	Behavioral symptoms (e.g., inappropriate sexual or aggressive behavior, mood lability, impaired judgment)	Autonomic hyperactivity (e.g., sweating, fast pulse)
Benzodiazepines	Sleepiness	Hand tremor
Barbiturates	Slurred speech	Insomnia
	Incoordination	Nausea or vomiting
	Unsteady gait	Transient hallucinations or illusions
	Involuntary eye movement	Psychomotor agitation
	Impairment in attention or memory	Anxiety
	Stupor or coma	Seizures

Drinking alcohol with food leads to a slower absorption rate of the alcohol. *Philip Lee Harvey/Stone+/Getty Images*

for the events that occurred while they were intoxicated (Ruiz & Strain, 2014).

One critical determinant of how quickly people become intoxicated with alcohol is whether their stomach is full or empty. An empty stomach speedily delivers alcohol to the small intestine, where it is rapidly absorbed into the body. A person with a full stomach may ingest significantly more drinks before reaching a dangerous blood-alcohol level or showing clear signs of intoxication (Brick, 2008). People in countries where alcohol is usually consumed with meals, such as France, show lower rates of alcohol use disorders than do people in countries where alcohol often is consumed on an empty stomach.

The legal definition of alcohol intoxication is much narrower than the criteria for a diagnosis of alcohol intoxication. Most U.S. states consider a person to be under the influence of alcohol if their blood-alcohol level is 0.08 or above. As Table 3 indicates, it does not take many drinks for most people to reach this level. It takes less alcohol to reach a high

TABLE 3 Relationships Among Sex, Weight, Oral Alcohol Consumption, and Blood-Alcohol Level

It doesn't take very many drinks for most people to reach a blood-alcohol level of 0.08, which is the legal definition of intoxication in most states.

Total Alcohol Content (Ounces)	Beverage Intake*	Blood-Alcohol Level (Percent)					
		Female (100 lb)	Male (100 lb)	Female (150 lb)	Male (150 lb)	Female (200 lb)	Male (200 lb)
1/2	1 oz spirits† 1 glass wine 1 can beer	0.045	0.037	0.03	0.025	0.022	0.019
1	2 oz spirits 2 glasses wine 2 cans beer	0.090	0.075	0.06	0.050	0.045	0.037
2	4 oz spirits 4 glasses wine 4 cans beer	0.180	0.150	0.12	0.100	0.090	0.070
3	6 oz spirits 6 glasses wine 6 cans beer	0.270	0.220	0.18	0.150	0.130	0.110
4	8 oz spirits 8 glasses wine 8 cans beer	0.360	0.300	0.24	0.200	0.180	0.150
5	10 oz spirits 10 glasses wine 10 cans beer	0.450	0.370	0.30	0.250	0.220	0.180

*In 1 hour
†100-proof spirits (50 percent alcohol)

Source: Data from Ray, O., & Ksir, C., *Drugs, society, and human behavior*. St. Louis: C. V. Mosby, 1993, 194.

blood-alcohol level in women than in men because women generally are smaller and have a lower body water content than men, leading to higher concentrations of alcohol in the blood for a given dose. Deficits in attention, reaction time, and coordination arise even with the first drink and can interfere with the ability to operate a car or machinery safely and to perform other tasks requiring a steady hand, coordination, clear thinking, and clear vision. These deficits are not always readily observable, even to trained eyes. People often leave parties or bars without appearing drunk but having a blood-alcohol level well above the legal limit (Brick, 2008).

Heavy drinking can be part of the culture of a peer group, but it still can lead to alcohol use disorder in some members. Drinking large quantities of alcohol can be fatal, even in people who are not chronic alcohol abusers. About one-third of such deaths result from respiratory paralysis, usually due to a final large dose of alcohol in people who are already intoxicated. Alcohol can also interact fatally with a number of substances, including some antidepressant drugs (Brick, 2008).

Excessive alcohol use is responsible for more than 95,000 deaths in the United States each year and is a leading cause of preventable death in the United States. Worldwide, approximately 3 million deaths per year result from harmful alcohol use which represents about 5% of all deaths worldwide. Alcohol misuse is one of the leading causes of preventable mortality around the world (Clay & Parker, 2020; WHO, 2020).

Unintentional alcohol-related injuries due to automobile accidents, drowning, burns, poisoning, and falls account for approximately 600,000 deaths per year internationally (WHO, 2014). Even being a little "buzzed" (i.e., having a blood-alcohol level of 0.02 percent) is associated with a significantly increased risk of having an automobile accident compared to being completely sober (Phillips & Brewer, 2011). There is a strong relationship between heavy alcohol use and suicide attempt among adolescents and young adults suggesting that many often do so under the influence of alcohol (Grazioli et al., 2018).

The symptoms of alcohol withdrawal manifest in three stages (Brick, 2008). The first, which usually begins within a few hours after drinking has been stopped or sharply curtailed, includes tremulousness (the "shakes"), weakness, and profuse perspiration. The person may complain of anxiety (the "jitters"), headache, nausea, and abdominal cramps and may retch and vomit. They are flushed, restless, and easily startled but alert. The EEG pattern may be mildly abnormal. The person may begin to see or hear things, at first only with eyes shut but later also with eyes open. Those whose alcohol use disorder is moderate may experience only this first stage of withdrawal, and the symptoms may disappear within a few days.

The second stage includes convulsive seizures, which may begin as soon as 12 hours after drinking stops but more often appear during the second or third day. The third stage of withdrawal is characterized by **delirium tremens,** or **DTs.** Auditory, visual, and tactile hallucinations occur. The person also may develop bizarre, terrifying delusions, such as the belief that monsters are attacking. They may sleep little and may become agitated and disoriented (Jesse et al., 2017). Fever, profuse perspiration, and an irregular heartbeat may develop. DTs is fatal in approximately 10 percent of cases. Death may occur from hyperthermia (extremely high body temperature) or the collapse of the peripheral vascular system. Fortunately, only about 10 percent of individuals with severe alcohol use disorder ever experience seizures or DTs (Mirijello et al., 2015). These symptoms are more common in people who drink large amounts in a single sitting and have an existing medical illness.

Alcohol Use Disorder

As noted in Substance Use Along the Continuum, alcohol use and misuse span a broad range from people who completely abstain from drinking alcohol to those who drink alcohol occasionally in social situations, to those who drink more frequently and heavily, and finally to those for whom alcohol use creates significant social, occupational, and health problems. **Alcohol Use disorder** involves a problematic pattern of alcohol use that creates significant impairment or distress. Those with alcohol use disorder show this impairment in a variety of behaviors such as consuming large amounts of alcohol, persistent desire and failed attempts to reduce the quantity of alcohol consumed, strong desire to use alcohol (craving), tolerance, and withdrawal (American Psychiatric Association, 2013).

Near the maladaptive end of the continuum are people who engage in *binge drinking,* which is defined as consuming five or more drinks within a 2-hour period for men, and four or more drinks in a 2-hour period for women resulting in a blood-alcohol content (BAC) of at least 0.08 percent for most individuals. Heavy drinking is also on the dysfunctional end of the spectrum in which individuals consume alcohol on 5 or more days in a month. Binge drinking among young adults has concerned researchers and educators for decades resulting in various long-term studies on alcohol use among this population. Multiple studies have found a steady decline in self-reported binge-drinking behaviors among college students from 1980 (44 percent), 1993 (40 percent) through 2014 (35 percent). The Substance Abuse and Mental Health Services Administration's (SAMHSA) National Survey on Drug Use and Health (NSDUH) found a slight decrease in binge drinking from 44.6 percent in 1998 to 37.7 percent in 2014 for young adults (18 to 25 years). In 2014, estimates for extreme binge drinking among college students, defined as consuming 10 or more drinks on one occasion, varied from 14 percent in 2005 to 20 percent. Although rates of binge drinking among college students may be decreasing, this is still an at-risk population as multiple studies consistently find higher rates of heavy drinking and alcohol-related problems among college students than among noncollege peers. Research has found small differences between male and female drinking rates and modest decreases over time, but a gender gap does exist. In 2014, female binge drinking (i.e., four plus drinks) decreased from 31 percent in 1988 to 26 percent and male binge drinking (i.e., five plus drinks) substantially decreased from 52 to 43 percent (Krieger, Young, Anthenien, & Neighbors, 2018).

Binge drinking and heavy drinking are associated with significant health problems (Paul, Grubaugh, Frueh, Ellis, & Egede, 2011). Large nationwide studies in the United States find that about 24 percent of adults report binge drinking at least once in the last month, and 6 percent of adults are heavy drinkers (Paul et al., 2011; SAMHSA, 2017). Binge drinking on college campuses is common. Nationwide, 35 percent of college students report binge drinking in the past month, compared to 32 percent of 18- to 22-year-olds not in college (Johnston, O'Malley, Bachman, & Schulenberg, 2012). Binge drinking is especially common among members of fraternities and sororities, with 75 percent of members saying they binge drink (Wechsler et al., 2002).

Gender and Age Differences In most nations of the world, men are more likely to drink alcohol than women, and also are more likely to drink heavily or binge drink (Hughes, Wilsnack, & Kantor, 2016; WHO, 2014). Similarly, across all age groups, males are much more likely to develop alcohol use disorders than are females, as can be seen in Figure 2. The gender gap in alcohol use is much greater among men and women who subscribe to traditional gender roles, which condone drinking for men but not for women (Hughes et al., 2016). Similarly, the gender gap is greater among U.S. ethnic minority groups that more widely accept traditional gender roles, such as Hispanics and recent Asian immigrants, than among European Americans, due largely to high percentages of minority women who completely abstain from alcohol. Sex differences have also been noted in help-seeking patterns with women less likely to seek help for alcohol use than men. Whites are proportionately more likely to utilize services than are Blacks and Hispanics (Tucker, Chandler, & Witkiewitz, 2020). We discuss other contributors to the gender differences in substance use later in this chapter.

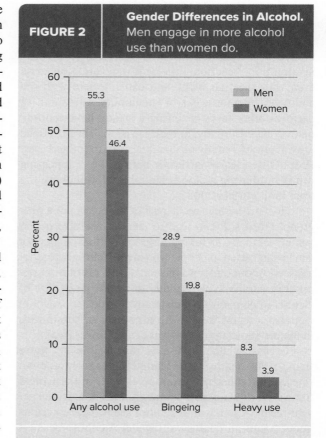

FIGURE 2   **Gender Differences in Alcohol.** Men engage in more alcohol use than women do.

Source: SAMHSA, 2017, Table 2.35B, 816 for any alcohol use, 2.36B, 818 for binge, 2.37B, 820 for heavy use. https://www.samhsa.gov/data/sites/default/files/NSDUH-DetTabs-2016/NSDUH-DetTabs-2016.pdf.

Note: Bingeing is defined as five or more drinks on the same occasion at least once in the past 30 days. Heavy use is defined as five or more drinks on the same occasion on at least 5 different days in the past 30 days.

Strong age differences in alcohol use disorders decline with age. There are many reasons for this decline. First, with age the liver metabolizes alcohol at a slower rate, and the lower percentage of body water increases the absorption of alcohol. As a result, older people become intoxicated faster and experience the negative effects of alcohol more severely and more quickly. Second, as people grow older, they may become more mature in their choices, including choices about drinking alcohol to excess. Third, older people have grown up under stronger prohibitions against alcohol use and abuse than have younger people. Fourth, people who have used alcohol excessively for many years may die from alcohol-related diseases before they reach old age (Sher, Grekin, & Williams, 2005).

Although alcohol use is illegal for persons under 21 years of age in the United States, one-third of 8th-graders and 70 percent of 12th-graders have tried

As people grow older, they may become more mature in their choices, including choices about drinking alcohol to excess.
Ariel Skelley/Getty Images

alcohol (Johnston et al., 2012). Of particular concern, 22 percent of 12th-graders report having engaged in binge drinking in the last year. Several studies suggest that the use of alcohol and the prevalence of alcohol-related problems have been increasing among young people in recent decades and that the age at which alcohol is first consumed is decreasing (e.g., Grucza, Bucholz, Rice, & Bierut, 2008; Keyes, Grant, & Hasin, 2008; Keyes, Martins, Blanco, & Hasin, 2010). The earlier the age of onset of drinking and drinking-related problems, the more likely individuals are to develop alcohol use disorders. Alcohol use before age 21 predicts persistence and severity of harmful use throughout the life span. Research has found that drinking to intoxication, binge drinking, and alcohol-related problems increase during adolescence and early adulthood often peaking between ages 18 and 22. In 2018, 5 percent of persons age 12 or older were identified as having alcohol use disorder which makes this the most prevalent substance use disorder. Alcohol use disorder is most prevalent (19 percent) during the early 20s and then decreases in the mid-20s and continuing well after early adulthood (Alvanzo, Storr, La Flair, Green, & Wagner, 2011; Tucker et al., 2020). Studies suggest that approximately 70 percent of persons with alcohol use disorder improve without professional intervention (natural recovery), and less than 25 percent of affected individuals access alcohol-focused services, in part because seeking treatment is associated with higher problem severity (Chandler, & Witkiewitz, 2020; Tucker et al., 2020).

Cultural and Ethnic/Racial Differences Cultures differ markedly in their use of alcohol and rates of alcohol-related problems. Consumption in the Russian Federation is high among both men and women, and the rates of negative health consequences due to alcohol are highest in this and surrounding countries (Rehm et al., 2009; WHO, 2014). Low rates of consumption in some African and Middle Eastern countries are tied to Islam's prohibitions against alcohol.

Ethnic groups within the United States differ substantially in their alcohol use. One group at high risk for alcohol-related problems is Native Americans, 43 percent of whom meet the criteria for alcohol abuse or alcohol dependence at some time in their life (Hasin, Stinson, Ogburn, & Grant, 2007). Deaths related to alcohol are more than twice as common among Native Americans than in the general U.S. population (Chartier & Caetano, 2010; Landen, Roeber, Naimi, Nielsen, & Sewell, 2014). This higher rate of alcohol-related problems has been tied to excessive rates of poverty and unemployment, lower levels of education, and a greater sense of helplessness and hopelessness.

SHADES OF GRAY

As you may have observed, binge drinking on the weekends is fairly common on college campuses. Read about Nick and his friends, who may resemble people you know.

Nick began drinking in high school, but his drinking escalated when he moved away from home for college. After just a couple of weeks there, Nick became friends with a group that liked to party on the weekends. On Thursday nights, they would drink and get so loud and obnoxious that their neighbors in the dorm would sometimes complain. They would sleep off their hangovers on Friday, miss classes, and then begin drinking again from Friday afternoon through Saturday, finally stopping on Sunday to sleep and recover. Nick was able to keep decent grades through his first year, despite missing many classes. In sophomore year, classes in his major were harder, and he would abstain from drinking from Sunday afternoon until noon on Thursday. But Thursday afternoon he would get the keg of beer for his friends, and the old pattern would kick in.

One night during a drinking game, Nick accidentally punched a hole in the wall of his dorm room and was kicked off campus as a result. Between this incident and his declining grades, his parents threatened to stop paying his college tuition.

Would you diagnose Nick with an alcohol use disorder? (Discussion appears at the end of this chapter.)

Long-Term Effects of Alcohol Misuse

Heavy and prolonged use of alcohol can have toxic effects on several systems of the body, including the stomach, esophagus, pancreas, and liver (Paul et al., 2011). One of the most common medical conditions associated with alcohol misuse is low-grade hypertension. This condition, combined with increases in the levels of triglycerides and low-density lipoprotein (or "bad") cholesterol, puts alcohol abusers at increased risk for heart disease. Heavy alcohol use increases the risk of cancer, particularly breast cancer in women (Chen, Rosner, Hankinson, Colditz, & Willett, 2011). People with alcohol use disorders often are malnourished, in part because chronic alcohol ingestion decreases the absorption of critical nutrients from the gastrointestinal system and in part because they tend to "drink their meals." Some show a chronic thiamine (Vitamin B_1) deficiency, which can lead to several disorders of the central nervous system, including numbness and pain in the extremities, deterioration in the muscles, and the loss of visual acuity for both near and far objects (Osiezagha et al., 2013). Heavy prolonged use of alcohol is a risk factor for dementia, a permanent substance-induced major neurocognitive disorder involving loss of intellectual abilities, including memory, abstract thinking, judgment, and problem solving, and often accompanied by personality changes such as increased paranoia (see the chapter "Neurodevelopmental and Neurocognitive Disorders"). Subtler deficits due to central nervous system damage (e.g., substance-induced mild neurocognitive disorder) are observed in many chronic abusers of alcohol, even after they quit drinking.

As noted earlier, binge drinking is relatively common among adolescents and young adults. There is increasing evidence that heavy and prolonged use of alcohol during adolescence and early adulthood may have permanent negative effects on the brain, which is undergoing massive developmental changes during these periods of life (Jacobus & Tapert, 2013). Neuroimaging studies show changes in the structure and functioning of several areas of the brain in adolescents and young adults who binge-drink frequently or are chronic heavy drinkers, changes associated with deficits in performance on a variety of cognitive tests. The few longitudinal studies that have been done suggest that these deleterious effects of alcohol consumption may persist even after people stop drinking.

Some studies indicate that moderate alcohol consumption, particularly of red wine, carries health benefits. Red wine contains antioxidants that can increase good cholesterol, along with other chemicals that can help prevent damage to blood vessels and reduce bad cholesterol, producing positive cardiac effects (Fillmore, Kerr, Stockwell, Chikritzhs, & Bostrom, 2006; Le Strat & Gorwood, 2011). Several studies suggest that individuals who consume one or two drinks a day have better physical health and lower mortality rates than individuals who abstain from alcohol (Corrao, Bagnardi, Zambon, & La Vecchia, 2004; Rehm, Greenfield, & Rogers, 2001). However, abstainers and moderate drinkers differ on many other variables that can affect health. Abstainers are more likely than moderate drinkers to be older, less well educated, physically inactive, and overweight and to have diabetes, hypertension, and high cholesterol (Naimi et al., 2005). Some people classified as abstainers drank heavily earlier in life and have quit due to negative health effects (Fillmore et al., 2006). These factors make the potential health benefits of moderate drinking less clear.

Benzodiazepines and Barbiturates

Like alcohol, benzodiazepines and barbiturates depress the central nervous system. Intoxication with and withdrawal from these substances are similar to alcohol intoxication and withdrawal. Users may initially feel euphoric and become disinhibited but then experience depressed moods, lethargy, perceptual distortions, loss of coordination, and other signs of central nervous system depression.

Benzodiazepines (such as Xanax, Valium, Halcion, Librium, and Klonopin) and **barbiturates** (such as Seconal) are legally manufactured and sold by prescription, usually as sedatives for the treatment of anxiety and insomnia. Benzodiazepines are also used as muscle relaxants and antiseizure medicines. In the United States, approximately 90 percent of people hospitalized for medical care or surgery are prescribed sedatives (Procyshyn, Bezchlibnyk-Butler, & Jeffries, 2017). Large quantities of these substances end up on the black market, however. They are especially likely to be abused in combination with other psychoactive substances to produce greater feelings of euphoria or to relieve the agitation created by other substances. Abuse of prescription sedatives and tranquilizers has increased in recent years. Nationwide studies find that about 9 percent of adults, 9.6 percent of college students, and close to 5 percent of teenagers report using prescription sedatives or tranquilizers in the last year for nonmedical purposes (Johnston et al., 2012; McCabe, Cranford, & West, 2008; see also SAMHSA, 2017). *DSM-5* classifies problematic misuse of these drugs as sedative, hypnotic, or anxiolytic use disorders.

Barbiturates and benzodiazepines cause decreases in blood pressure, respiratory rate, and heart rate. In overdose, they can be extremely dangerous and even cause death from respiratory arrest or cardiovascular collapse. Overdose is especially likely when people take these substances (particularly benzodiazepines) with alcohol. These were among the drugs that Heath Ledger overdosed on (see this chapter's Extraordinary People).

STIMULANTS

Stimulants activate the central nervous system, causing feelings of energy, happiness, and power; a decreased desire for sleep; and a diminished appetite (see Table 4). Cocaine and the amphetamines (including the related methamphetamines) are the two types of stimulants associated with severe substance use disorders. Both impart a psychological lift or rush. They cause dangerous increases in blood pressure and heart rate, alter the rhythm and electrical activity of the heart, and constrict the blood vessels, which can lead to heart attacks, respiratory arrest, and seizures. In the United States, over half of drug-related emergency room visits involve use of cocaine or the amphetamines (SAMHSA, 2013). Prescription stimulants, including Dexedrine and Ritalin, are used to treat asthma and other respiratory problems, obesity, neurological disorders, attention-deficit/hyperactivity disorder (ADHD; see the chapter "Neurodevelopmental

TABLE 4   Intoxication with and Withdrawal from Stimulants

The stimulants activate the central nervous system.

Drug	Intoxication Symptoms	Withdrawal Symptoms
Cocaine and amphetamines	Behavioral changes (e.g., euphoria or affective blunting; changes in sociability; hypervigilance; interpersonal sensitivity; anxiety, tension, or anger; impaired judgment) Rapid heartbeat Dilation of pupils Elevated or lowered blood pressure Perspiration or chills Nausea or vomiting Weight loss Psychomotor agitation or retardation Muscular weakness Slowed breathing Chest pain Confusion, seizures, coma	Dysphoric mood Fatigue Vivid, unpleasant dreams Insomnia or hypersomnia Increased appetite Psychomotor retardation or agitation
Nicotine	Not a diagnosis in the *DSM-5*	Dysphoria or depressed mood Insomnia Irritability, frustration, or anger Anxiety Difficulty concentrating Restlessness Decreased heart rate Increased appetite or weight gain
Caffeine	Restlessness Nervousness Excitement Insomnia Flushed face Frequent urination Stomach upset Muscle twitching Rambling flow of thought or speech Rapid or irregular heartbeat Periods of inexhaustibility Psychomotor agitation	Marked fatigue or drowsiness Dysphoric mood or irritability Flulike symptoms (e.g., nausea or vomiting)

and Neurocognitive Disorders"), and a variety of other conditions. Use of these prescription stimulants for nonmedical purposes has increased sharply in recent decades and according to results from National Survey on Drug Use and Health (2017), more than 1 million people annually misuse prescription stimulants (McCabe et al., 2008; SAMHSA, 2018). Caffeine and nicotine also are stimulants, and although their psychological effects are not as severe as those of cocaine and amphetamines, these drugs—particularly nicotine—can have long-term negative effects.

Cocaine

Cocaine, a white powder extracted from the coca plant, is one of the most addictive substances known. People snort the powder or inject it intravenously. In the 1970s, even more powerful freebase cocaine appeared when users developed a method for separating the most potent chemicals in cocaine by heating it with ether. Freebase cocaine is usually smoked in a water pipe or mixed in a tobacco or marijuana cigarette. *Crack* is a form of freebase cocaine boiled down into tiny chunks, or rocks, and usually smoked.

Cocaine use causes dangerous increases in blood pressure and heart rate, alterations in the rhythm and electrical activity of the heart, and constricted blood vessels, which can lead to heart attacks, respiratory arrest, and seizures. *Medioimages/ Photodisc/Getty Images*

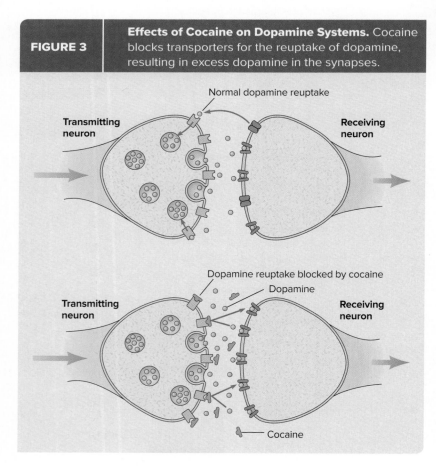

| FIGURE 3 | **Effects of Cocaine on Dopamine Systems.** Cocaine blocks transporters for the reuptake of dopamine, resulting in excess dopamine in the synapses. |

Normal dopamine reuptake

Transmitting neuron

Receiving neuron

Dopamine reuptake blocked by cocaine

Dopamine

Transmitting neuron

Receiving neuron

Cocaine

Initially, cocaine produces an instant rush of intense euphoria, followed by heightened self-esteem, alertness, energy, and feelings of competence and creativity. Users crave increasing amounts of the substance, for both its physiological and its psychological effects (Ruiz & Strain, 2014). When taken repeatedly or at high doses, however, it leads to grandiosity, impulsiveness, hypersexuality, compulsive behavior, agitation, and anxiety reaching the point of panic and paranoia. Stopping cocaine use can induce exhaustion and depression.

Cocaine activates those areas of the brain that register reward and pleasure. Normally, a pleasurable event releases dopamine into the synapses in these areas. Dopamine then binds to receptors on neighboring synapses (Figure 3). Cocaine blocks the reuptake of dopamine into the transmitting neuron, causing it to accumulate in the synapse and maintaining the pleasurable feeling (Ruiz & Strain, 2014). The rapid, strong effects of cocaine on the brain's reward centers make this substance more likely than most to lead to a stimulant use disorder. The following case study illustrates this process.

CASE STUDY

Dr. Arnie Rosenthal is a 31-year-old white male dentist, married for 10 years with two children. His wife insisted he see a psychiatrist because of uncontrolled use of cocaine, which over the past year had made it increasingly difficult for him to function as a dentist. During the previous 5 years he used cocaine virtually every day, with only occasional 1- or 2-week periods of abstinence. For the past 4 years Rosenthal wanted to stop, but his desire was overridden by a "compulsion" to take the drug.

He began using marijuana after being married a year, smoking a joint each day after school and spending the evening staring at TV. When he graduated from dental school his wife was pregnant, and he was "scared to death" at the prospect of being a father. His deepening depression was characterized by social isolation, increased loss of interests, and frequent temper outbursts. He needed intoxication with marijuana, or occasionally sedatives, for sex, relaxation, and socialization. Following the birth of the child he "never felt so crazy," and his marijuana and sedative use escalated. Two years later, a second child was born. Dr. Rosenthal was financially successful, had moved to an expensive suburban home with a swimming pool, and had two cars and "everything my parents wanted for me." He was 27 years old, felt he had nothing to look forward to, and felt painfully isolated; drugs were no longer providing relief.

Rosenthal tried cocaine for the first time and immediately felt good. "I was no longer depressed. I used cocaine as often as possible because all my problems seemed to vanish, but I had to keep doing it. The effects were brief and it was very expensive, but I didn't care. When the immediate effects wore off, I'd feel even more miserable and depressed so that I did as much cocaine as I was able to obtain." He is now continuously nervous and irritable. (Adapted from Spitzer, R. L., Skodol, A. E., Gibbon, M., & Williams, J. B. W., *Psychopathology: A case book*, New York, McGraw Hill, 1983, pp. 81–83.)

Cocaine's effects wear off quickly, and the dependent person must take frequent doses to maintain a high. Tolerance also can develop, and the individual must obtain larger and larger amounts to experience a high (Ruiz & Strain, 2014). People with cocaine-related stimulant use disorder spend huge amounts of money on the substance and may engage in theft, prostitution, or drug dealing to obtain enough money to purchase it. Desperation can lead frequent users to participate in extremely dangerous behaviors. Many contract HIV, the virus that causes AIDS, by sharing needles with infected users or by having unprotected sex in exchange for money or cocaine (Ruiz & Strain, 2014).

Other frequent medical complications of cocaine use are heart rhythm disturbances and heart attacks; respiratory failure; neurological effects, including strokes, seizures, and headaches; and gastrointestinal complications, including abdominal pain and nausea. Physical symptoms include chest pain, blurred vision, fever, muscle spasms, convulsions, and coma (Ruiz & Strain, 2014).

A large percentage of people who grew up in the 1960s and 1970s have tried cocaine, but these percentages are much lower in more recent generations: A nationwide study in the United States found that 48 percent of individuals who graduated from high school in 1979 had tried cocaine at some time in their life, compared to about 20 percent of individuals who had graduated from high school between 1980 and 1995 (Johnston et al., 2012). Among U.S. college students, 5.5 percent report ever having used cocaine, whereas 12 percent of 18- to 22-year-olds not in college report ever having used cocaine; among high school students, about 3.5 percent report ever having used cocaine (Johnston et al., 2012). In 2018, an estimated 5.5 million people aged 12 or older (2 percent of the U.S. population) used cocaine which includes approximately 757,000 users of crack (SAMHSA, 2019).

Amphetamines

Amphetamines and the related *methamphetamines* are stimulants prescribed for the treatment of attention problems (e.g., Ritalin, Adderall), narcolepsy, and chronic fatigue. They also are found in antihistamines

On the street, amphetamines are known as "speed," "meth," and "chalk." They are most often swallowed as pills but can be injected intravenously, and methamphetamine can be snorted ("crank") or smoked ("crystal meth" or "ice"). Serious health problems can result from their use. Shown here is a kitchen used as a methamphetamine lab.
The Washington Times/ZUMAPRESS/Newscom

(e.g., Sudafed) and diet drugs. Many stimulants are used appropriately under the supervision of a physician, but a great many doses are diverted to illegal use and abuse (Ruiz & Strain, 2014). Because of the potential for abuse, most states regulate over-the-counter sales of diet drugs and antihistamines. On the street, amphetamines are known as "speed," "meth," and "chalk." They are most often swallowed as pills but can be injected intravenously, and methamphetamine can be snorted ("crank") or smoked ("crystal meth" or "ice"). Owing in part to the easy and inexpensive manufacture of methamphetamine, its use is widespread in the United States. As of 2016, nearly 700,000 Americans reported using the drug within the last month (SAMHSA, 2017).

Amphetamines release the neurotransmitters dopamine and norepinephrine and block their reuptake. The symptoms of intoxication are similar to those of cocaine intoxication: euphoria, self-confidence, alertness, agitation, and paranoia (Ruiz & Strain, 2014). Like cocaine, amphetamines can produce perceptual illusions. The movement of other people and objects may seem distorted or exaggerated. Users may hear frightening voices making derogatory statements about them, see sores all over their body, or feel snakes crawling on their arms. They may have delusions of being stalked that lead them to act out violently. Some users know that these experiences are not real, but others lose their grip on reality and develop amphetamine-induced psychotic disorders (Ruiz & Strain, 2014). In 2018, approximately 1.9 million people aged 12 or older reported methamphetamine use during the past year which represents 0.7 percent of the population. The percentage of individuals who used methamphetamine in the past year was similar to the percentages reported in 2015 and 2017, but it was slightly higher than the percentage in 2016 (0.5 percent) (SAMHSA, 2019).

Legal problems typically arise for amphetamine abusers due to aggressive or inappropriate behavior while intoxicated or as a result of buying the drug illegally. Tolerance develops quickly, as does physical dependence. Users may switch from swallowing pills to injecting amphetamines intravenously. Some go on a *speed run,* in which they inject amphetamines frequently over several days without eating or sleeping. Then they crash into a devastating depression. Acute withdrawal symptoms typically subside within a few days, but chronic users may experience mood instability, memory loss, confusion, paranoid thinking, and perceptual abnormalities for weeks, months, or even years. They often battle the withdrawal symptoms with another speed run (Ruiz & Strain, 2014).

Abuse of amphetamines and methamphetamines can lead to a number of medical issues, particularly cardiovascular problems—including rapid or irregular heartbeat, increased blood pressure, and irreversible, stroke-producing damage to the small blood vessels in the brain. Elevated body temperature and convulsions can occur during overdoses, leading to death. People who share needles to inject amphetamines risk contracting HIV or hepatitis (Brick, 2008). With extended use, people become irritable and hostile and need more stimulants to avoid withdrawal symptoms. Their personal relationships and health decline. Emergency room visits involving amphetamines and methamphetamines increased drastically between 1995 and 2002, and after some decreases in the mid-2000s, began increasing again. Between 2009 and 2011 visits increased by 71 percent (SAMHSA, 2013).

Abuse of these drugs has risen in recent years. In 2011, 8.2 percent of 12th-graders reported using amphetamines or methamphetamines (Johnston et al., 2012). College students trying to stay up late to study may take them; nationwide studies find that 13.4 percent of college students report ever having used amphetamines or methamphetamines, with 9.3 percent reporting their use in the last year (Johnston et al., 2012). Employers may even provide amphetamines to their employees to increase productivity.

Nicotine

All the substances discussed thus far, except alcohol, are illegal for nonprescription use, and many laws regulate the use of alcohol. One of the most addictive substances known, however, is fully legal for use by adults and readily available to adolescents—**nicotine.**

Nicotine is an alkaloid found in tobacco. Cigarettes, the most popular nicotine delivery device, move this substance to the brain within seconds. In the United States, 70 percent of people over age 12 have smoked cigarettes at some time in their life, and about 23 percent currently are smokers (Johnston et al., 2012;

While the rate of cigarette smoking has decreased in the United States, it is on the rise in many developing countries around the world. *KAMBOU SIA/AFP/Getty Images*

SAMHSA, 2017). Smoking usually begins in the early teens, but fewer than 1 in 6 people reported cigarette use and there has been an observed decline across all age groups between 2002 and 2018. This decline may reflect, at least in part, the increased use of electronic vaporizing devices ("vaping"), such as e-cigarettes, as a substitute for delivering nicotine (SAMHSA, 2019). The rapid increased use of e-cigarettes or vaping among adolescents during the past decade has led to public safety concerns due to the potential links between vaping and acute lung injury. Research has found that more adolescents are vaping at higher rates each year with prevalence more than doubling from 2017 to 2019. Studies have found that 1 in 4 students in the 12th grade, more than 1 in 5 in the 10th grade, and more than 1 in 11 in the 8th grade report vaping. The number of students who reported vaping nicotine over the last year or longer also significantly increased within each grade from 2018 to 2019 (Miech et al., 2019).

Rates of cigarette use are much higher in Europe and many developing nations (Danielsson, Wennberg, Hibell, & Romelsjö 2012). Over two-thirds of people who begin smoking become dependent on nicotine, a rate much higher than is found with most other psychoactive substances (Lopez-Quintero et al., 2011). Tobacco use has declined in the United States and other industrialized countries over the past few decades, thanks in part to significantly increased taxes on tobacco products, laws restricting their use in public places, and lawsuits limiting tobacco companies' ability to advertise. In contrast, tobacco use is increasing in developing countries.

Nicotine operates on both the central and the peripheral nervous systems. It helps release several biochemicals in the brain, including dopamine, norepinephrine, serotonin, and the endogenous opioids. Although people often say they smoke to reduce stress, nicotine's physiological effects actually resemble the fight-or-flight response (see the chapter "Trauma, Anxiety, Obsessive-Compulsive, and Related Disorders")—several systems in the body are aroused, including the cardiovascular and respiratory systems. The subjective sense that smoking reduces stress actually may reflect the reversal of the tension and irritability that signal nicotine withdrawal. In other words, nicotine addicts need nicotine to feel normal to counteract its effects on the body and the brain (Ruiz & Strain, 2014). *DSM-5* recognizes nicotine dependence as a tobacco use disorder.

In 1964, based on a review of 6,000 empirical studies, the surgeon general of the United States concluded that smoking, particularly cigarette smoking, causes lung cancer, bronchitis, and probably coronary heart disease. Mortality rates for smokers are 70 percent greater than for nonsmokers, meaning that a person between ages 30 and 35 who smokes two packs a day will die 8 to 9 years earlier than a nonsmoker. Each year, an estimated 480,000 people in the United States (about one in five deaths) die prematurely from smoking-related coronary heart disease, lung cancer, emphysema, or chronic bronchitis or from exposure to secondhand smoke. An additional 16 million people have an illness related to smoking (CDC, 2018a). Women who smoke while pregnant give birth to smaller babies. The longer a person smokes and the more they smoke each day, the greater the health risks.

When chronic heavy smokers try to quit or are prohibited from smoking for an extended period, such as while at work or on an airplane, they show severe withdrawal symptoms. They become depressed, irritable, angry, anxious, frustrated, restless, and hungry; they have trouble concentrating; and they desperately crave another cigarette. These symptoms are immediately relieved by smoking, another sign of physiological dependence (Ruiz & Strain, 2014).

Because nicotine is relatively cheap and available, dependents tend not to spend much time trying to obtain it. They may panic, however, if they run out of cigarettes and replacements are not available. They also may spend a large part of their day smoking or chewing tobacco, and they continue to use nicotine even though it is damaging their health (e.g., after they have been diagnosed with emphysema). They may skip social activities where smoking is not allowed or recreational activities such as sports because they have trouble breathing.

Electronic cigarettes, also called e-cigarettes, first appeared in 2004 and are now used by millions around the world. The e-cigarette is an electronic device that vaporizes a flavored liquid that is inhaled, a practice called vaping. The fluid usually includes nicotine (Miech et al., 2019). The long-term health effects are not known and there are serious concerns about vaping-induced respiratory distress. Based on a multitude of cases, the Centers for Disease Control and Prevention (CDC) has identified a syndrome currently referred to as e-cigarette, or vaping, associated lung injury (EVALI). In January of 2020, the CDC reported that a total of 2711 patients had been hospitalized with EVALI throughout the entire United States, as well as Puerto Rico and the U.S. Virgin Islands and 60 deaths were confirmed (Christiani, 2020). There is some evidence that e-cigarettes may help cigarette smokers to quit, but this must be done in conjunction with stop smoking service support which is identified as the most effective type of support. Behavioral support in combination with electronic cigarettes may be an effective treatment used to help individuals quit smoking, although regulated replacement products and medications are generally viewed as safer (McNeill, Brose, Calder, Bauld &

Robson, 2019; McRobbie, Bullen, Hartmann-Boyce, & Hajek, 2014). The rising popularity of e-cigarettes has been especially noticeable among younger people, just as their rates of cigarette smoking have declined. E-cigarettes are now the most commonly used tobacco product among youth in the United States, with 4 percent of middle school students and 11 percent of high school students reporting using them (CDC, 2018c).

Nearly 70 percent of people who smoke say they want to quit (Babb, Malarcher, Shauer, Asman, & Jamal, 2017), and in fact rates of smoking have decreased consistently since 2005 (CDC, 2018a). Quitting is difficult, however, in part because the withdrawal syndrome is difficult to withstand. Fewer than 10 percent of smokers who try to stop smoking each year are successful, and most relapse within a few days of quitting (Babb et al., 2017). Cravings can remain after a smoker quits, with 50 percent of people who quit smoking reporting they have desired cigarettes in the past 24 hours (Goldstein, 2001). Nicotine patches and gum can help fight this urge.

Caffeine

Caffeine is by far the most heavily used stimulant, with 75 percent of it ingested in coffee (Chou, 1992). A cup of brewed coffee has about 100 milligrams of caffeine, and the average U.S. adult drinks about two cups per day. Other sources include tea (about 40 milligrams of caffeine per 6 ounces), caffeinated soda (45 milligrams per 12 ounces), over-the-counter analgesics and cold remedies (25 to 50 milligrams per tablet), weight-loss drugs (75 to 200 milligrams per tablet), and chocolate and cocoa (5 milligrams per bar).

Caffeine stimulates the central nervous system, increasing the levels of dopamine, norepinephrine, and serotonin. It also increases metabolism, body temperature, and blood pressure. People's appetite wanes, and they feel more alert. But in doses equivalent to just two to three cups of coffee, caffeine can cause unpleasant symptoms, including restlessness, nervousness, and hand tremors. People may experience an upset stomach and feel their heart beating rapidly or irregularly. They may have trouble going to sleep later on and may need to urinate frequently. These are symptoms of caffeine intoxication. Extremely large doses of caffeine can cause extreme agitation, seizures, respiratory failure, and cardiac problems.

The *DSM-5* specifies that a diagnosis of caffeine intoxication should be given only if an individual experiences significant distress or impairment in functioning as a result of the symptoms. Someone who drinks too much coffee for several days in a row during exam week, for example, might be so agitated that they cannot sit through the exams and so shaky that they cannot drive a car; such a person could be given a diagnosis of caffeine intoxication.

Some heavy coffee drinkers who joke that they are "caffeine addicts" actually cannot be diagnosed with caffeine use disorder, according to the *DSM-5*, because dependence on the drug seems not to cause significant social and occupational problems. Still, caffeine users can develop tolerance and undergo withdrawal if they stop ingesting caffeine. They may require several cups of coffee in the morning to feel "normal" and may experience significant headaches, fatigue, and anxiety if they do not get their coffee (American Psychiatric Association, 2013).

OPIOIDS

Morphine, heroin, codeine, and methadone are all **opioids.** They are derived from the sap of the opium poppy, which has been used for thousands of years to relieve pain. Our bodies produce natural opioids, including endorphins and enkephalins, to cope with pain. For example, a sports injury induces the body to produce endorphins to reduce pain and avoid shock. Doctors also may prescribe synthetic opioids, such as hydrocodone (Lorcet, Lortab, Vicodin) or oxycodone (Percodan, Percocet, OxyContin) for pain.

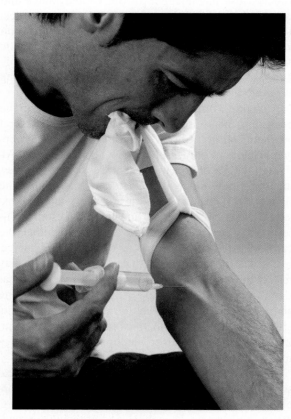

Severe intoxication from heroin use can lead to unconsciousness, coma, and seizures. *Michaela Begsteiger/ Getty Images*

Morphine was widely used as a pain reliever in the nineteenth century, until it was found to be highly addictive. Heroin was developed from morphine in the late nineteenth century and was used for a time for medicinal purposes. By 1917, however, it was clear that heroin and all the opioids have dangerous addictive properties, and Congress passed a law making heroin illegal and banning the other opioids except for specific medical needs. Heroin remained widely available on the street, however (Winger, Hoffmann, & Woods, 2004).

When used illegally, opioids often are injected into the veins (mainlining), snorted, or smoked. The initial symptom of opioid intoxication often is euphoria (see Table 5). People describe a sensation in the abdomen like a sexual orgasm, referring to it as a thrill, kick, or flash. They may have a tingling sensation and a pervasive sense of warmth. They pass into a state of drowsiness, during which they are lethargic, their speech is slurred, and their mind may be clouded. They may experience periods of light sleep with vivid dreams. Pain is reduced (Ruiz & Strain, 2014). A person in this state is referred to as being *on the nod*. Severe intoxication can lead to unconsciousness, coma, and seizures.

Opioids can suppress the respiratory and cardiovascular systems to the point of death. The drugs are especially dangerous when combined with depressants, such as alcohol or sedatives. Withdrawal symptoms include dysphoria, an achy feeling in the back and legs, increased sensitivity to pain, and a craving for more opioids. The person may experience nausea, vomiting, profuse sweating and goose bumps, diarrhea, and fever (Ruiz & Strain, 2014).

These symptoms usually appear within 8 to 16 hours of last use and peak within 36 to 72 hours. In chronic or heavy users, they may continue in strong form for 5 to 8 days and in a milder form for weeks to months.

Most street heroin is cut with other substances, so users do not know the actual strength of the drug or its true contents, leaving them at risk for overdose or death. Users also risk contracting HIV through contaminated needles or through unprotected sex, which many opioid abusers exchange for more heroin. In some areas of the United States, up to 60 percent of chronic heroin users are infected with HIV. Intravenous users also can contract hepatitis, tuberculosis, serious skin abscesses, and deep infections. Women who use heroin during pregnancy risk miscarriage and premature delivery, and children born to mothers with opioid use disorders are at increased risk for sudden infant death syndrome (Brady, Back, & Greenfield, 2009).

One of the biggest developments in the substance abuse area has been an explosion of opioid use and abuse in the United States in recent years, which has been dubbed a national epidemic. The use and misuse of prescription opioid pain relievers such as oxycodone or Vicodin increased significantly in the past two decades. In 2016 alone, 11.5 million people over the age of 12 misused these drugs, a prevalence of over 4 percent (SAMHSA, 2017). The rate among young adults was 7 percent. Opioids are the most common cause of drug overdoses; over 40,000 deaths in the United States in 2016 involved opioids, five times as many as in 1999 (CDC, 2018b). This stunning increase and severity of the opioid epidemic is partially attributable to increased use of illegally made

TABLE 5   Intoxication with and Withdrawal from Opioids

The opioids include morphine, heroin, codeine, and methadone.

Drug	Intoxication Symptoms	Withdrawal Symptoms
Opioids	Behavioral changes (e.g., initial euphoria followed by apathy, dysphoria, psychomotor agitation or retardation; impaired judgment)	Dysphoric mood
		Nausea or vomiting
		Muscle aches
	Constriction of pupils	Tearing or nasal mucus discharge
	Drowsiness or coma	Dilation of pupils
	Slurred speech	Goose bumps
	Attention and memory problems	Sweating
		Diarrhea
		Yawning
		Fever
		Insomnia

synthetic opioids like fentanyl (CDC, 2018c). The crisis presents severe challenges to local authorities, first responders, state and federal governments, and millions of families.

HALLUCINOGENS AND PCP

Most of the substances discussed so far can produce perceptual illusions and distortions when used in large doses. The category of **hallucinogens** include several drugs including lysergic acid diethylamide (LSD), phencyclidine (PCP), peyote, mescaline, psilocybin mushrooms, "Ecstasy" (also known as MDMA or "Molly"), and ketamine which produce perceptual changes even in small doses (see Table 6). In 2018, an estimated 5.6 million people aged 12 or older reported hallucinogen use which represents about 2percent of the U.S. population. This data indicate an increase in hallucinogen users identified in 2015 and 2016 (SAMHSA, 2019).

TABLE 6   Intoxication with Hallucinogens and PCP

The hallucinogens and PCP cause a variety of perceptual and behavioral changes.

Drug	Intoxication Symptoms
Hallucinogens	Behavioral changes (e.g., marked anxiety or depression, the feeling that others are talking about you, fear of losing your mind, paranoia, impaired judgment)
	Perceptual changes while awake (e.g., intensification of senses, depersonalization, illusions, hallucinations)
	Dilation of pupils
	Rapid heartbeat
	Sweating
	Palpitations
	Blurring of vision
	Tremors
	Incoordination
PCP	Behavioral changes (e.g., belligerence, assaultiveness, impulsiveness, unpredictability, psychomotor agitation, impaired judgment)
	Involuntary rapid eyeball movement
	Hypertension
	Numbness
	Loss of muscle coordination
	Problems speaking due to poor muscle control
	Muscle rigidity
	Seizures or coma
	Exceptionally acute hearing
	Perceptual disturbances

The psychoactive effects of LSD were first discovered in 1943 when Dr. Albert Hoffman accidentally swallowed a minute amount and experienced visual hallucinations. He later purposefully swallowed a small amount of LSD and reported its effects.

As Hoffman describes, one symptom of intoxication from LSD and other hallucinogens is *synesthesia,* the overflow from one sensory modality to another. People say they hear colors and see sounds (Liechti, Dolder, & Schmid, 2017). They feel at one with their surroundings, and time seems to pass very slowly. Moods also may shift from depression to elation to fear. Some people become anxious. Others feel a sense of detachment and a great sensitivity for art, music, and feelings. These experiences lent the drugs the label *psychedelic,* from the Greek words for "soul" and "to make manifest." LSD was used in the 1960s as part of the consciousness-expanding movement (Winger et al., 2004).

The hallucinogens are dangerous drugs, however. Although LSD was legal for use in the early 1960s, by 1967 reports of "bad acid trips," or "bummers," had become common, particularly in the Haight-Ashbury district of San Francisco, where many LSD enthusiasts from around the United States congregated (Smith & Seymour, 1994). Symptoms included severe anxiety, paranoia, and loss of control. Some people on bad trips would walk off a roof or jump out a window, believing they could fly, or walk into the sea, believing they were "one with the universe." For some, the anxiety and hallucinations were severe enough to produce psychosis requiring hospitalization and long-term treatment. Some people reexperience their psychedelic experiences, especially visual disturbances, long after the drug has worn off and may develop a distressing or impairing hallucinogen persisting perception disorder.

Phencyclidine (PCP) is a dissociative sedative hallucinogen originally used as a veterinary tranquilizer. Low doses of PCP can produce euphoria, slowed reaction times, and involuntary movements. Disorganized thinking, feelings of unreality, and hostility are often displayed at intermediate doses and amnesia, respiratory problems, and changes in body temperature occur at high doses. PCP was a very popular drug in the 1970s, known by the street names *angel dust, peace pills, hog*, and *tranq,* which was manufactured as a powder to be snorted or smoked. Over the last 40 years the use of PCP has declined, as evidenced by a reduction in hospital visits and poison center reports. However, in recent years, PCP use has risen again, increasing from 0.16 percent of law enforcement drug seizures in 2007 to 1.0 percent in 2015 within one metropolitan area. Liquid PCP is often applied to marijuana cigarettes by spraying or dipping them, which is referred to as smoking "wet," "embalming fluid," "illy," or "fry" (Farley, Anderson, & Feller, 2017).

At lower doses, it produces a sense of intoxication, euphoria or affective dulling, talkativeness, lack of concern, slowed reaction time, vertigo, eye twitching, mild hypertension, abnormal involuntary movements, and weakness. At intermediate doses, it leads to disorganized thinking, distortions of body image (e.g., feeling that one's arms are not part of one's body), depersonalization, and feelings of unreality. A user may become hostile, belligerent, and even violent. Confusion, disorientation, and slow or slurred speech, as well as an increased pain threshold are also common. At higher doses, PCP produces amnesia and coma, analgesia sufficient to allow surgery, seizures, severe respiratory problems, hypothermia, and hyperthermia. The effects begin immediately after injecting, snorting, or smoking and peak within minutes. Symptoms of severe intoxication can persist for several days; people with PCP intoxication may be misdiagnosed as having a psychotic disorder unrelated to substance use. The powerful effects of PCP warp an individual's perception of reality, creating a volatile situation in which the individual has little or no control (Hendricks, Daugherty, & Dang, 2017; Morrison, 1998).

PCP or other hallucinogen use disorder is diagnosed when individuals repeatedly fail to fulfill major role obligations at school, work, or home due to intoxication with these drugs. They may use the drugs in dangerous situations, such as while driving a car, and they may have legal troubles due to their possession of the drugs. Because the drugs can cause paranoia or aggressive behavior, frequent users may find their work and social relationships affected. About 11 percent of the U.S. population reports having tried a hallucinogen or PCP, but only 0.5 percent report having used it in the past month (Johnston et al., 2012; SAMHSA, 2017). Use is higher among teenagers and young adults, however, with 5.8 percent of 12th-graders, 4.1 percent of college students, and 6.4 percent of 18- to 22-year-olds not in college reporting use of a hallucinogen in the past year (Johnston et al., 2012).

CANNABIS

The leaves of the **cannabis** (or hemp) plant can be cut, dried, and rolled into cigarettes or inserted into food and beverages. In North America, the result is known as marijuana, weed, pot, grass, reefer, and Mary Jane. Cannabis is the most commonly used illegal drug, with 42 percent of adults in the United States and 23 percent of Europeans having used the drug (Degenhardt et al., 2008; European Monitoring Centre for Drugs and Drug Action, 2011; Johnston et al., 2012). In 2018, 43.5 million marijuana users were identified among individuals 12 years or older (15.9 percent) in the United States which was higher than previous estimates from 2002 to 2017. Over the last decade, there have been unprecedented shifts in the cannabis policy within the United States with many states moving to legalize or decriminalize this drug. This shift is not surprisingly since more than 60 percent of U.S. adults in 2018 supported the legalization of cannabis for recreational purposes which is a dramatic increase from only 32 percent in favor in 2006 (Smart & Pacula, 2019). These shifting attitudes and federal policies about cannabis use have led researchers to investigate the impact of both recreational and medical marijuana laws (MMLs) among adolescents and adult users. While many studies have produced mixed findings, it has consistently been found that states with MMLs have increased rates of marijuana use among adults, but not adolescents. Increases in marijuana use among individuals 21 years and older are observed in states with MMLs as compared to states without MMLs (Williams, Santaella-Tenorio, Mauro, Levin, & Martins, 2017).

Intoxication usually begins with a "high" feeling of well-being, relaxation, and tranquility (see Table 7). Users may feel dizzy, sleepy, or dreamy. They may become more aware of their environment, and everything may seem funny. They may become grandiose or lethargic. People who already are very anxious, depressed, or angry may become more so (Ruiz & Strain, 2014). The symptoms of cannabis intoxication may develop within minutes if the drug is smoked but may take a few hours to develop if it is taken orally. The acute symptoms last 3 to 4 hours, but some symptoms may linger or recur for 12 to 24 hours.

TABLE 7   Intoxication and Withdrawal Symptoms with Cannabis

Cannabis is the most commonly used illegal drug in the United States.

Drug	Intoxication Symptoms	Withdrawal Symptoms
Cannabis	Behavioral changes (e.g., impaired motor coordination, euphoria, anxiety, sensation of slowed time, impaired judgment)	Irritability, anger, or aggression Nervousness or anxiety Sleep difficulty Decreased appetite or weight loss
	Red eyes	Restlessness
	Increased appetite	Depressed mood
	Dry mouth	Stomach pain, shakiness, sweating, fever, chills, headache
	Rapid heartbeat	

Although people often view cannabis as a benign or safe drug, it can significantly affect cognitive and motor functioning. People taking cannabis may believe they are thinking profound thoughts, but their short-term memory is impaired to the point that they cannot remember thoughts long enough to express them in sentences. Motor performance also is impaired. People's reaction times are slower and their concentration and judgment are deficient, putting them at risk for accidents. The cognitive impairments caused by cannabis can last up to a week after heavy use stops (Pope, Gruber, Hudson, Huestis, & Yurgelun-Todd, 2001). These effects appear to be greater in women than in men (Pope, Jacobs, Mialet, Yurgelun-Todd, & Gruber, 1997).

The physiological symptoms of cannabis intoxication include increased or irregular heartbeat, increased appetite, and dry mouth. Cannabis smoke is irritating and increases the risk of chronic cough, sinusitis, bronchitis, and emphysema. It contains even larger amounts of known carcinogens than does tobacco and thus creates a high risk of cancer. The chronic use of cannabis lowers sperm count in men and may cause irregular ovulation in women (Ruiz & Strain, 2014).

At moderate to large doses, cannabis users experience perceptual distortions, feelings of depersonalization, and paranoid thinking. Some find these hallucinogenic effects pleasant, but others become frightened. Some users may have severe anxiety episodes resembling panic attacks. Several studies have found that cannabis use significantly increases the risk of developing a psychotic disorder (e.g., Kuepper et al., 2011; van Winkel & Kuepper, 2014). Physical tolerance to cannabis can develop, with users needing greater amounts to avoid the symptoms of withdrawal, which include irritability, difficulty sleeping, loss of appetite, hot flashes, runny nose, sweating, diarrhea,

Seven to 10 percent of the U.S. population would qualify for a diagnosis of cannabis use disorder. *belchonock/123RF*

and hiccups (Schlienz, Budney, Lee, & Vandrey, 2017). About 2 percent of the U.S. population would qualify for a diagnosis of cannabis use disorder (Hasin et al., 2015; SAMHSA, 2017).

In recent years several states have legalized the medicinal and recreational use of cannabis, although it remains illegal at the federal level. The federal government allows exemptions on the basis of mandated regulation. Thirty-one states and the District of Columbia have legalized the use of cannabis in some form for medical reasons (see Pacula & Smart, 2017). As of 2018, recreational cannabis is fully legal in Alaska, California, Colorado, Maine, Massachusetts, Nevada, Oregon, and Washington State and in several smaller jurisdictions. According to a Pew Research Center survey, 61 percent of Americans are in favor of complete or partial legalization of cannabis (Pew Research Center, 2018). As marijuana has come to be perceived to have lower risks over the last decade, the rate and frequency of use has increased (Compton, Han, Jones, Blanco, & Hughes, 2016).

INHALANTS

Inhalants are volatile substances that produce chemical vapors, which can be inhaled and which depress the central nervous system (see Table 8; Procyshyn et al., 2017). Inhalants include a variety of substances and products, such as nitrous oxide, cleaning fluids, gasoline, spray paint, paint thinners, computer keyboard cleaner, and other aerosol sprays (SAMHSA, 2019). Users may inhale vapors directly from the can or bottle containing the substance, soak a rag with the substance, and hold the rag to their mouth and nose, or place the substance in a paper or plastic bag and inhale the gases from the bag. The chemicals rapidly reach the lungs, bloodstream, and brain. Another group of inhalants is medical anesthetic gases, such as nitrous oxide ("laughing gas"), which also can be found in whipped cream dispensers and products that boost octane levels. Nitrites, another class of inhalants, dilate blood vessels and relax muscles and are used as sex enhancers. Illegally packaged nitrites are called "poppers" or "snappers" on the street. In diagnosing an inhalant use disorder, *DSM-5* recommends specifying the particular substance involved when possible (e.g., solvent use disorder).

In 2018, approximately 2 million people (12 years and older) were identified as users of inhalants which represented 0.7 percent of the population, a slight increase in recent years (SAMSHA, 2019). A nationwide study of adults found that less than 2 percent reported ever having used inhalants, with about 75 percent of users being male (Howard, Perron, Vaughn, Bender, & Garland, 2010). Adolescents report higher levels of inhalants use than any other age group. Recent data found that 662,000 adolescents (12 to 17 years) were users of inhalants within the past year, which represents 2.7 percent of this population (Johnston et al., 2012; SAMSHA, 2019).

Chronic users of inhalants may have a variety of respiratory irritations and rashes. Inhalants can cause permanent damage to the central nervous system, including degeneration and lesions of the brain; this damage can lead to cognitive deficits, including severe dementia. Recurrent use can also cause hepatitis and other liver and kidney disease. Death can occur from depression of the respiratory or cardiovascular system. Sudden sniffing death is due to acute heartbeat irregularities or loss of oxygen. Users sometimes suffocate when they fall unconscious with an inhalant-filled plastic bag over their nose and mouth. Users also can die or be seriously injured when the inhalants induce the delusion that users can do fantastic things, such as fly, and they then jump off a cliff or a tall building to test their perceived ability (Procyshyn et al., 2017).

OTHER DRUGS OF ABUSE

Drug sellers are creative in coming up with new psychoactive substances. Often these substances initially have legitimate medicinal purposes and then are hijacked or transformed into street drugs. In this section, we discuss ecstasy (3,4-methylenedioxymethamphetamine, or MDMA), GHB (gamma-hydroxybutyrate), ketamine, and rohypnol (flunitrazepam).

*Ecstasy (*MDMA*),* also known as *Molly,* has the stimulant effects of an amphetamine along with occasional hallucinogenic properties. The widespread recreational use of MDMA in the rave culture of the late 1980s and 1990s made this drug one of the four most widely used illicit drugs in the United States, United Kingdom, and other European countries. MDMA is no longer a subculture drug and is used recreationally around the world by a wide range of young adults in nightlife settings and social events. MDMA remains popular due to its low rates of dependence and the desired sensory and psychedelic effects. This substance facilitates sociability, empathy, affection, and bonding with intensified energy that allows for vigorous and long-term dancing. Worldwide, the use of ecstasy was 0.1 percent to 7.4 percent among European adults ages 15 to 64 years. Recent surveys suggest an increasing trend of MDMA usage among various countries in Europe who reported higher estimates

TABLE 8   Intoxication with Inhalants

Inhalants have a variety of effects depending on the specific drug.

Drug	Intoxication Symptoms
Inhalants	Behavioral changes (e.g., belligerence, assaultiveness, apathy, impaired judgment)
	Dizziness
	Nystagmus
	Incoordination
	Slurred speech
	Unsteady gait
	Lethargy
	Depressed reflexes
	Psychomotor retardation
	Tremor
	Generalized muscle weakness
	Blurred vision or diplopia
	Stupor or coma
	Euphoria

than in previous years (van Amsterdam, Pennings, & van den Brink, 2020). It is fairly popular with young adults; 6.8 percent of college students and 13.0 percent of 18- to 22-year-olds not in college report having used ecstasy at some time (Johnston et al., 2012). Even short-term use can have long-term negative effects on cognition and health, however.

People who use ecstasy score lower on tests related to attention, memory, learning, and general intelligence than do people who do not use the drug. The euphoric effects of ecstasy, and some of the brain damage, may be due to alterations in the functioning of serotonin in the brain—serotonin levels in ecstasy users are half those in people who are not users (Gold, Tabrah, & Frost-Pineda, 2001). Long-term users risk several cardiac problems and liver failure and show increased rates of anxiety, depression, psychotic symptoms, and paranoia (Gold et al., 2001). Another effect of ecstasy is teeth-grinding; some users suck a baby pacifier at parties to relieve this effect. The health risks associated with MDMA use are the subject of heated debate with some suggesting that one dose will cause irreversible health damage and others believing that MDMA is relatively harmless (van Amsterdam et al., 2020).

GHB is a central nervous system depressant approved for the treatment of the sleep disorder narcolepsy. At low doses, it can relieve anxiety and promote relaxation. At higher doses, it can result in sleep, coma, or death. In the 1980s, GHB was widely used by bodybuilders and athletes to lose fat and build muscle and was available over the counter in health food stores. In 1990, it was banned except under the supervision of a physician due to reports of severe side effects, including high blood pressure, wide mood swings, liver tumors, and violent behavior. Other side effects include sweating, headache, decreased heart rate, nausea, vomiting, impaired breathing, loss of reflexes, and tremors (National Institute on Drug Abuse [NIDA], 2018). GHB is also considered a *date-rape drug* because it has been associated with sexual assaults (NIDA, 2018). It goes by the street names Grievous Bodily Harm, G., Liquid Ecstasy, and Georgia Home Boy.

Ketamine is a rapid-acting anesthetic that produces hallucinogenic effects ranging from rapture to paranoia to boredom (NIDA, 2018). Ketamine can elicit an out-of-body or near-death experience. It also can render the user comatose. It has effects similar to those of PCP, including numbness, loss of coordination, a sense of invulnerability, muscle rigidity, aggressive or violent behavior, slurred or blocked speech, an exaggerated sense of strength, and a blank stare. Because ketamine is an anesthetic, users feel no pain, which can lead them to injure themselves (NIDA, 2018).

A ketamine high usually lasts 1 hour but can last as long as 4 to 6 hours, and it takes 24 to 48 hours for users to feel normal again. Large doses can produce vomiting and convulsions and may lead to oxygen starvation in the brain and muscles. One gram can cause death. Ketamine is another date-rape drug used to anesthetize victims (NIDA, 2018).

A widely known date-rape drug is *rohypnol,* which goes by the slang names Roofies, Rophies, Roche, and the Forget-Me Pill, among others. It is a benzodiazepine and has sedative and hypnotic effects (NIDA, 2018). Users may experience a high, as well as muscle relaxation, drowsiness, impaired judgment, blackouts, hallucinations, dizziness, and confusion. Rohypnol tablets can easily be crushed and slipped into someone's drink. Rohypnol is odorless, colorless, and tasteless, so victims often don't notice that their drink has been altered. Side effects can include headaches, muscle pain, and seizures. In combination with alcohol or other depressants, rohypnol can be fatal (NIDA, 2018).

THEORIES OF SUBSTANCE USE DISORDERS

All the substances we have discussed have powerful effects on the brain that determine their rewarding effects. Whether individuals ever use substances, and whether their use progresses into a substance use disorder, depends on a complex interplay of biological, psychological, and social vulnerabilities (Volkow & Boyle, 2018).

Biological Factors

The brain appears to have its own "pleasure pathway" that affects our experience of reward. This pathway begins in the ventral tegmental area in the midbrain, then progresses through an area of the limbic system called the nucleus accumbens and on to the frontal cortex. It is particularly rich in neurons sensitive to the neurotransmitter dopamine (Volkow & Boyle, 2018).

Some drugs, such as amphetamines and cocaine, directly increase the availability of dopamine in this pathway, producing a strong sense of reward or a "high." Cocaine clears out of the brain more rapidly than do amphetamines, which explains why users on a binge need to use cocaine much more frequently to maintain a high than do those using amphetamines (Volkow & Boyle, 2018). Snorting, smoking, or injecting drugs delivers them to the brain much faster than taking them orally and thus produces a quicker, more intense reaction. Other drugs increase the availability of dopamine more indirectly. For example, the neurons in the ventral tegmental area are inhibited from continuously firing by GABA neurons, so the firing of GABA neurons reduces the high caused by activity in the dopamine neurons. The opiate drugs inhibit GABA, which stops the GABA neurons from

The brain's "pleasure pathway" begins in the ventral tegmental area, then goes through the nucleus accumbens and on to the frontal cortex. It is rich in neurons sensitive to dopamine.

inhibiting dopamine, making dopamine available in the reward center (Volkow & Boyle, 2018).

Other areas of the frontal cortex, including the orbitofrontal cortex, the dorsolateral frontal cortex, and the inferior frontal gyrus, play important roles in controlling the urge to drink alcohol or use drugs (Bechara, 2005; Goldstein & Volkow, 2002). Individuals whose reward network overpowers their control network may be more likely to use substances (Goldstein & Volkow, 2002; Hutchison, 2010).

The chronic use of psychoactive substances alters the reward centers, creating a craving for these substances (Berridge & Robinson, 2016). The repeated use of substances such as cocaine, heroin, and amphetamines causes the brain to reduce its production of dopamine, with the result that dopamine receptors in the brain become less sensitive. As the brain produces less dopamine, more of the drug is needed to produce the desired effects. If the individual stops taking the drug, the brain does not immediately compensate for the loss of dopamine, and withdrawal symptoms occur. Also, because the brain is not producing its typical amount of dopamine, the person may feel sad and unmotivated and may have difficulty experiencing pleasure from other sources, such as food or happy events. Craving for the drug sets in because only the drug can produce pleasure (Berridge & Robinson, 2016).

Psychoactive drugs also affect a number of other biochemical (including glutamate) and brain systems. Alcohol produces sedative and antianxiety effects largely by enhancing the activity of the neurotransmitter GABA in the septal/hippocampal system. Alcohol also affects serotonin systems, which are associated with changes in mood (Brick, 2008).

Although individuals who have used a substance for an extended period experience decreased sensitivity to the rewarding aspects of the substance, they become more sensitive to cues associated with their substance use, such as the locations where they typically use the substance or the paraphernalia associated with it. These conditioned responses to drug cues can induce powerful cravings that can lead to relapse (Volkow & Boyle, 2018). Stress also activates reward systems, creating cravings. In addition, chronic use of drugs seems to lead to disrupted activity in frontal regions of the brain involved in impulse control, making it even more difficult for individuals to resist cravings.

Genetic factors regulate the functioning of the neurotransmitter systems involved in the rewarding effects of substance use. Family history, adoption, and twin studies all suggest that genetics plays a substantial role in determining who is at risk for substance use disorders, with about 50 percent of the variation in risk for substance use disorders attributable to genetic factors (see reviews by Urbanoski & Kelly, 2012; Young-Wolff, Kendler, Ericson, & Prescott, 2011). There seems to be a common underlying genetic vulnerability to substance use disorders in general, rather than to use of specific substances, perhaps accounting for the fact that individuals who use one substance are likely to use several.

Much research has focused on the genes that control the dopamine system, given its importance in the reinforcing properties of substances. Genetic variation in the dopamine receptor gene (labeled DRD2) and the dopamine transporter gene (labeled SLC6A3) influences how the brain processes dopamine, thereby affecting how reinforcing a person finds substances such as nicotine (Nemoda, Szekely, & Sasvari-Szekely, 2011). In addition, the genes that control GABA have also been implicated in substance use disorders, particularly alcohol use disorders (AUDs).

Psychological Factors

Social learning theories (see the chapter "Theories and Treatment of Abnormality") suggest that children and adolescents may learn substance use behaviors from the modeling of their parents and important others in their culture. Even as preschoolers, the children of heavy drinkers are more likely than other children to be able to identify alcoholic drinks and view alcohol use as a part of daily life (Zucker,

Children may learn substance-related behaviors from their parents. *Elena Kouptsova -Vasic/Shutterstock*

Kincaid, Fitzgerald, & Bingham, 1995). Children whose parents abuse alcohol by frequently getting drunk or by driving while intoxicated learn that these are acceptable behaviors and thus are more likely to engage in them (Chassin, Pitts, DeLucia, & Todd, 1999; Hussong, Huang, Serrano, Curran, & Chassin, 2012).

Studies suggest that there are various motives associated with the initiation and continuation of substance use. Among men, peer pressure, desire to appear more masculine, improve sexual performance, and pleasure-seeking have all been identified as significant factors related to the development of substance use disorders. The peer effect has been found to one of the most influential factors on substance use, particularly among young adults. Studies have found that a majority (65 to 89 percent) of those who consumed drugs did so under the influence of their peers (Moustafaa, Garamib, Soliemanc, Eissac, & Shakird, 2020).

The cognitive theories of AUDs have focused on people's expectations of alcohol's effects and their beliefs about the appropriateness of using it to cope with stress (Cooper, Kuntsche, Levitt, Barber, & Wolf, 2016). People who expect alcohol to reduce their distress and who do not have more adaptive means of coping (e.g., problem-solving skills or supportive friends or family) are more likely than others to drink alcohol when they are upset and to have social problems related to drinking (Cooper et al., 2016). In long-term studies of the sons of parents with AUDs, men

who used alcohol to cope and relax were more likely to develop AUDs themselves (Handley & Chassin, 2009; Schuckit, 1998).

One personality characteristic consistently related to an increased risk of substance use disorders is behavioral undercontrol, or the tendency to be impulsive, sensation-seeking, and prone to antisocial behaviors such as violating laws. People with high levels of behavioral undercontrol take psychoactive drugs at an earlier age, ingest more psychoactive drugs, and are more likely to be diagnosed with substance use disorders (McGue, Iacono, Legrand, Malone, & Elkins, 2001; White, Xie, & Thompson, 2001; Zucker, Heitzeg, & Nigg, 2011). Behavioral undercontrol runs strongly in families, and twin studies suggest that this may be due in part to genes (Rutter, Silberg, O'Connor, & Simonoff, 1999). Thus, genetics may influence behavioral undercontrol, which in turn influences the risk that individuals will develop substance use disorders.

Sociocultural Factors

The reinforcing effects of substances—the highs produced by stimulants, the calming and "zoning out" effects of the depressants and the opioids—can be more attractive to people under chronic stress. Thus, rates of substance use disorders are higher among people living in poverty, areas where there is more access to drugs, women in abusive relationships, and adolescents whose parents fight frequently and violently (Hughes, McCabe, Wilsnack, West, & Boyd, 2010; Moustafaa et al., 2020; SAMHSA, 2017). For these people, the effects of substances may be especially reinforcing. They also may think that they have little to lose.

Subtler environmental reinforcements and punishments clearly influence people's substance use habits. Some societies discourage any use of alcohol, often due to religious beliefs, and alcohol abuse and dependence are rare in these societies. Other societies, including many European cultures, allow the drinking of alcohol but strongly discourage excessive drinking and irresponsible behavior while intoxicated. Alcohol-related disorders are less common in these societies than in societies with few restrictions, either legal or cultural, on alcohol use (Sher et al., 2005; WHO, 2014).

Gender Differences

Substance use, particularly alcohol consumption, has been a male-dominated activity and generally more socially acceptable for men throughout history. Heavy drinking was part of what "masculine" men do and modeled by heroes and cultural icons. In contrast,

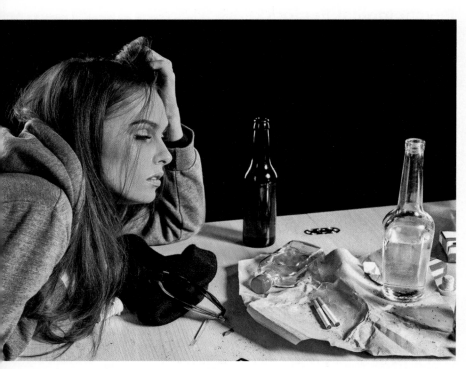

Women suffer the effects of excessive alcohol use at lower doses than men.
poznyakov/123RF

until recently heavy drinking in some Western cultures signified that a woman was "not a lady." However, in the last century, differences in alcohol use and related harms between males and females in the United States have diminished considerably. Societal acceptance of heavy drinking by women has increased in recent generations, as has the rate of alcohol use among young women (Nolen-Hoeksema, 2004; SAMHSA, 2017; White, 2020).

Overall, males still consume more alcohol and experience and cause more alcohol-related injuries and deaths than females do, but the gaps are narrowing. Among adolescents and young adults, the gender gaps in alcohol consumption have narrowed as a result of decreased use among males more so than females. Among adults, alcohol use is increasing for women but not for men (White, 2020). Recent data show increases in AUD prevalence rates among women, which includes higher rates of binge drinking and heavy drinking behaviors. (Guinle & Sinha, 2020). Studies have found that females are more susceptible than males to alcohol-induced liver inflammation, cardiovascular disease, memory blackouts, hangovers, and certain cancers (White, 2020). In addition, heavy alcohol use is associated with reproductive problems in women. Women may be more likely to experience greater cognitive and motor impairment due to alcohol than do men and to suffer physical harm and sexual assault following alcohol use (Lorenz & Ullman, 2016).

Although gender gaps in alcohol use seemingly are universal, the size of the gaps varies between countries and their respective cultures. For example, in New Zealand and Norway the male to female ratio for drinking is 1:1, but the ratio is significantly higher in India at 12:1. Large variations between countries suggest that culturally prescribed gender roles, that are more influential than physiological sex differences, are central in cultivating gender-specific patterns of alcohol consumption (White, 2020).

When women become substance abusers, their patterns and reasons for use tend to differ from those of men. Research shows that stress, trauma, victimization, negative affect, and mood and anxiety disorders in women represent a specific risk pathway for the onset and development substance use disorders (Guinle & Sinha, 2020). Men tend to begin using substances in the context of socializing with male friends, while women most often are initiated by family members, partners, or lovers (McCrady, Epstein, Cook, Jensen, & Hildebrandt, 2009). Perhaps because women's drug use is more closely tied to their intimate relationships, studies have found that treatments that include their partners tend to be more effective in reducing substance use disorders in women (McCrady et al., 2009).

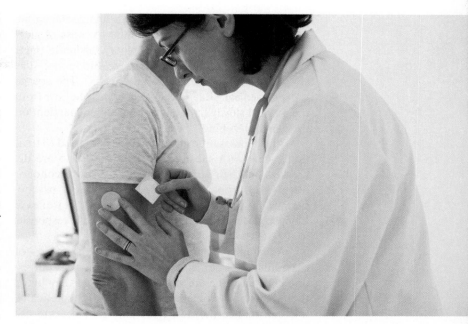

Nicotine replacement therapy aims to decrease substance abuse over time by weaning the user to lower doses, as well as breaking links between the behavior of smoking and its perceived positive physiological consequences. *Image Point Fr/Shutterstock*

TREATMENTS FOR SUBSTANCE USE DISORDERS

The treatment of substance-related disorders is challenging, and media accounts of celebrity drug abusers who are in rehab 1 month, out the next, and back a short time later suggest that it seldom is effective. Meta-analyses and reviews of existing treatments suggest that, as a whole, they help only about 17 to 35 percent of people with substance use disorders abstain for up to 1 year (Hutchison, 2010). Here we review the most common and best-supported biological and psychosocial treatments.

Biological Treatments

Medications can help wean individuals off a substance, reduce their desire for it, and maintain their use at a controlled level (Douaihy, Kelly, & Sullivan, 2013). Substance use disorder is often riddled with stigmatizing language and labels which can become barriers to treatment. Many substance use treatments have overlapping components and confusing labels that can limit patient access (Robinson & Adinoff, 2018).

Antianxiety Drugs, Antidepressants, and Drug Antagonists

Although many people with substance use disorders can withstand withdrawal symptoms if given emotional support, others may require medication. For people dependent on alcohol, a benzodiazepine, which has depressant effects similar to those of alcohol, can reduce tremors and anxiety, decrease pulse and respiration rate, and stabilize blood pressure (Ntais, Pakos, Kyzas, & Ioannidis, 2005). The dosage is decreased each day so that a patient withdraws from the alcohol slowly but does not become dependent on the benzodiazepine.

Antidepressant drugs sometimes are used to treat individuals with substance dependence who are depressed, but their efficacy in treating either alcohol or other drug problems or depression without psychotherapy has not been consistently supported (Nunes & Levin, 2004). People have widely different responses to the SSRIs.

Antagonist drugs block or change the effects of the addictive drug, reducing the desire for it. Naltrexone and naloxone are opioid antagonists—they block the effects of opioids such as heroin. Theoretically, this can reduce the desire for and therefore the use of the addictive drug. The opioid antagonists must be administered very carefully, however, because they can cause severe withdrawal reactions in people addicted to opioids (Douaihy et al., 2013).

Naltrexone has also proven useful in treating alcohol dependents and abusers, possibly because it blocks the effects of endorphins during drinking. People dependent on alcohol who take naltrexone report a diminished craving for alcohol and thus drink less (Douaihy et al., 2013).

The drug acamprosate affects glutamate and GABA receptors in the brain, which are involved in the craving for alcohol. Some clinical trials show that acamprosate can help people maintain abstinence from alcohol better than a placebo, although others do not, suggesting the need for additional research (Douaihy et al., 2013).

A drug that can make alcohol actually punishing is disulfiram, commonly called Antabuse. Just one alcoholic drink can make people taking disulfiram feel sick and dizzy and can make them vomit, blush, and even faint. People must be very motivated to remain on disulfiram, and it works to reduce their alcohol consumption only as long as they continue to take it.

The pharmacological treatment of nicotine dependence uses two general approaches. Most common is nicotine replacement therapy—the use of nicotine gum or a nicotine patch, nasal spray, or inhaler to prevent withdrawal effects. It is hoped that the individual will gradually reduce use of the nicotine replacement while slowly being weaned off nicotine's physiological effects.

The other approach is the use of prescription medication that reduces the craving for nicotine. One drug approved for this use is the antidepressant bupropion (marketed for smoking cessation as Zyban). A

drug called varenicline (Chantix), which binds to and partially stimulates nicotine receptors, also has been shown to reduce cravings for nicotine products, decrease their pleasurable effects (Ebbert et al., 2015; Jorenby et al., 2006).

Methadone Maintenance Programs

Medications for opioid use disorder (OUD) can facilitate recovery and prevent deaths. At this time, only three medications are approved by the Food and Drug Administration (FDA) for treating OUD: methadone, buprenorphine, and naltrexone. Both methadone and buprenorphine decrease opioid use, increase treatment retention, and significantly reduce deaths from overdose and are more effective than counseling alone. However, as a result of poor access to treatment and stigma, it is estimated that only 20-40 percent of the more than 2 million individuals with OUD in the U.S receive these life-saving treatments. **Methadone,** a synthetic opioid, is one of the oldest and most effective medications used for opioid treatment that provides less potent and shorter-acting effects than heroin and provides gradual withdrawal (Samet, Botticelli, & Bharel, 2018). The affected individual receives methadone to reduce extreme negative withdrawal symptoms. Those who take heroin while on methadone do not experience heroin's intense psychological effects, because methadone blocks receptors for heroin (Douaihy et al., 2013). Methadone treatment provides significant benefits to both patients and communities by reducing opioid use and decreasing adverse health risks, such as overdoses and the risk of relapse to drug use. Studies have also shown that methadone treatment programs help to stabilize clients which provides them with a better chance to find and maintain employment, improve social and family relations, and enhance their quality of life (Khazaee-Pool et al., 2018).

By the 1970s, a methadone delivery system was developed in the United States that restricts methadone treatment to designated clinic sites which are separate from the general medical care system. These "methadone clinics" provide specialized, highly structured care which includes daily observed medication administration, periodic drug tests, and counseling. Among the 14,000 substance use treatment facilities in the United States identified by the National Survey of Substance Abuse Treatment Services, only 1,500 facilities dispense methadone. This limited access to methadone sites has contributed to a treatment gap calling for alternative models of methadone delivery. Alternative methadone delivery models currently exist in Great Britain, Canada, and Australia where primary care physicians prescribe methadone for opioid treatment and community pharmacies dispense the medication. This model is cost-effective and provides increased access for those in need of treatment; but the treatment of OUD in primary care settings in the United States is not available at this time. Additionally, studies have found that patient retention was greater for pharmacy-based methadone access as compared to hospital-based methadone programs in Australia (Joudrey et al., 2020; Samet et al., 2018).

Although the goal of treatment is for individuals eventually to withdraw from methadone, some patients use it for years under a physician's care. Such methadone maintenance programs are controversial. Some people believe they allow the heroin dependent to simply transfer dependency to another substance that is legal and provided by a physician. Others believe methadone maintenance is the only way to keep some heroin dependents from going back on the street and relapsing. Studies find that patients in such programs are much more likely to remain in psychological treatment than are patients who try to withdraw from heroin without methadone and also are less likely to relapse into heroin use (Khazaee-Pool et al., 2018; Mattick, Breen, Kimber, Davoli, & Breen, 2003).

Psychosocial Treatments

Several behavioral and cognitive techniques have proven helpful in the treatment of substance use disorders (Higgins, Sigmon, & Heil, 2014; McCrady, 2014). The techniques have certain goals in common. The first is to motivate the individual to stop using the addictive drug. People who enter treatment often are ambivalent about stopping use and may have been forced into treatment against their will. The second goal is to teach patients new coping skills to replace the use of substances to cope with stress and negative feelings. The third goal is to change the reinforcements for using substances—for example, an individual may need to disengage from social circles that encourage drug use. The fourth is to enhance the individual's support from nonusing friends and family members. The final goal often is to foster adherence to pharmacotherapies in conjunction with psychotherapy.

Behavioral Treatments

Behavioral treatments based on aversive classical conditioning are sometimes used alone or in combination with biological or other psychosocial therapies (Finney & Moos, 1998; Schuckit, 1995). Drugs such as disulfiram (Antabuse) that make the ingestion of alcohol unpleasant or toxic are given to people who are alcohol dependent. Eventually, through classical conditioning, people develop conditioned responses to alcohol—namely, nausea and vomiting. Then, through operant conditioning, they learn to avoid alcohol in order to avoid the aversive response. Aversive conditioning is effective in reducing alcohol consumption, at least in the short term (Schuckit, 1995). "Booster" sessions often are needed to reinforce this conditioning, because its effects tend to weaken with time.

Covert sensitization therapy uses imagery to create associations between thoughts of alcohol use and thoughts of highly unpleasant consequences. An example of a sensitization scene that a therapist might take a client through begins as described in the following profile.

PROFILES

You finish the first sip of beer, and you . . . notice a funny feeling in your stomach. . . . Maybe another drink will help. . . . As you tip back . . . that funny feeling in your stomach is stronger, and you feel like you have to burp. . . . You swallow again, trying to force it down, but it doesn't work. You can feel the gas coming up. . . . You swallow more, but suddenly your mouth is filled with a sour liquid that burns the back of your throat and goes up your nose. . . . [You] spew the liquid all over the counter and sink. (Rimmele, C. T., Miller, W. R., & Dougher, M. J. (1989). Aversion therapies. In R. K. Hester & W. R. Miller (Eds.), *Handbook of alcoholism treatment approaches: Effective alternatives* (pp. 128–140). New York: Pergamon Press.)

The imagery gets even more graphic. Covert sensitization techniques seem to be effective in creating conditioned aversive responses to the sight and smell of alcohol and in reducing alcohol consumption, particularly when paired with a 12-step recovery program (Suneel & Siddique, 2020).

Contingency management programs provide reinforcements for individuals to curtail their use of substances—for example, employment, housing, or vouchers for purchases at local stores. Studies show that individuals dependent on heroin, cocaine, marijuana, or alcohol will remain in treatment longer and be much more likely to become abstinent when they are provided with incentives contingent on submitting drug-free urine specimens (Higgins et al., 2014; McCrady, 2014).

Cognitive Treatments

Interventions based on the cognitive models of alcohol abuse and dependency help clients identify situations in which they are most likely to drink and lose control over their drinking, as well as their expectations that alcohol will help them cope in those situations (Carroll & Kiluk, 2017; Daley & Marlatt, 2006). Therapists work with clients to challenge these expectations by reviewing alcohol's negative effects on the clients' behavior. Perhaps a client was feeling anxious at a recent party and began to drink heavily. The therapist might have the client recount his embarrassing behavior while intoxicated, challenging the notion that the alcohol helped him cope effectively. Therapists also help clients learn to handle stressful situations in adaptive ways, such as seeking the help of others or engaging in active problem solving. Finally, therapists help clients learn to say "No, thanks" when they are offered a drink and to deal with social pressure by using assertiveness skills.

Following is an excerpt from a discussion between a therapist and a client with alcohol-related problems (adapted from Sobell & Sobell, 1978, pp. 97–98) in which the therapist is helping the client generate strategies for coping with the stress of a possible job promotion. The therapist encourages the client to brainstorm coping strategies and refrains from evaluating them for the moment so the client will feel free to generate as many strategies as possible.

> **Client:** I've been offered the job I've been telling you about. It's a huge promotion. But now I have to make the decision about whether or not to move my entire family across the country to take it. I know my wife and kids don't want to move. And now I am really nervous about whether or not I can even do this new job. I don't have all the skills.
>
> **Therapist:** Yes, that's a big decision for you and your family. But rather than worrying about the skills problem just now, why don't we explore the different options you have relating to the promotion and move. You know, for now, you don't have to evaluate your options, only list them. The point right now is to come up with as many alternatives as possible. You're not yet acting on anything, only considering your possibilities.
>
> **Client:** You know, I've been pretty tense and you know what has happened before when I get nervous. I've been drinking quite a lot. My wife is pretty angry about it. And I don't feel so well.
>
> **Therapist:** Well, in a way, drinking is one option. But what other ways can you think of to deal with the problem of the promotion and move?
>
> **Client:** I've been thinking that because the new company has an educational benefit, I could take courses to learn more about management. Maybe even get my MBA. But I have no idea about how I could hold down the job, go to school, and be in any way present to my family.
>
> **Therapist:** Well, remember. Right now we're not talking about how you would do any of this; we're only coming up with options. You're doing really well. Let's keep going.
>
> **Client:** I could always just stay where I am. The family would be happier, even if I might not be so happy at work. But it means a lot to me that they are happy too. Or I could ask my new boss to give me time to get up to speed with my new responsibilities.
>
> **Therapist:** Good. Keep going.
>
> **Client:** What would happen if I take the new job, settle my family in a new state, and then find out that I can't get that kind of support?
>
> **Therapist:** Well, what do you think would happen? What are your options?
>
> **Client:** I think I really want the job. Maybe I should just be in touch with the person who hired me and tell her about my concerns. After all, they are willing to move me across the country; they must really want me. I need some time and some more education.
>
> **Therapist:** You've identified a lot of options today. Why don't we spend some time evaluating each before you make a final decision? (Adapted from Sobell & Sobell, 1978, 97–98)

The therapist helps the client evaluate the effectiveness of each option and anticipate any negative consequences. In this case, the client decides to accept the promotion but to take some courses at the local college to increase his business background. The two discuss the stresses of managing a new job and classes, and they generate ways the client can manage these stresses other than by drinking.

Cognitive behavioral therapy (CBT) for the treatment of drug and alcohol use disorders has some of the highest levels of empirical support and is widely acknowledged as evidence-based approaches. CBT explores how to best convey cognitive and behavioral skills that can help individuals successfully modify addictive behaviors and how to reduce the risk of relapse (Carroll & Kiluk, 2017). In most cases, therapists using cognitive-behavioral approaches encourage their clients to abstain from alcohol, especially when they have a history of frequent relapses into abuse. When a client's goal is to learn to drink socially and the therapist believes the client can achieve this goal, therapy may focus on teaching the client to engage in social, or controlled, drinking. Studies have shown that cognitive-behavioral approaches are effective in treating abuse and dependence on alcohol, cannabis, nicotine, heroin, amphetamines, and cocaine (see Higgins et al., 2014; McCrady, 2014; McHugh, Hearon, & Otto, 2010).

Motivational Interviewing

If individuals are not motivated to curtail their substance use, no treatment will be effective. William Miller (1983; Miller & Rollnick, 2012; Miller & Rose, 2009) developed **motivational interviewing (MI)** to elicit and solidify clients' motivation and commitment to changing their substance use. MI is recognized as an effective treatment for substance use disorders that combines a person-centered approach with strategies to enhance an individual's motivation for change. MI has been shown to increase statements that favor change, called change talk, among clients. Overall, studies have found that this form of treatment improves client retention and substance use outcomes (Martino et al., 2016).

Rather than confronting the user, the motivational interviewer adopts an empathic interaction style, drawing out the user's statements of desire, ability, reasons, need, and, ultimately, commitment to change. The interviewer focuses on the client's ambivalence, helping the client voice their own arguments for change. Many controlled studies find that just four sessions of MI lead to sustained reductions in substance use, particularly alcohol use (e.g., Ball et al., 2007; Carroll et al., 2006; see reviews in Miller & Rollnick, 2012; Miller & Rose, 2009).

CBT is often combined with other empirically supported treatments for alcohol and drug use disorders, such as MI, to increase client engagement and adherence to treatment. Several studies have investigated the combination of CBT and MI for various drugs of abuse, including amphetamines cocaine, methamphetamines, and marijuana. Although the findings have been mixed with respect to drug use outcomes, there is some evidence to suggest that adding motivational enhancement to the early stages of CBT can be effective at increasing motivation and improving retention in treatment (Carroll & Kiluk, 2017).

COVID-19 and Telehealth Services

The COVID-19 pandemic has created many additional challenges for patients with substance use disorders. As a result of this crisis, many addiction treatment and harm reduction organizations have reduced their hours and services for people with substance use disorders, placing these individuals at increased risk of death. The social isolation that those with substance use disorder can experience as a result of pandemic restrictions can be dangerous due to increased risk of overdose death. Limited access to proper treatment, withdrawal and loss of tolerance, using alone, and resumed use among people in recovery are all significant concerns (Khatri & Perrone, 2020). The COVID-19 pandemic poses significant risks to marginalized individuals, particularly those with substance use disorders. Individuals with substance use disorder already represent an under-served and stigmatized population. Now, with hospitals and clinics focused on COVID-19, these individuals are more likely to encounter additional barriers to health care and effective treatment (Samuels et al., 2020).

In an effort to minimize barriers to care and prevent overdose deaths during the COVID-19 emergency, the Substance Abuse Mental Health Services Administration (SAMHSA), the US Drug Enforcement Administration, and the US Department of Health and Human Services issued guidance that allow for use of audio-only telehealth encounters for buprenorphine prescription without requiring an in-person evaluation or video interface. Loosening regulations and utilizing technology provide a unique opportunity to evaluate new alternative treatment models. These new models of treatment delivery challenge some of the current regulations and requirements that limit engagement and access to care (Samuels et al., 2020). Access to effective therapy and medications are critical components of substance use treatment, yet fewer than one in five individuals receives services. The COVID-19 crisis created the urgent need for socially distanced forms of therapy and highlighted other important factors that contribute to an existing treatment gap.

Telemedicine may be a solution for many people without proper access to mental health services by delivering mental health services through live video technology. This is supported as an effective tool in the diagnosis and assessment of mental health disorders in a variety of populations across different settings. Videoconferencing, a type of telemedicine, has the potential to increase access to medication-based treatment for OUD in underserved, remote rural areas by providing direct-to-client services from a distance. In the treatment of psychological disorders, such as substance use disorders, telemedicine use is growing dramatically and its effects are comparable to in-person treatment, but more research is needed. Various professional organizations are advocating for the expanded use of telemedicine for substance use treatment to facilitate access in areas with few providers or for those who lack of transportation or have physical barriers. It also may help address concerns about privacy and perceived stigma for those with substance use disorder. Research supports the effectiveness of prescribing medications via telemedicine which is associated with increased retention rates and reduction in substance use that are comparable to face-to-face treatment. Unfortunately, financial, legal, and regulatory barriers have prevented the widespread adoption of medication-based treatment through telemedicine. As a result, there are limited data about the effectiveness of this treatment approach (Huskamp et al., 2018; Weintraub et al., 2021).

Relapse Prevention

Unfortunately, the relapse rate for people undergoing any kind of treatment for an alcohol use disorder is high. The **abstinence violation effect** contributes to relapse. It has two components. The first is a sense of conflict and guilt when an abstinent alcohol abuser or dependent violates abstinence and has a drink. They may continue to drink to try to suppress the conflict and guilt. The second component is a tendency to attribute a violation of abstinence to a lack of willpower and self-control rather than to situational factors. Thus, the person may think, "I'm an alcoholic and there's no way I can control my drinking. The fact that I had a drink proves this." This type of thinking may pave the way to continued, uncontrolled drinking.

Relapse prevention programs teach people who abuse alcohol to view slips as temporary and situationally caused (Donovan & Witkiewitz, 2012). Therapists help clients identify high-risk situations, such as parties, and either avoid them or develop effective coping strategies for them. A client who decides to go to a party may first practice with the therapist some assertiveness skills for resisting friends' pressure to drink and write down other coping strategies to use if he or she feels tempted, such as starting a conversation with a supportive friend or practicing deep-breathing exercises. They also may decide that, if the temptation becomes too great, they will ask a supportive friend to leave the party and go somewhere for coffee until the urge to drink passes. Relapse prevention programs have been shown in many studies to reduce the rate of relapse in people with several types of substance use disorders (Donovan & Witkiewitz, 2012).

These cognitive and behavioral interventions have been combined with training in mindfulness meditation, the nonjudgmental acceptance of one's current emotional and physical state, in the treatment of people with substance use disorders (Bowen, Chawla, & Marlatt, 2010; Wilson et al., 2017). People are taught to be aware of their internal states and the external triggers for these states and to accept and "ride out" their negative states rather than reacting to them in a habitual manner (i.e., by using a substance). Studies of people with alcohol and other substance use disorders showed that adding mindfulness meditation training to the usual treatment led to significant reductions in craving and relapse during the follow-up period (e.g., Bowen et al., 2014).

Alcoholics Anonymous

Alcoholics Anonymous (AA) is an organization created by and for people with alcohol-related problems. Its philosophy is based on the disease model of alcoholism, which asserts that, because of biological, psychological, and spiritual deficits, some people will lose all control over their drinking once they have one drink. Therefore, the only way to control alcohol intake is to abstain completely. AA prescribes 12 steps that people dependent on alcohol must take toward recovery. The first step is to admit their dependence on alcohol and their inability to control its effects. AA encourages its members to seek help from a higher power, to admit their weaknesses, and to ask forgiveness. The goal for all members is complete abstinence.

PROFILES

I am Duncan. I am an alcoholic. . . . I know that I will always be an alcoholic, that I can never again touch alcohol in any form. It'll kill me if I don't keep away from it. In fact, it almost did. . . . I must have been just past my 15th birthday when I had that first drink everybody talks about. And like so many of them—and you—it was like a miracle. With a little beer in my gut, the world was transformed. I wasn't a weakling anymore, I could lick almost anybody on the block. So, like for so many of you, my friends in the Fellowship, alcohol became the royal road to love, respect, and self-esteem. . . .

Though it's obvious to me now that my drinking even then, in high school, and after I got to college, was a problem, I didn't think so at the time. A couple of minor auto accidents, one conviction for drunken driving, a few fights—nothing out of the ordinary, it seemed to me at the time. True, I was drinking quite a lot, even then, but my friends seemed to be able to down as much beer as I did. I guess the fact that I hadn't really had any blackouts and that I could go for days without having to drink reassured me that things hadn't gotten out of control.

[Later] on, the drinking began to affect both my marriage and my career. With enough booze in me and under the pressures of guilt over my failure to carry out my responsibilities to my wife and children, I sometimes got kind of rough physically with them. I would break furniture, throw things around, then rush out and drive off in the car. I had a couple of wrecks, lost my license for two years because of one of them. Worst of all was when I tried to stop. By then I was totally hooked, so every time I tried to stop drinking, I'd experience withdrawal in all its horrors. I never had DTs, but I came awfully close many times, with the vomiting and the "shakes" and being unable to sit still or to lie down. And that would go on for days at a time. . . . Then, about 4 years ago, with my life in ruins, my wife given up on me and the kids with her, out of a job, and way down on my luck, the Fellowship and I found each other. Jim, over there, bless his heart, decided to sponsor me—we'd been friends for a long time, and I knew he'd found sobriety through this group. I've been dry now for a little over two years, and with luck and support, I may stay sober. (Adapted from Spitzer, R. L., Skodol, A. E., Gibbon, M., & Williams, J. B. W., *Psychopathology: A case book*, New York: McGraw Hill, 1983, pp. 81–83.)

Group members provide moral and social support and make themselves available to one another in times of crisis. Once they are able, they are expected to devote themselves to helping others who are recovering from alcohol dependence. AA members believe that people are never completely cured of alcohol dependence—they are always "recovering alcoholics," with the potential for falling back into uncontrolled drinking after taking only one drink. To motivate others to abstain from alcohol, AA meetings include testimonials from members, as in the following profile.

The practices and philosophies of AA do not appeal to everyone. The emphases on one's powerlessness, need for a higher power, and complete abstinence turn away many. In addition, many people who subscribe to AA's philosophy still find it difficult to maintain complete abstinence, and they "fall off the wagon" throughout their lives. However, many believe that AA has been critical to their recovery from an alcohol use disorder, and it remains the most common source of treatment for people with alcohol-related problems. There are over 100,000 registered AA groups, and meetings take place all over the United States day and night, providing a supportive community as an alternative to drinking. Self-help groups modeled on AA—including Narcotics Anonymous, Cocaine Anonymous, and Marijuana Anonymous—assist people with dependence on other drugs.

Evaluations of AA's effectiveness are complicated by differences between people who might attend and those who would not, the self-help nature of the intervention, and the fact that outcomes often are self-reported (Kelly, 2003). Perhaps as a result, meta-analyses and reviews of studies of AA's effectiveness have produced mixed results, with some analyses suggesting that AA is effective and others suggesting that it is worse than no treatment (Ferri, Amato, & Davoli, 2006; Kaskutas, 2009; Tonigan, Pearson, Magill, & Hagler, 2018).

Substance Use Treatment for Older Adults

We tend to think of substance use disorders as problems of the young. Indeed, the use of hard drugs, such as cocaine or heroin, is quite rare among the elderly. Many chronic users of illicit substances die before they reach old age, and others outgrow their use. Certain types of substance abuse and dependence are a frequent problem among older people, however, including alcohol-related problems and the misuse of prescription drugs (Kuerbis, Sacco, Blazer, & Moore, 2014).

Approximately 4 percent of people over age 65 can be diagnosed with an alcohol use disorder, and about 10 percent can be considered heavy drinkers (Kuerbis & Sacco, 2013). One-third to one-half of abusers of alcohol first develop problems after age 65. Moreover, the abuse of and dependence on prescription drugs (e.g., sedative, hypnotic, or anxiolytic use disorders) is a substantial problem among the elderly. Although only 15 percent of the U.S. population is over age 65, this group accounts for one-third of all prescription drug expenditures. Ninety percent of older adults take at least one prescription drug, and 39 percent take at least five (AARP Public Policy Institute, 2018). The most commonly prescribed drugs are diuretics, cardiovascular drugs, and sedatives. Older people also are more likely than younger people to purchase over-the-counter drugs, including analgesics, vitamins, and laxatives.

The abuse of drugs such as the benzodiazepines may begin innocently. Physicians frequently prescribe them for older patients, and as many as one-third of older people take these drugs at least occasionally—for insomnia or after experiencing a loss, for example. As tolerance develops and the withdrawal effects of discontinuing the drug become evident, an individual may try to get more of the drug by copying prescriptions or seeing multiple physicians. Slurred speech and memory problems caused by drug use may be overlooked in the elderly as normal symptoms of old age. Older adults often can hide their drug abuse for a long period of time. Eventually, the side effects of the drugs, the withdrawal symptoms people experience when they try to go off the drugs cold turkey, or the effects of interaction with other medications may land them in a hospital emergency room.

Treatment for older substance abusers is similar to that for younger abusers, although withdrawal symptoms may be more dangerous for older abusers and therefore must be monitored more carefully (Kuerbis et al., 2014). Psychotherapies that have been shown to be useful tend to have the following characteristics (Schonfeld & Dupree, 2002):

- Elders are treated along with people their same age in a supportive, nonconfrontational approach.
- Negative emotional states (such as depression and loneliness) and their relationship to the substance abuse are a focus of the intervention.
- Social skills and social networks are rebuilt.
- Staff members are respectful and are interested in working with older adults.
- Linkages are made with medical facilities and community resources (such as housing services).

Due to increasing longevity and the size of the baby-boomer generation, the proportion of the population that is above age 65 will increase dramatically over the next few decades, and by 2030 all baby boomers will be over age 65 (U.S. Census Bureau, 2018). In addition, older Americans will become much more ethnically diverse in the future, and the proportion of older people who are of Hispanic and Asian descent will increase. Much more research is needed on the psychological health needs of older people, particularly older people in ethnic and racial minority groups with substance use disorders.

Comparing Treatments

A large, multi-site clinical trial called Project MATCH compared three interventions designed to help people with alcohol use disorder: cognitive-behavioral intervention, MI and enhancement, and a 12-step program based on the AA model but led by professional counselors (Project MATCH Research Group, 1998). Surprisingly, the study showed that the three interventions were equally effective in reducing drinking behavior and preventing relapse over the following year (Project MATCH Research Group, 1998; Witkiewitz, Van der Maas, Hufford, & Marlatt, 2007).

Another multi-site study of over 1,300 individuals with alcohol use disorder, Project COMBINE, indicated that combining psychosocial intervention with medications did not yield better outcomes than individual therapies (Anton et al., 2006). The psychosocial treatment was a combination of cognitive-behavioral therapy, MI, a 12-step program facilitated by a professional, and community support. The medications were either naltrexone, acamprosate, or a combination of the two. Both psychosocial treatment and naltrexone led to significant reductions in drinking, and the combination of the two was not superior to the individual therapies. Acamprosate did not perform better than a placebo either alone or combined with psychosocial treatment (Anton et al., 2006). A similar pattern was found in a 1-year follow-up of the same individuals, with indications that those who received psychosocial treatment were especially likely to have good outcomes whether or not they also received naltrexone (Donovan et al., 2008).

Prevention Programs

Only about 25 percent of people with alcohol use disorder seek treatment (Dawson et al., 2005). About 25 percent may recover on their own, often due to maturation or positive changes in their environment (e.g., getting a good job or having a supportive partner) that motivate them to control their drinking (Dawson et al., 2005). The remainder of people with significant alcohol problems carry these problems throughout their lives. Some become physically ill or unable to hold a job or maintain a relationship. Others hide or control their alcohol use disorder and may be in relationships with people who facilitate it. Often they have periods of abstinence, sometimes long, but then—perhaps when facing stressful events—they begin drinking again. Therefore, preventing the development of a substance use disorder is very important.

In the United States, young adults between 18 and 24 have the highest rates of alcohol consumption and make up the largest proportion of problem drinkers of any age group. Many colleges have programs to reduce drinking and drinking-related problems. Programs that emphasize alcohol's health-related consequences tend not to impress young people, who are more likely to focus on the short-term gains of alcohol use. Some college counselors refer students with drinking problems to abstinence programs, such as AA, but students often dislike admitting powerlessness and adopting lifelong abstinence. Finally, many colleges provide alternative activities that do not focus on alcohol. In general, however, prevention programs designed to stop drinking have had limited success.

Psychologist Alan Marlatt and his colleagues at the University of Washington (Marlatt, Blume, & Parks, 2001; Marlatt, Larimer, & Witkiewitz, 2011; Marlatt & Witkiewitz, 2010) argued that a more credible approach to college drinking is to recognize it as normative behavior and focus education on the immediate risks of excess (alcohol-related accidents) and the payoffs of moderation (avoidance of hangovers). They view young drinkers as relatively inexperienced in regulating their use of alcohol and in need of skills training to prevent abuse. Learning to drink safely is compared to learning to drive safely in that people must learn to anticipate hazards, avoid "unnecessary accidents," and reduce risks (Andreano, Ford, Karwoski, & Wilson, 2018).

Based on this **harm reduction model**, the Alcohol Skills Training Program (ASTP) targets heavy-drinking college students for intervention. In eight weekly sessions of 90 minutes each, participants learn to be aware of their drinking habits—including when, where, and with whom they are most likely to overdrink—by keeping daily records of their alcohol consumption and the situations in which they drink. They also are taught to calculate their blood-alcohol level. It often comes as a surprise to them how few drinks it takes to become legally intoxicated.

Next, beliefs about the "magical" effects of drinking on social skills and sexual prowess are challenged. Participants discuss hangovers and alcohol's negative effects on social behaviors, ability to drive, and weight gain. They are encouraged to set personal goals for limiting consumption based on their blood-alcohol level and their desire to avoid drinking's negative effects. They learn skills for limiting consumption, such as alternating alcoholic and nonalcoholic beverages and selecting drinks for quality rather than quantity (e.g., buying two good beers rather than a six-pack of generic). Later, members are taught alternative ways to reduce negative emotional states, such as using relaxation exercises or reducing sources of stress. Finally, via role playing, participants learn skills for resisting peer pressure and avoiding high-risk situations in which they are likely to overdrink.

Evaluations of ASTP have shown that participants decrease their consumption and alcohol-related problems and increase their social skill at resisting alcohol abuse (Marlatt et al., 2011). ASTP was designed for a group format, and the use of group pressure to encourage change and allow role playing has many advantages. Adaptations of this program, delivered in person or in written form as a self-help manual, also have shown positive results (Baer, Kivlahan, Blume, McKnight, & Marlatt, 2001).

GAMBLING DISORDER

More than three-quarters of U.S. adults report having gambled in the past year, but most gamble only occasionally and recreationally (Kessler et al., 2008). As noted earlier, *DSM-5* expanded its chapter on substance-related and addictive disorders to include gambling disorder, which some refer to as a behavioral addiction. The *DSM-5* criteria for gambling disorder are given in Table 9. Prevalence of problem gambling varies across studies from below 1 percent of the adult population, up to around 5 to 6 percent (Håkansson & Widinghoff, 2020). Within the United States less than 1 percent of the general population meet these criteria (Kessler et al., 2008; Petry et al., 2018), but for those who do, their gambling frequently leads to serious financial, relationship, and employment problems. The most common criteria are related to preoccupation with gambling and "chasing" losses. With new online technologies and smart phone gaming apps there have been significant increases in online gambling, which includes online casino games

New online and mobile gambling apps have drastically increased access to live sports betting and casino games which can negatively impact those with problem gambling behaviors. *Faizal Ramli/Shutterstock*

and live sports betting, that have raised concerns about the significant potential for gambling-related harm (Håkansson & Widinghoff, 2020).

Mobile gambling provides far more access and opportunities to place bets and engage with casinos than traditional land-based gambling. Mobile gambling can

---

TABLE 9 *DSM-5* Criteria for Gambling Disorder

A. Persistent and recurrent problematic gambling behavior leading to clinically significant impairment or distress, as indicated by the individual exhibiting four (or more) of the following in a 12-month period:

1. Needs to gamble with increasing amounts of money in order to achieve the desired excitement.

2. Is restless or irritable when attempting to cut down or stop gambling.

3. Has made repeated unsuccessful efforts to control, cut back, or stop gambling.

4. Is often preoccupied with gambling (e.g., having persistent thoughts of reliving past gambling experiences, handicapping or planning the next venture, thinking of ways to get money with which to gamble).

5. Often gambles when feeling distressed (e.g., helpless, guilty, anxious, depressed).

6. After losing money gambling, often returns another day to get even ("chasing" one's losses).

7. Lies to conceal the extent of involvement with gambling.

8. Has jeopardized or lost a significant relationship, job, or educational or career opportunity because of gambling.

9. Relies on others to provide money to relieve desperate financial situations caused by gambling.

B. The gambling behavior is not better explained by a manic episode.

Specify if:

Episodic: Meeting diagnostic criteria at more than one time point, with symptoms subsiding between periods of gambling for at least several months.

Persistent: Continuous symptoms for multiple years.

Current Severity: Mild (4–5 criteria met); Moderate (6–7 criteria met); Severe (8–9 criteria met).

be done quickly anytime, and anywhere with a few taps on a mobile device. Research has found that mobile gambling has reached new audiences especially younger people who utilize smartphone technology. Through the use of smartphones, mobile gambling apps are able to personalize gambling and advertise gaming incentives in ways that traditional or even other forms of online gambling cannot. Gambling through an app also removes any stigma or shame associated with placing a bet directly with another person, which has been linked to an increase in sports gambling among young men. Gambling apps prompt users of gambling opportunities and utilize data such as the users' location, list of contacts, credit card balance, and use history. These sophisticated apps have access to valuable information that prompts gambling behaviors that was not available in traditional land-based gaming. Research has found that simulated gambling games on mobile devices can encourage real money gambling (Whelan, Laato, Islam, & Billieux, 2021). Those who spend more time playing a simulated gambling game were more likely to engage in real money gambling. At this time, there is no evidence to support that playing the simulated gaming helped people reduce their gambling behaviors (Rockloff et al., 2020).

Concerns about COVID-19-related consequences of online gambling behavior have also been raised since increased time spent at home, online, and worry about the future may affect gambling behavior (Håkansson, 2020). Studies have found that both anxiety and boredom are associated with problem gambling, both of which can be expected to increase during uncertain and threatening times and in connection with social distancing procedures introduced to reduce COVID-19 transmission. To what extent new gamblers who had never previously wagered online began doing so during the COVID-19 outbreak is of particular interest to researchers (Lindner, Forsström, Jonsson, Berman, & Carlbring, 2020). Those classified as high-risk gamblers and those with past experience of online gambling displayed an increased likelihood of online gambling during the COVID-19 crisis. Among high-risk online gamblers, the most predictive risk factors included moderate and severe anxiety and depression, reduced work hours, gambling under the influence of cannabis or alcohol, belief that gambling would reduce feelings of anxiety or depression, chasing gambling losses and seeking to earn income (Price, 2020).

Pathological gamblers also tend to have problems with substance use, depression, and anxiety and a family history of substance abuse and gambling problems (Petry et al., 2018). Gambling disorder is more common among men than women, among non-Hispanic Blacks than other racial/ethnic groups, and among people with less than a college education (Dowling et al., 2017; Kessler et al., 2008). Men tend to develop the disorder earlier in life, while women are more likely to show mid- or later-life onset gambling disorder.

Gambling disorder appears to be related to the same brain areas (i.e., activation of the brain's reward system) as the substance use disorders and to disruption in systems regulating the neurotransmitter dopamine (Leeman & Potenza, 2012). People with gambling disorder also show high levels of impulsivity, as do people with substance use disorders, as well as poor performance on cognitive tasks assessing control over impulses (Petry et al., 2018; Potenza et al., 2003).

Cognitive-behavioral therapy (CBT) concentrates on changing the individual's distorted beliefs that they have more control than the average person over gambling (chance) outcomes, overconfidence, and superstitions and on developing new activities and coping strategies to replace gambling. Some controlled studies of CBT have shown that it can help reduce compulsive gambling, although more research is needed (Casey et al., 2017; Håkansson, 2020; Petry, Rash, & Alessi, 2016; Petry et al., 2018). Serotonin reuptake inhibitors and antipsychotic medications have shown only mixed success in treating pathological gambling (Yip & Potenza, 2014). Naltrexone, an opioid antagonist that affects reward sensitivity, shows more promise, but its efficacy is not yet well established (Yip & Potenza, 2014). Very few people with gambling disorder ever seek treatment, however (Kessler et al., 2008), and those that do typically have moderate to severe forms of the disorder.

Gambling disorder is not the only so-called behavioral addiction addressed by the *DSM-5*. **Internet gaming disorder,** while not listed in the *DSM* as an official disorder, appears in the section listing conditions requiring further study. Video games, including multiplayer games played over the Internet, have become wildly popular across the world (Kuss, Griffiths, & Pontes, 2017). For a minority of people, playing such games can take on a pathological quality, affecting their well-being and occupational and social lives. Criteria for Internet gaming disorder include persistent engagement and preoccupation with gaming, tolerance, withdrawal, loss of interest in other activities, and clinically significant impairment or distress (American Psychiatric Association, 2013). Research to define and study Internet gaming disorder is well underway, along with substantial differences of opinion in the field as to whether it is even a true mental disorder (Kuss et al., 2017; Petry et al., 2018). Nevertheless, the World Health Organization announced in 2018 that it would include it, as "gaming disorder," in the addictive disorders section of the *ICD-11*, the newest edition of the international classification system used worldwide (WHO, 2018d).

Some believe other behaviors may also qualify as behavioral addictions when they meet certain criteria and severity. These include Internet addiction, sex addiction, porn addiction, and food addiction (Petry et al., 2018). These are very controversial, not yet well defined, and do not appear in the *DSM-5* as conditions requiring further study. Nevertheless, they are likely to be of greater interest as gambling disorder and gaming disorder attract attention. These issues reflect the challenges in defining "addiction," defining "substance," and distinguishing frequent behavior from pathological abuse or dependence.

CHAPTER INTEGRATION

The substances discussed in this chapter are powerful biological agents. They affect the brain directly, producing changes in mood, thoughts, and perceptions. Some people may be genetically or biochemically predisposed to find these changes more positive or rewarding than other people do (Figure 4). Rewards and punishments in the environment clearly can affect an individual's choice to pursue the effects of substances, however. Even many long-term chronic substance abusers can abstain given strong environmental and social support for abstention.

People who find substances more rewarding, for biological and/or environmental reasons, develop expectations that the substances will be rewarding, which in turn enhance how rewarding they actually are. Likewise, heavy substance users choose friends and situations that support their substance use. They tend to find partners who are also heavy substance users, creating a biological and psychosocial environment for their children that increases vulnerability to substance use disorders. Thus, the cycle of familial transmission of substance misuse has intersecting biological and psychosocial components.

Similar processes may play out in gambling disorder, and potentially Internet gaming disorder as well. For example, biological factors may influence how rewarding an individual finds gambling. The person will then associate with other gamblers, who reinforce the gambling behavior, and eventually the impulse to gamble may become pathological.

The COVID-19 pandemic has created many additional challenges for patients with substance use

| FIGURE 4 | Integration of Biological and Psychosocial Factors in the Development of Substance-Related Disorders. |

disorders. As a result of this crisis, many addiction treatment and harm reduction organizations have had to reduce their hours and services for people with substance use disorders, placing these individuals at increased risk of death. Telemedicine may be a solution for many people without proper access to mental health services by delivering mental health services through live video technology. This is supported as an effective tool in the diagnosis and assessment of mental health disorders in a variety of populations across different settings.

SHADES OF GRAY DISCUSSION

Nick's behaviors definitely meet the criteria for an alcohol use disorder. He is failing to fulfill his obligations at school and is continuing to use alcohol despite social problems (ejection from the campus and his parents' threat to withdraw their support). His hangovers are a sign of withdrawal, he spends much time drinking and recovering, and his drinking is hurting his grades. We don't know whether Nick has developed tolerance to alcohol, although the escalation of his drinking suggests that he needs more alcohol to achieve the desired effect. Nick doesn't seem to have

any intention of cutting back on his drinking, so the criteria for attempting to control his substance use have not been met.

It may seem odd to think of a college student who drinks with his friends as having a psychiatric diagnosis. Some critics argue that the criteria for alcohol use disorders are too broad and that too many individuals meet them. Others argue that simply because a large percentage of the population meet the criteria for abuse or dependence doesn't mean we should ignore their behavior. What do you think?

CHAPTER SUMMARY

- A substance is any natural or synthesized product that has psychoactive effects. The five groups of substances most often leading to substance disorders are (1) central nervous system depressants, including alcohol, barbiturates, benzodiazepines, and inhalants; (2) central nervous system stimulants, including cocaine, amphetamines, nicotine, and caffeine; (3) opioids; (4) hallucinogens and phencyclidine; and (5) cannabis.

- Substance intoxication is indicated by a set of behavioral and psychological changes that occur as a direct result of the physiological effects of a substance on the central nervous system. Substance withdrawal is a set of physiological and behavioral symptoms that result from the cessation of or reduction in heavy and prolonged use of a substance. The specific symptoms of intoxication and withdrawal depend on the substance being used, the amount ingested, and the method of ingestion.

- Substance use disorders are characterized by a maladaptive pattern of substance use leading to significant problems in a person's life, tolerance to the substance, withdrawal symptoms if it is discontinued, and compulsive substance-taking behavior.

- At low doses, alcohol produces relaxation and mild euphoria. At higher doses, it produces classic signs of depression and cognitive and motor impairment. A large proportion of deaths due to accidents, murders, and suicides are alcohol-related. Withdrawal symptoms can be mild or so severe as to be life-threatening. People with alcohol use disorders experience a wide range of social and interpersonal problems and are at risk for many serious health problems.

- Benzodiazepines and barbiturates can cause an initial rush and a loss of inhibitions, followed by depressed mood, lethargy, and physical signs of central nervous system depression. These substances are dangerous in overdose and when mixed with other substances.

- Cocaine activates those parts of the brain that register reward and pleasure and produces an instant rush of euphoria, followed by increased self-esteem, alertness, and energy and a greater sense of competence, creativity, and social acceptability. The user also may experience frightening perceptual changes. The symptoms of withdrawal from cocaine include exhaustion, a need for sleep, and depression. Cocaine's extraordinarily rapid and strong effects on the brain's reward centers seem to make it more likely than most illicit substances to lead to abuse and dependence.

- Amphetamines are readily available by prescription to treat certain disorders but often end up available on the black market. They can make people feel euphoric, invigorated, self-confident, and gregarious, but they also can lead to restlessness, hypervigilance, anxiety, aggressiveness, and several dangerous physiological symptoms and changes.

- Nicotine is widely available. Smoking tobacco is legal, but it causes cancer, bronchitis, and coronary heart disease in users and low birth weights in the children of women who smoke when pregnant. People become physiologically dependent on nicotine and undergo withdrawal when they stop smoking.

- The opioids are developed from the juice of the poppy plant. The most commonly used illegal opioid is heroin. The initial symptom of opioid intoxication is euphoria, followed by drowsiness, lethargy, and periods of light sleep. Severe intoxication can lead to respiratory difficulties, unconsciousness, coma, and seizures. Withdrawal symptoms include dysphoria, anxiety, agitation, sensitivity to pain, and a craving for more of the substance.

- The hallucinogens, phencyclidine (PCP), and cannabis produce perceptual changes, including sensory distortions and hallucinations. These experiences are pleasant for some, frightening for others. Some people experience a sense of euphoria or relaxation from using these substances, and others become anxious and agitated.

- The inhalants are volatile agents that people sniff to produce a sense of euphoria, disinhibition, and increased aggressiveness or sexual performance. They are extremely dangerous; even casual use may cause permanent brain damage or serious disease.

- Some additional drugs of abuse are ecstasy (3,4-methylenedioxymethamphetamine, or MDMA), GHB (gamma-hydroxybutyrate), ketamine, and rohypnol (flunitrazepam). These drugs have several euphoric and sedative effects and are used at dance clubs and sometimes by perpetrators of date rape.

- All substances of abuse have powerful effects on areas of the brain involved in the processing of reward. Repeated use of substances can cause alterations in these brain areas that increase the need for more of the substance in order to experience rewarding effects.

- Evidence indicates that genes play a role in vulnerability to substance use disorders through their effects on the synthesis and metabolism of substances.

- Behavioral theories of alcoholism note that people are reinforced or punished for their alcohol-related behaviors and also engage in behaviors modeled by important others. Cognitive theories argue that people who develop alcohol-related problems have expectations that alcohol will help them feel better and cope better with stressful events. One personality characteristic associated with substance use disorders is behavioral undercontrol.

- Men may have more risk factors for substance use than women, and women may be more sensitive to the negative consequences of substance use than men.

- Medications can ease withdrawal symptoms and reduce cravings for many substances. The symptoms of opioid withdrawal can be so severe that dependents are given methadone as they try to discontinue heroin use. Methadone also blocks the effects of subsequent doses of heroin, reducing the desire to obtain heroin. Methadone maintenance programs are controversial.

- People with alcohol use disorder sometimes respond to behavior therapies based on aversive classical conditioning. They use a drug that makes them ill if they ingest alcohol or imagery that makes them develop a conditioned aversive response to the sight and smell of alcohol. Contingency management programs provide incentives for reducing substance use.

- Cognitive therapies focus on training people with alcohol use disorder in developing coping skills and in challenging positive expectations about alcohol's effects.

- Motivational interviewing attempts to empathetically draw out individuals' motivations and their commitment to change their substance use behavior.

- The abstinence violation effect comprises an individual's feeling of guilt over relapse and attribution of relapse to lack of self-control. Relapse prevention programs help identify triggers for relapse.

- The most common treatment for alcohol use disorder is Alcoholics Anonymous (AA), a self-help group that encourages alcoholics to admit their weaknesses and call on a higher power and on other group members to help them abstain from alcohol.

- Prevention programs based on a harm reduction model seek to teach the responsible use of alcohol.

- Gambling disorder is new to *DSM-5* and represents a behavioral addiction. It is characterized by compulsive gambling even in the face of significant social, financial, and psychological consequences. It seems to share many risk factors and clinical patterns with the substance use disorders.

- The COVID-19 pandemic has created significant risks to marginalized individuals, particularly those with substance use disorders. Individuals with substance use disorder already represent an underserved and stigmatized population. Now, with hospitals and clinics focused on COVID-19, these individuals are more likely to encounter additional barriers to healthcare and effective treatment.

- Telemedicine may be a solution for many people without proper access to mental health services by delivering mental health services through live video technology. This is supported as an effective tool in the diagnosis and assessment of mental health disorders in a variety of populations across different settings. Videoconferencing, a type of telemedicine, has the potential to increase access to treatment of psychological disorders, such as substance use disorders. Telemedicine use is growing dramatically and its effects are comparable to in-person treatment, but more research is needed. Various professional organizations are advocating for the expanded use of telemedicine for substance use treatment to facilitate access in areas with few providers or for those who lack of transportation or have physical barriers. It also may help address concerns about privacy and perceived stigma for those with substance use disorder.

KEY TERMS

substance use disorders

gambling disorder

substance

substance intoxication

tolerance

substance withdrawal

depressants

delirium tremens (DTs)

alcohol use disorder

benzodiazepines

barbiturates

stimulants

cocaine

amphetamines

nicotine

caffeine

opioids

hallucinogens

phencyclidine (PCP)

cannabis

inhalants

antagonist drugs

methadone

motivational interviewing

abstinence violation effect

relapse prevention programs

Alcoholics Anonymous (AA)

harm reduction model

Internet gaming disorder

Chapter 15

RichLegg/Getty Images

Health Psychology

CHAPTER OUTLINE

Stress Along the Continuum

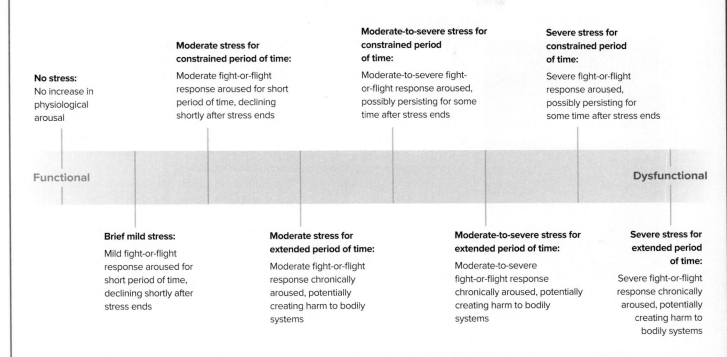

No stress:
No increase in physiological arousal

Brief mild stress:
Mild fight-or-flight response aroused for short period of time, declining shortly after stress ends

Moderate stress for constrained period of time:
Moderate fight-or-flight response aroused for short period of time, declining shortly after stress ends

Moderate stress for extended period of time:
Moderate fight-or-flight response chronically aroused, potentially creating harm to bodily systems

Moderate-to-severe stress for constrained period of time:
Moderate-to-severe fight-or-flight response aroused, possibly persisting for some time after stress ends

Moderate-to-severe stress for extended period of time:
Moderate-to-severe fight-or-flight response chronically aroused, potentially creating harm to bodily systems

Severe stress for constrained period of time:
Severe fight-or-flight response aroused, possibly persisting for some time after stress ends

Severe stress for extended period of time:
Severe fight-or-flight response chronically aroused, potentially creating harm to bodily systems

Functional — Dysfunctional

Anytime we face a stressor, a number of physiological responses kick in, as discussed in the chapter "Trauma, Anxiety, Obsessive-Compulsive, and Related Disorders." Known collectively as the *fight-or-flight response*, bodily changes such as increased heart rate and elevated blood pressure prepare the body to either face the threat or flee from it. The sympathetic system also stimulates the release of a number of hormones—including epinephrine (adrenaline) and norepinephrine—that keep the body ready to react. One of the primary stress hormones is cortisol, which is released by the adrenal cortex. Eventually, when the threatening stimulus has passed, the increase in cortisol signals the body to stop releasing these hormones. This process allows the body to adapt along a continuum of stress.

Even mild stressors trigger the fight-or-flight response. When the stressor is immediate, the response is activated and then subsides. This adaptation is called *allostasis*—the body learns how to react more efficiently to stress when it comes and goes, is not severe, and does not persist for long periods of time (McEwen, 2004; Schulkin & Sterling, 2019). But when a stressor is chronic—that is, when it lasts over a long period of time—and a person or animal cannot fight it or flee from it, then the chronic physiological arousal that results can be severely damaging to the body, a condition known as **allostatic load.**

Persistent uncontrollable and unpredictable stress can create allostatic load. Many factors, including gender, minority status, socioeconomic status, and culture, may affect an individual's exposure to uncontrollable and unpredictable events, perceptions of these events, and reactions to them (Chen & Miller, 2012). For example, many African Americans are exposed to excessive stress due to racism, discrimination, and lower socioeconomic status compared to many European Americans which causes an avalanche of biological processes. Perceived social exclusion and exposure to discrimination increases sympathetic nervous system and hypothalamic-pituitary-adrenal (HPA) axis activation. In turn, African Americans score higher on a number of indicators of chronic stress (*allostatic load*), such as persistent high blood pressure (Geronimus, Hicken, Keene, & Bound, 2006; Goosby, Cheadle, & Mitchell, 2018).

Culture can alter the very meaning of a stressor, even one as severe as homelessness. A study in Nepal found that homeless street children actually showed lower allostatic load than children living with their families in rural villages (Worthman & Panter-Brick, 2008). The homeless children had formed family groups with other street children, protecting one another and collectively finding food and shelter. The rural village children had stable homes, but these homes had poor sanitation, and the children received only subsistence nutrition and faced heavy physical workloads. In more developed countries such as the United States, in contrast, being a homeless street child is associated with more stress and poorer health than is living with family in a rural small town (Worthman & Panter-Brick, 2008).

Extraordinary People

Norman Cousins, *Healing with Laughter*

*Ron Galella/Ron Galella Collection/
Getty images*

In 1964, Norman Cousins, a successful writer at the *Saturday Review,* was diagnosed with ankylosing spondylitis, a painful collagen disease. After many medical tests and days in the hospital, doctors gave him a 1 in 500 chance of living. Cousins refused to believe that he would succumb to the disease and set out to find a course of action that might reverse its progression. His book *Anatomy of an Illness* describes his use of comedy and movies to raise his levels of positive emotions and thereby affect the functioning of his adrenal and endocrine systems:

> Allen Funt, producer of the spoofing television program "Candid Camera," sent films of some of his "CC" classics. It worked . . . I made the joyous discovery that ten minutes of genuine belly laughter had an anesthetic effect and would give me at least two hours of pain-free sleep.
>
> If laughter did in fact have a salutary [beneficial] effect on the body's chemistry, it seemed at least theoretically likely that it would enhance the system's ability to fight the inflammation. We took sedimentation-rate readings just before and hours after the laughter episodes. Each time, there was a drop of at least five points. The drop by itself was not substantial, but it held and was cumulative. I was elated that there is a physiological basis for the ancient theory that laughter is good medicine. (1985, pp. 55–66)*

Cousins eventually recovered from his illness. After returning to his career as a writer for several years, Cousins spent the last 12 years of his life at the UCLA Medical School, working with researchers to find scientific proof for his belief that positive emotions have healing properties. One of the leading institutes for the study of the impact of psychological factors on physical health is now named for him: The Cousins Center for Psychoneuroimmunology at UCLA.

*Source: Cousins, N. *Anatomy of an illness as perceived by the patient.* New York: W.W. Norton & Company, 1985, pp. 55–66.

In the years since Cousins' discovery that laughter was good medicine for him, a considerable number of studies have shown that positive emotions influence physiological functioning (Diener, Thapa, & Tay, 2020; Dockray & Steptoe, 2010). These findings evoke the ancient mind-body question: Does the mind affect the body, or does the body affect the mind? The answer now is clearly that the mind and the body affect each other reciprocally.

In this chapter, we review the research in *health psychology* (also referred to as *behavioral medicine*), a field that explores how biological, psychological, and social/environmental factors interact to influence physical health. Figure 1 illustrates the components of a biopsychosocial approach to physical health (Baum, Perry, & Tarbell, 2004). First, biological factors, such as genetic makeup, age, and sex, clearly have a major influence on our susceptibility to disease. For example, genetics plays a strong role in susceptibility to cancer, the risk of developing most cancers increases with age, and some forms of cancer, such as breast cancer, are much more common in women than in men. Second, social or environmental factors can directly impact health. The factor most often studied by health psychologists is stress, as we discuss in detail below. Another important social factor is culture, which influences our exposure to diseases and the treatments prescribed for these diseases. For example, the human immunodeficiency virus (HIV) is more widespread in sub-Saharan Africa than anywhere else in the world (UNAIDS, 2018), and cultural stigmas against condom use have played a role in the spread of HIV in this region. Third, a number of psychological factors can impact health. We can engage in behaviors that enhance our health, such as exercising regularly and brushing our teeth, or in behaviors that promote disease, such as smoking and eating fatty foods. When we are ill, we can seek treatment and follow our doctor's orders, or we can avoid treatment or not comply with the doctor's orders.

In addition to their individual direct effects on health, biological, psychological, and social/environmental factors all interact to influence health. Consider a few examples: Genetics not only influences our vulnerability to a particular disease but also influences how much stress we are exposed to in our life and our perceptions of stress (Kendler, Karkowski, & Prescott, 1999; Kendler et al., 2010). In turn, stress can make it more difficult to engage in healthy behaviors such as getting enough exercise. Our personalities influence how much stress we perceive in our lives, which in turn affects our health. What's more, our social experiences in day-to-day life can affect our internal biological functioning and contribute to mental heath problems and physical disease, as in the case of racial and ethnic discrimination (Lewis, Cogburn, & Williams, 2015). Throughout this chapter, we discuss how interactions among biological, psychological, and social/environmental factors promote or damage health.

As a field, health psychology has grown rapidly in recent decades as psychological and social/environmental factors have become increasingly important determinants of both the length and the quality of our lives. At the beginning of the twentieth century, the leading causes of death, in addition to cardiovascular disease, were primarily infectious diseases, including influenza, pneumonia, and tuberculosis (Table 1). Over the past century, advances in medicine have greatly reduced the number of deaths due to these diseases. In the twenty-first century, the five leading causes of death are diseases significantly influenced by psychological and social factors such as smoking, diet, and stress. Thus, understanding how psychological and social/environmental factors interact with each other and with biological vulnerabilities to create disease is a critical part of maintaining people's physical health.

FIGURE 1 Components in a Biopsychosocial Approach to Physical Health.

Source: Baum, A., Perry, N. W., Jr., & Tarbell, S. (2004). The development of psychology as a health science. In T. J. Ball, R. G. Frank, A. Baum, & J. L. Wallander (Eds.), *Handbook of clinical health psychology: Volume 3. Models and perspectives in health psychology* (pp. 9–28). Washington, DC: American Psychological Association.

PSYCHOLOGICAL FACTORS AND GENERAL HEALTH

We all know people who seem to be able to handle even severe stress extremely well—they bounce back from difficult times with renewed vigor, feeling as though they have grown psychologically from their stressful experiences. We call these people *resilient* (Johnson, 2016; Masten & Powell, 2003). Other people, however, are more fragile—even mild stresses overwhelm them and seem to lead to psychological and physical decline.

TABLE 1 Leading Causes of Death in the United States, 1900 and 2015

1900		2015	
Cause	Rate (per 100,000)	Cause	Rate (per 100,000)
1. Cardiovascular diseases (heart disease, stroke)	345	1. Heart disease	197
2. Influenza and pneumonia	202	2. Cancer	185
3. Tuberculosis	194	3. Chronic lower respiratory diseases	48
4. Gastritis, duodenitis, enteritis, and colitis	143	4. Accidents	46
5. Accidents	72	5. Cerebrovascular diseases	44

Source: Data for 1900: U.S. Bureau of the Census, *Historical Statistics of the United States: Colonial Times to 1970, I.* Washington, DC: U.S. Government Printing Office Table 1, 1975, 429; Data for 2015: Murphy, Xu, Kochanek, Curtin, & Aria. (2017). Deaths: Final data for 2015. *National Vital Statistics Reports, 66(4),* 2017.

Appraisals and Pessimism

One difference between resilient and fragile people is the way they appraise or interpret events. People who tend to have a pessimistic style of interpreting events—seeing negative events as their fault, likely to continue in the future, and having wide consequences—go through life seeing stress around every corner (Carver & Scheier, 2014; Peterson, Seligman, Yurko, Martin, & Friedman, 1998). Pessimism may contribute to poor health by causing chronic arousal of the body's fight-or-flight response, resulting in physiological damage. Several studies have found evidence for this explanation. In one study, the blood pressure of pessimists and optimists was monitored daily for 3 days. The pessimists had chronically higher blood pressure levels than the optimists across the 3 days (Raikkonen, Matthews, Flory, Owens, & Gump, 1999). Other studies find that adults who are pessimistic show poorer immune system functioning than those who are optimistic, even after researchers statistically control for differences between the pessimists and optimists on other measures of current health (see Carver & Scheier, 2014; Rasmussen, Scheier, & Greenhouse, 2009).

A pessimistic outlook also may lead people to engage in unhealthy behaviors. People who are more pessimistic are less likely to practice healthy behaviors, such as maintaining a proper diet, getting enough sleep, abstaining from smoking, and exercising (Carver & Scheier, 2014; Hingle et al., 2014). The effects of pessimism may be lifelong. In a long-term study of men in the Harvard classes of 1939 and 1940, those who were pessimistic in college were more likely to develop physical illness over the subsequent 35 years than were those who were more optimistic in college (Peterson, Seligman, & Vaillant, 1988).

In short, a pessimistic outlook may affect health directly by causing hyperarousal of the body's physiological response to stress or indirectly by reducing positive coping strategies and healthy behaviors. In contrast, an optimistic outlook, such as the outlook Norman Cousins attempted to create in himself through laughter, may promote physical health by reducing physiological stress responses and promoting positive coping strategies (Carver & Scheier, 2014; Scheier & Carver, 2018).

Coping Strategies

The ways people cope with illness and other stressful life circumstances can affect their health (Taylor & Stanton, 2007). One method of coping that can be bad for health is avoidance coping, that is, denying that you are ill or are facing other obvious stresses. Multiple meta-analyses have linked avoidance coping to several health-related problems, including postsurgical pain, poor adherence to medical regimens, and health-risk behaviors, as well as chronic disease progression and mortality for people with cancer, HIV/AIDS, and heart failure (Kvillemo & Bränström, 2014; Marroquín, Tennen, & Stanton, 2017).

In contrast, talking about negative emotions and important issues in one's life appears to have positive effects on health. Social media platforms, including online public health communities like Reddit, have become popular resources that enhance social support. Research has found that online health communities can help individuals to cope with and manage their illnesses while reducing barriers such as, geographical isolation, physical limitations, and disease stigma. For example, a recent study found that one in four Internet users living with a chronic condition desired peer support among those with a similar condition. Peers can also offer emotional support and advise on illness management that can provide positive benefits. Online interactions have been shown to improve depression, anxiety, stress, and negative mood, as well as facilitate coping and empowerment (Park, Conway, & Chen, 2018).

In a large series of studies, James Pennebaker (2007) found that encouraging people to reveal personal traumas in diaries or essays improves their health. In one study, 50 healthy college students were randomly assigned to write either about the most traumatic and upsetting events in their lives or about trivial topics for 20 minutes on 4 consecutive days. Blood samples were taken from the students on the day before they began writing, on the last day of writing, and 6 weeks after their writing. The students' blood was tested for several markers of immune system functioning. The number of times the students visited the college health center over the 6 weeks following the writing task was also recorded and was compared with the number of health center visits the students had made before the study. As Figure 2 shows, students who revealed their personal traumas in their essays showed more positive immune system functioning and visited the health center less frequently than did students in the control group (Pennebaker, Kiecolt-Glaser, & Glaser, 1988). In contrast, the group who wrote about trivial events experienced a slight increase in health center visits and a decrease in immune system functioning, for unknown reasons.

Pennebaker (2007) believes that writing helps people understand and find meaning in the events of their lives. Understanding and finding meaning in turn reduce people's negative emotions regarding events and therefore may reduce the physiological strain associated with chronic negative emotions. Indeed, multiple studies have found that coping by "approaching" one's emotions rather than avoiding them can have psychological and physical benefits, not only for healthy people but also for people coping

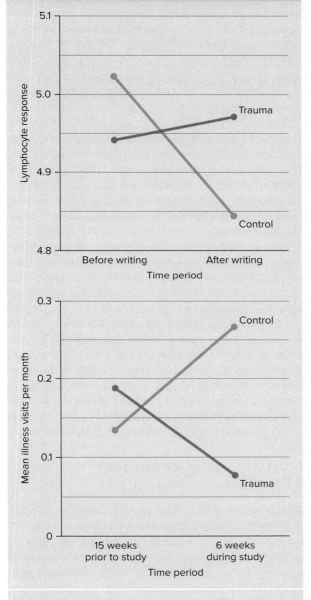

FIGURE 2

Students' Health After Writing About Traumas or Trivialities. Students who revealed personal traumas in a series of essays had stronger immune system functioning and fewer health care visits than students who wrote about trivial events in their essays.

Source: Pennebaker, J. W., Kiecolt-Glaser, J. K., & Glaser, R. (1988). Disclosure of traumas and immune function: Health implications for psychotherapy. *Journal of Consulting and Clinical Psychology, 56,* 239–245.

people who seek and receive positive emotional support from others show more positive health outcomes, both on microlevel measures such as immune system activity and on macrolevel outcomes such as the progression of major diseases (Robles, Slatcher, Trombello, & McGinn, 2014; Uchino, 2009). Shelley Taylor and colleagues found that young adults who had grown up in supportive families showed less reactivity in certain areas of the brain to emotionally provocative photos (Taylor, Eisenberger, Saxbe, Lehman, & Lieberman, 2006). This reduced emotional reactivity could reduce physiological reactivity to stress in these individuals. Social support can be soothing in itself, but it can also help facilitate other healthy coping behaviors by encouraging or assisting more effective actions (see Marroquín et al., 2017).

Gender Differences in Coping

Women and men appear to have different responses to stress. Taylor and colleagues (2000; Taylor & Master, 2011) have suggested that women faced with threats engage in a pattern termed *tend and befriend*. Throughout evolutionary history, women have not been as physically capable as men of fighting off aggressors; also, because they have had primary responsibility for their offspring, they have not always been able to run from an aggressor. Instead of attempting to fight a threat or flee from it, women join social groups for protection and resources (Robert, Virpi, & John, 2019). Underlying this behavioral response to stress by women is a different neurobiological response to stress: The physiological changes associated with the fight-or-flight response are less prominent in women than in men, but stressed women experience the release of the hormone oxytocin, which is associated with increased affiliative behavior such as seeking out and caring for others.

Women are indeed more likely than men to seek support from others in times of stress and to have larger social networks, including friends and extended family (Kiecolt-Glaser & Newton, 2001; Kiecolt-Glaser, & Wilson, 2017). Men, in contrast, typically have a much smaller network of people they turn to for support and also are less likely than women to share personal issues and concerns with friends and family members. Thus, women may have more opportunity than men to benefit from the positive health effects of social support.

A major source of support is a partner or spouse. Married people have less physical illness and are less likely to die from a variety of conditions, including cancer, heart disease, and surgery, than nonmarried people (see Kiecolt-Glaser & Newton, 2001; Robles et al., 2014). A conflictual marriage, however, can be a major detriment to health (Kiecolt-Glaser & Wilson, 2017; Robles et al., 2014). Experimental studies of

with illness, including cancer (Moreno, Wiley, & Stanton, 2017; Stanton et al., 2000).

A related positive coping strategy is seeking social support. A wide variety of studies have found that

SHADES OF GRAY

As you read the following case study, ask yourself whether it presents a healthful way of coping with a stressful event.

John Park is a 62-year-old engineer, originally from South Korea and now living in Columbus, Ohio. John recently received news from his physician that he has prostate cancer. The urologist John consulted recommended that he undergo radiation therapy to treat it. John told his wife about the diagnosis and treatment, but he did not tell his children, all of whom are grown and living in other cities. John also did not tell any of his co-workers about the cancer. He took vacation time to receive treatment and recover from its aftereffects. John and his wife seldom spoke about the cancer. He preferred to go on with his life, living as normally as possible. He did enjoy talking with his wife about their children's lives, their grandchildren's escapades, and upcoming visits with friends and family.

Is John coping in a healthful way with his cancer? (Discussion appears at the end of this chapter.)

married couples found that those who became hostile and negative toward each other while discussing marital problems showed greater decreases in four indicators of immune system functioning than couples who remained calm and nonhostile while discussing marital problems. Those who became hostile also showed elevated blood pressure for longer periods of time (Kiecolt-Glaser, Malarkey, Chee, & Newton, 1993).

Women are more physiologically reactive than men to marital conflict (Kiecolt-Glaser & Newton, 2001; Kiecolt-Glaser & Wilson, 2017). This may be because women's self-concepts, as well as their financial well-being, tend to be more closely tied to those of their spouse than are men's self-concepts (Cross & Madson, 1997). Women are also more emotionally attuned to their partners, more conscious of conflict in their relationships, and typically occupy a more subordinate societal role (Wanic & Kulik, 2011). For these reasons, women may be more emotionally, cognitively, and physiologically sensitive to marital conflict, and this sensitivity may counteract any positive health effects they might derive from support from their partner (Kiecolt-Glaser & Newton, 2017; Robles et al., 2014). In general, women can benefit physiologically from being in a close relationship, but only if that relationship is a positive one.

Cultural Differences in Coping

Different cultures have different norms for coping with stressful events. People from Asian cultures tend to be more reluctant than European Americans to reach out to others for social support or to express their personal concerns, because they are more concerned about potential harm to their relationships if they do so (Ford & Mauss, 2015; Kim, Sherman, & Taylor, 2008). People from Asian cultures instead may find ways to benefit from their social networks that don't involve revealing personal concerns or weaknesses or potentially burdening others. For example, they may remind themselves of their close relationships or simply enjoy the company of people they love. Studies of Asians and Asian Americans find that they derive more emotional and physiological benefit (in terms of lower cortisol levels) from this subtler, more implicit form of seeking social support than from explicitly asking others for support or revealing their needs (Kim et al., 2008). In contrast, European Americans benefit more from explicit forms of seeking social support than from implicit forms. Thus, while coping is important to health in all cultures, the specific forms of coping that are helpful may be influenced by cultural norms.

Another example of cultural differences involves religion and spirituality. Overall, people who describe themselves as religious or spiritual tend to have better physical health, partly because these factors are often linked with social support, coping, and optimism. These factors can be considered individual-level variables, but they also draw on particular cultural aspects of religion and spirituality (Masters & Hooker, 2013).

Psychological Disorders and Physical Health

People with psychological disorders have more physical health problems than people without psychological disorders. For example, a 20-year-long study of people who had been diagnosed with a psychological disorder found that they had more physical health problems throughout this period than people without a psychological disorder (Chen et al., 2009). Serious health problems included severe allergies, chronic respiratory disease, chronic gastrointestinal disease, cardiovascular disease, cancer, and diabetes. In particular, several studies have found links between depression and a variety of diseases, including cancer, heart disease, diabetes, arthritis, and asthma (Scott et al., 2016).

There may be many mechanisms linking psychological disorders with physical health problems. These include shared genetic causes; medical disorders contributing to psychological disorders; and psychological disorders contributing to medical disorders, elevated stress, impaired coping, or unhealthy behaviors. In some cases, psychopathology and medical illness may share a common genetic cause. For example, depression and cardiovascular disease are both related to genetic factors leading to dysfunction in serotonin systems (McCaffery et al., 2006). In other cases, medical disorders may create psychological disorders. Alzheimer's disease, a neurological disorder leading to dementia, also leads to depression, anxiety, personality changes, and psychotic symptoms such as hallucinations and delusions (see the chapter "Neurodevelopmental and Neurocognitive Disorders"). Thyroid diseases can cause depressive symptoms. Further, the social and psychological stress of having a serious medical illness can cause depression or anxiety (Hammen, 2018).

In still other cases, psychological disorders may contribute to medical disorders. Self-starvation in anorexia nervosa creates an increased risk of metabolic and autoimmune disorders, such as type 1 diabetes. This disorder can also lead to osteoporosis and loss of bone density as well as to cardiovascular problems (Johnson et al., 2021; Polivy & Herman, 2002). Substance abuse or dependence can cause many medical diseases, including hypertension and liver and kidney disease (see the chapter "Substance Use and Gambling Disorders").

Living with a psychological disorder is stressful in many ways. An individual may have difficulty holding down a job, face discrimination and social rejection, and have trouble obtaining medical care. People with many psychological disorders show signs of chronic arousal of the fight-or-flight response, including chronically elevated cortisol levels (McEwen, 2004). This excess allostatic load could in turn contribute to physical illness (Schulkin & Sterling, 2019). Having a psychological disorder also may lead a person to be more pessimistic and to have poorer skills for coping with stress, which could then increase the person's allostatic load. For example, one study found that the greater rate of physical illness in people with depressive disorders than in people with no psychological disorder was explained in part by higher levels of neuroticism in the depressed people (Rhebergen et al., 2010). Neuroticism is a personality trait characterized by hyperreactivity to stress and poor coping skills.

People with psychological disorders also appear to be less likely to engage in positive health-related behaviors (Zvolensky & Smits, 2008). The rate of smoking is two to three times higher in people with psychological disorders than in people without a psychological disorder (Grant, Hasin, Chou, et al., 2004; Lasser et al., 2000). A higher proportion of persons with serious mental illnesses, smoke cigarettes as compared with the general population. It is well documented that smoking contributes to the premature mortality of individuals with serious mental illness. Recent data have found that 64 percent of individuals with schizophrenia and 44 percent with bipolar disorder are current smokers (Dickerson et al., 2018). People with psychological disorders also appear to be less likely to exercise or to comply with medical regimens (Chen et al., 2009; Whooley et al., 2008). These health-related behaviors put the individual at risk for the development or worsening of a medical illness.

PSYCHOSOCIAL FACTORS IN SPECIFIC DISEASES

Health psychologists have intensively studied certain disease processes in which stress and psychological factors are expected to play a role. We consider two groups of diseases here: immune system diseases and cardiovascular diseases.

The Immune System

The **immune system** protects us from disease by identifying and killing pathogens and tumor cells. The immune system is divided into two branches, the *innate immune system* and the *specific immune system,* both of which have a number of cellular mechanisms for attacking invaders. The innate system reacts quickly and nonspecifically to any microorganism or toxin that enters the body, releasing cells that kill and ingest the invaders. The specific immune system is slower to respond, but its response is tailored to the particular type of pathogen present. The specific immune system remembers the pathogen so that if it attacks again the system is able to kill it more quickly and efficiently.

Due to the great strides made in neuroimmunological research, psychological stress has been identified as a significant factor in the development and progression of many physical diseases, such as cancer. Stress can be present in short and intense periods lasting only a few minutes, or chronic lasting for hours or days. Chronic stress is associated with alternations in the hypothalamic-pituitary-adrenal (HPA) axis, activation of sympathetic nervous system (SNS) and other physiological adaptations like hormones secretion which have impacts on physical health (Zhang, Pan, Chen, Jiang, & Huang, 2020).

The gut microbiota has received much recent attention for its influence on human behavior. This diverse collection of microorganisms that inhabit the gastrointestinal tract has been found to profoundly influence many aspects of physiology, including metabolism, resistance to infection, and immune system development. Studies investigating the gut–brain axis

People with relatively high levels of stress are more susceptible to coming down with colds. Stress also contributes to higher levels of herpes, mononucleosis, and other infectious diseases. *tomwang/123RF*

suggest that the gut microbiota play a critical role in the coordination of brain development and behavior, with the immune system emerging as an important regulator of these interactions. Aspects of immune function are influenced by stress and microbiota that result in changes in brain function via the HPA axis (Fung, Olson, & Hsiao, 2017).

These intestinal microbes modulate the maturation and function of immune cells in the central nervous system. Additionally, these microbes also influence the activation of peripheral immune cells, which regulate responses to neuroinflammation, brain injury, autoimmunity, and neurogenesis. Research has found that both the gut microbiota and immune system are implicated in the development of neurodevelopmental, psychiatric, and neurodegenerative diseases, such as autism spectrum disorder, depression, and Alzheimer's disease (Fung, Olson, & Hsiao, 2017; Sanz & Aidy, 2019). For example, research suggests that depression is associated with the gut-brain axis. While the etiology of depression is not fully understood, it is hypothesized that stress-induced changes in neural circuitry and neuroendocrine pathways, activation of the immune system, and interactions between the host and microbiota are strongly associated (Fung, Olson, & Hsiao, 2017).

Stress may affect the immune system in several ways. Numerous studies have identified mechanisms and pathways through which chronic stress suppresses protective immunity (Antoni & Dhabhar, 2019). Although short-term stress appears to increase the potency

of immune responses, more chronic stress decreases immune functioning, in part because some of the biochemicals released as part of the fight-or-flight response, such as cortisol, suppress the immune system if a stressor persists for long periods (Segerstrom & Miller, 2004; Slavich & Irwin, 2014). The most controlled research linking stress and immune system functioning has been conducted with animals. The animals are experimentally exposed to stressors, and then the functioning of their immune system is measured directly. Studies have shown that immune system cells are suppressed in animals exposed to loud noise, electric shock, separation from their mothers as infants, separation from their peers, and a variety of other stressors (Segerstrom & Miller, 2004).

Animals are most likely to show impairment of their immune system if they are exposed to stressors that are uncontrollable. In one experiment, one group of rats was subjected to an electric shock that the rats could turn off by pressing a lever (Laudenslager, Ryan, Drugan, Hyson, & Maier, 1983). Another group received an identical sequence of shocks but could not control the shock. A third group received no shock. The investigators examined how well the rats' killer T-cells, components of the specific immune system that secrete chemicals that kill harmful cells, multiplied when challenged by invaders. They found that the T-cells in the rats that could control the shock multiplied, as did those in the rats that were not shocked at all (Figure 3). The T-cells in the rats exposed to uncontrollable shock increased less, however.

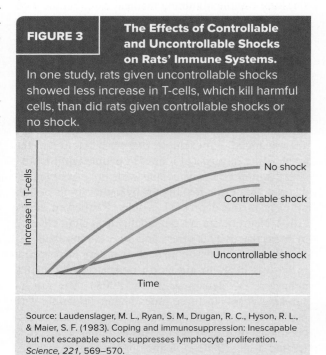

FIGURE 3   **The Effects of Controllable and Uncontrollable Shocks on Rats' Immune Systems.**

In one study, rats given uncontrollable shocks showed less increase in T-cells, which kill harmful cells, than did rats given controllable shocks or no shock.

Source: Laudenslager, M. L., Ryan, S. M., Drugan, R. C., Hyson, R. L., & Maier, S. F. (1983). Coping and immunosuppression: Inescapable but not escapable shock suppresses lymphocyte proliferation. *Science, 221,* 569–570.

In another study following the same experimental design, investigators implanted tumor cells into rats, gave them controllable or uncontrollable shocks, and examined whether the rats' natural defenses rejected the tumors. Only 27 percent of the rats given uncontrollable shocks rejected the tumors, whereas 63 percent of the rats given controllable shocks rejected the tumors (Visintainer, Volpicelli, & Seligman, 1982).

Uncontrollable stress also impairs immune system functioning in humans (Schneiderman, Ironson, & Siegel, 2005; Slavich & Irwin, 2014). The most common disease in which the immune system plays a role is the cold. You may have observed that you and your friends are more likely to get colds during times of stress. To test this common observation, investigators exposed about 400 healthy volunteers to a nasal wash containing either one of five cold viruses or an innocuous salt solution (Cohen, Tyrrell, & Smith, 1991). Participants received a stress score ranging from 3 (lowest stress) to 12 (highest stress) based on the number of stressful events they had experienced in the past year, the degree to which they felt able to cope with daily demands, and their frequency of negative emotions such as anger or depression. The participants were examined daily for cold symptoms and for the presence of cold viruses in their upper respiratory secretions. About 35 percent of the volunteers who reported the highest stress in their lives developed colds, compared to about 18 percent of those with the lowest stress scores.

Negative interpersonal events seem particularly likely to affect immune system functioning. Married couples who argue more show poorer immunological functioning than married couples who have fewer arguments (Kiecolt-Glaser & Wilson, 2017; Robles et al., 2014). Men and women who have recently been separated or divorced show poorer immune system functioning than married control subjects (Robles & Kiecolt-Glaser, 2003). However, the partner who has more control over the divorce or separation—that is, the partner who initiated it—shows better immune system functioning and better health than the other partner. This is another example of how perceptions of the controllability of a stressor can influence the impact of that stressor on health.

Cancer

Can psychosocial factors affect severe immune-related diseases such as cancer? Various studies have found strong support that the increased susceptibility and progression of cancer is associated with chronic stress (Antoni & Dhabhar, 2019; Zhang et al., 2020). One study of women with breast cancer found that those who felt they had little control over their cancer and other aspects of their lives were more likely to develop new tumors over a 5-year period than were women who felt more in control, even though the two groups of women did not differ in the type or initial seriousness of their cancers (Watson, Haviland, Greer, Davidson, & Bliss, 1999). Another study found that pessimistic cancer patients are more likely to die during the first few years after their diagnosis than are optimistic cancer patients (Schulz, Bookwala, Knapp, Scheier, & Williamson, 1996). Coping behaviors also may affect cancer: Studies of women with breast cancer have found that those who seek social support from others have greater immune system activity and lower mortality (Helgeson, Snyder, & Seltman, 2004; Kroenke et al., 2012; Turner-Cobb, Sephton, Koopman, Blake-Mortimer, & Spiegel, 2000).

If psychosocial factors such as social support and pessimism do influence the progression of cancer, this raises the possibility that the course of the disease can be affected by psychosocial interventions. Early studies gave hope. In a landmark study of women with advanced breast cancer who were expected to die within 2 years, one group of women participated in a series of weekly support groups and the other group did not (Spiegel, Bollm, Kraemer, & Gottheil, 1989). All the women received standard medical care for their cancer. The support groups focused on facing death and living their remaining days to the fullest. The researchers did not expect to alter the course of the cancer; they wanted only to improve the women's quality of life. To their surprise, 4 years later one-third of the women participating in the support groups had survived, whereas all the women who had not participated in the support groups had died. The average survival time for the women in the support groups was about 40 months, compared to about 19 months for the other women. Because no other differences between the two populations could explain the disparity in average survival times, it seems that the support groups helped prolong the participants' lives. The authors argued that the support groups reduced stress and distress for the women and thus reduced the release of corticosteroids, which can promote tumor growth (Spiegel, 2001). Having greater support also might help cancer patients engage in better health habits and adhere to difficult medical treatments such as chemotherapy.

Some studies also found that reducing stress can improve health in cancer patients since disease-related distress found across multiple types of cancer (breast, colorectal, prostate, leukemia, and lymphoma) is related to psychosocial adjustment and quality of life. Psychosocial interventions aimed at decreasing stress among cancer patients are helpful in managing and reducing the negative effects of cancer-related stressors. Mindfulness-based stress reduction has shown positive effects on quality of life and decreased stress symptoms in patients with varying cancer diagnoses by teaching clients to focus on what they are sensing and feeling in the moment, without interpretation or judgment (Rush & Sharma, 2017).

In a study of patients with malignant melanoma (skin cancer), some patients were given six weekly treatment sessions in which they were taught stress-management procedures, relaxation, and methods for coping with their illness. Six months after treatment, the group that received the stress-reduction intervention showed better immune system functioning than the control group, whose members received only customary medical care (Fawzy, Cousins, et al., 1990; Fawzy, Kemeny, et al., 1990). At a 5-year follow-up, patients who had received the intervention were less likely to have had recurrences of the cancer and were significantly less likely to have died (Fawzy et al., 1993). At a 10-year follow-up, there were no differences between the intervention group and the control group in recurrences of the cancer, but the intervention group had a higher survival rate than the control group when other risk factors were taken into account (Fawzy, Canada, & Fawzy, 2003).

A controlled trial tested an intervention that targeted stress reduction as well as medication adherence and healthy behaviors, finding that women with breast cancer who received the intervention had a lower risk of death over 11 years than a nonintervention control group (Andersen et al., 2008). Another trial, comparing cognitive-behavioral-based stress management to a psychoeducation-only condition found lower levels of breast cancer recurrence and mortality (Stagl et al., 2015).

It has been demonstrated that stress affects tumor emergence, progression, and metastasis. The immune system is a crucial mediator through which stress affects the course of cancer, although many immune independent mechanisms also are critical mediators of cancer related effects of stress. However, other studies have failed to find any effects of psychosocial interventions on the progression of cancer. For example, a large clinical trial attempting to replicate the effects in the breast cancer study described above (e.g., Fawzy et al., 2003) failed to find any effects of support groups on health in women with breast cancer (Goodwin et al., 2001; see also Kissane et al., 2007). Meta-analyses and reviews of the effects of psychosocial interventions on survival in cancer patients have found modest or no effects (Edwards, Hulbert-Williams, & Neal, 2008; Mustafa, Carson-Stevens, Gillespie, & Edwards, 2013). However, psychosocial interventions have been found to improve cancer patients' quality of life and depressive symptoms (Antoni & Dhabhar, 2019; Gudenkauf et al., 2015), and this is an important aspect of cancer treatment and survivorship. Researchers continue to hone interventions to target the factors that are most important in psychosocial interventions for cancer, such as cognition and coping strategies (Stanton, Luecken, MacKinnon, & Thompson, 2013).

HIV/AIDS

The Centers for Disease Control estimates that over a million people in the United States have been infected with the human immunodeficiency virus (HIV), which causes AIDS (CDC, 2018f). Worldwide, over 35 million people are infected with HIV (WHO, 2018b). The progression of illness in people infected with HIV varies greatly. Individuals may live for years with no symptoms, then begin to develop relatively minor health problems such as weight loss, fever, and night sweats. Eventually, they may develop a number of serious and potentially fatal diseases, including pneumocystis pneumonia, cancer, dementia, and a wasting syndrome in which the body withers away. When these diseases emerge, a diagnosis of AIDS may be given. Fortunately, antiretroviral drugs appear to suppress the virus in those infected and to slow the development of AIDS. Unfortunately, these drugs do not eliminate the virus, and their side effects lead many people to discontinue their use. Moreover, millions of people around the world who are infected do not have access to these drugs.

Approximately, 40 percent of people living with HIV do not sufficiently adhere to their medication therapy, which adversely affects their health (Spaan, van Luenen, Garnefski, & Kraaij, 2020). Some studies suggest that psychological factors can affect the progression of illness in people infected with HIV (Chida & Vedhara, 2009; Kołodziej, 2016; Leserman, 2008). Psychosocial factors that are associated with adverse health include depression, quality of life, social support, cognitive functioning, and coping skills. Research suggests that most psychosocial interventions have small to moderate effects on medication adherence and improving the psychosocial well-being of adults living with HIV or AIDS. Psychosocial interventions have significant implications since adherence to antiretroviral therapy (ART) is widely associated with disease suppression and lower transmission risk. These interventions may relieve significant stressors like stigma, depressive disorders, and lack of social support (Spaan, van Luenen, Garnefski, & Kraaij, 2020).

The development and widespread use of ART has enabled people with HIV to live longer, healthier lives. As a result, there is a large population of aging adults with HIV. In 2018, more than half of individuals living with HIV in the United States were 50 years and older, and it is estimated that by 2030 this number will increase to 64 percent. This rapidly growing segment of older adults living with HIV brings new and complex challenges. In addition to the biomedical risks such as cardiovascular disease, cancer, and osteoporosis, older adults with HIV report facing psychosocial challenges that include social isolation, stigma, and higher rates of depression as compared with their younger counterparts. Additionally, this group faces increased amounts of stigma that strongly affects the quality of life of older adults living with HIV. Many older adults living with HIV in the United States experience a "triple stigma" due to age, HIV status, and, for many, sexual and gender minority status. Therefore, the complications of aging with HIV present a unique set of physical and mental health-related challenges (Bhochhibhoya et al., 2020).

Experiencing more chronic stressors also appears to affect the progression of HIV in gay men. A study of HIV-positive gay men found that those who felt compelled to conceal their sexual orientation showed a faster progression of disease than those who did not (Cole, Kemeny, Taylor, Visscher, & Fahey, 1995). The differences in health between the men who were "out" and those who were "closeted" did not reflect differences in health-related behaviors (e.g., smoking, exercise). It may be that the stress of chronically hiding one's identity can have direct effects on health (e.g., Hatzenbuehler, 2009). More generally, researchers found that HIV-positive men who experienced declines in social support and increases in loneliness showed poorer immune system control over the virus (Dixon et al., 2001).

Stress also affects the progression of the disease in children and adolescents who have been infected with HIV. In a year-long study of 618 HIV-positive young people, those who experienced two or more stressful life events, such as a parent becoming seriously ill, a death in the family, or the loss of their home, were three times more likely than other participants to show immune system declines (Howland et al., 2000).

Even stressors experienced long before an individual is infected with HIV seem to increase the risk for disease progression. The Coping with HIV/AIDS in the Southeast (CHASE) Study followed 490 HIV-positive adult men and women from five rural southern U.S. states for up to 41 months (Leserman et al., 2007). Those with a history of trauma, including childhood physical or sexual abuse or neglect or the murder of a family member, showed faster development of opportunistic infections and were more likely to die of AIDS-related causes than those without a history of trauma (Mugavero et al., 2007).

Interpretations of stressors appear to be important moderators of their effects. In one study of 412 patients with HIV, those who scored high on questionnaires measuring pessimism at the beginning of the study had a greater load of the virus 18 months later than did those who initially were less pessimistic (Milam, Richardson, Marks, Kemper, & McCutchan, 2004). Similarly, a study of gay men who were HIV-positive found that those who blamed themselves for negative events and those who had more negative expectations showed a greater decline in immune system functioning and a greater development of HIV symptoms over time than did those who had more positive expectations (Reed, Kemeny, Taylor, & Visscher, 1999; Segerstrom, Taylor, Kemeny, Reed, & Visscher, 1996). In fact, a meta-analysis of 37 prospective studies suggests that psychological variables (including coping and personality) were better predictors of HIV progression than stressful events or social support (Chida & Vedhara, 2009).

Coronary Heart Disease and Hypertension

Orrin was having a *myocardial infarction*—a heart attack. A myocardial infarction is one end point of **coronary heart disease,** or **CHD.** CHD occurs when the blood vessels that supply the heart muscles are narrowed or closed by the gradual buildup of a hard, fatty substance called *plaque* and inflammation of the vessel walls, blocking the flow of oxygen and nutrients to the heart. This process is known as *atherosclerosis.* The blockage of vessels can lead to pain, called *angina pectoris,* that radiates across the chest and arm. When oxygen to the heart is completely blocked, a myocardial infarction can result.

CASE STUDY

Orrin was so mad he could scream. He had been told at 3:00 that afternoon to prepare a report on the financial status of his division of the company in time for a meeting of the board of directors the next morning. On the way home from work, someone rear-ended him at a stoplight and caused several hundred dollars in damage to his new car. When he got home from work, there was a message from his wife, saying she had been delayed at work and would not be home in time to cook dinner for the children, so Orrin would have to do it. Then, at dinner, Orrin's 12-year-old son revealed that he had flunked his math test that afternoon.

After finishing the dishes, Orrin went to his study to work on the report. The kids had the TV on so loud that he couldn't concentrate. Orrin yelled to the kids to turn off the TV but they couldn't hear him. Furious, he stalked into the family room and began yelling at the children about the television and anything else that came to his mind.

Then, suddenly, Orrin began to feel a tremendous pressure on his chest, as if a truck were driving across it. Pain shot through his chest and down his left arm. Orrin felt dizzy and terrified. He collapsed onto the floor. His 7-year-old began screaming. Luckily, his 12-year-old called 911 for an ambulance.

CHD is a leading cause of death and chronic illness around the world. Since 1990, more people have died from CHD than from any other cause (WHO, 2018a). In the United States, CHD accounts for 25 percent of all deaths (CDC, 2018e). CHD is also a chronic disease, and more than 15 million Americans live daily with its symptoms. Men are more prone to CHD than are women, but CHD still is the leading cause of death among women. African Americans and Hispanic Americans have higher rates of CHD than do European Americans. There seems to be a genetic contribution to CHD—people with family histories of CHD are at increased risk for the disease. However, 80 to 90 percent of people dying from CHD have one or more major risk factors that are affected by lifestyle choices, such as high blood pressure, high serum cholesterol, diabetes, smoking, and obesity (WHO, 2018a).

People who live in a chronically stressful environment over which they have little control appear to be at increased risk for CHD (Steptoe & Kivimäki, 2013). A study of 30,000 people in 52 countries found that

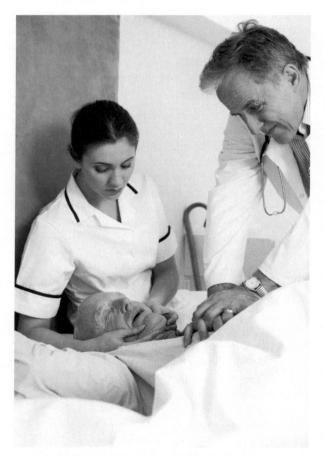

Coronary heart disease occurs when blood vessels supplying the heart are blocked by plaque; complete blockage causes a myocardial infarction—a heart attack. High levels of stress have been shown to increase rates of coronary heart disease. *Dean Mitchell/Getty Images*

about one-third of the risk for heart disease is connected to the stressfulness of people's environments (Rosengren et al., 2004; Yusuf et al., 2004). People in high-stress jobs are at increased risk for CHD, particularly if their jobs are highly demanding but provide them little control (Hintsanen et al., 2005; Schneiderman et al., 2005). For example, one study followed about 900 middle-aged men and women over 10 years and tracked the emergence of CHD (Karasek, Russell, & Theorell, 1982). The people in the study worked in a variety of jobs, and the researchers categorized these jobs in terms of how demanding they were and how much control they allowed a worker. Over the 10 years of this study, workers in jobs that were highly demanding but low in control, such as working on a factory production line, had a risk of CHD 1.5 times greater than that of workers in other occupations.

Experimental studies with animals have shown that disruption of the social environment can induce pathology that resembles coronary artery disease (Crestani, 2016; Sapolsky, 2007). Some of these experiments have been conducted with a type of macaque monkey whose social organization involves the establishment of stable hierarchies of dominance—dominant and submissive animals can be identified within a given group on the basis of the animals' social behavior. Introduction of unfamiliar monkeys into an established social group is a stressor that leads to increased aggressive behavior as group members attempt to reestablish a social dominance hierarchy (Sapolsky, 2007). In these studies, some monkey groups remained stable, with fixed memberships, and other groups were stressed by the repeated introduction of new members. After about 2 years under these conditions, the high-ranking or dominant males in the unstable social condition showed more extensive CHD than did the subordinate males (Sapolsky, 2007).

Hypertension, or high blood pressure, is a condition in which blood flows through vessels with excessive force, putting pressure on vessel walls. Hypertension can be caused by blood being pushed with too much force by the heart through vessels or by constriction of the vessel walls. Chronic high blood pressure can cause hardening of the arterial walls and deterioration of the cell tissue, leading eventually to CHD, kidney failure, and stroke. Almost one-third of the population of the United States has hypertension (Merai et al., 2016). As in CHD, genetics appears to play a role in the predisposition to hypertension, but only about 10 percent of all cases of hypertension can be traced to genetics or to specific organic causes, such as kidney dysfunction. The other 90 percent of cases are known as *essential hypertension,* meaning that the causes are unknown.

Because part of the body's response to stress—the fight-or-flight response—is to increase blood pressure, it is not surprising that people who live in chronically stressful circumstances are more likely to develop hypertension (Schneiderman et al., 2005; Steptoe & Kivimäki, 2013). As an example, people who move from quiet rural settings to crowded, noisy urban settings show increases in their rates of hypertension.

One group that lives in chronically stressful settings and has particularly high rates of hypertension is low-income African Americans (CDC, 2018e). They often lack adequate financial resources for daily living, may be poorly educated and have trouble finding good jobs, live in neighborhoods racked with violence, and frequently experience racism. All these conditions have been linked to higher blood pressure (Chen & Miller, 2012; Lehman, Taylor, Kiefe, & Seeman, 2009).

People with hypertension and the children of parents with hypertension tend to show a stronger blood pressure response to a wide variety of stressors. In experimental situations that have people solve arithmetic problems or immerse their hands in ice water, those with no personal or family history of hypertension show much less blood pressure response than do those with a history of hypertension (Harrell, 1980). In addition, it takes longer for the blood pressure of persons with hypertension to return to normal following exposure to stressors than it does the blood pressure of those without hypertension.

Thus, people with hypertension and people with family or genetic histories of hypertension may have a heightened physiological reactivity to stress. If they are exposed to chronic stress, their chronically elevated blood pressure can lead to hardening and narrowing of the arteries, creating a physiologically based hypertension. Low-income African Americans may have both this physiological predisposition to heightened reactivity to stress and chronic exposure to stressful environments, making them doubly vulnerable to hypertension (Lehman et al., 2009).

Personality and CHD

The personality factor traditionally linked to CHD is the **Type A behavior pattern.** The three components of the Type A pattern, according to the physicians who identified it (Friedman & Rosenman, 1974), are a sense of time urgency, easily aroused hostility, and competitive striving for achievement. People who are Type A are always in a hurry, setting unnecessary deadlines for themselves and trying to do multiple things at once. They are competitive, even in situations in which being competitive is ridiculous. They also are chronically hostile and will fly into a rage with little provocation.

One of the most compelling studies to demonstrate the relationship between the Type A pattern and CHD followed more than 3,000 healthy middle-aged men for 8½ years (Rosenman et al., 1976). Over the years of the study, Type A men had twice as many heart attacks or other forms of CHD as non–Type A men. These results held up even after diet, age, smoking, and other variables associated with CHD were taken into account. Other studies have confirmed this twofold risk and have linked Type A behavior to heart disease in both men and women (Myrtek, 2007; Schneiderman et al., 2005). In addition, Type A behavior is correlated with the severity of coronary artery blockage as determined at autopsy or in X-ray studies (Friedman, Rosenman, Straus, Wurm, & Kositcheck, 1968; Williams, Barefoot, Haney, & Harrell, 1988). Based on such evidence, in 1981 the American Heart Association classified Type A behavior as a risk factor for CHD.

Subsequent research suggests that the definition of Type A behavior as originally formulated is too diffuse. The crucial variable in predicting CHD may be hostility, particularly a cynical form of hostility characterized by suspiciousness, resentment, frequent anger, antagonism, and distrust of others (Chida &

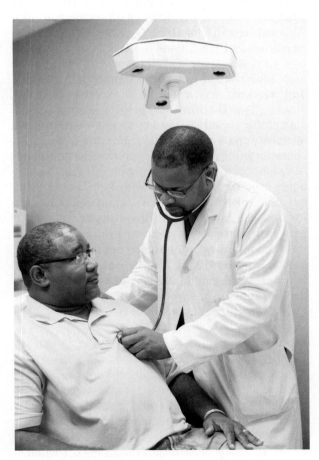

People who live in stressful settings are more likely to experience hypertension than are people who live in quieter and more secure surroundings. One group that disproportionately lives in chronically stressful settings and has particularly high rates of hypertension are low-income African Americans.
ERproductions Ltd/Blend Images/Getty Images

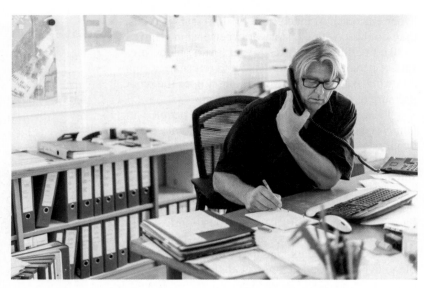

Individuals with Type A personalities often put heightened stress on themselves, which may put them at risk for coronary heart disease. *Westend61/Getty Images*

Steptoe, 2009; Miller, Smith, Turner, & Guijarro, 1996; Wong, Na, Regan, & Whooley, 2013). Time urgency and competitiveness appear to be less predictive of heart disease.

How does hostility lead to CHD? Again, over arousal of the SNS may play a role. Hostile people show greater physiological arousal in the anticipation of stressors and in the early stages of dealing with stressors. Their heart rates and blood pressures are higher, and they have greater secretion of the stress-related biochemicals known as catecholamines. They also return more slowly to baseline levels of SNS activity following stressors than do nonhostile people. This hyperreactivity may cause wear and tear on the coronary arteries, leading to CHD. Alternately, the excessive secretion of catecholamines in response to stress in hostile people may exert a direct chemical effect on blood vessels. The frequent rise and fall of catecholamine levels may cause frequent changes in blood pressure, reducing the resilience of the blood vessels. Hostile people also tend to engage in behaviors that increase their propensity for heart disease, including smoking, heavy drinking, and high-cholesterol diets (Schneiderman et al., 2005; Wong et al., 2013).

Some research has suggested that men are more likely than women to have the Type A personality pattern. Men also are more likely than women to carry three other risk factors for CHD: smoking, hypertension, and elevated cholesterol. Historically, far more men than women die of cardiovascular disease. In recent years, however, the number of women dying of cardiovascular disease has increased worldwide, while the number of men dying of cardiovascular disease has decreased (Sanchis-Gomar, Perez-Quilis, Leischik, R., & Lucia, 2016). Contrary to popular belief, women

carry as much anger and hostility as men—they just don't express it as readily (Brody, Hall, & Stokes, 2016; Lavoie, Miller, Conway, & Fleet, 2001). Excessive hostility and anger, whether expressed or suppressed, are associated with risk factors for CHD in both women and men (Matthews, Owens, Kuller, Sutton-Tyrrell, & Jansen-McWilliams, 1998; Wong et al., 2013).

Type-B individuals have a more relaxed, lower stress demeanor that is quite the reverse to Type-A individuals. Those with Type B traits tend to have less interpersonal conflicts and achieve goals in a steady way unlike Type As who generally work racing against the clock. These even-tempered and adaptable Type B traits tend allow these individuals to adjust and adapt to events in the environment and are not associated with any physical health problems (Lateef, Dahar, & Yousuf, 2019). While CHD-prone personality (Type A) is associated with neuroticism and extraversion, some research on Type C personality suggests that individuals with disordered self-image, impaired self-esteem, and behaviors associated with abnormal expression of emotions have higher risks of developing cancer. Although research on Type C personality traits is a heavily studied topic, there is a lack of agreement on how to define these specific type C traits and the associated risks of cancer development (Rymarczyk, Turbacz, Strus, & Cieciuch, 2020; Wei et al., 2019).

The **Type D (*Distressed*) behavior pattern** personality profile is characterized by high levels of negative affectivity and social inhibition. Negative affectivity is characterized by the tendency to experience feelings of dysphoria, anxiety, and irritability. The social inhibition experienced by people with Type D personality describes the tendency to inhibit emotions and behavior in social interactions. This distressed (Type D) personality profile is associated with emotional distress and negative cardiovascular outcomes. Research has found a strong association between type D personality traits and cardiovascular disease, hypertension and susceptibility to myocardial infarction (Kupper & Denollet, 2018; Timmermans et al., 2019).

Modifying Hostility to Improve Cardiovascular Functioning

A combination of cognitive and behavioral techniques has been shown to improve cardiovascular health by reducing Type A behavior, particularly hostility (Williams, 2008). One hallmark study included more than 1,000 individuals who had experienced at least one heart attack (Friedman et al., 1994). Treatment helped hostile participants learn to express themselves without exploding and to alter certain behaviors, such as interrupting others or talking or eating hurriedly. This treatment also targeted other aspects of Type A behavior, because the study was done before hostility was identified as the key factor. Participants were taught to overcome their sense of time urgency by practicing standing in line (which Type A individuals find irritating) and using the opportunity to reflect, to watch people, or to strike up a conversation with a stranger. Cognitive techniques helped participants reevaluate certain beliefs (such as the notion that success depends on the quantity of work produced) that might lead to urgent and hostile behavior. Also, participants found ways to make their home and work environments less stressful, such as by reducing unnecessary social engagements. By the end of the study 4½ years later, the intervention group had experienced half as many new heart attacks as the group whose participants were not taught to alter their lifestyles. Some cognitive-behavioral treatments that emphasize stress management and coping show effects on cardiovascular health (e.g., Gulliksson et al., 2011), but others do not. A meta-analysis of studies testing multiple types of psychological intervention found effects on mortality due to cardiac events, but not on other aspects of cardiovascular health (Whalley, Thompson, & Taylor, 2014).

Depression and Coronary Heart Disease

Major depression occurs in 15 to 20 percent of hospitalized patients with CHD, and up to 50 percent have some depressive symptoms (Steptoe, & Kivimäki, 2013; Whooley & Wong, 2013). There are several other variables that could account for the link between depression and CHD. The blocked arteries that lead to CHD also lead to reduced oxygen in the brain and the marshaling of the immune system, both of which can contribute to mood changes, including depression. Both CHD and depression may be caused by a relative deficiency in the polyunsaturated omega-3 fatty acids, found primarily in fatty fish (Ali et al., 2009). And, as noted earlier, both depression and CHD are linked to genes that alter the functioning of the serotonin system (Whooley & Wong, 2013).

Still, several studies suggest that depression doubles the risk of recurrent heart attacks and mortality in individuals with CHD (Whooley & Wong, 2013). For example, one study of patients with CHD found that those diagnosed with major depression were more than twice as likely to have a heart attack or some other major cardiac event (e.g., emergency heart surgery) over a 2-year follow-up period, even after taking into account a number of other risk factors for heart disease, such as age and high blood pressure (Frasure-Smith & Lesperance, 2008).

Depression could contribute to CHD through several pathways. Depression is associated with reduced heart rate variability (i.e., less variation from heartbeat to heartbeat), which is an indication of poorer functioning of the autonomic nervous system. In turn, low heart rate variability and other dysfunction of the SNS are risk factors for CHD. Other pathways include inflammation, activation of the HPA axis and stress hormones, and effects on blood vessels (Whooley & Wong, 2013).

Depressed people with CHD are less likely than nondepressed people with CHD to engage in behaviors that could reduce their risk of future cardiac events, such as eating a low-fat diet and increasing their exercise (Gehi, Haas, Pipkin, & Whooley, 2005; Whooley & Wong, 2013; Ziegelstein et al., 2000). In one longitudinal study of 1,017 adults with CHD, those who were depressed were more likely than those who were not depressed to smoke, to be less physically active, to not take prescribed medications, and to have a higher mean body mass index (Whooley et al., 2008). The depressed patients experienced 50 percent more cardiac events (e.g., heart attacks) over the 4-year follow-up than did the nondepressed patients. The depressed patients' poor health behaviors accounted for their increased risk of cardiac events even after controlling for a number of physiological risk factors and possible third variables. In particular, the depressed patients' lower level of physical exercise accounted for 31 percent of the difference in cardiac events between the depressed and the nondepressed patients.

These results suggest that increasing physical exercise is an important target of intervention for depressed patients with CHD. Exercise is effective in reducing both CHD and depression (Blumenthal et al., 2005, 2007). Attempts to reduce depression in CHD patients through the use of antidepressants or cognitive-behavioral therapy have had success in treating depression, but with limited effects on the CHD (Whalley et al., 2014; Whooley & Wong, 2013). Still, depression likely contributes to CHD and other cardiovascular diseases (such as stroke) through other mechanisms as well, including social isolation, smoking, and medication nonadherence (Whooley & Wong, 2013).

INTERVENTIONS TO IMPROVE HEALTH-RELATED BEHAVIORS

We know that our behaviors have a large influence on our health, yet most of us do not follow the recommendations of experts. Why? According to health psychologists, it takes more than information to change people's actions. People must have the motivation to change their behavior, believe they can change it, and have the skills to do so (Ajzen, 1991; Bandura, 2006; H. Leventhal, Weinman,

E. Leventhal, & Phillips, 2008). Here we consider some attempts to give people the tools they need to change their health-related behaviors.

Guided Mastery Techniques

Guided mastery techniques provide people with explicit information about how to engage in positive health-related behaviors and with opportunities to do so in increasingly challenging situations. The goals are to increase people's skills as well as their beliefs that they can engage in the behaviors, known as *self-efficacy beliefs* (Bandura, 2006; Bandura, 2019; Pirolli et al., 2021). The kinds of actions that might be targeted include using condoms during sex in order to prevent the spread of HIV and other sexually transmitted diseases (STDs), refusing alcohol when being pressured to drink, and starting an exercise program.

A guided mastery program for teaching women how to negotiate safe sexual practices might begin with information on condom use. A counselor then might model how a woman can ask a man to use a condom. The women would watch the counselor and then practice insisting on condom use in role-plays with the counselor or other group participants. In this role playing, the women would face increasingly difficult challenges to their insistence on condom use, learn strategies for meeting these challenges, and practice using those strategies. The women might also be taught to determine when it is useless to argue any longer and skills for removing themselves from unsafe sexual encounters.

Guided mastery techniques were used successfully in a program with African American women called Sister-to-Sister: The Black Women's Health Project Intervention (Jemmott, Jemmott, & O'Leary, 2007). In five short interventions, nurses gave women information about the cause, transmission, and prevention of STDs. The women then participated in guided mastery exercises to increase their skills and self-confidence for negotiating condom use by their male partners. The women also learned to eroticize condom use by incorporating putting on condoms into foreplay and intercourse in ways that increase positive attitudes toward their use. Compared to women who received only information, without guided mastery exercises, these women showed greater confidence in negotiating condom use and a stronger intention to use condoms (O'Leary, Jemmott, & Jemmott, 2008). Most important, the program resulted in lower sexual risk behavior and lower incidence of STDs over the 12 months following it.

Cultural norms regarding health behaviors can affect people's willingness to engage in them (Ajzen, 1991). Programs like the guided mastery program described above have been adapted to address cultural norms that might encourage or interfere with targeted health behaviors (Bandura, 2006). For example, a strong cultural value in many Hispanic groups is *familism,* or prioritizing the respect and care of one's family over one's individual needs. One study of Hispanic adolescents adapted a guided mastery program to include discussions of the impact of risky sexual behaviors on the loved ones of the adolescents (Koniak-Griffin et al., 2008). The adolescents in this program were all teen parents, so the program materials focused on cultural values of parental protectiveness, using traditional teachings of Chicano, Latino, and Native American ancestors. The adolescents who received this culturally adapted intervention showed greater increases in condom use than a comparison group of adolescents who received only general information about HIV prevention. This is an example of how culturally modified interventions and cultural sensitivity, as discussed in the chapter "Theories and Treatment of Abnormality," can also be important in interventions targeting physical health.

Internet-Based Health Interventions

Millions of people around the world get health information from the Internet every day. The Web can deliver high-quality health information and interventions to promote behaviors that improve health. Moreover, online interventions can be delivered to individuals who might not have access to in-person programs, either because none are available in their area or because they cannot afford them. More than half the world population has access to the Internet, and the majority of Internet users say they get health information off the Web (Vandelanotte et al., 2016; Vandelanotte, Spathonis, Eakin, & Owen, 2007). Controlled studies of the effectiveness of these

Fitness trackers, which are wearable electronic devices or computer applications that record an individual's daily physical activity, are used by many to motivate healthy lifestyle choices.
IGphotography/Getty Images

interventions offer hope that they can be effective in helping people change their behaviors and improve their health.

Many Internet-based behavioral interventions aim to increase people's exercise and improve their diet. Regular physical exercise significantly decreases the risk of cardiovascular disease, diabetes, and several forms of cancer (Ehrman, Gordon, Visich, & Keteyian, 2009). Yet most people do not exercise regularly. Similarly, while eating fresh fruits and vegetables every day reduces the risk of developing several major illnesses, the diets of people around the world increasingly are filled with high-fat, high-sugar, low-nutrition foods (Brownell & Walsh, 2017). As a result, obesity rates are skyrocketing, especially in developed countries. Intensive, in-person programs can spur people to increase their exercise and improve their diet. However, these programs are expensive, time-consuming, and unavailable to many people. The Internet provides the opportunity to deliver exercise and nutrition programs to large segments of the population for a relatively low cost.

One such program was designed by General Electric to improve the health of its workforce (Pratt, Jandzio, Tomlinson, Kang, & Smith, 2006). Employees were invited by e-mail to participate in the program, which involved increasing their daily exercise to 10,000 steps or 30 minutes of moderate-intensity physical exercise, eating five servings of fruits and vegetables a day, and losing weight if significantly overweight. Participating employees completed an online assessment of their current behaviors and physical needs. Based on their profile, they received regular e-mails about their progress in the program, as well as e-newsletters with health tips and case studies of employees who had made major lifestyle changes. They were given phone and e-mail access to nutrition and fitness coaches who could answer their questions and provide personalized advice. Participants discussed exercise and diet in chat rooms. The Weight Watchers program was made available online. The company even created a "video reality series" that followed two employees who were participating in the program.

An evaluation of 2,498 employees across 53 nations who participated in the program for about 8 months showed that these employees significantly increased their physical activity and their consumption of fruits and vegetables (Pratt et al., 2006). They also lost an average of 4 to 5 pounds over the duration of the program.

Reviews of Internet-based programs designed to improve physical activity and diet found that the majority resulted in positive outcomes for participants compared to control groups (Vandelanotte et al., 2016; Vandelanotte et al., 2007). Gains tend to be relatively modest, and they are short-lived if the programs are not continued. Across thousands or even millions of people, however, the potential public health impact of these programs is great. In addition to these interventions focused on health behaviors, other Internet-based self-help interventions are targeted toward people coping with chronic health conditions, like irritable bowel syndrome and chronic pain. A review of such interventions, which largely emphasize cognitive-behavioral techniques, showed that they can be effective in reducing physical symptoms and, to a lesser degree, psychological distress (Beatty & Lambert, 2013).

The new frontier in Internet-based health interventions capitalizes on the increased use of mobile devices, like smartphones and tablets. Such devices allow people to carry the tool with them, engage with social networks, and in some cases, record diet and physical activity data more accurately (Vandelanotte et al., 2016). Some trials suggest that interventions incorporating apps and social network components are more effective than traditional Internet-delivered interventions (Vandelanotte et al., 2017), although attrition tends to be high, and meta-analyses have found only small effects on health behavior (e.g., Maher et al., 2014). Vandelanotte and colleagues (2016) note that empirically based techniques for behavior change are currently not used in most popular apps, and that future development in this area may improve outcomes.

SLEEP AND HEALTH

Getting enough sleep is critically important to health. People who sleep fewer than 6 hours each night have a 70 percent higher mortality rate than those who sleep at least 7 or 8 hours each night (Ikehara et al., 2009; Kryger, Roth, & Dement, 2017). This is true for both men and women, for people of many ethnicities, and for people with many different health backgrounds. Lack of sleep weakens the immune system (Irwin, 2015; Irwin & Opp, 2017). Among middle-aged adults, those who sleep less show greater development of heart disease over time (King et al., 2008). People who work rotating shifts have higher rates of illness, including cardiovascular and gastrointestinal disease, than other people (Ohayon, Smolensky, & Roth, 2010).

Sleep deprivation also has many psychological effects: It impairs memory, learning, logical reasoning, arithmetic skills, complex verbal processing, and decision making. For example, reducing your amount of sleep to 5 hours each night for only 2 nights significantly reduces performance on math problems and creative-thinking tasks. This means that staying up to study for exams for only a couple of nights can significantly impair the ability to do well on those exams (Wolfson, 2010). Sleep deprivation also causes irritability, emotional ups and downs, and perceptual distortions, such as mild hallucinations (Harvey, 2008a). Sleep-deprived individuals are more reactive to both positive and negative emotional stimuli, but their emotional expressions and abilities to perceive others' emotions are blunted, which can cause problems during the day (Goldstein & Walker, 2014).

Sleep deprivation can literally kill. Each year in the United States, 7 percent of all car crashes and 16 percent of all car-crash deaths are due to driver sleepiness (National Transportation Safety Board, 2018). Over half of automobile drivers admit to having driven when drowsy at least once in the past year, and 28 percent say they have fallen asleep at the wheel (National Sleep Foundation, 2009). Medical professionals work longer hours than members of almost any other profession, and as many as 98,000 deaths occur annually in the United States due to medical errors—many associated with sleep deprivation. Some of the most serious disasters in modern history have been the result of mistakes made by sleepy people (M. Mitler & J. Miller, 1995). In 1979, the worst nuclear plant accident in the United States occurred when fatigued workers at Three Mile Island failed to respond to a mechanical problem at the plant. In 1986, the world's worst nuclear disaster happened in Chernobyl in Ukraine (then part of the Soviet Union) during a test conducted by an exhausted team of engineers. In 2008, a Boston trolley car crashed into a stopped trolley after the driver of the first vehicle ran a red light; the National Transportation Safety Board concluded that the driver went into a "microsleep"—falling asleep for only a few seconds—resulting in the crash and her death (Ahlers, 2009).

It is frightening to realize that sleep deprivation is so widespread. Over half of Americans say they chronically feel sleep deprived (Hirshkowitz et al., 2015; National Sleep Foundation, 2009); about 9 percent of men and 13 percent of women say they are chronically severely sleepy (Ohayon, 2012). Young adults need, on average, 9.2 hours of sleep each day. Yet most young adults sleep 7.5 or fewer hours each day (National Sleep Foundation, 2009). Similarly, most middle-aged adults need at least 7 or 8 hours of sleep each day, but most get fewer than 7 hours. People who work rotating shifts or in jobs demanding long periods of activity, such as nurses, doctors, firefighters, police, and rescue personnel, often are chronically sleep deprived (Chatzitheochari & Arber, 2009). Even when they have time to sleep, they have trouble falling asleep because their body's natural rhythms have been disrupted by their irregular schedule. The effects of sleep deprivation are cumulative. A person builds up an increasing "sleep debt" for every 24-hour period in which he or she does not get adequate sleep, and on average, Americans incur 26 minutes of sleep debt per day (Kryger et al., 2017; National Sleep Foundation, 2015).

Stress is a frequent contributor to sleep problems. A 2009 poll taken during a period of economic crisis found that one-third of Americans were losing sleep over the state of the U.S. economy and personal financial matters (National Sleep Foundation, 2009). A 2015 poll showed that 43 percent reported moderate, severe, or very severe stress, and the more stress people experienced, the shorter the duration and poorer the quality of their sleep (National Sleep Foundation, 2015). In general, Americans are sleeping less while trying to cram more and more into the day, including multiple jobs, exercise, socializing, and school. Similar patterns are found in other developed countries, including Great Britain (Chatzitheochari & Arber, 2009). Over the past century, the average night's sleep time in these societies has declined more than 20 percent (National Sleep Foundation, 2009).

Assessing Sleep

What is sleep? Analysis of brain-wave activity suggests that there are five stages of sleep: four differing depths of sleep and a fifth stage known as rapid eye movement (or REM) sleep (Figure 4). When a person

| FIGURE 4 | **EEG Recordings During Various Stages of Sleep.** |

The awake stage (relaxed with eyes closed) is characterized by alpha waves (8 to 12 hertz). Stage 1 is basically a transition from wakefulness to the deeper stages of sleep. Stage 2 is defined by the presence of sleep spindles (brief bursts of 12- to 16-hertz waves) and K-complexes (a sharp rise and fall in the brainwave pattern). Stages 3 and 4 are marked by the presence of delta waves (1 to 12 hertz), and the only difference between these two stages is the amount of delta waves found. Stage 3 is scored when 20 to 50 percent of the record contains delta waves, and Stage 4 when the percentage of delta waves is 50 percent or more.

Awake

Stage 1

Stage 2

Sleep spindle   K-complex

Stage 3

Delta wave

Stage 4

REM sleep

closes eyes and relaxes, the brain waves characteristically show a regular pattern of 8 to 12 hertz (cycles per second); these are known as *alpha waves.* As the individual drifts into Stage 1 sleep, the brain waves become less regular and have lower amplitude (in other words, they go up and down less, reflecting less electrical activity). Stage 2 includes spindles—short runs of higher-frequency activity of 12 to 16 hertz— and an occasional sudden sharp rise and fall in the amplitude of the entire EEG (this is referred to as a K-complex). The still deeper Stage 3 and Stage 4 are characterized by slow waves of 1 to 2 hertz, known as *delta waves.*

After an adult has been asleep for an hour or so, the EEG becomes very active. Electrodes near the person's eyes detect pronounced REMs. This stage is known as *REM sleep;* the other four stages are known as *non-REM* (or *NREM*) *sleep.* The stages alternate throughout the night, beginning with the NREM stages. Several sleep cycles occur, each containing some REM and some NREM sleep. There usually are four or five distinct REM periods over the course of an 8-hour night's sleep, with an occasional brief awakening as morning arrives. Dreaming occurs during REM sleep.

The pattern of the sleep cycles varies with a person's age. Newborn infants, for instance, spend about half their sleeping time in REM sleep. This drops to 20 to 25 percent of total sleep time by age 5 and remains fairly constant until old age, when it drops to 18 percent of total sleep time or less. Older people tend to experience less Stage 3 and Stage 4 sleep (sometimes these stages disappear) and more frequent and longer nighttime awakenings (Zdanys & Steffens, 2015).

A comprehensive assessment of how people sleep can be obtained by a *polysomnographic* (*PSG*) evaluation. This requires individuals to spend one or more nights in a sleep lab, connected to instruments that measure respiration and oxygen desaturation (a measure of airflow), leg movements, eye movements, brain-wave activity, and heart activity (Buysse, Ancoli-Israel, Edinger, Lichstein, & Morin, 2006). This evaluation gives the sleep specialist the data to determine what aspects of sleep may be irregular (for example, if a person is waking during REM of NREM sleep, or whether awakenings are related to low oxygen levels). An alternative is for individuals to wear a wristwatch-like device called an *actigraph,* which records movement (Irwin, 2015; Morgenthaler et al., 2007). The data it gathers can be compared to known patterns of movement during sleep to determine when individuals are awake or asleep.

These methods of assessing sleep are objective and detailed, but they also are expensive and require special equipment. More frequently, people are asked

Busy students are often sleep deprived. *Yellow Dog Productions/The Image Bank/Getty Images*

to keep a detailed diary of their sleep patterns (what time they go to bed, when they awaken during the night, and when they get up in the morning). Questionnaires may be used to assess people's sleep patterns even more quickly.

Sleep Disorders

Some people experience so much difficulty sleeping that they may be diagnosed with a sleep-wake disorder. Disturbances in sleeping or staying awake can occur for many reasons. They may be the result of another psychological disorder. In particular, insomnia is a symptom of unipolar depression and co-occurs at high rates in bipolar disorder, schizophrenia, attention-deficit/hyperactivity disorder, the anxiety disorders, and substance use disorder (Harvey, 2008a). The symptoms of these disorders, such as anxiety, can make it difficult to sleep. In turn, insomnia can worsen the symptoms of these other disorders, perhaps in part because people who are sleep deprived are more emotionally reactive and have more difficulty regulating their emotions. They also have more difficulty functioning in their daily life due to decreased concentration and performance, leading to the further accumulation of stressors (Harvey, 2008b). Sleep plays a key role in maintaining healthy functioning of the emotional parts of the brain for people in general, but a vicious cycle of psychological symptoms and insomnia among people with psychiatric conditions can make healthy sleep especially important (Goldstein & Walker, 2014).

Sleep disorders also often result from the physiological effects of a medical condition. Many medical conditions can disturb sleep, including degenerative neurological illnesses, such as Parkinson's disease; cerebrovascular disease, including strokes; endocrine conditions, such as hypo- or hyperthyroidism; viral and bacterial infections, such as viral encephalitis; pulmonary diseases, such as chronic bronchitis; and pain from musculoskeletal diseases, such as rheumatoid arthritis or fibromyalgia (Pack & Pien, 2011). In addition, substances such as illicit drugs, alcohol, or prescription drugs can lead to many sleep disturbances; in such cases, the diagnosis is **substance-induced sleep disorder** (Inkelis, Hasler, & Baker, 2020).

Insomnia

Probably the most familiar sleep-wake disorder is **insomnia disorder**—chronic difficulty initiating or maintaining sleep or sleep that does not restore energy and alertness. Insomnia is a major health issue associated with great psychological burden. People with insomnia usually report a combination of difficulty falling asleep and intermittent wakefulness during the night.

Occasional problems with insomnia are extremely common, with up to 50 percent of adults reporting they have had insomnia at some time in their life and one in three adults complaining they have had insomnia in the past year (National Sleep Foundation, 2015). Episodic insomnia is defined as difficulty falling asleep or staying asleep that lasts only a few days and is an isolated occurrence (Pack & Pien, 2011). This difficulty is often tied to a specific stressor, such as facing a major exam or being in an unfamiliar place, and it stops once the stressor has passed.

The COVID-19 global pandemic provided a new opportunity to explore psychological factors on sleep health. COVID-19-related worry, loneliness, and increased symptoms of depression were all found to be predictive of insomnia in a recent study in Greece. Increased rates of insomnia were reported during the COVID-19 pandemic which was attributed, in part, to rising stress levels and worry about health, financial consequences, changes in social life, and the daily routine during the outbreak. Reduced physical fatigue and exposure to the sun were identified as additional factors, as well as, increased use of electronic devices that may disrupt sleep. COVID-19-related worry, loneliness, uncertainty about viral exposure, and depressive symptoms were significantly associated with insomnia. Feelings of isolation, disruption of daily scheduled and reduced social contact may also contribute to an abnormal sleep-wake schedule (Voitsidis et al., 2020).

The COVID-19 outbreak also caused significant psychological distress and poor sleep quality for medical professionals. Among those frontline medical professionals working in isolated conditions, there was a 1.71-times higher probability of experiencing insomnia. Additionally, working in isolation during the COVID-19 outbreak predicted anger, avoidance behaviors, and more negative outcomes for medical professionals working in longer periods of isolation. Worry about COVID-19 exposure and concerns related to the safety of colleagues and family members, were strongly associated with anger, anxiety, insomnia, and stress among medical professionals. Factors related to insomnia included worry, perceived lack of psychological support through news or social media regarding the COVID-19 outbreak, and extreme uncertainty regarding effective COVID-19 disease control. (Zhang et al., 2020).

Stress increases psychological and physical activation and is associated with the dysregulation of the hypothalamic-pituitary-adrenal (HPA) axis resulting in sleep disorders. This may promote additional increases in the HPA system creating a vicious cycle of stress and insomnia. A longitudinal study showed that during the SARS outbreak, the sleep quality among medical staff was worst during the crisis and gradually improved after 2 weeks, suggesting that insomnia was related to contagion outbreak-induced stress (Zhang et al., 2020). Inflammation, genetic factors, and dysregulation of the circadian rhythm may be implicated in the pathophysiology of insomnia (Voitsidis et al., 2020).

To receive the diagnosis of insomnia disorder, the symptoms of insomnia must occur at least three nights per week for at least 3 months, and the sleep disturbance must cause significant distress or

A familiar sleep-wake order is insomnia, which usually involves a combination of falling asleep and intermittent wakefulness during the night. *Africa Studio/Shutterstock*

TABLE 2 *DSM-5* Criteria for Insomnia Disorder

A. A predominant complaint of dissatisfaction with sleep quantity or quality associated with one (or more) of the following symptoms:

  1. Difficulty initiating sleep. (In children, this may be manifested as difficulty initiating sleep without caregiver intervention.)

  2. Difficulty maintaining sleep, characterized by frequent awakenings or problems returning to sleep after awakenings. (In children this may be manifested as difficulty returning to sleep without caregiver intervention.)

  3. Early-morning awakening with inability to return to sleep.

B. The sleep disturbance causes clinically significant distress or impairment in social, occupational, educational, academic, behavioral, or other important areas of functioning.

C. The sleep difficulty occurs at least 3 nights per week.

D. The sleep difficulty is present for at least 3 months.

E. The sleep difficulty occurs despite adequate opportunity to sleep.

F. The insomnia is not better explained by and does not occur exclusively during the course of another sleep-wake disorder (a parasomnia).

G. The insomnia is not attributable to the physiological effects of a substance (e.g., a drug of abuse, a medication).

H. Coexisting mental disorders and medical conditions do not adequately explain the predominant complaint of insomnia.

Specify if:

With nonsleep disorder mental comorbidity, including substance use disorders

With other medical comorbidity

With other sleep disorder

impairment in functioning (Table 2). Chronic insomnia affects 10 to 15 percent of adults and is more frequent in women than in men and more common in older adults than in younger adults (Riemann et al., 2015; Zhang & Wing, 2006).

When we fall asleep and when we awaken are strongly influenced by our biological rhythms, particularly body temperature rhythms (Lack, Gradisar, Van Someren, Wright, & Lushington, 2008; Riemann et al., 2015). When we are on a schedule of sleeping at night and being awake and active during the day, our core body temperature typically reaches its minimum between 4 and 6 A.M.; falling asleep is easiest 5 to 6 hours before that minimum is reached (between about 11 P.M. and 1 A.M.). Awakening usually occurs 1 to 3 hours after the minimum core body temperature is reached. Some people have disruptions in this body temperature rhythm that interfere with their ability to fall asleep in the late evening or to stay asleep in the early morning (Lack et al., 2008).

Any major stressor can trigger an episode of insomnia, including relationship difficulties, job loss, the death of a loved one, and financial problems. In a vicious cycle, this episodic insomnia can become chronic insomnia. The longer the person lies in bed unable to go to sleep, the more distressed and restless they become. The person's wakefulness then becomes conditioned to the environment—to the bed and bedroom—leading to even more difficulty sleeping the next night.

Cognitive factors help maintain insomnia (Harvey, 2005). First, during the day and when trying to sleep, individuals with insomnia worry about whether they will sleep. They may monitor the clock while trying to fall asleep, worrying more as time passes (Tang, Schmidt, & Harvey, 2007). This worry creates a cognitive and physiological arousal that keeps them awake. Second, they are hypervigilant for things that might keep them awake, such as noises in the environment or bodily aches and pains (Semler & Harvey, 2007). Third, they believe they get less sleep than they do and attribute daytime problems to their insomnia. This cognition feeds their anxiety about their insomnia. Fourth, they engage in counterproductive behaviors to try to help themselves sleep. They may drink alcohol, which can exacerbate insomnia, or avoid social engagements at night, which leaves them with more time alone to worry.

Cognitive-behavioral interventions for insomnia can be highly effective (Harvey et al., 2014; Harvey &

Buysse, 2017; Trauer, Qian, Doyle, Rajaratnam, & Cunnington, 2015). Cognitive techniques aim to reduce worries about sleep ("I wonder if I'm going to have a bad night again tonight!"), unhelpful beliefs about sleep ("Waking up during the night means I haven't slept well at all"), and misperceptions about the effects of sleep loss ("If I don't get 8 hours, I'll be a wreck tomorrow!"). The behavioral techniques include stimulus control, that is, controlling conditions around the person, the ways they prepare for sleep, that might interfere with sleep (Morin et al., 2006). A person experiencing insomnia would be told to do the following:

1. Go to bed only when sleepy.

2. Use the bed and bedroom only for sleep and sex, not for reading, television watching, eating, or working.

3. Get out of bed and go to another room if you are unable to sleep for 15 to 20 minutes, and do not return to bed until you are sleepy.

4. Get out of bed at the same time each morning.

5. Don't nap during the day.

Sleep restriction therapy involves initially restricting the amount of time individuals with insomnia can try to sleep in the night, and is typically part of cognitive-behavioral treatment (Morin et al., 2006). Once they are able to sleep when they are in bed, they are gradually allowed to spend more time in bed. In addition, people often are taught relaxation exercises and are given information about the effects of diet, exercise, and substance use on sleep.

Various medications are used in the treatment of insomnia, including antidepressants, antihistamines, tryptophan, delta-sleep-inducing peptide (DSIP), melatonin, and benzodiazepines (Buysse, Rush, & Reynolds, 2017; Neubauer, Pandi-Perumal, Spence, Buttoo, & Monti, 2018). All these have proven effective in at least some studies, although the number of studies done on most of these agents is small. Those that have the least clear benefit are antihistamines and tryptophan. Those that have proven most reliably effective are benzodiazepines and zolpidem (trade name Ambien). Individuals can become dependent on these sleep aids, however, and may experience withdrawal when they try to stop using them. Rare cases of sleep-eating have been reported among users of Ambien—these users get up during the night and consume large quantities of food, then don't remember doing so in the morning. Insomnia often returns after individuals stop taking the medications, and can even get worse. In contrast, the behavioral and cognitive interventions tend to have long-lasting positive effects (Buysse et al., 2017).

Hypersomnolence Disorders and Narcolepsy

Hypersomnolence disorders are characterized by excessive sleepiness, which can be expressed as an excessive quantity of sleep (also referred to as *hypersomnia*) or a low quality of wakefulness (see Table 3). People with a hypersomnolence disorder are chronically sleepy and sleep for long periods. They may sleep 12 hours at a stretch and still wake up sleepy.

TABLE 3   *DSM-5* Criteria for Hypersomnolence Disorder

A. Self-reported excessive sleepiness (hypersomnolence) despite a main sleep period lasting at least 7 hours, with at least one of the following symptoms:

    1. Recurrent periods of sleep or lapses into sleep within the same day

    2. A prolonged main sleep episode of more than 9 hours per day that is nonrestorative (i.e., unrefreshing)

    3. Difficulty being fully awake after abrupt awakening.

B. The hypersomnolence occurs at least three times per week, for at least 3 months.

C. The hypersomnolence is accompanied by significant distress or impairment in cognitive, social, occupational, or other important areas of functioning.

D. The hypersomnolence is not better explained by and does not occur exclusively during the course of another sleep disorder (e.g., narcolepsy, breathing-related sleep disorder, circadian rhythm sleep-wake disorder, or a parasomnia).

E. The hypersomnolence is not attributable to the physiological effects of a substance (e.g., a drug of abuse, a medication).

F. Coexisting mental and medical disorders do not adequately explain the predominant complaint of hypersomnolence.

A nap during the day may last an hour or more, and they may wake up unrefreshed. If their environment is not stimulating (e.g., during a boring lecture), they are sure to fall asleep. They may even fall asleep while driving. To qualify for a diagnosis, the hypersomnolence must be present at least three times per week for at least 3 months and must cause significant distress or impairment in functioning. Hypersomnolence is a chronic condition that most often begins in early adulthood (Barateau, Lopes, Franchi, & Dauvilliers, 2017; Lee & Kazaglis, 2015). It is estimated that only 1 percent of the population meet the full criteria for a hypersomnolence disorder, but its prevalence is much higher among people with mood disorders (Barateau et al., 2017; Ohayon, Dauvilliers, & Reynolds, 2012).

Narcolepsy involves recurrent attacks of an irrepressible need to sleep, lapses into sleep, or naps occurring within the same day. Sleep episodes generally last 10 to 20 minutes but can last up to 1 hour, and people with narcolepsy move into REM sleep within a few minutes. Most people with narcolepsy experience **cataplexy,** usually characterized by episodes of sudden loss of muscle tone lasting under 2 minutes, triggered by laughter or joking in people who have had narcolepsy for a long time. People with cataplexy may suddenly drop objects, buckle at the knees, or even fall to the ground, but they are not asleep—their hearing and awareness may be normal. More rarely, cataplexy may be characterized by spontaneous grimacing or jaw-opening episodes with tongue thrusting and by low muscle tone. These symptoms tend to occur in children who then go on to develop the more common characteristics of cataplexy (Plazzi et al., 2011). When people with narcolepsy awaken, they may experience brief periods when they can't move or speak, referred to as *sleep paralysis.*

There are two types of narcolepsy. The vast majority of people with symptoms of narcolepsy with cataplexy lack cells in the hypothalamus that secrete the neurotransmitter hypocretin, which promotes wakefulness (Mignot et al., 2002; Pack & Pien, 2011). In contrast, only a minority of people with symptoms of narcolepsy without cataplexy show low levels of hypocretin (Dauvilliers et al., 2003). The *DSM-5* defines narcolepsy as a disorder (see criteria in Table 4) and allows for the specification of whether hypocretin deficiency is involved as a subtype diagnosis. Researchers now believe that deficiencies in hypocretin in the hypothalamus may be due to autoimmune mechanisms—that is, the body's immune system acting against itself (Partinen et al., 2014).

Other biological factors have been implicated in hypersomnia and narcolepsy without cataplexy. Low levels of histamine, another neurotransmitter that promotes wakefulness, have been found in people with these disorders (Kanbayashi et al., 2009; Nishino et al., 2009). Also, hypersomnia and narcolepsy run in families. Specific genes have been implicated in narcolepsy, including genes linked to autoimmune

---

TABLE 4 *DSM-5* Criteria for Narcolepsy

A. Recurrent periods of irrepressible need to sleep, lapsing into sleep, or napping occurring within the same day. These must have been occurring at least three times per week over the last 3 months.

B. The presence of at least one of the following:

1. Episodes of cataplexy, defined as either (a) or (b), occurring at least a few times per month:

   a. In individuals with long-standing disease, brief (seconds to minutes) episodes of sudden bilateral loss of muscle tone with maintained consciousness that are precipitated by laughter or joking.

   b. In children or in individuals within 6 months of onset, spontaneous grimaces or jaw-opening episodes with tongue thrusting or a global hypotonia, without any obvious emotional triggers.

2. Hypocretin deficiency, as measured using cerebrospinal fluid (CSF) hypocretin-1 immunoreactivity values (less than or equal to one-third of values obtained in healthy subjects tested using the same assay, or less than or equal to 110 pgmL). Low CSF of hypocretin-1 must not be observed in the context of acute brain injury, inflammation, or infection.

3. Nocturnal sleep polysomnography showing rapid eye movement (REM) sleep latency less than or equal to 15 minutes, or a multiple sleep latency test showing a mean sleep latency less than or equal to 8 minutes and two or more sleep-onset REM periods.

functioning (Partinen et al., 2014). Hypersomnia often is related to other mental disorders, particularly depression (Barateau et al., 2017; Plante, 2017).

The stimulant modafinil is consistently effective in the treatment of daytime sleepiness in individuals with narcolepsy or hypersomnia (Kallweit & Bassetti, 2017). Other stimulants, including amphetamines, methamphetamine, and methylphenidate, are also used as treatments for daytime sleepiness due to narcolepsy or hypersomnia. Sodium oxybate and selegiline can reduce cataplexy, hallucinations, and sleep paralysis in narcolepsy. In addition, some physicians prescribe antidepressants, although their effectiveness in treating narcolepsy or hypersomnia is less clear (Kallweit & Bassetti, 2017).

Sleep-Related Breathing Disorders

It's difficult to sleep well if you can't breathe well. The *DSM-5* recognizes three sleep disorders related to problems in breathing: central sleep apnea, sleep-related hypoventilation, and obstructive sleep apnea/hypopnea (see Table 5). People with **central sleep apnea** experience complete cessation of respiratory activity for brief periods of time (20 seconds or more) yet do not have frequent awakenings and do not tend to feel tired during the day. Central sleep apnea occurs when the brain does not send the signal to breathe to the respiratory system. It can be caused by central nervous system disorders, including cerebral vascular disease and head trauma; heart disease; and chronic opioid use (Muza, 2015). It also occurs in premature infants. The first line of treatment is to treat the underlying disorder leading to central sleep apnea. **Sleep-related hypoventilation,** a new disorder in the *DSM-5*, is characterized by episodes of decreased breathing associated with high carbon dioxide levels. Unlike hyperventilation, which is breathing too much or too quickly, hypoventilation refers to breathing too little. It is frequently associated with lung disease or diseases of the chest wall (Böing & Randerath, 2015).

By far, the most common **breathing-related sleep disorder** is **obstructive sleep apnea/hypopnea syndrome.** You have probably heard it referred to simply as sleep apnea. As noted above, apneas are brief episodes of complete cessation of breathing.

TABLE 5 *DSM-5* Criteria for Sleep-Related Breathing Disorders

Disorder	*DSM-5* Criteria
Central Sleep Apnea	A. Evidence by polysomnography of five or more central apneas per hour of sleep. B. The disorder is not better explained by another current sleep disorder.
Sleep-Related Hypoventilation	A. Polysomnography demonstrates episodes of decreased respiration associated with elevated CO_2 levels. (Note: In the absence of objective measurement of CO_2, persistent low levels of hemoglobin oxygen saturation unassociated with apneic/hypopneic events may indicate hypoventilation.) B. The disturbance is not better explained by another current sleep disorder.

Obstructive Sleep Apnea/Hypopnea	Either (1) or (2):
	1. Evidence by polysomnography of at least five obstructive apneas or hypopneas per hour of sleep and either of the following sleep symptoms:
	  a. Nocturnal breathing disturbances: snoring, snorting/gasping, or breathing pauses during sleep.
	  b. Daytime sleepiness, fatigue, or unrefreshing sleep despite sufficient opportunities to sleep that is not better explained by another mental disorder (including a sleep disorder) and is not attributable to another medical condition.
	2. Evidence by polysomnography of 15 or more obstructive apneas and/or hypopneas per hour of sleep regardless of accompanying symptoms.
	
	Specify current severity:
	Mild: Apnea hypopnea index is less than 15.
	Moderate: Apnea hypopnea index is 15–30.
	Severe: Apnea hypopnea index is greater than 30.

The CPAP machine helps people with breathing-related sleep patterns. *Amy Walters/Shutterstock*

Hypopneas are episodes of abnormally shallow breathing or a low respiratory rate. To meet the criteria for this diagnosis, an individual has to have evidence from polysomnograph tests showing frequent apneas or hypopneas (see Table 5 for frequencies). People with this disorder may snore loudly, go silent, and stop breathing for several seconds at a time, and then gasp for air. Obstructive sleep apnea/hypopnea occurs when airflow is stopped due to a narrow airway or an obstruction (an abnormality or damage) in the airway. Although it is associated with obesity, hypertension, and diabetes, it also can occur in tonsillitis and other disorders that cause inflammation in the airway. Estimates of prevalence vary widely worldwide, from 9 percent to 38 percent (Lim & Pack, 2017; Senaratna et al., 2017). Higher rates are seen in men than women and at older ages (Senaratna et al., 2017). The dramatic increase in overweight and obesity in recent decades (see the chapter "Eating Disorders") is associated with a major increase in obstructive sleep apnea.

Obstructive sleep apnea/hypopnea syndrome can be treated with a device called a continuous positive air pressure (CPAP) machine. The CPAP machine delivers a stream of compressed air via a hose to a nasal mask, keeping the airway open under air pressure so that unobstructed breathing is possible. CPAP is an effective treatment for obstructive sleep apnea and hypopnea, but 25 to 50 percent of people reject it because it makes them uncomfortable or does not offer sufficient relief from their breathing problems (Veasey et al., 2006). CPAP also is sometimes used to treat central sleep apnea.

Other treatment options include medication and surgery. Drugs that affect the serotonin system, including the serotonin reuptake inhibitors, have shown mixed effects in the treatment of obstructive sleep apnea/hypopnea; stimulants such as modafinil can reduce the daytime sleepiness associated with the disorder (Veasey et al., 2006). Surgery to remove obstructive tissue blocking the airway or to increase the upper airway area can be done in extreme cases, but meta-analyses of the small number of studies on the effectiveness of such surgeries do not show them to be consistently effective in treating the disorder (Franklin et al., 2009).

Circadian Rhythm Sleep-Wake Disorders

As noted, insomnia can be caused by disruptions in biological rhythms, especially core body temperature. These biological rhythms, also known as *circadian rhythms,* are driven by mechanisms in the brain that keep people in sync with the regular patterns of light and dark over the course of the day. These mechanisms are located in a part of the hypothalamus called the superchiasmatic nucleus and modulate daily rhythms in many systems of the body, including sleep and alertness (Riemann et al., 2015; Sack et al., 2007). Circadian rhythms are on a roughly 24-hour clock but can be affected by environmental time signals, especially the solar light/dark signal. Some people have more difficulty than others in adjusting their circadian rhythms after a disruption. Individual differences appear to have genetic roots (Riemann et al., 2015; Sack et al., 2007). If sustained and distressing, such difficulty can be diagnosed as a **circadian rhythm sleep-wake disorder** (Table 6).

The *DSM-5* recognizes five circadian rhythm sleep-wake disorders, each defined by the unique pattern of disturbance. These types are referred to as delayed sleep phase type, advanced sleep phase type, irregular sleep-wake type, non-24-hour type, and shift-work type. *Delayed sleep phase type* involves a persistent pattern of delayed sleep onset and awakenings and an inability to go to sleep or wake up earlier if desired. Adolescents typically experience a phase in their biological clock that makes them want to stay up late and sleep late. Delayed sleep phase type circadian rhythm disorder is diagnosed only when it seriously interferes with the person's functioning and causes

TABLE 6   *DSM-5* Criteria for Circadian Rhythm Sleep-Wake Disorders

A. A persistent or recurrent pattern of sleep disruption that is primarily due to an alteration of the circadian system or to a misalignment between the endogenous circadian rhythm and the sleep-wake schedule required by an individual's physical environment, social, or professional.

B. The sleep disruption leads to excessive sleepiness or insomnia, or both.

C. The sleep disturbance causes clinically significant distress or impairment in social, occupational, or other important areas of functioning.

Specify whether:

Delayed Sleep Phase Type: A pattern of delayed sleep onset and awakening times, with an inability to fall asleep and awaken at a desired or conventionally acceptable earlier time.

Specify if:

Familial: A family history of delayed sleep phase is present.

Specify if:

Overlapping with non-24-hour sleep-wake type: Delayed sleep phase type may overlap with another circadian rhythm sleep-wake disorder, non-24-hour sleep-wake type.

Advanced Sleep Phase Type: A pattern of advanced sleep onset and awakening times, with an inability to remain awake or asleep until the desired or conventionally acceptable later sleep or wake times.

Specify if:

Familial: A family history of advanced sleep phase is present.

Irregular Sleep-Wake Type: A temporally disorganized sleep and wake pattern, such that the timing of sleep and wake periods is variable throughout the 24-hour period.

Non-24-Hour Sleep-Wake Type: A pattern of sleep and wake cycles that is not synchronized to the 24-hour environment, with a consistent daily drift (usually to later and later times) of sleep onset and times.

Shift Work Type: Insomnia during the major sleep period and/or excessive sleepiness (including inadvertent sleep) during the major awake period associated with shift work schedule (i.e., requiring unconventional work hours).

Unspecified type

Specify if:

Episodic: Symptoms last at least 1 month but less than 3 months.

Persistent: Symptoms last 3 months or longer.

Recurrent: Two or more episodes occur within the space of 1 year.

distress. It is the most common circadian rhythm disorder diagnosed in clinical settings.

In contrast, *advanced sleep phase type* involves a persistent pattern of sleep onset and awakenings that are 2 or more hours earlier than desired (i.e., they are "advanced" to an earlier time than preferred). This pattern results in symptoms of early-morning insomnia and excessive sleepiness during the day. Individuals with this disorder show evidence of earlier timing of circadian biomarkers, including melatonin and core body temperature changes (Abbott, Reid, & Zee, 2015).

People with *irregular sleep-wake type* do not have a discernable sleep-wake rhythm. Their sleep tends to be fragmented into at least three periods per 24 hours; they may have insomnia during the night but be very sleepy during periods of the day. This disorder can be associated with neurological disorders (Abbott et al., 2015). People with *non-24-hour type* circadian rhythm sleep-wake disorder appear to have a free-running sleep-wake cycle that is not calibrated with the light-dark cycle of the day. The disorder has been most frequently documented in people who cannot see—particularly those who perceive no light at all—but it also has been documented in sighted individuals (Flynn-Evans, Tabandeh, Skene, & Lockley, 2014). It may begin with a gradual movement of the onset of sleep to later and later at night until the individual sleeps during the day and is awake at night. Individuals with this disorder complain of sleepiness during daylight and show deficits in cognition and functioning.

Finally, *shift work type* circadian rhythm sleep-wake disorder is caused by working rotating shifts or irregular hours. In one study, 31 percent of night workers and 26 percent of rotating shift workers met the criteria for this disorder (Drake, Roehrs, Richardson, Walsh, & Roth, 2004).

Behavioral interventions can help treat circadian rhythm sleep-wake disorders. It is easier to stay up late than to go to sleep early, so rotating shift workers can more easily move their shifts clockwise than counterclockwise (Sack et al., 2007). Planned napping during night shifts also can help reduce worker sleepiness and associated accidents (Sallinen, Harma, Akerstedt, Rosa, & Lillqvist, 1998). Exposing shift workers to bright light during night shifts can help shift their circadian rhythms (Sack et al., 2007). Similarly, exposing individuals with the delayed sleep phase type disorder to bright lights early in the morning can help shift their circadian rhythms.

Administering melatonin at prescribed times during the day has been shown to enhance the shifting of circadian rhythms in individuals with the delayed sleep phase type, blind adults with non-24-hour type, and the shift work type circadian rhythm sleep-wake disorders (Auger et al., 2015). The dosage and timing of melatonin administration are tricky, however, and can vary from one individual to another. Stimulants, such as modafinil, can improve alertness during night shifts and after crossing time zones, as can caffeine.

Disorders of Arousal

Disorders of arousal involve recurrent episodes of incomplete awakening from sleep that seem to mix elements of wakefulness and NREM sleep (see Table 7). "Arousal" in this case does not mean sexual arousal, as in the sexual disorders, or physiological arousal, as in the anxiety disorders. It refers to being more awake than during normal sleep, but not really quite awake. There are three types: sleep terrors, sleepwalking, and confusional arousals.

Sleep terror disorder occurs most often in children during which the sleeping child appears to be awake, afraid, and screaming but they are asleep. In a typical attack, the child abruptly sits upright in or jumps out of bed, screams in terror, displays intense fear, and has a frightened expression. The child is often confused and any verbalizations are incoherent and disorganized. Tachycardia, flushed face, dilated pupils, agitation, and increased muscle tone are often displayed. In the majority of cases, the individual does not fully awake and settles back to quiet and deep sleep. Sleep terrors often occur within the first three hours of sleep, during stage three or four nonrapid eye movement (NREM) sleep. Since these episodes occur during NREM sleep, a sleep stage not associated with vivid dreams, these episodes are not related to

---

TABLE 7   *DSM-5* Criteria for Non-Rapid Eye Movement Sleep Arousal Disorders

A. Recurrent episodes of incomplete awakening from sleep, usually occurring during the first third of the major sleep episode accompanied by either one of the following:

  1. **Sleepwalking:** Repeated episodes of rising from bed during sleep and walking about. While sleepwalking, the person has a blank, staring face, is relatively unresponsive to the efforts of others to communicate with him or her, and can be awakened only with great difficulty.

  2. **Sleep terrors:** Recurrent episodes of abrupt terror arousals from sleep, usually beginning with a panicky scream. There is intense fear and signs of autonomic arousal, such as mydriasis, tachycardia, rapid breathing, and sweating, during each episode. There is relative unresponsiveness to efforts of others to comfort the person during the episode.

B. No or little (e.g., only a single visual scene) dream imagery is recalled.

C. Amnesia for the episode is present.

D. The episodes cause clinically significant distress or impairment in social, occupational, or other important areas of functioning.

E. The disturbance is not attributable to the physiological effects of a substance (e.g., a drug of abuse, a medication).

F. Coexisting mental and medical disorders do not explain the episodes of sleepwalking or sleep terrors.

nightmares or dream content. Sleep terrors are most commonly displayed in children between the ages of 4 and 12, with a peak between 5 and 7 years of age. Children experiencing a sleep terror cannot be easily awakened and usually do not remember their sleep terrors on awakening. Sleep terrors are estimated to occur in 1 to 6.5 percentage of children. Although the exact etiology is not known, developmental, environmental, organic, psychological, and genetic factors have been identified as potential causes of sleep terrors (A. K. Leung, A. A.Leung, Wong, & Hon, 2020). Adults can experience sleep terrors as well. One large epidemiological study in Norway found that 2.7 percent of adults had experienced sleep terrors at least once in the last 3 months and that 1.0 percent experienced sleep terrors at least once per week (Bjorvatn, Grønli, & Pallesen, 2010).

Like sleep terrors, **sleepwalking disorder** is relatively common in children, with 15 to 30 percent having experienced at least one episode (Neylan et al., 2007). In the study in Norway, about 22 percent of adults reported having sleepwalked at some time in their lives, but only 1.7 percent reported sleepwalking in the previous 3 months (Bjorvatn et al., 2010). Sleepwalking occurs during NREM sleep, so the person sleepwalking is not acting out a dream. Sleepwalkers may respond to others' questions or commands but cannot hold a conversation. They may engage in nocturnal eating, going to the kitchen and eating food while asleep. They can injure themselves by running into furniture or thrashing about, especially if they are also experiencing a sleep terror (American Psychiatric Association, 2013). Sleepwalkers are difficult to wake (although doing so is not dangerous, as popularly believed). People sometimes do not remember their sleepwalking activity, but some do (Zadra, Desautels, Petit, & Montplaisir, 2013).

Confusional arousals are episodes of incomplete awakening during NREM sleep that do not involve sleep terrors or sleepwalking. They involve foggy thinking, slow speech, and sometimes disorientation, and occur most commonly when a person is awoken by someone else. These episodes are relatively common in adults, and are typically of relatively brief duration before the person fully awakens. The study in Norway found that nearly 7 percent reported episodes of confusional arousal occurring in the previous 3 months, with nearly 2 percent having had an episode at least once per week (Bjorvatn et al., 2010).

Sleepwalking and sleep terrors tend to run in families (Petit et al., 2015). Twin studies of sleep terrors show higher concordance rates among monozygotic twins than among dizygotic twins, suggesting a genetic influence on sleep terrors (Hublin, Kaprio, Partinen, Heikkilä, & Koskenvuo, 1997; Nguyen et al., 2008).

Stress, previous sleep deprivation, extreme fatigue, and the use of sedative or hypnotic drugs have been associated with both sleep terrors and sleepwalking.

Antidepressants are sometimes used to treat sleep terrors, with mixed results (Neylan et al., 2007). Most children outgrow the disorder by late adolescence and in the majority of cases, there is no prescribed treatment other than reassurance and parent education. Waking the child (*anticipatory awakening*) can be performed approximately half an hour before the individual is most likely to experience a sleep terror episode which has been found to be an effective treatment. After a minimum of 1 week without a night terror the scheduled awakenings are gradually ended. One study showed that such scheduled awakenings quickly reduced the frequency of children's night terrors; in a 1-year follow-up after the scheduled awakenings ended, the reductions in sleep terror episodes were maintained (Durand & Mindell, 1999; Leung et al., 2020).

Rapid Eye Movement Sleep Behavior Disorder

Whereas sleepwalking, sleep terrors, and confusional arousals occur during NREM sleep, other people become active during REM sleep. When this happens, they may engage in complex and often dangerous or violent behaviors, such as thrashing or fighting while asleep. They may appear to be acting out dreams and engaging in conversations with people in their dreams. Most people engaging in violent behaviors report having vivid dreams at the time, often involving being attacked by a person or an animal or protecting a loved one from harm (Ohayon, Guilleminault, & Chokroverty, 2010). They may actually injure themselves or their bed partner with their behaviors. About 4 percent of adults report ever having injured themselves or another during sleep (Bjorvatn et al., 2010). When behaviors during REM sleep are frequent and impairing, the individual may be diagnosed with **REM sleep behavior disorder** (Table 8).

A substantial percentage of people with REM sleep behavior disorder develop neurodegenerative diseases such as Parkinson's disease (Barber et al., 2017; Iranzo, Santamaria, & Tolosa, 2016). For example, one study found that the risk of developing Parkinson's disease or a related neurodegenerative disease among people with REM sleep behavior disorder was 65 percent over a 10-year period (Schenck & Mahowald, 2003). Individuals with REM sleep behavior disorder show abnormalities in dopamine functioning in the brain similar to those shown by people with Parkinson's disease (see the chapter "Neurodevelopmental and Neurocognitive Disorders"), even when they have not yet developed any

TABLE 8   *DSM-5* Diagnostic Criteria for Rapid Eye Movement Sleep Behavior Disorder

A. Repeated episodes of arousal during sleep associated with vocalization and/or complex motor behaviors.

B. These behaviors arise during rapid eye movement (REM) sleep and therefore usually occur more than 90 minutes after sleep onset, are more frequent during the later portions of the sleep period, and uncommonly occur during daytime naps.

C. Upon awakening from these episodes, the individual is completely awake, alert, and not confused or disoriented.

D. Either of the following:

    1. REM sleep without atonia on polysomnographic recording.

    2. A history suggestive of REM sleep behavior disorder and an established synucleinopathy diagnosis (e.g., Parkinson's disease, multiple system atrophy).

E. The behaviors cause clinically significant distress or impairment in social, occupational, or other important areas of functioning (which may include injury to self or the bed partner).

F. The disturbance is not attributable to the physiological effects of a substance (e.g., a drug of abuse, a medication) or another medical condition.

G. Coexisting mental and medical disorders do not explain the episodes.

neurological symptoms. In addition, the violent behaviors characteristic of REM sleep behavior disorder are comorbid with other sleep-wake disorders, including sleepwalking, sleep terrors, confusional arousals, and obstructive sleep apnea (Ohayon et al., 2010), suggesting that these disorders share some common causes.

The drug most often used to treat REM sleep behavior disorder is clonazepam, a benzodiazepine also commonly used to treat anxiety disorders (Jung & Louis, 2016). Melatonin also shows some efficacy in treating the disorder, alone or in combination with clonazepam. In contrast, some antidepressants that influence levels of norepinephrine and serotonin, including venlafaxine and mirtazapine, have been shown to worsen REM sleep behavior disorder, as can caffeine and chocolate when consumed in excess.

Nightmare Disorder

Over two-thirds of adults have had nightmares, or terrifying dreams (Bjorvatn et al., 2010). People often awaken from nightmares frightened, sweating, and with their heart racing. They may have vivid memories of the dream, which often involve physical danger. Nightmares are common among people who have recently experienced a traumatic event (Nadorff, Lambdin, & Germain, 2014). Nightmares are more common in children than in adults, with 10 to 50 percent of children having a sufficient number of nightmares to disturb their parents (Neylan et al., 2007). For a diagnosis of **nightmare disorder,** the nightmares must be frequent enough to cause significant distress or impairment in functioning (Table 9). The epidemiologic study in Norway found

TABLE 9   *DSM-5* Criteria for Nightmare Disorder

A. Repeated occurrences of extended, extremely dysphoric, and well-remembered dreams that usually involve efforts to avoid threats to survival, security, or physical integrity and that generally occur during the second half of the major sleep episode.

B. On awakening from the dysphoric dreams, the individual rapidly becomes oriented and alert.

C. The sleep disturbance causes clinically significant distress or impairment in social, occupational, or other important areas of functioning.

D. The nightmare symptoms are not attributable to the physiological effects of a substance (e.g., a drug of abuse, a medication).

E. Coexisting mental and medical disorders do not adequately explain the predominant complaint of dysphoric dreams.

TABLE 10   *DSM-5* Diagnostic Criteria for Restless Legs Syndrome

A. An urge to move the legs, usually accompanied by or in response to uncomfortable and unpleasant sensations in the legs, characterized by all of the following:

 1. The urge to move the legs begins or worsens during periods of rest or inactivity.

 2. The urge to move the legs is partially or totally relieved by movement.

 3. The urge to move the legs is worse in the evening or at night than during the day, or occurs only in the evening or at night.

B. The symptoms in Criterion A occur at least three times per week and have persisted for at least 3 months.

C. The symptoms in Criterion A are accompanied by significant distress or impairment in social, occupational, educational, academic, behavioral, or other important areas of functioning.

D. The symptoms in Criterion A are not attributable to another mental disorder or medical condition (e.g., arthritis, leg edema, peripheral ischemia, leg cramps) and are not better explained by a behavioral condition (e.g., positional discomfort, habitual foot tapping).

E. The symptoms are not attributable to the physiological effects of a drug of abuse or medication (e.g., akathisia).

randomized controlled trials among people whose nightmares are related to posttraumatic stress disorder (Nadorff et al., 2014).

Restless Legs Syndrome

Imagine that you are lying in bed and having creeping, crawling, tingling, itching sensations in your legs that are prominent enough to keep you awake. You feel as though you just have to move your legs. You get up and walk around and shake out your legs, and the sensations go away. But then, when you go back to bed, if you don't soon go to sleep the creeping, crawling sensations are back, and you just have to move again. This is the nature of **restless legs syndrome (RLS).**

Many people experience RLS occasionally, usually, or only at night. In order to be diagnosed with RLS, the *DSM-5* stipulates that the symptoms must be frequent and severe enough to significantly interfere with sleep and cause fatigue, mental health problems, and difficulty functioning (Table 10). About 2 to 3 percent of the population have RLS to this degree (see Allen et al., 2014). People with this syndrome have significantly higher rates of depression and anxiety disorders than do people in the general population, as well as more physical comorbidities (Szentkirályi, Völzke, Hoffmann, Trenkwalder, & Berger, 2014).

Specific genetic loci have been associated with RLS (Winkelmann et al., 2007). Abnormalities in the dopamine system also are associated with the disorder, and treatment with drugs that alter dopamine levels can be effective in treating it (Zintzaras et al., 2010). Iron deficiencies also are associated with the disorder, and reversal of iron deficiencies reduces symptoms (Trotti & Rye, 2011).

that 2.8 percent of adults have nightmares at least once per week (Bjorvatn et al., 2010), and worldwide between 2 to 6 percent of people meet criteria for nightmare disorder (Nadorff et al., 2014). Cognitive-behavioral interventions for nightmare disorder include exposure-based techniques that desensitize individuals to their nightmares. The person records the content of the nightmare in detail and then reads it repeatedly while doing relaxation exercises. Such interventions have been shown in small controlled trials to reduce the frequency of nightmares as well as the anxiety, depression, and sleeplessness associated with them. These gains persisted in a 4-year follow-up (Grandi, Fabbri, Panatoni, Gonnella, & Marks, 2006). A medication called prazosin, which affects sympathetic nervous system activity, has been shown to be effective in multiple

CHAPTER INTEGRATION

This chapter amply illustrates the effects of the body, the mind, and the environment on one another (Figure 5). Psychological and social factors can have direct effects on the physiology of the body and indirect effects on health by leading people to engage in behaviors that either promote or impair health. In turn, physical health affects people's emotional health and self-concept. People with a life-threatening or debilitating physical illness are at a greatly increased risk for depression and other emotional problems. For these reasons, health psychologists begin with the assumption that biology, psychology, and the social environment have reciprocal influences on one another. They then attempt to characterize these influences and determine their relative importance. Health psychologists also study how physical health problems impact other people—for example, caregivers of people with cancer, who are themselves at risk for stress and mental health problems like depression because of their caregiving role (e.g., Kim, Shaffer, Carver, & Cannady, 2014). Health psychologists also examine larger systems from a behavioral perspective, including doctor–patient communication, hospital systems, prevention programs, and public policies.

Due to the great strides made in neuroimmunological research, psychological stress has been identified as a significant factor in the development and progression of many physical diseases, such as cancer. Stress can be present in short and intense periods lasting only a few minutes, or chronic lasting for hours or days. Chronic stress is associated with alternations in the hypothalamic-pituitary-adrenal (HPA) axis, activation of sympathetic nervous system (SNS) and other physiological adaptations like hormones secretion which have impacts on physical health.

The gut microbiota has received much recent attention for its influence on human behavior. This diverse collection of microorganisms that inhabit the gastrointestinal tract has been found to profoundly influence many aspects of physiology, including metabolism, resistance to infection and immune system development. Studies investigating the gut–brain axis suggest that the gut microbiota play a critical role in the coordination of brain development and behavior, with the immune system emerging as an important regulator of these interactions. Aspects of immune function are influenced by stress and microbiota that result in changes in brain function via the HPA axis.

FIGURE 5 | Reciprocal Effects of Psychological, Social, and Biological Factors in Stress-Related Disorders.

Social factors: traumas, chronic stress, culture

Psychological factors: personality, health behaviors, emotions

Disorder

Biological factors: physiological stress response, genetic predisposition to disease, weakened organ systems

SHADES OF GRAY DISCUSSION

At first glance you might think that John's avoidance of thinking or talking about his cancer is an unhealthy way of coping. He is not drawing on social support from his children or his co-workers. You might even wonder if he is living in denial of his serious illness. But look closer. John appears to be engaging in a subtler form of social support characteristic of Asian cultures. He enjoys talking with his wife about their children and grandchildren and about visiting friends and family. For John, this may be a more acceptable means of coping than overtly asking for support from people other than his wife.

CHAPTER SUMMARY

- Three dimensions that affect the level of stress in situations are uncontrollability, unpredictability, and duration.

- The fight-or-flight response is a set of physiological changes the body undergoes when it faces a threat. In the short term it is adaptive, but if it persists for a long time it can cause damage to the body, a condition called allostatic load.

- Psychological factors associated with poorer health include pessimism and avoidance coping, while expressive writing and seeking social support are associated with better health. People with psychological disorders, especially depression, are at increased risk for a number of physical health problems.

- The immune system protects us from disease by identifying and killing pathogens and tumor cells. Chronic, uncontrollable stress; pessimism; and avoidance coping are associated with impaired immune system functioning, and with worse health in individuals with cancer or HIV/AIDS. Whether interventions to reduce stress or improve cognitions about stress affect the progression of cancer is not clear, however.

- Chronic stress is also associated with coronary heart disease. The Type A behavior pattern, characterized by a sense of time urgency, easily aroused hostility, and competitive striving for achievement, predicts coronary heart disease. The component of Type A that is most predictive is hostility. Depression also is predictive of CHD.

- The Type D (*Distressed*) personality profile is characterized by high levels of negative affectivity and social inhibition. Negative affectivity is characterized by the tendency to experience feelings of dysphoria, anxiety, and irritability associated with emotional distress and negative cardiovascular outcomes. Research has found a strong association between type D personality traits and cardiovascular disease, hypertension and susceptibility to myocardial infarction.

- Guided mastery techniques help people increase their positive health-related behaviors. The Internet is being used to deliver guided mastery interventions worldwide.

- Substance-induced sleep disorders are due to the use of substances, including both prescription medications (e.g., medications that control hypertension or cardiac arrhythmias) and nonprescription substances (e.g., alcohol and caffeine).

- Insomnia is difficulty initiating or maintaining sleep or sleep that chronically does not restore energy and alertness. It can be caused by disruptions in body temperature rhythms, stress, and faulty cognitions and habits concerning sleep. Cognitive-behavioral therapy is effective in treating insomnia. A variety of medications also are prescribed for insomnia, but cognitive-behavioral therapy is the most effective treatment.

- Increased rates of insomnia were reported during the COVID-19 pandemic which was attributed, in part, to rising stress levels and worry about health, financial consequences, changes in social life and the daily routine during the outbreak. Reduced physical fatigue and exposure to the sun were identified as additional factors, as well as, increased use of electronic devices that may disrupt sleep. COVID-19-related worry, loneliness, uncertainty about viral exposure and depressive symptoms were significantly associated with insomnia. Feelings of isolation, disruption of daily scheduled and reduced social contact may also contribute to an abnormal sleep-wake schedule

- Hypersomnolence is chronic excessive sleepiness as evidenced by either prolonged sleep episodes or daytime sleep episodes that occur almost daily. Narcolepsy involves irresistible attacks of sleep; people with narcolepsy also have (1) cataplexy or (2) recurrent intrusions of elements of rapid eye movement (REM) sleep into the transition between sleep and wakefulness. Stimulants are prescribed for people with hypersomnia or narcolepsy.

- Sleep-related breathing disorders (central sleep apnea, obstructive sleep apnea/hypopnea syndrome, sleep-related hypoventilation) involve numerous brief sleep disturbances due to breathing problems. Continuous positive airway pressure (CPAP) machines are used to treat obstructive sleep apnea. Obstructive sleep apnea also is sometimes treated with weight loss and/or surgery. Serotonin reuptake inhibitors and stimulants are sometimes prescribed.

- Circadian rhythm sleep-wake disorder includes delayed sleep phase type, advanced sleep phase type, irregular sleep-wake type, non-24-hour sleep-wake type, and shift work type. Melatonin, stimulants, light therapy, and behavioral techniques to change sleep habits are used to treat circadian rhythm sleep-wake disorders.

- Disorders of arousal include sleep terrors, sleepwalking, and confusional arousal. These syndromes occur during NREM sleep.

- Rapid eye movement (REM) sleep behavior disorder is characterized by activity, sometimes violent or injurious, during REM sleep. It is associated with neurodegenerative diseases and can be treated with clonazepam, a benzodiazepine also commonly used to treat anxiety disorders.

- Nightmare disorder involves frequent experiences of nightmares during REM sleep.

- Restless legs syndrome is characterized by evening or nighttime feelings of creeping, crawling, and itching in the legs accompanied by a desire to move the legs. It can be caused by abnormalities in the dopamine system and by iron deficiencies, and treatment with drugs designed to reverse these factors can be effective.

KEY TERMS

allostatic load

immune system

coronary heart disease (CHD)

hypertension

Type A behavior pattern

Type D (*Distressed*) behavior pattern

guided mastery techniques

sleep disorders

substance-induced sleep disorder

insomnia disorder

hypersomnolence disorders

narcolepsy

cataplexy

central sleep apnea

sleep-related hypoventilation

breathing-related sleep disorder

obstructive sleep apnea/hypopnea syndrome

circadian rhythm sleep-wake disorder

disorders of arousal

sleep terror disorder

sleepwalking disorder

rapid eye movement (REM) sleep behavior disorder

nightmare disorder

restless legs syndrome (RLS)

Chapter 16

RichLegg/Getty Images

Mental Health and the Law

CHAPTER OUTLINE

Mental Health Law Along the Continuum

A person with mental health problems is suspected of having committed a crime

Legal decision must be informed by mental health experts

(Mental health worker advises if the individual is fit to stand trial or should be considered not guilty by reason of insanity)

A person with no mental health problems is suspected of having committed a crime

Legal decision does not need to take mental health into account

***DSM-5* diagnosis of mental disorder**

Functional   Dysfunctional

Mental health problems bring a person to the attention of the law, although the individual does not have a diagnosis and has not committed a crime

Legal decision may place the individual in a mental health facility involuntarily if he is a danger to himself or others

A person with a diagnosed mental health disorder commits a crime

Legal decision must take the diagnosis into account, but the diagnosis does not guarantee that the person will receive specific treatment under the law

(The individual may or may not be found not guilty by reason of insanity)

Think back to before you took this course, before you had a sense of how fuzzy our definitions and understanding of mental disorders can be. Imagine yourself hearing a report on the news about a college student who posted videos of himself on YouTube ranting about injustices done to him and then went on a shooting rampage on his college campus and was subsequently caught and jailed. Back then, you might have thought that it should have been obvious to campus authorities that there was something seriously wrong with this person. Once the person was incarcerated, you might have thought the authorities should simply determine whether he had a mental disorder that caused him to be violent and then take appropriate action. If his violence was the result of a mental disorder, he should be given treatment to overcome the mental disorder; if his violence was not due to a mental disorder but was voluntary and intentional, he should be incarcerated.

Now you understand that the situation is not that clear-cut. The *DSM* provides criteria for diagnosing mental disorders, but whether a particular individual's behaviors meet those criteria is often a judgment call. Furthermore, we are limited in our ability to generalize from the research literature to individual cases. For example, just because a person has a mental disorder that may be associated with an increased risk of aggression or violence, we cannot know for certain whether this particular individual will be violent in the future.

When someone who appears to have mental health problems interacts with the judicial system, these judgment calls become even more complex. The fuzziness in our diagnostic criteria and in our understanding of mental disorders combines with the difficult ethical and social issues these cases involve. A *DSM-5* diagnosis of a mental disorder does not ensure that an individual will be treated in a particular way by the law. For example, a diagnosed mental disorder is not enough to ensure that an individual receives needed treatment and may not exonerate an individual who has committed a crime. Mental health law is further complicated by the fact that the laws concerning people with mental health problems vary from region to region and have changed dramatically over the past 50 years.

Thus, the fuzziness in our diagnostic systems that is inherent in the fact that psychological problems fall along a continuum, combined with the fuzziness in laws and their application to people with mental health problems, means that a great deal of subjective judgment is involved in mental health law.

Extraordinary People

Greg Bottoms, *Angelhead*

William DiLillo

Michael Bottoms was driven to violent outbursts by psychotic beliefs that were symptoms of schizophrenia. He came to believe that any medications for his schizophrenia were part of a conspiracy to control his mind and usually refused them. His violence was often directed toward his family, to the point that his brother Greg and his parents would lock their bedroom doors at night to prevent Michael from attacking them in their sleep. As Greg Bottoms describes in his book *Angelhead* (2000), the family tried to have Michael institutionalized but was told they could not unless they proved he was an imminent danger to himself or others.

Eventually the family found an institution that would take their insurance and placed Michael there. He hated the place, though, refused his medications, and attempted suicide. This landed him in a state psychiatric hospital for a while. Later he "confessed" to a murder he had not committed, having been convinced by the voices in his head that he was guilty. He was jailed, but DNA evidence proved Michael couldn't have committed the murder.

After he was exonerated for this murder, Michael was back home again, on high doses of antipsychotic medications but delusional, believing that God spoke directly to him and that his family was evil. Indeed, he decided that his father was the Antichrist and that, to save his family's souls, he had to kill them. One night, as his father lay dying of cancer and his family slept behind locked doors, Michael set the house on fire. He rode his bicycle to the end of the street, then sat watching, expecting his family's souls to float past him on the way to heaven. The family escaped. As they stood watching the firefighters try to extinguish the fire, Mr. Bottoms told the other family members this was the best thing that could happen, because now Michael could really be put away. In the next instant, however, he feared that Michael had been in the house and was dying in the fire. He tried to run into the house to look for Michael, but the firefighters held him back. Meanwhile, Michael rode up on his bicycle, nonchalant. A police officer asked Michael if he could ask him some questions, and Michael held out his hands for the handcuffs. Then he turned to his mother and asked her casually what she was going to make for breakfast. Michael confessed to setting the fire with the purpose of killing his family. He was convicted for attempted murder and arson and was sent to prison for 30 years.

Mental health professionals are asked regularly to help families such as the Bottoms family deal with the laws and social systems that guide the treatment of people with psychological disorders. Fundamental questions about society's values confront the personal wishes of people with mental disorders and their families: Does society have a right to impose treatment on an individual who doesn't want it? Under what conditions should people be absolved of responsibility for behaviors that harm others? Should the diagnosis of a psychological disorder entitle a person to special services and protection against discrimination?

This chapter explores how the law becomes involved in the lives of people with mental health problems, focusing first on when a person can be committed to a mental health facility against their will. Then we examine how the law regards a person charged with a crime who might have a mental disorder. Finally, we discuss how society treats a person who has a mental disorder and is convicted of a crime.

CIVIL COMMITMENT

In the best circumstances, people who need treatment for a psychological disorder seek it themselves. They work with mental health professionals to find medication and/or psychotherapy to reduce their symptoms and keep their disorder under control. Many people who have serious psychological problems, however, do not recognize their need for treatment or may refuse treatment for a variety of reasons. For example, Michael Bottoms believed the doctors treating him were part of a conspiracy and refused to follow their prescriptions. A man experiencing a manic episode may enjoy many of the symptoms—the high energy, inflated self-esteem, and grandiose thoughts—and not want to take medication that would reduce those symptoms. A teenager who is abusing illegal drugs may believe that it is their right to do so and that there is nothing wrong with the abuse. Can these people be forced to enter mental institutions and to undergo treatment against their will? These are the questions we address in this section.

Criteria for Civil Commitment

Prior to the mid-twentieth century, in the United States the **need for treatment** was sufficient cause to hospitalize people against their will and force them to undergo treatment. Such involuntary hospitalization is called **civil commitment.** All that was needed for civil commitment was a certificate signed by two physicians stating that a person needed treatment and was not agreeing to it voluntarily. The person could then be confined, often indefinitely, without recourse to an attorney, a hearing, or an appeal (Mannekote, Pillai & Harbishettar, 2019; Meyer & Weaver, 2006).

The need for treatment alone is no longer sufficient legal cause for civil commitment in most states in the United States. This change came about as part of the patients' rights movement of the 1960s, which raised concerns about violations of the personal freedoms and civil liberties of mental patients. Opponents of the civil commitment process argued that it allowed people to be incarcerated simply for having alternative lifestyles or different political or moral values (Szasz, 1963, 1977). Certainly, there were many cases in the former Soviet Union and other countries of political dissidents being labeled mentally ill and in need of treatment and then being incarcerated in prisons for years. There also were disturbing cases of the misuse of civil commitment proceedings in the United States. In the 1860s, for example, Illinois law allowed a husband to have his wife involuntarily committed without evidence that she had lost touch with reality or was dangerous. For example, Mrs. E. P. W. Packard was committed by her husband for holding "unacceptable" and "sick" political or moral views (Weiner & Wettstein, 1993). Mrs. Packard remained hospitalized for 3 years before winning her release; she then began crusading against civil commitment.

Procedurally, most states now mandate that persons being considered for involuntary commitment have the right to a public hearing, the right to counsel, the right to call and confront witnesses, the right to appeal decisions, and the right to be placed in the least restrictive treatment setting. In practice, however, judges typically defer to the judgment of mental health professionals about a person's mental health and whether the criteria for commitment are met (Melton et al., 2017; Meyer & Weaver, 2006). Even attorneys who are supposed to be upholding an individual's rights tend to acquiesce to the judgment of mental health professionals, particularly if the attorney is court-appointed, as is often the case.

In the United States and many other countries, individuals must be judged to meet one of the following criteria in order to be committed to a psychiatric facility against their will: (1) grave disability, (2) dangerousness to self, or (3) dangerousness to others. In addition, most states require that the danger people pose to themselves or to others be imminent—in other words, if they are not immediately incarcerated, they or someone else will likely be harmed in the very near future. Finally, all persons committed to psychiatric facilities must be diagnosed with a mental disorder, although the definition of mental disorders or mental illnesses varies from state to state (Meyer & Weaver, 2006; Swanson, Tong, Robertson, & Swartz, 2020). In particular, some states exclude substance abuse or dependence and mental retardation from their list of mental disorders or mental illnesses.

Grave Disability

The **grave disability** criterion requires that people be so incapacitated by a mental disorder that they cannot provide for their basic needs of food, clothing, and shelter. This criterion is, in theory, much more severe than the need for treatment criterion because it requires that the person's survival be in immediate danger because of a mental disorder (Braslow & Messac, 2018).

You might think that the grave disability criterion could be used to hospitalize homeless people living on the streets who appear to be psychotic and unable to take care of their basic needs. In the winter of 1988, New York City Mayor Ed Koch invoked the legal principle of *parens patriae* (sovereign as parent) to have mentally ill homeless people taken to mental health facilities. Mayor Koch argued that it was the city's duty to protect these mentally ill homeless people from the ravages of the winter weather because they were unable to protect themselves. One of the homeless people who was involuntarily hospitalized was a 40-year-old Joyce Brown, who subsequently was diagnosed with paranoid schizophrenia. Brown had been living on the streets on and off for years, resisting efforts by her family to get her into psychiatric treatment. Brown and the American Civil Liberties Union contested her commitment and won her release on the grounds that the city had no right to incarcerate Brown if she had no intention of being treated (Kasindorf, 1988).

One legal precedent relevant to Joyce Brown's release was *O'Connor v. Donaldson* (1975). Kenneth Donaldson had been committed to a Florida state hospital for 14 years. Donaldson's father originally had him committed, believing that Donaldson was delusional and therefore a danger to himself. At the time, Florida law allowed people to be committed if their mental disorder might impair their ability to manage their finances or to protect themselves against being cheated by others. Throughout his hospitalization,

Donaldson refused medication because it violated his Christian Science beliefs. The superintendent, Dr. J. B. O'Connor, considered this refusal to be a symptom of Donaldson's mental disorder. Even though Donaldson had been caring for himself adequately before his hospitalization and had friends who offered to help care for him if he was released from the hospital, O'Connor and the hospital continually refused Donaldson's requests for release. Donaldson sued on the grounds that he had received only custodial care during his hospitalization and was not a danger to himself. He requested to be released to the care of his friends and family. The Supreme Court agreed, ruling that "a State cannot constitutionally confine . . . a nondangerous individual, who is capable of surviving safely in freedom by himself or with the help of willing and responsible family and friends" (*O'Connor v. Donaldson*, 1975, p. 4).

In practice, however, most people involuntarily committed because of grave disability do not have the ACLU championing their rights or the personal ability to file suit. Often, they are people with few financial resources or friends. Their family members may also have serious mental disorders. The elderly mentally ill are especially likely to be committed because of grave disability. Often, these people are committed to psychiatric facilities because their families are unable to care for them and there are not enough less restrictive treatment facilities available in their communities (Braslow & Messac, 2018; Turkheimer & Parry, 1992).

Dangerousness to Self

The criterion **dangerousness to self** is most often invoked when it is believed that a person is imminently suicidal. In such cases, the person often is held in an inpatient psychiatric facility for a few days while undergoing further evaluation and possibly treatment. Most states allow short-term commitments without a court hearing in emergency situations such as this. All that is needed is a certification by the attending mental health professionals that the individual is in imminent danger to him- or herself. If the mental health professionals judge that the person needs further treatment but the person does not voluntarily agree to treatment, they can go to court to request that the person be committed for a longer period of time.

Dangerousness to Others

Dangerousness to others is the third criterion under which people can be committed involuntarily. If a person with a mental disorder is going to hurt another person if set free, then society has claimed the right to protect itself. While this action may seem justified, the appropriateness of this criterion rests on predictions of who will be dangerous and who will not. It is

Adam Lanza, who had previously exhibited behavior potentially indicative of a mental disorder, killed 20 children and 6 adults before fatally shooting himself at the Sandy Hook Elementary School in Newtown, Connecticut. *Uncredited/AP Images*

exceedingly difficult to make such predictions accurately (Monahan & Walker, 2014). We can all recall incidents in which individuals with severe mental health problems became violent and the media and public cried "How could we not have seen this coming?" In 2007, college student Seung-Hui Cho, who had been diagnosed with multiple mental disorders, shot and killed 32 people and wounded 17 others on the campus of Virginia Polytechnic University (also known as Virginia Tech). Professors and students had raised alarms with university officials because of Cho's disturbing writings and behaviors, and Cho had been investigated for stalking a woman student. He was ordered by a court to undergo outpatient treatment for his behaviors but did not comply and was not forced to do so. In 2009, U.S. Army psychiatrist Major Nidal Hasan shot and killed 13 people at Fort Hood, Texas. Students and faculty at Walter Reed Hospital, where Hasan trained, called Hasan's behavior "disconnected, aloof, paranoid, belligerent, and schizoid" (Zwerdling, 2009). Still, no one connected the dots to predict that Hasan could be a danger to others, and no action was taken to remove him from his post.

If mental health professionals believe that an individual may harm another person, they have a duty to warn that person, even if this violates a client's confidentiality. This duty to warn was established in a decision in the case of *Tarasoff v. Regents of the University of California* (1974). Tatiana Tarasoff was a student at the University of California at Berkeley in the late 1960s. A graduate student named Prosenjit Poddar was infatuated with Tarasoff, who had rejected him. Poddar told his therapist in the student counseling service that he planned to kill Tarasoff when she returned to campus from vacation. The therapist informed the campus police, who picked up Poddar for questioning. Poddar agreed to leave Tarasoff alone, and the campus police released him. Two months later, Poddar killed Tarasoff. Tarasoff's parents sued the university, arguing that the therapist should have protected Tarasoff from Poddar. The California courts agreed and established the precedent that therapists have a duty to warn persons who are threatened by their clients during therapy sessions and to take actions to protect those persons (Meyer & Weaver, 2006).

After Seung-Hui Cho's shooting rampage, officials at Virginia Tech reevaluated their interpretation of federal privacy laws that had led them not to share information about Cho's behavior or diagnoses with concerned faculty and administrators prior to the shooting. In 2008, the U.S. Department of Education proposed changes in the regulations governing the balance between protecting students' privacy rights and public safety in light of the Cho incident. Virginia Tech also was criticized for delays in warning the campus of danger once the shooting rampage began. Since this incident, many universities have instituted new policies and alarm systems to alert students, faculty, and staff when a violent incident is erupting.

Violence by People with Mental Disorders

Incidents such as the shootings discussed above lead the public to believe that people with a mental disorder are much more prone to violence than people without a mental disorder. They also lead to public demands for more intervention with troubled youth, regardless of whether they and their parents want it. One group of researchers examined the public's beliefs about the potential for harm to self or others by youth with mental health problems and the public's willingness to coerce these youth to get treatment (Pescosolido, Fettes, Martin, Monahan, & McLeod, 2007). They asked over 1,100 adults to read vignettes depicting youth with attention-deficit/hyperactivity disorder (ADHD), major depression, asthma, or "daily troubles." Many more youth with ADHD or major depression were perceived as somewhat likely or very likely to be dangerous to themselves or others (33 percent for ADHD, 81 percent for major depression), compared to youth with asthma (15 percent) or "daily troubles" (13 percent). Over one-third of the adults in the study were willing to use legal means to force the youth with major depression to get mental health treatment. Adults who labeled the youth with ADHD or major depression "mentally ill" were twice as likely to see a potential for violence in these youth and five times more likely to support forced treatment, compared to adults who didn't apply the label "mentally ill" to the youth. These results suggest that the public associates diagnoses of mental disorders in

Tragedies like the shootings by Seung-Hui Cho at Virginia Tech University (pictured) and Adam Lanza at Sandy Hook Elementary School have led the public to call for more intervention for troubled, potentially violent youth. *MSNBC/ZUMA Press/Newscom*

youth with dangerousness and that a substantial portion of the public is ready to use the legal system to force youth with mental disorders into treatment (see Pescosolido, 2013).

Are people with a mental disorder actually more prone to violence than those without a mental disorder? Research suggests that the answer is complex (Monahan & Skeem, 2014). In one major study, researchers followed 1,136 men and women with mental disorders for 1 year after they were discharged from a psychiatric hospital, monitoring their self-reports of violent behaviors, reports in police and hospital records, and reports by other informants, such as family members (Steadman et al., 1998). Serious violent acts were defined as battery that resulted in physical injury, sexual assaults, assaultive acts that involved the use of a weapon, and threats made with a weapon in hand. The former psychiatric patients' records of violent activity were compared to those of 519 people living in the same neighborhoods the patients lived in after their hospital discharge. This community group was interviewed only once, at the end of the year-long study, and was asked about violent behavior in the past 10 weeks.

The likelihood that the former patients would commit a violent act was strongly related to their specific diagnosis and whether they had a substance abuse problem. About 18 percent of the former patients who had a diagnosis of a major mental disorder (e.g., schizophrenia, major depression, some other psychotic disorder) without a history of substance abuse committed a serious violent act in the year following discharge, compared to 31 percent of those with a major mental disorder and a history of substance abuse and 43 percent of those with a diagnosis of "other" mental disorder (i.e., a personality or adjustment disorder) and a

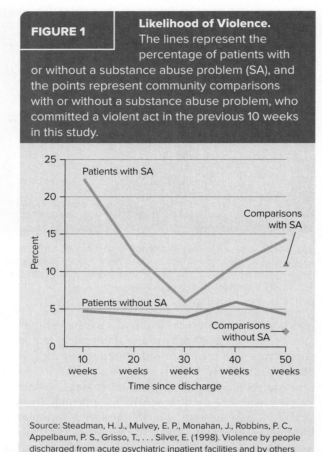

FIGURE 1

Likelihood of Violence. The lines represent the percentage of patients with or without a substance abuse problem (SA), and the points represent community comparisons with or without a substance abuse problem, who committed a violent act in the previous 10 weeks in this study.

Source: Steadman, H. J., Mulvey, E. P., Monahan, J., Robbins, P. C., Appelbaum, P. S., Grisso, T., . . . Silver, E. (1998). Violence by people discharged from acute psychiatric inpatient facilities and by others in the same neighborhoods. *Archives of General Psychiatry, 55,* 393–401.

co-occurring substance abuse problem (Steadman et al., 1998). The researchers were somewhat surprised to find that the former patients were most likely to commit a violent act in the first couple of months following their discharge and less likely to do so as the year wore on (Figure 1). They suggested that patients might still be in crisis shortly after their hospitalization and that it may take some months for social support systems and treatment to begin to affect their behavior (Steadman et al., 1998).

The rate of violence in the community sample was also strongly related to whether individuals had a history of substance abuse. Eleven percent of those with a substance abuse problem committed a violent act during the year of the study, compared to 3 percent of those with no substance abuse problem (Steadman et al., 1998). Although the overall rate of violence in the community sample was lower than in the patient sample, this difference was statistically significant only when the researchers considered violence committed by the former patients shortly after their discharge. By the end of that year, the former patients were no more likely to commit a violent act than were the people in the community comparison group.

The targets of violence by both the former patients and the community members most often were family members, followed by friends and acquaintances. The former patients actually were somewhat less likely than the comparison group to commit a violent act against a stranger (13.8 percent of the acts committed by former patients compared to 22.2 percent of the acts committed by the comparison group).

The rates of violence recorded in this study may seem high, for both the patient group and the comparison group. The patient group probably represented people with more serious psychological disorders who were facing acute crises in their lives. The comparison group consisted largely of people with low socioeconomic status living in impoverished neighborhoods. These contextual factors may account for the relatively high rates of violence in both groups.

The researchers who conducted this study emphasized that their data show how inappropriate it is to consider "former mental patients" to be a homogeneous group of people all prone to violence. The presence of substance abuse problems was a strong predictor of violent behavior both in this group and in the group of people who had not been mental patients; subsequent studies have also emphasized substance use as a key factor (see Swanson, McGinty, Fazel, & Mays, 2015). Moreover, the majority of people with serious mental disorders did not commit any violent acts in the year after their discharge, especially against random strangers, contrary to what media depictions of former mental patients often suggest.

Other research has suggested that violence by mentally ill women tends to be underestimated by clinicians (Coontz, Lidz, & Mulvey, 1994; Robbins, Monahan, & Silver, 2003). Clinicians do not expect mentally ill women to be violent to the same degree that they expect mentally ill men to be violent. As a result, they do not probe mentally ill women for evidence of a tendency toward violence as much as they do mentally ill men. In reality, however, mentally ill women and mentally ill men are equally likely to commit violent acts against others (Robbins et al., 2003; Sturup, Monahan, & Kristiansson, 2013). The victims of mentally ill women's violent acts are most likely to be family members; mentally ill men also are most often violent toward family members, but they commit violent acts against strangers more often than do mentally ill women (Newhill, Mulvey, & Lidz, 1995). Mentally ill men who commit violence are more likely to have been drinking before the violence and to be arrested following it than are mentally ill women who commit violence (Robbins et al., 2003).

Racial stereotypes lead people to expect mentally ill persons from ethnic minority groups to be more likely to commit acts of violence than white mentally ill people. However, there are no differences between ethnic groups in the rates of violence among mentally ill people (Kunst, Myhren, & Onyeador, 2018; Rueve & Welton, 2008).

Multiple meta-analyses and reviews have found that people with a mental disorder on average are more likely to commit violent acts than are those without a mental disorder, with rates varying depending on a number of factors (Choe, Teplin, & Abram, 2008; Fazel, Långström, Hjern, Grann, & Lichtenstein, 2009; Fazel, Lichtenstein, Grann, Goodwin, & Långström, 2010). Risk of violence is heightened with specific symptoms like hallucinations, delusions, and uncontrolled anger, but the most important factor is substance abuse (Swanson et al., 2015). It is important to note that people with mental disorders are much more likely to be the *victims* of violence than they are to be the perpetrators. They are also more likely to be victimized than people without a mental disorder.

Prevalence of Involuntary Commitment

How often are people involuntarily committed to a psychiatric facility? The data necessary to answer this question are sparse, but the available studies suggest that about 25 percent of admissions to inpatient psychiatric facilities in the United States are involuntary and that about 15 to 20 percent of inpatient admissions in European countries are involuntary (Monahan et al., 2001). Admissions to state and county mental hospitals are much more likely to be involuntary than are admissions to other types of hospitals (Table 1). In addition, 12 to 20 percent of patients of outpatient psychiatric facilities report having been ordered by civil courts to participate in outpatient treatment (Monahan et al., 2005). Court orders for outpatient care were more common among individuals who lived in residential psychiatric facilities and who had poor social support and poor psychosocial functioning, a recent history of violent behavior, recent police encounters, substance abuse problems, and higher rates of lifetime hospitalizations and involuntary hospitalizations (Swartz, Swanson, Kim, & Petrila, 2006). Involuntary commitment and court-ordered treatment rates also vary widely from state to state (Swartz, Bhattacharya, Robertson, & Swanson, 2017; Testa & West, 2010).

The numbers in Table 1 probably underestimate the number of people coerced into mental health care treatment, because parents and legal guardians often "volunteer" a protesting child or incompetent adult for admission (Monahan et al., 2001). In one study, nearly 50 percent of the adults admitted voluntarily to inpatient psychiatric facilities reported that someone other than themselves had initiated their going to the hospital, and 14 percent of the patients were under the custody of someone else at the time of admission (Hoge, et al., 1997; Segal, Laurie, &

TABLE 1 Frequency of Involuntary Admissions to Psychiatric Facilities

These data indicate the percent of all admissions to various types of psychiatric facilities that involve involuntary commitments. Data are from the United States in 1986.

Type of Facility	Percent of All Admissions That Are Involuntary
State and county hospitals	61.6%
Multiservice mental health organizations (e.g., community mental health centers)	46.1
Private psychiatric hospitals	15.6
Nonfederal general hospitals	14.8
Veterans Administration hospitals	5.6

Source: Monahan, J., Bonnie, R. J., Appelbaum, P. S., Hyde, P. S., Steadman, H. J., & Swartz, M. S. (2001). Mandated community treatment: Beyond outpatient commitment. *Psychiatric Services, 52,* 1198–1205.

Franskoviak, 2004). Nearly 40 percent of the voluntary patients believed they would have been involuntarily committed if they had not agreed to be hospitalized. Some of the patients felt they had been coerced by their therapists, who did not include them in the admissions process. Patients involuntarily committed often may need treatment that they cannot acknowledge they need. About half of those patients who felt they were coerced into treatment eventually acknowledge that they needed treatment, but about half continue to believe treatment was unnecessary (Gardner et al., 1999).

Marvin Swartz and colleagues (2010) evaluated the outcomes for individuals involuntarily committed to outpatient mental health care in New York over an 8-year period. Compared to the period before they were ordered to receive treatment, the involuntarily committed individuals had fewer hospitalizations, were more likely to have an adequate supply of medication appropriate for their diagnosis, and were more likely to be receiving intensive management of their condition. In addition, they had fewer hospitalizations than individuals with similar mental health problems who were receiving treatment voluntarily. Thus, it seems that involuntary treatment can result in several positive outcomes for individuals with serious mental health problems (Swartz et al., 2017).

PATIENTS' RIGHTS

Numerous court cases over the years have established that people committed to mental health institutions retain most of their civil rights. They also have certain additional rights, which we discuss in this section.

Right to Treatment

One basic right of people who have been committed is the **right to treatment.** In the past, mental patients, including both those involuntarily committed and those seeking treatment voluntarily, were often only warehoused. The conditions in which they lived were appalling, with little stimulation and few pleasantries, let alone treatment for their disorders. In *Wyatt v. Stickney* (1971), patient Ricky Wyatt and others filed a class action suit against a custodial facility in Alabama, charging that they received no useful treatment and lived in minimally acceptable living conditions. After 33 years in the courts, the case finally was settled in 2003. From the court ruling came four standards, known as the "Wyatt Standards," for the evaluation of care of psychiatric patients: (1) They must be provided with a humane psychological and physical environment, (2) there must be qualified and sufficient staff for the administration of treatment, (3) there must be individualized treatment plans, and (4) restrictions of patient freedoms must be kept to a minimum (Dvoskin, Knoll, & Silva, 2020; Sundram, 2009).

Right to Refuse Treatment

Another basic right is the **right to refuse treatment.** One of the greatest fears of people committed against their will is that they will be given drugs or other treatments that rob them of their consciousness and their free will.

One fundamental right of people committed to a mental health facility is the right to be treated rather than simply warehoused. *Oleksandr Rupeta/Alamy Stock Photo*

Many states now do not allow mental institutions or prisons to administer treatments without the informed consent of patients. **Informed consent** means that a patient accepts treatment after receiving a full and understandable explanation of the treatment being offered and making a decision based on his or her judgment of the risks and benefits of that treatment (Meyer & Weaver, 2006).

The right to refuse treatment is not recognized in some states, however, and in most states this right can be overruled in many circumstances (Monahan et al., 2001; Testa & West, 2010). Particularly if a patient is psychotic or manic, it may be judged that they cannot make a reasonable decision about treatment. Up to 45 percent of psychiatric inpatients may be incompetent to make decisions about their own treatment (Lepping, Stanly, & Turner, 2015). In some jurisdictions, the simple fact that patients have a psychiatric diagnosis is enough to have them declared incompetent to make decisions, especially if the diagnosis is schizophrenia (B. Appelbaum, P. Appelbaum, & Grisso, 1998; Scholten, Gather, & Vollmann, 2021). Yet studies using reliable measures of patients' ability to make rational decisions suggest that as many as 75 percent of those with schizophrenia and 90 percent of those with depression have adequate decision-making capacity (Grisso & Appelbaum, 1995; Larkin & Hutton, 2017).

Patients' psychiatrists or families may seek court rulings allowing them to administer treatment even if the patients refuse treatment. Judges most often agree with the psychiatrists' or families' requests to force treatment on patients. Most cases in which patients refuse treatment never go to court, however. Instead, clinicians and family members pressure patients to accept treatment, and most patients eventually agree to treatment after initially refusing (Griffin, Steadman, & Petrila, 2002; Monahan et al., 2001).

COMPETENCE TO STAND TRIAL

One fundamental principle of law is that, in order to stand trial, accused individuals must have a rational understanding of both the charges against them and the proceedings of the trial and must be able to participate in their defense. People who do not have an understanding of what is happening to them in a courtroom and who cannot participate in their defense are said to be **incompetent to stand trial.** Incompetence may involve impairment in several capacities, including the capacity to understand information, to think rationally about alternative courses of action, to make good choices, and to appreciate one's situation as a criminal defendant (Stafford & Sadoff, 2011; Scholten, Gather, & Vollmann, 2021).

Impaired competence may be a common problem. Defense attorneys suspect impaired competence

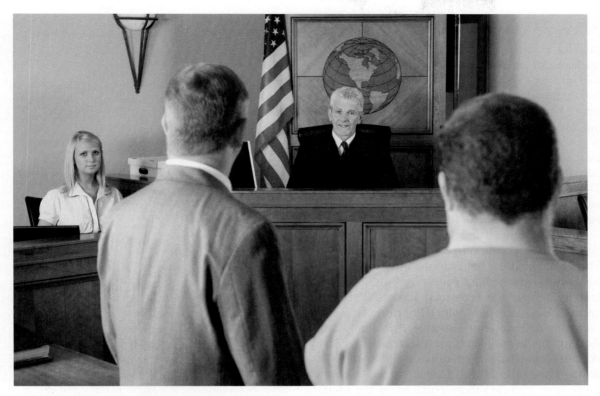

Competence to stand trial is one of the most common judgments psychologists are asked to help courts make.
RichLegg/Getty Images

in their clients in up to 10 percent of cases. Although only a handful of these clients are referred for formal evaluation, about 60,000 evaluations of criminal defendants for competence to stand trial are performed every year in the United States (Bonnie & Grisso, 2000). Competence judgments are one of the most frequent types of judgments that mental health professionals are asked to make for the courts. Judges appear to value the testimony of mental health experts concerning defendants' competence and rarely rule against these experts' recommendations.

The consequences of competence judgments for defendants are great. If defendants are judged incompetent, trials are postponed as long as there is reason to believe they will become competent in the foreseeable future, and defendants may be forced to receive treatment. On the other hand, incompetent defendants who are wrongly judged competent may not contribute adequately to their defense and may be wrongly convicted and incarcerated. Defendants who are suspected of being incompetent are described by their attorneys as much less helpful in establishing the facts of their case and much less actively involved in making decisions about their defense (MacArthur Research Network on Mental Health and the Law, 1998).

Not surprisingly, defendants with a long history of psychiatric problems, particularly schizophrenia or psychotic symptoms, are more likely than those without such a history to be referred for competence evaluations (Pirelli, Gottdiener, & Zapf, 2011). In a study of consultant liaison psychiatrists and psychologists, 70 percent of respondents rated it as common or very common for mental health practitioners to believe that if a person has a mental disorder such as schizophrenia, the person lacks competence to make any medical decisions (Scholten, Gather, & Vollmann, 2021). Defendants referred for competence evaluations also tend to have less education and to be poor, unemployed, and unmarried, compared to those not referred for evaluation. There is also some evidence that ethnic/racial minority individuals are more likely than whites to be judged incompetent to stand trial (Pirelli et al., 2011).

Psychologists have developed tests of those cognitive attributes important to the ability to follow legal proceedings, and people who perform poorly on these tests are more likely to be judged incompetent to stand trial. These tests have not been widely used, however (Appelbaum, 2007). Instead, judgments of incompetence usually are made for people who have existing diagnoses of psychotic disorders or who have symptoms indicating severe psychopathology, such as gross disorientation, delusions, hallucinations, and formal thought disorder (Cochrane, Grisso, & Frederick, 2001; Larkin & Hutton, 2017; Pirelli et al., 2011).

THE INSANITY DEFENSE

Insanity is a legal term rather than a psychological or medical term, and it has been defined in various ways. The **insanity defense** is based on the belief that people cannot be held fully responsible for illegal acts if they were so mentally incapacitated at the time of committing the acts that they could not conform to the rules of society (Kimonis, 2015; Meyer & Weaver, 2006). Note that people do not have to be chronically mentally incapacitated for the insanity defense to apply. They only have to be judged to have been incapacitated at the time they committed the illegal acts. This judgment can be difficult to make.

The insanity defense has been one of the most controversial applications of psychology to the law. The lay public often thinks of the insanity defense as a means by which guilty people "get off." When the insanity defense has been used successfully in celebrated cases—as when John Hinckley successfully used this defense after shooting President Ronald Reagan and the president's press secretary, Jim Brady, in 1981—there have been calls to eliminate it altogether (Kimonis, 2015). Indeed, these celebrated cases have often led to reappraisals of the insanity defense and redefinitions of the legal meaning of insanity.

The insanity defense actually is used much less often than the public tends to think. As shown in Table 2, fewer than 1 in 100 defendants in felony cases

John Hinckley was judged not guilty by reason of insanity in the shooting of President Ronald Reagan. This judgment inspired a reappraisal of the insanity defense. *FBI/ZUMA Press/ Newscom*

TABLE 2   Comparison of Public Perceptions of the Insanity Defense with Actual Use and Results

The public has the perception that many more accused persons use the insanity defense successfully than is actually the case.

	Public Perception	Reality
Percent of felony indictments for which an insanity plea is made	37%	1%
Percent of insanity pleas resulting in "not guilty by reason of insanity"	44	26
Percent of persons "not guilty by reason of insanity" sent to mental hospitals	51	85
Percent of persons "not guilty by reason of insanity" set free	26	15
Percent given conditional release		12
Percent assigned to outpatient treatment		3
Percent given unconditional release		1
Length of confinement of persons "not guilty by reason of insanity":		
All crimes		21.8 months
Murder		32.5 months

Source: Silver, E., Cirincione, C., & Steadman, H. J. (1994). Demythologizing inaccurate perceptions of the insanity defense. *Law & Human Behavior, 18,* 63–70.

files an insanity plea, and only 26 percent of these cases result in acquittal (Melton et al., 2017; Silver, Cirincione, & Steadman, 1994). This means that only about 1 in 400 people charged with a felony are judged not guilty by reason of insanity. About 265 of these people have diagnoses of schizophrenia, and most have a history of psychiatric hospitalizations and previous crimes (McGreevy, Steadman, & Callahan, 1991; Melton et al., 2017).

Almost 90 percent of the people who are acquitted after pleading the insanity defense are male, and 66 percent are white (McGreevy et al., 1991; Warren, Murrie, Chauhan, Dietz, & Morris, 2004). The reasons why men and whites are more likely to successfully plead the insanity defense are unclear but may have to do with their greater access to competent attorneys who can effectively argue the insanity defense. In the past decade or two, as society has become more aware of the plight of abused and battered women, increasing numbers of women are pleading the insanity defense after injuring or killing a partner who had been abusing them.

One such case is that of Lorena Bobbitt. According to Bobbitt, her husband, John, had sexually and emotionally abused her for years. One night in 1994, John returned home drunk and raped Lorena. In what her attorneys described as a brief psychotic episode, Lorena cut off her husband's penis and threw it away. She was acquitted of charges of malicious injury by reason of temporary insanity. She was referred to a mental institution for further evaluation and was released a few months later.

Even when a defendant is judged not guilty by reason of insanity, they usually are not set free. Of those people acquitted because of insanity, about 85 percent are sent to mental hospitals, and all but 1 percent are put under some type of supervision and care. Of those who are sent to mental hospitals, the average length of stay (or incarceration) in the hospital is almost 3 years when all types of crimes are considered, and over 6 years for those who have been accused of murder (and acquitted by reason of insanity) (McGreevy et al., 1991; Silver et al., 1994). Some states stipulate that people judged not guilty by reason of insanity cannot be incarcerated in mental institutions for longer than they would have served in prison had they been judged guilty of their crimes, but not all states have this rule. In short, there is little evidence that the insanity defense is widely used to help people avoid incarceration for their crimes.

Insanity Defense Rules

Five rules have been used in modern history to evaluate defendants' pleas that they be judged not guilty by reason of insanity. These rules are listed in Table 3.

M'Naghten rule

The first insanity defense rule was the **M'Naghten rule** (Kimonis, 2015; Melton et al., 2017). Daniel M'Naghten lived in England in the mid-1800s and believed that the English Tory party was persecuting him. He set out to kill the Tory prime minister but mistakenly shot the prime minister's secretary. At his trial in 1843, the jury judged M'Naghten not guilty by reason of insanity. There was a public outcry at this verdict, leading the House of Lords to establish a rule formalizing when a person could be absolved from responsibility for their acts because of a mental

TABLE 3 Insanity Defense Rules

Five rules have been used in determining whether an individual was insane at the time they committed a crime and therefore should not be held responsible for the crime.

Rule	The Individual Is Not Held Responsible for a Crime If . . .
M'Naghten rule	At the time of the crime, the individual was so affected by a disease of the mind that they did not know the nature of the act they were committing or did not know it was wrong.
Irresistible impulse rule	At the time of the crime, the individual was driven by an irresistible impulse to perform the act or had a diminished capacity to resist performing the act.
Durham rule	The crime was a product of a mental disease or defect.
ALI rule	At the time of the crime, as a result of a mental disease or defect, the person lacked substantial capacity either to appreciate the criminality (wrongfulness) of the act or to conform their conduct to the law.
Insanity Defense Reform Act	At the time of the crime, as a result of mental disease or mental retardation, the person was unable to appreciate the wrongfulness of their conduct.

disorder. This rule, known as the M'Naghten rule, still is used in many jurisdictions today:

> To establish a defense on the ground of insanity, it must be clearly proved that at the time of committing the act, the party accused was labouring under such a defect of reason, from disease of the mind, as not to know the nature and quality of the act he was doing, or if he did know it, that he did not know he was doing what was wrong.

The M'Naghten rule reflects the doctrine that a person must have a "guilty mind"—in Latin, *mens rea*—or the intention to commit the illegal act in order to be held responsible for the act.

Applying the M'Naghten rule might seem to be a straightforward matter—one simply determines whether a person suffers from a disease of the mind and whether during the crime they understood that their actions were wrong. Unfortunately, it is not that simple. A major problem in applying the M'Naghten rule is determining what is meant by a "disease of the mind." The law has been unclear and inconsistent in what disorders it recognizes as diseases of the mind. The most consistently recognized diseases are psychoses. It has been relatively easy for the courts and the public to accept that someone experiencing severe delusions and hallucinations is suffering from a disease and, at times, may not know right from wrong. However, defendants have argued that several other disorders, including alcohol abuse, severe depression, and posttraumatic stress disorder, are diseases of the mind that impair judgments of right and wrong. It is much more difficult for courts, the lay public, and mental health professionals to agree on the validity of such claims (Meyer & Weaver, 2006; Kimonis, 2015).

Another major problem is that the M'Naghten rule requires that a person not know right from wrong at the time of the crime in order to be judged not guilty by reason of insanity (Meyer & Weaver, 2006). This is a difficult judgment to make because it is retrospective. Even when everyone agrees that a defendant suffers from a severe psychological disorder, it does not necessarily follow that at the time of the crime the person was incapable of knowing "right from wrong," as the M'Naghten rule requires. For example, serial killer Jeffrey Dahmer, who tortured, killed, dismembered, and ate his victims, clearly seemed to have a psychological disorder. Nevertheless, the jury denied his insanity defense in part because he took great care to hide his crimes from the local police, suggesting that he knew that what he was doing was wrong or against the law.

Irresistible Impulse Rule

The second rule used to judge the acceptability of the insanity defense is the **irresistible impulse rule.** First applied in Ohio in 1934, the irresistible impulse rule

broadened the conditions under which a criminal act could be considered the product of insanity to include "acts of passion." Even if a person knew that the act they were committing was wrong, the person could be absolved of responsibility for performing the act if they were driven by an irresistible impulse to perform the act or had a diminished capacity to resist performing it (Kimonis, 2015).

One of the most celebrated applications of the notion of diminished capacity was the "Twinkie Defense" of Dan White. As depicted in the 2008 movie *Milk,* in 1979 Dan White assassinated San Francisco Board of Supervisors member Harvey Milk and mayor George Moscone. White argued that he had had diminished capacity to resist the impulse to shoot Moscone and Milk due to the psychological

After Dan White (pictured) killed San Francisco supervisor and gay rights activist Harvey Milk and mayor George Moscone, his lawyers argued that he had diminished capacity due to the psychological effects of extreme stress and the consumption of large quantities of junk food. *AP Images*

effects of extreme stress and the consumption of large amounts of junk food. Using a particularly broad definition of diminished capacity in force in California law at the time, the jury convicted White of manslaughter instead of first-degree murder. Variations of the "Twinkie Defense" have rarely been attempted since White's trial.

Durham Rule

In 1954, Judge David Bazelon further broadened the criteria for the legal definition of insanity in his ruling on the case *Durham v. United States,* which produced the third rule for defining insanity—the **Durham rule.** According to the Durham rule, the insanity defense could be accepted for any crimes that were the "product of mental disease or mental defect." This rule allowed defendants to claim that the presence of any disorder recognized by mental health professionals was the "cause" of their crimes. The Durham rule did not require that defendants show they were incapacitated by their disorders or did not understand that their acts were illegal. The rule eventually was dropped by almost all jurisdictions by the early 1970s (Kimonis, 2015).

ALI Rule

The fourth rule for deciding the acceptability of the insanity defense was proposed by the American Law Institute (ALI) in 1962. Motivated by dissatisfaction with the existing legal definitions of insanity, a group of lawyers, judges, and scholars associated with the ALI worked to formulate a better definition, which eventually resulted in what is known as the **ALI rule:**

> A person is not responsible for criminal conduct if at the time of such conduct as the result of mental disease or defect he lacks substantial capacity either to appreciate the criminality (wrongfulness) of his conduct or to conform his conduct to the requirements of the law.

This rule is broader than the M'Naghten rule because it requires only that the defendants have a lack of appreciation of the criminality of their act, not an absence of understanding of the criminality of the act. The defendants' inability to conform their conduct to the requirements of the law can result from the emotional symptoms of a psychological disorder as well as from the cognitive deficits caused by the disorder. This expanded understanding incorporates some of the crimes recognized by the irresistible impulse rule. The ALI rule clearly is more restrictive than the Durham rule, however, because it requires some lack of appreciation of the criminality of an act, rather than the mere presence of a mental disorder (Kimonis, 2015). The ALI rule further restricts the types of mental disorders that can contribute to a successful insanity defense:

> As used in this Article, the term "mental disease or defect" does not include an abnormality manifested only by repeated criminal or otherwise antisocial conduct.

This restriction prohibits defense attorneys from arguing that a defendant's long history of antisocial acts is itself evidence of the presence of a mental disease or defect. Further, in 1977, in *Barrett v. United States,* it was ruled that "temporary insanity created by voluntary use of alcohol or drugs" also does not qualify a defendant for acquittal by reason of insanity.

The ALI rule was widely adopted in the United States, including in the jurisdiction in which John Hinckley was tried for shooting Ronald Reagan. Hinckley had a long-standing diagnosis of schizophrenia and an obsession with the actress Jodie Foster. Letters he wrote to Foster before shooting Reagan indicated that he committed the act under the delusion that it would impress Foster and cause her to return his love. Hinckley's defense attorneys successfully argued that he had a diminished capacity to understand the wrongfulness of shooting Reagan or to conform his behaviors to the requirements of the law. The public outcry over the judgment that Hinckley was "not guilty by reason of insanity" initiated another reappraisal of the legal definition of insanity and the use of the insanity defense (Kimonis, 2015).

Insanity Defense Reform Act

The reappraisal of the insanity defense after John Hinckley's shooting of President Reagan led to the fifth rule for defining legal insanity, codified in the **Insanity Defense Reform Act,** enacted by Congress in 1984. The Insanity Defense Reform Act adopted the 1983 **American Psychiatric Association definition of insanity.** This definition dropped the provision in the ALI rule that absolved people of responsibility for criminal acts if they were unable to conform their behavior to the law and retained the wrongfulness criterion initially proposed in the M'Naghten rule (Kimonis, 2015). The definition reads as follows:

> A person charged with a criminal offense should be found not guilty by reason of insanity if it is shown that, as a result of mental disease or mental retardation, he was unable to appreciate the wrongfulness of his conduct at the time of his offense.

This definition now applies in all cases tried in U.S. federal courts and in the courts of about half the states. Also following the Hinckley verdict, most states now require that a defendant pleading not guilty by reason of insanity proves that he or she was insane at the time of the crime. Previously, the burden of proof had been on the prosecution to prove that the defendant was sane at the time the crime was committed (Kimonis, 2015). The specific rules that are applied vary state to state, but some version of the M'Naghten, ALI, or federal rules is most common. As of 2018, all of the states except Kansas, Idaho, Montana, and Utah have some form of the insanity defense.

Problems with the Insanity Defense

Cases in which the insanity defense is pled often use mental health professionals to provide expert opinions. Despite their expertise, mental health professionals often disagree about the nature and causes of psychological disorders, the presence or absence of a psychological disorder, and the evaluation of defendants' states of mind at the time crimes were committed (Melton et al., 2017; Warren et al., 2004). Usually, lawyers on both sides of the case find a mental health professional who supports their point of view, and the two professionals inevitably are in disagreement with each other. This disagreement leads to confusion on the part of judges, juries, and the public.

Mental health professionals also have raised concerns about the rules used to determine the acceptability of the insanity defense (Meyer & Weaver, 2006). Behind these rules is the assumption that most people, including most people with a psychological disorder, have free will and usually can choose how they will act in any given situation. Many current models of both normal and abnormal behavior suggest that

people do not have that much control over their behaviors. Biological predispositions, early life experiences, or disordered patterns of thinking can make people act in irrational and perhaps uncontrolled ways. This view makes it more difficult to determine when individuals should or should not be held responsible for their behaviors.

Andrea Yates argued that severe psychosis and postpartum depression led her to drown her five young children in 2001.
8708/Gamma-Rapho/Getty Images

SHADES OF GRAY

Read the following case study.

On June 20, 2001, after her husband Rusty left for work, Andrea Yates methodically drowned all five of her young children in the bathtub. She then called 911 and asked that a police officer come to her house. She also called her husband at work and told him he needed to come home.

Andrea had a long history of psychotic depression. In the summer of 1999, she had tried to commit suicide and had been hospitalized twice. She had hallucinations and delusions that led her to believe she was evil and that her children were irreparably damaged and doomed to hell. Her psychiatrist diagnosed her with postpartum psychosis and successfully treated her but urged the couple not to have any more children, saying future episodes of psychotic depression were inevitable. The Yates conceived

their fifth child approximately 7 weeks after her discharge from the hospital.

Three months after the birth of her fifth child, Andrea's father died, and her condition worsened, leading her to be hospitalized. When she was discharged, her psychiatrist gave instructions that she be watched around the clock. On the day of the drowning, her husband left for work expecting his mother to arrive at the house soon to supervise Andrea and the children. It was then that Andrea drowned the children. She later told a psychiatrist, "My children weren't righteous. They stumbled because I was evil. The way I was raising them, they could never be saved. They were doomed to perish in the fires of hell." (*Houston Chronicle,* March 5, 2002)

Would you judge Andrea Yates "not guilty by reason of insanity"? Why or why not? (Discussion appears at the end of this chapter.)

Guilty but Mentally Ill

In a sixth and most recent reform of the insanity defense, some states have adopted as an alternative to the verdict "not guilty by reason of insanity" the verdict **guilty but mentally ill (GBMI)**. Defendants convicted as GBMI are incarcerated for the normal term designated for their crimes, with the expectation that they also will receive treatment for their mental illness (Kimonis, 2015). Proponents of the GBMI verdict argue that it recognizes the mental illness of defendants while still holding them responsible for their actions. Critics argue that the GBMI verdict is essentially a guilty verdict and a means of eliminating the insanity defense (Tanay, 1992). Juries may believe they are ensuring that a person gets treatment by judging them GBMI but there is no guarantee that a person convicted under GBMI will receive treatment. In most states, it is left to legal authorities to decide whether to incarcerate people judged GBMI in mental institutions or in prisons and, if they are sent to prisons, whether to provide them with treatment for their mental illness. As we discuss in the next section, people with mental disorders usually do not receive adequate—if any—treatment when they are incarcerated.

MENTAL HEALTH CARE IN THE JUSTICE SYSTEM

Since the 1970s, the number of prisoners in U.S. prisons has quadrupled. Over 20 million Americans are currently or have been incarcerated, the highest rate in the world. The mentally ill are overrepresented in correctional settings at estimates ranging from two to four times the general population which has resulted in ten times more individuals with Serious Mental Illnesses (SMI) in prisons and jails than there are in state mental hospitals (Al-Rousan, Rubenstein, Sieleni, Deol, & Wallace, 2017). Nearly one out of 100 Americans is in prison, a rate 5 to 10 times that of other industrialized democracies (National Research Council [NRC], 2014). This increase has largely to do with tougher enforcement of drug possession laws beginning in the 1980s and anti-crime initiatives in the 1990s, and disproportionately affects lower-income and ethnic minority individuals (Alexander, 2012; NRC, 2014). At the same time, the deinstitutionalization movement (see the chapter "Looking at Abnormality") has led to mentally ill and at-risk individuals living in their communities without adequate care. It is not surprising that these social and historical factors combine to affect mental health and the justice system for the worse.

A recent study found that almost half of inmates were diagnosed with a mental illness (48 percent) with higher rates among females (41 percent) than males (27 percent). Women were more likely to be diagnosed with both a mental illness and substance use disorder. Among this group, 29 percent had a SMI and 26 percent had a history of a substance use disorder. Almost all psychiatric diagnoses were assigned during the individual's first incarceration. Almost all mental illness diagnoses (99 percent) were first made during incarceration (Al-Rousan et al., 2017). Men with a mental disorder are four times more likely to be incarcerated than men without a mental disorder, and women with a mental disorder are eight times likelier to be incarcerated than women without a mental disorder (Teplin, Abram, & McClelland, 1996). Although a subset of the crimes committed by people with mental disorders involve violence or theft, many of their crimes involve drug possession and use (Osher & Steadman, 2007). Many of these individuals are repeat offenders, going through a revolving door between prison and a freedom characterized by joblessness, homelessness, and poverty.

As a result, the jail and prison systems have become the de facto mental health system for millions of people with mental disorders (NRC, 2014; Osher & Steadman, 2007). Multiple studies show very high rates of mental disorders in incarcerated populations, up to three times the rates in the general population (NRC, 2014; Prins, 2014). Rates are especially high for SMI like bipolar disorder and psychotic disorders (Steadman, Osher, Robbins, Case, & Samuels, 2009). Studies of detained youth find that 60 percent of boys and two-thirds of girls have a diagnosable mental disorder, even when conduct disorder is excluded (Teplin, Abram, McClelland, Dulcan, & Mericle, 2002). Over 50 percent of incarcerated adult males can be diagnosed with a mental disorder, most often a substance use disorder or antisocial personality disorder (James & Glaze, 2006; NRC, 2014). A study of women prison inmates found that 64 percent had a lifetime history of a major psychiatric disorder such as major depression, an anxiety disorder, a substance use disorder, or a personality disorder and that 46 percent had had symptoms of a major psychiatric disorder in the previous 6 months (Jordan, Schlenger, Fairbank, & Caddell, 1996). In addition, nearly 80 percent of these women had been exposed to an extreme trauma, such as sexual abuse, sometime in their life. Another study of 1,272 women jail detainees awaiting trial in Chicago found that over 80 percent had a lifetime history of a psychiatric disorder and that 70 percent had been symptomatic within the previous 6 months (Teplin et al., 1996). In these studies, the most common diagnosis the women received was substance abuse or dependence, but substantial percentages of the women also had been diagnosed with major depression and/or a borderline or antisocial personality disorder.

Numerous court decisions have mandated that prison inmates receive necessary mental health services, just as they should receive necessary medical services. Most inmates with mental disorders do not receive these services, however. About one-third of prison and jail inmates with significant mental health problems receive treatment while incarcerated, according to federal statistics (Bronson & Berzofsky, 2017). A study of male inmates found that only 37 percent of those with schizophrenia or a major mood disorder received treatment while in jail (Teplin, 1990), and a study of female inmates found that only 23.5 percent of these with schizophrenia or a major mood disorder received treatment in jail (Teplin, Abram, & McClelland, 1997). Only 15.4 percent of youth in detention facilities who have a mental disorder receive treatment (Teplin et al., 2002). Depression in inmates is particularly likely to go unnoticed and untreated, even though suicide is one of the leading causes of death among incarcerated people.

The services inmates do receive often are minimal. Substance abuse treatments may involve only the provision of information about drugs and perhaps Alcoholics Anonymous or Narcotics Anonymous meetings held in the prison. Treatment for schizophrenia or depression may involve only occasional visits with a prison physician who prescribes a standard drug treatment but has neither the time nor the expertise to follow individuals closely.

Comprehensive treatment programs focusing on the special needs of prison inmates with mental disorders can successfully reduce their symptoms of mental disorder, their substance abuse, and their repeat offense rates. Many of these treatment programs focus on male inmates, who greatly outnumber female inmates.

Female inmates may have different needs for services than male inmates (Teplin et al., 1997). Female inmates may be more likely than male inmates to have a history of sexual and physical abuse, which needs to be addressed in treatment. Also, female inmates are more likely than male inmates to be suffering from depression or anxiety and to have children for whom they will become caregivers after they are released from prison.

Increasingly, communities are developing systems to divert criminal offenders with mental disorders into community-based treatment programs rather than incarceration (Redlich, Steadman, Monahan, Robbins, & Petrila, 2006). The hope is that providing these individuals with comprehensive mental health treatment combined with occupational rehabilitation and social services will enable them to live in the community as healthy and productive citizens. Diversion from jail into community services is especially likely to be a goal when the offender is a youth (Steinberg, 2009).

Some states have developed mental health courts, in which the cases of offenders with mental disorders are reviewed by judges who specialize in working with mental health and social service professionals to divert offenders into treatment and rehabilitation. Courts that focus specifically on drug offenders often are called *drug courts*. Offenders diverted by mental health courts or drug courts into community treatment are still under the watchful eye of the court. If they do not cooperate with the plan developed by the mental health court for their treatment and rehabilitation, they can be diverted back into jail. This feature of mental health courts is controversial because it amounts to coercing offenders into treatment. Most courts attempt to avoid reincarceration and instead use milder sanctions, such as requiring offenders to reappear before the judge, to motivate them to cooperate with their treatment plan (Redlich et al., 2006). The effectiveness of mental health courts and drug courts in reducing recidivism and rehabilitating offenders into the community relies heavily on the availability of high-quality community services, services sorely lacking in many communities (Boothroyd, Mercado, Poythress, Christy, & Petrila, 2005).

CHAPTER INTEGRATION

There has perhaps been less integration of biological, social, and psychological viewpoints in the law's approach to issues of mental health than in the mental health field itself. The rules governing the insanity defense suggest that the law takes a biological perspective on psychological disorders, conforming to the belief that mental disorders are like medical diseases (Figure 2). Similarly, civil commitment rules require certification

FIGURE 2 | **Differences Between the Perspective of the Law and That of the Mental Health Profession.**

Perspective of the law

Does the individual have a mental disorder or disease?

Yes → Can be absolved from responsibility for a crime and can be committed to a mental health facility against his or her will

No → Will be held responsible for a crime and cannot be committed to a mental health facility against his or her will

Perspective of the mental health profession

Biological, psychological, or social vulnerabilities to mental health problems

Yes → More likely to commit a crime

No → Less likely to commit a crime

that a person has a mental disorder or disease before they can be committed, further legitimating psychiatric diagnostic systems based on medical models.

In each area discussed in this chapter, however, there are mental health professionals advocating a more integrated and complex view of mental disorders than that traditionally held by the legal system. These professionals are trying to educate judges, juries, and laypeople to help them understand that some people have biological, psychological, or social predispositions to disorders and that other biological, psychological, or social factors can interact with these predispositions to trigger the onset of mental disorders or certain manifestations of mental disorders. What is most difficult to explain is the probabilistic nature of the predictions that can be made about mental disorders and about the behavior of people with these disorders. While a predisposition or certain recent life experiences may make a person more likely to develop a disorder or to engage in a specific behavior (such as a violent behavior), they do not determine the disorder or the specific behavior.

We all prefer to have predictions about the future that are definite, especially when we are making decisions that will determine a person's freedom or confinement. That kind of definitiveness is not possible, however, given our present knowledge of the ways biological, psychological, and social forces interact to influence people's behavior.

SHADES OF GRAY   DISCUSSION

The first point you might note in making your decision is that Andrea Yates had a well-documented history of psychotic depressions—in fact, the psychiatrist who treated her in 1999 warned that she could harm her children as a result of her psychosis. Yates testified that on the morning of the drownings, her delusions and hallucinations led her to believe that she had to kill her children to "save" them. But consider the fact that Yates called 911 and her husband after the drownings. Would this affect your decision? For the jury in Yates' 2002 murder trial, it did. They rejected the insanity defense, accepting the assertion by the State of Texas that the fact that Yates called 911 proved she knew her actions were wrong despite her mental defect. Yates was convicted of murder and sentenced to life in prison. In 2005, Yates' conviction was overturned due to false testimony by one of the prosecution witnesses. In 2006, Yates was retried, and this time she was found not guilty by reason of insanity and committed to a Texas state mental hospital.

In making your judgment, you likely found yourself struggling with emotions related to accepting the killing of children by a parent. You are not alone. The public often cannot accept any excuse for such a crime, and therefore the plea of "not guilty by reason of insanity," supposedly as the result of psychotic postpartum depression, is highly controversial in such cases (Williamson, 1993). Severe postpartum depression with psychotic symptoms is very rare, and violence by these women against their newborns is even rarer (Nolen-Hoeksema, 1990). When such violence does occur, some courts have accepted that the mothers' behaviors are the result of the postpartum psychosis and have judged these women not guilty by reason of insanity, as the Texas courts finally did in Andrea Yates' case. At other times, however, even though the law is intended to be objective, its application can be influenced by people's emotional reactions to the behaviors of people with mental disorders.

CHAPTER SUMMARY

- Civil commitment is the procedure through which a person may be committed for treatment in a mental institution against their will. In most jurisdictions, three criteria are used to determine whether individuals may be committed: if they suffer from grave disability that impairs their ability to provide for their own basic needs, if they are an imminent danger to themselves, or if they pose an imminent danger to others. Each of these criteria requires a subjective judgment on the part of clinicians and, often, predictions about the future that clinicians may not be competent to make. In particular, the prediction of who will pose a danger to others in the future is difficult to make and often is made incorrectly.

- When being considered for commitment, patients have the right to have an attorney, to have a public hearing, to call and confront witnesses, to appeal decisions, and to be placed in the least restrictive treatment setting. (The right to a hearing is often waived for short-term commitments in emergency settings.) Once committed, patients have the right to be treated and the right to refuse treatment.

- People with mental disorders, particularly those who also have a history of substance abuse, are somewhat more likely to commit violent acts, especially against family members and friends, than are people without a mental disorder. The prevalence of violence among people with mental disorders is not as great as is often perceived by the public and the media, however.

- One fundamental principle of law is that, in order to stand trial, an accused individual must have a reasonable degree of rational understanding both of the charges against them and of the proceedings of the trial and must be able to participate in their defense. People who do not have an understanding of what is happening to them in a courtroom and who cannot participate in their defense are said to be incompetent to stand trial. Defendants who have a history of a psychotic disorder, who have current symptoms of psychosis, or who perform poorly on tests of important cognitive skills may be judged incompetent to stand trial.

- Five rules for judging the acceptability of the insanity defense have been used in recent history: the M'Naghten rule, the irresistible impulse rule, the Durham rule, the ALI rule, and the Insanity Defense Reform Act. Each of these rules requires that the defendant be diagnosed with a mental disorder, and most of them require that it be shown that the defendant did not appreciate the criminality of their act or could not control their behaviors at the time of the crime.

- The verdict "guilty but mentally ill" was introduced following public uproar over uses of the insanity defense in high-profile cases. Persons judged guilty but mentally ill are confined for the duration of a regular prison term but with the assumption that they will receive psychiatric treatment while incarcerated.

- Mental health professionals have raised a number of concerns about the insanity defense. For one thing, it requires after-the-fact judgments of a defendant's state of mind at the time of the crime. In addition, the rules governing the insanity defense presume that people have free will and usually can control their actions. These presumptions contradict some models of normal and abnormal behavior that suggest that behavior is strongly influenced by biological, psychological, and social forces.

- Communities are increasingly attempting to divert persons with mental disorders who commit crimes away from jail and into community-based treatment programs. Mental health courts and drug courts have been established specifically for this purpose.

KEY TERMS

need for treatment

civil commitment

grave disability

dangerousness to self

dangerousness to others

right to treatment

right to refuse treatment

informed consent

incompetent to stand trial

insanity

insanity defense

M'Naghten rule

irresistible impulse rule

Durham rule

ALI rule

Insanity Defense Reform Act

American Psychiatric Association definition of insanity

guilty but mentally ill (GBMI)

A

ABAB (reversal) design type of experimental design in which an intervention is introduced, withdrawn, and then reinstated, and the behavior of a participant is examined on and off the treatment

abstinence violation effect what happens when a person attempting to abstain from alcohol use ingests alcohol and then endures conflict and guilt by making an internal attribution to explain why he or she drank, thereby making him or her more likely to continue drinking in order to cope with the self-blame and guilt

acute stress disorder disorder similar to posttraumatic stress disorder but occurs within 1 month of exposure to the stressor and does not last more than 4 weeks; often involves dissociative symptoms

adjustment disorder stress-related disorder that involves emotional and behavioral symptoms (depressive symptoms, anxiety symptoms, and/or antisocial behaviors) that arise within 3 months of the onset of a stressor

adolescent-onset conduct disorder a conduct disorder characterized by aggression, destructiveness, deceitfulness, and rules violation beginning after age 10

adoption study study of the heritability of a disorder by finding adopted people with a disorder and then determining the prevalence of the disorder among their biological and adoptive relatives, in order to separate out contributing genetic and environmental factors

adrenal-cortical system the hormonal system situated in the adrenal cortex and activated by the hypothalamus, that responds to stress to determine fight-or-flight reactions

agnosia impaired ability to recognize objects or people

agoraphobia anxiety disorder characterized by fear of places and situations in which it would be difficult to escape, such as enclosed places, open spaces, and crowds

Alcohol Use disorder A problematic pattern of alcohol use that creates significant impairment or distress that is manifested in a variety of behaviors such as consuming large amounts of alcohol, persistent desire and failed attempts to reduce the quantity of alcohol consumed, strong desire to use alcohol (craving), tolerance, and withdrawal.

Alcoholics Anonymous (AA) an organization created by and for people with alcoholism involving a 12-step treatment program

ALI rule legal principle stating that a person is not responsible for criminal conduct if they lack the capacity to appreciate the criminality (wrongfulness) of the act or to conform their conduct to the requirements of the law as a result of mental disease

allostatic load physiological condition resulting from chronic arousal of the fight-or-flight response to stress

Alzheimer's disease (AD) progressive neurological disease that is the most common cause of dementia

amenorrhea cessation of the menses

American Psychiatric Association definition of insanity definition of insanity stating that people cannot be held responsible for their conduct if, at the time they commit crimes, as the result of mental disease or mental retardation they are unable to appreciate the wrongfulness of their conduct

amphetamines stimulant drugs that can produce symptoms of euphoria, self-confidence, alertness, agitation, paranoia, perceptual illusions, and depression

amygdala structure of the limbic system critical in emotions such as fear

animal studies studies that attempt to test theories of psychopathology using animals

animal-type phobias extreme fears of specific animals that may induce immediate and intense panic attacks and cause the individual to go to great lengths to avoid the animals

anorexia nervosa eating disorder in which people fail to maintain body weights that are normal for their age and height and have fears of becoming fat, distorted body images, and amenorrhea

antagonism hostility toward others

antagonist drugs drugs that block or change the effects of an addictive drug, reducing desire for the drug

anterograde amnesia deficit in the ability to learn new information

antianxiety drugs drugs used to treat anxiety, insomnia, and other psychological symptoms

anticonvulsants drugs used to treat mania and depression

antidepressant drugs drugs used to treat the symptoms of depression, such as sad mood, negative thinking, and disturbances of sleep and appetite; common types are tricyclics, selective serotonin reuptake inhibitors, and serotonin-norepinephrine reuptake inhibitors

antipsychotic drugs drugs used to treat psychotic symptoms, such as delusions, hallucinations, and disorganized thinking

antisocial personality disorder (ASPD) pervasive pattern of criminal, impulsive, callous, and/or ruthless behavior, predicated on disregard for the rights of others and an absence of respect for social norms

anxiety state of apprehension, tension, and worry

anxiety sensitivity belief that bodily symptoms have harmful consequences

aphasia impaired ability to produce and comprehend language

applied tension technique technique used to treat blood-injection-injury type phobias in which the therapist teaches the client to increase his or her blood pressure and heart rate, thus preventing the client from fainting

apraxia impaired ability to initiate common voluntary behaviors

arousal phase in the sexual response cycle, psychological experience of arousal and pleasure as well as physiological changes, such as the tensing of muscles and enlargement of blood vessels and tissues (also called the excitement phase)

assessment the process of evaluating psychological, social, and emotional functioning through a variety of clinical techniques to determine if a psychological disorder is present

association studies genetic studies in which researchers identify physical disorders associated with a target psychological disorder for which genetic abnormalities or markers are known; the DNA of individuals with the psychological disorder and their first-degree relatives is then examined to determine if they also have this genetic marker (one form of molecular genetic studies)

attention-deficit/hyperactivity disorder (ADHD) syndrome marked by deficits in controlling attention, inhibiting impulses, and organizing behavior to accomplish long-term goals

atypical anorexia nervosa disorder characterized by all the criteria for anorexia nervosa except that despite significant weight loss, the weight of the affected individual remains within or above the normal range

atypical antipsychotics drugs that seem to be even more effective in treating schizophrenia than phenothiazines without the same neurological side effects; they bind to a different type of dopamine receptor than other neuroleptic drugs

autism childhood disorder marked by deficits in social interaction (such as a lack of interest in one's family or other children), communication (such as failing to modulate one's voice to signify emotional expression), and activities and interests (such as engaging in bizarre, repetitive behaviors)

autism spectrum disorder (ASD) a spectrum of neurodevelopmental disorders characterized by disrupted social and language development (formerly referred to as autism)

autonomic nervous system the part of the nervous system that controls bodily functions not consciously directed, such as breathing, the heartbeat, and digestive processes

aversion therapy treatment that involves the pairing of unpleasant stimuli with deviant or maladaptive sources of pleasure in order to induce an aversive reaction to the formerly pleasurable stimulus

avoidant personality disorder (AVPD) pervasive anxiety, sense of inadequacy, and fear of being criticized that lead to the avoidance of most social interactions with others and to restraint and nervousness in social interactions

avolition inability to persist at common goal-directed activities

B

barbiturates drugs used to treat anxiety and insomnia that work by suppressing the central nervous system and decreasing the activity level of certain neurons

behavioral approaches approaches to psychopathology that focus on the influence of reinforcements and punishments in producing behavior; the two core principles or processes of learning according to behaviorism are *classical conditioning* and *operant conditioning*

behavioral genetics study of the processes by which genes affect behavior and the extent to which personality and abnormality are genetically inherited

behavioral inhibition set of behavioral traits including shyness, fearfulness, irritability, cautiousness, and introversion; behaviorally inhibited children tend to avoid or withdraw from novel situations, are clingy with parents, and become excessively aroused when exposed to unfamiliar situations

behavioral observation method for assessing the frequency of a client's behaviors and the specific situations in which they occur

behavioral theories of depression theories that view depression as resulting from negative life events that represent a reduction in positive reinforcement; sympathetic responses to depressive behavior then serve as positive reinforcement for the depression itself

behavioral therapies psychotherapeutic approaches that focus on identifying the reinforcements and punishments contributing to a person's maladaptive behaviors and on changing specific behaviors

behavioral therapy therapy that focuses on changing a person's specific behaviors by replacing unwanted behaviors with desired behaviors

behaviorism study of the impact of reinforcements and punishments on behavior

benzodiazepines drugs that reduce anxiety and insomnia

beta-amyloid class of proteins that accumulates in the spaces between neurons in the brain, contributing to Alzheimer's disease

binge-eating disorder eating disorder in which people compulsively overeat either continuously or on discrete binges but do not behave in ways to compensate for the overeating

binge/purge type of anorexia nervosa type of anorexia nervosa in which periodic bingeing or purging behaviors occur along with behaviors that meet the criteria for anorexia nervosa

bingeing eating a large amount of food in one sitting

biological approach view that biological factors cause and should be used to treat abnormality

biological theories theories of abnormality that focus on biological causes of abnormal behaviors

biopsychosocial approach approach to psychopathology that seeks to integrate biological, psychological, and social factors in understanding and treating psychopathology

bipolar disorders are defined by fluctuations in mood and activity levels.

bipolar I disorder form of bipolar disorder in which the full symptoms of mania are experienced; depressive aspects may be more infrequent or mild

bipolar II disorder form of bipolar disorder in which only hypomanic episodes are experienced and the depressive component is more pronounced

Black box warning a black box warning is the FDA's most stringent warning for drugs and medical devices on the market which notify the public and health care providers to serious side effects, such as injury or death

blood-injection-injury type phobias extreme fears of seeing blood or an injury or of receiving an injection or another invasive medical procedure, which cause a drop in heart rate and blood pressure and fainting

body dysmorphic disorder an obsessive-compulsive disorder, characterized by excessive concern about physical appearance which results in significant distress and the impairment of interpersonal situations

borderline personality disorder syndrome characterized by rapidly shifting and unstable mood, self-concept, and interpersonal relationships, as well as impulsive behavior and transient dissociative states

breathing-related sleep disorder group of sleep disorders characterized by numerous brief sleep disturbances due to problems breathing

brief psychotic disorder disorder characterized by the sudden onset of delusions, hallucinations, disorganized speech, and/or disorganized behavior that lasts only between 1 day and 1 month, after which the symptoms vanish completely

bulimia nervosa eating disorder in which people engage in bingeing and behave in ways to prevent weight gain from the binges, such as self-induced vomiting, excessive exercise, and abuse of purging drugs (such as laxatives)

C

caffeine chemical compound with stimulant effects

cannabis substance that causes feelings of well-being, perceptual distortions, and paranoid thinking

case studies in-depth analyses of individuals

cataplexy episodes of sudden loss of muscle tone lasting under 2 minutes, triggered by laughter or joking in people who have had narcolepsy for a long time

catatonia group of disorganized behaviors that reflect an extreme lack of responsiveness to the outside world

catharsis expression of emotions connected to memories and conflicts, which, according to Freud, leads to the release of energy used to keep these memories in the unconscious

causal attribution explanation for why an event occurred

central sleep apnea sleep disorder characterized by complete cessation of respiratory activity for brief periods of time (20 seconds or more); sufferers do not have frequent awakenings and do not tend to feel tired during the day; occurs when the brain does not send the signal to breathe to the respiratory system

cerebral cortex part of the brain that regulates complex activities, such as speech and analytical thinking

cerebrovascular disease disease that occurs when the blood supply to the brain is blocked, causing tissue damage to the brain

childhood-onset conduct disorder a conduct disorder characterized by aggression, destructiveness, deceitfulness, and rules violation beginning before age 10 that tends to worsen with age

childhood-onset fluency disorder disturbances of the normal fluency and motor production of speech, including repetitive sounds or syllables, prolongation of consonants or vowel sounds, broken words, blocking or words produced with an excess of physical tension; also known as stuttering

chlorpromazine antipsychotic drug

circadian rhythm sleep-wake disorder sleep disorder characterized by insomnia, excessive sleepiness, or both due to disruptions in circadian rhythms

civil commitment forcing of a person into a mental health facility against their will

classical conditioning form of learning in which a neutral stimulus becomes associated with a stimulus that naturally elicits a response, thereby making the neutral stimulus itself sufficient to elicit the same response

classification system set of syndromes and the rules for determining whether an individual's symptoms are part of one of these syndromes

client-centered therapy (CCT) Carl Rogers' form of psychotherapy, which consists of an equal relationship between therapist and client as the client searches for his or her inner self, receiving unconditional positive regard and an empathic understanding from the therapist

clinical interview a face-to-face conversation between a mental health professional and a client in which information is gathered about the client's behavior, attitudes, emotions, life history, and personality

cocaine central nervous system stimulant that causes a rush of positive feelings initially but that can lead to impulsiveness, agitation, and anxiety and can cause withdrawal symptoms of exhaustion and depression

cognitions thoughts or beliefs

cognitive theories theories that focus on belief systems and ways of thinking as the causes of abnormal behavior

cognitive therapies therapeutic approaches that focus on changing people's maladaptive thought patterns

cognitive-behavioral therapy (CBT) treatment focused on changing negative patterns of thinking and solving concrete problems through brief sessions in which a therapist helps a client challenge negative thoughts, consider alternative perspectives, and take effective actions

cohort effect effect that occurs when people born in one historical period are at different risk for a disorder than are people born in another historical period

collective unconscious according to Carl Jung, the wisdom accumulated by a society over hundreds of years of human existence and stored in the memories of individuals

communication disorders disorders characterized by persistent difficulties in the acquisition and use of language and other means of communicating

community mental health centers institutions for the treatment of people with mental health problems in the community; may include teams of social workers, therapists, and physicians who coordinate care

community mental health movement movement launched in 1963 that attempted to provide coordinated mental health services to people in community-based treatment centers

comorbidity meeting the criteria for two or more diagnostic categories simultaneously

compulsions repetitive behaviors or mental acts that an individual feels he or she must perform

computerized tomography (CT) method of analyzing brain structure by passing narrow X-ray beams through a person's head from several angles to produce measurements from which a computer can construct an image of the brain

concordance rate probability that both twins will develop a disorder if one twin has the disorder

conditioned avoidance response behavior that is reinforced because it allows individuals to avoid situations that cause anxiety

conditioned response (CR) in classical conditioning, response that first followed a natural stimulus but that now follows a conditioned stimulus

conditioned stimulus (CS) in classical conditioning, previously neutral stimulus that, through pairing with a natural stimulus, becomes sufficient to elicit a response

conduct disorder syndrome marked by chronic disregard for the rights of others, including specific behaviors such as stealing, lying, and engaging in acts of violence

conscious refers to mental contents and processes of which we are actively aware

continuous variable factor that is measured along a continuum (such as 0–100) rather than falling into a discrete category (such as "diagnosed with depression")

continuum model of abnormality model of abnormality that views mental disorders not as categorically different from "normal" experiences but as lying somewhere along a continuum from healthy, functional behaviors, thoughts, and feelings to unhealthy, dysfunctional behaviors, thoughts, and feelings

control group in an experimental study, group of subjects whose experience resembles that of the experimental group in all ways except that they do not receive the key manipulation

conversion disorder (functional neurological symptom disorder) syndrome marked by a sudden loss of functioning in a part of the body, usually following an extreme psychological stressor

coronary heart disease (CHD) chronic illness that is a leading cause of death in the United States, occurring when the blood vessels that supply the heart with oxygen and nutrients are narrowed or closed by plaque, resulting in a myocardial infarction (heart attack) when closed completely

correlation coefficient statistic used to indicate the degree of relationship between two variables

correlational studies method in which researchers assess only the relationship between two variables and do not manipulate one variable to determine its effects on another variable

cortisol hormone that helps the body respond to stressors, inducing the fight-or-flight response

cross-sectional type of research examining people at one point in time but not following them over time

cultural relativism view that norms among cultures set the standard for what counts as normal behavior, which implies that abnormal behavior can only be defined relative to these norms and that no universal definition of abnormality is therefore possible; only definitions of abnormality relative to a specific culture are possible

cyclothymic disorder milder but more chronic form of bipolar disorder that consists of alternation between hypomanic episodes and mild depressive episodes over a period of at least 2 years

D

dangerousness to others legal criterion for involuntary commitment that is met when a person would pose a threat or danger to other people if not incarcerated

dangerousness to self legal criterion for involuntary commitment that is met when a person is imminently suicidal or a danger to themselves as judged by a mental health professional

day treatment centers mental health facilities that provide more intensive psychiatric, occupational, and rehabilitative therapies for persons with mental illness during the day while clients live at home during recovery

deep brain stimulation procedure to treat depression in which electrodes are surgically implanted in specific areas of the brain and connected to a pulse generator that is placed under the skin and stimulates these brain areas

degradation process in which a receiving neuron releases an enzyme into the synapse, breaking down neurotransmitters into other biochemicals

deinstitutionalization movement in which thousands of mental patients were released from mental institutions; a result of the patients' rights movement, which was aimed at stopping the dehumanization of mental patients and at restoring their basic legal rights

delayed ejaculation marked delay, infrequency, or absence of ejaculation during sexual encounters

delirium cognitive disorder including disorientation and memory loss that is acute and usually transient

delirium tremens (DTs) symptoms that result during severe alcohol withdrawal, including hallucinations, delusions, agitation, and disorientation

delusion of reference false belief that external events, such as other people's actions or natural disasters, relate somehow to oneself

delusional disorder disorder characterized by delusions lasting at least 1 month regarding situations that occur in real life, such as being followed, poisoned, or deceived by a spouse or having a disease; people with this disorder do not show any other symptoms of schizophrenia

delusions fixed beliefs with no basis in reality

delusions of thought insertion beliefs that one's thoughts are being controlled by outside forces

demand characteristics factors in an experiment that suggest to participants how the experimenter would like them to behave

dementia cognitive disorder in which a gradual and usually permanent decline of intellectual functioning occurs; can be caused by a medical condition, substance intoxication, or withdrawal; also known as *major neurocognitive disorder*

dependent personality disorder people suffering from this disorder are anxious about interpersonal interactions, but their anxiety stems from a deep need to be cared for by others, rather than from a concern that they will be criticized

dependent variable factor that an experimenter seeks to predict

depersonalization/derealization disorder syndrome marked by frequent episodes of feeling detached from one's own body and mental processes, as if one were an outside observer of oneself; symptoms must cause significant distress or interference with one's ability to function

depressants drugs that slow the nervous system

depressive disorders a set of disorders characterized by depressed mood and/or anhedonia (and not mania)

detachment the inability to connect with others

developmental coordination disorder disorder involving deficits in the ability to walk, run, or hold on to objects

diagnosis label given to a set of symptoms that tend to occur together

Diagnostic and Statistical Manual of Mental Disorders (DSM) official manual for diagnosing mental disorders in the United States, containing a list of specific criteria for each disorder, how long a person's symptoms must be present to qualify for a diagnosis, and requirements that the symptoms interfere with daily functioning in order to be called disorders

dialectical behavior therapy cognitive-behavioral intervention aimed at teaching problem-solving skills, interpersonal skills, and skill at managing negative emotions

diathesis-stress model model that asserts that only when a diathesis or vulnerability interacts with a stress or trigger will a disorder emerge

disinhibition lack of restraint

disorders of arousal sleep disorders that involve recurrent episodes of incomplete awakening from sleep that seem to mix elements of wakefulness and NREM sleep

disruptive mood dysregulation disorder a disorder in children characterized by immature and inappropriate temper outbursts that are grossly out of proportion to a situation in intensity and duration

dissociation process whereby different facets of an individual's sense of self, memories, or consciousness become disconnected from one another

dissociative amnesia loss of memory for important facts about a person's own life and personal identity, usually including the awareness of this memory loss

dissociative disorders Disorders that are characterized by a disruption of and/or discontinuity in the normal integration of consciousness, memory, identity, emotion, perception, body representation, motor control, or behavior.

dissociative fugue disorder in which a person moves away and assumes a new identity, with amnesia for the previous identity

dissociative identity disorder (DID) syndrome in which a person develops more than one distinct identity or personality, each of which can have distinct facial and verbal expressions, gestures, interpersonal styles, attitudes, and even physiological responses

dizygotic (DZ) twins twins who average only 50 percent of their genes in common because they developed from two separate fertilized eggs

dopamine neurotransmitter in the brain, excess amounts of which have been thought to cause schizophrenia

double-blind experiment study in which both the researchers and the participants are unaware of which experimental condition the participants are in, in order to prevent demand effects

Durham rule legal principle stating that the presence of a mental disorder is sufficient to absolve an individual of responsibility for a crime

dysphoria an intense feeling of unease, discontent, or sadness

E

early or premature ejaculation recurrent ejaculation within 1 minute of initiation of partnered sexual activity when not desired

echolalia communication abnormality in which an individual simply repeats back what they hear rather than generating their own speech

effectiveness in therapy outcome research, how well a therapy works in real-world settings

efficacy in therapy outcome research, how well a therapy works in highly controlled settings with a narrowly defined group of people

ego psychology branch of psychodynamic theory emphasizing the importance of the individual's ability to regulate defenses in ways that allow healthy functioning within the realities of society

electroconvulsive therapy (ECT) treatment for depression that involves the induction of a brain seizure by passing electrical current through the patient's brain while he or she is anesthetized

electroencephalogram (EEG) procedure in which multiple electrodes are placed on the scalp to detect low-voltage electrical current produced by the firing of specific neurons in the brain

endocrine system system of glands that produces many different hormones

epidemiology study of the frequency and distribution of a disorder, or a group of disorders, in a population

epigenetics study of how environmental conditions can change the expression of genes without changing the gene sequence

erectile disorder in men, recurrent inability to attain or maintain an erection until the completion of sexual activity

executive functions functions of the brain that involve the ability to sustain concentration; use abstract reasoning and concept formation; anticipate, plan, and program; initiate purposeful behavior; self-monitor; and shift from maladaptive patterns of behavior to more adaptive ones

exhibitionist disorder obtainment of sexual gratification by exposing one's genitals to involuntary observers

experimental group in an experimental study, group of participants that receive the key manipulation

experimental studies studies in which the independent variables are directly manipulated and the effects on the dependent variable are examined

exposure and response prevention type of therapy in which individuals with anxiety symptoms are exposed repeatedly to the focus of their anxiety but prevented from avoiding it or engaging in compulsive responses to the anxiety

expressed emotion family interaction style in which families are overinvolved with each other, are overprotective of the disturbed family member, voice self-sacrificing attitudes to the disturbed family member, and simultaneously are critical, hostile, and resentful of this member

external validity extent to which a study's results can be generalized to phenomena in real life

F

factitious disorder disorder marked by deliberately faking physical or mental illness to gain medical attention

factitious disorder imposed on another disorder in which the individual creates an illness in another individual in order to gain attention

family history study study of the heritability of a disorder involving identifying people with the disorder and people without the disorder and then determining the disorder's frequency within each person's family

family systems theories theories that see the family as a complex system that works to maintain the status quo

family systems therapy psychotherapy that focuses on the family, rather than the individual, as the source of problems; family therapists challenge communication styles, disrupt pathological family dynamics, and challenge

defensive conceptions in order to harmonize relationships among all members and within each member

family-focused therapy (FFT) treatment for people with bipolar disorder in which patients and their families are given education about bipolar disorder and training in communication and problem-solving skills

female orgasmic disorder in women, recurrent delay in or absence of orgasm after having reached the excitement phase of the sexual response cycle (also called anorgasmia)

female sexual interest/arousal disorder in women, recurrent inability to attain or maintain the swelling-lubrication response of sexual excitement

fetal alcohol syndrome (FAS) syndrome that occurs when a mother abuses alcohol during pregnancy, causing the baby to have lowered IQ, increased risk for mental retardation, distractibility, and difficulties with learning from experience

fetishistic disorder paraphilic disorder in which a person uses inanimate objects as the preferred or exclusive source of sexual arousal

fight-or-flight response physiological changes in the human body that occur in response to a perceived threat, including the secretion of glucose, endorphins, and hormones as well as the elevation of heart rate, metabolism, blood pressure, breathing, and muscle tension

five-factor model a dimensional perspective that posits that everyone's personality is organized along five broad personality traits: negative emotionality, extraversion, openness to experience, agreeableness, and conscientiousness

flashbacks vivid, sensory experiences during which, a person may experience images, sounds, body sensations, tastes, or smells that mirror what they experienced during the traumatic moment

formal thought disorder state of highly disorganized thinking (also known as loosening of associations)

free association method of uncovering unconscious conflicts in which the client is taught to talk about whatever comes to mind, without censoring any thoughts

frotteuristic disorder disorder characterized by obtainment of sexual gratification by rubbing one's genitals against or fondling the body parts of a nonconsenting person

G

gambling disorder a disorder, similar to substance abuse, characterized by the inability to resist the impulse to gamble

gender dysphoria condition in which a person believes that they were born with the wrong sex's genitals and is fundamentally a person of the opposite sex

gender identity one's perception of oneself as male or female

general paresis disease that leads to paralysis, insanity, and eventually death; discovery of this disease helped establish a connection between biological diseases and mental disorders

generalizability extent to which the results of a study generalize to, or inform us about, people other than those who were studied

generalized anxiety disorder (GAD) anxiety disorder characterized by chronic anxiety in daily life

genito-pelvic pain/penetration disorder marked difficulty having vaginal penetration; pain or tightening of pelvic floor muscles during penetration

global assumptions fundamental beliefs that encompass all types of situations

grandiose delusions false, persistent beliefs that one has superior talents and traits

grave disability legal criterion for involuntary commitment that is met when a person is so incapacitated by a mental disorder that he or she cannot provide his or her own basic needs, such as food, clothing, or shelter, and his or her survival is threatened as a result

group comparison study study that compares two or more distinct groups on a variable of interest

guided mastery techniques interventions designed to increase health-promoting behaviors by providing explicit information about how to engage in these behaviors, as well as opportunities to engage in the behaviors in increasingly challenging situations

guilty but mentally ill (GBMI) verdict that requires a convicted criminal to serve the full sentence designated for their crime, with the expectation that they will also receive treatment for mental illness

H

hair-pulling disorder (trichotillomania) disorder characterized by recurrent pulling out of the hair resulting in noticeable hair loss; these individuals report tension immediately before or while attempting to resist the impulse, and pleasure or relief when they are pulling out their hair (also known as trichotillomania)

halfway houses living facilities that offer people with long-term mental health problems the opportunity to live in a structured, supportive environment while they are trying to reestablish employment and ties to family and friends

hallucinations false or inaccurate perceptions and that affect the senses

hallucinogens substances, including LSD and MDMA (ecstasy), that produce perceptual illusions and distortions even in small doses

harm reduction model approach to treating substance use disorders that views alcohol use as normative behavior and focuses education on the immediate risks of the excessive use of alcohol (such as alcohol-related accidents) and on the payoffs of moderation (such as avoidance of hangovers)

hippocampus structure of the brain involved in memory and in the stress response

histrionic personality disorder sharing features with borderline personality disorder, including rapidly shifting emotions and intense, unstable relationships, people with this disorder also behave in ways to draw attention to themselves across situations

hoarding a compulsive disorder characterized by the inability to throw away unneeded possessions (such as trash)

hopelessness sense that the future is bleak and there is no way to make it more positive

hormone chemical that carries messages throughout the body, potentially affecting a person's mood, level of energy, and reaction to stress

human laboratory study experimental study involving human participants

humanistic theories views that people strive to develop their innate potential for goodness and self-actualization; abnormality arises as a result of societal pressures to conform to unchosen dictates that clash with a person's self-actualization needs and from an inability to satisfy more basic needs, such as hunger

humanistic therapy type of therapy in which the goal is to help the client discover his or her place in the world and to accomplish self-actualization through self-exploration; based on the assumption that the natural tendency for humans is toward growth (also called person-centered therapy)

hypersomnolence disorders disorders characterized by excessive sleepiness, which can be expressed as either an excessive quantity of sleep (also referred to as hypersomnia) or a low quality of wakefulness

hypertension condition in which the blood supply through the blood vessels is excessive and can lead to deterioration of the cell tissue and hardening of the arterial walls

hypomania state in which an individual shows mild symptoms of mania

hypothalamic-pituitary-adrenal axis (HPA axis) three key components of the neuroendocrine system that work together in a feedback system interconnected with the limbic system and the cerebral cortex

hypothalamus component of the brain that regulates eating, drinking, sex, and basic emotions; abnormal behaviors involving any of these activities may be the result of dysfunction in the hypothalamus

hypothesis testable statement about two or more variables and the relationship between them

I

illness anxiety disorder a form of anxiety characterized by a preoccupation with fears of having a serious medical illness based on misinterpretations of bodily sensations (formerly called hypochondriasis)

immune system system that protects the body from disease-causing microorganisms and affects susceptibility to diseases

impulsivity difficulty controlling behaviors; acting without thinking first

incidence number of new cases of a specific disorder that develop during a specific period of time

incompetent to stand trial legal status of an individual who lacks a rational understanding of the charges against them, an understanding of the proceedings of their trial, or the ability to participate in their defense

independent variable factor that is manipulated by an experimenter or used to predict the dependent variable

informed consent procedure (often legally required prior to treatment administration) in which a patient receives a full and understandable explanation of the treatment being offered and makes a decision about whether to accept or refuse the treatment

inhalants solvents, such as gasoline, glue, or paint thinner, that one inhales to produce a high and that can cause permanent central nervous system damage as well as liver and kidney disease

insanity legal term denoting a state of mental incapacitation during the time a crime was committed

insanity defense defense used by people accused of a crime in which they state that they cannot be held responsible for their illegal acts because they were mentally incapacitated at the time of the act

Insanity Defense Reform Act 1984 law, affecting all federal courts and about half the state courts, that finds a person not guilty by reason of insanity if it is shown that, as a result of mental disease or mental retardation, the accused was unable to appreciate the wrongfulness of their conduct at the time of the offense

insomnia disorder a disorder characterized by chronic difficulty initiating or maintaining sleep or by sleep that does not restore energy and alertness

intellectual disability (ID) a spectrum of neurodevelopmental disorders characterized by impaired general intellectual functioning (formerly referred to as mental retardation)

intelligence tests tests that assess a person's intellectual strengths and weaknesses

intermittent explosive disorder disorder characterized by (a) several episodes of failure to resist aggressive impulses that result in serious assaultive acts or destruction of property, (b) a degree of aggressiveness grossly out of proportion to the situation, and (c) symptoms not better explained by another mental disorder (such as antisocial personality disorder), the effects of substances, or a medical condition (e.g., a head trauma)

internal validity extent to which all factors that could extraneously affect a study's results are controlled within a laboratory study

Internet gaming disorder Persistent engagement and preoccupation with Internet and video gaming, with symptoms of tolerance, withdrawal, loss of interest in other activities, and clinically significant impairment or distress

interoceptive awareness sensitivity to stimuli arising from within the body, such as heart rate

interoceptive conditioning process by which symptoms of anxiety that have preceded panic attacks become the signals for new panic attacks

interpersonal and social rhythm therapy (ISRT) treatment for people with bipolar disorder that helps them manage their social relationships and daily rhythms to try to prevent relapse

interpersonal theories of depression theories that view the causes of depression as rooted in interpersonal relationships

interpersonal therapy (IPT) more structured, short-term version of psychodynamic therapies

irresistible impulse rule legal principle stating that even a person who knowingly performs a wrongful act can be absolved of responsibility if he or she was driven by an irresistible impulse to perform the act or had a diminished capacity to resist performing the act

L

language disorder a communication disorder characterized by difficulties with spoken and written language and other language modalities (e.g., sign language)

learned helplessness theory view that exposure to uncontrollable negative events leads to a belief in one's inability to control important outcomes and a subsequent loss of motivation, indecisiveness, and failure of action

life-course-persistent antisocial behavior a form of conduct disorder involving aggression, destructiveness, deceitfulness, and rules violation that persists into adulthood

light therapy treatment for seasonal affective disorder that involves exposure to bright lights during the winter months

limbic system part of the brain that relays information from the primitive brain stem about changes in bodily functions to the cortex, where the information is interpreted

linkage analysis genetic study that looks for associations between psychological disorders and physical disorders for which genetic causes are known

lithium drug used to treat manic and depressive symptoms

locus ceruleus area of the brain stem that plays a part in the emergency response and may be involved in panic attacks

longitudinal type of research evaluating the same group(s) of people for an extended period of time

M

magnetic resonance imaging (MRI) method of measuring both brain structure and brain function through the construction of a magnetic field that affects hydrogen atoms in the brain, emitting signals that a computer then records and uses to produce a three-dimensional image of the brain

major depressive disorder disorder involving a sad mood or anhedonia plus four or more of the following symptoms: weight loss or a decrease in appetite, insomnia or hypersomnia, psychomotor agitation or retardation, fatigue, feelings of worthlessness or severe guilt, trouble concentrating, and suicidal ideation; these symptoms must be present for at least 2 weeks and must produce marked impairments in normal functioning

major neurocognitive disorder a brain disorder characterized by a deteriorating course of deficits in neurocognitive functioning (e.g., memory, attention) that interferes significantly with independent living

male hypoactive sexual desire disorder condition in which a man's desire for sex is diminished to the point that it causes him significant distress or interpersonal difficulties and is not due to transient life circumstances or another sexual dysfunction

malingering feigning of a symptom or a disorder for the purpose of avoiding an unwanted situation, such as military service

managed care health care system in which all necessary services for an individual patient are supposed to be coordinated by a primary care provider; the goals are to coordinate services for an existing medical problem and to prevent future medical problems

mania a distinct period of abnormally and persistently elevated or irritable mood and abnormally and persistently increased goal-directed activity or energy lasing for at least one week.

mental hygiene movement movement to treat mental patients more humanely and to view mental disorders as medical diseases

Mental Status Exam used to organize the information collected during the interview and systematically evaluate the client through a series of questions that assess to determine the patient's mental status at that moment

mentalization-based treatment a form of psychodynamic treatment for borderline personality disorder based on attachment

mesmerism treatment for hysterical patients based on the idea that magnetic fluids in the patients' bodies are affected by the magnetic forces of other people and objects; the patients' magnetic forces are thought to be realigned by the practitioner through his or her own magnetic force

mesolimbic pathway subcortical part of the brain involved in cognition and emotion

meta-analysis statistical technique for summarizing results across several studies

methadone opioid that is less potent and longer-lasting than heroin; taken by heroin users to decrease their cravings and help them cope with negative withdrawal symptoms

mild neurocognitive disorder a mental disorder manifesting a slight abnormal decrease in mental function involving memory, thought, communication, behavior, or the completion of tasks

mindfulness a state of consciousness in which attention is focused on present-moment phenomena.

modeling process of learning behaviors by imitating others, especially authority figures or people like oneself

molecular genetic studies studies of the structure and function of genes that help in understanding how genetic mutations can lead to disease

monoamines neurotransmitters, including catecholamines (epinephrine, norepinephrine, and dopamine) and serotonin, that have been implicated in the mood disorders

monoamine oxidase inhibitors (MAOIs) class of antidepressant drugs

monozygotic (MZ) twins twins who share 100 percent of their genes because they developed from a single fertilized egg

moral treatment type of treatment delivered in mental hospitals in which patients were treated with respect and dignity and were encouraged to exercise self-control

motivational interviewing intervention for sufferers of substance use disorders to elicit and solidify individuals' motivation and commitment to changing their substance use; rather than confronting the user, the motivational interviewer adopts an empathic interaction style, drawing out the user's own statements of desire, ability, reasons, need, and, ultimately, commitment to change

motor disorders a group of disorders characterized by motor symptoms such as tics, stereotypic movements, or dyscoordination

multiculturalism the recognition and inclusion of of cultural factors, such as client and counselor worldviews, ethnicity/race, gender, sexual orientation, religion, and social justice.

multiple baseline design type of study in which an intervention is given to the same individual but begun in different settings or is given to different individuals but at different points in time and in which the effects of the intervention are systematically observed

M'Naghten rule legal principle stating that, in order to claim a defense of insanity, accused persons must have been burdened by such a defect of reason, from disease of the mind, as not to know the nature and quality of the act they were doing or, if they did know it, as not to know what they were doing was wrong

N

narcissistic personality disorder syndrome marked by grandiose thoughts and feelings of one's own worth as well as an obliviousness to others' needs and an exploitative, arrogant demeanor

narcolepsy sleep disorder characterized by irresistible attacks of sleep plus (1) cataplexy or (2) recurrent intrusions of elements of rapid eye movement (REM) sleep into the transition between sleep and wakefulness

natural environment type phobias extreme fears of events or situations in the natural environment that cause impairment in one's ability to function normally

need for treatment legal criterion operationalized as a signed certificate by two physicians stating that a person requires treatment but will not agree to it voluntarily; formerly a sufficient cause to hospitalize the person involuntarily and force him or her to undergo treatment

negative affectivity a dimension of personality characterized by negative mood states

negative cognitive triad perspective seen in depressed people in which they have negative views of themselves, of the world, and of the future

negative reinforcement process in which people avoid being exposed to feared objects and their avoidance is reinforced by the subsequent reduction of their anxiety

negative symptoms in schizophrenia, deficits in functioning that indicate the absence of a capacity present in people without schizophrenia, such as restricted affect

neurocognitive disorders behavioral disorders known or presumed to result from disruptions of brain structure and functioning

neurodevelopmental disorders behavioral disorders with onset during childhood known or presumed to result at least in part from disruption of brain development

neurofibrillary tangles twists or tangles of filaments within nerve cells, especially prominent in the cerebral cortex and hippocampus, common in the brains of Alzheimer's disease patients

neuroinflammation inflammatory response within the brain or spinal cord that occurs in response to disease, injury, infection, or stress

neuroleptics drugs used to treat psychotic symptoms

neuropsychological tests tests of cognitive, sensory, and/or motor skills that attempt to differentiate people with deficits in these areas from normal subjects

neurotransmitters biochemicals, released from a sending neuron, that transmit messages to a receiving neuron in the brain and nervous system

nicotine alkaloid found in tobacco; operates on both the central and peripheral nervous systems, resulting in the release of biochemicals, including dopamine, norepinephrine, serotonin, and the endogenous opioids

night eating disorder an eating disorder characterized by the regular intake of excessive amounts of food after dinner and into the night

nightmare disorder sleep disorder characterized by nightmares frequent enough to cause significant distress or impairment in functioning

nonsuicidal self-injury (NSSI) act of deliberately cutting, burning, puncturing, or otherwise significantly injuring one's skin with no intent to die

norepinephrine neurotransmitter that is involved in the regulation of mood

norepinephrine-dopamine reuptake inhibitors drugs used to treat depression; inhibit the reuptake of both norepinephrine and dopamine

null hypothesis alternative to a primary hypothesis, stating that there is no relationship between the independent variable and the dependent variable

O

obesity condition of being significantly overweight, defined by the Centers for Disease Control and Prevention as a body mass index (BMI) of 30 or over, where BMI is calculated as weight in pounds multiplied by 703, then divided by the square of height in inches

object relations view held by a group of modern psychodynamic theorists that one develops a self-concept and appraisals of others in a four-stage process during childhood and retains them throughout adulthood; psychopathology consists of an incomplete progression through these stages or an acquisition of poor self- and other concepts

observational learning learning that occurs when a person observes the rewards and punishments of another's behavior and then behaves in accordance with the same rewards and punishments

obsessions uncontrollable, persistent thoughts, images, ideas, or impulses that an individual feels intrude on his or her consciousness and that cause significant anxiety or distress

obsessive-compulsive disorder (OCD) anxiety disorder characterized by obsessions (persistent thoughts) and compulsions (rituals)

obsessive-compulsive personality disorder pervasive rigidity in one's activities and interpersonal relationships; includes qualities such as emotional constriction, extreme perfectionism, and anxiety resulting from even slight disruptions in one's routine

obstructive sleep apnea hypopnea syndrome sleep disorder characterized by repeated episodes of upper-airway obstruction during sleep

operant conditioning form of learning in which behaviors lead to consequences that either reinforce or punish the organism, leading to an increased or a decreased probability of a future response

operationalization specific manner in which variables in a study are measured or manipulated

opioids substances, including morphine and heroin, that produce euphoria followed by a tranquil state; in severe intoxication, can lead to unconsciousness, coma, and seizures; can cause withdrawal symptoms of emotional distress, severe nausea, sweating, diarrhea, and fever

oppositional defiant disorder syndrome of chronic misbehavior in childhood marked by belligerence, irritability, and defiance, although not to the extent found in a diagnosis of conduct disorder

organic amnesia loss of memory caused by brain injury resulting from disease, drugs, accidents (blows to head), or surgery

orgasm discharge of neuromuscular tension built up during sexual activity; in men, entails rhythmic contractions of the prostate, seminal vesicles, vas deferens, and penis and seminal discharge; in women, entails contractions of the orgasmic platform and uterus

other specified feeding or eating disorder presentations of an eating disorder that cause clinically significant distress or impairment but do not meet the full diagnostic criteria for any of the eating disorders otherwise identified

P

palilalia continuous repetition of sounds and words

panic attacks short, intense periods during which an individual experiences physiological and cognitive symptoms of anxiety, characterized by intense fear and discomfort

panic disorder disorder characterized by recurrent, unexpected panic attacks

paranoid personality disorder personality disorder characterized by a pervasive pattern of mistrust and suspiciousness of others' motives

paraphilic disorder disorder characterized by atypical sexual activity that involves one of the following: (1) nonhuman objects, (2) nonconsenting adults, (3) the suffering or humiliation of oneself or one's partner, or (4) children

pathogenic Disease causing exposure to bacterium, virus, or other microorganism.

patients' rights movement movement to ensure that mental patients retain their basic rights and to remove them from institutions and care for them in the community

pedophilic disorder disorder characterized by adult obtainment of sexual gratification by engaging in sexual activities with young children

performance anxiety anxiety over sexual performance that interferes with sexual functioning

peripartum onset subtype of major depressive or manic episode used when the episode occurs during pregnancy or in the 4 weeks after childbirth

persecutory delusions false, persistent beliefs that one is being pursued by other people

persistent depressive disorder a chronic form of depression with symptoms lasting for at least 2 years

persistent motor or vocal tic disorder (PMVTD) a condition involving quick and uncontrollable movements or vocal outbursts (but not both)

personality patterns of thinking, emotions, and behavior that tend to be enduring

personality disorder chronic pattern of maladaptive cognition, emotion, and behavior that begins by adolescence or early adulthood and continues into later adulthood

personality inventories questionnaires that assess people's typical ways of thinking, feeling, and behaving; used to obtain information about people's well-being, self-concept, attitudes, and beliefs

personality trait a facet of personality on which people differ from one another

phencyclidine (PCP) substance that produces euphoria, slowed reaction times, and involuntary movements at low doses; disorganized thinking, feelings of unreality, and hostility at intermediate doses; and amnesia, analgesia, respiratory problems, and changes in body temperature at high doses

phenothiazines drugs that reduce the functional level of dopamine in the brain and tend to reduce the symptoms of schizophrenia

pituitary major endocrine gland that lies partly on the outgrowth of the brain and just below the hypothalamus; produces the largest number of different hormones and controls the secretions of other endocrine glands

placebo control group in a therapy outcome study, group of people whose treatment is an inactive substance (to compare with the effects of a drug) or a nontheory-based therapy providing social support (to compare with the effects of psychotherapy)

plaques deposits of amyloid protein that accumulate in the extracellular spaces of the cerebral cortex, hippocampus, and other forebrain structures in people with Alzheimer's disease

plateau phase in the sexual response cycle, period between arousal and orgasm, during which excitement remains high but stable

polygenic combination of many genes, each of which makes a small contribution to an inherited trait

positive symptoms in schizophrenia, hallucinations, delusions, and disorganization in thought and behavior

positron-emission tomography (PET) method of localizing and measuring brain activity by detecting photons that result from the metabolization of an injected isotope

posttraumatic stress disorder (PTSD) anxiety disorder characterized by (1) repeated mental images of experiencing a traumatic event, (2) emotional numbing and detachment, and (3) hypervigilance and chronic arousal

premenstrual dysphoric disorder a set of symptoms occurring immediately prior to onset of menses characterized by a mixture of depression, anxiety and tension, and irritability and anger; may occur in mood swings during the week before onset of menses and subside once menses has begun

prepared classical conditioning theory that evolution has prepared people to be easily conditioned to fear objects or situations that were dangerous in ancient times

presenting problem typically refers to the specific problem that brought the person in for help

prevalence proportion of the population who have a specific disorder at a given point or period in time

primary prevention prevention of the development of psychological disorders before they start

prodromal symptoms in schizophrenia, milder symptoms prior to an acute phase of the disorder, during which behaviors are unusual and peculiar but not yet psychotic or completely disorganized

projective test presentation of an ambiguous stimulus, such as an inkblot, to a client, who then projects unconscious motives and issues onto the stimulus in his or her interpretation of its content

psychic epidemics phenomena in which large numbers of people begin to engage in unusual behaviors that appear to have a psychological origin

psychoanalysis form of treatment for psychopathology involving alleviating unconscious conflicts driving psychological symptoms by helping people gain insight into their conflicts and finding ways of resolving these conflicts

psychodynamic theories theories developed by Freud's followers but usually differing somewhat from Freud's original theories

psychodynamic therapies therapies focused on uncovering and resolving unconscious conflicts that drive psychological symptoms

psychogenic amnesia loss of memory in the absence of any brain injury or disease and thought to have psychological causes

psychological approach approach to abnormality that focuses on personality, behavior, and ways of thinking as possible causes of abnormality

psychological theories theories that view mental disorders as caused by psychological processes, such as beliefs, thinking styles, and coping styles

psychopathology the scientific study of psychological disorders which focuses on the assessment, treatment, and prevention of maladaptive behavior

psychopathy set of broad personality traits including superficial charm, a grandiose sense of self-worth, a tendency toward boredom and need for stimulation, pathological lying, an ability to be cunning and manipulative, and a lack of remorse

psychophysiological tests tests in which instruments are attached to the periphery of the body to record changes due to activity in the nervous system

psychosis state involving a loss of contact with reality as well as an inability to differentiate between reality and one's subjective state

psychosurgery rare treatment for mental disorders in which a neurosurgeon attempts to destroy small areas of the brain thought to be involved in a patient's symptoms

psychoticism proneness to psychotic-like symptoms, such as illusions

PTSD with prominent dissociative (depersonalization/derealization) symptoms a form of posttraumatic stress disorder in which the individual experiences feelings of being detached from their mental processes or body and of the unreality of the surroundings

R

random assignment assignment of participants in an experiment to groups based on a random process

rapid cycling bipolar disorder diagnosis given when a person has four or more cycles of mania and depression within 1 year

rapid eye movement (REM) sleep behavior disorder frequent and impairing behaviors such as sleepwalking, sleep terrors, and confusional episodes during REM sleep

Reactive Attachment Disorder trauma and stressor-related disorder that results from significant neglect and/or trauma. Affected children have difficulty forming emotional attachments to others, they are emotionally withdrawn and show little positive affect

receptors molecules on the membranes of neurons to which neurotransmitters bind

reflection method of responding in which a therapist expresses his or her attempt to understand what the client is experiencing and trying to communicate

reformulated learned helplessness theory view that people who attribute negative events to internal, stable, and global causes are more likely than other people to experience learned helplessness deficits following such events and thus are predisposed to depression

rejection sensitivity tendency to be hypervigilant and overreactive to signs of rejection from others

relapse prevention programs treatments that seek to offset continued alcohol use by identifying high-risk situations for those attempting to stop or cut down on drinking and teaching them either to avoid those situations or to use assertiveness skills when in them, while viewing setbacks as temporary

relational psychoanalysis a subfield of psychoanalysis that emphasizes internalized relationships with other people based on the influences of early formative relationships with parents and other attachment figures

reliability degree of consistency in a measurement—that is, the extent to which it yields accurate measurements of a phenomenon across several trials, across different populations, and in different forms

repetitive transcranial magnetic stimulation (rTMS) biological treatment that exposes patients to repeated, high-intensity magnetic pulses that are focused on particular brain structures in order to stimulate those structures

repression defense mechanism in which the ego pushes anxiety-provoking material back into the unconscious

residual symptoms symptoms associated with schizophrenia, such as unusual beliefs or strange perceptual experiences, that are present for at least 6 months

resistance in psychodynamic therapy, when a client finds it difficult or impossible to address certain material; the client's resistance signals an unconscious conflict, which the therapist then tries to interpret

resolution in the sexual response cycle, state of deep relaxation following orgasm in which a man loses his erection and a woman's orgasmic platform subsides

restless legs syndrome (RLS) creeping, crawling, tingling, itching sensations in the legs that are prominent enough to interfere with sleep

restricted affect a symptom in which emotional expression is reduced or absent

restricting type of anorexia nervosa type of anorexia nervosa in which weight gain is prevented by refusal to eat

retrograde amnesia deficit in the ability to recall previously learned information or past events

reuptake process in which a sending neuron reabsorbs some of the neurotransmitter in the synapse, decreasing the amount left in the synapse

right to refuse treatment right, not recognized by all states, of involuntarily committed people to refuse drugs or other treatment

right to treatment fundamental right of involuntarily committed people to receive active treatment for their disorders rather than shelter alone

risk factors conditions or variables associated with a higher risk of having a disorder

rumination focusing on one's personal concerns and feelings of distress repetitively and passively

S

sadomasochism pattern of sexual rituals between a sexually sadistic "giver" and a sexually masochistic "receiver"

sample group of people taken from a population of interest to participate in a study

schizoaffective disorder disorder in which individuals simultaneously experience schizophrenic symptoms (i.e., delusions, hallucinations, disorganized speech and behavior, and/or negative symptoms) and mood symptoms meeting the criteria for a major depressive episode, a manic episode, or an episode of mixed mania/depression

schizoid personality disorder personality disorder characterized by pervasive detachment from social relationships and a restricted range of emotional expression

schizophrenia spectrum the set of psychiatric disorders related to schizophrenia that vary along a severity continuum

schizophreniform disorder disorder in which individuals meet the primary criteria for schizophrenia but show symptoms lasting only 1 to 6 months

schizotypal personality disorder chronic pattern of inhibited or inappropriate emotion and social behavior as well as aberrant cognitions and disorganized speech

scientific method systematic method of obtaining and evaluating information relevant to a problem

seasonal affective disorder (SAD) disorder identified by a 2-year period in which a person experiences major depression during winter months and then recovers fully during the summer; some people with this disorder also experience mild mania during summer months

secondary prevention detection of psychological disorders in their earliest stages and treatment designed to reduce their development

selective serotonin reuptake inhibitors (SSRIs) class of antidepressant drugs

selective serotonin-norepinephrine reuptake inhibitors (SNRIs) drugs that affect both the serotonin system and the norepinephrine system and are used to treat anxiety and depression

self psychology a form of psychoanalytic theory and therapy developed by Heinz Kohut in which psychopathology is viewed as being the result of disrupted or unmet developmental needs

self-actualization fulfillment of one's potential for love, creativity, and meaning

self-efficacy beliefs beliefs that one can engage in the behaviors necessary to overcome a situation

self-monitoring method of assessment in which a client records the number of times per day that he or she engages in a specific behavior and the conditions surrounding the behavior

Semi-structured interviews This format combines standardized with open-ended questions which allow clinicians to follow up with specific questions in order to gather more personalized information.

sensate focus therapy treatment for sexual dysfunction in which partners alternate between giving and receiving stimulation in a relaxed, openly communicative atmosphere in order to reduce performance anxiety and concern over achieving orgasm by learning each partner's sexual fulfillment needs

sensorium our general awareness to our surroundings

separation anxiety disorder syndrome of childhood and adolescence marked by the presence of abnormal fear or worry over becoming separated from one's caregiver(s) as well as clinging behaviors in the presence of the caregiver(s)

serotonin neurotransmitter involved in the regulation of mood and impulsive responses

sexual desire in the sexual response cycle, an urge or inclination to engage in sexual activity

sexual dysfunctions problems in experiencing sexual arousal or carrying through with sexual acts to the point of sexual arousal

sexual functioning the ability and capacity to engage in sexual behavior

sexual masochism disorder disorder characterized by obtaining sexual gratification through experiencing pain and humiliation at the hands of one's partner

sexual sadism disorder disorder characterized by obtaining sexual gratification through inflicting pain and humiliation on one's partner

simple control group consists of participants who do not receive the experimental therapy but are tracked for the same period of time as the participants who do receive the therapy

single photon emission computed tomography (SPECT) procedure to assess brain functioning in which a tracer substance is injected into the bloodstream and then travels to the brain, where it can indicate the activity level of specific areas of the brain when viewed through a SPECT scanner

single-case experimental design experimental design in which an individual or a small number of individuals are studied intensively; the individual is put through some sort of manipulation or intervention, and his or her behavior is examined before and after this manipulation to determine the effects

situational type phobias extreme fears of situations such as public transportation, tunnels, bridges, elevators, flying, driving, or enclosed spaces

skin-picking disorder a disorder characterized by recurrent picking at scabs or places on the skin, creating significant lesions that often become infected and cause scars

sleep disorders disturbances in sleeping or staying awake, such as insomnia and narcolepsy

sleep terror disorder disorder of arousal in which the individual screams, sweats, and has a racing heart during NREM sleep; the person cannot be easily wakened and usually does not remember the episode on awakening

sleep-related hypoventilation episodes of decreased breathing associated with high carbon dioxide levels

sleepwalking disorder of arousal characterized by repeated episodes of walking during NREM sleep

social anxiety disorder an anxiety disorder in which the individual experiences intense fear of public humiliation or rejection and therefore tends to avoid social situations

social communication disorder a communication disorder characterized by difficulty using language and other modalities for communicating in social situations

social drift a theory that suggests that cumulative exposure to environmental risk factors in deprived and urban areas over time increases risk of psychological disorders, particularly for individuals with genetic predispositions.

sociocultural approach approach to psychopathology focusing on the role of the environment, stress, and culture in producing psychopathology

somatic symptom disorder syndrome marked by health concerns that are excessive given actual physical health, that persist despite contrary evidence, and that interfere with daily functioning

specific learning disorder disrupted or delayed development in a specific domain of cognition, such as reading

specific phobias extreme fears of specific objects or situations that cause an individual to routinely avoid those objects or situations

speech sound disorder a communication disorder characterized by difficulties in producing speech

squeeze technique sex therapy technique used for premature ejaculation; the man's partner stimulates him to an erection, and then when he signals that ejaculation is imminent, the partner applies a firm but gentle squeeze to his penis, either at the glans or at the base, for 3 or 4 seconds; the goal of this technique is for the man to learn to identify the point of ejaculatory inevitability and to control his arousal level at that point

statistical significance likelihood that a study's results have occurred only by chance

stereotypic movement disorder a motor disorder characterized by repetitive, seemingly driven, and apparently purposeless motor behavior, such as hand waving or head banging

stigma a mark of shame or discredit

stimulants drugs that activate the nervous system

stop-start technique sex therapy technique used for premature ejaculation; the man or his partner stimulates his penis until he is about to ejaculate; the man then relaxes and concentrates on the sensations in his body until his level of arousal declines; the goal of this technique is for the man to learn to identify the point of ejaculatory inevitability and to control his arousal level at that point

stress-inoculation therapy a form of cognitive-behavior therapy that focuses on developing skills that allow the individual to cope with stress

stroke sudden damage to the brain due to blockage of blood flow or hemorrhaging

structured interview meeting between a clinician and a client or a client's associate(s) in which the clinician asks questions that are standardized and are usually designed to determine whether a diagnosis is warranted

substance naturally occurring or synthetically produced product that alters perceptions, thoughts, emotions, and behaviors when ingested, smoked, or injected

substance intoxication experience of significantly maladaptive behavioral and psychological symptoms due to the effect of a substance on the central nervous system that develops during or shortly after use of the substance

substance use disorders disorders characterized by inability to use a substance in moderation and/or the intentional use of a substance to change one's thoughts, feelings, and/or behaviors, leading to impairment in work, academic, personal, or social endeavors

substance withdrawal experience of clinically significant distress in social, occupational, or other areas of functioning due to the cessation or reduction of substance use

substance-induced sexual dysfunction problems in sexual functioning caused by substance use

substance-induced sleep disorder sleep disturbance due to the use of substances, including prescription medications (e.g., medications that control hypertension or cardiac arrhythmias) and nonprescription substances (e.g., alcohol and caffeine)

suicidal ideation thoughts about killing oneself

suicide purposeful taking of one's own life

suicide attempts behaviors engaged in with some intent to kill oneself

suicide cluster when two or more suicides or attempted suicides nonrandomly occur closely together in space or time

supernatural theories theories that see mental disorders as the result of supernatural forces, such as divine intervention, curses, demonic possession, and/or personal sins; mental disorders then can be cured through religious rituals, exorcisms, confessions, and/or death

symptom questionnaire questionnaire that assesses what symptoms a person is experiencing

synapse space between a sending neuron and a receiving neuron into which neurotransmitters are first released (also known as the synaptic gap)

syndrome set of symptoms that tend to occur together

systematic desensitization therapy type of behavior therapy that attempts to reduce client anxiety through relaxation techniques and progressive exposure to feared stimuli

T

tardive dyskinesia neurological disorder marked by involuntary movements of the tongue, face, mouth, or jaw, resulting from taking neuroleptic drugs

tertiary prevention program focusing on people who already have a disease with the aim of preventing relapse and reducing the impact of the disease on the person's quality of life

thalamus structure of the brain that directs incoming information from sense receptors (such as vision and hearing) to the cerebrum

theory set of assumptions about the likely causes of abnormality and appropriate treatments

therapy outcome studies experimental studies that assess the effects of an intervention designed to reduce psychopathology in an experimental group, while performing no intervention or a different type of intervention on another group

third variable problem possibility that variables not measured in a study are the real cause of the relationship between the variables measured in the study

third-wave approaches modern psychotherapeutic techniques that combine elements of the first- and second-wave approaches—behavioral therapy and cognitive therapy, respectively—with mindfulness meditation practices derived from Zen Buddhism to help people accept, understand, and better regulate their emotions

tolerance condition of experiencing less and less effect from the same dose of a substance

Tourette's disorder a motor disorder characterized by multiple motor tics and one or more vocal tics

transference in psychodynamic therapies, the client's reaction to the therapist as if the therapist were an important person in his or her early development; the client's feelings and beliefs about this other person are transferred onto the therapist

transference-focused therapy a highly structured psychodynamic treatment for borderline personality disorder that uses the relationship between patient and therapist to help patients develop a more realistic and healthier understanding of their interpersonal relationships

transgender a term for the broad spectrum of individuals who identify with a gender different from their natal (born) biological sex

transvestic disorder paraphilic disorder in which a heterosexual man dresses in women's clothing as his primary means of becoming sexually aroused

traumatic brain injury injury to the brain resulting from traumatic force; often associated with loss of consciousness

trephination procedure in which holes were drilled in the skulls of people displaying abnormal behavior, presumably to allow evil spirits to depart their bodies; performed in the Stone Age

tricyclic antidepressants class of antidepressant drugs

twin studies studies of the heritability of a disorder by comparing concordance rates between monozygotic and dizygotic twins

Type A behavior pattern personality pattern characterized by time urgency, hostility, and competitiveness

Type D (*Distressed*) behavior pattern The Type D (Distressed) personality profile is characterized by high levels of negative affectivity and social inhibition associated with emotional distress and negative cardiovascular outcomes

U

unconditioned response (UR) in classical conditioning, response that naturally follows when a certain stimulus appears, such as a dog salivating when it smells food

unconditioned stimulus (US) in classical conditioning, stimulus that naturally elicits a reaction, as food elicits salivation in dogs

unstructured interview A process in which a clinician uses open-ended questions to gather information about the client. This process is not standardized and the questions are directed by the based on the client's responses.

V

vagus nerve stimulation (VNS) treatment in which the vagus nerve—the part of the autonomic nervous system that carries information from the head, neck, thorax, and abdomen to several areas of the brain, including the hypothalamus and amygdala—is stimulated by a small electronic device much like a cardiac pacemaker, which is surgically implanted under a patient's skin in the left chest wall

validity the accuracy of a test, measurement, or instrument

variable measurable factor or characteristic that can vary within an individual, between individuals, or both

vascular neurocognitive disorder a form of dementia resulting from multiple strokes and/or ischemic events

voyeuristic disorder disorder characterized by obtainment of sexual arousal by compulsively and secretly watching another person undressing, bathing, engaging in sex, or being naked

W

wait list control group in a therapy outcome study, group of people that functions as a control group while an experimental group receives an intervention and then receives the intervention itself after a waiting period

working through method used in psychodynamic therapies in which the client repeatedly goes over and over painful memories and difficult issues as a way to understand and accept them

A

Aaronson, S. T., Sears, P., Ruvuna, F., Bunker, M., Conway, C. R., Dougherty, D. D., & Zajecka, J. M. (2017). A 5-year observational study of patients with treatment-resistant depression treated with vagus nerve stimulation or treatment as usual: Comparison of response, remission, and suicidality. *American Journal of Psychiatry, 174*(7), 640–648.

AARP Public Policy Institute. (2018). Prescription drug abuse among older adults. https://www.aarp.org/ppi/info-2017/prescription-drug-abuse-among-older-adults.html. Retrieved July 4, 2018.

Aarsland, D., & Kurz, M. W. (2009). The epidemiology of dementia associated with Parkinson disease. *Journal of the Neurological Sciences, 289,* 18–22.

Abasi, I., Dolatshahi, B., Farazmand, S., Pourshahbaz, A., & Tamanaeefar, S. (2018). Emotion Regulation in Generalized Anxiety and Social Anxiety: Examining the Distinct and Shared Use of Emotion Regulation Strategies. *Iranian journal of psychiatry, 13*(3), 160–167.

Abbott, S. M., Reid, K. J., & Zee, P. C. (2015). Circadian rhythm sleep-wake disorders. *Psychiatric Clinics, 38*(4), 805–823.

Abdolhosseinzadeh, S., Sina, M., Ahmadiani, A., Asadi, S., & Shams, J. (2019). Genetic and pharmacogenetic study of glutamate transporter (SLC1A1) in Iranian patients with obsessive-compulsive disorder. *Journal of Clinical Pharmacy & Therapeutics, 44*(1), 39–48.

Abera, M., Robbins, J. M., & Tesfaye, M. (2015). Parents' perception of child and adolescent mental health problems and their choice of treatment option in southwest Ethiopia. *Child and Adolescent Psychiatry and Mental Health, 9,* 40.

Abi-Dargham, A., Kegeles, L. S., Zea-Ponce, Y., Mawlawi, O., Martinez, D., Mitropoulou, V., . . . Siever, L. J. (2004). Striatal amphetamine-induced dopamine release in patients with schizotypal personality disorder studied with single photon emission computed tomography and [123I] Iodobenzamide. *Biological Psychiatry, 55,* 1001–1006.

Abramowitz, J. S., & Jacoby, R. J. (2015). Obsessive-compulsive and related disorders: A critical review of the new diagnostic class. *Annual Review of Clinical Psychology, 11,* 165–186.

Abramson, L. Y., Alloy, L. B., Hankin, B. L., Haeffel, G. J., MacCoon, D. G., & Gibb, B. E. (2002). Cognitive vulnerability-stress models of depression in a self-regulatory and psychobiological context. In I. H. Gotlib & C. L. Hammen (Eds.), *Handbook of depression* (pp. 268–294). New York: Guilford Press.

Abramson, L. Y., Bardone-Cone, A. M., Vohs, K. D., Joiner, T. E., Jr., & Heatherton, T. F. (2006). Cognitive vulnerability to bulimia. In L. B. Alloy & J. H. Riskind (Eds.), *Cognitive vulnerability to emotional disorders* (pp. 329–364). Mahwah, NJ: Erlbaum.

Abramson, L. Y., Metalsky, G. I., & Alloy, L. B. (1989). Hopelessness depression: A theory-based subtype of depression. *Psychological Review, 96,* 358–372.

Abramson, L. Y., Seligman, M. E. P., & Teasdale, J. (1978). Learned helplessness in humans: Critique and reformulation. *Journal of Abnormal Psychology, 87,* 49–74.

Achilli, C., Pundir, J., Ramanathan, P., Sabatini, L., Hamoda, H., & Panay, N. (2017). Efficacy and safety of transdermal testosterone in postmenopausal women with hypoactive sexual desire disorder: A systematic review and meta-analysis. *Fertility and Sterility, 107*(2), 475–482.

Adams, C. E., Awad, G., Rathbone, J., & Thornley, B. (2007). Chlorpromazine versus placebo for schizophrenia. *Cochrane Database of Systematic Reviews, 2,* CD000284.

Addis, M. E. (2008). Gender and depression in men. *Clinical Psychology: Science and Practice, 15,* 153–168.

Adler, C. M., Adams, J., DelBello, M. P., Holland, S. K., Schmithorst, V., Levine, A., . . . Strakowski, S. M. (2006). Evidence of white matter pathology in bipolar disorder adolescents experiencing their first episode of mania: A diffusion tensor imaging study. *American Journal of Psychiatry, 163,* 322–324.

Afifi, T. O., Mather, A., Boman, J., Fleisher, W., Enns, M. W., MacMillan, H., & Sareen, J. (2011). Childhood adversity and personality disorders: Results from a nationally representative population-based study. *Journal of Psychiatric Research, 45,* 814–822.

Agarwal, S. & Landon, B. (2019, January 25). Patterns in Outpatient Benzodiazepine Prescribing in the United States. Retrieved November 03, 2020, from https://jamanetwork.com/journals/jamanetworkopen/article-abstract/2722576

Ágh, T., Kovács, G., Pawaskar, M., Supina, D., Inotai, A., & Vokó, Z. (2015). Epidemiology, health-related quality of life and economic burden of binge eating disorder: A systematic literature review. *Eating and Weight Disorders—Studies on Anorexia, Bulimia and Obesity, 20*(1), 1–12.

Agras, W. S., Fitzsimmons-Craft, E. E., & Wilfley, D. E. (2017). Evolution of cognitive-behavioral therapy for eating disorders. *Behaviour Research and Therapy, 88,* 26–36.

Agras, W. S., Walsh, B. T., Fairburn, C. C., Wilson, G. T., & Kraemer, H. C. (2000). A multicenter comparison of cognitive-behavioral therapy and interpersonal psychotherapy for bulimia nervosa. *Archives of General Psychiatry, 57,* 459–466.

Agrawal, A., Heath, A. C., & Lynskey, M. T. (2011). *DSM-IV* to *DSM-5*: The impact of proposed revisions on diagnosis of alcohol use disorders. *Addiction, 106,* 1935–1943.

Ahlers, M. M. (2009, July 14). NTSB: Sleep disorder may have contributed to Boston train crash. http://www.cnn.com/2009/US/07/14/ntsb.train.crash/index.html (accessed July 23, 2009).

Ahmad, S. I., & Hinshaw, S. P. (2016). Attention-deficit/hyperactivity disorder: Similarities to and differences from other externalizing disorders. In T. P. Beauchaine & S. P. Hinshaw (Eds.), *The Oxford handbook of externalizing spectrum disorders* (pp. 19–37). New York: Oxford University Press.

Ahmed, A. O., Buckley, P. F., & Mabe, P. A. (2012). Latent structure of psychotic experiences in the general population. *Acta Psychiatrica Scandinavica, 125,* 54–65.

Ajdacic-Gross, V., Killias, M., Hepp, U., Gadola, E., Bopp, M., Lauber, C., . . . Rossler, W. (2006). Changing times: A longitudinal analysis of international firearm suicide data. *American Journal of Public Health, 96,* 1752–1755.

Ajzen, I. (1991). The theory of planned behavior. *Organizational Behavior and Human Decision Processes, 50,* 179–211.

Alarcon, R. D., Becker, A. E., Lewis-Fernandez, R., Like, R. C., Desai, P., Foulks, E., Gonzales, J., Hansen, H., Kopelowicz, A., Lu, F. G., Oquendo, M. A., & Primm, A. (2009). Issues for *DSM-V*: The role of culture in psychiatric diagnosis. *Journal of Nervous and Mental Disease, 197,* 559–560.

Albert, P. R., Benkelfat, C., & Descarries, L. (2012). The neurobiology of depression—revisiting the serotonin hypothesis. I. Cellular and molecular mechanisms. *Philosophical Transactions of the Royal Society, 367,* 2378–2381.

Albert, U., Pellegrini, L., Maina, G., Atti. A. R., De Ronchi, D., & Rhimer, Z. (2019). Suicide in obsessive-compulsive related disorders: Prevalence rates and psychopathological risk factors. *Journal of Psychopathology, 25,* 139–148.

Albuquerque, D., Stice, E., Rodríguez-López, R., Manco, L., & Nóbrega, C. (2015). Current review of genetics of human obesity: From molecular mechanisms to an evolutionary perspective. *Molecular Genetics and Genomics, 290*(4), 1191–1221

Aldao, A., Mennin, D. S., Linardatos, E., & Fresco, D. M. (2010). Differential patterns of physical symptoms and subjective processes in generalized anxiety disorder and unipolar depression. *Journal of Anxiety Disorders, 24,* 250–259.

Alegría, M., Álvarez, K., & DiMarzio, K. (2017). Immigration and mental health. *Current Epidemiology Reports, 4*(2), 145–155.

Alegría, M., Canino, G., Shrout, P. E., Woo, M., Duan, N., Vila, D., et al. (2008). Prevalence of mental illness in immigrant and nonimmigrant U.S. Latino groups. *American Journal of Psychiatry, 165,* 359–369.

Alegria, M., Nakash, O., & Johnson, K. (2018). Effectiveness of the DECIDE interventions on shared decision making and perceived quality of care in behavioral health with multicultural patients: A randomized clinical trial. *JAMA Psychiatry, 75*(4), 325–335.

Alexander, M. (2012). *The new Jim Crow: Mass incarceration in the age of colorblindness.* New York: New Press.

Al-Haddad, B., Jacobsson, B., Chabra, S., Modzelewska, D., Olson, E. M., Bernier, R., . . . Sengpiel, V. (2019). Long-term risk of neuropsychiatric disease after exposure to infection in utero. *JAMA Psychiatry, 76*(6), 594–602. https://doi.org/10.1001/jamapsychiatry.2019.0029

Alim, T. N., Feder, A., Graves, R. E., Wang, Y., Weaver, J., Westphal, M., . . . Charney, D. S. (2008). Trauma, resilience, and recovery in a high-risk African-American population. *The American Journal of Psychiatry, 165*(12), 1566–1575.

Ali, S., Garg, S., Cohen, B. E., Bhave, P., Harris, W. S., & Whooley, M. A. (2009). Association between omega-3 fatty acids and depressive symptoms among patients with established coronary artery disease: Data from the Heart and Soul Study. *Psychotherapy and Psychosomatics, 78,* 125–127.

Alix, S., Cossette, L., Hébert, M., Cyr, M., & Frappier, J. Y. (2017). Posttraumatic stress disorder and suicidal ideation among sexually abused adolescent girls: The mediating role of shame. *Journal of Child Sexual Abuse, 26*(2), 158–174.

Alldridge, P. (1979). Hospitals, madhouses and asylums: Cycles in the care of the insane. *British Journal of Psychiatry, 134,* 321–334.

Allen, J. J., Anderson, C. A., & Bushman, B. J. (2018). The general aggression model. *Current Opinion in Psychology, 19,* 75–80. https://doi.org/10.1016/j.copsyc.2017.03.034

Allen, M. S., Robson, D. A., & Laborde, S. (2020). Normal variations in personality predict eating behavior, oral health, and partial syndrome bulimia nervosa in adolescent girls. *Food Science & Nutrition, 8*(3), 1423–1432.

Allen, R. P., Picchietti, D. L., Garcia-Borreguero, D., Ondo, W. G., Walters, A. S., Winkelman, J. W., & International Restless Legs Syndrome Study Group. (2014). Restless legs syndrome/Willis–Ekbom disease diagnostic criteria: Updated International Restless Legs Syndrome Study Group (IRLSSG) consensus criteria—history, rationale, description, and significance. *Sleep Medicine, 15*(8), 860–873.

Allison, K. C. (2017). Night eating syndrome. In K. D. Brownell & B. T. Walsh (Eds.), *Eating disorders and obesity: A comprehensive handbook* (3rd ed., pp. 203–208). New York: Guilford Press.

Allison, S., Bastiampillai, T., Licinio, J., Fuller, D. A., Bidargaddi, N., & Sharfstein, S. S. (2018). When should governments increase the supply of psychiatric beds? *Molecular Psychiatry, 23*(4), 796–800.

Alloy, L. B., Abramson, L. Y., & Francis, E. L. (1999). Do negative cognitive styles confer vulnerability to depression? *Current Directions in Psychological Science, 8,* 128–132.

Alloy, L. B., Abramson, L. Y., Walshaw, P. D., Cogswell, A., Grandin, L. D., Hughes, M. E., . . . Hogan, M. E. (2008). Inhibition system sensitivities and bipolar spectrum disorders: Prospective prediction of bipolar mood episodes. *Bipolar Disorders, 10,* 310–322.

Alloy, L. B., Hamilton, J. L., Hamlat, E. J., & Abramson, L. Y. (2016). Pubertal development, emotion regulatory styles, and the emergence of sex differences in internalizing disorders and symptoms in adolescence. *Clinical Psychological Science, 4*(5), 867–881.

Alloy, L. B., Ng, T. H., Titone, M. K., & Boland, E. M. (2017). Circadian rhythm dysregulation in bipolar spectrum disorders. *Current Psychiatry Reports, 19*(4), 21.

Alloy, L. B., Nusslock, R., & Boland, E. M. (2015). The development and course of bipolar spectrum disorders: An integrated reward and circadian rhythm dysregulation model. *Annual Review of Clinical Psychology, 11,* 213.

Alloy, L. B., Olino, T., Freed, R. D., & Nusslock, R. (2016). Role of reward sensitivity and processing in major depressive and bipolar spectrum disorders. *Behavior Therapy, 47*(5), 600–621.

Al-Rousan, T., Rubenstein, L., Sieleni, B., Deol, H., & Wallace, R. B. (2017). Inside the nation's largest mental health institution: A prevalence study in a state prison system. *BMC public health, 17*(1), 1–9.

Althof, S. E. (1995). Pharmacologic treatment of rapid ejaculation. *Psychiatric Clinics of North America, 18,* 85–94.

Altintaş, E., & Taşkintuna, N. (2015). Factors associated with depression in obsessive-compulsive disorder: A cross-sectional study. *Noro psikiyatri arsivi, 52*(4), 346–353.

Altman, S., Haeri, S., Cohen, L. J., Ten, A., Harron, E., Galynker, I. I., & Duhamel, K. N. (2006). Predictors of relapse in bipolar disorder: A review. *Journal of Psychiatric Practice, 12,* 269–282.

Alvanzo, A. A. H., Storr, C. L., La Flair, L., Green, K. G., & Wagner, F. A. (2011). Race/ethnicity and sex differences in progression from drinking initiation to the development of alcohol dependence. *Drug and Alcohol Dependence, 118,* 375–382.

Alvarez-Tomás, I., Soler, J., Bados, A., Martín-Blanco, A., Elices, M., Carmona, C., . . . & Pascual, J. C. (2017). Long-term course of borderline personality disorder: A prospective 10-year follow-up study. *Journal of Personality Disorders, 31*(5), 590–605.

Alzheimer's Association. (2018). Alzheimer's disease facts and figures. *Alzheimer's & Dementia, 14*(3), 367–429.

American Psychiatric Association (APA). (2013). *Diagnostic and statistical manual of mental disorders* (5th ed.). Arlington, VA: American Psychiatric Publishing.

American Psychiatric Association (APA). (2013). *Diagnostic and statistical manual of mental disorders* (5th ed.). Washington, DC: Author.

American Psychological Association. (2009). *Report of the American Psychological Association task force on appropriate therapeutic responses to sexual orientation.* Washington, DC: Author.

American Psychological Association. (2015). Guidelines for psychological practice with transgender and gender nonconforming people. *American Psychologist, 70*(9), 832–864.

Andersen, A. E., & DiDomenico, L. (1992). Diet vs. shape content of popular male and female magazines: A dose-response relationship to the incidence of eating disorders? *International Journal of Eating Disorders, 11,* 283–287.

Andersen, B. L., Yang, H. C., Farrar, W. B., Golden-Kreutz, D. M., Emery, C. F., Thornton, L. M., . . . Carson III, W. E. (2008). Psychologic intervention improves survival for breast cancer patients: A randomized clinical trial. *Cancer, 113,* 3450-3458.

Anderson, D. K., Liang, J. W., & Lord, C. (2014). Predicting young adult outcome among more and less cognitively able individuals with autism spectrum disorders. *Journal of Child Psychology and Psychiatry, 55*(5), 485-494.

Anderson, E. R., & Mayes, L. C. (2010). Race/ethnicity and internalizing disorders in youth: A review. *Clinical Psychology Review, 30,* 338-348.

Anderson, M. C., Ochsner, K. N., Kuhl, B., Cooper, J., Robertson, E., Gabrieli, S. W., . . . Gabrieli, J. D. (2004). Neural systems underlying the suppression of unwanted memories. *Science 303,* 232-235. doi: 10.1126/science.1089504

Anderson, P. L., Price, M., Edwards, S. M., Obasaju, M. A., Schmertz, S. K., Zimand, E., & Calamaras, M. R. (2013). Virtual reality exposure therapy for social anxiety disorder: A randomized controlled trial. *Journal of Consulting and Clinical Psychology, 81,* 751-760.

Andersson, G. (2016). Internet-delivered psychological treatments. *Annual Review of Clinical Psychology, 12,* 157-179.

Andreano, G. M., Ford, A., Karwoski, A. L., & Wilson, C. K. (2018). Bros & booze: Assessing the impact of alcohol skills training program on fraternity drinking. *Journal of the Student Personnel Association at Indiana University.*

Andreasen, N. C. (1998). Jeff: A difficult case of schizophrenia. In R. P. Halgin & S. K. Whitbourne (Eds.), *A casebook in abnormal psychology from the files of experts* (pp. 197-210). New York: Oxford University Press.

Andreasen, N. C., Flaum, M., Swayze, V. W., Tyrrell, G., & Arndt, S. (1990). Positive and negative symptoms in schizophrenia: A critical reappraisal. *Archives of General Psychiatry, 47,* 615-621.

Andrews, G., Hobbs, M. J., Borkovec, T. D., Beesdo, K., Craske, M. G., Heimberg, R. G.,... Stanley, M. A. (2010). Generalized worry disorder: A review of *DSM-IV* generalized anxiety disorder and options for *DSM-V*. *Depression and Anxiety,* 1-14.

Anestis, M. D., & Anestis, J. C. (2015). Suicide rates and state laws regulating access and exposure to handguns. *American Journal of Public Health, 105*(10), 2049-2058.

Anestis, M. D., Soberay, K. A., Gutierrez, P. M., Hernández, T. D., & Joiner, T. E. (2014). Reconsidering the link between impulsivity and suicidal behavior. *Personality and Social Psychology Review, 18*(4), 366-386.

Angold, A., Costello, E. J., & Worthman, C. M. (1998). Puberty and depression: The roles of age, pubertal status, and pubertal timing. *Psychological Medicine, 28,* 51-61.

Angold, A., Erkanli, A., Egger, H. L., & Costello, J. (2000). Stimulant treatment for children: A community perspective. *Journal of the American Academy of Child & Adolescent Psychiatry, 39,* 975-994.

Angst, J., Gamma, A., Endrass, J., Goodwin, R., Ajdacic, V., Eich, D., & Rossler, W. (2004). Obsessive-compulsive severity spectrum in the community: Prevalence, comorbidity, and course. *European Archives of Psychiatry & Clinical Neuroscience, 254,* 156-164.

Angst, J., Gamma, A., Pezawas, L., Ajdacic-Gross, V., Eich, D., Rossler, W., & Altamura, C. (2007). Parsing the clinical phenotype of depression: The need to integrate brief depressive episodes. *Acta Psychiatrica Scandinavica, 115,* 221-228.

Anonymous. (1992). First-person account: Portrait of a schizophrenic. *Schizophrenia Bulletin, 18,* 333-334.

Antoni, M. H., & Dhabhar, F. S. (2019). The impact of psychosocial stress and stress management on immune responses in patients with cancer. *Cancer, 125*(9), 1417-1431.

Anton, R. F., O'Malley, S. S., Ciraulo, D. A., Cisler, R. A., Couper, D., Donovan, D. M . . . Zweben, A. (2006). Combined pharmacotherapies and behavioral interventions for alcohol dependence: The combine study: A randomized controlled trial. *JAMA, 295,* 2003-2017.

Antypa, N., Serretti, A., & Rujescu, D. (2013). Serotonergic genes and suicide: A systematic review. *European Neuropsychopharmacology, 23*(10), 1125-1142.

Apostolopoulos, A., Michopoulos, I., Zachos, I., Rizos, E., Tzeferakos, G., Manthou, V., . . . Douzenis, A. (2018). Association of schizoid and schizotypal personality disorder with violent crimes and homicides in Greek prisons. *Annals of General Psychiatry, 17.*

Appelbaum, B. C., Appelbaum, P. S., & Grisso, T. (1998). Competence to consent to voluntary psychiatric hospitalization: A test of a standard proposed by APA. *Psychiatric Services, 49,* 1193-1196.

Appelbaum, P. S. (2007). Assessment of patients' competence to consent to treatment. *New England Journal of Medicine, 357*(18), 1834-1840.

Arcelus, J., Bouman, W. P., Van Den Noortgate, W., Claes, L., Witcomb, G., & Fernandez-Aranda, F. (2015). Systematic review and meta-analysis of prevalence studies in transsexualism. *European Psychiatry, 30*(6), 807-815.

Arcelus, J., Mitchell, A. J., Wales, J., & Nielson, S. (2011). Mortality rates in patients with anorexia nervosa and other eating disorders. *Archives of General Psychiatry, 68,* 724-731.

Ardito, R. B., & Rabellino, D. (2011). Therapeutic alliance and outcome of psychotherapy: Historical excursus, measurements, and prospects for research. *Frontiers in Psychology, 2,* 270. https://doi.org/10.3389/fpsyg.2011.00270

Arias, J. M. C., Palacio Acosta, C. A., Valencia, J. G., Montoya, G. J., Arango Viana, J. C., Nieto, O. C., . . . Andres Ruiz-Linares, A. (2011). Exploring epistasis in candidate genes for antisocial personality disorder. *Psychiatric Genetics, 21,* 115-124.

Arntz, A., Weertman, A., & Salet, S. (2011). Interpretation bias in Cluster-C and borderline personality disorders. *Behaviour Research and Therapy, 49,* 472-481.

Arroyo, A., Segrin, C., & Andersen, K. K. (2017). Intergenerational transmission of disordered eating: Direct and indirect maternal communication among grandmothers, mothers, and daughters. *Body Image, 20,* 107-115.

Arshanapally, S., Werner, K. B., Sartor, C. E., & Bucholz, K. K. (2017). The association between racial discrimination and suicidality among African-American adolescents and young adults. *Archives of Suicide Research, 22*(4), 584-595.

Asarnow, J. R., Hughes, J. L., Babeva, K. N., & Sugar, C. A. (2017). Cognitive-behavioral family treatment for suicide attempt prevention: A randomized controlled trial. *Journal of the American Academy of Child & Adolescent Psychiatry, 56*(6), 506-514.

Asher, M., Asnaani, A., & Aderka, I. M. (2017). Gender differences in social anxiety disorder: A review. *Clinical Psychology Review, 56,* 1-12.

Asherson, P., Buitelaar, J., Faraone, S. V., & Rohde, L. A. (2016). Adult attention-deficit hyperactivity disorder: Key conceptual issues. *Lancet Psychiatry, 3*(6), 568-578.

Ashok, A. H., Marques, T. R., Jauhar, S., Nour, M. M., Goodwin, G. M., Young, A. H., & Howes, O. D. (2017). The dopamine hypothesis of bipolar affective disorder: The state of the art and implications for treatment. *Molecular Psychiatry, 22*(5), 666-679.

Asmundson, G., & Taylor, S. (2020). Coronaphobia: Fear and the 2019-nCoV outbreak. *Journal of anxiety disorders, 70,* 102196.

Asmundson, G., & Taylor, S. (2020). Coronaphobia: Fear and the 2019-nCoV outbreak. *Journal of anxiety disorders, 70,* 102196. https://doi.org/10.1016/j.janxdis.2020.102196

A-Tjak, J. G., Davis, M. L., Morina, N., Powers, M. B., Smits, J. A., & Emmelkamp, P. M. (2015). A meta-analysis of the efficacy of acceptance and commitment therapy for clinically relevant mental and physical health problems. *Psychotherapy and Psychosomatics, 84*(1), 30-36.

Attia, E., & Roberto, C. A. (2009). Should amenorrhea be a diagnostic criterion for anorexia nervosa? *International Journal of Eating Disorders, 42,* 581-589.

Attia, E., & Walsh, B. T. (2007). Anorexia nervosa. *American Journal of Psychiatry, 164,* **1805**-1810.

Attwells, S., Setiawan, E., Wilson, A. A., Rusjan, P. M., Mizrahi, R., Miler, L., . . . Meyer, J. H. (2017). Inflammation in the neurocircuitry of obsessive-compulsive disorder. *JAMA Psychiatry, 74*(8), 833-840.

Auger, R. R., Burgess, H. J., Emens, J. S., Deriy, L. V., Thomas, S. M., & Sharkey, K. M. (2015). Clinical practice guideline for the treatment of intrinsic circadian rhythm sleep-wake disorders: advanced sleep-wake phase disorder (ASWPD), delayed sleep-wake phase disorder (DSWPD), non-24-hour sleep-wake rhythm disorder (N24SWD), and irregular sleep-wake rhythm disorder (ISWRD). An update for 2015. *Journal of Clinical Sleep Medicine, 11*(10), 1199-1236.

Aybek, S., & Vuilleumier, P. (2016). Imaging studies of functional neurologic disorders. *Handbook of Clinical Neurology, 139,* 73-84.

Ayers, C. R., Saxena, S., Golshan, S., & Wetherell, J. L. (2009). Age at onset and clinical features of late life compulsive hoarding. *International Journal of Geriatric Psychiatry, 25,* 142-149.

Azevedo, J., Vieira-Coelho, M., Castelo-Branco, M., Coelho, R., & Figueiredo-Braga, M. (2020). Impulsive and premeditated aggression in male offenders with antisocial personality disorder. *Plos One, 15*(3), e0229876.

Azrin, N. H., & Nunn, R. G. (1973). Habit-reversal: A method of eliminating nervous habits and tics. *Behaviour Research and Therapy, 11,* 619-628.

Azrin, N. H., Nunn, R. G., & Frantz, S. E. (1980). Treatment of hair-pulling (trichotillomania): A comparative study of habit reversal and negative practice training. *Journal of Behavior Therapy and Experimental Psychiatry, 11,* 13-20.

B

Başbuğ, S., Cesur, G., & Durak Batıgün, A. (2017). Perceived parental styles and adult separation anxiety. Algılanan Ebeveynlik Biçimi ve Yetişkin Ayrılma Anksiyetesi: Kişilerarası Bilişsel Çarpıtmaların Aracı Rolü. *Turk psikiyatri dergisi = Turkish Journal of Psychiatry, 28*(4), 255-267.

Baba, T., Endo, T., Honnma, H., Kitajima, Y., Hayashi, T., Ikeda, H., Saito, T. (2007). Association between polycystic ovary syndrome and female-to-male transsexuality. *Human Reproduction, 22,* 1011-1016.

Babb, S., Malarcher, A., Shauer, G., Asman, K., & Jamal, A. (2017). Quitting smoking among adults—United States, 2000-2015. *Morbidity and Mortality Weekly Report, 65,* 1457-1464.

Bachhuber, M. A., Hennessy, S., Cunningham, C. O., & Starrels, J. L. (2016). Increasing benzodiazepine prescriptions and overdose mortality in the United States, 1996-2013. *American Journal of Public Health, 106*(4), 686-688.

Baer, J. S., Kivlahan, D. R., Blume, A. W., McKnight, P., & Marlatt, G. A. (2001). Brief intervention for heavy-drinking college students: 4-year follow-up and natural history. *American Journal of Public Health, 91,* 1310-1316.

Baer, R. A., Peters, J. R., Eisenlohr-Moul, T. A., Geider, P. J., & Sauer, S. E. (2012). Emotion-related cognitive processes in borderline personality disorder: A review of the empirical literature. *Clinical Psychology, 32,* 359-369.

Baker, D., Hunter, E., Lawrence, E., Medford, N., Patel, M., Senior, C., . . . David, A. S. (2003). Depersonalisation disorder: Clinical features of 204 cases. *British Journal of Psychiatry, 182,* 428-433.

Baker, S. C., Konova, A. B., Daw, N. D., & Horga, G. (2019). A distinct inferential mechanism for delusions in schizophrenia. *Brain, 142*(6), 1797-1812.

Balasuriya, L., Buelt, E., & Tsai, J. (2020). The never-ending loop: Homelessness, psychiatric disorder, and mortality. *Psychiatric Times, 37,* 11-14.

Balia, C., Carucci, S., Coghill, D., & Zuddas, A. (2018). The pharmacological treatment of aggression in children and adolescents with conduct disorder: Do callous-unemotional traits modulate the efficacy of medication? *Neuroscience & Biobehavioral Reviews, 91,* 218-238.

Ballenger, J. C., Davidson, J. R. T., Lecrubier, Y., Nutt, D. J., Marshall, R. D., Nemeroff, C. B., . . . Yehuda, R. (2004). Consensus statement update on posttraumatic stress disorder from the International Consensus Group on Depression and Anxiety. *Journal of Clinical Psychiatry, 65* (Suppl. 1), 55-62.

Ball, S. A., Martino, S., Nich, C., Frankforter, T. L., Van Horn, D., Crits-Christoph, P., . . . Carroll, K. M. (2007). Site matters: Multisite randomized trial of motivational enhancement therapy in community drug abuse clinics. *Journal of Consulting and Clinical Psychology, 75,* 556-567.

Balon, R., Segraves, R. T., & Clayton, A. (2007). Issues for *DSM-V*: Sexual dysfunction, disorder, or variation along normal distribution: Toward rethinking *DSM* criteria of sexual dysfunctions. *American Journal of Psychiatry, 164,* 198-200.

Bandelow, B., Michaelis, S., & Wedekind, D. (2017). Treatment of anxiety disorders. *Dialogues in Clinical Neuroscience, 19*(2), 93-107. https://doi.org/10.31887/DCNS.2017.19.2/bbandelow

Bandura, A. (1969). *Principles of behavior modification.* New York: Holt, Rinehart & Winston.

Bandura, A. (2006). Going global with social cognitive theory: From prospect to paydirt. In S. I. Donaldson, D. E. Berger, & K. Pezdek (Eds.), *Applied psychology: New frontiers and rewarding careers* (pp. 53-79). Mahwah, NJ: Erlbaum.

Bandura, A. (2019). Applying theory for human betterment. *Perspectives on Psychological Science, 14*(1), 12-15.

Barateau, L., Lopez, R., Franchi, J. A. M., & Dauvilliers, Y. (2017). Hypersomnolence, hypersomnia, and mood disorders. *Current Psychiatry Reports, 19*(2), 13.

Barber, T. R., Lawton, M., Rolinski, M., Evetts, S., Baig, F., Ruffmann, C., et al. (2017). Prodromal Parkinsonism and neurodegenerative risk stratification in REM sleep behavior disorder. *Sleep, 40*(8).

Barch, D. M., Csernansky, J. G., Conturo, T., & Snyder, A. Z. (2002). Working and long-term memory deficits in schizophrenia: Is there a common prefrontal mechanism? *Journal of Abnormal Psychology, 111,* 478-494.

Barch, D. M., & Sheffield, J. M. (2017). Cognitive control in schizophrenia. In T. Egner (Ed.), *Wiley handbook of cognitive control* (pp. 556-580). Chichester, UK: Wiley.

Barker, E. D., Walton, E., & Cecil, C. A. (2018). Annual research review: DNA methylation as a mediator in the association between risk exposure and child and adolescent psychopathology. *Journal of Child Psychology and Psychiatry, 59*(4), 303-322.

Barkhof, E., Meijer, C. J., de Sonneville, L. M. J., Linszen, D. H., & de Haan, L. (2012). Interventions to improve adherence to antipsychotic medication in patients with schizophrenia: A review of the past decade. *European Psychiatry, 27,* 9–18.

Barkley, R. A. (2014). *Attention-deficit hyperactivity disorder: A handbook for diagnosis and treatment* (4th ed.). New York: Guilford Press.

Barlow, D. H. (2011). The development and evaluation of psychological treatments for panic disorder. In M. Gernsbacher, D. Pew, & L. Hough (Eds.), *Psychology and the real world: Essays illustrating fundamental contributors to society* (pp. 198–204). New York: Worth.

Barlow, D. H., Farchione, T. J., Bullis, J. R., Gallagher, M. W., Murray-Latin, H., Sauer-Zavala, S., . . . Cassiello-Robbins, C. (2017). The Unified protocol for transdiagnostic treatment of emotional disorders compared with diagnosis-specific protocols for anxiety disorders: A randomized clinical trial. *JAMA Psychiatry, 74,* 875–884.

Barlow, D. H., Farchione, T. J., Sauer-Zavala, S., Latin, H. M., Ellard, K. K., Bullis, J. R., . . . Cassiello-Robbins, C. (2018). *Unified protocol for transdiagnostic treatment of emotional disorders: Therapist guide.* New York: Oxford University Press.

Barlow, D. H., Gorman, J. M., Shear, M. K., & Woods, S. W. (2000). Cognitive-behavioral therapy, imipramine, or their combination for panic disorder: A randomized controlled trial. *Journal of the American Medical Association, 283,* 2529–2536.

Barlow, D. H., Sakheim, D. K., & Beck, J. G. (1983). Anxiety increases sexual arousal. *Journal of Abnormal Psychology, 92,* 49–54.

Barnes, L. L., Wilson, R. S., Bienias, J. L., Schneider, J. A., Evans, D. A., & Bennett, D. A. (2005). Sex differences in the clinical manifestations of Alzheimer disease pathology. *Archives of General Psychiatry, 62,* 685–691.

Barrio, C., & Yamada, A. M. (2010). Culturally based intervention development: The case of Latino families dealing with schizophrenia. *Research on Social Work Practice, 20*(5), 483–492.

Barsaglini, A., Sartori, G., Benetti, S., Pettersson-Yeo, W., & Mechelli, A. (2014). The effects of psychotherapy on brain function: A systematic and critical review. *Progress in Neurobiology, 114,* 1–14.

Bartley, C. M., & Ross, D. A. (2020). Schizophrenia: A Homecoming. *Biological Psychiatry, 88*(4), e15–e17.

Baruch, I. (2020). Paraphillic disorders. *International Journal of Advanced Studies in Sexology, 2*(2), 94–97.

Bas-Hoogendam, J. M., Blackford, J. U., Brühl, A. B., Blair, K. S., van der Wee, N. J., & Westenberg, P. M. (2016). Neurobiological candidate endophenotypes of social anxiety disorder. *Neuroscience & Biobehavioral Reviews, 71,* 362–378.

Bassett, A. M., & Baker, C. (2015). Normal or abnormal? 'Normative uncertainty' in psychiatric practice. *Journal of Medical Humanities, 36*(2), 89–111.

Basson, R., Berman, J., Burnett, A., Derogatis, L., Ferguson, D., Fourcroy, J., . . . Whippie, B. (2001). Report of the international consensus development conference on female sexual dysfunction: Definitions and classifications. *Journal of Sex & Marital Therapy, 27,* 83–94.

Bastiampillai, T., Sharfstein, S. S., & Allison, S. (2016). Increase in US suicide rates and the critical decline in psychiatric beds. *Journal of the American Medical Association, 316*(24): 2591–2592.

Batelaan, N. M., Van Balkom, A. J. L. M., & Stein, D. J. (2012). Evidence-based pharmacotherapy of panic disorder: An update. *International Journal of Neuropsychopharmacology, 15,* 403–415.

Bateman, A., & Fonagy, P. (2008). 8-year follow-up of patients treated for borderline personality disorder: Mentalization-based treatment versus treatment as usual. *American Journal of Psychiatry, 165,* 631–638.

Bateson, G., Jackson, D. D., Haley, J., & Weakland, J. (1956). Toward a theory of schizophrenia. *Behavioral Science, 1,* 251–264.

Baum, A., Perry, N. W., Jr., & Tarbell, S. (2004). The development of psychology as a health science. In T. J. Ball, R. G. Frank, A. Baum, & J. L. Wallander (Eds.), *Handbook of clinical health psychology: Volume 3. Models and perspectives in health psychology* (pp. 9–28). Washington, DC: American Psychological Association.

Baweja, R., Mayes, S. D., Hameed, U., & Waxmonsky, J. G. (2016). Disruptive mood dysregulation disorder: Current insights. *Neuropsychiatric Disease and Treatment, 12,* 2115–2124.

Beards, S., Gayer-Anderson, C., Borges, S., Dewey, M. E., Fisher, H. L., & Morgan, C. (2013). Life events and psychosis: A review and meta-analysis. *Schizophrenia Bulletin, 39*(4), 740–747.

Beatty, L., & Lambert, S. (2013). A systematic review of Internet-based self-help therapeutic interventions to improve distress and disease-control among adults with chronic health conditions. *Clinical Psychology Review, 33,* 609–622.

Beauchaine, T. P., & Constantino, J. N. (2017). Redefining the endophenotype concept to accommodate transdiagnostic vulnerabilities and etiological complexity. *Biomarkers in Medicine, 11*(9), 769–780.

Beauchaine, T. P., Hinshaw, S. P., & Pang, K. L. (2010). Comorbidity of attention-deficit/hyperactivity disorder and early-onset conduct disorder: Biological, environmental, and developmental mechanisms. *Clinical Psychology: Science and Practice, 17,* 327–336.

Bechara, A. (2005). Decision making, impulse control and loss of willpower to resist drugs: A neurocognitive perspective. *Nature Neuroscience, 8,* 1458–1463.

Beck, A. T. (1967). *Depression: Clinical, experimental, and theoretical aspects.* New York: Harper & Row.

Beck, A. T. (1976). *Cognitive therapy and the emotional disorders.* New York: International Universities Press.

Beck, A. T., & Beck, R. W. (1972). Screening depressed patients in family practice: A rapid technique. *Postgraduate Medicine, 52,* 81–85.

Beck, A. T., & Bredemeier, K. (2016). A unified model of depression: Integrating clinical, cognitive, biological, and evolutionary perspectives. *Clinical Psychological Science, 4*(4), 596–619.

Beck, A. T., Butler, A. C., Brown, G. K., Dahlsgaard, K. K., Newman, C. F., & Beck, J. S. (2001). Dysfunctional beliefs discriminate personality disorders. *Behaviour Research & Therapy, 39,* 1213–1225.

Beck, A. T., Davis, D. D., & Freeman, A. (Eds.). (2015). *Cognitive therapy of personality disorders* (3rd ed.). New York: Guilford Press.

Beck, A. T., & Emery, G. (1985). *Anxiety disorders and phobias: A cognitive perspective.* New York: Basic Books.

Beck, A. T., & Rector, N. A. (2005). Cognitive approaches to schizophrenia: Theory and therapy. *Annual Review of Clinical Psychology, 1,* 577–606.

Beck, A. T., Rush, A. J., Shaw, B. F., & Emery, G. (1979). *Cognitive therapy of depression.* New York: Guilford Press.

Beck, A. T., Steer, R. A., Kovacs, M., & Garrison, B. (1985). Hopelessness and eventual suicide: A 10-year prospective study of patients hospitalized with suicidal ideation. *American Journal of Psychiatry, 142,* 559–563.

Beck, A. T., Ward, C. H., Mendelson, M., Moch, J. E., & Erbaugh, J. (1962). Reliability of psychiatric diagnosis: II. A study of consistency of clinical judgments and ratings. *American Journal of Psychiatry, 119,* 351–357.

Beck, A. T., Weissman, A., Lester, D., & Trexler, L. (1974). The measurement of pessimism: The Hopelessness Scale. *Journal of Consulting & Clinical Psychology, 42,* 861–865.

Becker, A. E., Fay, K. E., Agnew-Blais, J., Kahn, A. N., Striegel-Moore, R. H., & Gilman, S. E. (2011). Social network media exposure and adolescent eating pathology in Fiji. *British Journal of Psychiatry, 198,* 43–50.

Becker-Blease, K. A., Deater-Deckard, K., Eley, T., Freyd, J. J., Stevenson, J., & Plomin, R. (2004). A genetic analysis of individual differences in dissociative behaviors in childhood and adolescence. *Journal of Child Psychology & Psychiatry, 45,* 522–532.

Becker, C. B., & Stice, E. (2017). From efficacy to effectiveness to broad implementation: Evolution of the Body Project. *Journal of Consulting and Clinical Psychology, 85*(8), 767.

Bednarchik, C. L., Kottwitz, M., & Geiger, S. W. (2016). Self-injection, transurethral, and topical therapy in erectile dysfunction. In T. S. Köhler & K. T. McVary (Eds.), *Contemporary treatment of erectile dysfunction: A clinical guide* (pp. 187–207). Cham: Springer.

Beech, A. R., Miner, M. H., & Thornton, D. (2016). Paraphilias in the DSM-5. *Annual Review of Clinical Psychology, 12,* 383–406.

Bekhuis, E., Schoevers, R. A., van Borkulo, C. D., Rosmalen, J. G. M., & Boschloo, L. (2016). The network structure of major depressive disorder, generalized anxiety disorder and somatic symptomatology. *Psychological Medicine, 46*(14), 2989–2998.

Belle, D., & Doucet, J. (2003). Poverty, inequality, and discrimination as sources of depression among U.S. women. *Psychology of Women Quarterly, 27,* 101–113.

Bender, D. S. (2012). Mirror, mirror on the wall: Reflecting on narcissism. *Journal of Psychology, 68,* 877–885.

Bender, L. (1938). *A visual motor gestalt test and its clinical use.* New York: American Orthopsychiatric Association.

Benet-Martinez, V., & John, O. P. (1998). Los Cinco Grandes across cultures and ethnic groups: Multitrait-multimethod analyses of the Big Five in Spanish and English. *Journal of Personality & Social Psychology, 75,* 729–750.

Benjet, C., Bromet, E., Karam, E. G., Kessler, R. C., McLaughlin, K. A., Ruscio, A. M., . . . Koenen, K. C. (2016). The epidemiology of traumatic event exposure worldwide: Results from the World Mental Health Survey Consortium. *Psychological Medicine, 46*(2), 327–343.

Bennett, A., & Johnson, D. (2017). Co-morbidity of personality disorder and clinical syndrome in high-risk incarcerated offenders. *Journal of Forensic Practice, 19*(3), 207–216. doi: http://dx.doi.org.mccc.idm.oclc.org/10.1108/JFP-05-2016-0026

Bennett, N. E. (2016). Oral prescription therapy for erectile dysfunction. In T. S. Köhler & K. T. McVary (Eds.), *Contemporary treatment of erectile dysfunction: A clinical guide* (pp. 163–173). Cham: Springer.

Benson, L., & Christensen, A. (2016). Empirically supported couple therapies. In K. T. Sullivan & E. Lawrence (Eds.), *The Oxford handbook of relationship science and couple interventions* (pp. 177–192). New York: Oxford University Press.

Bentall, R. P., Rouse, G., Kinderman, P., Blackwood, N., Howard, R., Moore, R., . . . Corcoran, R. (2008). Paranoid delusions in schizophrenia spectrum disorders and depression: The transdiagnostic role of expectations of negative events and negative self-esteem. *Journal of Nervous and Mental Disease, 196,* 375–383.

Bentley, K. H., Cassiello-Robbins, C. F., Vittorio, L., Sauer-Zavala, S., & Barlow, D. H. (2015). The association between nonsuicidal self-injury and the emotional disorders: A meta-analytic review. *Clinical Psychology Review, 37,* 72–88.

Bentley, K. H., Franklin, J. C., Ribeiro, J. D., Kleiman, E. M., Fox, K. R., & Nock, M. K. (2016). Anxiety and its disorders as risk factors for suicidal thoughts and behaviors: A meta-analytic review. *Clinical Psychology Review, 43,* 30–46.

Berger, W., Coutinho, E. S. F., Figueira, I., Marques-Portella, C., Luz, M. P., Neylan, T. C., . . . & Mendlowicz, M. V. (2012). Rescuers at risk: A systematic review and meta-regression analysis of the worldwide current prevalence and correlates of PTSD in rescue workers. *Social Psychiatry and Psychiatric Epidemiology, 47*(6), 1001–1011.

Berkowitz, R. I., Wadden, T. A., Gehrman, C. A., Bishop-Gilyard, C. T., Moore, R. H., Womble, L. G., . . . Xanthopoulos, M. S. (2011). Meal replacements in the treatment of adolescent obesity: A randomized control trial. *Obesity, 19,* 1193–1199.

Berlin, F. S. (2019). Paraphilic disorders: A better understanding. *Current Psychiatry, 18*(4), 22–28.

Berlin, L. J., Brooks-Gunn, J., McCartoon, C., & McCormick, M. C. (1998). The effectiveness of early intervention: Examining risk factors and pathways to enhanced development. *Preventive Medicine, 27,* 238–245.

Berman, M. (2020, July 15). Understanding Kanye West's bipolar disorder. Retrieved December 23, 2020, from https://www.medpagetoday.com/blogs/celebritydiagnosis/87581

Berridge, K. C., & Robinson, T. E. (2016). Liking, wanting, and the incentive-sensitization theory of addiction. *American Psychologist, 71*(8), 670–679.

Berry, S. M., Broglio, K., Bunker, M., Jayewardene, A., Olin, B., & Rush, A. J. (2013). A patient-level meta-analysis of studies evaluating vagus nerve stimulation therapy for treatment-resistant depression. *Medical Devices (Auckland, N.Z.), 6,* 17–35. https://doi.org/10.2147/MDER.S41017

Berthoud, H. R., & Morrison, C. (2008). The brain, appetite, and obesity. *Annual Review of Psychology, 59,* 55–92.

Bettelheim, B. (1967). *The empty fortress: Infantile autism and the birth of the self.* New York: Free Press.

Beurel, E., Toups, M., & Nemeroff, C. B. (2020). The bidirectional relationship of depression and inflammation: Double trouble. *Neuron, 107*(2), 234–256.

Bewernick, B., & Schlaepfer, T. E. (2015). Update on Neuromodulation for Treatment-Resistant Depression. *F1000Research, 4,* F1000 Faculty Rev-1389. https://doi.org/10.12688/f1000research.6633.1

Bezerra de Carvalho, A., de Azevedo Cardoso, T., Campos Mondin,T., Azevedo da Silva, T., Dias de Mattos Souza, L., Vieira da Silva Magalhães, P., & Jansen, K. (2018). Prevalence and factors associated with premenstrual dysphoric disorder: A community sample of young adult women. *Psychiatry Research, 268,* 42–45.

Bögels, S. M., Alden, L., Beidel, D. C., Clark, L. A., Pine, D. S., Stein, M. B., & Voncken, M. (2010). Social anxiety disorder: Questions and answers for the *DSM-V. Depression and Anxiety, 27,* 168–189.

Bögels, S. M., Knappe, S., & Clark, L. A. (2013). Adult separation anxiety disorder in *DSM-5. Clinical Psychology Review, 33,* 663–674.

Bhati, K. S. (2014). Effect of client-therapist gender match on the therapeutic relationship: An exploratory analysis. *Psychological Reports, 115*(2), 565–583.

Bhochhibhoya, A., Harrison, S., Yonce, S., Friedman, D. B., Ghimire, P. S., & Li, X. (2020). A systematic review of psychosocial interventions for older adults living with HIV. *AIDS care,* 1–12.

Biederman, J., Faraone, S. V., Hirschfeld-Becker, D. R., Friedman, D., Robin, J. A., & Rosenbaum, J. F. (2001). Patterns of psychopathology and dysfunction in high-risk children of parents with panic disorder and major depression. *American Journal of Psychiatry, 158,* 49-57.

Böing, S., & Randerath, W. J. (2015). Chronic hypoventilation syndromes and sleep-related hypoventilation. *Journal of Thoracic Disease, 7*(8), 1273-1285.

Birmaher, B., Axelson, D., Strober, M., Gill, M. K., Valeri, S., Chiappetta, L., . . . Keller, M. (2006). Clinical course of children and adolescents with bipolar spectrum disorders. *Archive of General Psychiatry, 63,* 175-183.

Biron, M., Risch, N., Hamburger, R., Mandel, B., Kushner, S., Newman, M., . . . Belmaker, R. H. (1987). Genetic linkage between X-chromosome markers and bipolar affective illness. *Nature, 326,* 289-292.

Bizic, M. R., Jeftovic, M., Pusica, S., Stojanovic, B., Duisin, D., Vujovic, S., . . . & Djordjevic, M. L. (2018). Gender dysphoria: Bioethical aspects of medical treatment. *Biomed Research International, 2018, 1-6.*

Bjorvatn, B., Grønli, J., & Pallesen, S. (2010). Prevalence of different parasomnias in the general population. *Sleep Medicine Reviews, 11,* 1031-1034.

Black, D. W. (2017). The treatment of antisocial personality disorder. *Current Treatment Options in Psychiatry, 4*(4), 295-302.

Black, D. W., Blum, N., & Allen, J. (2018). STEPPS treatment programme for borderline personality disorder: Which scale items improve? An item-level analysis. *Personality and Mental Health, 12*(4), 345-354.

Black, D. W., Zanarini, M. C., Romine, A., Shaw, M., Allen, J., & Schulz, S. C. (2014). Comparison of low and moderate dosages of extended-release quetiapine in borderline personality disorder: A randomized, double-blind, placebo-controlled trial. *American Journal of psychiatry, 171*(11), 1174-1182.

Blaney, P. H. (1986). Affect and memory: A review. *Psychological Bulletin, 99,* 229-246.

Blank, R., Smits-Engelsman, B., Polatajko, H., & Wilson, P. (2012). European Academy for Childhood Disability (EACD): Recommendations on the definition, diagnosis and intervention of developmental coordination disorder (long version). *Developmental Medicine and Child Neurology, 54,* 54-93.

Blashfield, R. K., Reynolds, S. M., & Stennett, B. (2012). The death of histrionic personality disorder. In T. A. Widiger (Ed.), *The Oxford handbook of personality disorders* (pp. 603-627). New York: Oxford University Press.

Blond, A. (2008). Impacts of exposure to images of ideal bodies on male body dissatisfaction: A review. *Body Image, 5,* 244-250.

Blöte, A. W., Miers, A. C., Heyne, D. A., & Westenberg, P. M. (2015). Social anxiety and the school environment of adolescents. In K. Ranta, A. M. La Greca, L. J. Garcia-Lopez, & M. Marttunen (Eds.), *Social anxiety and phobia in adolescents* (pp. 151-181). Cham: Springer.

Bölte, S., & Poustka, F. (2004). Comparing the intelligence profiles of savant and nonsavant individuals with autistic disorder. *Intelligence, 32,* 121-131.

Blumenthal, J. A., Babyak, M. A., Doraiswamy, P. M., Watkins, L., Hoffman, B. M., Barbour, K. A., Herman, S., Craighead, W. E., Brosse, A. L., Waugh, R., Hinderliter, A., & Sherwood, A. (2007). Exercise and pharmacotherapy in the treatment of major depressive disorder. *Psychosomatic Medicine, 69,* 587-596.

Blumenthal, J. A., Sherwood, A., Babyak, M. A., Watkins, L. L., Waugh, R., Georgiades, A., . . . Hinderliter, A. (2005). Effects of exercise and stress management training on markers of cardiovascular risk in patients with ischemic heart disease: A randomized controlled trial. *JAMA, 293,* 1626-1634.

Blum, N., St. John, D., Pfohl, B., Stuart, S., McCormick, B., Allen, J., Arndt, S., & Black, D. W. (2008). Systems training for emotional predictability and problem solving (STEPPS) for outpatients with borderline personality disorder: A randomized controlled trial and 1-year follow-up. *American Journal of Psychiatry, 165,* 468-478.

Bockting, C. L., Hollon, S. D., Jarrett, R. B., Kuyken, W., & Dobson, K. (2015). A lifetime approach to major depressive disorder: The contributions of psychological interventions in preventing relapse and recurrence. *Clinical Psychology Review, 41,* 16-26.

Bohart, A. C. (1995). The person-centered psychotherapies. In A. S. Gurman (Ed.), *Essential psychotherapies: Theory and practice* (pp. 55-84). New York: Guilford Press.

Bohlken, M., Hugdahl, K., & Sommer, I. (2017). Auditory verbal hallucinations: Neuroimaging and treatment. *Psychological Medicine, 47*(2), 199-208. doi: 10.1017/S003329171600115X

Bohus, M., Haaf, B., Simms, T., Limberger, M. F., Schmahl, C., Unckel, C., . . . Linehan, M. M. (2004). Effectiveness of inpatient dialectical behavioral therapy for borderline personality disorder: A controlled trial. *Behaviour Research & Therapy, 42,* 487-499.

Boileau, B. (2011). A review of obsessive-compulsive disorder in children and adolescents. *Dialogues in Clinical Neuroscience, 13*(4), 401-411.

Bonanno, G. A., Neria, Y., Mancini, A., Coifman, K. G., Litz, B., & Insel, B. (2007). Is there more to complicated grief than depression and posttraumatic stress disorder? A test of incremental validity. *Journal of Abnormal Psychology, 116,* 342-351.

Bonanno, G. A., Westphal, M., & Mancini, A. D. (2011). Resilience to loss and potential trauma. *Annual Review of Clinical Psychology, 7,* 511-535.

Bonnie, R. J., & Grisso, T. (2000). Adjudicative competence and youthful offenders. In T. Grisso & R. G. Schwartz (Eds.), *Youth on trial: A developmental perspective on juvenile justice.* Chicago: University of Chicago Press.

Book, A. S., Starzyk, K. B., & Quinsey, V. L. (2001). The relationship between testosterone and aggression: A meta-analysis. *Aggression & Violent Behavior, 6,* 579-599.

Boone, L., Soenens, B., & Luyten, P. (2014). When or why does perfectionism translate into eating disorder pathology? A longitudinal examination of the moderating and mediating role of body dissatisfaction. *Journal of Abnormal Psychology, 123*(2), 412.

Boothroyd, R. A., Mercado, C. C., Poythress, N. G., Christy, A., & Petrila, J. (2005). Clinical outcomes of defendants in mental health court. *Psychiatric Services, 56,* 829-834.

Borges, G., Angst, J., Nock, M. K., Ruscio, A. M., & Kessler, R. C. (2008). Risk factors for the incidence and persistence of suicide-related outcomes: A 10-year follow-up study using the national comorbidity surveys. *Journal of Affective Disorders, 105,* 25-33.

Borges, G., Nock, M. K., Haro Abad, J. M., Hwang, I., Sampson, N. A., Alonso, J., . . . Kessler, R. C. (2010). Twelve-month prevalence of and risk factors for suicide attempts in the World Health Organization World Mental Health Surveys. *Journal of Clinical Psychiatry, 71,* 1617-1628.

Borkovec, T. D., Alcaine, O., & Behar, E. (2004). Avoidance theory of worry and generalized anxiety disorder. In R. G. Heimberg, C. L. Turk, & D. S. Mennin (Eds.), *Generalized anxiety disorder: Advances in research and practice* (pp. 77-108). New York: Guilford Press.

Borkovec, T. D., Newman, M. G., & Castonguay, L. G. (2003). Cognitive-behavioral therapy for generalized anxiety disorder with integrations from interpersonal and experiential therapies. *CNS Spectrums, 8,* 382-389.

Borkovec, T. D., Newman, M. G., Pincus, A. L., & Lytle, R. (2002). A component analysis of cognitive-behavioral therapy for generalized anxiety disorder and the role of interpersonal problems. *Journal of Consulting & Clinical Psychology, 70,* 288-298.

Borkovec, T. D., & Ruscio, A. M. (2001). Psychotherapy for generalized anxiety disorder. *Journal of Clinical Psychiatry, 62* (Suppl. 11), 37–42.

Bornstein, R. F. (2012). Illuminating a neglected clinical issue: Societal costs of interpersonal dependency and dependent personality disorder. *Journal of Clinical Psychology, 68,* 766–781.

Bortolon, C., Yazbek, H., Norton, J., Capdevielle, D., & Raffard, S. (2019). The contribution of optimism and hallucinations to grandiose delusions in individuals with schizophrenia. *Schizophrenia Research, 210,* 203–206.

Boschloo, L., Bekhuis, E., Weitz, E. S., Reijnders, M., DeRubeis, R. J., Dimidjian, S., . . . & Jarrett, R. B. (2019). The symptom-specific efficacy of antidepressant medication vs. cognitive behavioral therapy in the treatment of depression: Results from an individual patient data meta-analysis. *World Psychiatry, 18*(2), 183–191.

Bouton, M. E., Mineka, S., & Barlow, D. H. (2001). A modern learning theory perspective on the etiology of panic disorder. *Psychological Review, 108,* 4–32.

Bowen, S., Chawla, N., & Marlatt, G. A. (2010). *Mindfulness-based relapse prevention for the treatment of substance-use disorders: A clinician's guide.* New York: Guilford Press.

Bowen, S., Witkiewitz, K., Clifasefi, S. L., Grow, J., Chawla, N., Hsu, S. H., . . . Larimer, M. E. (2014). Relative efficacy of mindfulness-based relapse prevention, standard relapse prevention, and treatment as usual for substance use disorders: A randomized clinical trial. *JAMA Psychiatry, 71*(5), 547–556.

Bowie, C. R., Leung, W. W., Reichenberg, A., McClure, M. M., Patterson, T., Heaton, R. K., & Harvey, P. D. (2008). Predicting schizophrenia patients' real-world behavior with specific neuropsychological and functional capacity measures. *Biological Psychiatry, 63,* 505–511.

Braden, A., Rhee, K., Peterson, C. B., Rydell, S. A., Zucker, N., & Boutelle, K. (2014). Associations between child emotional eating and general parenting style, feeding practices, and parent psychopathology. *Appetite, 80,* 35–40.

Brady, K. T., Back, S. E., & Greenfield, S. F. (Eds.). (2009). *Women and addiction: A comprehensive handbook.* New York: Guilford Press.

Brady, R. O., Jr., Tandon, N., Masters, G. A., Margolis, A., Cohen, B. M., Keshavan, M., & Öngür, D. (2017). Differential brain network activity across mood states in bipolar disorder. *Journal of Affective Disorders, 207,* 367–376.

Brand, B. L., Loewenstein, R. J., & Spiegel, D. (2014). Dispelling myths about dissociative identity disorder treatment: An empirically based approach. *Psychiatry: Interpersonal and Biological Processes, 77*(2), 169–189.

Brand, B. L., McNary, S. W., Myrick, A. C., Classen, C. C., Lanius, R., . . . Putnam, F. W. (2013). A longitudinal naturalistic study of patients with dissociative disorders treated by community clinicians. *Psychological Trauma: Theory, Research, Practice, and Policy, 5*(4), 301–308. https://doi-org. mccc.idm.oclc.org/10.1037/a0027654.supp (Supplemental)

Brand, B., Sar, V., Stavropoulos, P., Krüger, C., Korzekwa, M., Martínez-Taboas, A., & Middleton, W. (2016). Separating fact from fiction: An empirical examination of six myths about dissociative identity disorder. *Harvard Review of Psychiatry, 24*(4), 257–270. doi: 10.1097/HRP.0000000000000100

Braslow, J. T., & Messac, L. (2018). Medicalization and demedicalization-A gravely disabled homeless man with psychiatric illness. *The New England Journal of Medicine, 379*(20), 1885–1888.

Bratiotis, C., Davidow, J., Glossner, K., & Steketee, G. (2016). Requests for help with hoarding: Who needs what from whom? *Practice Innovations, 1*(1), 82–88.

Breaux, R. P., Harvey, E. A., & Lugo-Candelas, C. I. (2014). The role of parent psychopathology in the development of preschool children with behavior problems. *Journal of Clinical Child and Adolescent Psychology: The Official Journal for the Society of Clinical Child and Adolescent Psychology, American Psychological Association, Division 53, 43*(5), 777–790.

Brenner, L., Köllner, V., & Bachem, R. (2019). Symptom burden and work-related impairment among patients with PTSD and complex PTSD. *European Journal of Psychotraumatology, 10*(1).

Brent, D. A., & Bridge, J. (2003). Firearms availability and suicide. *American Behavioral Scientist, 46*(9), 1192–1210.

Brent, D. A., Oquendo, M., Birmaher, B., Greenhill, L., Kolko, D., Stanley, B., . . . Mann, J. J. (2002). Familial pathways to early-onset suicide attempt. *Archives of General Psychiatry, 59,* 801–807.

Brent, D. A., Oquendo, M., Birmaher, B., Greenhill, L., Kolko, D., Stanley, B., Zelazny, J., Brodsky, B., Firinciogullari, S., Ellis, S. P., & Mann, J. J. (2003). Peripubertal suicide attempts in offspring of suicide attempters with siblings concordant for suicidal behavior. *American Journal of Psychiatry, 160,* 1486–1493.

Brewin, C. R., & Andrews, B. (2017). Creating memories for false autobiographical events in childhood: A systematic review. *Applied Cognitive Psychology, 31*(1), 2–23.

Brick, J. (Ed.). (2008). *Handbook of the medical consequences of alcohol and drug abuse* (2nd ed.). New York: Haworth Press/ Taylor & Francis Group.

Bridley, A., & Daffin, L. W., Jr. (2018, January 05). *Abnormal psychology* (2nd ed.). Retrieved November 12, 2020, from https://opentext.wsu.edu/abnormal-psych/chapter/module-3-clinical-assessment-diagnosis-and-treatment/

Brignell, A., Morgan, A. T., Woolfenden, S., Klopper, F., May, T., Sarkozy, V., & Williams, K. (2018). A systematic review and meta-analysis of the prognosis of language outcomes for individuals with autism spectrum disorder. *Autism & Developmental Language Impairments, 3,* 2396941518767610.

Briley, D. A., & Tucker-Drob, E. M. (2012). Broad bandwidth or high fidelity? Evidence from the structure of genetic and environmental effects on the facets of the five factor model. *Behavior Genetics, 42,* 743–763.

Britton, J. C., & Rauch, S. L. (2009). Neuroanatomy and neuroimaging of anxiety disorders. In M. M. Antony & M. B. Stein (Eds.), *Oxford handbook of anxiety and related disorders* (pp. 97–110). New York: Oxford University Press.

Brody, L. R., Hall, J. A., & Stokes, L. R. (2016). Gender and emotion: Theory, findings, and context. In L. F. Barrett, M. Lewis, & J. M. Haviland-Jones (Eds.), *Handbook of emotions,* 4th ed. (pp. 369–392). New York: Guilford.

Bronson, J., & Berzofsky, M. (2017). *Indicators of mental health problems reported by prisoners and jail inmates, 2011-12.* Washington, DC: Bureau of Justice Statistics.

Brosschot, J. F., Van Dijk, E., & Thayer, J. F. (2007). Daily worry is related to low heart rate variability during waking and the subsequent nocturnal sleep period. *International Journal of Psychophysiology, 63,* 39–47.

Brotman, M. A., Sharif-Askary, B., Dickstein, D. P., & Leibenluft, E. (2016). Biological factors in bipolar disorder in childhood and adolescence. In J. C. Soares & A. H. Young (Eds.), *Bipolar disorders: Basic mechanisms and therapeutic implications* (pp. 219–233). Cambridge: Cambridge University Press.

Brotto, L. A. (2017). Evidence-based treatments for low sexual desire in women. *Frontiers in Neuroendocrinology, 45,* 11–17.

Brown, C. H., IV. (2014). Delirium in the cardiac surgical intensive care unit. *Current Opinion in Anaesthesiology, 27*(2), 117–122.

Brown, C. W., Olson, H. C., & Croninger, R. G. (2010). Maternal alcohol consumption during pregnancy and infant social, mental, and motor development. *Journal of Early Intervention, 32,* 110–126.

Browne, K. O. (2001). Cultural formulation of psychiatric diagnoses. *Culture, Medicine, & Psychiatry, 25,* 411–425.

Brownell, K. D., & Horgen, K. B. (2004). *Food fight: The inside story of the food industry, America's obesity crisis, and what we can do about it.* New York: McGraw-Hill.

Brownell, K. D., & Walsh, B. T. (2017). *Eating disorders and obesity: A comprehensive handbook* (3rd ed.). New York: Guilford Press.

Brownley, K. A., Berkman, N. D., Peat, C. M., Lohr, K. N., Cullen, K. E., Bann, C. M., & Bulik, C. M. (2016). Binge-eating disorder in adults: A systematic review and meta-analysis. *Annals of Internal Medicine, 165*(6), 409–420.

Bruch, H. (1973). *Eating disorders: Obesity, anorexia nervosa, and the person within.* New York: Basic Books.

Bruch, H. (1982). Anorexia nervosa: Therapy and theory. *American Journal of Psychiatry, 139,* 1531–1538.

Bruffaerts, R., Demyttenaere, K., Borges, G., Haro, J. M., Chiu, W. T., Hwang, I., . . . Nock, M. K. (2010). Childhood adversities as risk factors for onset and persistence of suicidal behaviour. *British Journal of Psychiatry, 197*(1), 20–27.

Bruffaerts, R., Demyttenaere, K., Hwang, I., Chiu, W. T., Sampson, N., Kessler, R. C., . . . Nok, K. M. (2011). Treatment of suicidal people around the world. *British Journal of Psychiatry, 199*(1), 64–70.

Bruno, A., Celebre, L., Torre, G., Pandolfo, G., Mento, C., Cedro, C., . . . Muscatello, M. (2019, June 01). *Focus on disruptive mood dysregulation disorder: A review of the literature.* Retrieved December 16, 2020, from https://www.sciencedirect.com/science/article/abs/pii/S0165178119300290

Bryant, C., Jackson, H., & Ames, D. (2008). The prevalence of anxiety in older adults: Methodological issues and a review of the literature. *Journal of Affective Disorders, 109,* 233–250.

Bryant, R. A., & Das, P. (2012). The neural circuitry of conversion disorder and its recovery. *Journal of Abnormal Psychology, 121,* 289–296.

Bryant, R. A., Friedman, M. J., Spiegel, D., Ursano, R., & Strain, J. (2011). A review of acute stress disorder in *DSM-5. Depression and Anxiety, 28,* 802–817.

Buckman, J. E. J., Underwood, A., Clarke, K., Saunders, R., Hollon, S. D., Fearon, P., & Pilling, S. (2018). Risk factors for relapse and recurrence of depression in adults and how they operate: A four-phase systematic review and meta-synthesis. *Clinical Psychology Review, 64,* 13–38.

Budisteanu, M., Andrei, E., Linca, F., Hulea, D. S., Velicu, A. C., Mihailescu, I., . . . Rad, F. (2020). Predictive factors in early onset schizophrenia. *Experimental and Therapeutic Medicine, 20*(6), 210. https://doi.org/10.3892/etm.2020.9340

Buerger, A., Ernst, V., Wolter, V., Huss, M., Kaess, M., & Hammerle, F. (2019). Treating eating disorders in the real world—MaiStep: A skill-based universal prevention for schools. *Preventive Medicine, 123,* 324–332.

Buka, S. L., Cannon, T. D., Torrey, E. F., Yolken, R. H., & the Collaborative Study Group on the Perinatal Origins of Severe Psychotic Disorders. (2008). Maternal exposure to herpes simplex virus and risk of psychosis among adult offspring. *Biological Psychiatry, 63,* 809–815.

Bulantika, S., Wibowo, M., & Jafar, M. (2018). Group Counseling with Systematic Desensitization Techniques and Thought-Stopping Techniques to Reduce Social Anxiety. Retrieved November 06, 2020, from https://journal.unnes.ac.id/sju/index.php/jubk/article/view/25494

Bulik, C. M., Sullivan, P. F., & Kendler, K. S. (2003). Genetic and environmental contributions to obesity and binge eating. *International Journal of Eating Disorders, 33,* 293–298.

Bulik, C. M., Sullivan, P. F., Tozzi, F., Furberg, H., Lichtenstein, P., & Pedersen, N. L. (2006). Prevalence, heritability, and prospective risk factors for anorexia nervosa. *Archives of General Psychiatry, 63,* 305–312.

Bulik, C. M., Thornton, L. M., Root, T. L., Pisetsky, E. M., Lichtenstein, P., & Pedersen, N. L. (2010). Understanding the relation between anorexia nervosa and bulimia nervosa in a Swedish national twin sample. *Biological Psychiatry, 67,* 71–77.

Burcusa, S. L., & Iacono, W. G. (2007). Risk for recurrence in depression. *Clinical Psychology Review, 27*(8), 959–985.

Burhan, A. M., Moradizadeh, M., & Marlatt, N. E. (2018). Major or mild vascular neurocognitive disorder. In A. Hategan, J. Bourgeois, C. Hirsch, & C. Giroux (Eds.), *Geriatric psychiatry* (pp. 445–466). New York: Springer International.

Busfield, J. (1986). *Managing madness: Changing ideas and practice.* London: Unwin Hyman.

Bustillo, J. R., Lauriello, J., Horan, W. P., & Keith, S. J. (2001). The psychosocial treatment of schizophrenia: An update. *American Journal of Psychiatry, 158,* 163–175.

Buysse, D. J., Ancoli-Israel, S., Edinger, J. D., Lichstein, K. L., & Morin, C. M. (2006). Recommendations for a standard research assessment of insomnia. *Sleep, 29,* 1155–1173.

Buysse, D. J., Rush, A. J., & Reynolds, C. F. (2017). Clinical management of insomnia disorder. *JAMA, 318*(20), 1973–1974.

Byne, W., Bradley, S. J., Coleman, E., Eyler, A. E., Green, R., Menvielle, E., . . . Tompkins, D. A. (2012). Treatment of gender identity disorder. *American Journal of Psychiatry, 169,* 875–876.

Byrne, S., Wade, T., Hay, P., Touyz, S., Fairburn, C. G., Treasure, J., . . . Crosby, R. D. (2017). A randomised controlled trial of three psychological treatments for anorexia nervosa. *Psychological Medicine, 47*(16), 2823–2833.

Bystritsky, A., Ackerman, D. L., Rosen, R. M., Vapnik, T., Gorvis, E., Maidment, K. M., & Saxena, S. (2004). Augmentation of serotonin reuptake inhibitors in refractory obsessive-compulsive disorder using adjunctive olanzapine: A placebo-controlled trial. *Journal of Clinical Psychiatry, 65,* 565–568.

C

Căndel, O. S., & Constantin, T. (2017). Antisocial and schizoid personality disorder scales: Conceptual bases and preliminary findings. *Romanian Journal of Psychology, 19*(1).

Cai, N., Choi, K. W., & Fried, E. I. (2020). Reviewing the genetics of heterogeneity in depression: Operationalizations, manifestations and etiologies. *Human Molecular Genetics, 29*(R1), R10–R18.

Calear, A. L., Christensen, H., Freeman, A., Fenton, K., Grant, J. B., Van Spijker, B., & Donker, T. (2016). A systematic review of psychosocial suicide prevention interventions for youth. *European Child & Adolescent Psychiatry, 25*(5), 467–482.

Cale, E. M., & Lilienfeld, S. O. (2002). Sex differences in psychopathy and antisocial personality disorder: A review and integration. *Clinical Psychology Review, 22,* 1179–1207.

Callaghan, G. M., Summers, C. J., & Weidman, M. (2003). The treatment of histrionic and narcissistic personality disorder behaviors: A single-subject demonstration of clinical improvement using functional-analytic psychotherapy. *Journal of Contemporary Psychotherapy, 33,* 321–339.

Campos, S. & Link, D. (June 2016). Pseudocyesis. *The Journal for Nurse Practitioners, 12*(6), 390–394.

Canino, G., Polanczyk, G., Bauermeister, J. J., Rohde, L. A., Frick, P. J. (2010). Does the prevalence of CD and ODD vary across cultures? *Social Psychiatry and Psychiatric Epidemiology, 45*, 695–704.

Cannon, B. J., & Kramer, L. M. (2012). Delusion content across the 20th century in an American psychiatric hospital. *International Journal of Social Psychiatry, 58*(3), 323–327.

Cannon, T. D. (2009). What is the role of theories in the study of schizophrenia? *Schizophrenia Bulletin, 35*, 563–567.

Cannon, T. D., Hennah, W., van Erp, T. G., Thompson, P. M., Lonnqvist, J., Huttunen, M., . . . Peltonen, L. (2005). Association of DISC1/TRAX haplotypes with schizophrenia, reduced prefrontal gray matter, and impaired short- and long-term memory. *Archives of General Psychiatry, 62*, 1205–1213.

Cannon, T. D., van Erp, T. G. M., Bearden, C. E., Loewy, R., Thompson, P., Toga, A. W., . . . Tsuang, M. T. (2003). Early and late neurodevelopmental influences in the prodrome to schizophrenia: Contributions of genes, environment, and their interactions. *Schizophrenia Bulletin, 29*, 653–669.

Cannon, T. D., van Erp, T. G. M., & Glahn, D. C. (2002). Elucidating continuities and discontinuities between schizotypy and schizophrenia in the nervous system. *Schizophrenia Research, 54*, 151–156.

Caramanica, K., Brackbill, R. M., Stellman, S. D., & Farfel, M. R. (2015). Posttraumatic stress disorder after hurricane sandy among persons exposed to the 9/11 disaster. *International Journal of Emergency Mental Health, 17*(1), 356–362.

Cardeña, E., & Carlson, E. (2011). Acute stress disorder revisited. *Annual Review of Clinical Psychology, 7*, 245–267.

Cardeña, E., van Duijl, M., Weiner, L. A., & Terhune, D. B. (2009). Possession/trance phenomena. In P. F. Dell & J. A. O'Neil (Eds.), *Dissociation and the dissociative disorders: DSM-V and beyond* (pp. 171–184). New York: Routledge.

Cardozo, B. L., Kaiser, R., Gotway, C. A., & Agani, F. (2003). Mental health, social functioning, and feelings of hatred and revenge in Kosovar Albanians one year after the war in Kosovo. *Journal of Traumatic Stress, 16*, 351–360.

Carlo, G., Knight, G. P., Roesch, S. C., Opal, D., & Davis, A. (2014). Personality across cultures: A critical analysis of Big Five research and current directions. In F. T. L. Leong, L. Comas-Díaz, G. C. Nagayama Hall, V. C. McLoyd, & J. E. Trimble (Eds.), *APA handbook of multicultural psychology: Vol. 1. Theory and research* (pp. 285–298). Washington, DC: American Psychological Association.

Carlyle, K. E., Guidry, J. P., Williams, K., Tabaac, A., & Perrin, P. B. (2018). Suicide conversations on Instagram™: contagion or caring?. *Journal of Communication in Healthcare, 11*(1), 12–18.

Carmassi, C., Gesi, C., Massimetti, E., Shear, M. K., & Dell'Osso, L. (2015). Separation anxiety disorder in the DSM-5 era. *Journal of Psychopathology, 21*, 365–371.

Carmichael, V., & Whitley, R. (2019). Media coverage of Robin Williams' suicide in the United States: A contributor to contagion? *PLoS ONE, 14*(5), 1–13.

Carpenter, K. M., Williams, K., & Worly, B. (2017). Treating women's orgasmic difficulties. In Z. D. Peterson (Ed.), *The Wiley handbook of sex therapy* (pp. 57–71). Oxford: Wiley.

Carpenter, R. W., & Trull, T. J. (2013). Components of emotion dysregulation in borderline personality disorder: A review. *Current Psychiatry Reports, 15*(1), 335.

Carr, A. (2014). The evidence base for family therapy and systemic interventions for child-focused problems. *Journal of Family Therapy, 36*(2), 107–157.

Carr, A. (2019). Family therapy and systemic interventions for child-focused problems: The current evidence base. *Journal of Family Therapy, 41*(2), 153–213.

Carrion-Castillo, A., Franke, B., & Fisher, S. E. (2013). Molecular genetics of dyslexia: An overview. *Dyslexia, 19*(4), 214–240.

Carroll, K. M., Ball, S. A., Nich, C., Martino, S., Frankforter, T. L., Farentinos, C., . . . Woody, G. E. (2006). Motivational interviewing to improve treatment engagement and outcome in individuals seeking treatment for substance abuse: A multisite effectiveness study. *Drug and Alcohol Dependence, 81*, 301–312.

Carroll, K. M., & Kiluk, B. D. (2017). Cognitive behavioral interventions for alcohol and drug use disorders: Through the stage model and back again. *Psychology of Addictive Behaviors: Journal of the Society of Psychologists in Addictive Behaviors, 31*(8), 847–861. https://doi.org/10.1037/adb0000311

Carter, J. C., Mercer-Lynn, K. B., Norwood, S. J., Bewll-Weiss, C. V., Crosby, R. D., Woodside, D. B., & Olmstead, M. P. (2012). A prospective study of predictors of relapse in anorexia nervosa: Implications for relapse prevention. *Psychiatry Research, 200*, 518–523.

Carver, C. S., & Scheier, M. F. (2014). Dispositional optimism. *Trends in Cognitive Sciences, 18*(6), 293–299.

Casey, B. J., Tottenham, N., Liston, C., & Durston, S. (2005). Imaging the developing brain: What have we learned about cognitive development? *Trends in Cognitive Sciences, 9*, 104–110.

Casey, L. J., Wootton, B. M., & McAloon, J. (2020). Mental health, minority stress, and the Australian Marriage Law postal survey: A longitudinal study. *American Journal of Orthopsychiatry, 90*(5), 546–556. https://doi.org/10.1037/ort0000455

Casey, L. M., Oei, T. P., Raylu, N., Horrigan, K., Day, J., Ireland, M., & Clough, B. A. (2017). Internet-based delivery of cognitive behaviour therapy compared to monitoring, feedback and support for problem gambling: A randomised controlled trial. *Journal of Gambling Studies, 33*(3), 993–1010.

Caspi, A., Harrington, H., Milne, B., Amell, J. W., Theodore, R. F., & Moffitt, T. E. (2003). Children's behavioral styles at age 3 are linked to their adult personality traits at age 26. *Journal of Personality, 71*, 495–513.

Caspi, A., McClay, J., Moffitt, T. E., Mill, J., Martin, J., Craig, I. W., . . . Poulton, R. (2002). Role of genotype in the cycle of violence in maltreated children. *Science, 297*, 851–854.

Caspi, A., Sugden, K., Moffitt, T. E., Taylor, A., Craig, I. W., Harrington, H., . . . Poulton, R. (2003). Influence of life stress on depression: Moderation by a polymorphism in the 5-HTT gene. *Science, 301*, 386–389.

Castiajo, P., & Pinheiro, A. P. (2017). On "hearing" voices and "seeing" things: Probing hallucination predisposition in a Portuguese nonclinical sample with the Launay-Slade Hallucination Scale-revised. *Frontiers in Psychology, 8*, 1138.

Castiglioni, A. (1946). *Adventures of the mind* (1st American ed.). New York: Knopf.

Catala-Lopez, F., Hutton, B., Núñez-Beltrán, A., Page, M. J., Ridao, M., Saint-Gerons, D. M., . . . Moher, D. (2017). The pharmacological and non-pharmacological treatment of attention deficit hyperactivity disorder in children and adolescents: A systematic review with network meta-analyses of randomised trials. *PLoS One, 12*(7), e0180355.

Ceci, S. J., & Bruck, M. (1995). *Jeopardy in the courtroom.* Washington, DC: American Psychological Association.

Center for Behavioral Health Statistics and Quality. Results from the 2017 National Survey on Drug Use and Health: Detailed Tables. Rockville (MD): SAMHSA; 2018. https://www.samhsa.gov/data/report/2017-nsduh-detailed-tables. Accessed February 22, 2021.

Center for Substance Abuse Treatment (US). (2013). *Behavioral health services for people who are homeless: A review of the literature.* Rockville, MD: Substance Abuse and Mental Health Services Administration (US). Retrieved from https://www.ncbi.nlm.nih.gov/books/NBK138716/

Center for Substance Abuse Treatment (US). (2014). Understanding the impact of trauma. In *Trauma-informed care in behavioral health services.* Rockville, MD: Substance Abuse and Mental Health Services Administration (US). (Treatment Improvement Protocol (TIP) Series, No. 57.) Retrieved from https://www.ncbi.nlm.nih.gov/books/NBK207191/

Centers for Disease Control (CDC). (2015). Suicide: Facts at a glance. Retrieved May 14, 2018, from www.cdc.gov/ncipc/dvp/suicide/SuicideDataSheet.pdf

Centers for Disease Control (CDC). (2018a). Current cigarette smoking among adults in the United States. https://www.cdc.gov/tobacco/data_statistics/fact_sheets/adult_data/cig_smoking/index.htm. Retrieved July 3, 2018.

Centers for Disease Control (CDC). (2018b). Drug overdose death data. Retrieved July 4, 2018, from https://www.cdc.gov/drugoverdose/data/statedeaths.html

Centers for Disease Control (CDC). (2018c). Electronic cigarettes. https://www.cdc.gov/tobacco/basic_information/e-cigarettes/index.htm. Retrieved July 3, 2018.

Centers for Disease Control (CDC). (2018d). Fetal alcohol spectrum disorders (FASDs). https://www.cdc.gov/ncbddd/fasd/facts.html (accessed June 11, 2018).

Centers for Disease Control (CDC). (2018e). Heart disease fact sheet. https://www.cdc.gov/dhdsp/data_statistics/fact_sheets/fs_heart_disease.htm. Retrieved July 5, 2018.

Centers for Disease Control (CDC). (2018f). HIV/AIDS Basic Statistics. https://www.cdc.gov/hiv/basics/statistics.html. Retrieved July 5, 2018.

Chamberlain, S. R., Redden, S. A., Stein, D. J., Lochner, C., & Grant, J. E. (2017). Impact of obsessive-compulsive personality disorder symptoms in Internet users. *Annals of Clinical Psychiatry: Official Journal of the American Academy of Clinical Psychiatrists, 29*(3), 173–181.

Chan, E., Fogler, J. M., & Hammerness, P. G. (2016). Treatment of attention-deficit/hyperactivity disorder in adolescents: A systematic review. *JAMA, 315*(18), 1997–2008.

Chang, S. H., Stoll, C. R., Song, J., Varela, J. E., Eagon, C. J., & Colditz, G. A. (2014). The effectiveness and risks of bariatric surgery: An updated systematic review and meta-analysis, 2003–2012. *JAMA Surgery, 149*(3), 275–287.

Chard, K. M., Schuster, J. L., & Resick, P., A. (2012). Empirically supported psychological treatments: Cognitive processing therapy. In J. G. Beck & D. M. Sloan (Eds.), *The Oxford handbook of traumatic stress disorders* (pp. 439–448). New York: Oxford University Press.

Charlson, F. J., Ferrari, A. J., Santomauro, D. F., Diminic, S., Stockings, E., Scott, J. G., . . . Whiteford, H. A. (2018). Global epidemiology and burden of schizophrenia: findings from the global burden of disease study 2016. *Schizophrenia Bulletin, 44*(6), 1195–1203.

Charney, D. S. (2004). Psychobiological mechanisms of resilience and vulnerability: Implications for successful adaptation to extreme stress. *American Journal of Psychiatry, 161,* 195–216.

Charney, D. S., Nagy, L. M., Bremner, J. D., Goddard, A. W., Yehuda, R., & Southwick, S. M. (2000). Neurobiologic mechanisms of human anxiety. In B. S. Fogel (Ed.), *Synopsis of neuropsychiatry* (pp. 273–288). Philadelphia: Lippincott Williams & Wilkins.

Chartier, K., & Caetano, R. (2010). Ethnicity and health disparities in alcohol research. *Alcohol Research & Health, 33*(1–2), 152–160.

Chassin, L., Pitts, S. C., DeLucia, C., & Todd, M. (1999). A longitudinal study of children of alcoholics: Predicting young adult substance use disorders, anxiety, and depression. *Journal of Abnormal Psychology, 108,* 106–119.

Chatzitheochari, S., & Arber, S. (2009). Lack of sleep, work and the long hours culture: Evidence from the UK time use survey. *Work, Employment and Society, 23,* 30–48.

Chavira, D. A., Grilo, C. M., Shea, M. T., Yen, S., Gunderson, J. G., Morey, L. C., . . . Mcglashan, T. H. (2003). Ethnicity and four personality disorders. *Comprehensive Psychiatry, 44,* 483–491.

Checknita, D., Maussion, G., Labonté, B., Comai, S., Tremblay, R. E., Vitaro, F., . . . Turecki, G. (2015). Monoamine oxidase: A gene promoter methylation and transcriptional downregulation in an offender population with antisocial personality disorder. *British Journal of Psychiatry, 206*(3), 216–222.

Chenausky, K., Brignell, A., Morgan, A., & Tager-Flusberg, H. (2019). Motor speech impairment predicts expressive language in minimally verbal, but not low verbal, individuals with autism spectrum disorder. *Autism & Developmental Language Impairments, 4,* 2396941519856333.

Chen, E., & Miller, G. E. (2012). "Shift-and-persist" strategies: Why being low in socioeconomic status isn't always bad for health. *Perspectives on Psychological Science, 7,* 135–158.

Cheng-Ta, L., Chia-Feng, L., Hui-Ching, L., Ying-Zu, H., Chi-Hung, J., Tung-Ping, . . . Wei-Chen, L. (2017). Cortical inhibitory and excitatory function in drug-naive generalized anxiety disorder. *Brain Stimulation, 10*(3) 604–608.

Chen, H., Cohen, P., Crawford, T. N., Kasen, S., Guan, B., & Gordon, K. (2009). Impact of early adolescent psychiatric and personality disorder on long-term physical health: A 20-year longitudinal follow-up study. *Psychological Medicine, 39,* 865–874.

Chen, J. A., Peñagarikano, O., Belgard, T. G., Swarup, V., & Geschwind, D. H. (2015). The emerging picture of autism spectrum disorder: Genetics and pathology. *Annual Review of Pathology: Mechanisms of Disease, 10,* 111–144.

Chen, L., Shi, G. R., Huang, D. D., Li, Y., Ma, C. C., Shi, M., . . . & Shi, G. J. (2019). Male sexual dysfunction: a review of literature on its pathological mechanisms, potential risk factors, and herbal drug intervention. *Biomedicine & Pharmacotherapy, 112,* 108585.

Chen, L., Staubli, S. E., Schneider, M. P., Kessels, A. G., Ivic, S., Bachmann, L. M., & Kessler, T. M. (2015). Phosphodiesterase 5 inhibitors for the treatment of erectile dysfunction: a trade-off network meta-analysis. *European Urology, 68*(4), 674–680.

Chen, W. Y., Rosner, B., Hankinson, S. F., Colditz, G. A., & Willett, W. C. (2011). Moderate alcohol consumption during adult life, drinking patterns, and breast cancer risk. *JAMA, 306,* 1884–1890.

Cherepkova, E. V., Maksimov, V. V., & Aftanas, L. I. (2018). Polymorphism of serotonin transporter gene in male subjects with antisocial behavior and MMA fighters. *Translational Psychiatry, 8*(1), 1–9.

Cherry, M. G., Taylor, P. J., Brown, S. L., Rigby, J. W., & Sellwood, W. (2017). Guilt, shame and expressed emotion in carers of people with long-term mental health difficulties: A systematic review. *Psychiatry Research, 249,* 139–151.

Chew, D., Anderson, J., Williams, K., May, T., & Pang, K. (2018). Hormonal treatment in young people with gender dysphoria: A systematic review. *Pediatrics, 141*(4), e20173742.

Chida, Y., & Steptoe, A. (2009). The association of anger and hostility with future coronary heart disease: A meta-analytic review of prospective evidence. *Journal of the American College of Cardiology, 53*(11), 936–946.

Chida, Y., & Vedhara, K. (2009). Adverse psychosocial factors predict poorer prognosis in HIV disease: A meta-analytic review of prospective investigations. *Brain, Behavior, and Immunity, 23*(4), 434–445.

Chilvers, R., Macdonald, G. M., & Hayes, A. A. (2006). Supported housing for people with severe mental disorders. *Cochrane Database of Systematic Reviews, 4*, CD000453.

Chin, A. L., Negash, S., & Hamilton, R. (2011). Diversity and disparity in dementia: The impact of ethnoracial differences in Alzheimer's disease. *Alzheimer's Disease and Associated Disorders, 25*, 187–195.

Choe, J. Y., Teplin, L. A., & Abram, K. M. (2008). Perpetration of violence, violent victimization, and severe mental illness: Balancing public health concerns. *Psychiatric Services, 59*, 153–164.

Choi-Kain, L. W., Finch, E. F., Masland, S. R., Jenkins, J. A., & Unruh, B. T. (2017). What works in the treatment of borderline personality disorder. *Current Behavioral Neuroscience Reports, 4*(1), 21–30.

Cho, J., Hayes, R. D., Jewell, A., Kadra, G., Shetty, H., MacCabe, J. H., & Downs, J. (2019). Clozapine and all-cause mortality in treatment-resistant schizophrenia: A historical cohort study. *Acta Psychiatrica Scandinavica, 139*(3), 237–247.

Chokhawala, K. (2020, July 10). Lithium. Retrieved November 03, 2020, from https://www.ncbi.nlm.nih.gov/books/NBK519062/

Chou, I. J., Kuo, C. F., Huang, Y. S., Grainge, M. J., Valdes, A. M., See, L. C., . . . Doherty, M. (2017). Familial aggregation and heritability of schizophrenia and co-aggregation of psychiatric illnesses in affected families. *Schizophrenia Bulletin, 43*(5), 1070–1078. https://doi.org/10.1093/schbul/sbw159

Chou, T. (1992). Wake up and smell the coffee: Caffeine, coffee, and the medical consequences. *Western Journal of Medicine, 157*, 544–553.

Chou, W. Y. S., Oh, A., & Klein, W. M. (2018). Addressing health-related misinformation on social media. *Journal of the American Medical Association, 320*(23), 2417–2418.

Christiani, D. (2020). New England Journal of Medicine. *Vaping-Induced Acute Lung Injury, 382*, 960–962. DOI: 10.1056/NEJMe1912032

Chu, J., & Leino, A. (2017). Advancement in the maturing science of cultural adaptations of evidence-based interventions. *Journal of Consulting and Clinical Psychology, 85*, 45–57.

Chu, J., Leino, A., Pflum, S., & Sue, S. (2016). A model for the theoretical basis of cultural competency to guide psychotherapy. *Professional Psychology: Research and Practice, 47*(1), 18–29.

Chumpalova, P., Iakimova, R., Stoimenova-Popova, M., Aptalidis, D., Pandova, M., Stoyanova,M., & Fountoulakis, K. N. (2020). Prevalence and clinical picture of premenstrual syndrome in females from Bulgaria. *Annals of General Psychiatry, 19*, 3.

Chung, W. C., De Vries, G. J., & Swaab, D. F. (2002). Sexual differentiation of the bed nucleus of the striaterminalis in humans may extend into adulthood. *Journal of Neuroscience, 22*, 1027–1033.

Cicchetti, D., & Rogosch, F. A. (2001). Diverse patterns of neuroendocrine activity in maltreated children. *Development & Psychopathology, 13*, 677–694.

Cicchetti, D., & Toth, S. L. (2005). Child maltreatment. *Annual Review of Clinical Psychology, 1*, 409–438.

Cicchetti, D., & Toth, S. L. (2016). Child maltreatment and developmental psychopathology: A multilevel perspective. In D. Cicchetti (Ed.), *Developmental psychopathology: Vol. 3. Maladaptation and psychopathology* (3rd ed., pp. 457–512). Hoboken, NJ: Wiley.

Clancy, S. A., McNally, R. J., Schacter, D. L., Lenzenweger, M. F., & Pitman, R. K. (2002). Memory distortion in people reporting abduction by aliens. *Journal of Abnormal Psychology, 111*, 455–461.

Clancy, S. A., Schacter, D. L., McNally, R. J., & Pitman, R. (2000). False recognition in women reporting recovered memories of sexual abuse. *Psychological Science, 11*, 26–31.

Clark, D. M., & Wells, A. (1995). A cognitive model of social phobia. In R. G. Heimberg, M. R. Liebowitz, D. A. Hope, & F. R. Schneier (Eds.), *Social phobia: Diagnosis, assessment and treatment* (pp. 69–93). New York: Guilford Press.

Clark, I., Holmes, E., Woolrich, M., & Mackay, C. (2016). Intrusive memories to traumatic footage: The neural basis of their encoding and involuntary recall. *Psychological Medicine, 46*(3), 505–518.

Clarkin, J. F., Levy, K. N., Lenzenweger, M. F., & Kernberg, O. F. (2007). Evaluating three treatments for borderline personality disorder: A multiwave study. *American Journal of Psychiatry, 164*, 922–928.

Clark, L. A., Cuthbert, B., Lewis-Fernández, R., Narrow, W. E., & Reed, G. M. (2017). Three approaches to understanding and classifying mental disorder: *ICD-11, DSM-5*, and the National Institute of Mental Health's Research Domain Criteria (RDoC). *Psychological Science in the Public Interest, 18*(2), 72–145.

Clark, L. A., Vanderbleek, E. N., Shapiro, J. L., Nuzum, H., Allen, X., Daly, E., . . . Ro, E. (2015). The brave new world of personality disorder-trait specified: Effects of additional definitions on coverage, prevalence, and comorbidity. *Psychopathology Review, 2*(1), 52–82.

Clay, J. M., & Parker, M. O. (2020). Alcohol use and misuse during the COVID-19 pandemic: a potential public health crisis?. *The Lancet Public Health, 5*(5), e259.

Clayton, A. H. (2007). Epidemiology and neurobiology of female sexual dysfunction. *Journal of Sexual Medicine, 4*, 260–268.

Cleckley, H. M. (1941/1982). *The mask of sanity: An attempt to reinterpret the so-called psychopathic personality.* St. Louis: Mosby.

Cloninger, C. R., & Gottesman, I. I. (1987). Genetic and environmental factors in antisocial behavior disorders. In S. A. Mednick, T. E. Moffitt, & S. A. Stack (Eds.), *The causes of crime: New biological approaches* (pp. 92–109). New York: Cambridge University Press.

Coccaro, E. F. (2012). Intermittent explosive disorder as a disorder of impulsive aggression for DSM-5. *American Journal of Psychiatry, 169*(6), 577–588.

Coccaro, E. F., Fanning, J. R., & Lee, R. (2017). Intermittent explosive disorder and substance use disorder: Analysis of the National Comorbidity Survey Replication sample. *Journal of Clinical Psychiatry, 78*(6), 697–702.

Coccaro, E. F., Lee, R., & Kavoussi, R. J. (2010). Aggression, suicidality, and intermittent explosive disorder: Serotonergic correlates in personality disorder and healthy control subjects. *Neuropsychopharmacology, 35*, 435–444.

Cocchetti, C., Ristori, J., Mazzoli, F., Vignozzi, L., Maggi, M., & Fisher, A. D. (2021). Management of hypoactive sexual desire disorder in transgender women: A guide for clinicians. *International Journal of Impotence Research, 1–7.*

Cochrane, M., Petch, I., & Pickering, A. D. (2012). Aspects of cognitive functioning in shizotypy and schizophrenia: Evidence for a continuum model. *Psychiatry Research, 196*, 230–234.

Cochrane, R. E., Grisso, T., & Frederick, R. I. (2001). The relationship between criminal charges, diagnoses, and psycholegal opinions among federal pretrial defendants. *Behavioral Sciences & the Law, 19*, 565–582.

Cocores, J., Pottash, A. C., & Gold, M. S. (1991). Cocaine. In N. S. Miller (Ed.), *Comprehensive handbook of drug and alcohol addiction* (pp. 341–352). New York: Marcel Dekker.

Cohen, J. R., Thakur, H., Burkhouse, K. L., & Gibb, B. E. (2019). A multimethod screening approach for pediatric depression onset: An incremental validity study. *Journal of Consulting and Clinical Psychology, 87*(2), 184–197.

Cohen, K. M., & Savin-Williams, R. C. (2017). Treating sexual problems in lesbian, gay, and bisexual clients. In Z. D. Peterson (Ed.), *The Wiley handbook of sex therapy* (pp. 269–290). Oxford: Wiley.

Cohen, S., Tyrrell, D. A., & Smith, A. P. (1991). Psychological stress and susceptibility to the common cold. *New England Journal of Medicine, 325,* 606–612.

Coid, J. W., Kirkbride, J. B., Barker, D., Cowden, F., Stamps, R., Yang, M., & Jones, P. B. (2008). Raised incidence rates of all psychoses among migrant groups. *Archives of General Psychiatry, 65,* 1250–1258.

Colapinto, J. (2000). *As nature made him: The boy who was raised as a girl.* New York: HarperCollins.

Colapinto, J. (2004, June 3). Gender gap: What were the real reasons behind David Reimer's suicide? *Slate.* http://www.slate.com/articles/health_and_science/medical_examiner/2004/06/gender_gap.html

Cole, J., Costafreda, S. G., McGuffin, P., & Fu, C. H. (2011). Hippocampal atrophy in first episode depression: A meta-analysis of magnetic resonance imaging studies. *Journal of Affective Disorders, 134*(1), 483–487.

Cole, M. G., Ciampi, A., Belzile, E., & Zhong, L. (2009). Persistent delirium in older hospital patients: A systematic review of frequency and prognosis. *Age Ageing, 38,* 19–26.

Coles, A. S., Kozak, K., & George, T. P. (2018). A review of brain stimulation methods to treat substance use disorders. *American Journal on Addictions, 27,* 71–91.

Cole, S. W., Kemeny, M. E., Taylor, S. E., Visscher, B. R., & Fahey, J. L. (1995). Accelerated course of human immunodeficiency virus infection in gay men who conceal their homosexual identity. *Psychosomatic Medicine, 58,* 219–238.

Colizzi, M., Bortoletto, R., Silvestri, M., Mondini, F., Puttini, E., Cainelli, C., . . . Zoccante, L. (2020). Medically unexplained symptoms in the times of COVID-19 pandemic: A case-report. *Brain, Behavior, & Immunity - Health, 5,* 1–4. https://doi.org/10.1016/j.bbih.2020.100073.

Coltheart, M., Langdon, R., & McKay, R. (2011). Delusional belief. *Annual Review of Psychology, 62,* 271–298.

Coman, E. N., & Wu, H. Z. (2018). Examining differential resilience mechanisms by comparing 'tipping points' of the effects of neighborhood conditions on anxiety by race/ethnicity. *Healthcare (Basel, Switzerland), 6*(1), 18.

Compton, M., & Shim, R. (2020, September 01). Mental Illness Prevention and Mental Health Promotion: When, Who, and How. Retrieved 2020, from https://ps.psychiatryonline.org/doi/10.1176/appi.ps.201900374

Compton, W. M., Han, B., Jones, C. M., Blanco, C., & Hughes, A. (2016). Marijuana use and use disorders in adults in the USA, 2002–14: Analysis of annual cross-sectional surveys. *Lancet Psychiatry, 3*(10), 954–964.

Conduct Problems Prevention Research Group. (2002). Evaluation of the first 3 years of the Fast Track Prevention Trial with children at high risk for adolescent conduct problems. *Journal of Abnormal Child Psychology, 30,* 19–35.

Conduct Problems Prevention Research Group. (2007). The Fast Track randomized controlled trial to prevent externalizing psychiatric disorders: Findings from grades 3 to 9. *Journal of the American Academy of Child and Adolescent Psychiatry, 46,* 1250–1262.

Conduct Problems Prevention Research Group. (2015). Impact of early intervention on psychopathology, crime, and well-being at age 25. *American Journal of Psychiatry, 172,* 59–70.

Conwell, Y., & Thompson, C. (2008). Suicidal behavior in elders. *Psychiatric Clinics of North America, 31,* 333–356.

Cook, B. L., Zuvekas, S. H., Carson, N., Wayne, G. F., Vesper, A., & McGuire, T. G. (2014). Assessing racial/ethnic disparities in treatment across episodes of mental health care. *Health Services Research, 49*(1), 206–229.

Coolidge, F. L., Thede, L., & Jang, K. L. (2004). Are personality disorders psychological manifestations of executive function deficits? Bivariate heritability evidence from a twin study. *Behavior Genetics, 34,* 75–84.

Coolidge, F. L., Thede, L. L., & Young, S. E. (2002). The heritability of gender identity disorder in a child and adolescent twin sample. *Behavior Genetics, 32,* 251–257.

Coon, K. D., Myers, A. J., Craig, D. W., Webster, J. A., Pearson, J. V., Lince, D. H., . . . Stephan, D. A. (2007). A high-density whole-genome association study reveals that APOE is the major susceptibility gene for sporadic late-onset Alzheimer's disease. *Journal of Clinical Psychiatry, 68,* 613–618.

Coons, P. M. (1980). Multiple personality: Diagnostic considerations. *Journal of Clinical Psychiatry, 41,* 330–336.

Coons, P. M. (1984). *Childhood antecedents of multiple personality.* Paper presented at the Meeting of the American Psychiatric Association, Los Angeles.

Coons, P. M., & Milstein, V. (1990). Self-mutilation associated with dissociative disorders. *Dissociation: Progress in the Dissociative Disorders, 3,* 81–87.

Coontz, P. D., Lidz, C. W., & Mulvey, E. P. (1994). Gender and the assessment of dangerousness in the psychiatric emergency room. *International Journal of Law & Psychiatry, 17,* 369–376.

Cooper, M. L., Kuntsche, E., Levitt, A., Barber, L. L., & Wolf, S. (2016). Motivational models of substance use: A review of theory and research on motives for using alcohol, marijuana, and tobacco. In K. Sher (Ed.), *The Oxford handbook of substance use and substance use disorders,* vol. 1 (pp. 375–421). Oxford: Oxford University Press.

Cooper, S. E., Campbell, L. F., & Barnwell, S. S. (2019). Telepsychology: A Primer for Counseling Psychologists. *The Counseling Psychologist, 47*(8), 1074–1114. doi: 10.1177/0011000019895276

Corlett, P. R., Horga, G., Fletcher, P. C., Alderson-Day, B., Schmack, K., & Powers III, A. R. (2019). Hallucinations and strong priors. *Trends in Cognitive Sciences, 23*(2), 114–127.

Cornelius, M. D., Goldschmidt, L., Day, N. L., & Larkby, C. (2002). Alcohol, tobacco and marijuana use among pregnant teenagers: 6-year follow-up of offspring growth effects. *Neurotoxicology & Teratology, 24,* 703–710.

Coronado, V. G., Haileyesus, T., Cheng, T. A., Bell, J. M., Haarbauer-Krupa, J., Lionbarger, M. R., . . . Gilchrist, J. (2015). Trends in sports- and recreation-related traumatic brain injuries treated in US emergency departments: The National Electronic Injury Surveillance System–All Injury Program (NEISS-AIP) 2001–2012. *Journal of Head Trauma Rehabilitation, 30*(3), 185–197.

Corrao, G., Bagnardi, V., Zambon, A., & La Vecchia, C. (2004). A meta-analysis of alcohol consumption and the risk of 15 diseases. *Prevention by Medicine, 38,* 613–619.

Costanza, A., D'Orta, I., Perroud, N., Burkhardt, S., Malafosse, A., Mangin, P., & La Harpe, R. (2014). Neurobiology of suicide: Do biomarkers exist? *International Journal of Legal Medicine, 128*(1), 73–82.

Costello, E. J., Compton, S. N., Keeler, G., & Angold, A. (2003). Relationships between poverty and psychopathology: A natural experiment. *JAMA, 290,* 2023–2029.

Courtet, P., Picot, M. C., Bellivier, F., Torres, S., Jollant, F., Michelon, C., . . . Malafosse, A. (2004). Serotonin transporter gene may be involved in short-term risk of subsequent suicide attempts. *Biological Psychiatry, 55,* 46–51.

Courtney, D., Watson, P., Battaglia, M., Mulsant, B. H., & Szatmari, P. (2020). COVID-19 impacts on child and youth anxiety and depression: Challenges and opportunities. *The Canadian Journal of Psychiatry, 65*(10), 688–691.

Cowan H. R. (2020). Is schizophrenia research relevant during the COVID-19 pandemic?. *Schizophrenia Research, 220,* 271–272. https://doi.org/10.1016/j.schres.2020.04.002

Cox, B. J., Turnbull, D. L., Robinson, J. A., Grant, B. F., & Stein, M. B. (2011). The effect of avoidant personality disorder on the persistence of generalized social anxiety disorder in the general population: Results from a longitudinal, nationally representative mental health survey. *Depression and Anxiety, 28,* 250–255.

Coyne, J. C. (1976). Toward an interactional description of depression. *Psychiatry, 39,* 28–40.

Craddock, N., & Sklar, P. (2013). Genetics of bipolar disorder. *Lancet, 381*(9878), 1654–1662.

Craske, M. G. (2017). *Cognitive-behavioral therapy.* Washington, DC: American Psychological Association.

Craske, M. G., & Barlow, D. H. (2014). Panic disorder and agoraphobia. In D. H. Barlow (Ed.), *Clinical handbook of psychological disorders: A step-by-step treatment manual* (pp. 1–61). New York: Guilford Press.

Craske, M. G., Kircanski, K., Epstein, A., Wittchen, H.-U., Pine, D. S., Lewis-Fernández, R., Hinton, D., & DSM-V OC Spectrum, Posttraumatic and Dissociative Disorder Work Group. (2010). Panic disorder: A review of DSM-IV panic disorder and proposals for DSM-V. *Depression and Anxiety, 27,* 93–112.

Craske, M. G., Niles, A. N., Burklund, L. J., Wolitzky-Taylor, K. B., Vilardaga, J. C. P., Arch, J. J., . . . Lieberman, M. D. (2014). Randomized controlled trial of cognitive behavioral therapy and acceptance and commitment therapy for social phobia: Outcomes and moderators. *Journal of Consulting and Clinical Psychology, 82,* 1034–1048.

Craske, M. G., Treanor, M., Conway, C. C., Zbozinek, T., & Vervliet, B. (2014). Maximizing exposure therapy: An inhibitory learning approach. *Behaviour Research and Therapy, 58,* 10–23.

Craske, M. G., & Waters, A. M. (2005). Panic disorder, phobias, and generalized anxiety disorder. *Annual Review of Clinical Psychology, 1,* 197–226.

Crestani, C. C. (2016). Emotional stress and cardiovascular complications in animal models: A review of the influence of stress type. *Frontiers in Physiology, 7,* 251.

Crick, N. R., Ostrov, J. M., & Kawabata, Y. (2007). Relational aggression and gender: An overview. In D. J. Flannery, A. T. Vazsonyi, & I. D. Waldman (Eds.), *The Cambridge handbook of violent behavior and aggression* (pp. 245–259). New York, NY: Cambridge University Press.

Crisp, H., & Gabbard, G. O. (2020). Principles of psychodynamic treatment for patients with narcissistic personality disorder. *Journal of Personality Disorders, 34,* 143–158.

Cristea, I. A., Gentili, C., Cotet, C. D., Palomba, D., Barbui, C., & Cuijpers, P. (2017). Efficacy of psychotherapies for borderline personality disorder: A systematic review and meta-analysis. *JAMA Psychiatry, 74*(4), 319–328.

Critelli, J. W., & Bivona, J. M. (2008). Women's erotic rape fantasies: An evaluation of theory and research. *Journal of Sex Research, 45*(1), 57–70.

Crnic, K. A., Neece, C. L., McIntyre, L. L., Blacher, J., & Baker, B. L. (2017). Intellectual disability and developmental risk: Promoting intervention to improve child and family well-being. *Child Development, 88*(2), 436–445.

Cromby, J., Chung, E., Papadopoulos, D., & Talbot, C. (2016). Reviewing the epigenetics of schizophrenia. *Journal of Mental Health,* 1–9.

Cronbach, L. J., & Meehl, P. E. (1955). Construct validity in psychological tests. *Psychological Bulletin, 52,* 281–302.

Cross, S. E., & Madson, L. (1997). Models of the self: Self-construals and gender. *Psychological Bulletin, 122,* 5–37.

Crouch, T., Lewis, J., Erickson, T., & Newman, M. (2017). Prospective investigation of the contrast avoidance model of generalized anxiety and worry. *Behavior Therapy, 48*(4), 544–556.

Crowther, J. H., Armey, M., Luce, K. H., Dalton, G. R., & Leahey, T. (2008). The point prevalence of bulimic disorders from 1990 to 2004. *International Journal of Eating Disorders, 41,* 491–497.

Csaszar-Nagy, N., Scholkmann, F., Kapócs, G., Bokkon, I. (2016). The "Hidden Observer" as the Cognitive Unconscious During Hypnosis. *Activitas Nervosa Superior, 58,* 51–61. DOI10.1007/BF03379735

Csillik, A. (2015). Positive motivational interviewing: Activating clients' strengths and intrinsic motivation to change. *Journal of Contemporary Psychotherapy, 45*(2), 119–128. doi: http://dx.doi.org.mccc.idm.oclc.org/10.1007/s10879-014-9288-6

Cubillo, A., Halari, R., Smith, A., Taylor, E., & Rubia, K. (2012). A review of fronto-cortico brain abnormalities in children and adults with attention deficit hyperactivity disorder (ADHD) and new evidence for dysfunction in adults with ADHD during motivation and attention. *Cortex, 8,* 194–215.

Cui, H., Zhang, J., Liu, Y., Li, Q., Li, H., Zhang, L., Hu, Q., Cheng, W., Luo, Q., Li, J., Li, W., Wang, J., Feng, J., Li, C., & Northoff, G. (2016). Differential alterations of resting-state functional connectivity in generalized anxiety disorder and panic disorder. *Human brain mapping, 37*(4), 1459–1473. https://doi.org/10.1002/hbm.23113

Cuijpers, P., Donker, T., Weissman, M. M., Ravitz, P., & Cristea, I. A. (2016). Interpersonal psychotherapy for mental health problems: A comprehensive meta-analysis. *American Journal of Psychiatry, 173*(7), 680–687.

Cuijpers, P., Sijbrandij, M., Koole, S., Huibers, M., Berking, M., & Andersson, G. (2014). Psychological treatment of generalized anxiety disorder: A meta-analysis. *Clinical Psychology Review, 34,* 130–140.

Cuijpers, P., van Straten, A., van Oppen, P., & Andersson, G. (2008). Are psychological and pharmacological interventions equally effective in the treatment of adult depressive disorders? A meta-analysis of comparative studies. *Journal of Clinical Psychiatry, 69,* 1675–1685.

Culbert, K. M., Racine, S. E., & Klump, K. L. (2015). Research review: What we have learned about the causes of eating disorders—a synthesis of sociocultural, psychological, and biological research. *Journal of Child Psychology and Psychiatry, 56*(11), 1141–1164.

Cummings, J., Aisen, P. S., DuBois, B., Frölich, L., Jack, C. R., Jones, R. W., . . . Scheltens, P. (2016). Drug development in Alzheimer's disease: The path to 2025. *Alzheimer's Research & Therapy, 8*(1), 39.

Curry, J., Silva, S., Rohde, P., Ginsburg, G., Kratochvil, C., Simons, A., . . . & March, J. (2011). Recovery and recurrence following treatment for adolescent major depression. *Archives of General Psychiatry, 68*(3), 263–269.

Cusack, K., Jonas, D. E., Forneris, C. A., Wines, C., Sonis, J., Middleton, J. C., . . . Gaynes, B. N. (2016). Psychological treatments for adults with posttraumatic stress disorder: A systematic review and meta-analysis. *Clinical Psychology Review, 43,* 128–141.

Cuthbert, B. N., & Insel, T. R. (2013). Toward the future of psychiatric diagnosis: The seven pillars of RDoC. *BMC Medicine, 11*(1), 126.

D

Dagöö, J., Persson, R., Helene, A., Bsenko, A., Hjerling, S., Holmberg, A., . . . Andersson, G. (2014). Cognitive behavior therapy versus interpersonal psychotherapy for social anxiety disorder delivered via smartphone and computer: A randomized controlled trial. *Journal of Anxiety Disorders, 28*(4); 410-417.

Daley, D. C., & Marlatt, G. A. (2006). *Overcoming your alcohol or drug problem: Effective recovery strategies: Therapist guide* (2nd ed.). New York: Oxford University Press.

Damasio, H., Grabowski, T., Frank, R., Galaburda, A. M., & Damasio, A. R. (1994). The return of Phineas Gage: Clues about the brain from the skull of a famous patient. *Science, 264,* 1102-1105.

Dana, R. H. (2005). *Multicultural assessment: Principles, applications, and examples.* Mahwah, NJ: Routledge.

Daniels, R. A., Holdsworth, E., & Tramontano, C. (2017). Relating therapist characteristics to client engagement and the therapeutic alliance in an adolescent custodial group substance misuse treatment program. *Substance Use & Misuse, 52*(9), 1139-1150. https://doi.org/10.1080/10826084.2017.1299181

Danielsson, A. K., Wennberg, P., Hibell, B., & Romelsjö, A. (2012). Alcohol use, heavy episodic drinking and subsequent problems among adolescents in 23 European countries: Does the prevention paradox apply? *Addiction, 107,* 71-80.

Dansinger, M. L., Gleason, J. A., Griffith, J. L., Selker, H. P., & Schaefer, E. J. (2005). Comparison of the Atkins, Ornish, Weight Watchers, and Zone diets for weight loss and heart disease risk reduction: A randomized trial. *Journal of the American Medical Association, 293,* 43-53.

Darcangelo, S. (2008). Fetishism: Psychopathology and treatment. In D. R. Laws & W. T. O'Donohue (Eds.), *Sexual deviance: Theory, assessment, and treatment* (pp. 108-119). New York: Guilford Press.

Darcangelo, S., Hollings, A., & Paladino, G. (2008). Fetishism: Assessment and treatment. In D. R. Laws & W. T. O'Donohue (Eds.), *Sexual deviance: Theory, assessment, and treatment* (pp. 119-131). New York: Guilford Press.

Dauvilliers, Y., Baumann, C. R., Carlander, B., Bischof, M., Blatter, T., Lecendreux, M., ... Bassetti, C. L. (2003). CSF hypocretin-1 levels in narcolepsy, Kleine-Levin syndrome, and other hypersomnias and neurological conditions. *Journal of Neurology, Neurosurgery, and Psychiatry, 74,* 1667.

Davidson, J. R. T. (2001). Pharmacotherapy of generalized anxiety disorder. *Journal of Clinical Psychiatry, 62* (Suppl. 11), 46-50.

Davidson, K., Norrie, J., Tyrer, P., Gumley, A., Tata, P., Murray, H., & Palmer, S. (2006). The effectiveness of cognitive behavior therapy for borderline personality disorder: Results from the borderline personality disorder of cognitive therapy (BOSCOT) trial. *Journal of Personality Disorders, 20,* 450-465.

Davidson, R. J., Pizzagalli, D. A., & Nitschke, J. B. (2009). Representation and regulation of emotion in depression: Perspectives from affective neuroscience. In I. H. Gotlib & C. L. Hammen (Eds.), *Handbook of depression* (2nd ed., pp. 218-248). New York: Guilford Press.

Davidson, R. J., Pizzagalli, D., Nitschke, J. B., & Putnam, K. (2002). Depression: Perspectives from affective neuroscience. *Annual Review of Psychology, 53,* 545-574.

Davis, K. L., Kahn, R. S., Ko, G., & Davidson, M. (1991). Dopamine in schizophrenia: A review and conceptualization. *American Journal of Psychiatry, 148,* 1474-1486.

Davis, O. S. P., Haworth, C. M. A., & Plomin, R. (2009). Learning abilities and disabilities: Generalist genes in early adolescence. *Cognitive Neuropsychiatry, 14,* 312-331.

Davis, T. E., III, Ollendick, T. H., & Öst, L. G. (2009). Intensive treatment of specific phobias in children and adolescents. *Cognitive and Behavioral Practice, 16,* 294-303.

Davis, T. S., Mauss, I. B., Lumian, D., Troy, A. S., Shallcross, A. J., Zarolia, P., . . . McRae, K. (2014). Emotional reactivity and emotion regulation among adults with a history of self-harm: Laboratory self-report and functional MRI evidence. *Journal of Abnormal Psychology, 123,* 499-509.

Dawson, D. A., Grant, B. F., Stinson, F. S., Chou, P. S., Huang, B., & Ruan, W. J. (2005). Recovery from *DSM-IV* alcohol dependence: United States, 2001-2002. *Addiction, 100,* 281-292.

Deary, V., Chalder, T., & Sharpe, M. (2007). The cognitive behavioural model of medically unexplained symptoms: A theoretical and empirical review. *Clinical Psychology Review, 27,* 781-797.

Deeny, S. P., Poeppel, D., Zimmerman, J. B., Roth, S. M., Brandauer, J., Witkoswki, S., . . . Hatfield, B. D. (2008). Exercise, APOE, and working memory: MEG and behavioral evidence for benefit of exercise in epsilon4 carriers. *Biological Psychology, 78,* 179-187.

De Fruyt, F., & De Clercq, B. (2014). Antecedents of personality disorder in childhood and adolescence: Toward an integrative developmental model. *Annual Review of Clinical Psychology, 10,* 449-476.

Degenhardt, L., Chiu, W. T., Sampson, N., Kessler, R. C., Anthony, J. C., Angermeyer, M., . . . Wells, J. E. (2008). Toward a global view of alcohol, tobacco, cannabis, and cocaine use: Findings from the WHO World Mental Health Surveys. *PLoS Med., 5,* e141.

De Genna, N. M., & Feske, U. (2013). Phenomenology of borderline personality disorder: The role of race and socioeconomic status. *Journal of Nervous and Mental Disease, 201*(12), 1027-1034.

de Gusmão, C. M., Guerriero, R. M., Bernson-Leung, M. E., Pier, D., Ibeziako, P. I., Bujoreanu, S., . . . Waugh, J. L.. (2014). Functional neurological symptom disorders in a pediatric emergency room: Diagnostic accuracy, features, and outcome. *Pediatric Neurology, 51*(2), 233-238.

Dela Peña, I., Gevorkiana, R., & Shi, W. X. (2015). Psychostimulants affect dopamine transmission through both dopamine transporter-dependent and independent mechanisms. *European Journal of Pharmacology, 764,* 562-570. https://doi.org/10.1016/j.ejphar.2015.07.044

del Campo, N., Chamberlain, S. R., Sahakian, B. J., & Robbins, T. W. (2011). The roles of dopamine and noradrenaline in the pathophysiology and treatment of attention-deficit/hyperactivity disorder. *Biological Psychiatry, 69,* e146-e157.

DeLisi, M., Drury, A. J., & Elbert, M. J. (2019). The etiology of antisocial personality disorder: The differential roles of adverse childhood experiences and childhood psychopathology. *Comprehensive Psychiatry, 92,* 1-6.

Dell, P. F. (2018). Reconsidering the autohypnotic model of the dissociative disorders. *Journal of Trauma & Dissociation,* 1-31.

Dell, P. F., & Eisenhower, J. W. (1990). Adolescent multiple personality disorder: A preliminary study of eleven cases. *Journal of the American Academy of Child & Adolescent Psychiatry, 29,* 359-366.

De Los Reyes, A., Augenstein, T. M., Wang, M., Thomas, S. A., Drabick, D. A., Burgers, D. E., & Rabinowitz, J. (2015). The validity of the multi-informant approach to assessing child and adolescent mental health. *Psychological Bulletin, 141*(4), 858-900.

Denis, C., Fatséas, M., & Auriacombe, M. (2012). Analyses related to the development of *DSM-5* criteria for substance use related disorders: 3. An assessment of pathological gambling criteria. *Drug and Alcohol Dependence, 122,* 22-27.

DePrince, A. P. & Freyd, J. J. (2014). Trauma-induced dissociation. In M. J. Friedman, T. M. Keane, & P. A. Resick (Eds.), *Handbook of PTSD: Science and practice* (2nd ed., pp 219–233). New York: Guilford Press.

De Raedt, R., Vanderhasselt, M. A., & Baeken, C. (2015). Neurostimulation as an intervention for treatment resistant depression: From research on mechanisms towards targeted neurocognitive strategies. *Clinical Psychology Review, 41,* 61–69.

Derenne, J., & Beresin, E. (2018). Body image, media, and eating disorders—A 10-year update. *Academic Psychiatry, 42*(1), 129–134.

DeRubeis, R. J., Gelfand, L. A., Tang, T. Z., & Simons, A. D. (1999). Medications versus cognitive behavior therapy for severely depressed outpatients: Mega-analysis of four randomized comparisons. *American Journal of Psychiatry, 156,* 1001–1013.

DeRubeis, R. J., Hollon, S. D., Amsterdam, J. D., Shelton, R. C., Young, P. R., Salomon, R. M., . . . Gallop, R. (2005). Cognitive therapy vs. medications in the treatment of moderate to severe depression. *Archives of General Psychiatry, 62,* 409–416.

deSilva, P., Rachman, S., & Seligman, M. (1977). Prepared phobias and obsessions. *Behaviour Research & Therapy, 15,* 65–77.

de Snyder, V. N. S., Diaz-Perez, M. D., & Ojeda, V. D. (2000). The prevalence of nervios and associated symptomatology among inhabitants of Mexican rural communities. *Culture, Medicine & Psychiatry, 24,* 453–470.

Deutsch, Albert. (1937). *The mentally ill in America* (1st ed.). New York: Doubleday.

Dewaraja, R., & Sasaki, Y. (1991). Semen-loss syndrome: A comparison between Sri Lanka and Japan. *American Journal of Psychotherapy, 45,* 14–20.

Dhawan, N., Kunik, M. E., Oldham, J., & Coverdale, J. (2010). Prevalence and treatment of narcissistic personality disorder in the community: A systematic review. *Comprehensive Psychiatry, 51,* 333–339.

Diaconescu, A. O., Hauke, D. J., & Borgwardt, S. (2019). Models of persecutory delusions: A mechanistic insight into the early stages of psychosis. *Molecular Psychiatry, 24*(9), 1258–1267. doi: http://dx.doi.org.mccc.idm.oclc.org/10.1038/s41380-019-0427-z

Dick, D. M., Agrawal, A., Keller, M. C., Adkins, A., Aliev, F., Monroe, S., . . . Sher, K. J. (2015). Candidate gene–environment interaction research: Reflections and recommendations. *Perspectives on Psychological Science, 10*(1), 37–59.

Dickerson, F., Schroeder, J., Katsafanas, E., Khushalani, S., Origoni, A. E., Savage, C., . . . & Yolken, R. H. (2018). Cigarette smoking by patients with serious mental illness, 1999–2016: An increasing disparity. *Psychiatric Services, 69*(2), 147–153.

Dickey, R., & Stephens, J. (1995). Female-to-male transsexualism, heterosexual type: Two cases. *Archives of Sexual Behavior, 24,* 439–445.

Diedrich, A., & Voderholzer, U. (2015). Obsessive–compulsive personality disorder: A current review. *Current Psychiatry Reports, 17*(2), 2.

Diener, E., Thapa, S., & Tay, L. (2020). Positive emotions at work. *Annual Review of Organizational Psychology and Organizational Behavior, 7,* 451–477.

Dimidjian, S., Arch, J. J., Schneider, R. L., Desormeau, P., Felder, J. N., & Segal, Z. V. (2016). Considering meta-analysis, meaning, and metaphor: A systematic review and critical examination of "third wave" cognitive and behavioral therapies. *Behavior Therapy, 47(6),* 886–905.

Dimidjian, S., Barrera, M., Jr., Martell, C., Muñoz, R. F., & Lewinsohn, P. M. (2011). The origins and current status of behavioral activation treatments for depression. *Annual Review of Clinical Psychology, 7,* 1–38.

Dimidjian, S., Hollon, S. D., Dobson, K. S., Schmaling, K. B., Kohlenberg, R. J., Addis, M. E., . . . Jacobson, N. S. (2006). Randomized trial of behavioral activation, cognitive therapy, and antidepressant medication in the acute treatment of adults with major depression. *Journal of Consulting and Clinical Psychology, 74,* 658–670.

Dindelegan, C. M., Faur, D., Purza, L., Bumbu, A., & Sabau, M. (2020). Distress in neurocognitive disorders due to Alzheimer's disease and stroke. *Experimental and Therapeutic Medicine, 20*(3), 2501–2509.

DiSabato, D. J., Quan, N., & Godbout, J. P. (2016). Neuroinflammation: The devil is in the details. *Journal of Neurochemistry, 139* (Suppl. 2), 136–153.

Dishion, T. J., & Patterson, G. R. (1997). The timing and severity of antisocial behavior: Three hypotheses within an ecological framework. In D. M. Stoff, J. Breiling, & J. D. Maser (Eds.), *Handbook of antisocial personality disorder* (pp. 205–217). New York: Wiley.

Disney, K. L., Weinstein, Y., & Oltmanns, T. F. (2012). Personality disorder symptoms are differentially related to divorce frequency. *Journal of Family Psychology, 26,* 959–965.

Distel, M. A., Rebollo-Mesa, I., Willemsen, G., Derom, C. A., Trull, T. J., Martin, N. G., & Boomsma, D. I. (2009). Familial resemblance of borderline personality disorder features: Genetic or cultural transmission? *PLoS One, 4,* e5334.

Diwadkar, V. A., Bustamante, A., Rai, H., & Uddin, M. (2014). Epigenetics, stress, and their potential impact on brain network function: A focus on the schizophrenia diatheses. *Frontiers in Psychiatry, 5,* 71.

Dixon, D., Cruess, S., Kilbourn, K., Klimas, N., Fletcher, M. A., Ironson, G., . . . Antoni, M. H. (2001). Social support mediates loneliness and human herpes virus Type 6 (HHV-6) antibody titers. *Journal of Applied Social Psychology, 31,* 1111–1132.

Dobrescu, S. R., Dinkler, L., Gillberg, C., Råstam, M., Gillberg, C., & Wentz, E. (2020). Anorexia nervosa: 30-year outcome. *The British Journal of Psychiatry, 216*(2), 97–104.

Dochnal, R. B., Vetró, Á., Kiss, E., Baji, I., Lefkovics, E., Bylsma, L. M., . . . & Kapornai, K. (2019). Emotion regulation among adolescents with pediatric depression as a function of anxiety comorbidity. *Frontiers in Psychiatry, 10,* 722.

Dockray, S., & Steptoe, A. (2010). Positive affect and psychobiological processes. *Neuroscience & Biobehavioral Reviews, 35*(1), 69–75.

Dodge, K. A. (2009). Mechanisms of gene-environment interaction effects in the development of conduct disorder. *Perspectives on Psychological Science, 4,* 408–414.

Doenyas, C. (2018). Gut microbiota, inflammation, and probiotics on neural development in autism spectrum disorder. *Neuroscience, 374,* 271–286

Dohrenwend, B. P. (2000). The role of adversity and stress in psychopathology: Some evidence and its implications for theory and research. *Journal of Health and Social Behavior, 41,* 1–19.

Dominguez, M. L. (2017). LGBTQIA people of color: Utilizing the cultural psychology model as a guide for the mental health assessment and treatment of patients with diverse identities. *Journal of Gay & Lesbian Mental Health, 21*(3), 203–220.

Donegan, N. H., Sanislow, C. A., Blumberg, H. P., Fulbright, R. K., Lacadie, C., Skudlarski, P., Gore, J. C., Olson, I. R., McGlashan, T. H., & Wexler, B. E. (2003).

Amygdala hyperreactivity in borderline personality disorder: Implications for emotional dysregulation. *Biological Psychiatry, 54*, 1284–1293.

Dong-Bin, C., Zheng, W., Zhang Qing-E, Ng, C. H., Ungvari, G. S., Huang, X., & Yu-Tao, X. (2020). Minocycline for depressive symptoms: A meta-analysis of randomized, double-blinded, placebo-controlled trials. *Psychiatric Quarterly, 91*(2), 451–461.

Donnelly, B., Touyz, S., Hay, P., Burton, A., Russell, J., & Caterson, I. (2018). Neuroimaging in bulimia nervosa and binge eating disorder: A systematic review. *Journal of Eating Disorders, 6*(1), 1–24.

Donovan, D. M., Anton, R. F., Miller, W. R., Longabaugh, R., Hosking, J. D., & Youngblood, M. (2008). Combined pharmacotherapies and behavioral interventions for alcohol dependence (the COMBINE study): Examination of posttreatment drinking outcomes. *Journal of Studies on Alcohol and Drugs, 69*, 5–13.

Donovan, D., & Witkiewitz, K. (2012). Relapse prevention: From radical idea to common practice. *Addiction Research & Theory, 20*, 204–217.

Dorahy, M. J., Brand, B. L., Şar, V., Krüger, C., Stavropoulos, P., Martínez-Taboas, A., . . . Middleton, W. (2014). Dissociative identity disorder: An empirical overview. *Australian & New Zealand Journal of Psychiatry, 48*(5), 402–417.

Douaihy, A. B., Kelly, T. M., & Sullivan, C. (2013). Medications for substance use disorders. *Social Work in Public Health, 28*(3–4), 264–278.

Dougherty, D. D., & Rauch, S. L. (2007). Brain correlates of antidepressant treatment outcome from neuroimaging studies in depression. *Psychiatric Clinics of North America, 30*, 91–103.

Dowling, N. A., Merkouris, S. S., Greenwood, C. J., Oldenhof, E., Toumbourou, J. W., & Youssef, G. J. (2017). Early risk and protective factors for problem gambling: A systematic review and meta-analysis of longitudinal studies. *Clinical Psychology Review, 51*, 109–124.

Downey, G., & Feldman, S. I. (1996). Implications of rejection sensitivity for intimate relationships. *Journal of Personality and Social Psychology, 70*, 1327–1343.

Drake, C. L., Roehrs, T., Richardson, G., Walsh, J. K., & Roth, T. (2004). Shift work sleep disorder: Prevalence and consequences beyond that of symptomatic day workers. *Sleep, 27*, 1453–1462.

Drake, K. L., & Ginsburg, G. S. (2012). Family factors in the development, treatment, and prevention of childhood anxiety disorders. *Clinical Child and Family Psychology Review, 15*(2), 144–162.

Drayna, D., & Kang, C. (2011). Genetic approaches to understanding the causes of stuttering. *Journal of Neurodevelopment Disorders, 3*, 374–380.

Driessen, E., Van, H. L., Peen, J., Don, F. J., Twisk, J. W., Cuijpers, P., & Dekker, J. J. (2017). Cognitive-behavioral versus psychodynamic therapy for major depression: Secondary outcomes of a randomized clinical trial. *Journal of Consulting and Clinical Psychology, 85*(7), 653.

Driessen, J., Blom, J. D., Muris, P., Blashfield, R., & Molendijk, M. (2020). Anxiety in children with selective mutism: A meta-analysis. *Child Psychiatry & Human Development, 51*, 330–341.

Druss, B. G., & Goldman, H. H. (2018). Integrating health and mental health services: A past and future history. *American Journal of Psychiatry, 175*(12), 1199–1204.

Ducharme, E. (2017). Best practices in working with complex trauma and dissociative identity disorder. *Practice Innovations, 2*(3), 150 –161.

Dudley, R., Aynsworth, C., Cheetham, R., McCarthy-Jones, S., & Collerton, D. (2018). Prevalence and characteristics of multi-modal hallucinations in people with psychosis who experience visual hallucinations. *Psychiatry Research, 269*, 25–30.

Duffy, A., Carlson, G., Dubicka, B., & Hillegers, M. H. J. (2020). Pre-pubertal bipolar disorder: Origins and current status of the controversy. *International Journal of Bipolar Disorders, 8*, 1–10.

Duffy, J. D. (1995). General paralysis of the insane: Neuropsychiatry's first challenge. *Journal of Neuropsychiatry, 7*, 243–249.

Dukart, J., Regen, F., Kherif, F., Colla, M., Bajbouj, M., Heuser, I., . . . Daganski, B. (2014). Electroconvulsive therapy-induced brain plasticity determines therapeutic outcome in mood disorders. *Proceedings of the National Academy of Sciences, 111*(3), 1156–1161.

Duncan, L. E., Ostacher, M., & Ballon, J. (2019). How genome-wide association studies (GWAS) made traditional candidate gene studies obsolete. *Neuropsychopharmacology, 44*(9), 1518–1523

Duncan, L., Yilmaz, Z., Gaspar, H., Walters, R., Goldstein, J., Anttila, V., . . . & Bulik, C. M. (2017). Significant locus and metabolic genetic correlations revealed in genome-wide association study of anorexia nervosa. *American Journal of Psychiatry, 174*(9), 850–858.

Dunn, E. C., Brown, R. C., Dai, Y., Rosand, J., Nugent, N. R., Amstadter, A. B., & Smoller, J. W. (2015). Genetic determinants of depression: Recent findings and future directions. *Harvard Review of Psychiatry, 23*(1), 1–18.

Durand, V. M., & Mindell, J. A. (1999). Behavioral intervention for childhood sleep terrors. *Behavior Therapy, 30*, 705–715.

Dutra, S. J., Cunningham, W. A., Kober, H., & Gruber, J. (2015). Elevated striatal reactivity across monetary and social rewards in bipolar I disorder. *Journal of Abnormal Psychology, 124*, 890–904.

Duval, E. R., Javanbakht, A., & Liberzon, I. (2015). Neural circuits in anxiety and stress disorders: A focused review. *Therapeutics and Clinical Risk Management, 11*, 115–126.

Dvoskin, J. A., Knoll, J. L., & Silva, M. (2020). A brief history of the criminalization of mental illness. *CNS spectrums, 25*(5), 638–650.

E

Eaton, N. R., Krueger, R. F., Keyes, K. M., Skodol, A. E., Markon, K. E., Grant, B. F., & Hasin, D. S. (2011). Borderline personality disorder co-morbidity: Relationship to the internalizing-externalizing structure of common mental disorders. *Psychological Medicine, 41*, 1041–1050.

Eaton, W. W., Bienvenu, O. J., & Miloyan, B. (2018). Specific phobias. *The lancet. Psychiatry, 5*(8), 678–686.

Eaton, W. W., Moortensenk, P. B., Herrman, H., & Freeman, H. (1992). Long-term course of hospitalization for schizophrenia: I. Risk for rehospitalization. *Schizophrenia Bulletin, 18*, 217–228.

Ebbert, J. O., Hughes, J. R., West, R. J., Rennard, S. I., Russ, C., McRae, T. D., . . . Park, P. W. (2015). Effect of varenicline on smoking cessation through smoking reduction: A randomized clinical trial. *JAMA, 313*(7), 687–694.

Ebner-Priemer, U. W., Houben, M., Santangelo, P., Kleindienst, N., Tuerlinckx, F., Oravecz, Z., . . . Kuppens, P. (2015). Unraveling affective dysregulation in borderline personality disorder: A theoretical model and empirical evidence. *Journal of Abnormal Psychology, 124*, 186–198.

Edinger, D. (1963). *Bertha Pappenheim—Freud's Anna O.* Highland Park, IL: Congregation Solel.

Edwards, A. G. K., Hulbert-Williams, S., & Neal, R. D. (2008). Psychological interventions for women with metastatic breast cancer. *Cochrane Database of Systematic Reviews, 3,* CD004253.

Efthymiou, A. G., & Goate, A. M. (2017). Late onset Alzheimer's disease genetics implicates microglial pathways in disease risk. *Molecular Neurodegeneration, 12*(1), 1–12.

Ehlers, A. (2010). Understanding and treating unwanted trauma memories in posttraumatic stress disorder. *Zeitschrift fur Psychologie, 218*(2), 141–145.

Ehlers, A., Clark, D. M., Hackmann, A., Grey, N., Liness, S., Wild, J., . . . McManus, F. (2010). Intensive cognitive therapy for PTSD: A feasibility study. *Behavioral and Cognitive Psychotherapy, 38,* 383–398.

Ehring, T., Ehlers, A., Cleare, A., & Glucksman, E. (2008). Do acute psychological and psychobiological responses to trauma predict subsequent symptom severities and PTSD and depression? *Psychiatry Research, 161,* 67–75.

Ehrman, J. K., Gordon, P. M., Visich, P. S., & Keteyian, S. J. (Eds.). (2009). *Clinical exercise physiology* (2nd ed.). Champaign, IL: Human Kinetics.

Eilenberg, T., Fink, P., Jensen, J. S., Rief, W., & Frostholm, L. (2016). Acceptance and commitment group therapy (ACT-G) for health anxiety: A randomized controlled trial. *Psychological Medicine, 46*(1), 103–115.

Eisenberg, N., Spinrad, T. L., & Eggum, N. D. (2010). Emotion-related self-regulation and its relation to children's maladjustment. *Annual Review of Clinical Psychology, 6,* 495–525.

Eldevik, S., Hastings, R. P., Hughes, J. C., Jahr, E., Eikeseth, S., & Cross, S. (2009). Meta-analysis of early intensive behavioral intervention for children with autism. *Journal of Clinical Child & Adolescent Psychology, 38,* 439–450.

Eley, T. C., Bolton, D., O'Connor, T. G., Perrin, S., Smith, P., & Plomin, R. (2003). A twin study of anxiety-related behaviours in pre-school children. *Journal of Child Psychology & Psychiatry, 44,* 945–960.

Eley, T. C., McAdams, T. A., Rijsdijk, F. V., Lichtenstein, P., Narusyte, J., Reiss, D., . . . Neiderhiser, J. M. (2015). The intergenerational transmission of anxiety: A children-of-twins study. *The American Journal of Psychiatry, 172*(7), 630–637.

Ellason, J. W., & Ross, C. A. (1997). Two-year follow-up of inpatients with dissociative identity disorder. *American Journal of Psychiatry, 154,* 832–839.

Ellason, J. W., Ross, C. A., & Fuchs, D. L. (1996). Lifetime Axis I and II comorbidity and childhood trauma history in dissociative identity disorder. *Psychiatry, 59,* 255–266.

Ellepola, A., & Abayaweera, C. A. (2020). Expressed emotion, medication adherence and association with disease prognosis in patients with schizophrenia at Teaching Hospital, Anuradhapura. *Sri Lanka Journal of Psychiatry, 11*(1).

Elliott, R., Greenberg, L. S., Lietaer, G. (2004). Research on experiential therapies. In M. J. Lambert (Ed.), *Bergin and Garfield's handbook of psychotherapy and behavior change* (5th ed.), pp. 493–539. New York: John Wiley.

Ellis, A. (1997). The evolution of Albert Ellis and emotive behavior therapy. In J. K. Zeig (Ed.), *The rational evolution of psychotherapy: The third conference* (pp. 69–78). New York: Brunner/Mazel.

Ellis, A., & Harper, R. A. (1961). *A guide to rational living.* Englewood Cliffs, NJ: Prentice Hall.

Ellis, E. E., & Saadabadi, A. (2020, January). Reactive attachment disorder. In *StatPearls* [Internet]. Treasure Island, FL: StatPearls Publishing. Retrieved from https://www.ncbi.nlm.nih.gov/books/NBK537155/

Ellison, J. W., Rosenfeld, J. A., & Shaffer, L. G. (2013). Genetic basis of intellectual disability. *Annual Review of Medicine, 64,* 441–450.

Ellman, L. M., & Cannon, T. D. (2008). Environmental pre- and perinatal influences on etiology. In K. T. Mueser & D. V. Jeste (Eds.), *Clinical handbook of schizophrenia* (pp. 65–73). New York: Guilford Press.

Emerson, E., Shahtahmasebi, S., Lancaster, G., & Berridge, D. (2010). Poverty transitions among families supporting a child with intellectual disability. *Journal of Intellectual & Developmental Disability, 35,* 224–234.

Emmelkamp, P. M. G., Benner, A., Kuipers, A., Feiertag, G. A., Koster, H. C., & van Apeldoorn, F. J. (2006). Comparison of brief dynamic and cognitive-behavioural therapies in avoidant personality disorder. *British Journal of Psychiatry, 189,* 60–64.

Epperson, C. N., Steiner, M., Hartlage, S. A., Eriksson, E., Schmidt, P. J., Jones, I., & Yonkers, K. A. (2012). Premenstrual dysphoric disorder: Evidence for a new category for DSM-5. *American Journal of Psychiatry, 169,* 465–475.

Erdelyi, M. H. (1992). Psychodynamics and the unconscious. *American Psychologist, 47,* 784–787.

Erskine, H. E., Norman, R. E., Ferrari, A. J., Chan, G. C., Copeland, W. E., Whiteford, H. A., & Scott, J. G. (2016). Long-term outcomes of attention-deficit/hyperactivity disorder and conduct disorder: A systematic review and meta-analysis. *Journal of the American Academy of Child & Adolescent Psychiatry, 55*(10), 841–850.

Escobar, J. I. (1993). Psychiatric epidemiology. In A. C. Gaw (Ed.), *Culture, ethnicity, and mental illness* (pp. 43–73). Washington, DC: American Psychiatric Press.

e Silva, L. F. S., Brito, M. D., Yuzawa, J. M. C., & Rosenstock, T. R. (2019). Mitochondrial Dysfunction and Changes in High-Energy Compounds in Different Cellular Models Associated to Hypoxia: Implication to Schizophrenia. *Scientific Reports, 9*(1), 1–19.

Eslami, B., Di Rosa, M., Barros, H., Torres-Gonzalez, F., Stankunas, M., Ioannidi-Kapolou, E., Lindert, J., Soares, J., Lamura, G., & Melchiorre, M. G. (2019). Lifetime abuse and somatic symptoms among older women and men in Europe. *PloS one, 14*(8), e0220741. https://doi.org/10.1371/journal.pone.0220741

European Monitoring Centre for Drugs and Drug Addiction (EMCDDA). (2011, November). *2011 Annual report on the state of the drugs problem in Europe.* Lisbon, Portugal: Author.

Eusei, D., & Delcea, C. (2019). Fetishistic disorder. *Theoretical-experimental models in sexual and paraphilic dysfunctions, 1*(2), 73–77.

Evans, S. W., Owens, J. S., Wymbs, B. T., & Ray, A. R. (2018). Evidence-based psychosocial treatments for children and adolescents with attention deficit/hyperactivity disorder. *Journal of Clinical Child & Adolescent Psychology, 47*(2), 157–198.

Everson-Rose, S. A., & Lewis, T. T. (2005). Psychosocial factors and cardiovascular diseases. *Annual Review of Public Health, 26,* 469–500.

Exner, J., Levy, A., Exner, J., Groth-Marnat, G., Wood, J. M., & Garb, H. N. (2008). *The Rorschach: A comprehensive system. Volume 1: The Rorschach, basic foundations and principles of interpretation.* New York: Wiley.

Eysenck, H. J. (1994). The biology of morality. In B. Puka (Ed.), *Defining perspectives in moral development* (pp. 212–229). New York: Garland.

F

Fabiano, G. A., Pelham Jr, W. E., Coles, E. K., Gnagy, E. M., Chronis-Tuscano, A., & O'Connor, B. C. (2009). A meta-analysis of behavioral treatments for attention-deficit/hyperactivity disorder. *Clinical Psychology Review, 29*(2), 129–140.

Fabrega, H. (1993). Toward a social theory of psychiatric phenomena. *Behavioral Science, 38,* 75–100.

Fabrega, H., Ulrich, R., Pilkonis, P., & Mezzich, J. (1991). On the homogeneity of personality disorder clusters. *Comprehensive Psychiatry, 32,* 373–386.

Fairburn, C. G. (2005). Evidence-based treatment of anorexia nervosa. *International Journal of Eating Disorders, 37,* 526–530.

Fairburn, C. G., Bailey-Straebler, S., Basden, S., Doll, H. A., Jones, R., Murphy, R., et al. (2015). A transdiagnostic comparison of enhanced cognitive behaviour therapy (CBT-E) and interpersonal psychotherapy in the treatment of eating disorders. *Behaviour Research and Therapy, 70,* 64–71.

Fairburn, C. G., Cooper, Z., Doll, H. A., O'Connor, M. E., Bohn, K., Hawker, D. M., Wales, J. A., & Palmer, R. L. (2009). Transdiagnostic cognitive-behavioral therapy for patients with eating disorders: a two-site trial with 60-week follow-up. *The American journal of psychiatry, 166*(3), 311–319. https://doi.org/10.1176/appi.ajp.2008.08040608

Fairburn, C. G., Cooper, Z., Shafra, R., Bohn, K., & Hawker, D. M. (2008). Clinical perfectionism, core low self-esteem and interpersonal problems. In C. G. Fairburn (Ed.), *Cognitive behavior therapy and eating disorders* (pp. 197–220). New York: Guilford Press.

Fairweather, G. W., Sanders, D. H., Maynard, H., & Cressler, D. L. (1969). *Community life for the mentally ill: An alternative to institutional care.* Chicago: Aldine.

Famitafreshi, H., & Karimian, M. (2020). Overview of withdrawal syndrome mechanisms in different substance abuse addictions: Neuronal circuits and transmitters. *Journal of Addiction Medicine and Therapeutic Science, 6*(1), 070–076.

Fang, A., & Wilhelm, S. (2015). Clinical features, cognitive biases, and treatment of body dysmorphic disorder. *Annual Review of Clinical Psychology, 11,* 187–212.

Fanning, J. R., Coleman, M., Lee, R., & Coccaro, E. F. (2019). Subtypes of aggression in intermittent explosive disorder. *Journal of Psychiatric Research, 109,* 164–172. https://doi.org/10.1016/j.jpsychires.2018.10.013

Fanous, A. H., Prescott, C. A., & Kendler, K. S. (2004). The prediction of thoughts of death or self-harm in a population-based sample of female twins. *Psychological Medicine, 34,* 301–312.

Fanti, K. A. (2018). Understanding heterogeneity in conduct disorder: A review of psychophysiological studies. *Neuroscience & Biobehavioral Reviews, 91,* 4–20.

Fariba, K., & Sapra, A.(2020). Avoidant Personality Disorder. StatPearls [Internet]. Treasure Island (FL): StatPearls Publishing. https://www.ncbi.nlm.nih.gov/books/NBK559325/

Farley, T. M., Anderson, E. N., & Feller, J. N. (2017). False-positive phencyclidine (PCP) on urine drug screen attributed to desvenlafaxine (Pristiq) use. *BMJ Case Reports, 2017,* bcr2017222106. https://doi.org/10.1136/bcr-2017-222106

Farmer, M. A., Kao, A., & Binik, Y. M. (2009). Dyspareunia and vaginismus. In R. Balon & E. R. Segraves (Eds.), *Clinical manual of sexual disorders* (pp. 305–334). Arlington, VA: American Psychiatric Publishing.

Farmer, M. A., Kukkonen, T., & Binik, Y. M. (2008). Female genital pain and its treatment. In D. L. Rowland & L. Incrocci (Eds.), *Handbook of sexual and gender identity disorders* (pp. 220–250). Hoboken, NJ: Wiley.

Fawzy, F. I., Canada, A. L., & Fawzy, N. W. (2003). Malignant melanoma: Effects of a brief, structured psychiatric intervention on survival and recurrence at 10-year follow-up. *Archives of General Psychiatry, 60,* 100–103.

Fawzy, F. I., Cousins, N., Fawzy, N. W., Kemeny, M. E., Elashoff, R., & Morton, D. (1990). A structured psychiatric intervention for cancer patients: I. Changes over time in methods of coping and affective disturbance. *Archives of General Psychiatry, 47,* 720–725.

Fawzy, F. I., Fawzy, N. W., Huyn, C. S., Elashoff, R., Morton, D., Cousins, N., & Fahey, J. L. (1993). Effects of an early structured psychiatric intervention, coping and affective state on recurrence and survival 6 years later. *Archives of General Psychiatry, 50,* 681–689.

Fawzy, F. I., Kemeny, M. E., Fawzy, N. W., Elashoff, R., Morton, D., Cousins, N., & Fahey, J. L. (1990). A structured psychiatric intervention for cancer patients: II. Changes over time in immunological measures. *Archives of General Psychiatry, 47,* 729–735.

Fazel, S., & Danesh, J. (2002). Serious mental disorder in 23,000 prisoners: A systematic review of 62 surveys. *Lancet, 359,* 545–550.

Fazel, S., Långström, N., Hjern, A., Grann, M., & Lichtenstein, P. (2009). Schizophrenia, substance abuse, and violent crime. *JAMA, 301*(19), 2016–2023.

Fazel, S., Lichtenstein, P., Grann, M., Goodwin, G. M., & Långström, N. (2010). Bipolar disorder and violent crime: New evidence from population-based longitudinal studies and systematic review. *Archives of General Psychiatry, 67*(9), 931–938.

Feder, A., Olfson, M., Fuentes, M., Shea, S., Lantigua, R. A., & Weissman, M. M. (2001). Medically unexplained symptoms in an urban general medicine practice. *Psychosomatics, 42,* 261–268.

Feingold, A. (1994). Gender differences in personality: A meta-analysis. *Psychological Bulletin, 116,* 429–456.

Feinstein, A. (2011). Conversion disorder: Advances in our understanding. *Canadian Medical Association Journal, 183,* 915–920.

Feldman, M. A. (Ed.). (2004). *Early intervention: The essential readings.* Malden, MA: Blackwell.

Feldman, R. P., & Goodrich, J. T. (2001). Psychosurgery: A historical overview. *Neurosurgery, 48,* 647–659.

Fenn, K., & Byrne, M. (2013). The key principles of cognitive behavioural therapy. *InnovAiT: Education and Inspiration for General Practice, 6*(9), 579–585. doi: 10.1177/1755738012471029

Ferri, C. P., Prince, M., Brayne, C., Brodaty, H., Fratiglioni, L., Ganguli, M., . . . Scazufca, M. (2005). Global prevalence of dementia: A Delphi consensus study. *Lancet, 366,* 2112–2117.

Ferrier, I. N. (2019). *ECT in the Treatment of Depression.* RCPsych Publications.

Ferri, M., Amato, L., & Davoli, M. (2006). Alcoholics Anonymous and other 12-step programmes for alcohol dependence. *Cochrane Database of Systematic Reviews 2006,* Issue 3.

Ficks, C. A., & Waldman, I. D. (2014). Candidate genes for aggression and antisocial behavior: A meta-analysis of association studies of the 5HTTLPR and MAOA-uVNTR. *Behavior Genetics, 44*(5), 427–444.

Fillmore, K. M., Kerr, W. C., Stockwell, T., Chikritzhs, T., & Bostrom, A. (2006). Moderate alcohol use and reduced mortality risk: Systematic error in prospective studies. *Addiction Research and Theory, 14,* 101–132.

Fink, M. (2001). Convulsive therapy: A review of the first 55 years. *Journal of Affective Disorders, 63,* 1–15.

Finney, G. R., Minagar, A., & Heilman, K. M. (2016). Assessment of mental atatus. *Neurologic Clinics, 34*(1), 1–16.

Finney, J. W., & Moos, R. H. (1998). Psychosocial treatments for alcohol use disorders. In P. E. Nathan (Ed.), *A guide to treatments that work* (pp. 156–166). New York: Oxford University Press.

First, M. B. (2010). Paradigm shifts and the development of the *Diagnostic and Statistical Manual of Mental Disorders*: Past experiences and future aspirations. *Canadian Journal of Psychiatry, 55,* 692–700.

Fischer, M., & Barkley, R. (2006). Young adult outcomes of children with hyperactivity: Leisure, financial, and social activities. *International Journal of Disability, Development and Education, 53,* 229–245.

Fisher, K.A., & Hany, M. (2020). Antisocial Personality Disorder. StatPearls [Internet]. Treasure Island (FL): StatPearls Publishing; 2020 Jan-. Available from: https://www.ncbi.nlm.nih.gov/books/NBK546673/

Fiske, A., Wetherell, J. L., & Gatz, M. (2009). Depression in older adults. *Annual Review of Clinical Psychology, 9,* 363–391.

Fitzsimmons, S., & Buettner, L. L. (2002). Therapeutic recreation interventions for need-driven dementia-compromised behaviors in community-dwelling elders. *American Journal of Alzheimer's Disorder and Other Dementias, 17,* 367–381.

Flament, M. F., Bissada, H., & Spettigue, W. (2012). Evidence-based pharmacotherapy of eating disorders. *International Journal of Neuropsychopharmacology, 15,* 189–207.

Flegal, K. M., Carroll, M. D., Ogden, C. L., & Johnson, C. L. (2002). Prevalence and trends in obesity among U.S. adults, 1999–2000. *Journal of the American Medical Association, 288,* 1723–1727.

Flessner, C. A. (2011). Cognitive-behavioral therapy for childhood repetitive behavior disorders: Tic disorders and trichotillomania. *Child and Adolescent Psychiatric Clinics of North America, 20,* 319–328.

Fletcher, J. M., Lyon, G. R., Fuchs, L. S., & Barnes, M. A. (2018). *Learning disabilities: From identification to intervention* (2nd ed.). New York: Guilford Press.

Flint, J., & Kendler, K. S. (2014). The genetics of major depression. *Neuron, 81*(3), 484–503.

Flora, K. (2018). THE THERAPEUTIC RELATIONSHIP IN BORDERLINE PERSONALITY DISORDER: A COGNITIVE PERSPECTIVE. *Journal of Evidence - Based Psychotherapies, 18*(2), 19. Retrieved from https://mccc.idm.oclc.org/login?url=https://www-proquest-com.mccc.idm.oclc.org/scholarly-journals/therapeutic-relationship-borderline-personality/docview/2160706974/se-2?accountid=40611

Flores, A. R., Herman, J. L., Gates, G. J., & Brown, T. N. T. (2016). *How many adults identify as transgender in the United States?* Los Angeles: Williams Institute.

Flores, A. R., Mallory, C., & Conron, K. J. (2020). Public attitudes about emergent issues in LGBTQ rights: Conversion therapy and religious refusals. *Research & Politics, 7*(4), 2053168020966874.

Flynn-Evans, E. E., Tabandeh, H., Skene, D. J., & Lockley, S. W. (2014). Circadian rhythm disorders and melatonin production in 127 blind women with and without light perception. *Journal of Biological Rhythms, 29*(3), 215–224.

Foa, E. B., & McLean, C. P. (2016). The efficacy of exposure therapy for anxiety-related disorders and its underlying mechanisms: The case of OCD and PTSD. *Annual Review of Clinical Psychology, 12,* 1–28.

Fombonne, E. (1999). The epidemiology of autism: A review. *Psychological Medicine, 29,* 769–786.

Fonagy, P., & Bateman, A. (2008). The development of borderline personality disorder: A mentalizing model. *Journal of Personality Disorders, 22,* 4–21.

Fong, T. G., Vasunilashorn, S. M., Libermann, T., Marcantonio, E. R., & Inouye, S. K. (2019). Delirium and Alzheimer disease: A proposed model for shared pathophysiology. *International Journal of Geriatric Psychiatry, 34*(6), 781–789. https://doi.org/10.1002/gps.5088

Fontaine, R. G., & Dodge, K. A. (2006). Real-time decision making and aggressive behavior in youth: A heuristic model of response evaluation and decision (RED). *Aggressive Behavior, 32*(6), 604–624.

Fonteille, V., Redouté, J., Lamothe, P., Straub, D., Lavenne, F., Le Bars, D., . . . & Stoléru, S. (2019). Brain processing of pictures of children in men with pedophilic disorder: A positron emission tomography study. *NeuroImage: Clinical, 21,* 101647.

Fontenelle, L. F., Coutinho, E. S., Lins-Martins, N. M., Fitzgerald, P. B., Fujiwara, H., & Yucel, M. (2015). Electroconvulsive therapy for obsessive-compulsive disorder: A systematic review. *A Journal of Clinical Psychiatry, 76,* 949–957. doi: 10.4088/JCP.14r09129

Forbes, M. K., Rapee, R. M., Camberis, A. L., & McMahon, C. A. (2017). Unique associations between childhood temperament characteristics and subsequent psychopathology symptom trajectories from childhood to early adolescence. *Journal of Abnormal Child Psychology, 45*(6), 1221–1233.

Ford, B. Q., & Mauss, I. B. (2015). Culture and emotion regulation. *Current Opinion in Psychology, 3,* 1–5.

Forscher, P. S., Taylor, V. J., Cavagnaro, D., Lewis, N. A., Jr., Buchanan, E. M., Moshontz, H., ... Chartier, C. R. (2019, July 17). Stereotype threat in Black college students across many operationalizations. *PsyArXiv.* Retrieved from https://doi.org/10.31234/osf.io/6hju9

Forslund, T., Brocki, K. C., Bohlin, G., Granqvist, P., & Eninger, L. (2016). The heterogeneity of attention-deficit/hyperactivity disorder symptoms and conduct problems: Cognitive inhibition, emotion regulation, emotionality, and disorganized attachment. *British Journal of Developmental Psychology, 34*(3), 371–387.

Fosse, R., Joseph, J., & Jones, M. (2016). Schizophrenia: A critical view on genetic effects. *Psychosis, 8*(1), 72–84.

Foulkes, L. (2019). Sadism: Review of an elusive construct. *Personality and Individual Differences, 151*(1), 1–9.

Fournier, J. C., DeRubeis, R. J., Hollon, S. D., Dimidjian, S., Amsterdam, J. D., Shelton, R. C., & Fawcett, J. (2010). Antidepressant drug effect and depression severity: A patient-level meta-analysis. *Journal of the American Medical Association, 303,* 47–53.

Fox, A. B., Earnshaw, V. A., Taverna, E. C., & Vogt, D. (2018). Conceptualizing and measuring mental illness stigma: The mental illness stigma framework and critical review of measures. *Stigma and Health, 3*(4), 348.

Fox, K. R., Franklin, J. C., Ribeiro, J. D., Kleiman, E. M., Bentley, K. H., & Nock, M. K. (2015). Meta-analysis of risk factors for nonsuicidal self-injury. *Clinical Psychology Review, 42,* 156–167.

Fox, K. R., Toole, K. E., Franklin, J. C., & Hooley, J. M. (2017). Why does nonsuicidal self-injury improve mood? A preliminary test of three hypotheses. *Clinical Psychological Science, 5*(1), 111–121.

Frías, Á., Palma, C., Farriols, N., & González, L. (2015). Comorbidity between obsessive-compulsive disorder and body dysmorphic disorder: Prevalence, explanatory theories, and clinical characterization. *Neuropsychiatric Disease and Treatment, 11,* 2233–2244.

Frühauf, S., Gerger, H., Schmidt, H. M., Munder, T., & Barth, J. (2013). Efficacy of psychological interventions for sexual dysfunction: A systematic review and meta-analysis. *Archives of Sexual Behavior, 42*(6), 915–933.

Frances, A. (2013). The new somatic symptom disorder in DSM-5 risks mislabeling many people as mentally ill. *BMJ: British Medical Journal (Online), 346.*

Frances, A., & First, M. B. (2011). Paraphilia NOS, nonconsent: Not ready for the courtroom. *Journal of the American Academy of Psychiatry and the Law, 39,* 555–561.

Frances, A. J., & Widiger, T. (2012). Psychiatric diagnosis: Lessons from the *DSM-IV* past and cautions for the *DSM-5* future. *Clinical Psychology, 8,* 109–130.

Frank, E., Kupfer, D. J., Thase, M. E., Mallinger, A. G., Swartz, H. A., Fagiolini, A. M., . . . Monk, T. (2005). Two-year outcomes for interpersonal and social rhythm therapy in individuals with bipolar I disorder. *Archives of General Psychiatry, 62,* 996-1004.

Frank, G. K., DeGuzman, M. C., & Shott, M. E. (2019). Motivation to eat and not to eat–The psycho-biological conflict in anorexia nervosa. *Physiology & behavior, 206,* 185-190.

Franklin, J. C., Fox, K. R., Franklin, C. R., Kleiman, E. M., Ribeiro, J. D., Jaroszewski, A. C., . . . Nock, K. M. (2016). A brief mobile app reduces nonsuicidal and suicidal self-injury: Evidence from three randomized controlled trials. *Journal of Consulting and Clinical Psychology, 84*(6), 544-557.

Franklin, K. A., Anttila, H., Axelsson, S., Gislason, T., Maasita, P., Myhre, K. I., & Rehnqvist, N. (2009). Effects and side-effects of surgery for snoring and obstructive sleep apnea–a systematic review. *Sleep, 32,* 27-36.

Frasure-Smith, N., & Lesperance, F. (2008). Depression and anxiety as predictors of 2-year cardiac events in patients with stable coronary artery disease. *Archives of General Psychiatry, 65,* 62-71.

Frazier, J. A., Breeze, J. L., Papadimitriou, G., Kennedy, D. M., Hodge, S. M., Moore, C. M., . . . Makris, N. (2007). White matter abnormalities in children with and at risk for bipolar disorder. *Bipolar Disorders, 9,* 799-809.

Freedman, D., & Woods, G. W. (2013). Neighborhood effects, mental illness and criminal behavior: A Review. *Journal of Politics and Law, 6*(3), 1-16. https://doi.org/10.5539/jpl.v6n3p1

Freeman, A., & Chen, Y. (2019, March 01). Interpreting pediatric intelligence tests: A framework from evidence-based medicine. Retrieved November 13, 2020, from https://www.sciencedirect.com/science/article/pii/B9780128022030000031?via=ihub

Freeman, A., & Reinecke, M. A. (1995). Cognitive therapy. In A. S. Gurman (Ed.), *Essential psychotherapies: Theory and practice* (pp. 182-225). New York: Guilford Press.

Freeman, D., & Garety, P. (2014). Advances in understanding and treating persecutory delusions: A review. *Social Psychiatry and Psychiatric Epidemiology, 49*(8), 1179-1189. https://doi.org/10.1007/s00127-014-0928-7

French, J., & Hameed, S. (2020, June 27). Illness Anxiety Disorder. Retrieved December 07, 2020, from https://www.ncbi.nlm.nih.gov/books/NBK554399/

French, J., & Shrestha, S. (2020). Histrionic personality disorder. In *StatPearls [Internet].* Treasure Island, FL: StatPearls Publishing. Retrieved from https://www.ncbi.nlm.nih.gov/books/NBK542325/

Frenda, S. J., Nichols, R. M., & Loftus, E. F. (2011). Current issues and advances in misinformation research. *Current Directions in Psychological Science, 20,* 20-23.

Freyd, J. J., Martorella, S. R., Alvarado, J. S., Hayes, A. E., & Christman, J. C. (1998). Cognitive environments and dissociative tendencies: Performance on the standard Stroop task for high versus low dissociators. *Applied Cognitive Psychology, 12,* S91-S103.

Frick, P. J. (2012). Developmental pathways to conduct disorder: Implications for future directions in research, assessment, and treatment. *Journal of Clinical Child and Adolescent Psychology, 41,* 378-389.

Frick, P. J. (2016). Current research on conduct disorder in children and adolescents. *South African Journal of Psychology, 46*(2), 160-174.

Frick, P. J., & Nigg, J. T. (2012). Current issues in the diagnosis of attention deficit hyperactivity disorder, oppositional defiant disorder, and conduct disorder. *Clinical Psychology, 8,* 77-107.

Friedman, M. J., Resik, P. A., Bryant, R. A., Strain, J., Horowitz, M., & Spiegel, D. (2011). Classification of trauma and stressor-related disorders in *DSM-5. Depression and Anxiety, 28,* 737-749.

Friedman, M., & Rosenman, R. H. (1974). *Type A behavior and your heart.* New York: Knopf.

Friedman, M., Rosenman, R. H., Straus, R., Wurm, M., & Kositcheck, R. (1968). The relationship of behavior pattern A to the state of coronary vasculature. *American Journal of Medicine, 44,* 525-537.

Friedman, M., Thoresen, C. E., Gill, J. J., Ulmer, D., Powell, L. H., Price, V., . . . Dixon, T. (1994). Alteration of Type A behavior and its effect on cardiac recurrences in post myocardial infarction patients: Summary results of the recurrent coronary prevention project. In A. Steptoe (Ed.), *Psychosocial processes and health: A reader.* Cambridge, England: Cambridge University Press.

Friedman, R. A. (2014). Antidepressants' black-box warning–10 years later. *New England Journal of Medicine, 371,* 1666-1668.

Frith, M. (2009). *Beckham reveals his battle with obsessive disorder.* Retrieved January 24, 2021, from https://www.independent.co.uk/news/uk/this-britain/beckham-reveals-his-battle-obsessive-disorder-6104728.html

Fromm-Reichmann, F. (1948). Notes on the development of treatments of schizophrenia by psychoanalytic psychotherapy. *Psychiatry, 2,* 263-273.

Frost, R. O., Steketee, G., & Tolin, D. F. (2012). Diagnosis and assessment of hoarding disorder. *Annual Review of Clinical Psychology, 8,* 219-242.

Fuller, D. A., Sinclair, E., Geller, J., Quanbeck, C., & Snook, J. (2016). *Going, going, gone: Trends and consequences of eliminating state psychiatric beds.* Arlington, VA: Treatment Advocacy Center.

Fung, T. C., Olson, C. A., & Hsiao, E. Y. (2017). Interactions between the microbiota, immune and nervous systems in health and disease. *Nature Neuroscience, 20*(2), 145-155. doi: http://dx.doi.org.mccc.idm.oclc.org/10.1038/nn.4476

G

Gabrieli, J. D. (2009). Dyslexia: A new synergy between education and cognitive neuroscience. *Science, 325*(5938), 280-283.

Galderisi, S., Mucci, A., Bitter, I., Libiger, J., Bucci, P., Fleischhacker, W. W., & Kahn, R. S. (2012). Persistent negative symptoms in first episode patients with schizophrenia: Results from the European First Episode Schizophrenia Trial. *European Neuropsychopharmacology, 23,* 196-204.

Galea, S., Ahern, J., Resnick, H., Kilpatrick, D., Bucuvalas, M., Gold, J., & Vlahov, D. (2002). Psychological sequelae of the September 11 terrorist attacks in New York City. *New England Journal of Medicine, 346,* 982-987.

Galea, S., Tracy, M., Norris, F., & Coffey, S. F. (2008). Financial and social circumstances and the incidence and course of PTSD in Mississippi during the first two years after Hurricane Katrina. *Journal of Traumatic Stress, 21,* 357-368.

Gallegos, A. M., Crean, H. F., Pigeon, W. R., & Heffner, K. L. (2017). Meditation and yoga for posttraumatic stress disorder: A meta-analytic review of randomized controlled trials. *Clinical Psychology Review, 15,* 115-124.

Galván, A., & Tottenham, N. (2016). Adolescent brain development. In Cicchetti, D. (Ed.), *Developmental psychopathology: Vol. 2. Developmental neuroscience* (3rd ed., pp. 684-719). Hoboken, NJ: Wiley

Gao, K., Kemp, D.E., Wu, R., and Calabrese, J.R. (2015). Mood stabilizers. In A. Tasman, J. Kay, A. Lieberman, M.B. First & M.B. Riba (Eds.), *Psychiatry.* Chichester: John Wiley & Sons, Ltd.

García-Batista, Z. E., Guerra-Peña, K., Cano-Vindel, A., Herrera-Martínez, S. X., & Medrano, L. A. (2018). Validity and reliability of the Beck Depression Inventory (BDI-II) in general and hospital population of Dominican Republic. *PLoS ONE, 13*(6), e0199750.

García-Molina A. (2012). Phineas Gage y el enigma del córtex prefrontal [Phineas Gage and the enigma of the prefrontal cortex]. *Neurologia (Barcelona, Spain), 27*(6), 370–375. https://doi.org/10.1016/j.nrl.2010.07.015

Garcia-Falgueras, A., & Swaab, D. F. (2008). A sex difference in the hypothalamic uncinate nucleus: Relationship to gender identity. *Brain, 131*(12), 3132–3146.

Garcia, F. D., Delavenne, H. G., Assumpção, A. D. F. A., & Thibaut, F. (2013). Pharmacologic treatment of sex offenders with paraphilic disorder. *Current Psychiatry Reports, 15*(5), 356.

Gardner, C. D., Kiazand, A., Alhassan, S., Kim, S., Stafford, R. S., Balise, R. R., et al. (2007). Comparison of the Atkins, Zone, Ornish, and LEARN diets for change in weight and related risk factors among overweight premenopausal women, the A to Z weight loss story: A randomized trial. *Journal of the American Medical Association, 297,* 969–977.

Gardner, H. (2008). *Multiple intelligences: New horizons in theory and practice.* New York: Basic Books.

Gardner, W., Lidz, C. W., Hoge, S. K., Monahan, J., Eisenberg, M. M., Bennett, N. S., Mulvey, E. P., & Roth, L. H. (1999). Patients' revisions of their beliefs about the need for hospitalization. *American Journal of Psychiatry, 156,* 1385–1391.

Garety, P. A., & Freeman, D. (2013). The past and future of delusions research: From the inexplicable to the treatable. *British Journal of Psychiatry, 203*(5), 327–333.

Garfin, D. R., Holman, E. A., & Silver, R. C. (2015). Cumulative exposure to prior collective trauma and acute stress responses to the Boston marathon bombings. *Psychological Science, 26*(6), 675–683.

Garland, E. J., Kutcher, S., Virani, A., & Elbe, D. (2016). Update on the use of SSRIs and SNRIs with children and adolescents in clinical practice. *Journal of the Canadian Academy of Child and Adolescent Psychiatry, 25*(1), 4–10.

Garner, D. M., & Garfinkel, P. E. (1980). Sociocultural factors in the development of anorexia nervosa. *Psychological Medicine, 10,* 647–656.

Garrett, A. S., Reiss, A. L., Howe, M. E., Kelley, R. G., Singh, M. K., Adleman, N. E., . . . Chang, K. D. (2012). Abnormal amygdala and prefrontal cortex activation to facial expressions in pediatric bipolar disorder. *Journal of the American Academy of Child & Adolescent Psychiatry, 51*(8), 821–831.

Gatov, E., Rosella, L., Chiu, M., & Kurdyak, P. A. (2017). Trends in standardized mortality among individuals with schizophrenia, 1993–2012: A population-based, repeated cross-sectional study. *CMAJ: Canadian Medical Association Journal = journal de l'Association medicale canadienne, 189*(37), E1177–E1187. https://doi.org/10.1503/cmaj.161351

Gatz, M. (2007). Genetics, dementia, and the elderly. *Current Directions in Psychological Science, 16,* 123–127.

Gatz, M., Prescott, C. A., & Pedersen, N. L. (2006). Lifestyle risk and delaying factors. *Alzheimer Disease and Associated Disorders, 20,* S84–S88.

Gatz, M., Reynolds, C. A., Fratiglioni, L., Johansson, B., Mortimer, J. A., Berg, . . . Pedersen, N. L. (2006). Role of genes and environments for explaining Alzheimer disease. *Archives of General Psychiatry, 63,* 168–174.

Gauntlett-Gilbert, J., & Kuipers, E. (2003). Phenomenology of visual hallucinations in psychiatric conditions. *Journal of Nervous and Mental Disease, 191,* 203–205.

Gautam, S., Jain, A., Gautam, M., Vahia, V. N., & Gautam, A. (2017). Clinical practice guidelines for the management of generalized anxiety disorder (GAD) and panic disorder (PD). *Indian Journal of Psychiatry, 59*(1), S67–S73.

Gazdag, G., & Ungvari, G. S. (2019). Electroconvulsive therapy: 80 years old and still going strong. *World Journal of Psychiatry, 9*(1), 1–6.

Gearhardt, A. N., Bragg, M. A., Pearl, R. L., Schvey, N. A., Roberto, C. A., & Brownell, K. D. (2012). Obesity and public policy. *Annual Review of Clinical Psychology, 8,* 405–430.

Gearhardt, A. N., Davis, C., Kuschner, R., & Brownell, K. D. (2011). The addiction potential of hyperpalatable foods. *Current Drug Abuse Review, 4,* 140–145.

Gearhardt, A. N., Yokum, S., Orr, P., Stice, E., Corbin, W., & Brownell, K. (2011). Neural correlates of food addiction. *Archive of General Psychiatry, 68,* 808–816.

Gearing, R. E., & Alonzo, D. (2018). Religion and suicide: New findings. *Journal of Religion and Health,* 1–22.

Geddes, J. R., Burgess, S., Hawton, K., Jamison, K., & Goodwin, G. M. (2004). Long-term lithium therapy for bipolar disorder: Systematic review and meta-analysis of randomized controlled trials. *American Journal of Psychiatry, 161,* 217–222.

Gehi, A., Haas, D., Pipkin, S., & Whooley, M. A. (2005). Depression and medication adherence in outpatients with coronary heart disease: Findings from the Heart and Soul Study. *Archives of Internal Medicine, 165,* 2508–2513.

Gelauff, J., & Stone, J. (2016). Prognosis of functional neurologic disorders. *Handbook of Clinical Neurology, 139,* 523–541.

Geoffroy, P. A., Bellivier, F., Scott, J., Boudebesse, C., Lajnef, M., Gard, S., . . . Etain, B. (2013). Bipolar disorder with seasonal pattern: Clinical characteristics and gender influences. *Chronobiology International, 30*(9), 1101–1107.

Gerardin, P., & Thibaut, F. (2004). Epidemiology and treatment of juvenile sexual offending. *Pediatric Drugs, 6,* 79–91.

Geronimus, A. T., Hicken, M., Keene, D., & Bound, J. (2006). "Weathering" and age patterns of allostatic load scored among blacks and whites in the United States. *American Journal of Public Health, 96,* 826–833.

Geschwind, D. H., & Flint, J. (2015). Genetics and genomics of psychiatric disease. *Science, 349*(6255), 1489–1494.

Ghasemi, A., Seifi, M., Baybordi, F., Danaei, N., & Rad, B. S. (2018). Association between serotonin 2A receptor genetic variations, stressful life events and suicide. *Gene, 658,* 191–197.

Ghirardi, L., Brikell, I., Kuja-Halkola, R., Freitag, C. M., Franke, B., Asherson, P., . . . & Larsson, H. (2018). The familial co-aggregation of ASD and ADHD: a register-based cohort study. *Molecular psychiatry, 23*(2), 257–262.

Gibbons, R. D., Hooker, G., Finkelman, M. D., Weiss, D. J., Pilkonis, P. A., Frank, E., . . . Kupfer, D. J. (2013). The computerized adaptive diagnostic test for major depressive disorder (CAD-MDD): A screening tool for depression. *The Journal of Clinical Psychiatry, 74*(7), 669–674. Retrieved from https://doi.org/10.4088/JCP.12m08338

Gibbons, R. D., Weiss, D. J., Frank, E., & Kupfer, D. (2016). Computerized adaptive diagnosis and testing of mental health disorders. *Annual Review of Clinical Psychology, 12,* 83–104.

Gibson, D., Workman, C., & Mehler, P. S. (2019). Medical complications of anorexia nervosa and bulimia nervosa. *The Psychiatric Clinics of North America, 42*(2), 263–274.

Giesen-Bloo, J., van Dyck, R., Spinhoven, P., van Tilburg, W., Dirksen, C., van Asselt, T., . . . Arntz, A. (2006). Outpatient psychotherapy for borderline personality disorder: Randomized trial of schema-focused therapy vs. transference-focused psychotherapy. *Archives of General Psychiatry, 63,* 649–658.

Gilman, S. E., Cochran, S. D., Mays, V. M., Hughes, M., Ostrow, D., & Kessler, R. C. (2001). Risk of psychiatric disorders among individuals reporting same-sex sexual partners in the National Comorbidity Survey. *American Journal of Public Health, 91,* 933-939.

Giraldi, A., Kristensen, E., & Sand, M. (2015). Endorsement of models describing sexual response of men and women with a sexual partner: An online survey in a population sample of Danish adults ages 20-65 years. *Journal of Sexual Medicine, 12*(1), 116-128.

Gitlin, M. J. (2015). Pharmacotherapy and other somatic treatments for depression. In I. H. Gotlib & C. L. Hammen (Eds.), *Handbook of depression* (3rd ed., pp. 492-512). New York: Guilford.

Gitlin, M., Nuechterlein, K., Subotnik, K. L., Ventura, J., Mintz, J., Fogelson, D. L., Bartzokis, G., & Aravagiri, M. (2001). Clinical outcome following neuroleptic discontinuation in patients with remitted recent-onset schizophrenia. *American Journal of Psychiatry, 158,* 1835-1842.

Glassman, A. (1969). Indoleamines and affective disorders. *Psychosomatic Medicine, 31,* 107-114.

Gleaves, D. H., Hernandez, E., & Warner, M. S. (2003). The etiology of dissociative identity disorder: Reply to Gee, Allen, and Powell (2003). *Professional Psychology: Research & Practice, 34,* 116-118.

Gleaves, D. H., Smith, S. M., Butler, L. D., & Spiegel, D. (2004). False and recovered memories in the laboratory and clinic: A review of experimental and clinical evidence. *Clinical Psychology: Science & Practice, 11,* 3-28.

Glenn, C. R., Franklin, J. C., & Nock, M. K. (2015). Evidence-based psychosocial treatments for self-injurious thoughts and behaviors in youth. *Journal of Clinical Child and Adolescent Psychology, 44,* 1-29.

Glowinski, A. L., Bucholz, K. K., Nelson, E. C., Fu, Q., Madden, P. A. F., Reich, W., & Heath, A. C. (2001). Suicide attempts in an adolescent female twin sample. *Journal of the American Academy of Child & Adolescent Psychiatry, 40,* 1300-1307.

Godfrey, J. R., & Brownell, K. (2008). Toward optimal health: The influence of the environment on obesity. *Journal of Women's Health, 17,* 325-330.

Goikolea, J. M., Colom, F., Martinez-Aran, A., Sanchez-Moreno, J., Giordano, A., Bulbena, A., & Vieta, E. (2007). Clinical and prognostic implications of seasonal pattern in bipolar disorder: A 10-year follow-up of 302 patients. *Psychological Medicine, 37,* 1595-1599.

Goldberg, E. M., & Morrison, S. L. (1963). Schizophrenia and social class. *British Journal of Psychiatry, 109,* 785-802.

Goldin, P. R., & Gross, J. J. (2010). Effects of mindfulness-based stress reduction (MBSR) on emotion regulation in social anxiety disorder. *Emotion, 10,* 83-91.

Gold, M. S., Tabrah, H., & Frost-Pineda, K. (2001). Psychopharmacology of MDMA (ecstasy). *Psychiatric Annals, 31,* 675-681.

Goldschmidt, A. B., Conceição, E. M., Thomas, J. G., Mitchell, J. E., Raynor, H. A., & Bond, D. S. (2016). Conceptualizing and studying binge and loss of control eating in bariatric surgery patients—time for a paradigm shift? *Surgery for Obesity and Related Diseases, 12*(8), 1622-1625.

Goldstein, A. (2001). *Addiction: From biology to drug policy* (2nd ed.). New York: W. H. Freeman.

Goldstein, A. N., & Walker, M. P. (2014). The role of sleep in emotional brain function. *Annual Review of Clinical Psychology, 10,* 679-708.

Goldstein, M. J., Talovic, S. A., Nuechterlein, K. H., & Fogelson, D. L. (1992). Family interaction versus individual psychopathology: Do they indicate the same processes in the families of schizophrenia? *British Journal of Psychiatry, 161,* 97-102.

Goldstein, R. Z., & Volkow, N. D. (2002). Drug addiction and its underlying neurobiological basis: Neuroimaging evidence for the involvement of the frontal cortex. *American Journal of Psychiatry, 159,* 1642-1652.

Goldston, D. B., Daniel, S. S., Erkanli, A., Heilbron, N., Doyle, O., Weller, B., & Sapyta, J. (2015). Suicide attempts in a longitudinal sample of adolescents followed through adulthood: Evidence of escalation. *Journal of Consulting and Clinical Psychology, 83,* 253-264.

Gomes, V. M. G. M., Compte, E. J., Almeida, M., Campos, P. F., Queiroz, A. C. C., Pereira, L. F., . . . de Carvalho, P. H. B. (2020). Psychometric properties of the Muscle Dysmorphic Disorder Inventory among physically active Brazilian college men. *Psychology of Men & Masculinities, 21*(4), 622-631.

Gomez, W., Morales, R., Maracaja-Coutinho, V., Parra, V., & Nassif, M. (2020). Down syndrome and Alzheimer's disease: common molecular traits beyond the amyloid precursor protein. *Aging (Albany NY), 12*(1), 1011.

Gone, J. P. (2010). Psychotherapy and traditional healing for American Indians: Exploring the prospects for therapeutic integration. *Counseling Psychologist, 38,* 166-235.

González, H. M., Tarraf, W., Whitfield, K. E., & Vega, W. A. (2010). The epidemiology of major depression and ethnicity in the United States. *Journal of Psychiatric Research, 44*(15), 1043-1051.

Goodlad, J. K., Marcus, D. K., & Fulton, J. J. (2013). Lead and attention-deficit/hyperactivity disorder (ADHD) symptoms: A meta-analysis. *Clinical Psychology Review, 33*(3), 417-425.

Goodwin, P. J., Leszcz, M., Ennis, M., Koopmans, J., Vincent, L., Guther, H., . . . & Hunter, J. (2001). The effect of group psychosocial support on survival in metastatic breast cancer. *New England Journal of Medicine, 345,* 1719-1726.

Goosby, B. J., Cheadle, J. E., & Mitchell, C. (2018). Stress-related biosocial mechanisms of discrimination and African American health inequities. *Annual Review of Sociology, 44,* 319-340.

Gordon, O. M., Salkovskis, P. M., Oldfield, V. B., & Carter, N. (2013). The association between obsessive compulsive disorder and obsessive compulsive personality disorder: Prevalence and clinical presentation. *British Journal of Clinical Psychology, 52,* 300-315.

Gordon, R. A. (2017). The history of eating disorders. In K. D. Brownell & B. T. Walsh (Eds.), *Eating disorders and obesity: A comprehensive handbook* (3rd ed., pp. 163-168). New York: Guilford Press.

Gordovez, F. J. A., & McMahon, F. J. (2020). The genetics of bipolar disorder. *Molecular Psychiatry,* 1-16.

Gorin-Lazard, A., Baumstarck, K., Boyer, L., Maquigneau, A., Penochet, J. C., Pringuey, D., . . . Auquier, P. (2013). Hormonal therapy is associated with better self-esteem, mood, and quality of life in transsexuals. *Journal of Nervous and Mental Disease, 201*(11), 996-1000.

Gorman, J. M. (2003). Treating generalized anxiety disorder. *Journal of Clinical Psychiatry, 64* (Suppl. 2), 24-29.

Gotlib, I. H., Krasnoperova, E., Yue, D. L., & Joormann, J. (2004). Attentional biases for negative interpersonal stimuli in clinical depression. *Journal of Abnormal Psychology, 113,* 127-135.

Gottesman, I. I., & Shields, J. (1976). A critical review of recent adoption, twin, and family studies of schizophrenia: Behavioral genetics perspectives. *Schizophrenia Bulletin, 2*(3), 360.

Gould, M. S., Greenberg, T., Velting, D. M., & Shaffer, D. (2003). Youth suicide risk and preventive interventions: A review of the past 10 years. *Journal of the American Academy of Child & Adolescent Psychiatry, 42,* 386-405.

Gould, M. S., Marrocco, F., Kleinman, M., Thomas, J. G., Mostkoff, K., Cote, J., & Davies, M. (2005). Evaluating iatrogenic risk of youth suicide screening programs: A randomized controlled trial. *Journal of the American Medical Association, 293,* 1635–1643.

Graber, R., Pichon, F., & Carabine, E. (2015). Psychological resilience. *London: Overseas Development Institute.*

Grabe, S., Ward, L. M., & Hyde, J. S. (2008). The role of the media in body image concerns among women: A meta-analysis of experimental and correlational studies. *Psychological Bulletin, 134,* 460–476.

Grandin, T. (1995). *Thinking in pictures and my other reports from my life with autism.* New York: Vintage Books.

Grandi, S., Fabbri, S., Panatoni, N., Gonnella, E., & Marks, I. (2006). Self-exposure treatment of recurrent nightmares: Waiting-list-controlled trial and 4-year follow-up. *Psychotherapy and Psychosomatics, 75,* 384–388.

Grant, B. F., Hasin, D. S., Chou, S. P., Stinson, F. S., & Dawson, D. A. (2004). Nicotine dependence and psychiatric disorders in the United States: Results from the National Epidemiologic Survey on Alcohol and Related Conditions. *Archives of General Psychiatry, 61,* 1107–1115.

Grant, B. F., Stinson, F., Dawson, D., Chou, P., Dufour, M., Compton, W., . . . Kaplan, K. (2004). Prevalence and co-occurrence of substance use disorders and independent mood and anxiety disorders: Results from the National Epidemiologic Survey on Alcohol and Related Conditions. *Archives of General Psychiatry, 61,* 807–816.

Grant, B. F., Stinson, F. S., Dawson, D. A., Chou, S. P., & Ruan, W. J. (2005). Co-occurrence of *DSM-IV* personality disorders in the United States: Results from the National Epidemiologic Survey on Alcohol and Related Conditions. *Comprehensive Psychiatry, 46,* 1–5.

Grant, J. E., & Chamberlain, S. R. (2016). Trichotillomania. *The American Journal of Psychiatry, 173*(9), 868–874.

Grant, N., Lawrence, M., Preti, A., Wykes, T., & Cella, M. (2017). Social cognition interventions for people with schizophrenia: a systematic review focussing on methodological quality and intervention modality. *Clinical Psychology Review, 56,* 55–64.

Gratz, K. L., Moore, K. E., & Tull, M. T. (2016). The role of emotion dysregulation in the presence, associated difficulties, and treatment of borderline personality disorder. *Personality Disorders: Theory, Research, and Treatment, 7*(4), 344–353.

Gratz, K. L., Rosenthal, M. Z., Tull, M. T., Lejuez, C. W., & Gunderson, J. G. (2010). An experimental investigation of emotional reactivity and delayed emotional recovery in borderline personality disorder: The role of shame. *Comprehensive Psychiatry, 51,* 275–285.

Grazioli, V. S., Bagge, C. L., Studer, J., Bertholet, N., Rougemont-Bücking, A., Mohler-Kuo, M., . . . & Gmel, G. (2018). Depressive symptoms, alcohol use and coping drinking motives: Examining various pathways to suicide attempts among young men. *Journal of Affective Disorders, 232,* 243–251.

Greaves, G. B. (1980). Multiple personality: 165 years after Mary Reynolds. *Journal of Nervous & Mental Disease, 168,* 577–596.

Green, M., Kern, R. S., Braff, D. L., & Mintz, J. (2000). Neurocognitive deficits and functional outcome in Schizophrenia: Are we measuring the "right stuff?" *Schizophrenia Bulletin, 18,* 119–136.

Green, R. (1987). *The "Sissy boy syndrome" and the development of homosexuality.* New Haven, CT: Yale University Press.

Grieve, F. G., & Bonneau-Kaya, C. M. (2007). Weight loss and muscle building content in popular magazines oriented toward women and men. *North American Journal of Psychology, 9*(1), 97–102.

Griffin, P. A., Steadman, H. J., & Petrila, J. (2002). The use of criminal charges and sanctions in mental health courts. *Psychiatric Services, 53,* 1285–1289.

Griffiths, S., Castle, D., Cunningham, M., Murray, S. B., Bastian, B., & Barlow, F. K. (2018). How does exposure to thinspiration and fitspiration relate to symptom severity among individuals with eating disorders? Evaluation of a proposed model. *Body Image, 27,* 187–195.

Grisso, T., & Appelbaum, P. S. (1995). The MacArthur Treatment Competence Study: III. Abilities of patients to consent to psychiatric and medical treatments. *Law & Human Behavior, 19,* 149–174.

Grob, G. N. (1994). *The mad among us: A history of the care of America's mentally ill.* Cambridge, MA: Harvard University Press.

Groesz, L. M., Levine, M. P., & Murnen, S. K. (2002). The effect of experimental presentation of thin media images on body satisfaction: A meta-analytic review. *International Journal of Eating Disorders, 31,* 1–16.

Grossman, L. S., Harrow, M., Rosen, C., Faull, R., & Strauss, G. P. (2008). Sex differences in schizophrenia and other psychotic disorders: A 20-year longitudinal study of psychosis and recovery. *Comprehensive Psychiatry, 49,* 523–529.

Gross, R. T., Brooks-Gunn, J., & Spiker, D. (1992). Efficacy of educational interventions for low birth weight infants: The Infant Health and Development Program. In S. L. Friedman & M. D. Sigman (Eds.), *The psychological development of low birth weight children: Advances in applied developmental psychology* (Vol. 6, pp. 411–433). Norwood, NJ: Ablex.

Groth-Marnat, G., & Wright, A. J. (2016). *Handbook of psychological assessment* (6th ed.). Hoboken, NJ: Wiley.

Grucza, R. A., Bucholz, K. K., Rice, J. P., & Bierut, L. J. (2008). Secular trends in the lifetime prevalence of alcohol dependence in the United States: A re-evaluation. *Alcoholism: Clinical and Experimental Research, 32,* 763–770.

Guérin, E., Dupuis, J. P., Jacob, J. D., & Prud'homme, D. (2019). Incorporating a physical activity program into an assertive community treatment team: Impact and strategies. *Community Mental Health Journal, 55*(8), 1293–1297.

Guarnaccia, P. J., Rivera, M., Franco, F., Neighbors, C., & Allende-Ramos, C. (1996). The experiences of *ataques de nervios:* Toward an anthropology of emotions in Puerto Rico. *Culture, Medicine, & Psychiatry, 15,* 139–165.

Gudenkauf, L. M., Antoni, M. H., Stagl, J. M., Lechner, S. C., Jutagir, D. R., Bouchard, L. C., . . . Carver, C. S. (2015). Brief cognitive-behavioral and relaxation training interventions for breast cancer: A randomized controlled trial. *Journal of Consulting and Clinical Psychology, 83,* 677–688.

Guinle, M., & Sinha, R. (2020). The role of stress, trauma, and negative affect in alcohol misuse and alcohol use disorder in women. *Alcohol Research: Current Reviews, 40*(2), 05. https://doi.org/10.35946/arcr.v40.2.05

Gulliksson, M., Burell, G., Vessby, B., Lundin, L., Toss, H., & Svärdsudd, K. (2011). Randomized controlled trial of cognitive behavioral therapy vs standard treatment to prevent recurrent cardiovascular events in patients with coronary heart disease: Secondary Prevention in Uppsala Primary Health Care project (SUPRIM). *Archives of Internal Medicine, 171*(2), 134–140.

Gunderson, J. G., Herpertz, S. C., Skodol, A. E., Torgersen, S., & Zanarini, M. C. (2018). Borderline personality disorder. *Nature Reviews Disease Primers, 4*(1), 1–20.

Gunderson, J. G., Stout, R. L., McGlashan, T. H., Shea, T., Morey, L. C., Grilo, C. M., . . . Skodol, A. E. (2011). Ten-year course of borderline personality disorder: Psychopathology and function from the Collaborative Longitudinal Personality Disorders Study. *Archive of General Psychiatry, 68,* 827–837.

Gunderson, J. G., Zanarini, M. C., Choi-Kain, L. W.; Mitchell, K. S., Jang, K. L., & Hudson, J. I. (2011). Family study of borderline personality disorder and its sectors of psychopathology. *Archives of General Psychiatry, 68,* 753–762.

Guo, X., Zhai, J., Liu, Z., Fang, M., Wang, B., Wang, C., . . . & Zhao, J. (2010). Effect of antipsychotic medication alone vs. combined with psychosocial intervention on outcomes of early-stage schizophrenia. *Archive of General Psychiatry, 67*(9): 895–904.

Gur, R. E., Calkins, M. E., Gur, R. C., Horan, W. P., Nuechterlein, K. H., Seidman, L. J., & Stone, W. S. (2007). The Consortium on the Genetics of Schizophrenia: Neurocognitive endophenotypes. *Schizophrenia Bulletin, 33,* 49–68.

Gustavsson, A., Svensson, M., Jacobi, F., Allgulander, C., Alonso, J., Beghi, E., . . . CDBE2010 Study Group., (2011). Cost of disorders of the brain in Europe 2010. *European Neuropsychopharmacology, 21,* 718–779.

H

Häfner, H. (2019). From onset and prodromal stage to a life-long course of schizophrenia and its symptom dimensions: how sex, age, and other risk factors influence incidence and course of illness. *Psychiatry Journal, 2019.* https://doi.org/10.1155/2019/9804836

Håkansson, A. (2020). Impact of COVID-19 on online gambling–a general population survey during the pandemic. *Frontiers in Psychology, 11,* 2588.

Håkansson, A., & Widinghoff, C. (2020). Over-Indebtedness and problem gambling in a general population sample of online gamblers. *Frontiers in Psychiatry, 11,* 7. https://doi.org/10.3389/fpsyt.2020.00007

Hachinski, V. (2008). World Stroke Day 2008: "Little strokes, big trouble." *Stroke, 39,* 2407–2420.

Haddad, P. M., & Correll, C. U. (2018). The acute efficacy of antipsychotics in schizophrenia: A review of recent meta-analyses. *Therapeutic Advances in Psychopharmacology, 8*(11), 303–318.

Hail, L., & Le Grange, D. (2018). Bulimia nervosa in adolescents: Prevalence and treatment challenges. *Adolescent Health, Medicine and Therapeutics, 9,* 11–16.

Haliczer, L. A., Dixon-Gordon, K. L., Law, K. C., Anestis, M. D., Rosenthal, M. Z., & Chapman, A. L. (2019). Emotion regulation difficulties and borderline personality disorder: The moderating role of race. *Personality Disorders: Theory, Research, and Treatment, 11*(4), 280–289.

Halldorsdottir, T., & Binder, E. B. (2017). Gene × environment interactions: From molecular mechanisms to behavior. *Annual Review of Psychology, 68,* 215–241.

Hall, G. C. N. (2001). Psychotherapy research with ethnic minorities: Empirical, ethical, and conceptual issues. *Journal of Consulting & Clinical Psychology, 69,* 502–510.

Hall, K. S. K. (2016). Multicultural sensitivity in the treatment of sexual dysfunction. In L. Lipshultz, A. Pastuszak, A. Goldstein, A. Giraldi, & M. Perelman (Eds.), *Management of sexual dysfunction in men and women* (pp. 25–29). New York: Springer.

Hall, K. S. K., & Graham, C. A. (2013). *The cultural context of sexual pleasure and problems: Psychotherapy with diverse clients.* New York: Routledge.

Hallmayer, J., Cleveland, S., Torres, A., Phillips, J., Cohen, B., Torigoe, T., . . . Risch, N. (2011). Genetic heritability and shared environmental factors among twin pairs with autism. *Archives of General Psychiatry, 68*(11), 1095–1102.

Halpern, A. L. (2011). The proposed diagnosis of hypersexual disorder for inclusion in *DSM-5*: Unnecessary and harmful. *Archives of Sexual Behavior, 40,* 487–488, author reply 489–490.

Hames, J. L., Hagan, C. R., & Joiner, T. E. (2013). Interpersonal processes in depression. *Annual Review of Clinical Psychology, 9,* 355–377.

Hammen, C. (2003). Social stress and women's risk for recurrent depression. *Archives of Women's Mental Health, 6,* 9–13.

Hammen, C. (2018). Risk factors for depression: An autobiographical review. *Annual Review of Clinical Psychology, 14.*

Hanachi, M., Pleple, A., Barry, C., Dicembre, M., Latour, E., Duquesnoy, M., . . . & Fayssoil, A. (2020). Echocardiographic abnormalities in 124 severely malnourished adult anorexia nervosa patients: Frequency and relationship with body composition and biological features. *Journal of Eating Disorders, 8*(1), 1–8.

Handley, E. D., & Chassin, L. (2009). Intergenerational transmission of alcohol expectancies in a high-risk sample. *Journal of Studies on Alcohol and Drugs, 70*(5), 675–682.

Haney, C. (2017). "Madness" and penal confinement: Some observations on mental illness and prison pain. *Punishment & Society, 19*(3), 310–326.

Hanson, R. F., Borntrager, C., Self-Brown, S., Kilpatrick, D. G., Saunders, B. E., Resnick, H. S., & Amstadter, A. (2008). Relations among gender, violence exposure, and mental health: The national survey of adolescents. *The American Journal of Orthopsychiatry, 78*(3), 313–321.

Hantoosh, S. F., Ameen, R. S., & Amin, S. S. (2021). Antisocial behavior etiologies. *Iraqi National Journal of Medicine, 3*(1), 49–61. DOI: https://doi.org/10.37319/iqnjm.3.1.6

Hantsoo, L., & Epperson, C. N. (2015). Premenstrual dysphoric disorder: Epidemiology and treatment. *Current Psychiatry Reports, 17*(11), 87.

Harbison, A. L., Woynaroski, T. G., Tapp, J., Wade, J. W., Warlaumont, A. S., & Yoder, P. J. (2018). A new measure of child vocal reciprocity in children with autism spectrum disorder. *Autism Research, 11*(6), 903–915.

Harding, D. (2019, November 13). Signs of depression. symptoms and treatment - patient. Retrieved December 15, 2020, from https://patient.info/doctor/depression-pro

Hare, R. D., & Hart, S. D. (1993). Psychopathy, mental disorder, and crime. In S. Hodgins (Ed.), *Mental disorder and crime* (pp. 104–115). Thousand Oaks, CA: Sage.

Hare, R. D., & Neumann, C. S. (2008). Psychopathy as a clinical and empirical construct. *Annual Review of Clinical Psychology, 4,* 217–246.

Harold, G. T., Leve, L. D., Barrett, D., Elam, K., Neiderhiser, J. M., Natsuaki, M. N., . . . Thapar, A. (2013). Biological and rearing mother influences on child ADHD symptoms: Revisiting the developmental interface between nature and nurture. *Journal of Child Psychology and Psychiatry, 54*(10), 1038–1046.

Harrell, J. P. (1980). Psychological factors and hypertension: A status report. *Psychological Bulletin, 87,* 482–501.

Harriger, J. A., Schaefer, L. M., Thompson, J. K., & Cao, L. (2019). You can buy a child a curvy Barbie doll, but you can't make her like it: Young girls' beliefs about Barbie dolls with diverse shapes and sizes. *Body Image, 30,* 107–113.

Harris, I. M., Beese, S., & Moore, D. (2019). Predicting future self-harm or suicide in adolescents: A systematic review of risk assessment scales/tools. *BMJ Open, 9*(9).

Harris, K., & Singer, H. S. (2006). Tic disorders: Neural circuits, neurochemistry, and neuroimmunology. *Journal of Child Neurology, 21,* 678–689.

Harrow, M., Grossman, L. S., Jobe, T. H., & Herbener, E. S. (2005). Do patients with schizophrenia ever show periods of recovery? A 15-year multi-follow-up study. *Schizophrenia Bulletin, 31,* 723–734.

Harvey, A. G. (2005). A cognitive theory and therapy for chronic insomnia. *Journal of Cognitive Psychotherapy, 19,* 41–59.

Harvey, A. G. (2008a). Insomnia, psychiatric disorders, and the transdiagnostic perspective. *Current Directions in Psychological Science, 17,* 299–303.

Harvey, A. G. (2008b). Sleep and circadian rhythms in bipolar disorder: Seeking synchrony, harmony, and regulation. *American Journal of Psychiatry, 165,* 820–829.

Harvey, A. G., Bélanger, L., Talbot, L., Eidelman, P., Beaulieu-Bonneau, S., Fortier-Brochu, É., et al. (2014). Comparative efficacy of behavior therapy, cognitive therapy, and cognitive behavior therapy for chronic insomnia: A randomized controlled trial. *Journal of Consulting and Clinical Psychology, 82*(4), 670–683.

Harvey, A. G., & Buysse, D. J. (2017). *Treating sleep problems: A transdiagnostic approach.* New York: Guilford.

Harvey, A. G., Soehner, A. M., Kaplan, K. A., Hein, K., Lee, J., Kanady, J. L., . . . Buysse, D. J. (2015). Treating insomnia improves mood state, sleep, and functioning in bipolar disorder: A pilot randomized controlled trial. *Journal of Consulting and Clinical Psychology, 83,* 564–577.

Harvey, A. G., Watkins, E., Mansell, W., & Shafran, R. (2004). *Cognitive behavioural processes across psychological disorders: A transdiagnostic approach to research and treatment.* Oxford: Oxford University Press.

Harwood, D. M. J., Hawton, K., Hope, T., & Jacoby, R. (2000). Suicide in older people: Mode of death, demographic factors, and medical contact before death. *International Journal of Geriatric Psychiatry, 15,* 736–743.

Hashimoto K. (2020). Risk of neuropsychiatric disorders in offspring of COVID-19-infected pregnant women and nutritional intervention. *European Archives of Psychiatry and Clinical Neuroscience,* 1–3. Advance online publication. https://doi.org/10.1007/s00406-020-01148-5

Hasin, D., Sarvet, A., Meyers, J., Saha, T., Ruan, J., Stohl, M., & Grant, B. (2018). Epidemiology of adult *DSM-5* major depressive disorder and its specifiers in the United States. *JAMA Psychiatry, 75*(4):336–346. doi: 10.1001/jamapsychiatry.2017.4602

Hasin, D. S., Fenton, M. C., Beseler, C., Park, J. Y., & Wall, M. M. (2012). Analysis related to the development of *DSM-5* criteria for substance use related disorders: 2. Proposed *DSM-5* criteria for alcohol, cannabis, cocaine, and heroin disorders in 663 substance abuse patients. *Drug and Alcohol Dependence, 122,* 28–37.

Hasin, D. S., Fenton, M. C., Skodol, A., Krueger, R., Keyes, K., Geier, T., . . . Grant, B. (2011). Personality disorders and the 3-year course of alcohol, drug, and nicotine use disorders. *Archives of General Psychiatry, 68,* 1158–1167.

Hasin, D. S., Saha, T. D., Kerridge, B. T., Goldstein, R. B., Chou, S. P., Zhang, H., . . . Grant, B. F. (2015). Prevalence of marijuana use disorders in the United States between 2001–2002 and 2012–2013. *JAMA Psychiatry, 72*(12), 1235–1242.

Hasin, D. S., Sarvet, A. L., Meyers, J. L., Saha, T. D., Ruan, W. J., . . . Grant, B. F. (2017). Epidemiology of adult *DSM-5* major depressive disorder and its specifiers in the United States. *JAMA Psychiatry, 75*(4), 336–346.

Hasin, D. S., Stinson, F. S., Ogburn, E., & Grant, B. F. (2007). Prevalence, correlates, disability and comorbidity of *DSM-IV* alcohol abuse and dependence in the United States: Results from the National Epidemiologic Survey on alcohol and related conditions. *Archives of General Psychiatry, 64,* 830–842.

Hatzenbuehler, M. L. (2009). How does sexual minority stigma "get under the skin"? A psychological mediation framework. *Psychological Bulletin, 135,* 707–730.

Hatzenbuehler, M. L. (2016). Structural stigma: Research evidence and implications for psychological science. *American Psychologist, 71*(8), 742–751.

Hauck, T. S., Lau, C., Wing, L. L. F., Kurdyak, P., & Tu, K. (2017). ADHD treatment in primary care: Demographic factors, medication trends, and treatment predictors. *The Canadian Journal of Psychiatry, 62*(6), 393–402.

Haukvik, U. K., Gurholt, T. P., Nerland, S., Elvsåshagen, T., Akudjedu, T. N., Alda, M., . . . & Benedetti, F. (2020). In vivo hippocampal subfield volumes in bipolar disorder—A mega-analysis from the enhancing neuro imaging genetics through meta-analysis bipolar disorder working group. *Human Brain Mapping.* doi: 10.1002/hbm.25249

Hausenblas, H. A., Campbell, A., Menzel, J. E., Doughty, J., Levine, M., & Thompson, J. K. (2013). Media effects of experimental presentation of the ideal physique on eating disorder symptoms: A meta-analysis of laboratory studies. *Clinical Psychology Review, 33*(1), 168–181.

Haw, C., Hawton, K., Niedzwiedz, C., & Platt, S. (2013). Suicide clusters: A review of risk factors and mechanisms. *Suicide and Life-Threatening Behavior, 43*(1), 97–108.

Hawton, K., Saunders, K. E., & O'Connor, R. C. (2012). Self-harm and suicide in adolescents. *Lancet, 379*(9834), 2373–2382.

Hayes, J. A., Petrovich, J., Janis, R. A., Yang, Y., Castonguay, L. G., & Locke, B. D. (2020). Suicide among college students in psychotherapy: Individual predictors and latent classes. *Journal of Counseling Psychology, 67*(1), 104–114.

Hayes, S. C., Luoma, J. B., Bond, F. W., Masuda, A., & Lillis, J. (2006). Acceptance and commitment therapy: Model, processes, and outcomes. *Behaviour Research and Therapy, 44,* 1–25.

Haynes, P. L., Gengler, D., & Kelly, M. (2016). Social rhythm therapies for mood disorders: An update. *Current Psychiatry Reports, 18*(8), 75.

Hayward, C., Killen, J. D., Kraemer, H. C., & Taylor, C. B. (2000). Predictors of panic attacks in adolescents. *Journal of the American Academy of Child & Adolescent Psychiatry, 39,* 207–214.

Hebert, L. E., Weuve, J., Scherr, P. A., & Evans, D. A. (2013). Alzheimer disease in the United States (2010–2050) estimated using the 2010 census. *Neurology, 80*(19), 1778–1783.

Heckers, S., Barch, D. M., Bustillo, J., Gaebel, W., Gur, R., Malaspina, D., . . . Carpenter, W. (2013). Structure of the psychotic disorders classification in *DSM 5. Schizophrenia Research, 13,* 255–257.

Hedley, A. A., Ogden, C. L., Johnson, C. L., Carroll, M. D., Curtin, L. R., & Flegal, K. M. (2004). Prevalence of overweight and obesity among U.S. children, adolescents, and adults, 1999–2002. *Journal of the American Medical Association, 291,* 2847–2850.

Hedman, E., & Axelsson, E. (2017). Severe health anxiety in the somatic symptom and related disorders. Treatments for psychological problems and syndromes. In D. McKay, J. S. Abramowitz, & E. A. Storch (Eds.), *Treatments for psychological problems and syndromes* (pp. 345–359). Hoboken, NJ: Wiley & Sons.

Hefter, D., Marti, H. H., Gass, P., & Inta, D. (2018). Perinatal hypoxia and ischemia in animal models of schizophrenia. *Frontiers in Psychiatry, 9,* 106.

Heiman, J. R. (2000). Orgasmic disorders in women. In S. R. Leiblum & R. C. Rosen (Eds.), Principles and practice of sex therapy (3rd ed., pp. 118–153). New York: Guilford Press.

Heimberg, R. G., Brozovich, F. A., & Rapee, R. M. (2010). A cognitive-behavioral model of social anxiety disorder: Update and extension. In S. G. Hofmann & P. M. DiBartolo (Eds.), *Social anxiety: Clinical, developmental, and social perspectives* (2nd ed., pp. 395–422). New York: Academic Press.

Heim, C., Meinlschmidt, G., & Nemeroff, C. B. (2003). Neurobiology of early-life stress. *Psychiatric Annals, 33,* 18–26.

Heim, C., & Nemeroff, C. B. (2001). The role of childhood trauma in the neurobiology of mood and anxiety disorders: Preclinical and clinical studies. *Biological Psychiatry, 49*, 1023-1039.

Heim, C., Plotsky, P. M., & Nemeroff, C. B. (2004). Importance of studying the contributions of early adverse experience to neurobiological findings in depression. *Neuropsychopharmacology, 29*, 641-648.

Heinz, A., Deserno, L., & Reininghaus, U. (2013). Urbanicity, social adversity and psychosis. *World Psychiatry, 12*(3), 187-197.

Heiser, N. A., Turner, S. M., & Beidel, D. C. (2003). Shyness: Relationship to social phobia and other psychiatric disorders. *Behaviour Research & Therapy, 41*, 209-221.

Heiss, J., Swavola, E., & Kang-Brown, J. (2015, October 20). Incarceration's Front Door. Retrieved October 21, 2020, from https://www.vera.org/publications/incarcerations-front-door-the-misuse-of-jails-in-america

Helgeland, M. I., & Torgersen, S. (2004). Developmental antecedents of borderline personality disorder. *Comprehensive Psychiatry, 45*, 138-147.

Helgesen, A. K., Adan, Y. H., Dybvik Bjørglund, C., Weberg-Haugen, C., Johannessen, M., Åsmul Kristiansen, K., . . . Abrahamsen Grøndahl, V. (2020). Nurses' experiences of delirium and how to identify delirium—A qualitative study. *Nursing Open*.

Helgeson, V. S., Snyder, P., & Seltman, H. (2004). Psychological and physical adjustment to breast cancer over 4 years: Identifying distinct trajectories of change. *Health Psychology, 23*, 3-15.

Helseth, S. A., Waschbusch, D. A., King, S., & Willoughby, M. T. (2015). Aggression in children with conduct problems and callous-unemotional traits: Social information processing and response to peer provocation. *Journal of Abnormal Child Psychology, 43*(8), 1503-1514.

Helzer, J. E., Kraemer, H. C., Krueger, R. F., Wittchen, H.-U., Sirovatka, P. J., & Regier, D. A. (2008). *Dimensional approaches in diagnostic classification: Refining the research agenda for DSM-V.* Arlington, VA: American Psychiatric Association.

Hendricks, L., Daugherty, J. L., & Dang, Q. (2017). Phencyclidine ("PCP"): A dangerous drug impacting youth. *Journal of Substance Abuse & Alcoholism, 5*(4), 1065.

Hengartner, M. P., & Moncrieff, J. (2018). Inconclusive evidence in support of the dopamine hypothesis of psychosis: Why neurobiological research must consider medication use, adjust for important confounders, choose stringent comparators, and use larger samples. *Frontiers in Psychiatry, 9*, 174.

Henningsen P. (2018). Management of somatic symptom disorder. *Dialogues in clinical neuroscience, 20*(1), 23-31. https://doi.org/10.31887/DCNS.2018.20.1/phenningsen

Henriksen, M. G., Nordgaard, J., & Jansson, L. B. (2017). Genetics of schizophrenia: overview of methods, findings and limitations. *Frontiers in Human Neuroscience, 11*, 322.

Herbenick, D., Bowling, J., Fu, T. J., Dodge, B., Guerra-Reyes, L., & Sanders, S. (2017). Sexual diversity in the United States: Results from a nationally representative probability sample of adult women and men. *PloS One, 12*(7), e0181198.

Herbert, J. D., Gaudiano, B. A., Rheingold, A. A., Myers, V. H., Dalrymple, K., & Nolan, E. M. (2005). Social skills training augments the effectiveness of cognitive behavioral group therapy for social anxiety disorder. *Behavior Therapy, 36*, 125-138.

Herman, J. P., McKlveen, J. M., Ghosal, S., Kopp, B., Wulsin, A., Makinson, R., . . . Myers, B. (2016). Regulation of the hypothalamic-pituitary-adrenocortical stress response. *Comprehensive Physiology, 6*(2), 603-621.

Hettema, J. M., Neale, M. C., & Kendler, K. S. (2001). A review and meta-analysis of the genetic epidemiology of anxiety disorders. *American Journal of Psychiatry, 158*, 1568-1578.

Hewage, K., Steel, Z., Mohsin, M., Tay, A. K., De Oliveira, J. C., Da Piedade, M., . . . & Silove, D. (2018). A wait-list controlled study of a trauma-focused cognitive behavioral treatment for intermittent explosive disorder in Timor-Leste. *American Journal of Orthopsychiatry, 88*(3), 282.

Heylens, G., De Cuypere, G., Zucker, K. J., Schelfaut, C., Elaut, E., VandenBossche, H., De Baere, E., & T'Sjoen, G. (2012). Gender identity disorder in twins: A review of the case report literature. *Journal of Sexual Medicine, 9*, 751-757.

Higgins, S. T., Sigmon, S. C., & Heil, S. H. (2014). Drug use disorders. In D. H. Barlow (Ed.), *Clinical handbook of psychological disorders: A step-by-step treatment manual* (pp. 588-616). New York: Guilford.

Higgins, S. & Wysong, A. (2017). Cosmetic surgery and body dysmorphic disorder – an update. *International Journal of Women's Dermatology, 4*(1), 43-48.

Hilbert, A., Pike, K. M., Goldschmidt, A. B., Wilfley, D. E., Fairburn, C. G., Dohm, F. A., . . . Weissman, R. S. (2014). Risk factors across the eating disorders. *Psychiatry Research, 220*(1), 500-506.

Hilbert, A., Wilfley, D. E., Dohm, F.-A., & Striegel-Moore, R. H. (2011). Characterization, significance, and predictive validity of binge size in binge eating disorder. In R. H. Striegel-Moore, S. A. Wonderlich, B. T. Walsh, & J. E. Mitchell (Eds.), *Developing an evidence-based classification of eating disorders: Scientific findings for DSM-5* (pp. 47-66). Washington, DC: American Psychiatric Association.

Hilgard, E. R. (1977/1986). *Divided consciousness: Multiple controls in human thought and action.* New York: Wiley.

Hilgard, E. R. (1992). Divided consciousness and dissociation. *Consciousness & Cognition: An International Journal, 1*, 16-31.

Hill, A. J., & Franklin, J. A. (1998). Mothers, daughters, and dieting: Investigating the transmission of weight control. *British Journal of Clinical Psychology, 37*, 3-13.

Hillman, J. (2017). Treating sexual problems in aging adults. In Z. D. Peterson (Ed.), *The Wiley handbook of sex therapy* (pp. 324-344). Oxford: Wiley.

Himmerich, H., Kan, C., Au, K., & Treasure, J. (2020). Pharmacological treatment of eating disorders, comorbid mental health problems, malnutrition and physical health consequences. *Pharmacology & Therapeutics*, 107667.

Hines, M., Ahmed, S. F., & Hughes, I. A. (2003). Psychological outcomes and gender-related development in complete androgen insensitivity syndrome. *Archives of Sexual Behavior, 32*, 93-101.

Hingle, M. D., Wertheim, B. C., Tindle, H. A., Tinker, L., Seguin, R. A., Rosal, M. C., & Thomson, C. A. (2014). Optimism and diet quality in the Women's Health Initiative. *Journal of the Academy of Nutrition and Dietetics, 114*(7), 1036-1045.

Hinshaw, S. P. (2018). Attention deficit hyperactivity disorder (ADHD): Controversy, developmental mechanisms, and multiple levels of analysis. *Annual Review of Clinical Psychology, 14*, 291-316.

Hintsanen, M., Kivimaki, M., Elovainio, M., Pulkki-Raback, L., Keskivaara, P., Juonala, M., . . . Keltikangas-Jarvinen, L. (2005). Job strain and early atherosclerosis: The cardiovascular risk in young finns study. *Psychosomatic Medicine, 67*, 740-747.

Hiroto, D. S., & Seligman, M. E. (1975). Generality of learned helplessness in man. *Journal of Personality and Social Psychology, 31*(2), 311-327. Retrieved from https://doi.org/10.1037/h0076270

Hirschtritt, M. E., Bloch, M. H., & Mathews, C. A. (2017). Obsessive-compulsive disorder: Advances in diagnosis and treatment. *Journal of the American Medical Association, 317*(13), 1358-1367.

Hirshkowitz, M., Whiton, K., Albert, S. M., Alessi, C., Bruni, O., DonCarlos, L., . . . Hillard, P. J. A. (2015). National Sleep Foundation's sleep time duration recommendations: Methodology and results summary. *Sleep Health, 1*(1), 40–43.

Hölzelab, B., Hogea, E., Grevea, D., Gardab, T., Creswel, T., Kirk, C., . . . Lazara, S. (2013). Neural mechanisms of symptom improvements in generalized anxiety disorder following mindfulness training. *NeuroImage: Clinical, 2,* 448–458.

Hobfoll, S. E., Blais, R. K., Stevens, N. R., Walt, L., & Gengler, R. (2016). Vets prevail online intervention reduces PTSD and depression in veterans with mild-to-moderate symptoms. *Journal of Consulting and Clinical Psychology, 84,* 31–42.

Hobson, C. W., Scott, S., & Rubia, K. (2011). Investigation of cool and hot executive function in ODD/CD independently of ADHD. *Journal of Child Psychology and Psychiatry, 52*(10), 1035–1043.

Hockenberry, M. S., & Masson P. (2016). Hormonal evaluation and therapy of erectile dysfunction. In T. S. Köhler & K. T. McVary (Eds.), *Contemporary treatment of erectile dysfunction: A clinical guide* (pp. 85–100). Cham: Springer.

Hoek, H. W., van Harten, P. N., Hermans, K. M. E., Katzman, M. A., Matroos, G. E., & Susser, E. S. (2005). The incidence of anorexia nervosa on Curaçao. *American Journal of Psychiatry, 162,* 748–752.

Hoge, C. W., Castro, C. A., Messer, S. C., McGurk, D., Cotting, D. I., & Koffman, R. L. (2004). Combat duty in Iraq and Afghanistan, mental health problems, and barriers to care. *New England Journal of Medicine, 351,* 13–22.

Hoge, E., Bickham, D., & Cantor, J. (2017). Digital media, anxiety, and depression in children. *Pediatrics, 140*(2), 76–80.

Hoge, S. K., Poythress, N., Bonnie, R. J., Monahan, J., Eisenberg, M., & Feucht-Haviar, T. (1997). The MacArthur Adjudicative Competence Study: Diagnosis, psychopathology, and competence-related abilities. *Behavioral Sciences & the Law, 15,* 329–345.

Holden, C. (1980). Identical twins reared apart. *Science, 207*(4437), 1323–1328.

Holland, K. M., Vivolo-Kantor, A. M., Logan, J. E., & Leemis, R. W. (2017). Antecedents of suicide among youth aged 11–15: A multistate mixed methods analysis. *Journal of Youth and Adolescence, 46*(7), 1598–1610.

Hollon, S. D., DeRubeis, R. J., Shelton, R. C., Amsterdam, J. D., Salomon, R. M., O'Reardon, J. P., . . . Gallop. R. (2005). Prevention or relapse following cognitive therapy versus medications in moderate to severe depression. *Archives of General Psychiatry, 62,* 417–422.

Hollon, S. D., & Dimidjian, S. (2015). Cognitive and behavioral treatment of depression. In I. H. Gotlib & C. L. Hammen (Eds.), *Handbook of depression* (3rd ed., pp. 513–531). New York: Guilford Press.

Holm-Denoma, J. M., Scaringi, V., Gordon, K. H., van Orden, K. A., & Joiner, T. E., Jr. (2009). Eating disorder symptoms among undergraduate varsity athletes, club athletes, independent exercisers, and nonexercisers. *International Journal of Eating Disorders, 42,* 47–53.

Holmes, S. E., Hinz, R., Conen, S., Gregory, C. J., Matthews, J. C., Anton-Rodriguez, J. M., . . . & Talbot, P. S. (2018). Elevated translocator protein in anterior cingulate in major depression and a role for inflammation in suicidal thinking: a positron emission tomography study. *Biological Psychiatry, 83*(1), 61–69.

Holoyda, B. J., & Kellaher, D. C. (2016). The biological treatment of paraphilic disorders: An updated review. *Current Psychiatry Reports, 18*(2), 19.

Holtom-Viesel, A., & Allan, S. (2014). A systematic review of the literature on family functioning across all eating disorder diagnoses in comparison to control families. *Clinical Psychology Review, 34*(1), 29–43.

Hoogman, M., Bralten, J., Hibar, D. P., Mennes, M., Zwiers, M. P., Schweren, L. S., et al. (2017). Subcortical brain volume differences in participants with attention deficit hyperactivity disorder in children and adults: A cross-sectional mega-analysis. *Lancet Psychiatry, 4*(4), 310–319.

Hooley, J. M. (2007). Expressed emotion and relapse of psychopathology. *Annual Review of Clinical Psychology, 3,* 329–352.

Hooley, J. M., & Campbell, C. (2002). Control and controllability: Beliefs and behaviour in high and low expressed emotion relatives. *Psychological Medicine, 32,* 1091–1099.

Hopkins, P. & Shook, N. (2017). A review of sociocultural factors that may underlie differences in African American and European American anxiety. *Journal of Anxiety Disorders, 49,* 104–113.

Hopko, D. R., Robertson, S. M. C., Widman, L., & Lejuez, C. W. (2008). Specific phobias. In M. Hersenand & J. Rosqvist (Eds.), *The handbook of assessment, conceptualization, and treatment (HACT)* (pp. 139–170). New York: John Wiley.

Hopper, K. (2008). Outcomes elsewhere: Course of psychosis in "other cultures." In C. Morgan, K. McKenzie, & P. Fearon (Eds.), *Society and psychosis* (pp. 198–216). Cambridge: Cambridge University Press.

Hopwood, T. L., & Schutte, N. S. (2017). A meta-analytic investigation of the impact of mindfulness-based interventions on post traumatic stress. *Clinical Psychology Review, 57,* 12–20.

Hornbacher, M. (1998). *Wasted.* New York: HarperPerennial.

Hornberger, L. L., & Lane, M. A. (2021). Identification and management of eating disorders in children and adolescents. *Pediatrics, 147*(1).

Houtsma, C., Butterworth, S. E., & Anestis, M. D. (2018). Firearm suicide: Pathways to risk and methods of prevention. *Current Opinion in Psychology, 22,* 7–11.

Howard, A. L., Robinson, M., Smith, G. J., Ambrosini, G. L., Piek, J. P., & Oddy, W. H. (2011). ADHD is associated with a "western" dietary pattern in adolescents. *Journal of Attention Disorders, 15,* 403–411.

Howard, D. M., Adams, M. J., Toni-Kim, C., Hafferty, J. D., Gibson, J., Masoud, S., . . . McIntosh, A. M. (2019). Genome-wide meta-analysis of depression identifies 102 independent variants and highlights the importance of the prefrontal brain regions. *Nature Neuroscience, 22*(3), 343–352.

Howard, M. O., Perron, B. E., Vaughn, M. G., Bender, K. A., & Garland, E. (2010). Inhalant use, inhalant-use disorders, and antisocial behavior: Findings from the National Epidemiologic Survey on Alcohol and Related Conditions (NESARC). *Journal of Studies on Alcohol and Drugs, 71,* 201–209.

Howell, E. F. (2011). Understanding and treating dissociative identity disorder: A relational approach. Routledge. ISBN 1135845832. 4

Howell, P. (2007). Signs of developmental stuttering up to age eight and at 12 plus. *Clinical Psychology Review, 27,* 287–306.

Howes, O. D., McCutcheon, R., Owen, M. J., & Murray, R. M. (2017). The role of genes, stress, and dopamine in the development of schizophrenia. *Biological Psychiatry, 81*(1), 9–20.

Howes, O. D., & Murray, R. M. (2014). Schizophrenia: An integrated sociodevelopmental-cognitive model. *Lancet, 383*(9929), 1677–1687.

Howes, O., McCutcheon, R., & Stone, J. (2015). Glutamate and dopamine in schizophrenia: An update for the 21st century. *Journal of Psychopharmacology, 29*(2), 97–115.

Howland, L. C., Gortmaker, S. L., Mofenson, L. M., Spino, C., Gardner, J. D., Gorski, H., . . . Oleske, J. (2000). Effects of negative life events on immune suppression in children and youth infected with human immunodeficiency virus type 1. *Pediatrics, 106,* 540–546.

Howlin, P., Goode, S., Hutton, J., & Rutter, M. (2004). Adult outcome for children with autism. *Journal of Child Psychology & Psychiatry, 45,* 212–229.

How P.C., Lo P., Xiong G.L. (2018) Major or Mild Neurocognitive Disorders with Lewy Bodies. In: Hategan A., Bourgeois J., Hirsch C., Giroux C. (eds) *Geriatric psychiatry*. Springer, Cham. https://doi.org/10.1007/978-3-319-67555-8_20

Hoza, B., Mrug, S., Verdes, A. C., Hinshaw, S. P., Bukowski, W. M., Gold, J. A., . . . Arnold, L. E. (2005). What aspects of peer relationships are impaired in children with attention-deficit/hyperactivity disorder? *Journal of Consulting and Clinical Psychology, 73,* 411–423.

Hua, A., & Major, N. (2016, February). Selective mutism. *Current Opinion in Pediatrics, 28*(1) 114–120.

Hua, A., Major, N. (February 2016). Selective mutism. *Current Opinion in Pediatrics,* 28(1) 114–120. doi: 10.1097/MOP.0000000000000300

Huang, Y., Wang, Y., Zeng, L., Yang, J., Song, X., Rao, W., . . . Zhang, X. (2020, August 14). Prevalence and Correlation of Anxiety, Insomnia and Somatic Symptoms in a Chinese Population During the COVID-19 Epidemic. Retrieved December 07, 2020, from https://www.frontiersin.org/articles/10.3389/fpsyt.2020.568329/full

Hublin, C., Kaprio, J., Partinen, M., Heikkilä, K., & Koskenvuo, M. (1997). Prevalence and genetics of sleepwalking: A population-based twin study. *Neurology, 48,* 177–181.

Hucker, S. J. (2008). Sexual masochism: Psychopathology and theory. In D. R. Laws & W. T. O'Donohue (Eds.), *Sexual deviance: Theory, assessment, and treatment* (pp. 250–264). New York: Guilford Press.

Hudson, J. I., Hiripi, E., Pope, H. G., & Kessler, R. C. (2007). The prevalence and correlates of eating disorders in the National Comorbidity Survey Replication. *Biological Psychiatry, 61,* 348–358.

Hudziak, J. J., van Beijsterveldt, C. E. M., Althoff, R. R., Stanger, C., Rettew, D. C., Nelson, E. C., . . . Boomsma, D. I. (2004). Genetic and environmental contributions to the Child Behavior Checklist Obsessive-Compulsive Scale: A cross-cultural twin study. *Archives of General Psychiatry, 61,* 608–616.

Huerta, M., Bishop, S. L., Duncan, A., Hus, V., & Lord, C. (2012). Application of *DSM-5* criteria for autism spectrum disorder to three samples of children with *DSM-IV* diagnoses of pervasive developmental disorders. *American Journal of Psychiatry, 169* (10), 1056–1064.

Hugdahl K. (2017). Auditory hallucinations as translational psychiatry: Evidence from magnetic resonance imaging. *Balkan Medical Journal, 34*(6), 504–513. https://doi.org/10.4274/balkanmedj.2017.1226

Hugdahl, K., & Ohman, A. (1977). Effects of instruction on acquisition and extinction of electrodermal response to fear-relevant stimuli. *Journal of Experimental Psychiatry: Human Learning & Memory, 3,* 608–618.

Hugdahl, K., & Sommer, I. E. (2018). Auditory verbal hallucinations in schizophrenia from a levels of explanation perspective. *Schizophrenia Bulletin, 44*(2), 234–241.

Hughes, A., Brewer, G., & Khan, R. (2020). Sexual coercion by women: The influence of pornography and narcissistic and histrionic personality disorder traits. *Archives of Sexual Behavior, 49*(3), 885–894.

Hughes, T. L., Wilsnack, S. C., & Kantor, L. W. (2016). The influence of gender and sexual orientation on alcohol use and alcohol-related problems: Toward a global perspective. *Alcohol Research: Current Reviews, 38*(1), 121–132.

Hughes, T., McCabe, S. E., Wilsnack, S. C., West, B. T., & Boyd, C. J. (2010). Victimization and substance use disorders in a national sample of heterosexual and sexual minority women and men. *Addiction, 105,* 2130–2140.

Hultman, C. M., Sandin, S., Levine, S. Z., Lichtenstein, P., & Reichenberg, A. (2011). Advancing paternal age and risk of autism: New evidence from a population-based study and a meta-analysis of epidemiological studies. *Molecular Psychiatry, 16*(12), 1203–1212.

Humeau, Y., Gambino, F., Chelly, J., & Vitale, N. (2009). X-linked mental retardation: Focus on synaptic function and plasticity. *Neurochemistry, 109,* 1–14.

Humphreys, K., Nelson, C., Fox, N., & Zeanah, C. (2017). Signs of reactive attachment disorder and disinhibited social engagement disorder at age 12 years: Effects of institutional care history and high-quality foster care. *Development and Psychopathology, 29*(2), 675–684.

Hur, J., DeYoung, K. A., Islam, S., Anderson, A. S., Barstead, M. G., & Shackman, A. J. (2020). Social context and the real-world consequences of social anxiety. *Psychological Medicine, 50*(12), 1989–2000.

Hurley, R. A., Saxena, S., Rauch, S. L., Hoehn-Saric, R., & Taber, K. H. (2008). Predicting treatment response in obsessive-compulsive disorder. In R. A. Hurley & K. H. Taber (Eds.), *Windows to the brain: Insights from neuroimaging* (pp. 213–219). Arlington, VA: American Psychiatric Publishing.

Huskamp, H. A., Busch, A. B., Souza, J., Uscher-Pines, L., Rose, S., Wilcock, A., Landon, . . . Mehrotra, A. (2018). How is telemedicine being used in opioid and other substance use disorder treatment?. *Health Affairs (Project Hope), 37*(12), 1940–1947. https://doi.org/10.1377/hlthaff.2018.05134

Hussein, H. A., Jacoob, S., & Sharour, L. A. (2016). Impact of Life Events on the Relapse of Schizophrenic Patients. *Journal of Education and Practice, 7*(10), 40–47.

Hussong, A. M., Huang, W., Serrano, D., Curran, P. J., & Chassin, L. (2012). Testing whether and when parent alcoholism uniquely affects various forms of adolescent substance use. *Journal of Abnormal Child Psychology, 40*(8), 1265–1276.

Hutchison, K. E. (2010). Realizing the promise of pharmacogenomics and personalized medicine. *Annual Review of Clinical Psychology, 6,* 577–589.

Hutsebaut, J., Videler, A. C., Verheul, R., & Van Alphen, S. (2019). Managing borderline personality disorder from a life course perspective: Clinical staging and health management. *Personality Disorders, 10*(4), 309–316.

Hwang, K. S., Jang, S. H., Soh, M. J., Lee, H. J., & Lee, S. Y. (2019). Cognitive decline in korean patients with neurocognitive disorder due to traumatic brain injury: a control for premorbid intelligence. *Psychiatry investigation, 16*(12), 889.

Hyman, S. E. (2010). The diagnosis of mental disorders: The problem of reification. *Clinical Psychology, 6,* 155–179.

I

Iacovino, J. M., Jackson, J. J., & Oltmanns, T. F. (2014). The relative impact of socioeconomic status and childhood trauma on Black-White differences in paranoid personality disorder symptoms. *Journal of Abnormal Psychology, 123,* 225–230.

Iimori, T., Nakajima, S., Miyazaki, T., Tarumi, R., Ogyu, K., Wada, M., & Noda, Y. (2018, June 25). Effectiveness of the prefrontal repetitive transcranial magnetic stimulation on cognitive profiles in depression, schizophrenia, and Alzheimer's disease: A systematic review. Retrieved November 03, 2020, from https://www.sciencedirect.com/science/article/abs/pii/S0278584618302525

Ikehara, S., Iso, H., Date, C., Kikuchi, S., Watanabe, Y., Wada, Y., . . . JACC Study Group. (2009). Association of sleep duration with mortality from cardiovascular disease and other causes for Japanese men and women: The JACC Study. *Sleep, 32,* 259–301.

Infant Health and Development Program. (1990). Enhancing the outcome of low-birth-weight, premature infants: A multisite randomized trial. *JAMA, 263,* 3035–3042.

Inkelis, S. M., Hasler, B. P., & Baker, F. C. (2020). Sleep and alcohol use in women. *Alcohol Research: Current Reviews, 40*(2), 13. https://doi.org/10.35946/arcr.v40.2.13

Inouye, S. K., Westendorp, R. G., & Saczynski, J. S. (2014). Delirium in elderly people. *Lancet, 383*(9920), 911–922.

Insel, T. R. (Ed.). (1984). *New findings in obsessive-compulsive disorder.* Washington, DC: American Psychiatric Press.

Institute of Medicine. (2008). *Treatment of posttraumatic stress disorder: An assessment of the evidence.* Washington, DC: National Academies Press.

International Society for the Study of Trauma and Dissociation (ISSTD). (2011). Guidelines for treating dissociative identity disorder in adults (3rd Rev.: Summary version). *Journal of Trauma & Dissociation, 12,* 188–212.

Ioannou, M., Argyrides, M., & Mousoulidou, M. (2020). Effects of family dynamics on disordered eating patterns and behaviors: Evidence from Cyprus. *The European Journal of Counselling Psychology, 8*(1), 64–77.

Ionescu, D. F., & Papakostas, G. I. (2017). Experimental medication treatment approaches for depression. *Translational Psychiatry, 7*(3), e1068-e1068.

Iranzo, A., Santamaria, J., & Tolosa, E. (2016). Idiopathic rapid eye movement sleep behaviour disorder: Diagnosis, management, and the need for neuroprotective interventions. *Lancet Neurology, 15*(4), 405–419.

Ironside, R. N., & Batchelor, I. R. C. (1945). *Aviation neuropsychiatry.* Baltimore: Williams & Wilkins.

Irwin, M. R. (2015). Why sleep is important for health: A psychoneuroimmunology perspective. *Annual Review of Psychology, 66,* 143–172.

Irwin, M. R., & Opp, M. R. (2017). Sleep health: Reciprocal regulation of sleep and innate immunity. *Neuropsychopharmacology, 42*(1), 129–155.

Isham, L., Griffith, L., Boylan, A. M., Hicks, A., Wilson, N., Byrne, R., . . . & Freeman, D. (2019). Understanding, treating, and renaming grandiose delusions: A qualitative study. *Psychology and Psychotherapy: Theory, Research and Practice, 94*(1), 119–140.

Isidori, A. M., Buvat, J., Corona, G., Goldstein, I., Jannini, E. A., Lenzi, A., . . . Maggi, M. (2014). A critical analysis of the role of testosterone in erectile function: From pathophysiology to treatment—a systematic review. *European Urology, 65*(1), 99–112.

Iversen, A. C., Fear, N. T., Ehlers, A., Hacker Hughes, J., Hull, L., Earnshaw, M., . . . Hotopf, M. (2008). Risk factors for post-traumatic stress disorder among UK Armed Forces personnel. *Psychological Medicine, 38,* 511–522.

Ivey-Stephenson, A. Z., Crosby, A. E., Jack, S., Haileyesus, T., & Kresnow-Sedacca, M. J. (2017). Suicide trends among and within urbanization levels by sex, race/ethnicity, age group, and mechanism of death - United States, 2001-2015. *Morbidity and Mortality Weekly Report. Surveillance Summaries (Washington, DC: 2002), 66*(18), 1–16.

Izadi, E. (2018, April 02). *'You are not alone': Dwayne 'The Rock' Johnson opens up about depression.* Retrieved December 15, 2020, from https://www.washingtonpost.com/news/arts-and-entertainment/wp/2018/04/02/you-are-not-alone-dwayne-the-rock-johnson-opens-up-about-depression/

J

Jablensky, A. (2000). Epidemiology of schizophrenia: The global burden of disease and disability. *European Archives of Psychiatry & Clinical Neuroscience, 250,* 274–285.

Jack, C. R., Jr., Petersen, R. C., Grundman, M., Jin, S., Gamst, A., Ward, C. P., . . . Thal, L. J. (2007). Longitudinal MRI findings from the vitamin E and donepezil treatment study for MCI. *Neurobiology of Aging, 29,* 1285–1295.

Jack, D. C. (1991). *Silencing the self: Women and depression.* New York: Harper Perennial.

Jacobi, F., Wittchen, H.-U., Hölting, C., Höfler, M., Pfister, H., Muller, N., & Lieb, R. (2004). Prevalence, co-morbidity and correlates of mental disorders in the general population: Results from the German Health Interview and Examination Survey (GHS). *Psychological Medicine, 34,* 597–611.

Jacobson, C. M., & Gould, M. (2009). Suicide and nonsuicidal self-injurious behaviors among youth: Risk and protective factors. In S. Nolen-Hoeksema & L. Hilt (Eds.), *Handbook of depression in adolescents* (pp. 207–236). New York: Routledge.

Jacobson, E. (1964). *The self and the object world.* New York: International Universities Press.

Jacobson, S. W., & Jacobson, J. L. (2000). Teratogenic insult and neurobehavioral function in infancy and childhood. In C. A. Nelson (Ed.), *The Minnesota symposia on child psychology: Vol. 31. The effects of early adversity on neurobehavioral development* (pp. 61–112). Mahwah, NJ: Erlbaum.

Jacobus, J., & Tapert, S. F. (2013). Neurotoxic effects of alcohol in adolescence. *Annual Review of Clinical Psychology, 9,* 703–721.

Jacoby, R. J., & Abramowitz, J. S. (2016). Inhibitory learning approaches to exposure therapy: A critical review and translation to obsessive-compulsive disorder. *Clinical Psychology Review, 49,* 28–40.

Jacoby, R. J., Leonard, R. C., Riemann, B. C., & Abramowitz, J. S. (2016). Self-punishment as a maladaptive thought control strategy mediates the relationship between beliefs about thoughts and repugnant obsessions. *Cognitive Therapy and Research, 40*(2), 179–187.

Jahnke, S. (2018). The stigma of pedophilia: Clinical and forensic implications. *European Psychologist, 23*(2), 144–153.

James, D. J., & Glaze, L. E. (2006). *Mental health problems of prison and jail inmates.* Washington, DC: Bureau of Justice Statistics (BJS), U.S. Dept. of Justice, Office of Justice Programs.

Jamison, K. R. (1993). *Touched with fire: Manic-depressive illness and the artistic temperament.* New York: Free Press.

Jamison, K. R. (1995). *An unquiet mind: A memoir of moods and madness.* New York: Knopf.

Jang, K. L., Livesley, W. J., Ando, J., Yamagata, S., Suzuki, A., Angleitner, A., . . . Spinath, F. (2006). Behavioral genetics of the higher-order factors of the Big Five. *Personality and Individual Differences, 41,* 261–272

Jangmo, A., Stålhandske, A., Chang, Z., Chen, Q., Almqvist, C., Feldman, I., . . . & Larsson, H. (2019). Attention-deficit/hyperactivity disorder, school performance, and effect of medication. *Journal of the American Academy of Child & Adolescent Psychiatry, 58*(4), 423–432.

Jauhar, S., McKenna, P. J., Radua, J., Fung, E., Salvador, R., & Laws, K. R. (2014). Cognitive-behavioural therapy for the symptoms of schizophrenia: Systematic review and meta-analysis with examination of potential bias. *British Journal of Psychiatry, 204*(1), 20–29.

Jefferson, J. W. (2001). Benzodiazepines and anticonvulsants for social phobia (social anxiety disorder). *Journal of Clinical Psychiatry, 62* (Suppl. 1), 50–53.

Jellinger, K. A., & Korczyn, A. D. (2018). Are dementia with Lewy bodies and Parkinson's disease dementia the same disease? *BMC Medicine, 16*(1), 1–16.

Jelovac, A., Kolshus, E., & McLoughlin, D. M. (2013). Relapse following successful electroconvulsive therapy for major depression: A meta-analysis. *Neuropsychopharmacology, 38*, 2467–2474.

Jemberie, W. B., Stewart Williams, J., Eriksson, M., Grönlund, A. S., Ng, N., Blom Nilsson, M., . . . Lundgren, L. M. (2020). Substance use disorders and COVID-19: Multi-faceted problems which require multi-pronged solutions. *Frontiers in Psychiatry, 11*, 714. https://doi.org/10.3389/fpsyt.2020.00714

Jemmott, L. S., Jemmott, J. B., III, & O'Leary, A. (2007). A randomized controlled trial of brief HIV/STD prevention interventions for African American women in primary care settings: Effects on sexual risk behavior and STD incidence. *American Journal of Public Health, 97*, 1034–1040.

Jenkins, J. H., & Karno, M. (1992). The meaning of expressed emotion: Theoretical issues raised by cross-cultural research. *American Journal of Psychiatry, 149*, 9–21.

Jenkins, J. H., Kleinman, A., & Good, B. J. (1991). Cross-cultural studies of depression. In J. Becker (Ed.), *Psychosocial aspects of depression* (pp. 67–99). Hillsdale, NJ: Erlbaum.

Jenkins, T. A. (2013). Perinatal complications and schizophrenia: involvement of the immune system. *Frontiers in Neuroscience, 7*, 110.

Jenks, D. & Oka, M. (2020) Breaking hearts: Ethically handling transference and countertransference in therapy. *The American Journal of Family Therapy,* DOI: 10.1080/01926187.2020.1830732

Jennings, W. G., Perez, N. M., & Reingle Gonzalez, J. M. (2018). Conduct disorders and neighborhood effects. *Annual Review of Clinical Psychology, 14*, 317–341.

Jensen, P. S., Arnold, E., Swanson, J. M., Vitiello, B., Abikoff, H. B., Greenhill, L. L., . . . Hur, K. (2007). Three-year follow-up of the NIMH MTA study. *Journal of the American Academy of Child and Adolescent Psychiatry, 46*, 989–1002.

Jensen, P. S., Hinshaw, S. P., Swanson, J. M., Greenhill, L. L., Conners, C. K., Arnold, L. E., . . . Wigal, T. (2001). Findings from the NIMH Multimodal Treatment Study of ADHD (MTA): Implications and applications for primary care providers. *Journal of Developmental & Behavioral Pediatrics, 22*, 60–73.

Jesse, S., Bråthen, G., Ferrara, M., Keindl, M., Ben-Menachem, E., Tanasescu, R., . . . & Ludolph, A. C. (2017). Alcohol withdrawal syndrome: Mechanisms, manifestations, and management. *Acta Neurologica Scandinavica, 135*(1), 4–16.

Jiang, N. M., Cowan, M., Moonah, S. N., & Petri Jr, W. A. (2018). The impact of systemic inflammation on neurodevelopment. *Trends in Molecular Medicine, 24*(9), 794–804.

Jin, H., & Mosweu, I. (2017). The societal cost of schizophrenia: A systematic review. *Pharmacoeconomics, 35*(1), 25–42.

Jobe, T. H., & Harrow, M. (2010). Schizophrenia course, long-term outcome, recovery, and prognosis. *Current Directions in Psychological Science, 19*(4), 220–225.

Joe, S., & Kaplan, M. S. (2001). Suicide among African American men. *Suicide & Life-Threatening Behavior, 31*, 106–121.

Johnson, J. (2016). Resilience: The bi-dimensional framework. In E. M. Wood & J. Johnson (Eds.), *Wiley handbook of positive clinical psychology* (pp. 73–88). Oxford: Wiley.

Johnson, J. S., Cote, A. C., Dobbyn, A., Sloofman, L. G., Xu, J., Cotter, L., . . . & Huckins, L. M. (2021). The Phenome-wide Consequences of Anorexia Nervosa Genes. *medRxiv.*

Johnson, K. V. A. (2020). Gut microbiome composition and diversity are related to human personality traits. *Human Microbiome Journal, 15*, 100069.

Johnson, P. M., & Kenny, P. J. (2010). Dopamine D2 receptors in addiction-like reward dysfunction and compulsive eating in obese rats. *Nature Neuroscience, 13*, 635–641.

Johnson, S. L., Fulford, D., & Carver, C. S. (2012). The double-edged sword of goal engagement: Consequences of goal pursuit in bipolar disorder. *Clinical Psychology and Psychotherapy, 19*, 352–362.

Johnson, S. M., Simakhodskaya, Z. & Moran, M. (2018). Addressing issues of sexuality in in couples therapy: Emotionally focused therapy meets sex therapy. *Current Sexual Health Reports, 10*, 65–71.

Johnston, L. D., O'Malley, P. M., Bachman, J. G., & Schulenberg, J. E. (2012). *Monitoring the Future national survey results on drug use, 1975–2011. Volume 2. College students and adults ages 19–50.* Ann Arbor: Institute for Social Research, University of Michigan.

Joiner, T. E. (2005). *Why people die by suicide.* Cambridge, MA: Harvard University Press.

Joiner, T. E., Brown, J. S., & Wingate, L. R. (2005). The psychology and neurobiology of suicidal behavior. *Annual Review of Psychology, 56*, 287–314.

Joiner, T. E., & Timmons, K. A. (2009). Depression in its interpersonal context. In I. H. Gotlib & C. L. Hammen (Eds.), *Handbook of depression* (2nd ed., pp. 322–339). New York: Guilford Press.

Jones, D., Godwin, J., Dodge, K. A., Bierman, K. L., Coie, J. D., Greenberg, M. T., . . . Pinderhughes, E. E. (2010). Impact of the fast track program on health services use by conduct-problem youth. *Pediatrics, 125*, 130–136.

Jones-Smith, E. (2019). *Culturally diverse counseling: Theory and practice.* SAGE Publications.

Joormann, J. (2004). Attentional bias in dysphoria: The role of inhibitory processes. *Cognition and Emotion, 18*, 125–147.

Joormann, J., & Vanderlind, W. M. (2014). Emotion regulation in depression: The role of biased cognition and reduced cognitive control. *Clinical Psychological Science, 2*(4), 402–421.

Jordan, B. K., Schlenger, W. E., Fairbank, J. A., & Caddell, J. M. (1996). Prevalence of psychiatric disorders among incarcerated women: II. Convicted felons entering prison. *Archives of General Psychiatry, 53*, 513–519.

Jordan, J. C. First person account: Schizophrenia - Adrift in an anchorless reality. *Schizophrenia Bulletin, 21*(3), 1995, 502.

Jordan, K., Fromberger, P., Stolpmann, G., & Müller, J. L. (2011). The role of testosterone in sexuality and paraphilia—a neurobiological approach. Part II: Testosterone and paraphilia. *Journal of Sexual Medicine, 8*, 3008–3029.

Jorenby, D. E., Hays, J. T., Rigotti, N. A., Azoulay, S., Watsky, E. J., Williams, K. E., Billing, C. B., Gong, J., & Reeves, K. R. (2006). Efficacy of varenicline, an alpha 4 beta 2 nicotinic acetylcholine receptor partial agonist, vs. placebo or sustained-release bupropion for smoking cessation: A randomized controlled trial. *JAMA, 296*, 56–63.

Joseph, S. M., & Siddiqui, W. (2020). Delusional Disorder. *StatPearls [Internet].*

Joudrey, P. J., Chadi, N., Roy, P., Morford, K. L., Bach, P., Kimmel, S., . . . & Calcaterra, S. L. (2020). Pharmacy-based methadone dispensing and drive time to methadone treatment in five states within the United States: A cross-sectional study. *Drug and Alcohol Dependence, 211*, 107968.

Joyal, C. C., Cossette, A., & Lapierre, V. (2015). What exactly is an unusual sexual fantasy?. *The Journal of Sexual Medicine, 12*(2), 328–340.

Joy, E., Kussman, A., & Nattiv, A. (2016). 2016 update on eating disorders in athletes: A comprehensive narrative review with a focus on clinical assessment and management. *British Journal of Sports Medicine, 50*(3), 154–162.

Joyner, M. A., Kim, S., & Gearhardt, A. N. (2017). Investigating an incentive-sensitization model of eating behavior: Impact of a simulated fast-food laboratory. *Clinical Psychological Science, 5*(6), 1014–1026.

Jules, A., Ajdacic-Gross, V., & Rössler, W. (2020). Bipolar disorders in ICD-11: Current status and strengths. *International Journal of Bipolar Disorders, 8*(1).

Jung, Y., & Louis, E. K. S. (2016). Treatment of REM sleep behavior disorder. *Current Treatment Options in Neurology, 18*(11), 50.

K

Kılıç, F., Coşkun, M., Bozkurt, H., Kaya, İ., & Zoroğlu, S. (2017). Self-injury and suicide attempt in relation with trauma and dissociation among adolescents with dissociative and non-dissociative disorders. *Psychiatry investigation, 14*(2), 172–178. https://doi.org/10.4306/pi.2017.14.2.172

Kafantaris, V., Kingsley, P., Ardekani, B., Saito, E., Lencz, T., Lim, K., & Szeszko, P. (2009). Lower orbital frontal white matter integrity in adolescents with bipolar I disorder. *Journal of the American Academy of Child & Adolescent Psychiatry, 48*(1), 79–86.

Kafka, M. P. (2010). Hypersexual disorder: A proposed diagnosis for *DSM-V. Archives of Sexual Behavior, 39,* 377–400.

Kafka, M. P., & Hennen, J. (2003). Hypersexual desire in males: Are males with paraphilias different from males with paraphilia-related disorders? *Sexual Abuse: A Journal of Research and Treatment, 15,* 307–321.

Kallweit, U., & Bassetti, C. L. (2017). Pharmacological management of narcolepsy with and without cataplexy. *Expert Opinion on Pharmacotherapy, 18*(8), 809–817.

Kamenov, K., Twomey, C., Cabello, M., Prina, A., & Ayuso-Mateos, J. (2017). The efficacy of psychotherapy, pharmacotherapy and their combination on functioning and quality of life in depression: A meta-analysis. *Psychological Medicine, 47*(3), 414–425.

Kanbayashi, T., Kodama, T., Kondo, H., Satoh, S., Inoue, U., Chiba, S., Shimizu, T., & Nishino, S. (2009). CSF histamine contents in narcolepsy, idiopathic hypersomnia and obstructive sleep apnea syndrome. *Sleep, 32,* 181–187.

Kanherkar, R. R., Bhatia-Dey, N., & Csoka, A. B. (2014). Epigenetics across the human lifespan. *Frontiers in Cell and Developmental Biology, 2,* 49. https://doi.org/10.3389/fcell.2014.00049

Kanner, L. (1943). Autistic disturbances of affective contact. *Nervous Child, 21,* 217–250.

Kany, S., Vollrath, J. T., & Relja, B. (2019). Cytokines in inflammatory disease. *International Journal of Molecular Sciences, 20*(23), 6008.

Kaplan, M. S., & Krueger, R. B. (2012). Cognitive-behavioral treatment of the paraphilias. *Israeli Journal of Psychiatry and Relationship Science, 49*(4), 291–296.

Kapsalis, T. (2019, April 12). Hysteria, Witches, and The Wandering Uterus: A Brief History. Retrieved from https://lithub.com/hysteria-witches-and-the-wandering-uterus-a-brief-history/

Karasek, R. A., Russell, R. S., & Theorell, T. (1982). Physiology of stress and regeneration in job related cardiovascular illness. *Journal of Human Stress, 8,* 29–42.

Karazsia, B. T., Murnen, S. K., & Tylka, T. L. (2017). Is body dissatisfaction changing across time? A cross-temporal meta-analysis. *Psychological Bulletin, 143*(3), 293–320.

Karg, K., Burmeister, M., Shedden, K., & Sen, S. (2011). The serotonin transporter promoter variant (5-HTTLPR), stress and depression meta-analysis revisited. *Archives of General Psychiatry, 68,* 444–454.

Karlsgodt, K. H., Niendam, T. A., Bearden, C. E., & Cannon, T. D. (2009). White matter integrity and prediction of social and role functioning in subjects at ultra-high risk for psychosis. *Biological Psychiatry, 66,* 562–569.

Karlsgodt, K. H., Sun, D., & Cannon, T. D. (2010). Structural and functional brain abnormalities in schizophrenia. *Current Directions in Psychological Science, 19*(4), 226–231.

Karlsgodt, K. H., van Erp, T. G., Poldrack, R. A., Bearden, C. E., Nuechterlein, K. H., & Cannon, T. D. (2008). Diffusion tensor imaging of the superior longitudinal fasciculus and working memory in recent-onset schizophrenia. *Biological Psychiatry, 63,* 512–518.

Karno, M., & Jenkins, J. H. (1993). Cross-cultural issues in the course and treatment of schizophrenia. *Psychiatric Clinics of North America, 16,* 339–350.

Kartheiser, P. H., Ursano, A. M., & Barnhill, L. J. (2007). Communication disorders. In R. Fletcher, E. Loschen, C. Stavrakaki, & M. First (Eds.), *Diagnostic manual of intellectual disability: A textbook of diagnosis of mental disorders in persons with intellectual disability* (pp. 97–106). Kingston, NY: National Association for the Dually Diagnosed.

Kasindorf, J. (1988, May 2). *The real story of Billie Boggs: Was Koch right—or the civil libertarians? New York,* pp. 35–44. Retrieved from https://www.abajournal.com/magazine/article/joyce_patricia_brown_billie_boggs_1988

Kaskutas, L. A. (2009). Alcoholics Anonymous effectiveness: Faith meets science. *Journal of Addictive Diseases, 28,* 145–157.

Katon, W. (2003). Clinical and health services relationships between major depression, depressive symptoms, and general medical illness. *Biological Psychiatry, 54,* 216–226.

Katon, W., Sullivan, M., & Walker, E. (2001). Medical symptoms without identified pathology: Relationship to psychiatric disorders, childhood and adult trauma, and personality traits. *Annals of International Medicine, 134,* 917–925.

Kaufman, J., Yang, B. Z., Douglas-Palumberi, H., Grasso, D., Lipschitz, D., et al. (2006). Brain-derived neurotrophic factor-5-HTTLPR gene interactions and environmental modifiers of depression in children. *Biological Psychiatry, 59,* 673–680.

Kaufman, J., Yang, B. Z., Douglas-Palumberi, H., Houshyar, S., Lipschitz, D., Krystal, J. H., & Gelernter, J. (2004). Social supports and serotonin transporter gene moderate depression in maltreated children. *Proceedings of the National Academy of Sciences, 101,* 17316–17321.

Kazdin, A. E. (2015). Psychosocial treatments for conduct disorder in children and adolescents. In P. E. Nathan & J. M. Gorman (Eds.), *A guide to treatments that work* (4th ed., pp. 141–173). New York: Oxford University Press.

Kazdin, A. E. (2017). Parent management training and problem-solving skills training for child and adolescent conduct problems. In J. R. Weisz & A. E. Kazdin (Eds.), *Evidence-based psychotherapies for children and adolescents,* 3rd ed. (pp. 142–158). New York: Guilford.

Kazdin, A. E. (2018). Implementation and evaluation of treatments for children and adolescents with conduct problems: Findings, challenges, and future directions. *Psychotherapy Research, 28*(1), 3–17.

Kazdin, A. E., & Blase, S. L. (2011). Rebooting psychotherapy research and practice to reduce the burden of mental illness. *Perspectives on Psychological Science, 6,* 21–37.

Kazdin, A. E., Fitzsimmons-Craft, E. E., & Wilfley, D. E. (2017). Addressing critical gaps in the treatment of eating disorders. *International Journal of Eating Disorders, 50,* 170–189.

Keel, P. K., Brown, T. A., Holland, L. A., & Bodell, L. P. (2012). Empirical classification of eating disorders. *Annual Review of Clinical Psychology, 8,* 381–404.

Keel, P. K., & Forney, K. J. (2013). Psychosocial risk factors for eating disorders. *International Journal of Eating Disorders, 46*(5), 433–439.

Keel, P. K., & Klump, K. L. (2003). Are eating disorders culture-bound syndromes? Implications for conceptualizing their etiology. *Psychological Bulletin, 129,* 747–769.

Keeton, C. P., Teetsel, R. N., Dull, N. M., & Ginsburg, G. S. (2015). Parent psychopathology and children's psychological health: Moderation by sibling relationship dimensions. *Journal of Abnormal Child Psychology, 43*(7), 1333–1342.

Keles, B., McCrae, N., & Grealish, A. (2020). A systematic review: The influence of social media on depression, anxiety and psychological distress in adolescents. *International Journal of Adolescence and Youth, 25*(1), 79–93.

Kellett, S. (2007). A time series evaluation of the treatment of histrionic personality disorder with cognitive analytic therapy. *Psychology and Psychotherapy: Theory, Research, and Practice, 80,* 389–405.

Kellett, S., & Lees, S. (2020). Quasi-experimental N = 1 evaluation of the effectiveness of cognitive analytic therapy for dependent personality disorder. *Journal of Psychotherapy Integration, 30*(3), 458–475. https://doi.org/10.1037/int0000170

Kelly, J. F. (2003). Self-help for substance-use disorders: History, effectiveness, knowledge gaps, and research opportunities. *Clinical Psychological Revue, 23,* 639–663.

Kemp, K. C., Bathery, A. J., Barrantes-Vidal, N., & Kwapil, T. R. (2020). A brief questionnaire measure of multidimensional schizotypy predicts interview-rated symptoms and impairment. *PloS One, 15*(8), e0237614. https://doi.org/10.1371/journal.pone.0237614

Kendall, P. C., Crawford. E. A., Kagan, E. R., Furr, J. M., & Podell, J. L. (2017). Child-focused treatment for anxiety. In A. E. Kazdin & J. R. Weisz (Eds.), *Evidence-based psychotherapies for children and adolescents* (pp. 17–34). New York: Guilford.

Kendall, P. C., Hudson, J. L., Gosch, E., Flannery-Schroeder, E., & Suveg, C. (2008). Cognitive-behavioral therapy for anxiety disordered youth: A randomized clinical trial evaluating child and family modalities. *Journal of Consulting and Clinical Psychology, 76,* 282–297.

Kendler, K. S. (2017). The clinical features of mania and their representation in modern diagnostic criteria. *Psychological Medicine, 47*(6), 1013–1029.

Kendler, K. S. (2019). The genealogy of dementia praecox I: Signs and symptoms of delusional psychoses from 1880 to 1900. *Schizophrenia Bulletin, 45*(2), 296–304.

Kendler, K. S. (2020). Maternal bacterial infection during pregnancy: A potential causal risk factor for psychosis in offspring. *American Journal of Psychiatry, 177*(1), 14–16. https://doi.org/10.1176/appi.ajp.2019.19111150

Kendler, K. S., & Engstrom, E. J. (2016). Kahlbaum, Hecker, and Kraepelin and the transition from psychiatric symptom complexes to empirical disease forms. *American Journal of Psychiatry, 174*(2), 102–109.

Kendler, K. S., Karkowski, L. M., & Prescott, C. A. (1999). Causal relationship between stressful life events and the onset of major depression. *American Journal of Psychiatry, 156,* 837–848.

Kendler, K. S., Kessler, R. C., Walters, E. E., MacLean, C., Neale, M. C., Heath, A. C., & Eaves, L. J. (2010). Stressful life events, genetic liability, and onset of an episode of major depression in women. *Focus, 8*(3), 459–470.

Kendler, K. S., Neale, M. C., Kessler, R. C., Heath, A. C., & Eaves, L. J. (1993). A test of the equal-environment assumption in twin studies of psychiatric illness. *Behavior Genetics, 23,* 21–28.

Kennedy, S. H., Evans, K. R., Kruger, S., Mayberg, H. S., Meyer, J. H., McCann, S. . . . Vaccarino, F. J. (2001). Changes in regional brain glucose metabolism measured with positron emission tomography after paroxetine treatment of major depression. *American Journal of Psychiatry, 158,* 899–905.

Kerckhof, M. E., Kreukels, B. P., Nieder, T. O., Becker-Hébly, I., van de Grift, T. C., Staphorsius, A. S., . . . & Elaut, E. (2019). Prevalence of sexual dysfunctions in transgender persons: results from the ENIGI follow-up study. *The Journal of Sexual Medicine, 16*(12), 2018–2029.

Kerekes, N., Zouini, B., Karlsson, E., Cederholm, E., Lichtenstein, P., Anckarsäter, H., & Råstam, M. (2020). Conduct disorder and somatic health in children: A nationwide genetically sensitive study. *BMC Psychiatry, 20*(1), 1–14.

Kernberg, O. F. (1979). Psychoanalytic profile of the borderline adolescent. *Adolescent Psychiatry, 7,* 234–256.

Kernberg, O. F. (1993). *Severe personality disorders: Psychotherapeutic strategies.* New Haven, CT: Yale University Press.

Keshavan, M. S., DeLisi, L. E., & Seidman, L. J. (2011). Early and broadly defined psychosis risk mental states. *Schizophrenia Research, 126*(1–3), 1–10. https://doi.org/10.1016/j.schres.2010.10.006

Kessler, A., Sollie, S., Challacombe, B., Briggs, K., & Van Hemelrijck, M. (2019). The global prevalence of erectile dysfunction: A review. *BJU International, 124,* 587–599.

Kessler, D. S., MacNeill, S. J., Tallon, D., Lewis, G., Peters, T. J., Hollingworth, W., . . . & Shepherd, T. (2018). Mirtazapine added to SSRIs or SNRIs for treatment resistant depression in primary care: Phase III randomised placebo controlled trial (MIR). *British Medical Journal, 363.*

Kessler, R., Aguilar-Gaxiola, S., Alonso, J., Benjet, C., Bromet, E., Cardoso, G., . . . Koenen, C. (2017). Trauma and PTSD in the WHO World Mental Health Surveys. *European Journal of Psychotraumatology, 8*(5).

Kessler, R. C. (2003). The impairments caused by social phobia in the general population: Implications for intervention. *Acta Psychiatrica Scandinavica, 108* (Suppl. 417), 19–27.

Kessler, R. C., Adler, L., Barkley, R., Biederman, J., Conners, C. K., Demler, O., Faraone, S. V., Greenhill, L. L., Howes, M. J., Secnik, K., Spencer, T., Ustun, T. B., Walters, E. E., & Zaslavsky, A. M. (2006). The prevalence and correlates of adult ADHD in the United States: Results from the National Comorbidity Survey Replication. *American Journal of Psychiatry, 163,* 716–723.

Kessler, R. C., Aguilar-Gaxiola, S., Alonso, J., Chatterji, S., Lee, S., Ormel, J., . . . Wang, P. S. (2009). The global burden of mental disorders: An update from the WHO World Mental Health (WMH) Surveys. *Epidemiologia e Psichiatria Sociale, 18,* 23–33.

Kessler, R. C., Berglund, P. A., Bruce, M. L., Koch, J. R., Laska, E. M., Leaf, P. J., . . . Wang, P. S. (2001). The prevalence and correlates of untreated serious mental illness. *Health Services Research, 36,* 987–1007.

Kessler, R. C., Berglund, P. A., Chiu, W. T., Deitz, A. C., Hudson, J. I., Shahly, V., . . . Xavier, M. (2013). The prevalence and correlates of binge eating disorder in the World Health Organization World Mental Health Surveys. *Biological Psychiatry, 73*(9), 904–914.

Kessler, R. C., Berglund, P., Demler, O., Jin, R., Merikangas, M. R., & Walters, E. E. (2005). Lifetime prevalence and age-of-onset distributions of *DSM-IV* disorders in the National Comorbidity Survey Replication. *Archives of General Psychiatry, 62,* 593–602.

Kessler, R. C., Chiu, W. T., Jin, R., Ruscio, A. M., Shear, K., & Walters, E. E. (2006). The epidemiology of panic attacks, panic disorder, and agoraphobia in the National Comorbidity Survey Replication. *Archives of General Psychiatry, 63,* 415–424.

Kessler, R. C., Coccaro, E. F., Fava, M., Jaeger, S., Jin, R., & Walters, E. (2006). The prevalence and correlates of *DSM-IV* intermittent explosive disorder in the National Comorbidity Survey Replication. *Archives of General Psychiatry, 63,* 669–678.

Kessler, R. C., Heeringa, S., Lakoma, M. D., Petukhova, M., Rupp, A. E., Schoenbaum, M., . . . Zaslavsky, A. M. (2008). Individual and societal effects of mental disorders on earnings in the United States: Results from the National Comorbidity Survey Replication. *American Journal of Psychiatry, 165,* 703–711.

Kessler, R. C., Merikangas, K. R., & Wang, P. S. (2007). Prevalence, comorbidity, and service utilization for mood disorders in the United States at the beginning of the twenty-first century. *Annual Review of Clinical Psychology, 3,* 137–158.

Kessler, R. C., & Wang, P. S. (2008). The descriptive epidemiology of commonly occurring mental disorders in the United States. *Public Health, 29,* 115–129.

Ketter, T. A., Miller, S., Dell'Osso, B., & Wang, P. W. (2016). Treatment of bipolar disorder: Review of evidence regarding quetiapine and lithium. *Journal of Affective Disorders, 191,* 256–273.

Kety, S. S., Wender, P. H., Jacobsen, B., Ingraham, L. J., Jansson, L., Faber, B., & Kinney, D. K. (1994). Mental illness in the biological and adoptive relative of schizophrenic adoptees: Replication of the Copenhagen study in the rest of Denmark. *Archives of General Psychiatry, 51,* 442–455.

Keyes, K. M., Eaton, N. R., Krueger, R. F., McLaughlin, K. A., Wall, M. M., Grant, B. F., & Hasin, D. S. (2012). Childhood maltreatment and the structure of common psychiatric disorders. *British Journal of Psychiatry, 200*(2), 107–115.

Keyes, K. M., Grant, B. F., & Hasin, D. S. (2008). Evidence for a closing gender gap in alcohol use, abuse, and dependence in the United States population. *Drug and Alcohol Dependence, 93,* 21–29.

Keyes, K. M., Martins, S. S., Blanco, C., & Hasin, D. S. (2010). Telescoping and gender differences in alcohol dependence: New evidence from two national surveys. *American Journal of Psychiatry, 167,* 969–976.

Keyes, K. M., Schulenberg, J. E., O'Malley, M., Johnston, L. D., Bachman, J. G., Li, G., & Hasin, D. (2011). The social norms of birth cohorts and adolescent marijuana use in the United States, 1976–2007. *Addiction, 106,* 1790–1800.

Khan, A., Leventhal, R. M., Khan, S. R., & Brown, W. A. (2002). Severity of depression and response to antidepressants and placebo: An analysis of the Food and Drug Administration database. *Journal of Clinical Psychopharmacology, 22,* 40–45.

Khanna, A., & Sharma, M. K. (2017). Selfie use: The implications for psychopathology expression of body dysmorphic disorder. *Industrial Psychiatry Journal, 26*(1), 106–109.

Khatri, U. G., & Perrone, J. (2020). Opioid use disorder and COVID-19: Crashing of the crises. *Journal of Addiction Medicine, 14*(4), e6–e7. https://doi.org/10.1097/ADM.0000000000000684

Khawaja, I. S., & Westermeyer, J. J. (2010). Providing crisis-oriented and recovery-based treatment in partial hospitalization programs. *Psychiatry (Edgmont (Pa.: Township)), 7*(2), 28–31.

Khazaee-Pool, M., Moeeni, M., Ponnet, K., Fallahi, A., Jahangiri, L., & Pashaei, T. (2018). Perceived barriers to methadone maintenance treatment among Iranian opioid users. *International Journal for Equity in Health, 17*(1), 1–10.

Köhler, T. S., & McVary, K. T. (2016). *Contemporary treatment of erectile dysfunction: A clinical guide.* Cham: Springer.

Kiecolt-Glaser, J. K., Malarkey, W. B., Chee, M., & Newton, T. (1993). Negative behavior during marital conflict is associated with immunological down-regulation. *Psychosomatic Medicine, 55,* 395–409.

Kiecolt-Glaser, J. K., & Newton, T. L. (2001). Marriage and health: His and hers. *Psychological Bulletin, 127,* 472–503.

Kiecolt-Glaser, J. K., & Wilson, S. J. (2017). Lovesick: How couples' relationships influence health. *Annual Review of Clinical Psychology, 13,* 421–443.

Kihlstrom, J. F. (2001). Dissociative disorders. In P. B. Sutker (Ed.), *Comprehensive handbook of psychopathology* (3rd ed., pp. 259–276). New York: Kluwer Academic/Plenum.

Kihlstrom, J. F. (2005). Dissociative disorders. *Annual Review of Clinical Psychology, 1,* 227–254.

Kihlstrom, J. F., & Couture, L. J. (1992). Awareness and information processing in general anesthesia. *Journal of Psychopharmacology, 6,* 410–417.

Kihlstrom, J. F., Glisky, M. L., & Angiulo, M. J. (1994). Dissociative tendencies and dissociative disorders. *Journal of Abnormal Psychology, 103,* 117–124.

Kimble, M., Boxwala, M., Bean, W., Maletsky, K., Halper, J., Spollen, K., & Fleming, K. (2014). The impact of hypervigilance: Evidence for a forward feedback loop. *Journal of Anxiety Disorders, 28*(2), 241–245.

Kim-Cohen, J., Caspi, A., Rutter, M., Polo Tomas, M., & Moffitt, T. E. (2006). The caregiving environments provided to children by depressed mothers with or without an antisocial history. *American Journal of Psychiatry, 163,* 1009–1018.

Kim, H. S., Sherman, D. K., & Taylor, S. E. (2008). Culture and social support. *American Psychologist, 63,* 518–526.

Kim, J., & Lopez, S. R. (2014). The expression of depression in Asian Americans and European Americans. *Journal of Abnormal Psychology, 123,* 754–763.

Kim, L. I. C. (1993). Psychiatric care of Korean Americans. In A. C. Gaw (Ed.), *Culture, ethnicity, and mental illness* (pp. 347–375). Washington, DC: American Psychiatric Press.

Kimonis, E. R. (2015). Insanity defense/guilty but mentally ill. In *The encyclopedia of clinical psychology* (pp. 1–6). Chichester, UK: Wiley Blackwell.

Kim, Y., Shaffer, K. M., Carver, C. S., & Cannady, R. S. (2014). Prevalence and predictors of depressive symptoms among cancer caregivers 5 years after the relative's cancer diagnosis. *Journal of Consulting and Clinical Psychology, 82,* 1–8.

King, B. H., Hodapp, R. M., & Dykens, E. M. (2005). Mental retardation. In B. J. Sadock & V. A. Sadock (Eds.), *Kaplan & Sadock's comprehensive textbook of psychiatry* (pp. 3076–3206). Philadelphia: Lippincott Williams & Wilkins.

King, C. R., Knutson, K. L., Rathouz, P. J., Sidney, S., Liu, K., & Lauderdale, D. S. (2008). Short sleep duration and incident coronary artery calcification. *Jama, 300*(24), 2859–2866.

Kirchner, S. K., Roeh, A., Nolden, J., & Hasan, A. (2018). Diagnosis and treatment of schizotypal personality disorder: Evidence from a systematic review. *NPJ Schizophrenia, 4*(1), 1–18.

Kirmayer, L. J. (2001). Cultural variations in the clinical presentation of depression and anxiety: Implications for diagnosis and treatment. *Journal of Clinical Psychiatry, 62* (Suppl. 13), 22–30.

Kirsch, I., Deacon, B. J., Huedo-Medina, T. B., Scoboria, A., Moore, T. J., & Johnson, B. T. (2008). Initial severity and antidepressant benefits: A meta-analysis of data submitted to the Food and Drug Administration. *PLoS Medicine, 5,* e45.

Kissane, D. W., Grabsch, B., Clarke, D. M., Smith, G. C., Love, A. W., Bloch, S., Snyder, R. D., & Li, Y. (2007). Supportive-expressive group therapy for women with metastatic breast cancer: Survival and psychosocial outcome from a randomized controlled trial. *Psycho-Oncology, 16,* 277–286.

Klang, N., Göransson, K., Lindqvist, G., Nilholm, C., Hansson, S., & Bengtsson, K. (2020). Instructional Practices for Pupils with an Intellectual Disability in Mainstream and Special Educational Settings. *International journal of disability, development and education, 67*(2), 151–166.

Klassen, L. J., Katzman, M. A., & Chokka, P. (2010). Adult ADHD and its comorbidities, with a focus on bipolar disorder. *Journal of Affective Disorders, 124,* 1–8.

Klein, C., & Gorzalka, B. B. (2009). Sexual functioning in transsexuals following hormone therapy and genital surgery: A review. *Journal of Sexual Medicine, 6,* 2922–2939.

Kleine Deters, R., Naaijen, J., Rosa, M., Aggensteiner, P. M., Banaschewski, T., Saam, M. C., . . . & Dietrich, A. (2020). Executive functioning and emotion recognition in youth with oppositional defiant disorder and/or conduct disorder. *The World Journal of Biological Psychiatry, 21*(7), 539–551.

Klein, M. (1952). Notes on some schizoid mechanisms. In M. Klein, P. Heimann, S. Isaacs, & J. Riviere (Eds.), *Developments in psychoanalysis* (pp. 292–320). London: Hogarth Press.

Klerman, G. L., & Weissman, M. M. (1989). Increasing rates of depression. *Journal of the American Medical Association, 261,* 2229–2235.

Klerman, G. L., Weissman, M. M., Rounsaville, B., & Chevron, E. (1984). *Interpersonal psychotherapy of depression.* New York: Basic Books.

Klonsky, E. D., May, A. M., & Saffer, B. Y. (2016). Suicide, suicide attempts, and suicidal ideation. *Annual Review of Clinical Psychology, 12,* 307–330.

Klorman, R., Cicchetti, D., Thatcher, J. E., & Ison, J. R. (2003). Acoustic startle in maltreated children. *Journal of Abnormal Child Psychology, 31,* 359–370.

Klump, K. L., Culbert, K. M., Slane, J. D., Burt, S. A., Sisk, C. L., & Nigg, J. T. (2012). The effects of puberty on genetic risk for disordered eating: Evidence for a sex difference. *Psychological Medicine, 42,* 627–637.

Knable, M. B., Barci, B. M., Webster, M. J., Meador-Woodruff, J., & Torrey, E. F. (2004). Molecular abnormalities of the hippocampus in severe psychiatric illness: Postmortem findings from the Stanley Neuropathology Consortium. *Molecular Psychiatry, 9,* 609–620.

Kneeland, R. E., & Fatemi, S. H. (2013). Viral infection, inflammation and schizophrenia. *Progress in Neuro-Psychopharmacology and Biological Psychiatry, 42,* 35–48.

Knight, R. A. (2010). Is a diagnostic category for paraphilic coercive disorder defensible? *Archives of Sexual Behavior, 39,* 419–426.

Knouse, L. E., Teller, J., & Brooks, M. A. (2017). Meta-analysis of cognitive-behavioral treatments for adult ADHD. *Journal of Consulting and Clinical Psychology, 85*(7), 737–750.

Kołodziej, J. (2016). Effects of stress on HIV infection progression. *HIV & AIDS Review, 15,* 13–16.

Kober, H., & Boswell, R. G. (2018). Potential psychological and neural mechanisms in binge eating disorder: Implications for treatment. *Clinical Psychology Review, 60,* 32–44.

Koenen, K. C., Harley, R., Lyons, M. J., Wolfe, J., Simpson, J. C., Goldberg, J., . . . Tsuang, M. (2002). A twin registry study of familial and individual risk factors for trauma exposure and posttraumatic stress disorder. *Journal of Nervous and Mental Disease, 190,* 209–218.

Kohut, H. (1977). *The restoration of the self.* New York: International Universities Press.

Kolar, D. (2017). Current status of electroconvulsive therapy for mood disorders: A clinical review. *Evidence - Based Mental Health, 20*(1), 12.

Kong, L. L., Allen, J. J. B., & Glisky, E. L. (2008). Interidentity memory transfer in dissociative identity disorder. *Journal of Abnormal Psychology, 117,* 686–692.

Koniak-Griffin, D., Lesser, J., Henneman, T., Huang, R., Huang, X., Kappos, B., . . . Cumberland, W. G. (2008). HIV prevention for Latino adolescent mothers and their partners. *Western Journal of Nurse Research, 30,* 724.

Koopman, C., Drescher, K., Bowles, S., Gusman, F., Blake, D., Dondershine, H., . . . & Spiegel, D. (2001). Acute dissociative reactions in veterans with PTSD. *Journal of trauma & dissociation, 2*(1), 91–111.

Koskela, M., Chudal, R., Luntamo, T., Suominen, A., Steinhausen, H. C., & Sourander, A. (2020). The impact of parental psychopathology and sociodemographic factors in selective mutism - a nationwide population-based study. *BMC Psychiatry, 20,* 221.

Koss-Chioino, J. D. (2000). Traditional and folk approaches among ethnic minorities. In J. F. Aponte & J. Wohl (Eds.), *Psychological intervention and cultural diversity* (2nd ed., pp. 149–166). Needham Heights, MA: Allyn & Bacon.

Kotlicka-Antczak, M., Pawełczyk, A., Pawełczyk, T., Strzelecki, D., Żurner, N., & Karbownik, M. S. (2017). A history of obstetric complications is associated with the risk of progression from an at risk mental state to psychosis. *Schizophrenia Research, 197,* 498–503.

Koukoui, S. D., & Chaudhuri, A. (2007). Neuroanatomical, molecular, genetic, and behavioral correlates of fragile X syndrome. *Brain Research Reviews, 53,* 27–38.

Krakowsky, Y., & Grober, E. D. (2016). Hypoactive sexual desire in men. In L. Lipshultz, A. Pastuszak, A. Goldstein, A. Giraldi, & M. Perelman (Eds.), *Management of sexual dysfunction in men and women* (pp. 171–187). New York: Springer.

Kratochvil, C. J., Michelson, D., Newcorn, J. H., Weiss, M. D., Busner, J., Moore, R. J., . . . The Atomoxetine High-Dose Study Group. (2007). High-dose atomoxetine treatment of ADHD in youths with limited response to standard doses. *Journal of the American Academy of Child and Adolescent Psychiatry, 46,* 1128–1137.

Kraus, G., & Reynolds, D. J. (2001). The "A-B-C's" of the Cluster B's: Identifying, understanding, and treating Cluster B personality disorders. *Clinical Psychology Review, 21,* 345–373.

Krentz, E. M., & Warschburger, P. (2011). Sport-related correlates of disordered eating: A comparison between aesthetic and ballgame sports. *International Journal of Sport Psychology, 42,* 548–564.

Kreukels, B. P., & Guillamon, A. (2016). Neuroimaging studies in people with gender incongruence. *International Review of Psychiatry, 28*(1), 120–128.

Krieger, H., Young, C. M., Anthenien, A. M., & Neighbors, C. (2018). The epidemiology of binge drinking among college-age individuals in the United States. *Alcohol Research: Current Reviews, 39*(1), 23–30.

Kring, A. M., & Elis, O. (2013). Emotion deficits in people with schizophrenia. *Annual Review of Clinical Psychology, 9,* 409–433.

Kring, A. M., & Moran, E. K. (2008). Emotional response deficits in schizophrenia: Insights from affective science. *Schizophrenia Bulletin, 34,* 819–834.

Kring, A. M., & Neale, J. M. (1996). Do schizophrenic patients show a disjunctive relationship among expressive, experiential, and psychophysiological components of emotion? *Journal of Abnormal Psychology, 105,* 249–257.

Kring, A. M., & Sloan, D. S. (Eds.). (2009). *Emotion regulation and psycho-pathology: A transdiagnostic approach to etiology and treatment.* New York: Guilford Press.

Kroenke, C. H., Kwan, M. L., Neugut, A. I., Ergas, I. J., Wright, J. D., Caan, B. J., . . . Kushi, L. H. (2012). Social networks, social support mechanisms, and quality of life after breast cancer diagnosis. *Breast Cancer Research and Treatment, 139*(2), 515–527.

Kroll, J. (1973). A reappraisal of psychiatry in the Middle Ages. *Archives of General Psychiatry, 29,* 276-283.

Krueger, R. F., & Eaton, N. R. (2015). Transdiagnostic factors of mental disorders. *World psychiatry: official journal of the World Psychiatric Association (WPA), 14*(1), 27-29. https://doi.org/10.1002/wps.20175

Krueger, R. F., & Markon, K. E. (2014). The role of the DSM-5 personality trait model in moving toward a quantitative and empirically based approach to classifying personality and psychopathology. *Annual Review of Clinical Psychology, 10,* 477-501.

Krug, O. (2016). Existential, humanistic, experiential psychotherapies in historical perspective. In A. J. Consoli, L. E. Beutler, & B. Bongar (Eds.), *Comprehensive textbook of psychotherapy: Theory and practice* (2nd ed.), pp. 91-105. New York: Oxford University Press.

Kryger, M. H., Roth, T., & Dement, W. C. (Eds.). (2017). *Principles and practice of sleep medicine* (6th ed.). Philadelphia: Elsevier.

Kuepper, R., van Os, J., Lieb, R., Wittchen, H. U., Höfler, M., & Henquet, C. (2011). Continued cannabis use and risk of incidence and persistence of psychotic symptoms: 10 year follow-up cohort study. *British Medical Journal, 342,* d738.

Kuerbis, A., & Sacco, P. (2013). A review of existing treatments for substance abuse among the elderly and recommendations for future directions. *Substance Abuse: Research and Treatment, 7,* 13-37.

Kuerbis, A., Sacco, P., Blazer, D. G., & Moore, A. A. (2014). Substance abuse among older adults. *Clinics in Geriatric Medicine, 30*(3), 629-654.

Kuester, A., Niemeyer, H., & Knaevelsrud, C. (2016). Internet-based interventions for posttraumatic stress: A meta-analysis of randomized controlled trials. *Clinical Psychology Review, 43,* 1-16.

Kujawa, A., Proudfit, G. H., & Klein, D. N. (2014). Neural reactivity to rewards and losses in offspring of mothers and fathers with histories of depressive and anxiety disorders. *Journal of Abnormal Psychology, 123,* 287-297.

Kunst, J. R., Myhren, L. S., & Onyeador, I. N. (2018). Simply insane? Attributing terrorism to mental illness (versus ideology) affects mental representations of race. *Criminal Justice and Behavior, 45*(12), 1888-1902.

Kupper, N., & Denollet, J. (2018). Type D personality as a risk factor in coronary heart disease: A review of current evidence. *Current Cardiology Reports, 20*(11), 1-8.

Kurlansik, S., & Maffei, M. (2016, January 01). Somatic Symptom Disorder. Retrieved December 08, 2020, from https://www.aafp.org/afp/2016/0101/p49.html?utm_cmpid=aafp

Kuss, D. J., Griffiths, M. D., & Pontes, H. M. (2017). Chaos and confusion in DSM-5 diagnosis of Internet Gaming Disorder: Issues, concerns, and recommendations for clarity in the field. *Journal of Behavioral Addictions, 6*(2), 103-109.

Kvillemo, P., & Bränström, R. (2014). Coping with breast cancer: A meta-analysis. *PLoS One, 9,* e112733.

Kwapil, T. R., & Barrantes-Vidal, N. (2012). Schizotypal personality disorder: An integrative review. In T. A. Widiger (Ed.), *The Oxford handbook of personality disorders* (pp. 437-477). New York: Oxford University Press.

L

Lack, L. C., Gradisar, M., Van Someren, E. J. W., Wright, H. R., & Lushington, K. (2008). The relationship between insomnia and body temperatures. *Sleep Medicine Reviews, 12,* 307-317.

Ladwig, K. H., Martin-Mittag, B., Lacruz, M. E., Henningsen, P., & Creed, F. (2010). Screening for multiple somatic complaints in a population-based survey: Does excessive symptom reporting capture the concept of somatic symptom disorders? *Journal of Psychosomatic Research, 68,* 427-437.

Laird, K., Lavretsky, H., Paholpak, P., Vlasova, R., Roman, M., St. Cyr, N., & Siddarth, P. (2019). Clinical correlates of resilience factors in geriatric depression. *International Psychogeriatrics, 31*(2), 193-202.

Lamb, H. R., & Weinberger, L. E. (2016). Rediscovering the concept of asylum for persons with serious mental illness. *Journal of the American Academy of Psychiatry and the Law, 44*(1), 106-110.

Lamb, H. R., & Weinberger, L. E. (2017). Understanding and treating offenders with serious mental illness in public sector mental health. *Behavioral Sciences & the Law, 35*(4), 303-318.

Lampe, L., & Malhi, G. S. (2018). Avoidant personality disorder: Current insights. *Psychology Research and Behavior Management, 11,* 55-66. doi: http://dx.doi.org.mccc.idm.oclc.org/10.2147/PRBM.S121073

Landen, M., Roeber, J., Naimi, T., Nielsen, L., & Sewell, M. (2014). Alcohol-attributable mortality among American Indians and Alaska natives in the United States, 1999-2009. *American Journal of Public Health, 104*(S3), S343-S349.

Landgren, V., Malki, K., Bottai, M., Arver, S., & Rahm, C. (2020). Effect of gonadotropin-releasing hormone antagonist on risk of committing child sexual abuse in men with pedophilic disorder: A randomized clinical trial. *JAMA Psychiatry, 77*(9), 897-905.

Lane, R. (2020, July 23). Kanye West says he's done with Trump-opens up about White House Bid, damaging biden and everything in between. Retrieved December 23, 2020, from https://www.forbes.com/sites/randalllane/2020/07/08/kanye-west-says-hes-done-with-trump-opens-up-about-white-house-bid-damaging-biden-and-everything-in-between/?sh=5dcf48c947aa

Laney, C., & Loftus, E. F. (2013). Recent advances in false memory research. *South African Journal of Psychology, 43*(2), 137-146.

Langberg, J. M., Molina, B. S. G., Arnold, L. E., Epstein, J. N., Altaye, M., Hinshaw, S. P., . . . Hechtman, L. (2012). Patterns and predictors of adolescent academic achievement and performance in a sample of children with attention-deficit/hyperactivity disorder. *Journal of Clinical Child & Adolescent Psychology, 40,* 519-531.

Langhoff, C., Baer, T., Zubraegel, D., & Linden, M. (2008). Therapist–patient alliance, patient–therapist alliance, mutual therapeutic alliance, therapist–patient concordance, and outcome of CBT in GAD. *Journal of Cognitive Psychotherapy, 22*(1), 68-79.

Langlois, J. A., Rutland-Brown, W., & Wald, M. M. (2006). The epidemiology and impact of traumatic brain injury: A brief overview. *Journal of Head Trauma Rehabilitation 21,* 375-378.

Langstrom, N. (2009, November 19). The *DSM* diagnostic criteria for exhibitionism, voyeurism, and frotteurism. *Archives of Sexual Behavior, 39*(2), 317-324.

Langstrom, N., & Seto, M. C. (2006). Exhibitionistic and voyeuristic behavior in a Swedish national population survey. *Archives of Sexual Behavior, 35,* 427-435.

Langstrom, N., & Zucker, K. J. (2005). Transvestic fetishism in the general population: Prevalence and correlates. *Journal of Sex and Marital Therapy, 31,* 87-95.

Larøi, F., Luhrmann, T. M., Bell, V., Christian W. A., Jr., Deshpande, S., Fernyhough, C., . . . Woods, A. (2014). Culture and hallucinations: Overview and future directions. *Schizophrenia Bulletin, 40*(Suppl. 4), S213-S220.

Larkin, A., & Hutton, P. (2017). Systematic review and meta-analysis of factors that help or hinder treatment decision-making capacity in psychosis. *British Journal of Psychiatry, 211*(4), 205-215.

Larsson, H., Chang, Z., D'Onofrio, B. M., & Lichtenstein, P. (2014). The heritability of clinically diagnosed attention deficit hyperactivity disorder across the lifespan. *Psychological Medicine, 44*(10), 2223–2229.

Larsson, H., Tuvblad, C., Rijsdijk, F. V., Andershed, H., Grann, M., & Lichtenstein, P. (2007). A common genetic factor explains the association between psychopathic personality and antisocial behavior. *Psychological Medicine, 37,* 15–26.

Lasser, K., Boyd, J. W., Woolhandler, S., Himmelstein, D. U., McCormick, D., & Bor, D. H. (2000). Smoking and mental illness: A population-based prevalence study. *JAMA, 284,* 2606–2610.

Lataster, J., Myin-Germeys, I., Lieb, R., Wittchen, H. U., & van Os, J. (2011). Adversity and psychosis: A 10-year prospective study investigating synergism between early and recent adversity in psychosis. *Acta Psychiatrica Scandinavica, 125*(5), 388–399.

Lateef, A., Dahar, M. A., & Yousuf, M. I. (2019). Influence of Type A and Type B personality on academic achievement of university students. *Global Social Sciences Review, 4*(2), 109–118.

Latvala, A., Kuja-Halkola, R., Almqvist, C., Larsson, H., & Lichtenstein, P. (2015). A longitudinal study of resting heart rate and violent criminality in more than 700,000 men. *JAMA Psychiatry, 72*(10), 971–978.

Laudenslager, M. L., Ryan, S. M., Drugan, R. C., Hyson, R. L., & Maier, S. F. (1983). Coping and immunosuppression: Inescapable but not escapable shock suppresses lymphocyte proliferation. *Science, 221,* 569–570.

Laumann, E. O., Gagnon, J. H., Michael, R. T., & Michaels, S. (1994). *The social organization of sexuality: Sexual practices in the United States.* Chicago: University of Chicago Press.

Laumann, E. O., Paik, A., & Rosen, R. C. (1999). Sexual dysfunction in the United States. *Journal of the American Medical Association, 281,* 537–544.

Laursen, T. M., Nordentoft, M., & Mortensen, P. B. (2014). Excess early mortality in schizophrenia. *Annual Review of Clinical Psychology, 10,* 425–448.

Lavin, M. (2008). Voyeurism: Psychopathology and theory. In D. R. Laws & W. T. O'Donohue (Eds.), *Sexual deviance: Theory, assessment, and treatment* (pp. 305–320). New York: Guilford Press.

Lavoie, K. L., Miller, S. B., Conway, M., & Fleet, R. P. (2001). Anger, negative emotions, and cardiovascular reactivity during interpersonal conflict in women. *Journal of Psychosomatic Research, 51,* 503–512.

Lavretsky, H. (2008). History of schizophrenia as a psychiatric disorder. In K. T. Mueser & D. V. Jeste (Eds.), *Clinical handbook of schizophrenia* (pp. 3–13). New York: Guilford Press.

Lawrence, A. A. (2008). Gender identity disorders in adults: Diagnosis and treatment. In D. L. Rowland & L. Incrocci (Eds.), *Handbook of sexual and gender identity disorders* (pp. 423–456). Hoboken, NJ: Wiley.

Lawrence, M. B. (2020). Parity is not enough! Mental health, managed care, and Medicaid. *Journal of Law, Medicine & Ethics, 48*(3), 480–484.

Lawrie, S. M., McIntosh, A. M., Hall, J., Owens, D. G. C., & Johnstone, E. C. (2008). Brain structure and function changes during the development of schizophrenia: The evidence from studies of subjects at increased genetic risk. *Schizophrenia Bulletin, 34,* 330–340.

Laws, K. R., Irvine, K., & Gale, T. M. (2016). Sex differences in cognitive impairment in Alzheimer's disease. *World Journal of Psychiatry, 6*(1), 54–65. https://doi.org/10.5498/wjp.v6.i1.54

Lazarus, S. A., Cheavens, J. S., Festa, F., & Rosenthal, M. Z. (2014). Interpersonal functioning in borderline personality disorder: A systematic review of behavioral and laboratory-based assessments. *Clinical Psychology Review, 34,* 193–205.

Leadbeater, B. J., Kuperminc, G. P., Blatt, S. J., & Herzog, C. (1999). A multivariate model of gender differences in adolescents' internalizing and externalizing problems. *Developmental Psychology, 35,* 1268–1282.

Leaver, A. M., Wade, B., Vasavada, M., Hellemann, G., Joshi, S. H., Espinoza, R., & Narr, K. L. (2018). Fronto-temporal connectivity predicts ECT outcome in major depression. *Frontiers in Psychiatry, 9,* 92.

LeBeau, R. T., Glenn, D., Liao, B., Wittchen, H.-U., Beesdo-Baum, K., Ollendick, T., & Craske, M. G. (2010). Specific phobia: A review of *DSM-IV* specific phobia and preliminary recommendations for *DSM-V*. *Depression and Anxiety, 27,* 148–167.

Lebowitz, M. S., & Ahn, W. K. (2012). Combining biomedical accounts of mental disorders with treatability information to reduce mental illness stigma. *Psychiatric Services, 63,* 496–499.

Leckman, J. F., Denys, D., Simpson, H. B., Mataix-Cols, D., Hollander, E., Saxena, S., . . . Stein, D. S. (2010). Obsessive-compulsive disorder: A review of the diagnostic criteria and possible subtypes and dimensional signifiers for *DSM-V*. *Depression and Anxiety, 27,* 507–527.

Lee, E. K., & Kazaglis, L. (2015). Hypersomnolence disorders in DSM-5: A review for clinicians. *Psychiatric Annals, 45*(1), 25–29.

Leehr, E. J., Krohmer, K., Schag, K., Dresler, T., Zipfel, S., & Giel, K. E. (2015). Emotion regulation model in binge eating disorder and obesity—a systematic review. *Neuroscience & Biobehavioral Reviews, 49,* 125–134.

Lee, J. K. P., Jackson, H. J., Pattison, P., & Ward, T. (2002). Developmental risk factors for sexual offending. *Child Abuse & Neglect, 26,* 73–92.

Leeman, R. F., & Potenza, M. N. (2012). Similarities and differences between pathological gambling and substance use disorders: A focus on impulsivity and compulsivity. *Psychopharmacology, 219,* 469–490.

Lee, R. (2017). Mistrustful and misunderstood: A review of paranoid personality disorder. *Current Behavioral Neuroscience Reports, 4*(2), 151–165.

Lee, S. (2020). Coronavirus Anxiety Scale: A brief mental health screener for COVID-19 related anxiety. *Death Studies, 44,* 7, 393–401.

Lee, S. C., DelPozo-Banos, M., Lloyd, K., Jones, I., Walters, J. T., Owen, M. J., . . . & John, A. (2020). Area deprivation, urbanicity, severe mental illness and social drift—A population-based linkage study using routinely collected primary and secondary care data. *Schizophrenia Research, 220, 130–140.* https://doi.org/10.1016/j.schres.2020.03.044

Lee, S., Mathis, A., Jobe, M., & Pappalardo, E. (2020). Clinically significant fear and anxiety of COVID-19: A psychometric examination of the Coronavirus Anxiety Scale. *Psychiatry Research, 290,* 112–113.

Lehman, B. J., Taylor, S. E., Kiefe, C., & Seeman, T. E. (2009). Relationship of early life stress and psychological functioning to blood pressure in the CARDIA study. *Health Psychology, 28,* 338–346.

Lehn, A., Gelauff, J., Hoeritzauer, I., Ludwig, L., McWhirter, L., Williams, S., . . . Stone, J. (2016). Functional neurological disorders: Mechanisms and treatment. *Journal of Neurology, 263*(3), 611–620.

Leiblum, S. R. (Ed.). (2010). *Treating sexual desire disorders: A clinical casebook.* New York: Guilford Press.

Leiblum, S. R., Koochaki, P. E., Rodenberg, C. A., Barton, I. P., & Rosen, R. C. (2006). Hypoactive sexual desire disorder in postmenopausal women: U.S. results from the Women's International Study of Health and Sexuality (WISHeS). *Menopause, 13,* 46–56.

Leichsenring, F., & Steinert, C. (2018). Towards an evidence-based unified psychodynamic protocol for emotional disorders. *Journal of Affective Disorders, 232,* 400–416.

Lei, H., Huang, L., Li, J., Liu, W., Fan, J., Zhang, X., . . . & Rao, H. (2020). Altered spontaneous brain activity in obsessive-compulsive personality disorder. *Comprehensive Psychiatry, 96,* 152144.

Leiknes, K. A., Jarosh-von Schweder, L., & Høie, B. (2012). Contemporary use and practice of electroconvulsive therapy worldwide. *Brain and Behavior, 2*(3), 283–344.

Le, L. K. D., Barendregt, J. J., Hay, P., & Mihalopoulos, C. (2017). Prevention of eating disorders: A systematic review and meta-analysis. *Clinical Psychology Review, 53,* 46–58.

Lemmens, L. H., Galindo-Garre, F., Arntz, A., Peeters, F., Hollon, S. D., DeRubeis, R. J., & Huibers, M. J. (2017). Exploring mechanisms of change in cognitive therapy and interpersonal psychotherapy for adult depression. *Behaviour Research and Therapy, 94,* 81–92.

Lengel, G. J. (2020). Histrionic personality disorder. *The Wiley Encyclopedia of Personality and Individual Differences: Clinical, Applied, and Cross-Cultural Research,* 187–191.

Leonard, H. L., Ale, C. M., Freeman, J. B., Garcia, A. M., & Ng, J. S. (2005). Obsessive-compulsive disorder. *Child and Adolescent Psychiatric Clinics of North America, 14*(4), 727–743.

Leon, G. R., Fulkerson, J. A., Perry, C. L., & Early-Zald, M. B. (1995). Prospective analysis of personality and behavioral vulnerabilities and gender influences in the later development of disordered eating. *Journal of Abnormal Psychology, 104,* 140–149.

Lepping, P., Stanly, T., & Turner, J. (2015). Systematic review on the prevalence of lack of capacity in medical and psychiatric settings. *Clinical Medicine, 15*(4), 337–343.

Lerner, A., Wassermann, E., & Tamir, D. (2019, April 06). Seizures from transcranial magnetic stimulation 2012–2016: Results of a survey of active laboratories and clinics. Retrieved November 03, 2020, from https://www.sciencedirect.com/science/article/pii/S1388245719301105

Lescai, E. (2020). The transvestic disorder. *International Journal of Advanced Studies in Sexology, 2*(1), 25–31.

Leserman J. (2008). Role of depression, stress, and trauma in HIV disease progression. *Psychosomatic Medicine, 70,* 539–545.

Leserman, J., Pence, B. W., Whetten, K., Mugavero, M. J., Thielman, N. M., Swartz, M. S., & Stangl, D. (2007). Relation of lifetime trauma and depressive symptoms to mortality in HIV. *American Journal of Psychiatry, 164,* 1707–1713.

Le Strat, Y., & Gorwood, P. (2011). Hazardous drinking is associated with lower risk of coronary heart disease: Results from a national representative sample. *American Journal on Addictions, 20*(3), 257–263.

Leung, A. K., Leung, A. A., Wong, A. H., & Hon, K. L. (2020). Sleep terrors: An updated review. *Current Pediatric Reviews, 16*(3), 176–182.

Leventhal, H., Weinman, J., Leventhal, E. A., & Phillips, L. A. (2008). Health psychology: The search for pathways between behavior and health. *Annual Review of Psychology, 59,* 477–506.

Levi-Belz, Y., Gvion, Y., Levi, U., & Apter, A. (2019). Beyond the mental pain: A case-control study on the contribution of schizoid personality disorder symptoms to medically serious suicide attempts. *Comprehensive Psychiatry, 90,* 102–109.

Levine, S., Rabinowitz, J., Ascher-Svanum, H., Faries, D. E., & Lawson, A. H. (2011). Extent of attaining and maintaining symptom remission by antipsychotic medication in the treatment of chronic schizophrenia: Evidence from the CATIE study. *Schizophrenia Research, 133,* 42–46.

Levinson, D. F. (2006). The genetics of depression: A review. *Biological Psychiatry, 60,* 84–92.

Lewinsohn, P. M. (1974). A behavioral approach to depression. In R. J. Friedman & M. M. Katz (Eds.), *The psychology of depression: Contemporary theory and research* (pp. 157–178). Washington, DC: Winston-Wiley.

Lewinsohn, P. M., & Gotlib, I. H. (1995). Behavioral therapy and treatment of depression. In E. E. Beckham & W. R. Leber (Eds.), *Handbook of depression* (2nd ed., pp. 352–375). New York: Guilford Press.

Lewinsohn, P. M., Muñoz, R. F., Youngren, M. A., & Zeiss, A. M. (1986). *Control your depression.* Englewood Cliffs, NJ: Prentice Hall.

Lewinsohn, P. M., Striegel-Moore, R. H., & Seeley, J. R. (2000). Epidemiology and natural course of eating disorders in young women from adolescence to young adulthood. *Journal of the American Academy of Child & Adolescent Psychiatry, 39,* 1284–1292.

Lewis-Fernandez, R., Hinton, D. E., Laria, A. J., Patterson, E. H., Hofmann, S. G., Craske, M. G., . . . Liao, B. (2010). Culture and the anxiety disorders: Recommendations for the *DSM-V. Depression and Anxiety, 27,* 212–229.

Lewis, K. C., & Ridenour, J. M. (2020). Paranoid personality disorder. *Encyclopedia of Personality and Individual Differences,* 3413–3421.

Lewis, R. W., Fugl-Meyer, K. S., Corona, G., Hayes, R. D., Laumann, E. O., Moreira, E. D., . . . Segraves, T. (2010). Definitions/epidemiology/risk factors for sexual dysfunction. *Journal of Sexual Medicine, 7* (4, pt. 2), 1598–1607.

Lewis, R. W., Yuan, J., & Wangt, R. (2008). Male sexual arousal disorder. In D. L. Rowland & L. Incrocci (Eds.), *Handbook of sexual and gender identity disorders* (pp. 32–67). Hoboken, NJ: Wiley.

Lewis, T. T., Cogburn, C. D., & Williams, D. R. (2015). Self-reported experiences of discrimination and health: Scientific advances, ongoing controversies, and emerging issues. *Annual Review of Clinical Psychology, 11,* 407–440.

Leys, C., Kotsou, I., Goemanne, M., & Fossion, P. (2017). The influence of family dynamics on eating disorders and their consequence on resilience: A mediation model. *The American Journal of Family Therapy, 45*(2), 123–132.

Liang, J., Matheson, B. E., & Douglas, J. M. (2016). Mental health diagnostic considerations in racial/ethnic minority youth. *Journal of Child and Family Studies, 25*(6), 1926–1940.

Liberman, R. P. (2008). *Recovery from disability: Manual of psychiatric rehabilitation.* Washington, DC: American Psychiatric Publishing.

Liberman, R. P., Glynn, S., Blair, K. E., Ross, D., & Marder, S. R. (2002). In vivo amplified skills training: Promoting generalization of independent living skills for clients with schizophrenia. *Psychiatry: Interpersonal & Biological Processes, 65,* 137–155.

Lichtenstein, P., Yip, B. H., Björk, C., Pawitan, Y., Cannon, T. D., Sullivan, P. F., & Hultman, C. M. (2009). Common genetic determinants of schizophrenia and bipolar disorder in Swedish families: A population-based study. *Lancet, 373*(9659), 234–239.

Lieberman, J. A., Girgis, R. R., Brucato, G., Moore, H., Provenzano, F., Kegeles, L., . . . Small, S. A. (2018). Hippocampal dysfunction in the pathophysiology of schizophrenia: A selective review and hypothesis for early detection and intervention. *Molecular Psychiatry, 23* (8): 1764–1772.

Liechti, M. E., Dolder, P. C., & Schmid, Y. (2017). Alterations of consciousness and mystical-type experiences after acute LSD in humans. *Psychopharmacology, 234*(9–10), 1499–1510.

Lilienfeld, S. O., & Treadway, M. T. (2016). Clashing diagnostic approaches: DSM-ICD versus RDoC. *Annual Review of Clinical Psychology, 12,* 435–463.

Lim, D. C., & Pack, A. I. (2017). Obstructive sleep apnea: Update and future. *Annual Review of Medicine, 68,* 99–112.

Linardon, J., Wade, T. D., de la Piedad Garcia, X., & Brennan, L. (2017). The efficacy of cognitive-behavioral therapy for eating disorders: A systematic review and meta-analysis. *Journal of Consulting and Clinical Psychology, 85*(11), 1080–1094.

Lindau, S. T., Schumm, L. P., Laumann, E. O., Levinson, W., O'Muircheartaigh, C. A., & Waite, L. J. (2007). A study of sexuality and health among older adults in the United States. *New England Journal of Medicine, 357*(8), 762–774.

Lindner, P., Forsström, D., Jonsson, J., Berman, A. H., & Carlbring, P. (2020). Transitioning between online gambling modalities and decrease in total gambling activity, but no indication of increase in problematic online gambling intensity during the first phase of the COVID-19 outbreak in Sweden: A time series forecast study. *Frontiers in Public Health, 8,* 554542. https://doi.org/10.3389/fpubh.2020.554542

Lindsay, S. D., Hagen, L., Read, J. D., Wade, K. A., & Garry, M. (2004). True photographs and false memories. *Psychological Science, 15,* 149–154.

Linehan, M. M. (1999). Standard protocol for assessing and treating suicidal behaviors for patients in treatment. In D. G. Jacobs (Ed.), *The Harvard Medical School guide to suicide assessment and intervention* (pp. 146–187). San Francisco: Jossey-Bass.

Linehan, M. M. (2018). *Cognitive-behavioral treatment of borderline personality disorder.* Guilford Publications.

Linehan, M. M., Comtois, K. A., Murray, A. M., Brown, M. Z., Gallop, R. J., Heard, H. L., . . . Lindenboim, N. (2006). Two-year randomized controlled trial and follow-up of dialectical behavior therapy vs therapy by experts for suicidal behaviors and borderline personality disorder. *Archives of General Psychiatry, 63*(7), 757–766.

Links, P. S., & Eynan, R. (2013). The relationship between personality disorders and Axis I psychopathology: Deconstructing comorbidity. *Annual Review of Clinical Psychology, 9,* 529–554.

Linschoten, M., Weiner, L., & Avery-Clark, C. (2016). Sensate focus: A critical literature review. *Sexual and Relationship Therapy, 31*(2), 230–247.

Linscott, R. J., Allardyce, J., & van Os, J. (2009). Seeking verisimilitude in a class: A systematic review of evidence that the criterial clinical symptoms of schizophrenia are taxonic. *Schizophrenia Bulletin.* doi: 10.1093

Linscott, R. J., & van Os, J. (2010). Systematic reviews of categorical versus continuum models in psychosis: Evidence for discontinuous subpopulations underlying a psychometric continuum. Implications for *DSM-V, DSM-VI,* and *DSM-VII. Annual Review of Clinical Psychology, 6,* 391–419.

Lipari, R. N., Hughes, A., & Bose, J. (2016). *Driving under the influence of alcohol and illicit drugs. The CBHSQ Report: December 27, 2016.* Rockville, MD: Center for Behavioral Health Statistics and Quality, Substance Abuse and Mental Health Services Administration.

Li, R., Ma, X., Wang, G., Yang, J., & Wang, C. (2016). Why sex differences in schizophrenia?. *Journal of Translational Neuroscience, 1*(1), 37–42.

Little, K., Olsson, C. A., Youssef, G. J., Whittle, S., Simmons, J. G., Yücel, M., . . . Allen, N. B. (2015). Linking the serotonin transporter gene, family environments, hippocampal volume and depression onset: A prospective imaging gene × environment analysis. *Journal of Abnormal Psychology, 124,* 834–849.

Liu, H. Y., Potter, M. P., Woodsworth, K. Y., Yorks, D. M., Petty, C. R., Wozniak, J. R., . . . Biederman, J. (2011). Pharmacologic treatments for pediatric bipolar disorder: A review and meta-analysis. *Journal of the American Academy of Child & Adolescent Psychiatry, 50,* 749–762.

Liu, R. T. (2013). Stress generation: Future directions and clinical implications. *Clinical Psychology Review, 33,* 406–416.

Liu, W., Ge, T., Leng, Y., Pan, Z., Fan, J., Yang, W., & Cui, R. (2017). The role of neural plasticity in depression: From hippocampus to prefrontal cortex. *Neural Plasticity, 2017,* 6871089.

Li, Z., Chang, S. H., Zhang, L. Y., Gao, L., & Wang, J. (2014). Molecular genetic studies of ADHD and its candidate genes: A review. *Psychiatry Research, 219,* 10–24.

Llabre, M. M., Schneiderman, N., Gallo, L. C., Arguelles, W., Daviglus, M. L., Gonzalez, F., 2nd, . . . Penedo, F. J. (2017). Childhood trauma and adult risk factors and disease in Hispanics/Latinos in the U.S.: Results from the Hispanic Community Health Study/Study of Latinos (HCHS/SOL) sociocultural ancillary study. *Psychosomatic Medicine.*

Llabre, M. M., Schneiderman, N., Gallo, L. C., Arguelles, W., Daviglus, M. L., Gonzalez, F., 2nd, . . . Penedo, F. J. (2017). Childhood trauma and adult risk factors and disease in Hispanics/Latinos in the US: Results from the Hispanic Community Health Study/Study of Latinos (HCHS/SOL) sociocultural ancillary study. *Psychosomatic Medicine, 79*(2), 172–180.

Loas, G., Cormier, J., & Perez-Diaz, F. (2011). Dependent personality disorder and physical abuse. *Psychiatry Research, 185,* 167–170.

Locher, C., Meier, S., & Gaab, J. (2019). Psychotherapy: A World of Meanings. *Frontiers in psychology, 10,* 460. https://doi.org/10.3389/fpsyg.2019.00460

Lochner, C., Roos, A., & Stein, D. J. (2017). Excoriation (skin-picking) disorder: A systematic review of treatment options. *Neuropsychiatric Disease and Treatment, 13,* 1867–1872.

Lochner, C., Serebro, P., van der Merwe, L., Hemmings, S., Kinnear, C., Seedat, S., & Stein, D. J. (2011). Comorbid obsessive-compulsive personality disorder in obsessive-compulsive disorder (OCD): A marker of severity. *Progress in Neuropsychopharmacology & Biological Psychiatry, 35,* 1087–1092.

Locke, A. B., Kirst, N., & Shultz, C. G. (2015). Diagnosis and management of generalized anxiety disorder and panic disorder in adults. *American Family Physician, 91*(9), 617–624.

Lock, J., Agras, W. S., Bryson, S., & Kraemer, H. C. (2005). A comparison of short- and long-term family therapy for adolescent anorexia nervosa. *Journal of the American Academy of Child and Adolescent Psychiatry, 44,* 632–639.

Lock, J., & le Grange D. (2013). *Treatment manual for anorexia nervosa: A family-based approach* (2nd ed.). New York: Guilford Press.

Loebel, J. P., Loebel, J. S., Dager, S. R., Centerwall, B. S., & Reay, D. T. (1991). Anticipation of nursing home placement may be a precipitant of suicide among the elderly. *Journal of the American Geriatric Society, 39,* 407–408.

Loeber, R., & Burke, J. D. (2011). Developmental pathways in juvenile externalizing and internalizing problems. *Journal of Research on Adolescence, 21,* 34–46.

Loeber, R., Burke, J., & Pardini, D. A. (2009a). Development and etiology of disruptive and delinquent behavior. *Clinical Psychology, 5,* 291–310.

Loeber, R., Burke, J., & Pardini, D. A. (2009b). Perspectives on oppositional defiant disorder, conduct disorder, and psychopathic features. *Journal of Child Psychology and Psychiatry, 50,* 133–142.

Loehlin, J. C. (2009). History of behavior genetics. In Y.-K. Kim (Ed.), *Handbook of behavior genetics* (pp. 3–11). New York: Spring Science & Business Media.

Loftus, E. F. (1993). The reality of repressed memories. *American Psychologist, 48,* 518–537.

Loftus, E. F. (2003). Make-believe memories. *American Psychologist, 58,* 867–873.

Loftus, E. F. (2011). Crimes of memory: False memories and societal justice. In M. A. Gernsbacher, R. W. Pew, L. M. Hough, & J. R. Pomerantz (Eds., FABBS Foundation), *Psychology and the real world: Essays illustrating fundamental contributions to society* (pp. 83–88). New York: Worth.

Longpré, N., Guay, J. P., Knight, R. A., & Benbouriche, M. (2018). Sadistic offender or sexual sadism? Taxometric evidence for a dimensional structure of sexual sadism. *Archives of Sexual Behavior, 47*(2), 403–416.

Lopez-Quintero, C., Pérez de los Cobos, J., Hasin, D. S., Okuda, M., Wang, S., Grant, B. F., & Blanco, C. (2011). Probability and predictors of transition from first use to dependence on nicotine, alcohol, cannabis, and cocaine: Results of the National Epidemiologic Survey on Alcohol and Related Conditions (NESARC). *Drug and Alcohol Dependence, 115*(1–2), 120–130.

Lopez, S. R., & Guarnaccia, P. J. J. (2000). Cultural psychopathology: Uncovering the social world of mental illness. *Annual Review of Psychology, 51,* 571–598.

Lopez, S. R., Kopelowicz, A., & Canive, J. M. (2002). Strategies in developing culturally congruent family interventions for schizophrenia: The case of Hispanics. In H. P. Lefley & D. L. Johnson (Eds.), *Family interventions in mental illness: International perspectives* (pp. 61–90). Westport, CT: Praeger.

Lord, C., & Bishop, S. L. (2015). Recent advances in autism research as reflected in DSM-5 criteria for autism spectrum disorder. *Annual Review of Clinical Psychology, 11,* 53–70.

Lorenz, K., & Ullman, S. E. (2016). Alcohol and sexual assault victimization: Research findings and future directions. *Aggression and Violent Behavior, 31,* 82–94.

Lotspeich, L. J., Kwon, H., Schumann, C. M., Fryer, S. L., Goodlin-Jones, B. L., Buonocore, M. H., . . . Reiss, A. L. (2004). Investigation of neuroanatomical differences between autism and Asperger syndrome. *Archives of General Psychiatry, 61,* 291–298.

Lou, W. J., Chen, B., Zhu, L., Han, S. M., Xu, T., Lang, J. H., & Zhang, L. (2017). Prevalence and factors associated with female sexual dysfunction in Beijing, China. *Chinese Medical Journal, 130*(12), 1389–1394.

Lowe, S. R., & Galea, S. (2017). The mental health consequences of mass shootings. *Trauma, Violence, & Abuse, 18*(1), 62–82.

Luborsky, L., & Barrett, M. S. (2006). The historical and empirical status of key psychoanalytic concepts. *Annual Review of Clinical Psychology, 2,* 1–20.

Ludwig, A. M. (1992). Creative achievement and psychopathology: Comparison among professions. *American Journal of Psychotherapy, 46,* 330–356.

Ludwig, L., Pasman, J. A., Nicholson, T., Aybek, S., David, A. S., Tuck, S., Stone, J. (2018). Stressful life events and maltreatment in conversion (functional neurological) disorder: Systematic review and meta-analysis of case-control studies. *Lancet Psychiatry, 5*(4), 307–320.

Lund, C., & Cois, A. (2018). Simultaneous social causation and social drift: Longitudinal analysis of depression and poverty in South Africa. *Journal of Affective Disorders, 229,* 396–402.

Luo, Y., Chen, L., Li, H., Dong, Y., Zhou, X., Qiu, L., . . . Wang, K. (2020). Do individuals with obsessive-compulsive disorder and obsessive-compulsive personality disorder share similar neural mechanisms of decision-making under ambiguous circumstances?. *Frontiers in Human Neuroscience, 14,* 585086. https://doi.org/10.3389/fnhum.2020.585086

Luria, A. (1973). *The working brain.* New York: Basic Books.

Lussier, P., & Pichè, L. (2008). Frotteurism: Psychopathology and theory. In D. R. Laws & W. T. O'Donohue (Eds.), *Sexual deviance: Theory, assessment, and treatment* (pp. 131–150). New York: Guilford Press.

Lutter, M. (2017). Emerging treatments in eating disorders. *Neurotherapeutics: The Journal of the American Society for Experimental NeuroTherapeutics, 14*(3), 614–622.

Löwe, B., Spitzer, R. L., Williams, J. B., Mussell, M., Schellberg, D., & Kroenke, K. (2008). Depression, anxiety and somatization in primary care: Syndrome overlap and functional impairment. *General Hospital Psychiatry, 30*(3), 191–199.

Lydon, S., Healy, O., O'Callaghan, O., Mulhern, T., & Holloway, J. (2015). A systematic review of the treatment of fears and phobias among children with autism spectrum disorders. *Review Journal of Autism and Developmental Disorders, 2,* 141–154.

Lyketsos, C. G., Miller, D. S., & Neuropsychiatric Syndromes Professional Interest Area of the International Society to Advance Alzheimer's Research and Treatment. (2012). Addressing the Alzheimer's disease crisis through better understanding, treatment, and eventual prevention of associated neuropsychiatric syndromes. *Alzheimer's & Dementia: The Journal of the Alzheimer's Association, 8,* 60–64.

Lynam, D. R., Caspi, A., Moffitt, T. E., Wikstrom, P. H., Loeber, R., & Novak, S. (2000). The interaction between impulsivity and neighborhood context on offending: The effects of impulsivity are stronger in poorer neighborhoods. *Journal of Abnormal Psychology, 109,* 563–574.

Lynn, S. J., Lilienfeld, S. O., Merckelbach, H., Giesbrecht, T., & van der Kloet, D. (2012). Dissociation and dissociative disorders: Challenging conventional wisdom. *Current Directions in Psychological Science, 21*(1), 48–53.

Lyons-Ruth, K., Holmes, B. M., Sasvari-Szekely, M., Ronai, Z., Nemoda, Z., & Pauls, D. (2007). Serotonin transporter polymorphism and borderline or antisocial traits among low-income young adults. *Psychiatric Genetics, 17,* 339–343.

M

Münch, R., Walter, H., & Müller, S. (2020). Should behavior harmful to others be a sufficient criterion of mental disorders? Conceptual problems of the diagnoses of antisocial personality disorder and pedophilic disorder. *Frontiers in Psychiatry, 11,* 954.

Maïmoun, L., Guillaume, S., Lefebvre, P., Bertet, H., Seneque, M., Philibert, P., . . . & Sultan, C. (2018). Effects of the two types of anorexia nervosa (binge eating/purging and restrictive) on bone metabolism in female patients. *Clinical Endocrinology, 88*(6), 863–872.

MacArthur Research Network on Mental Health and the Law. (1998). Executive summary. http://ness.sys.Virginia.EDU/macarthur/violence.html (accessed June 1, 2006).

Maciejewski, P. K., Maercker, A., Boelen, P. A., & Prigerson, H. G. (2016). "Prolonged grief disorder" and "persistent complex bereavement disorder", but not "complicated grief," are one and the same diagnostic entity: An analysis of data from the Yale Bereavement Study. *World Psychiatry, 15*(3), 266–275.

Madden, J. M., Lakoma, M. D., Lynch, F. L., Rusinak, D., Owen-Smith, A. A., Coleman, K. J., . . . Croen, L. A. (2017). Psychotropic medication use among insured children with autism spectrum disorder. *Journal of Autism and Developmental Disorders, 47*(1), 144–154.

Maeng, L. Y., & Milad, M. R. (2015). Sex differences in anxiety disorders: Interactions between fear, stress, and gonadal hormones. *Hormones and Behavior, 76,* 106–117.

Maher, B. A. (1966). *Principles of psychotherapy: An experimental approach*. New York: McGraw-Hill.

Maher, C. A., Lewis, L. K., Ferrar, K., Marshall, S., De Bourdeaudhuij, I., & Vandelanotte, C. (2014). Are health behavior change interventions that use online social networks effective? A systematic review. *Journal of Medical Internet Research, 16*(2), e40.

Maher, W. B., & Maher, B. A. (1985). Psychopathology: I. From ancient times to eighteenth century. In G. A. Kimble & K. Schlesinger (Eds.), *Topics in the history of psychology* (Vol. 2). Hillsdale, NJ: Erlbaum.

Mahler, M. (1968). *On human symbiosis and the vicissitudes of individuation: Vol. 1. Infantile psychosis*. New York: International Universities Press.

Maiorino, M. I., Bellastella, G., & Esposito, K. (2014). Diabetes and sexual dysfunction: Current perspectives. *Diabetes, Metabolic Syndrome and Obesity: Targets and Therapy, 7*, 95–105.

Ma-Kellams, C., Baek, J. H., & Or, F. (2018). Suicide contagion in response to widely publicized celebrity deaths: The roles of depressed affect, death-thought accessibility, and attitudes. *Psychology of Popular Media Culture, 7*(2), 164–170.

Makwana N. (2019). Disaster and its impact on mental health: A narrative review. *Journal of Family Medicine and Primary Care, 8*(10), 3090–3095. https://doi.org/10.4103/jfmpc.jfmpc_893_19

Maletzky, B. (1998). The paraphilias: Research and treatment. In P. E. Nathan (Ed.), *A guide to treatments that work* (pp. 472–500). New York: Oxford University Press.

Maletzky, B. M., & Field, G. (2003). The biological treatment of dangerous sexual offenders, a review and preliminary report of the Oregon pilot depo-Provera program. *Aggression and Violent Behavior, 8*, 391–412.

Malhi, G. S., Tanious, M., Das, P., Coulston, C. M., & Berk, M. (2013). Potential mechanisms of action of lithium in bipolar disorder. *CNS drugs, 27*(2), 135–153.

Malhotra, S., & Sahoo, S. (2017). Rebuilding the brain with psychotherapy. *Indian Journal of Psychiatry, 59*(4), 411–419. https://doi.org/10.4103/0019-5545.217299

Mandel, H. (2009). *Here's the deal: Don't touch me*. New York: Bantam Books

Mandell, D., Siegle, G. J., Shutt, L., Feldmiller, J., & Thase, M. E. (2014). Neural substrates of trait ruminations in depression. *Journal of Abnormal Psychology, 123*, 35–48.

Manicavasagar, V., Silove, D., Rapee, R., Waters, F., & Momartin, S. (2001). Parent-child concordance for separation anxiety: A clinical study. *Journal of Affective Disorders, 65*, 81–84.

Mannarini, S., & Rossi, A. (2019). Assessing mental illness stigma: A complex issue. *Frontiers in Psychology, 9*, 2722.

Mannekote, S., Pillai, A., & Harbishettar, V. (2019). Civil commitment of persons with mental illness: Comparison of the Mental Healthcare Act 2017 with corresponding legislations of the USA. *Indian Journal of Psychiatry, 61*(Suppl 4), S821–S826. https://doi.org/10.4103/psychiatry.IndianJPsychiatry_81_19

Mann, J. J. (2013). The serotonergic system in mood disorders and suicidal behaviour. *Philosophical Transactions of the Royal Society B, 368*(1615), 20120537.

Marangell, L. B. (2004). The importance of subsyndromal symptoms in bipolar disorder. *Journal of Clinical Psychiatry, 65*(Suppl. 10), 24–27.

Marazziti, D., Catena, M., & Pallanti, S. (2006). Pharmacologic treatment of obsessive-compulsive disorder. *Psychiatric Annals, 36*, 454–462.

March, D., Hatch, S. L., Morgan, C., Kirkbride, J. B., Bresnahan, M., Fearon, P., & Susser, E. (2008). Psychosis and place. *Epidemiologic Reviews, 30*(1), 84–100.

Marchis, D. M. (2019). Sexual sadism disorder. *Transtheoretical Approaches to Paraphilic Disorders, 1*(2), 105–106.

Marcks, B. A., Weisberg, R. B., Dyck, I., & Keller, M. B. (2011). Longitudinal course of obsessive-compulsive disorder in patients with anxiety disorders: a 15-year prospective follow-up study. *Comprehensive psychiatry, 52*(6), 670–677. https://doi.org/10.1016/j.comppsych.2011.01.001

Marder, S. R., & Galderisi, S. (2017). The current conceptualization of negative symptoms in schizophrenia. *World Psychiatry, 16*(1), 14–24.

Marlatt, G. A., Blume, A. W., & Parks, G. A. (2001). Integrating harm reduction therapy and traditional substance abuse treatment. *Journal of Psychoactive Drugs, 33*, 13–21.

Marlatt, G. A., Larimer, M. E., & Witkiewitz, K. (Eds.). (2011). *Harm reduction: Pragmatic strategies for managing high-risk behaviors*. New York: Guilford.

Marlatt, G. A., & Witkiewitz, K. (2010). Update on harm reduction policy and intervention research. *Annual Review of Clinical Psychology, 6*, 591–606.

Marques, J. K., Wiederanders, M., Day, M., Nelson, C., & van Ommeren, A. (2005). Effects of a relapse prevention program on sexual recidivism: Final results from California's Sex Offender Treatment Evaluation Project (SOTEP). *Sex Abuse, 17*, 79–107.

Marroquín, B., & Nolen-Hoeksema, S. (2015). Emotion regulation and depressive symptoms: Close relationships as context and influence. *Journal of Personality and Social Psychology, 109*, 836–855.

Marroquín, B., Tennen, H., & Stanton, A. L. (2017). Coping, emotion regulation, and well-being: Intrapersonal and interpersonal processes. In M. D. Robinson & M. Eid (Eds.), *The happy mind: Cognitive contributions to well-being* (pp. 253–274). Cham: Springer.

Marshall, G. N., & Orlando, M. (2002). Acculturation and peritraumatic dissociation in young adult Latino survivors of community violence. *Journal of Abnormal Psychology, 111*, 166–174.

Marshall, S. (2020). Conversion Disorders. Retrieved December 08, 2020, from https://emedicine.medscape.com/article/287464-overview

Marshall, W. L., & Marshall, L. E. (2015). Psychological treatment of the paraphilias: A review and an appraisal of effectiveness. *Current Psychiatry Reports, 17*(6), 47.

Martínez-Taboas, A. (2005). Psychogenic seizures in an espiritismo context: The role of culturally sensitive psychotherapy. *Psychotherapy: Theory, Research, Practice, Training, 42*, 6–13.

Martinez, K. B., Leone, V., & Chang, E. B. (2017). Western diets, gut dysbiosis, and metabolic diseases: Are they linked?. *Gut Microbes, 8*(2), 130–142.

Martino, S., Paris, M., Jr, Añez, L., Nich, C., Canning-Ball, M., Hunkele, K., . . . Carroll, K. M. (2016). The effectiveness and cost of clinical supervision for motivational interviewing: A randomized controlled trial. *Journal of Substance Abuse Treatment, 68*, 11–23. https://doi.org/10.1016/j.jsat.2016.04.005

Martins, C. M. S., de Carvalho Tofoli, S. M., Von Werne Baes, C., & Juruena, M. (2011). Analysis of the occurrence of early life stress in adult psychiatric patients: A systematic review. *Psychology & Neuroscience, 4*, 219–227.

Martland, N., Martland, R., Cullen, A. E., & Bhattacharyya, S. (2020). Are adult stressful life events associated with psychotic relapse? A systematic review of 23 studies. *Psychological Medicine, 50*(14), 2302–2316.

Martorana, A., Esposito, Z., & Koch, G. (2010). Beyond the cholinergic hypothesis: Do current drugs work in Alzheimer's disease? *CNS Neuroscience & Therapeutics, 16*, 235–245.

Marzilli, E., Cerniglia, L., & Cimino, S. (2018). A narrative review of binge eating disorder in adolescence: Prevalence, impact, and psychological treatment strategies. *Adolescent Health, Medicine and Therapeutics, 9,* 17–30.

Masheb, R. M., Grilo, C. M., & White, M. A. (2011). An examination of eating patterns in community women with bulimia nervosa and binge eating disorder. *International Journal of Eating Disorders, 44,* 618–624.

Masten, A. S., & Powell, J. L. (2003). A resilience framework for research, policy, and practice. In S. E. Luthar (Ed.), *Resilience and vulnerability: Adaptation in the context of childhood adversities* (pp. 1–25). New York: Cambridge University Press.

Masters, K. S., & Hooker, S. A. (2013). Religiousness/spirituality, cardiovascular disease, and cancer: Cultural integration for health research and intervention. *Journal of Consulting and Clinical Psychology, 81,* 206–216.

Masters, W. H., & Johnson, V. E. (1970). *Human sexual inadequacy.* Boston: Little, Brown.

Mataix-Cols, D., Frost, R. O., Pertusa, A., Clark, L. A., Saxena, S., Leckman, J. F., . . . Wilhelm, S. (2010). Hoarding disorder: A new diagnosis for *DSM-V*? *Depression and Anxiety, 27,* 556–572.

Matarazzo, J. D. (1985). Psychotherapy. In G. A. Kimble & K. Schlesinger (Eds.), *Topics in the history of psychology* (pp. 219–250). Hillsdale, NJ: Erlbaum.

Mathews, A., & MacLeod, C. (2005). Cognitive vulnerability to emotional disorders. *Annual Review of Clinical Psychology, 1,* 167–196.

Matson, J. L., & Neal, D. (2009). Psychotropic medication use for challenging behaviors in persons with intellectual disabilities: An overview. *Research in Developmental Disabilities, 30,* 572–586.

Matt, G. E., Vasquez, C., & Campbell, W. K. (1992). Mood-congruent recall of affectively toned stimuli: A meta-analytic review. *Clinical Psychology Review, 12,* 227–255.

Matthews, K. A., Owens, J. F., Kuller, L. H., Sutton-Tyrrell, K., & Jansen-McWilliams, L. (1998). Are hostility and anxiety associated with carotid atherosclerosis in healthy postmenopausal women? *Psychosomatic Medicine, 5,* 633–638.

Matthiasdottir, E., Jonsson, S. H., & Kristjansson, A. L. (2012). Body weight dissatisfaction in the Icelandic adult population: A normative discontent? *European Journal of Public Health, 22,* 116–121.

Matthys, W., Vanderschuren, L. J., & Schutter, D. J. (2013). The neurobiology of oppositional defiant disorder and conduct disorder: Altered functioning in three mental domains. *Development and Psychopathology, 25*(1), 193–207.

Mattick, R. P., Breen, C., Kimber, J., Davoli, M., & Breen, R. (2003). Methadone maintenance therapy versus no opioid replacement therapy for opioid dependence. *Cochrane Database of Systematic Reviews, 2,* CD002209.

Mattila, M.-L., Kielinen, M., Linna, S.-S., Jussila, K., Ebeling, H., Bloigu, R., . . . & Moilanen, I. (2011). Autism spectrum disorders according to *DSM-IV-TR* and comparison with *DSM-5* draft criteria: An epidemiological study. *Journal of the American Academy of Child and Adolescent Psychiatry, 50,* 583–592.

Mattila, T., Koeter, M., Wohlfarth, T., Storosum, J., van den Brink, W., de Haan, L., . . . Denys, D. (2015). Impact of DSM-5 changes on the diagnosis and acute treatment of schizophrenia. *Schizophrenia Bulletin, 41*(3), 637–643. https://doi.org/10.1093/schbul/sbu172

Maughan, B., Pickles, A., Rowe, R., Costello, E. J., & Angold, A. (2000). Developmental trajectories of aggressive and non-aggressive conduct problems. *Journal of Quantitative Criminology, 16,* 199–221.

Maurer, D. M., Raymond, T. J., & Davis, B. N. (2018). Depression: Screening and diagnosis. *American Family Physician, 98*(8), 508–515.

Mausbach, B. T., Coon, D. W., Depp, C., Rabinowitz, Y. G., Wilson-Arias, E., Kraemer, H. C., . . . Gallagher-Thompson, D. (2004). Ethnicity and time to institutionalization of dementia patients: A comparison of Latina and Caucasian female family caregivers. *Journal of the American Geriatrics Society, 52,* 1077–1084.

Mayberg, H. S., Lozano, A. M., Voon, V., et al. (2005). Deep brain stimulation for treatment-resistant depression. *Neuron, 45,* 651–660.

Mayo, D., Corey, S., Kelly, L. H., Yohannes, S., Youngquist, A. L., Stuart, B. K., . . . & Loewy, R. L. (2017). The role of trauma and stressful life events among individuals at clinical high risk for psychosis: a review. *Frontiers in psychiatry, 8,* 55.

Mayou, R., Bryant, B., & Ehlers, A. (2001). Prediction of psychological outcomes one year after a motor vehicle accident. *American Journal of Psychiatry, 158,* 1231–1238.

Mayo-Wilson, E., Dias, S., Mavranezouli, I., Kew, K., Clark, D. M., Ades, A. E., & Pilling, S. (2014). Psychological and pharmacological interventions for social anxiety disorder in adults: A systematic review and network meta-analysis. *Lancet Psychiatry, 1*(5), 368–376.

Mazzoni, G., & Loftus, E. F. (1998). Dream interpretations can change beliefs about the past. *Psychotherapy, 35,* 177–187.

McCabe, M. P., Sharlip, I. D., Lewis, R., Atalla, E., Balon, R., Fisher, A. D., . . . Segraves, R. T. (2016). Incidence and prevalence of sexual dysfunction in women and men: A consensus statement from the Fourth International Consultation on Sexual Medicine 2015. *Journal of Sexual Medicine, 13*(2), 144–152.

McCabe, R., Antony, M., Summerfeldt, L., Liss, A., & Swinson, R. (2003). Preliminary examination of the relationship between anxiety disorders in adults and self-reported history of teasing or bullying experiences. *Cognitive Behaviour Therapy, 32,* 187–193.

McCabe, S. E., Cranford, J. A., & West, B. T. (2008). Trends in prescription drug abuse and dependence, co-occurrence with other substance use disorders, and treatment utilization: Results from two national surveys. *Addictive Behaviors, 33,* 1297–1305.

McCaffery, J. M., Frasure-Smith, N., Dubé, M. P., Théroux, P., Rouleau, G. A., Duan, Q., & Lesperance, F. (2006). Common genetic vulnerability to depressive symptoms and coronary artery disease: A review and development of candidate genes related to inflammation and serotonin. *Psychosomatic Medicine, 68,* 187–200.

McCarthy, B., & Ross, L. W. (2018). Maintaining sexual desire and satisfaction in securely bonded couples. *Family Journal: Counseling and Therapy for Couples and Families.*

McCarthy, B. W. (2001). Relapse prevention strategies and techniques with erectile dysfunction. *Journal of Sex & Marital Therapy, 27,* 1–8.

McCarthy, B. W., & Ross, L. W. (2017). Integrating sexual concepts and interventions into couple therapy. In J. Fitzgerald (Ed.), *Foundations for couples' therapy: Research for the real world* (pp. 355–364). New York: Routledge.

McCarthy-Jones, S., Castro Romero, M., McCarthy-Jones, R., Dillon, J., Cooper-Rompato, C., Kieran, K., . . . Blackman, L. (2015). Hearing the unheard: An interdisciplinary, mixed methodology study of women's experiences of hearing voices (Auditory verbal hallucinations). *Frontiers in Psychiatry, 6,* 181. https://doi.org/10.3389/fpsyt.2015.00181

McCarthy, M. (1990). The thin ideal, depression and eating disorders in women. *Behaviour Research & Therapy, 28,* 205–215.

McCloskey, M. S., Noblett, K. L., Deffenbacher, J. L., Gollan, J. K., & Coccaro, E. F. (2008). Cognitive-behavioral therapy for intermittent explosive disorder: A pilot randomized clinical trial. *Journal of Consulting and Clinical Psychology, 76,* 876-886.

McCormick, M. C., McCarton, C., Brooks-Gunn, J., Belt, P., & Gross, R. T. (1998). The Infant Health and Development Program: Interim summary. *Developmental & Behavioral Pediatrics, 19,* 359-370.

McCrady, B. S. (2014). Alcohol use disorders. In D. H. Barlow (Ed.), *Clinical handbook of psychological disorders: A step-by-step treatment manual* (pp. 533-587). New York: Guilford.

McCrady, B. S., Epstein, E. E., Cook, S., Jensen, N., & Hildebrandt, T. (2009). A randomized trial of individual and couple behavioral alcohol treatment for women. *Journal of Consulting and Clinical Psychology, 77,* 243-256.

McCrae, R. R., & Costa, P. T. (1999). A five-factor theory of personality. In L. A. Pervin (Ed.), *Handbook of personality: Theory and research* (2nd ed., pp. 139-153). New York: Guilford Press.

McCrae, R. R., & Costa, P. T. (2013). Introduction to the empirical and theoretical status of the five-factor model of personality traits. In T. A. Widiger & P. T. Costa (Ed.), *Personality disorders and the five-factor model of personality* (3rd ed., pp. 15-27). Washington, DC: American Psychological Association.

McCrae, R. R., & Terracciano, A. (2005). Universal features of personality traits from the observer's perspective: Data from 50 cultures. *Journal of Personality and Social Psychology, 88,* 547-561.

McEwen, B. S. (2004). Protection and damage from acute and chronic stress: Allostasis and allostatic overload and relevance to the pathophysiology of psychiatric disorders. *Annals of the New York Academy of Sciences, 1032*(1), 1-7.

McFarlane, A. C., Barton, C. A., Yehuda, R., & Wittert, G. (2011). Cortisol response to acute trauma and risk of posttraumatic stress disorder. *Psychoneuroendocrinology, 36,* 720-727.

McFarlane, W. R. (2016). Family interventions for schizophrenia and the psychoses: A review. *Family Process, 55*(3), 460-482.

McGovern, C. M. (1985). *Masters of madness.* Hanover, NH: University Press of New England.

McGreevy, M. A., Steadman, H. J., & Callahan, L. A. (1991). The negligible effects of California's 1982 reform of the insanity defense test. *American Journal of Psychiatry, 148,* 744-750.

McGue, M., Iacono, W. G., Legrand, L. N., Malone, S., & Elkins, I. (2001). Origins and consequences of age at first drink: I. Associations with substance-use disorders, disinhibitory behavior and psychopathology, and P3 amplitude. *Alcoholism: Clinical & Experimental Research, 25,* 1156-1165.

McGuffin, P., Rijsdijk, F., Andrew, M., Sham, P., Katz, R., & Cardno, A. (2003). The heritability of bipolar affective disorder and the genetic relationship to unipolar depression. *Archives of General Psychiatry, 60,* 497-502.

McGuire, J. F., Piacentini, J., Brennan, E. A., Lewin, A. B., Murphy, T. K., Small, B. J., & Storch, E. A. (2014). A meta-analysis of behavior therapy for Tourette syndrome. *Journal of Psychiatric Research, 50,* 106-112.

McGurk, S. R., Mueser, K. T., Mischel, R., Adams, R., Harvey, P. D., McClure, M. M., . . . Siever, L. J. (2013). Vocational functioning in schizotypal and paranoid personality disorders. *Psychiatry Research, 210*(2), 498-504.

McHugh, R. K., Hearon, B. A., & Otto, M. W. (2010). Cognitive behavioral therapy for substance use disorders. *Psychiatric Clinics, 33*(3), 511-525.

McIntosh, J. L. (1995). Suicide prevention in the elderly (age 65-99). *Suicide & Life-Threatening Behaviors, 25,* 180-192.

McKenzie, S. K., Jenkin, G., Steers, D., Magill, R., & Collings, S. (2020). Young people's perspectives and understanding of the suicide story in 13 reasons why. *Crisis,* 1-7.

McKinnon, D. H., McLeod, S., & Reilly, S. (2008). The prevalence of stuttering, voice, and speech-sound disorders in primary school students in Australia. *Language, Speech, and Hearing Services in Schools, 38,* 5-15.

McLaughlin, J., O'Carroll, R. E., & O'Connor, R. C. (2012). Intimate partner abuse and suicidality: A systematic review. *Clinical Psychology Review, 32*(8), 677-689.

McLaughlin, K., & Kar, J. A. (2019). Aftermath of the parkland shooting: A case report of post-traumatic stress disorder in an adolescent survivor. *Cureus, 11*(11).

McMahon, P. (2018, June 16). Years after case, Jennifer Bush says she wasn't a victim of Munchausen or abuse by her mom. Retrieved December 09, 2020, from https://www.sun-sentinel.com/local/broward/fl-jennifer-bush-munchausen-20150415-story.html

McMillan, T. M., & Rachman, S. J. (1987). Fearlessness and courage: A laboratory study of paratrooper veterans of the Falklands War. *British Journal of Psychology, 78,* 375-383.

McNally, R. J. (2002). Anxiety sensitivity and panic disorder. *Biological Psychiatry, 52*(10), 938-946.

McNally, R. J. (2003). Recovering memories of trauma: A view from the laboratory. *Current Directions in Psychological Science, 12,* 32-35.

McNally, R. J. (2017). False memories in the laboratory and in life: Commentary on Brewin and Andrews (2016). *Applied Cognitive Psychology, 31*(1), 40-41.

McNally, R. J., Clancy, S. A., & Schacter, D. L. (2001). Directed forgetting of trauma cues in adults reporting repressed or recovered memories of childhood sexual abuse. *Journal of Abnormal Psychology, 110,* 151-156.

McNally, R. J., Clancy, S. A., Schacter, D. L., & Pitman, R. K. (2000a). Cognitive processing of trauma cues in adults reporting repressed, recovered, or continuous memories of childhood sexual abuse. *Journal of Abnormal Psychology, 109,* 355-359.

McNally, R. J., Clancy, S. A., Schacter, D. L., & Pitman, R. K. (2000b). Personality profiles, dissociation, and absorption in women reporting repressed, recovered, or continuous memories of childhood sexual abuse. *Journal of Consulting Clinical Psychology, 68,* 1033-1037.

McNeill, A., Brose, L. S., Calder, R., Bauld, L., & Robson, D. (2019). Vaping in England: An evidence update February 2019. *A Report Commissioned by Public Health England.* London: Public Health England.

McPartland, J., Reichow, B., & Volkmar, F. R. (2012). Sensitivity and specificity of proposed *DSM-5* diagnostic criteria for autism spectrum disorder. *Journal of the American Academy of Child & Adolescent Psychiatry, 51,* 368-383.

McRobbie, H., Bullen, C., Hartmann-Boyce, J., & Hajek, P. (2014). Electronic cigarettes for smoking cessation and reduction. Cochrane Library 12: CD010216.

McWilliams, N. (2011). *Psychoanalytic diagnosis: Understanding personality structure in the clinical process.* Guilford Press.

Mechanic, D., & Olfson, M. (2016). The relevance of the Affordable Care Act for improving mental health care. *Annual Review of Clinical Psychology, 12,* 515-542.

Mednick, B., Reznick, C., Hocevar, D., & Baker, R. (1987). Long-term effects of parental divorce on young adult male crime. *Journal of Youth & Adolescence, 16,* 31-45.

Mehta, K. M., & Yeo, G. W. (2017). Systematic review of dementia prevalence and incidence in United States race/ethnic populations. *Alzheimer's & Dementia, 13*(1), 72-83.

Melton, G. B., Petrila, J., Poythress, N. G., Slobogin, C., Otto, R. K., Mossman, D., & Condie, L. O. (2017). *Psychological evaluations for the courts: A handbook for mental health professionals and lawyers.* New York: Guilford.

Mendrek, A., & Mancini-Marie, A. (2016). Sex/gender differences in the brain and cognition in schizophrenia. *Neuroscience & Biobehavioral Reviews, 67,* 57–78.

Menezes, N. M., Arenovich, T., & Zipursky, R. B. (2006). A systematic review of longitudinal outcomes studies of first-episode psychosis. *Psychological Medicine, 36,* 1349–1362.

Mennin, D. S., Fresco, D. M., O'Toole, M. S., & Heimberg, R. G. (2018). A randomized controlled trial of emotion regulation therapy for generalized anxiety disorder with and without co-occurring depression. *Journal of Consulting and Clinical Psychology, 86*(3), 268–281.

Merai, R., Siegel, C., Rakotz, M., Basch, P., Wright, J., Wong, B., & Thorpe, P. (2016). CDC grand rounds: A public health approach to detect and control hypertension. *Morbidity and Mortality Weekly Report, 65*(45), 1261–1264.

Merikangas, K. R., Akiskal, H. S., Angst, J., Greenberg, P. E., Hirschfield, R. M. A., Petukhova, M., & Kessler, R. C. (2007). Lifetime and 12-month prevalence of bipolar spectrum disorder in the national comorbidity survey replication. *Archives of General Psychiatry, 64,* 543–552.

Merikangas, K. R., Jin, R., He, J. P., Kessler, R. C., Lee, S., Sampson, N. A., . . . Zarkov, Z. (2011). Prevalence and correlates of bipolar spectrum disorder in the World Mental Health Survey Initiative. *Archive of General Psychiatry, 68*(3), 241–251.

Merikangas, K. R., Lieb, R., Wittchen, H.-U., & Avenevoli, S. (2003). Family and high-risk studies of social anxiety disorder. *Acta Psychiatrica Scandinavica, 108* (Suppl. 417), 28–37.

Merrill, L. L., Thomsen, C. J., Sinclair, B. B., Gold, S. R., & Milner, J. S. (2001). Predicting the impact of child sexual abuse on women: The role of abuse severity, parental support, and coping strategies. *Journal of Consulting & Clinical Psychology, 69,* 992–1006.

Meston, C. M., & Bradford, A. (2007). Sexual dysfunctions in women. *Annual Review of Clinical Psychology, 3,* 233–256.

Meuret, A. E., Kroll, J., & Ritz, T. (2017). Panic disorder comorbidity with medical conditions and treatment implications. *Annual Review of Clinical Psychology, 13,* 209–240.

Meyer, I. H. (2003). Prejudice, social stress, and mental health in lesbian, gay, and bisexual populations: Conceptual issues and research evidence. *Psychological Bulletin, 129,* 674–697.

Meyer, R. G., & Weaver, C. M. (2006). *Law and mental health: A case-based approach.* New York: Guilford Press.

Mian, M., Shah, J., Dalpiaz, A., Schwamb, R., Miao, Y., Warren, K., & Khan, S. (2015). Shaken baby syndrome: A review. *Fetal and Pediatric Pathology, 34*(3), 169–175.

Micallef, J., & Blin, O. (2001). Neurobiology and clinical pharmacology of obsessive-compulsive disorder. *Clinical Neuropharmacology, 24,* 191–207.

Michael, R. T., Gagnon, J. H., Laumann, E., & Kolata, G. (1994). *Sex in America: A definitive survey.* Boston: Little, Brown.

Micheau, J., & Marighetto, A. (2011). Acetylcholine and memory: A long, complex and chaotic but still living relationship. *Behavioural Brain Research, 221,* 24–29.

Miech, R., Johnston, L., O'Malley, P. M., Bachman, J. G., & Patrick, M. E. (2019). Trends in adolescent vaping, 2017–2019. *New England Journal of Medicine, 381*(15), 1490–1491.

Mier, D., Lis, S., Esslinger, C., Sauer, C., Hagenhoff, M., Ulferts, J., et al. (2012). Neuronal correlates of social cognition in borderline personality disorder. *Social Cognitive and Affective Neuroscience, 8*(5), 531–537.

Mignot, E., Lammers, G. J., Ripley, B., Okun, M., Nevsimalova, S., Overeem, S., . . . Nishino, S. (2002). The role of cerebrospinal fluid hypocretin measurement in the diagnosis of narcolepsy and other hypersomnias. *Archives of Neurology, 59,* 1553.

Mihura, J. L., Meyer, G. J., Dumitrascu, N., & Bombel, G. (2013). The validity of individual Rorschach variables: Systematic reviews and meta-analyses of the comprehensive system. *Psychological Bulletin, 139*(3), 548–605.

Miklowitz, D. J. (2010). *The bipolar disorder survival guide* (2nd ed.). New York: Guilford Press.

Miklowitz, D. J., & Chung, B. (2016). Family-focused therapy for bipolar disorder: Reflections on 30 years of research. *Family Process, 55*(3), 483–499.

Miklowitz, D. J., Schneck, C. D., Singh, M. K., Taylor, D. O., George, E. L., Cosgrove, V. E., et al. (2013). Early intervention for symptomatic youth at risk for bipolar disorder: A randomized trial of family-focused therapy. *Journal of the American Academy of Child & Adolescent Psychiatry, 52*(2), 121–131.

Milad, M. R., & Rauch, S. L. (2012). Obsessive-compulsive disorder: Beyond segregated cortico-striatal pathways. *Trends in Cognitive Sciences, 16,* 43–51.

Milam, J. E., Richardson, J. L., Marks, G., Kemper, C. A., & McCutchan, A. J. (2004). The roles of dispositional optimism and pessimism in HIV disease progression. *Psychology & Health, 19,* 167–181.

Miller, J. D., Campbell, W. K., & Pilkonis, P. A. (2007). Narcissistic personality disorder: Relations with distress and functional impairment. *Comprehensive Psychiatry, 48,* 170–177.

Miller, J. D., Lynam, D. R., Hyatt, C. S., & Campbell, W. K. (2017). Controversies in narcissism. *Annual Review of Clinical Psychology, 13,* 291–315.

Miller, M., & Hemenway, D. (2008). Guns and suicide in the United States. *New England Journal of Medicine, 359,* 989–991.

Miller, T. Q., Smith, T. W., Turner, C. W., & Guijarro, M. L. (1996). Meta-analytic review of research on hostility and physical health. *Psychological Bulletin, 119,* 322–348.

Miller, W. R., & Rollnick, S. (2012). *Motivational interviewing: Helping people change* (3rd ed.). New York: Guilford.

Miller, W. R., & Rose, G. S. (2009). Toward a theory of motivational interviewing. *American Psychologist, 64,* 527–537.

Millon, T., Grossman, S., Millon, C., Meagher, S., & Ramnath, R. (2004). *Personality disorders in modern life* (2nd ed.). Hoboken, NJ: Wiley.

Mineka, S. (1985). Animal models of anxiety based disorders: Their usefulness and limitations. In A. H. Tuma & J. Maser (Eds.), *Anxiety and the anxiety disorders* (pp. 199–244). Hillsdale, NJ: Erlbaum.

Mineka, S., Davidson, M., Cook, M., & Keir, R. (1984). Observational conditioning of snake fear in rhesus monkeys. *Journal of Abnormal Psychology, 93,* 355–372.

Mineka, S., Gunnar, M., & Champoux, M. (1986). Control and early socioemotional development: Infant rhesus monkeys reared in controllable versus uncontrollable environments. *Child Development, 57,* 1241–1256.

Mineka, S., & Zinbarg, R. (2006). A contemporary learning theory perspective on the etiology of anxiety disorders: It's not what you thought it was. *American Psychologist, 61,* 10–26.

Minor, K. S., & Cohen, A. S. (2010). Affective reactivity of speech disturbances in schizotypy. *Journal of Psychiatric Research, 44,* 99–105.

Minuchin, S., Rosman, B. L., & Baker, L. (1978). *Psychosomatic families: Anorexia nervosa in context.* Cambridge, MA: Harvard University Press.

Miranda, J., Bernal, G., Lau, A., Kohn, L., Hwang, W. C., & La Fromboise, T. (2005). State of the science on psychosocial interventions for ethnic minorities. *Annual Review of Clinical Psychology, 1,* 113–142.

Mirica, I. (2020). Paraphilias and paraphilic behaviours. *International Journal of Advanced Studies in Sexology, 2*(1), 54–57.

Mirijello, A., D'Angelo, C., Ferrulli, A., Vassallo, G., Antonelli, M., Caputo, F., . . . Addolorato, G. (2015). Identification and management of alcohol withdrawal syndrome. *Drugs, 75,* 353–365.

Mirsky, A. E., Bieliauskas, L. A., French, L. M., Van Kammen, D. P., Joensson, E., & Sedvall, S. (2000). A 39-year follow-up on the Genain quadruplets. *Schizophrenia Bulletin, 26,* 699–708.

Mitler, M. M., & Miller, J. C. (1995). Some practical considerations and policy implications of studies and sleep patterns. *Behavioral Medicine, 21,* 184–185.

Mitropoulou, V., Barch, D., Harvey, P., Maldari, L., New, B., Cornblatt, B., & Siever, L. (2003). Two studies of attentional processing in schizotypal personality disorder. *Schizophrenia Research, 60,* S148.

Mittal, V. A., Willhite, R., Daley, M., Bearden, C. E., Niendam, T., Ellman, L. M., & Cannon, T. D. (2009). Obstetric complications and risk for conversion to psychosis among individuals at high clinical risk. *Early Intervention in Psychiatry, 3,* 226–230.

Moffitt, T. E. (1993). The neuropsychology of conduct disorder. *Development & Psychopathology, 5,* 135–151.

Moffitt, T. E. (2006). Life-course persistent versus adolescence-limited antisocial behavior. In D. Cicchetti & D. J. Cohen (Eds.), *Developmental psychopathology: Vol. 3. Risk, disorder, and adaptation* (2nd ed., pp. 570–598). New York: Wiley.

Moffitt, T. E., Arseneault, L., Jaffee, S. R., Kim-Cohen, J., Koenen, K. C., Odgers, C. L., Slutske, W. S., & Viding, E. (2008). Research review: *DSM-V* conduct disorder: Research needs for an evidence base. *Journal of Child Psychology and Psychiatry, 49,* 3–33.

Moffitt, T. E., Brammer, G. L., Caspi, A., Fawcet, J. P., Raleigh, M., Yuwiler, A., & Silva, P. A. (1998). Whole blood serotonin relates to violence in an epidemiological study. *Biological Psychiatry, 43,* 446–457.

Moffitt, T. E., Caspi, A., Harrington, H., & Milne, B. J. (2002). Males on the life-course-persistent and adolescence-limited antisocial pathways: Follow-up at age 26 years. *Development and Psychopathology, 14,* 179–207.

Moffitt, T. E., Caspi, A., Rutter, M., & Silva, P. A. (2001). *Sex differences in antisocial behaviour: Conduct disorder, delinquency, and violence in the Dunedin Longitudinal Study.* Cambridge: Cambridge University Press.

Molina, B. S., Hinshaw, S. P., Swanson, J. M., Arnold, L. E., Vitiello, B., Jensen, P. S., . . . Houck, P. R. (2009). The MTA at 8 years: Prospective follow-up of children treated for combined-type ADHD in a multisite study. *Journal of the American Academy of Child and Adolescent Psychiatry, 48,* 484–500.

Molina, O., Yegidis, B., & Jacinto, G. (2019). The pulse nightclub mass shooting and factors affecting community resilience following the terrorist attack. *Best Practices in Mental Health, 15*(2), 1–15. Retrieved from https://mccc.idm.oclc.org/login?url=https://search-proquest-com.mccc.idm.oclc.org/docview/2371576794?accountid=40611

Molnar, B. E., Berkman, L. F., & Buka, S. L. (2001). Psychopathology, childhood sexual abuse and other childhood adversities: Relative links to subsequent suicidal behavior in the U.S. *Psychological Medicine, 31,* 965–977.

Monaco, K. (2018, June 14). Suicide rate in women jumps by 50%. Retrieved December 28, 2020, from https://www.medpagetoday.com/psychiatry/depression/73485

Monahan, J., Bonnie, R. J., Appelbaum, P. S., Hyde, P. S., Steadman, H. J., & Swartz, M. S. (2001). Mandated community treatment: Beyond outpatient commitment. *Psychiatric Services, 52,* 1198–1205.

Monahan, J., Redlich, A. D., Swanson, J., Robbins, P. C., Appelbaum, P. S., Petrila, J., . . . & McNiel, D. E. (2005). Use of leverage to improve adherence to psychiatric treatment in the community. *Psychiatric Services, 56*(1), 37–44.

Monahan, J., & Skeem, J. L. (2014). The evolution of violence risk assessment. *CNS Spectrums, 19*(5), 419–424.

Monahan, J., & Walker, L. (2014). *Social science in law: Cases and materials* (8th ed.). Westbury, NY: Foundation Press.

Monroe, S. M. (2010). Recurrence in major depression: Assessing risk indicators in the context of risk estimates. In C. S. Richards & M. G. Perri (Eds.), *Relapse prevention for depression* (pp. 27–49). Washington, DC: American Psychological Association.

Montejo, A. L., Montejo, L., & Navarro-Cremades, F. (2015). Sexual side-effects of antidepressant and antipsychotic drugs. *Current Opinion in Psychiatry, 28*(6), 418–423.

Moore, A. A., Lapato, D. M., Brotman, M. A., Leibenluft, E., Aggen, S. H., Hettema, J. M., . . . Roberson, N. R. (2019). Heritability, stability, and prevalence of tonic and phasic irritability as indicators of disruptive mood dysregulation disorder. *Journal of Child Psychology & Psychiatry, 60*(9), 1032–1041.

Moore, A. A., Silberg, J. L., Roberson-Nay, R., & Mezuk, B. (2017). Life course persistent and adolescence limited conduct disorder in a nationally representative US sample: Prevalence, predictors, and outcomes. *Social Psychiatry and Psychiatric Epidemiology, 52*(4), 435–443. https://doi.org/10.1007/s00127-017-1337-5

Moorkath, F., Vranda, M. N., & Naveenkumar, C. (2018). Lives without roots: Institutionalized homeless women with chronic mental illness. *Indian Journal of Psychological Medicine, 40*(5), 476–481.

Mora, G. (2008). Renaissance conceptions and treatments of madness. In E. Wallace, IV, & J. Gach (Eds.), *History of psychiatry and medical psychology: With an epilogue on psychiatry and the mind-body relation* (pp. 199–226). New York: Springer Science.

Moran, E. K., & Kring, A. M. (2018). Anticipatory emotion in schizophrenia. *Clinical Psychological Science, 6*(1), 63–75.

Moreno-Küstner, B., Martín, C., & Pastor, L. (2018). Prevalence of psychotic disorders and its association with methodological issues. A systematic review and meta-analyses. *PloS One, 13*(4), e0195687. https://doi.org/10.1371/journal.pone.0195687

Moreno, P. I., Wiley, J. F., & Stanton, A. L. (2017). Coping through emotional approach: The utility of processing and expressing emotions in responding to stressors. In S. R. Snyder, S. J. Lopez, L. Edwards, & S. Marques (Eds.), *Oxford handbook of positive psychology* (3rd ed.). New York: Oxford University Press.

Morey, L. C., Benson, K. T., Busch, A. J., & Skodol, A. E. (2015). Personality disorders in DSM-5: Emerging research on the alternative model. *Current Psychiatry Reports, 17*(4), 24.

Morgado, P., Freitas, D., Bessa, J. M., Sousa, N., & Cerqueira, J. J. (2013). Perceived stress in obsessive-compulsive disorder is related with obsessive but not compulsive symptoms. *Frontiers in Psychiatry, 4,* 21.

Morgenthaler, T., Alessi, C., Friedman, L., Owens, J., Kapur, V., Boehlecke, B., . . . Swick, T. J. (2007). Practice parameters for the use of actigraphy in the assessment of sleep and sleep disorders: An update for 2007. *Sleep, 30,* 519–529.

Morina, N., Schnyder, U., Klaghofer, R., Müller, J., & Martin-Soelch, C. (2018). Trauma exposure and the mediating role of posttraumatic stress on somatic symptoms in civilian war victims. *BMC Psychiatry, 18*(1), 92. https://doi.org/10.1186/s12888-018-1680-4

Morin, C. M., Bootzin, R., Buysse, D., Edinger, J. D., Espie, C. A., & Lichstein, K. L. (2006). Psychological and behavioral treatment of insomnia: Update of the recent evidence (1998–2004). *Sleep, 29,* 1398–1414.

Morin, L., & Franck, N. (2017). Rehabilitation interventions to promote recovery from schizophrenia: A systematic review. *Frontiers in Psychiatry, 8,* 100.

Morrison, A. S., & Heimberg, R. G. (2013). Social anxiety and social anxiety disorder. *Annual Review of Clinical Psychology, 9,* 249–274.

Morrison, N. K. (1998). Behavioral pharmacology of hallucinogens. In R. E. Tarter (Ed.), *Handbook of substance abuse: Neurobehavioral pharmacology* (pp. 229–240). New York: Plenum Press.

Moser, C. (2011). Hypersexual disorder: Just more muddled thinking. *Archives of Sexual Behavior, 40,* 227–229, author reply 231–232.

Moustafaa, A. A., Garamib, J., Soliemanc, A., Eissac, A. M., & Shakird, M. (2020). Causes and clinical characteristics of drug abuse. *Cognitive, Clinical, and Neural Aspects of Drug Addiction, 239.*

Mowlem, F., Agnew-Blais, J., Taylor, E., & Asherson, P. (2019). Do different factors influence whether girls versus boys meet ADHD diagnostic criteria? Sex differences among children with high ADHD symptoms. *Psychiatry Research, 272,* 765–773.

Mowrer, O. H. (1939). A stimulus-response analysis of anxiety and its role as a reinforcing agent. *Psychological Review, 46,* 553–566.

Muñoz, R. F., Beardslee, W. R., & Leykin, Y. (2012). Major depression can be prevented. *American Psychologist, 67,* 287–295.

Muñoz, R. F., Bunge, E. L., Chen, K., Schueller, S. M., Bravin, J. I., Shaughnessy, E. A., & Pérez-Stable, E. J. (2016). Massive open online interventions: A novel model for delivering behavioral-health services worldwide. *Clinical Psychological Science, 4,* 194–205.

Muñoz, R. F., Cuijpers, P., Smit, F., Barrera, A., & Leykin, Y. (2010). Prevention of onset and recurrence of major depression. *Annual Review of Clinical Psychology, 6,* 181–212.

Muehlenkamp, J. J., Claes, L., Havertape, L., & Plener, P. L. (2012). International prevalence of adolescent non-suicidal self-injury and deliberate self-harm. *Child and Adolescent Psychiatry and Mental Health, 6*(1), 10–18.

Mueser, K. T., Deavers, F., Penn, D. L., & Cassisi, J. E. (2013). Psychosocial treatments for schizophrenia. *Annual Review of Clinical Psychology, 9,* 465–497.

Mueser, K. T., & Jeste, D. V. (Eds.). (2008). *Clinical handbook of schizophrenia.* New York: Guilford Press.

Mugavero, M. J., Pence, B. W., Whetten, K., Leserman, J., Swartz, M., Stangl, D., & Thielman, N. M. (2007). Predictors of AIDS-related morbidity and mortality in a southern U.S. cohort. *AIDS Patient Care STDs, 21,* 681–690.

Mukherjee, A. S. M., Hollins, S., & Turk, J. (2006). Fetal alcohol spectrum disorder: An overview. *Journal of the Royal Society of Medicine, 99,* 298–302.

Mullen, S. (2018). Major depressive disorder in children and adolescents. *The Mental Health Clinician, 8*(6), 275–283.

Muller, C. L., Anacker, A. M., & Veenstra-VanderWeele, J. (2016). The serotonin system in autism spectrum disorder: From biomarker to animal models. *Neuroscience, 321,* 24–41.

Mullins, N., & Lewis, C. M. (2017). Genetics of depression: progress at last. *Current Psychiatry Reports, 19*(8), 43.

Mundo, E., Zanoni, S., & Altamura, A. C. (2006). Genetic issues in obsessive-compulsive disorder and related disorders. *Psychiatric Annals, 36,* 495–512.

Munsch, S., Meyer, A. H., Quartier, V., & Wilhelm, F. H. (2012). Binge eating in binge eating disorder: A breakdown of emotion regulatory process? *Psychiatry Research, 195,* 118–124.

Murad, M. H., Elamin, M. B., Garcia, M. Z., Mullan, R. J., Murad, A., Erwin, P. J., & Montori, V. M. (2010). Hormonal therapy and sex reassignment: A systematic review and meta-analysis of quality of life and psychosocial outcomes. *Clinical Endocrinology (Oxf), 72,* 214–231.

Murphy, J. M. (1976). Psychiatric labeling in cross-cultural perspective. *Science, 191,* 1019–1028.

Murphy, W. D., & Page, I. J. (2008). Exhibitionism: Psychopathology and theory. In D. R. Laws & W. T. O'Donohue (Eds.), *Sexual deviance: Theory, assessment, and treatment* (pp. 61–76). New York: Guilford Press.

Murray, H. A. (1943). *Thematic apperception test manual.* Cambridge, MA: Harvard University Press.

Murray, L. K., Nguyen, A., & Cohen, J. A. (2014). Child sexual abuse. *Child and Adolescent Psychiatric Clinics, 23*(2), 321–337.

Murray, S. B., Nagata, J. M., Griffiths, S., Calzo, J. P., Brown, T. A., Mitchison, D., . . . Mond, J. M. (2017). The enigma of male eating disorders: A critical review and synthesis. *Clinical Psychology Review, 57,* 1–11.

Murray, S. B., Quintana, D. S., Loeb, K. L., Griffiths, S., & Le Grange, D. (2019). Treatment outcomes for anorexia nervosa: A systematic review and meta-analysis of randomized-controlled trials–Corrigendum. *Psychological Medicine, 49*(4), 701–704.

Musser, E. D., Karalunas, S. L., Dieckmann, N., Peris, T. S., & Nigg, J. T. (2016). Attention-deficit/hyperactivity disorder developmental trajectories related to parental expressed emotion. *Journal of Abnormal Psychology, 125*(2), 182.

Mustafa, M., Carson-Stevens, A., Gillespie, D., & Edwards, A. G. (2013). Psychological interventions for women with metastatic breast cancer. *Cochrane Database of Systematic Reviews, 6.*

Muza, R. T. (2015). Central sleep apnoea—a clinical review. *Journal of Thoracic Disease, 7*(5), 930–937.

Myrick, A. C., Webermann, A. R., Loewenstein, R. J., Lanius, R., Putnam, F. W., & Brand, B. L. (2017). Six-year follow-up of the treatment of patients with dissociative disorders study. *European Journal of Psychotraumatology, 8*(1), 1344080.

Myrseth, H., & Pallesen, S. (2010). Pharmacological treatments of impulse control disorders. In M. Hertzman & L. Adler (Eds.), *Clinical trials in psychopharmacology: A better brain* (2nd ed., pp. 289–308). Hoboken, NJ: Wiley-Blackwell.

Myrtek, M. (2007). Type A behavior and hostility as independent risk factors for coronary heart disease. In J. Jordan, B. Barden, & A. M. Zeiher (Eds.), *Contributions toward evidence-based psychocardiology: A systematic review of the literature* (pp. 159–183). Washington, DC: American Psychological Association.

N

Nadorff, M. R., Lambdin, K. K., & Germain, A. (2014). Pharmacological and non-pharmacological treatments for nightmare disorder. *International Review of Psychiatry, 26*(2), 225–236.

Nagata, J. M., Golden, N. H., Peebles, R., Long, J., Murray, S. B., Leonard, M. B., & Carlson, J. L. (2017). Assessment of sex differences in body composition among adolescents with anorexia nervosa. *The Journal of Adolescent Health: Official Publication of the Society for Adolescent Medicine, 60*(4), 455–459.

Nahata, L., Chelvakumar, G., & Leibowitz, S. (2017). Gender-affirming pharmacological interventions for youth with gender dysphoria: When treatment guidelines are not enough. *Annals of Pharmacotherapy, 51*(11), 1023–1032.

Naimi, T. S., Brown, D. W., Brewer, R. D., Giles, W. H., Mensah, G., Serdula, M. K., . . . Stroup, D. F. (2005). Cardiovascular risk factors and confounders among nondrinking and moderate-drinking U.S. adults. *American Journal of Prevention Medicine, 28*, 369–373.

Naj, A. C., Schellenberg, G. D., & Alzheimer's Disease Genetics Consortium (ADGC). (2017). Genomic variants, genes, and pathways of Alzheimer's disease: An overview. *American Journal of Medical Genetics Part B: Neuropsychiatric Genetics, 174*(1), 5–26.

Nasar, S. (1998). *A beautiful mind.* New York: Simon & Schuster.

Nath, A., Schless, N., Venkatesan, A., Rumbaugh, J., Sacktor, N., & McArthur, J. (2008). Evolution of HIV dementia with HIV infection. *International Review of Psychiatry, 20*, 25–31.

National Child Traumatic Stress Network (NCTSN). (2010). *Early childhood trauma.* Los Angeles, CA & Durham, NC: National Center for Child Traumatic Stress.

National Institute of Mental Health (NIMH). (2017c). *Bipolar disorder.* Retrieved from https://www.nimh.nih.gov/health/statistics/bipolar-disorder.shtml#part_155458

National Institute of Mental Health (NIMH). (2017). *Major Depression.* https://www.nimh.nih.gov/health/statistics/major-depression.shtml

National Institute on Drug Abuse (NIDA). (2018). Club drugs. https://www.drugabuse.gov/drugs-abuse/club-drugs. Retrieved July 3, 2018.

National LGBT Health Education Center. (2018*). Suicide risk and prevention for LGBTQ people.* Retrieved from https://www.lgbtqiahealtheducation.org/wp-content/uploads/2018/10/Suicide-Risk-and-Prevention-for-LGBTQ-Patients-Brief.pdf

National Research Council (NRC). (2014). *The growth of incarceration in the United States: Exploring causes and consequences.* Washington, DC: National Academies Press.

National Scientific Council on the Developing Child. (2005/2014). *Excessive stress disrupts the architecture of the developing brain: Working paper 3.* Updated Edition. Retrieved from http://www.developingchild.harvard.edu

National Sleep Foundation. (2009). *2009 Sleep in America poll.* Washington, DC: Author.

National Sleep Foundation. (2015). *2015 Sleep in America poll.* Washington, DC: Author.

National Transportation Safety Board. (2018). Drowsy driving. https://www.nhtsa.gov/risky-driving/drowsy-driving. Retrieved July 6, 2018.

Neacsiu, A. D, Eberle, J. W., Kramer, R., Wiesmann, T., & Linehan, M. M. (2014). Dialectical behavior therapy skills for transdiagnostic emotion dysregulation: A pilot randomized controlled trial. *Behaviour Research and Therapy, 59,* 40–51.

Neacsiu, A. D., & Linehan, M. M. (2014). Borderline personality disorder. In D. H. Barlow (Ed.), *Clinical handbook of psychological disorders: A step-by-step treatment manual* (pp. 394–461). New York: Guilford Press.

Neighbors, H. W., Trierweiler, S. J., Ford, B. C., & Muroff, J. R. (2003). Racial differences in *DSM* diagnosis using a semi-structured instrument: The importance of clinical judgment in the diagnosis of African Americans. *Journal of Health & Social Behavior, 43,* 237–256.

Neighbors, L. A., & Sobal, J. (2007). Prevalence and magnitude of body weight and shape dissatisfaction among university students. *Eating Behaviors, 9,* 429–439.

Nelson, B., & Yung, A. (2008). Treatment of the schizophrenia prodrome. In K. T. Mueser & D. V. Jeste (Eds.), *Clinical handbook of schizophrenia* (pp. 380–389). New York: Guilford Press.

Nelson, M. T., Seal, M. L., Pantelis, C., & Phillips, L. J. (2013). Evidence of a dimensional relationship between schizotypy and schizophrenia: A systematic review. *Neuroscience & Biobehavioral Reviews, 37*(3), 317–327.

Nelson, S., Baldwin, N., & Taylor, J. (2012). Mental health problems and medically unexplained physical symptoms in adult survivors of childhood sexual abuse: An integrative literature review. *Journal of Psychiatric and Mental Health Nursing, 19*(3), 211–220.

Nemeroff, C. B. (2004). Neurobiological consequences of childhood trauma. *Journal of Clinical Psychiatry, 65* (Suppl. 1), 18–28.

Nemeroff, C. B., Kalali, A., Keller, M. B., Charney, D. S., Lendarts, S. E., Cascade, E. F., . . . Schatzberg, A. F. (2007). Impact of publicity concerning pediatric suicidality data on physician practice patterns in the United States. *Archives of General Psychiatry, 64,* 466–472.

Nemoda, Z., Szekely, A., & Sasvari-Szekely, M. (2011). Psychopathological aspects of dopaminergic gene polymorphisms in adolescence and young adulthood. *Neuroscience & Biobehavioral Reviews, 35,* 1665–1686.

Nestadt, P. S., MacKrell, K., McCourt, A. D., Fowler, D. R., & Crifasi, C. K. (2020). Prevalence of long gun use in Maryland firearm suicides. *Injury epidemiology, 7*(1), 4.

Neubauer, D. N., Pandi-Perumal, S. R., Spence, D. W., Buttoo, K., & Monti, J. M. (2018). Pharmacotherapy of insomnia. *Journal of Central Nervous System Disease, 10,* 1–7.

Neueder, D., Andreatta, M., & Pauli, P. (2019). Contextual fear conditioning and fear generalization in individuals with panic attacks. *Frontiers in Behavioral Neuroscience, 13,* 152.

Neugebauer, R. (1979). Medieval and early modern theories of mental illness. *Archives of General Psychiatry, 36,* 477–483.

Newby, J., Hobbs, M., Mahoney, A., Shiu, W., Andrews, G. (2017). DSM-5 illness anxiety disorder and somatic symptom disorder: Comorbidity, correlates, and overlap with DSM-IV hypochondriasis. *Journal of Psychosomatic Research, 101,* 31–37. https://doi.org/10.1016/j.jpsychores.2017.07.010.

Newby, J. M., Hobbs, M. J., Mahoney, A. E., Wong, S. K., & Andrews, G. (2017). DSM-5 illness anxiety disorder and somatic symptom disorder: Comorbidity, correlates, and overlap with DSM-IV hypochondriasis. *Journal of Psychosomatic Research, 101,* 31–37.

Newby, J. M., Smith, J., Uppal, S., Mason, E., Mahoney, A. E., & Andrews, G. (2018). Internet-based cognitive behavioral therapy versus psychoeducation control for illness anxiety disorder and somatic symptom disorder: A randomized controlled trial. *Journal of Consulting and Clinical Psychology, 86*(1), 89–98.

Newhill, C. E., Mulvey, E. P., & Lidz, C. W. (1995). Characteristics of violence in the community by female patients seen in a psychiatric emergency service. *Psychiatric Services, 46,* 785–789.

Newman, M. G., & Llera, S. J. (2011). A novel theory of experiential avoidance in generalized anxiety disorder: A review and synthesis of research supporting a contrast avoidance model of worry. *Clinical Psychology Review, 31,* 371–382.

Newman, M. G., Llera, S. J., Erickson, T. M., Przeworski, A., & Castonguay, L. G. (2013). Worry and generalized anxiety disorder: A review and theoretical synthesis of research on its nature, etiology, mechanisms, and treatment. *Annual Review of Clinical Psychology, 9,* 275–297.

Newring, K. A. B., Wheeler, J., & Draper C. (2008). Transvestic fetishism: Assessment and treatment. In D. R. Laws & W. T. O'Donohue (Eds.), *Sexual deviance: Theory, assessment, and treatment* (pp. 285–304). New York: Guilford Press.

Neylan, T. C., Reynolds, C. F., III, & Kupfer, D. J. (2007). Sleep disorders. In J. A. Bourgeois, R. E. Hales, & S. C. Yudofsky (Eds.), *The American Psychiatric Publishing Board prep and review guide for psychiatry* (pp. 275–280). Arlington, VA: American Psychiatric Publishing.

Ng, T. H., Chung, K., Ho, F. Y.-Y, Yeung, W., Yung, K., & Lam, T. (2015). Sleep-wake disturbance in interepisode bipolar disorder and high-risk individuals: A systematic review and meta-analysis. *Sleep Medicine Review, 20C,* 46–58.

Nguyen, B. H., Pérusse, D., Paquet, J., Petit, D., Boivin, M., Tremblay, R. E., & Montplaisir, J. (2008). Sleep terrors in children: A prospective study of twins. *Pediatrics, 122*(6), e1164–e1167.

Nguyen, H. M. T., Gabrielson, A. T., & Hellstrom, W. J. (2017). Erectile dysfunction in young men—a review of the prevalence and risk factors. *Sexual Medicine Reviews, 5*(4), 508–520.

Nguyen, S. A., & McAloon, J. (2018). A cross-cultural comparison of parental perceptions of childhood separation anxiety disorder symptoms and likelihood to seek help. *Journal of Cross-Cultural Psychology, 49*(3), 453–469.

Nienhuis, J. B., Owen, J., Valentine, J. C., Winkeljohn Black, S., Halford, T. C., Parazak, S. E., Budge, S., & Hilsenroth, M. (2018). Therapeutic alliance, empathy, and genuineness in individual adult psychotherapy: A meta-analytic review. *Psychotherapy research: journal of the Society for Psychotherapy Research, 28*(4), 593–605. https://doi.org/10.1080/10503307.2016.1204023

Nigg, J. T., Lewis, K., Edinger, T., & Falk, M. (2012). Meta-analysis of attention-deficit/hyperactivity disorder or attention-deficit/hyperactivity disorder symptoms, restriction diet, and synthetic food color additives. *Journal of the American Academy of Child and Adolescent Psychiatry, 51,* 86–97.

Nijhof, A. D., Dhar, M., Goris, J., Brass, M., & Wiersema, J. R. (2018). Atypical neural responding to hearing one's own name in adults with ASD. *Journal of Abnormal Psychology, 127*(1), 129–138.

Nikolas, M. A., & Burt, S. A. (2010). Genetic and environmental influences on ADHD symptom dimensions of inattention and hyperactivity: A meta-analysis. *Journal of Abnormal Psychology, 119,* 1–17.

Nikulina, V., Bautista, A., & Brown, E. J. (2019). Negative responses to disclosure of sexual victimization and victims' symptoms of PTSD and depression: The protective role of ethnic identity. *Journal of Interpersonal Violence, 34*(21–22), 4638–4660.

Nishino, S., Sakurai, E., Nevsimalova, S., Yoshida, Y., Watanabe, T., Yanai, K., & Mignot, E. (2009). Decreased CSF histamine in narcolepsy with and without low CSF hypocretin-1 in comparison to healthy controls. *Sleep, 32,* 175–180.

Nobakht, H. & Dale, K. (2017) The prevalence of deliberate self-harm and its relationships to trauma and dissociation among Iranian young adults, Journal of *Trauma & Dissociation, 18*(4), 610–623, DOI: 10.1080/15299732.2016.1246397

Nobre, P. J., & Pinto-Gouveia, J. (2006). Dysfunctional sexual beliefs as vulnerability factors for sexual dysfunction. *Journal of Sex Research, 43,* 68–75.

Nock, M. K. (2008). Actions speak louder than words: An elaborated theoretical model of the social functions of self-injury and other harmful behaviors. *Applied and Preventive Psychology, 12*(4), 159–168.

Nock, M. K. (2010). Self-injury. *Annual Review of Clinical Psychology, 6,* 339–363.

Nock, M. K., & Kazdin, A. E. (2001). Parent expectancies for child therapy: Assessment and relation to participant in treatment. *Journal of Child & Family Studies, 10,* 155–180.

Nock, M. K., & Kessler, R. C. (2006). Prevalence of and risk factors for suicide attempts versus suicide gestures: Analysis of the national comorbidity survey. *Journal of Abnormal Psychology, 115,* 616–623.

Nolen-Hoeksema, S. (2004). Gender differences in risk factors and consequences for alcohol use and problems. *Clinical Psychology Review, 24,* 981–1010.

Nolen-Hoeksema, S., & Hilt, L. M. (2013). *Handbook of depression in adolescents.* London: Routledge.

Nolen-Hoeksema, S., & Watkins, E. R. (2011). A heuristic for developing transdiagnostic models of psychopathology: Explaining multifinality and divergent trajectories. *Perspectives on Psychological Science, 6,* 589–609.

Nolen-Hoeksema, S., Wisco, B. E., & Lyubomirsky, S. (2008). Rethinking rumination. *Perspectives on Psychological Science, 3,* 400–424.

Norcross, J. C. (2002). Empirically supported therapy relationships. In J. C. Norcross (Ed.), *Psychotherapy relationships that work: Therapist contributions and responsiveness to patients* (pp. 3–16). London: Oxford University Press.

Norcross, J. C., & Lambert, M. (Eds.). (2019). *Psychotherapy relationships that work.* Oxford University Press.

Norman, R. M., & Malla, A. K. (1993). Stressful life events and schizophrenia: II. Conceptual and methodological issues. *British Journal of Psychiatry, 162,* 166–174.

Norris, D., Clark, M. S., & Shipley, S. (2016). The mental status examination. *American Family Physician, 94*(8), 635–641.

Novak, N. L., & Brownell, K. D. (2011). Obesity: A public health approach. *Psychiatric Clinics of North America, 34,* 895–909.

Ntais, C., Pakos, E., Kyzas, P., & Ioannidis, J. P. A. (2005). Benzodiazepines for alcohol withdrawal. *Cochrane Database of Systematic Reviews, 3,* CD005063.

Nunes, E. V., & Levin, F. R. (2004). Treatment of depression in patients with alcohol or other drug dependence: A meta-analysis. *JAMA, 291,* 1887–1896.

Nusslock, R., Abramson, L. Y., Harmon-Jones, E., Alloy, L. B., & Hogan, M. E. (2007). A goal-striving life event and the onset of bipolar episodes: Perspective from the behavioral approach system (BAS) dysregulation theory. *Journal of Abnormal Psychology, 116,* 105–115.

Nusslock, R., Almeida, J. R., Forbes, E. E., Versace, A., Frank, E., LaBarbara, E. J., . . . Phillips, M. L. (2012). Waiting to win: Elevated striatal and orbitofrontal cortical activity during reward anticipation in euthymic bipolar disorder adults. *Bipolar Disorders, 14*(3), 249–260.

O

O'Connor, K., Hallam, R., & Rachman, S. (1985). Fearlessness and courage: A replication experiment. *British Journal of Psychology, 76,* 187–197.

O'Connor, R. C., & Nock, M. K. (2014). The psychology of suicidal behaviour. *Lancet Psychiatry, 1*(1), 73–85.

O'Connor v. Donaldson. (1975). 422 U.S. 563.

O'Donnell, L., O'Donnell, C., Wardlaw, D. M., & Stueve, A. (2004). Risk and resiliency factors influencing suicidality among urban African American and Latino youth. *American Journal of Community Psychology, 33,* 37–49.

O'Driscoll, C., Sener, S. B., Angmark, A., & Shaikh, M. (2019). Caregiving processes and expressed emotion in psychosis, a cross-cultural, meta-analytic review. *Schizophrenia Research, 208,* 8–15.

Odgers, C. L., Moffitt, T. E., Broadbent, J. M., Dickson, N., Hancox, R. J., Harrington, H., Poulton, R., Sears, M. R., Thomson, W. M., & Caspi, A. (2008). Female and male antisocial trajectories: From childhood origins to adult outcomes. *Development and Psychopathology, 20,* 673–716.

Ogden, C. L., Carroll, M. D., Kit, B. K., & Flegal, K. M. (2012). Prevalence of obesity in the United States, 2009–2010. National Center for Health Statistics, *Data Brief, 82,* 1–7.

Ogden, C. L., Flegal, K. M., Carroll, M. D., & Johnson, C. L. (2002). Prevalence and trends in overweight among US children and adolescents, 1999–2000. *Journal of the American Medical Association, 288,* 1728–1732.

Ogilvie, J. M., Stewart, A. L., Chan, R. C., & Shum, D. H. (2011). Neuropsychological measures of executive function and antisocial behavior: A meta-analysis. *Criminology, 49*(4), 1063–1107.

O'Hara, M. W., & McCabe, J. E. (2013). Postpartum depression: Current status and future directions. *Annual Review of Clinical Psychology, 9,* 379–407.

Ohayon, M. M. (2012). Determining the level of sleepiness in the American population and its correlates. *Journal of Psychiatric Research, 46,* 422–427.

Ohayon, M. M., Dauvilliers, Y., & Reynolds, C. F. (2012). Operational definitions and algorithms for excessive sleepiness in the general population: Implications for *DSM-5* nosology. *Archives of General Psychiatry, 69,* 71–79.

Ohayon, M. M., Guilleminault, C., & Chokroverty, S. (2010). Sleep epidemiology 30 years later: Where are we? *Sleep Medicine, 11,* 961–962.

Ohayon, M. M., Smolensky, M. H., & Roth, T. (2010). Consequences of shift working on sleep duration, sleepiness, and sleep attacks. *Chronobiology International, 27,* 575–589.

Ohi, K., Hashimoto, R., Nakazawa, T., Okada, T., Yasuda, Y., Yamamori, H., . . . Takeda, M. (2012). The p250GAP gene is associated with risk for schizophrenia and schizotypal personality traits. *PLoS ONE, 7*(4), e35696.

Ohman, A., Fredrikson, M., Hugdahl, K., & Rimmo, P. (1976). The premise of equipotentiality in human classical conditioning: Conditioned electrodermal responses to potentially phobic stimuli. *Journal of Experimental Psychology: General, 105,* 313–337.

Ohman, A., & Mineka, S. (2001). Fears, phobias, and preparedness: Toward an evolved module of fear and fear learning. *Psychological Review, 108,* 483–522.

Okhuijsen-Pfeifer, C., Huijsman, E. A. H., Hasan, A., Sommer, I. E. C., Leucht, S., Kahn, R. S., & Luykx, J. J. (2018). Clozapine as a first-or second-line treatment in schizophrenia: A systematic review and meta-analysis. *Acta Psychiatrica Scandinavica, 138*(4), 281–288.

Olatunji, B. O., Kauffman, B. Y., Meltzer, S., Davis, M. L., Smits, J. A., & Powers, M. B. (2014). Cognitive-behavioral therapy for hypochondriasis/health anxiety: A meta-analysis of treatment outcome and moderators. *Behaviour Research and Therapy, 58,* 65–74.

Olatunji, B. O., & Wolitzky-Taylor, K. B. (2009). Anxiety sensitivity and the anxiety disorders: A meta-analytic review and synthesis. *Psychological Bulletin, 135,* 974–999.

Oldershaw, A., Lavender, T., Sallis, H., Stahl, D., & Schmidt, U. (2015). Emotion generation and regulation in anorexia nervosa: A systematic review and meta-analysis of self-report data. *Clinical Psychology Review, 39,* 83–95.

O'Leary, A., Jemmott, L. S., & Jemmott, J. B., III. (2008). Mediation analysis of an effective sexual risk-reduction intervention for women: The importance of self-efficacy. *Health Psychology, 27,* S180–S184.

Oliffe, J. L., Rossnagel, E., Seidler, Z. E., Kealy, D., Ogrodniczuk, J. S., & Rice, S. M. (2019). Men's depression and suicide. *Current Psychiatry Reports, 21*(10), 1–6.

Olivier, I. S., Cacabelos, R., & Naidoo, V. (2018). Risk factors and pathogenesis of HIV-associated neurocognitive disorder: the role of host genetics. *International Journal of Molecular Sciences, 19*(11), 3594.

Ollendick, T. H., & Davis III, T. E. (2013). One-session treatment for specific phobias: A review of Öst's single-session exposure with children and adolescents. *Cognitive Behaviour Therapy, 42*(4), 275–283.

Olmsted, M. P., McFarlane, T. L., Carter, J. C., Trottier, K., Woodside, D. B., & Dimitropoulos, G. (2010). Inpatient and day hospital treatment for anorexia nervosa. In C. M. Grilo & J. E. Mitchell (Eds.), *The treatment of eating disorders: A clinical handbook* (pp. 198–211). New York: Guilford Press.

Olson, K. R. (2016). Prepubescent transgender children: What we do and do not know. *Journal of the American Academy of Child & Adolescent Psychiatry, 55*(3), 155–156.

Olweus, D. (2011). Bullying at school and later criminality: Findings from three Swedish community samples of males. *Criminal Behavior and Mental Health, 21,* 151–156.

Ono, M., Devilly, G. J., & Shum, D. H. (2016). A meta-analytic review of overgeneral memory: The role of trauma history, mood, and the presence of posttraumatic stress disorder. *Psychological Trauma: Theory, Research, Practice, and Policy, 8*(2), 157–164.

Opara, I., Assan, M. A., Pierre, K., Gunn III, J. F., Metzger, I., Hamilton, J., & Arugu, E. (2020). Suicide among Black children: An integrated model of the interpersonal-psychological theory of suicide and intersectionality theory for researchers and clinicians. *Journal of Black Studies, 51*(6), 611–631.

Oquendo, M. A., Ellis, S. P., Greenwald, S., Malone, K. M., Weissman, M. M., & Mann, J. J. (2001). Ethnic and sex differences in suicide rates relative to major depression in the United States. *American Journal of Psychiatry, 158,* 1652–1658.

Orefici, G., Cardona, F., Cox, C. J., & Cunningham, M. W. (2016, February 10). Pediatric autoimmune neuropsychiatric disorders associated with streptococcal infections (PANDAS). In J. J. Ferretti, D. L. Stevens, V. A. Fischetti (Eds.), *Streptococcus pyogenes: Basic biology to clinical manifestations [Internet]*. Oklahoma City, OK: University of Oklahoma Health Sciences Center. Retrieved from https://www.ncbi.nlm.nih.gov/books/NBK333433/

Orgilés, M., Penosa, P., Morales, A., Fernández-Martínez, I., & Espada, J. P. (2018). Maternal anxiety and separation anxiety in children aged between 3 and 6 years: The mediating role of parenting style. *Journal of Developmental and Behavioral Pediatrics: JDBP, 39*(8), 621–628.

Orri, M., Galera, C., Turecki, G., Forte, A., Renaud, J., Boivin, M., . . . & Geoffroy, M. C. (2018). Association of childhood irritability and depressive/anxious mood profiles with adolescent suicidal ideation and attempts. *JAMA Psychiatry, 75*(5), 465-473.

Ortiz, J., & Raine, A. (2004). Heart rate and antisocial behavior in children and adolescents: A meta-analysis. *Journal of the American Academy of Child and Adolescent Psychiatry, 43,* 154-162.

Osher, F. C., & Steadman, H. J. (2007). Adapting evidence-based practices for persons with mental illness involved with the criminal justice system. *Psychiatric Services, 58,* 1472-1478.

Osiezagha, K., Ali, S., Freeman, C., Barker, N. C., Jabeen, S., Maitra, S., . . . Bailey, R. K. (2013). Thiamine deficiency and delirium. *Innovations in Clinical Neuroscience, 10*(4), 26-32.

Ost, J., Granhag, P. A., Udell, J., Roos, A. F., & Hjelmsater, E. (2008). Familiarity breeds distortion: The effects of media exposure on false reports concerning media coverage of the terrorist attacks in London on 7 July 2005. *Memory, 16,* 76-85.

Öst, L.-G. (2014). The efficacy of Acceptance and Commitment Therapy: An updated systematic review and meta-analysis. *Behaviour Research and Therapy, 61,* 105-121.

Öst, L.-G., Havnen, A., Hansen, B., & Kvale, G. (2015). Cognitive behavioral treatments of obsessive-compulsive disorder: A systematic review and meta-analysis of studies published 1993-2014. *Clinical Psychology Review, 40,* 156-169.

Öst, L. S., & Sterner, U. (1987). Applied tension: A specific behavioral method for treatment of blood phobia. *Behaviour Research & Therapy, 25,* 25-29.

Ougrin, D., Tranah, T., Stahl, D., Moran, P., & Asarnow, J. R. (2015). Therapeutic interventions for suicide attempts and self-harm in adolescents: Systematic review and meta-analysis. *Journal of the American Academy of Child & Adolescent Psychiatry, 54*(2), 97-107.

Overmier, J. B., & Seligman, M. E. (1967). Effects of inescapable shock upon subsequent escape and avoidance responding. *Journal of Comparative & Physiological Psychology, 63,* 28-33.

Ozbay, F., Johnson, D. C., Dimoulas, E., Morgan, C. A., Charney, D., & Southwick, S. (2007). Social support and resilience to stress: From neurobiology to clinical practice. *Psychiatry (Edgmont (Pa.: Township)), 4*(5), 35-40.

Öztürk, E., & Sar, V. (2016). Formation and functions of alter personalities in dissociative identity disorder: A theoretical and clinical elaboration. *J Psychol Clin Psychiatry, 6*(6), 00385.

P

Pack, A. I., & Pien, G. W. (2011). Update on sleep and its disorders. *Annual Review of Medicine, 62,* 447-460.

Pacula, R. L., & Smart, R. (2017). Medical marijuana and marijuana legalization. *Annual Review of Clinical Psychology, 13,* 397-419.

Padgett, D. K., & Henwood, B. F. (2011). Moving into the fourth decade of ACT. *Psychiatric Services, 62,* 605.

Pae C. U. (2020). Antipsychotic Polypharmacy in treatment of schizophrenia; should or should not?. *Chonnam Medical Journal, 56*(3), 157-165. https://doi.org/10.4068/cmj.2020.56.3.157

Pakenham, K. I., Landi, G., Boccolini, G., Furlani, A., Grandi, S., & Tossani, E. (2020). The moderating roles of psychological flexibility and inflexibility on the mental health impacts of COVID-19 pandemic and lockdown in Italy. *Journal of Contextual Behavioral Science, 17,* 109-118.

Paniagua, F. A., & Yamada, A. M. (2013). *Handbook of multicultural mental health: Assessment and treatment of diverse populations* (2nd ed.). San Diego: Academic Press.

Pankow, A., Katthagen, T., Diner, S., Deserno, L., Boehme, R., Kathmann, N., . . . & Schlagenhauf, F. (2016). Aberrant salience is related to dysfunctional self-referential processing in psychosis. *Schizophrenia bulletin, 42*(1), 67-76.

Panos, P. T., Jackson, J. W., Hasan, O., & Panos, A. (2014). Meta-analysis and systematic review assessing the efficacy of dialectical behavior therapy (DBT). *Research on Social Work Practice, 24*(2), 213-223.

Pappadopulos, E., Woolston, S., Chait, A., Perkins, M., Connor, D. F., & Jensen, P. S. (2006). Pharmacotherapy of aggression in children and adolescents: Efficacy and effect size. *Journal of the Canadian Academy of Child and Adolescent Psychiatry, 15,* 27-39.

Parish, S. J., & Hahn, S. R. (2016). Hypoactive sexual desire disorder: A review of epidemiology, biopsychology, diagnosis, and treatment. *Sexual Medicine Reviews, 4*(2), 103-120.

Paris, J. (1998). *Working with traits: Psychotherapy of personality disorders.* Northvale, NJ: Jason Aronson.

Park, A., Conway, M., & Chen, A. T. (2018). Examining Thematic Similarity, Difference, and Membership in Three Online Mental Health Communities from Reddit: A Text Mining and Visualization Approach. *Computers in human behavior, 78,* 98-112. https://doi.org/10.1016/j.chb.2017.09.001

Park, D. C., & Reuter-Lorenz, P. (2009). The adaptive brain: Aging and neurocognitive scaffolding. *Annual Review of Psychology, 60,* 173-196.

Parke, E. M., Thaler, N. S., Etcoff, L. M., & Allen, D. N. (2020). Intellectual profiles in children with ADHD and comorbid learning and motor disorders. *Journal of Attention Disorders, 24*(9), 1227-1236.

Parmar, A., & Kaloiya, G. (2018). Comorbidity of Personality Disorder among Substance Use Disorder Patients: A Narrative Review. *Indian Journal of Psychological Medicine, 40*(6), 517-527. https://doi.org/10.4103/IJPSYM.IJPSYM_164_18

Parrow, K. K., Sommers-Flanagan, J., Cova, J. S., & Lungu, H. (2019). Evidence-based relationship factors: A new focus for mental health counseling research, practice, and training. *Journal of Mental Health Counseling, 41*(4), 327-342. doi: http://dx.doi.org.mccc.idm.oclc.org/10.17744/mehc.41.4.04

Partinen, M., Kornum, B. R., Plazzi, G., Jennum, P., Julkunen, I., & Vaarala, O. (2014). Narcolepsy as an autoimmune disease: The role of H1N1 infection and vaccination. *Lancet Neurology, 13*(6), 600-613.

Patel, K. R., Cherian, J., Gohil, K., & Atkinson, D. (2014). Schizophrenia: Overview and treatment options. *P & T: A Peer-Reviewed Journal for Formulary Management, 39*(9), 638-645.

Patel, R. S., Amaravadi, N., Bhullar, H., Lekireddy, J., & Win, H. (2018). Understanding the demographic predictors and associated comorbidities in children hospitalized with conduct disorder. *Behavioral Sciences (Basel, Switzerland), 8*(9), 80. https://doi.org/10.3390/bs8090080

Patrick, D. L., Althof, S. E., Pryor, J. L., Rosen, R., Rowland, D. L., Ho, K. F., . . . Jamieson, C. (2005). Premature ejaculation: An observational study of men and their partners. *Journal of Sexual Medicine, 2,* 358-367.

Patriquin, M. A., & Mathew, S. J. (2017). The neurobiological mechanisms of generalized anxiety disorder and chronic stress. *Chronic stress (Thousand Oaks, Calif.), 1,* 2470547017703993.

Paul, L. A., Grubaugh, A. L., Frueh, B. C., Ellis, C., & Egede, L. E. (2011). Associations between binge and heavy drinking and health behaviors in a nationally representative sample. *Addictive Behaviors, 36,* 1240-1245.

Paulus, F. W., Backes, A., Sander, C. S., Weber, M., & von Gontard, A. (2015). Anxiety disorders and behavioral inhibition in preschool children: A population-based study. *Child Psychiatry & Human Development, 46,* 150-157.

Pearce, J., Jovev, M., Hulbert, C., McKechnie, B., McCutcheon, L., Betts, J., & Chanen, A. M. (2017). Evaluation of a psychoeducational group intervention for family and friends of youth with borderline personality disorder. *Borderline Personality Disorder and Emotion Dysregulation, 4*(1), 1–7.

Pearl, R. L. (2018). Weight bias and stigma: Public health implications and structural solutions. *Social Issues and Policy Review, 12*(1), 146–182.

Pearl, R. L., Puhl, R. M., & Brownell, K. D. (2012). Positive media portrayals of obese persons: Impact on attitudes and image preferences. *Health Psychology, 31,* 821–829.

Peat, C., Mitchell, J. E., Hoek, H. W., & Wonderlich, S. A. (2009). Validity and utility of subtyping anorexia nervosa. *International Journal of Eating Disorders, 42,* 590–594.

Peixoto, M. M., & Nobre, P. (2014). Dysfunctional sexual beliefs: A comparative study of heterosexual men and women, gay men, and lesbian women with and without sexual problems. *Journal of Sexual Medicine, 11*(11), 2690–2700.

Pelsser, L. M., Frankena, K., Toorman, J., & Rodrigues Pereira, R. (2017). Diet and ADHD, reviewing the evidence: A systematic review of meta-analyses of double-blind placebo-controlled trials evaluating the efficacy of diet interventions on the behavior of children with ADHD. *PloS One, 12*(1), e0169277.

Pennebaker, J. W. (2007). Current issues and new directions in psychology and health: Listening to what people say—the value of narrative and computational linguistics in health psychology. *Psychology & Health, 22,* 631–635.

Pennebaker, J. W., Kiecolt-Glaser, J. K., & Glaser, R. (1988). Disclosure of traumas and immune function: Health implications for psychotherapy. *Journal of Consulting and Clinical Psychology, 56,* 239–245.

Perelman, M. A., & Rowland, D. L. (2008). Retarded and inhibited ejaculation. In D. L. Rowland & L. Incrocci (Eds.), *Handbook of sexual and gender identity disorders* (pp. 100–121). Hoboken, NJ: Wiley.

Perelman, M. A., & Watter, D. N. (2016). Psychological aspects of erectile dysfunction. In T. S. Köhler & K. T. McVary (Eds.), *Contemporary treatment of erectile dysfunction: A clinical guide* (pp. 29–43). Cham: Springer.

Perepletchikova, F., Nathanson, D., Axelrod, S., Merrill, C., Walker, A., Grossman, M., . . . Walkup, J. (2017). Randomized clinical trial of dialectical behavior therapy for preadolescent children with disruptive mood dysregulation disorder: Feasibility and outcomes. *Journal of the American Academy of Child & Adolescent Psychiatry, 56*(10), 832–840.

Perepletchikova, F., Nathanson, D., Axelrod, S. R., Merrill C., Walker, A., Grossman, M., . . . Walkup. J. (2017). Randomized clinical trial of Dialectical Behavior Therapy for pre-adolescent children with disruptive mood dysregulation disorder: Feasibility and outcomes. *Journal of the American Academy of Child & Adolescent Psychiatry, 56,* 832–840.

Perez, M., Ohrt, T. K., & Hoek, H. W. (2016). Prevalence and treatment of eating disorders among Hispanics/Latino Americans in the United States. *Current Opinion in Psychiatry, 29*(6), 378–382.

Perez, S., Brown, C., & Binik, Y. M. (2016). Vaginismus: When genito-pelvic pain/penetration disorder makes intercourse seem impossible. In L. Lipshultz, A. Pastuszak, A. Goldstein, A. Giraldi, & M. Perelman (Eds.), *Management of sexual dysfunction in men and women* (pp. 273–285). New York: Springer.

Perneczky, R., Alexopoulos, P., Wagenpfeil, S., & Kurz, A. (2012). Head circumference, apolipoprotein E genotype and cognition in the Bavarian School Sisters study. *European Psychiatry, 27,* 219–222.

Perneczky, R., Drzezga, A., Diehl-Schmid, J., Li, Y., & Kurz, A. (2007). Gender differences in brain reserve: An (18)F-FDG PET study in Alzheimer's disease. *Journal of Neurology, 254,* 1395–1400.

Perry, A., Koudys, J., & Blacklock, K. (2016). Early intensive behavioral intervention. In N. N. Singh (Ed.), *Handbook of evidence-based practices in intellectual and developmental disabilities* (pp. 511–535). Cham: Springer.

Perugi, G., Medda, P., Toni, C., Mariani, M. G., Socci, C., & Mauri, M. (2017). The role of electroconvulsive therapy (ect) in bipolar disorder: Effectiveness in 522 patients with bipolar depression, mixed-state, mania and catatonic features. *Current Neuropharmacology, 15,* 359–371.

Pescosolido, B. A. (2013). The public stigma of mental illness: What do we think; what do we know; what can we prove? *Journal of Health and Social Behavior, 54*(1), 1–21.

Pescosolido, B. A., Fettes, D. L., Martin, J. K., Monahan, J., & McLeod, J. D. (2007). Perceived dangerousness of children with mental health problems and support for coerced treatment. *Psychiatric Services, 58,* 619–625.

Peters, A. T., West, A. E., Eisner, L., Baek, J., & Deckersbach, T. (2016). The burden of repeated mood episodes in bipolar I disorder: Results from the National Epidemiological Survey on alcohol and related conditions. *The Journal of Nervous and Mental Disease, 204*(2), 87–94.

Peterson, C., & Seligman, M. E. (1984). Causal explanations as a risk factor for depression: Theory and evidence. *Psychological Review, 91,* 347–374.

Peterson, C., Seligman, M. E. P., Yurko, K. H., Martin, L. R., & Friedman, H. S. (1998). Catastrophizing and untimely death. *Psychological Science, 9,* 127–130.

Peterson, C., Seligman, M. E., & Vaillant, G. E. (1988). Pessimistic explanatory style is a risk factor for physical illness: A thirty-five-year longitudinal study. *Journal of Personality & Social Psychology, 55,* 23–27.

Peterson, R. L., & Pennington, B. F. (2015). Developmental dyslexia. *Annual Review of Clinical Psychology, 11,* 283–307.

Peterson, Z. D. (2017). *The Wiley handbook of sex therapy.* Oxford: Wiley.

Petit, D., Pennestri, M. H., Paquet, J., Desautels, A., Zadra, A., Vitaro, F., . . . Montplaisir, J. (2015). Childhood sleepwalking and sleep terrors: A longitudinal study of prevalence and familial aggregation. *JAMA Pediatrics, 169*(7), 653–658.

Petronis, A., Gottesman, I. I., Kan, P., Kennedy, J. L., Basile, V. S., Paterson, A. D., & Popendikyte, V. (2003). Monozygotic twins exhibit numerous epigenetic differences: Clues to twin discordance? *Schizophrenia Bulletin, 29,* 168–178.

Petry, N. M., Rash, C. J., & Alessi, S. M. (2016). A randomized controlled trial of brief interventions for problem gambling in substance abuse treatment patients. *Journal of Consulting and Clinical psychology, 84*(10), 874–886.

Petry, N. M., Zajac, K., & Ginley, M. K. (2018). Behavioral addictions as mental disorders: To be or not to be? *Annual Review of Clinical Psychology, 14,* 399–423.

Pew Research Center. (2018). About six-in-ten Americans support marijuana legalization. http://www.pewresearch.org/fact-tank/2018/01/05/americans-support-marijuana-legalization/ Retrieved July 3, 2018

Pharoah, F., Mari, J. J., Rathbone, J., & Wong, W. (2010). Family intervention for schizophrenia. *The Cochrane Library.*

Phillips, D. P., & Brewer, K. M. (2011). The relationship between serious injury and blood alcohol concentration (BAC) in fatal motor vehicle accidents: BAC = 0.01% is associated with significantly more dangerous accidents than BAC = 0.00%. *Addiction, 106,* 1614–1622.

Phillips K. A. (2007). Suicidality in body dysmorphic disorder. *Primary Psychiatry, 14*(12), 58–66.

Phillips, K. A., Didie, E. R., Feusner, J., & Wilhelm, S. (2008). Body dysmorphic disorder: Treating an underrecognized disorder. *American Journal of Psychiatry, 165,* 1111–1118.

Phillips, K. A., Wilhelm, S., Koran, L. M., Didie, E. R., Fallon, B. A., Feusner, J., & Stein, D. J. (2010). Body dysmorphic disorder: Some key issues for *DSM-V. Depression and Anxiety, 27,* 573–591.

Phillips, M. L., & Swartz, H. A. (2014). A critical appraisal of neuroimaging studies of bipolar disorder: Toward a new conceptualization of underlying neural circuitry and a road map for future research. *American Journal of Psychiatry, 171*(8), 829–843.

Pieper, S., Brosschot, J. F., van der Leeden, R., & Thayer, J. F. (2010). Prolonged cardiac effects of momentary assessed stressful events and worry episodes. *Psychosomatic Medicine, 72*(6), 570–577.

Pieper, S., Out, D., Bakermans-Kranenburg, M. J., & van IJzendoorn, M. H. (2011). Behavioral and molecular genetics of dissociation: The role of the serotonin transporter gene promoter polymorphism (5-HTTLPR). *Journal of Traumatic Stress, 24*(4), 373–380.

Pincus, A. L., Ansell, E. B., Pimentel, C. A., Cain, N. M., Wright, A. G. C., & Levy, K. N. (2009). Initial construction and validation of the Pathological Narcissism Inventory. *Psychological Assessment, 21,* 365–379.

Pincus, A. L., & Lukowitsky, M. R. (2010). Pathological narcissism and narcissistic personality disorder. *Clinical Psychology, 6,* 421–426.

Pingault, J. B., Viding, E., Galéra, C., Greven, C. U., Zheng, Y., Plomin, R., & Rijsdijk, F. (2015). Genetic and environmental influences on the developmental course of attention-deficit/hyperactivity disorder symptoms from childhood to adolescence. *JAMA Psychiatry, 72*(7), 651–658.

Pini, S., Abelli, M., Shear, K. M., Cardini, A., Lari, L., Gesi, C., . . . Cassano, G. B. (2010). Frequency and clinical correlates of adult separation anxiety in a sample of 508 outpatients with mood and anxiety disorders. *Acta Psychiatrica Scandinavica, 122,* 40–46.

Pipher, M. (1994). *Reviving Ophelia: Saving the selves of adolescent girls.* New York: Putnam.

Pirelli, G., Gottdiener, W. H., & Zapf, P. A. (2011). A meta-analytic review of competency to stand trial research. *Psychology, Public Policy, and Law, 17,* 1–53.

Pirolli, P., Youngblood, G. M., Du, H., Konrad, A., Nelson, L., & Springer, A. (2021). Scaffolding the mastery of healthy behaviors with Fittle+ systems: Evidence-based interventions and theory. *Human-Computer Interaction, 36*(2), 73–106.

Pittenger, C., & Duman, R. S. (2008). Stress, depression, and neuroplasticity: A convergence of mechanisms. *Neuropsychopharmacology Reviews, 33,* 88–109.

Pizzagalli, D. A. (2014). Depression, stress, and anhedonia: Toward a synthesis and integrated model. *Annual Review of Clinical Psychology, 10,* 393–423.

Plante, D. T. (2017). Sleep propensity in psychiatric hypersomnolence: A systematic review and meta-analysis of multiple sleep latency test findings. *Sleep Medicine Reviews, 31,* 48–57.

Platt, S., & Hawton, K. (2000). Suicidal behaviour and the labour market. In K. Hawton & K. van Heeringen (Eds.), *The international handbook of suicide and attempted suicide.* New York: Wiley.

Plazzi, G., Pizza, F., Palaia, V., Franceschini, C., Poli, F., Moghadam, K. V., . . . Bhatia, K. P. (2011). Complex

movement disorders in childhood narcolepsy with cataplexy at disease onset. *Brain, 134*(pt. 12), 3480–3492.

Plöderl, M., & Tremblay, P. (2015). Mental health of sexual minorities: A systematic review. *International Review of Psychiatry, 27*(5), 367–385.

Plimpton, E., Frost, R., Abbey, B., & Dorer, W. (2009). Compulsive hoarding in children: Six case studies. *International Journal of Cognitive Therapy, 2*(1), 88–104.

Poewe, W., Seppi, K., Tanner, C. M., Halliday, G. M., Brundin, P., Volkmann, J., . . . Lang, A. E. (2017). Parkinson disease. *Nature Reviews Disease Primers, 3,* 17013.

Poggi, A., Richetin, J., & Preti, E. (2019). Trust and rejection sensitivity in personality disorders. *Current Psychiatry Reports, 21*(8), 69.

Polanco-Roman, L., Anglin, D. M., Miranda, R., & Jeglic, E. L. (2019). Racial/ethnic discrimination and suicidal ideation in emerging adults: The role of traumatic stress and depressive symptoms varies by gender not race/ethnicity. *Journal of Youth and Adolescence, 48*(10), 2023–2037.

Polanczyk, G. V., Willcutt, E. G., Salum, G. A., Kieling, C., & Rohde, L. A. (2014). ADHD prevalence estimates across three decades: An updated systematic review and meta-regression analysis. *International Journal of Epidemiology, 43*(2), 434–442.

Poland, S., Lieberman, R., & Niznik, M. (2019). Suicide contagion and clusters—Part 1: What school psychologists should know. *Communique, 47*(5), 1–21.

Polderman, T. J., Benyamin, B., De Leeuw, C. A., Sullivan, P. F., Van Bochoven, A., Visscher, P. M., & Posthuma, D. (2015). Meta-analysis of the heritability of human traits based on fifty years of twin studies. *Nature Genetics, 47*(7), 702.

Pole, N., Neylan, T. C., Otte, C., Metzler, T. J., Best, S. R., & Henn-Haase, C. (2007). Associations between childhood trauma and emotion-modulated psychophysiological responses to startling sounds: A study of police cadets. *Journal of Abnormal Psychology, 116,* 352–361.

Polivy, J., & Herman, C. P. (2002). Causes of eating disorders. *Annual Review of Psychology, 53,* 187–213.

Pope, H. G., Gruber, A. J., Hudson, J. I., Huestis, M. A., & Yurgelun-Todd, D. (2001). Neuropsychological performance in long-term cannabis users. *Archives of General Psychiatry, 58,* 909–915.

Pope, H. G., Jacobs, A., Mialet, J., Yurgelun-Todd, D., & Gruber, S. (1997). Evidence for a sex-specific residual effect of cannabis on visuospatial memory. *Psychotherapy & Psychosomatics, 66,* 179–184.

Pope, H. G., Jr., Lalonde, J. K., Pindyck, L. J., Walsh, B. T., Bulik, C. M., Crow, S., . . . Hudson, J. I. (2006). Binge eating disorder: A stable syndrome. *American Journal of Psychology, 163,* 2181–2183.

Popova, S., Lange, S., Probst, C., Gmel, G., & Rehm, J. (2017). Estimation of national, regional, and global prevalence of alcohol use during pregnancy and fetal alcohol syndrome: A systematic review and meta-analysis. *The Lancet Global Health, 5*(3), e290–e299.

Popovic, D., Schmitt, A., Kaurani, L., Senner, F., Papiol, S., Malchow, B., . . . & Falkai, P. (2019). Childhood trauma in schizophrenia: Current findings and research perspectives. *Frontiers in Neuroscience, 13,* 274.

Potenza, M. N., Steinberg, M. A., Skudlarski, P., Fulbright, R. K., Lacadie, C. M., Wilbur, M. K., . . . Wexler, B. E. (2003). Gambling urges in pathological gambling: A functional magnetic resonance imaging study. *Archives of General Psychiatry, 60,* 828–836.

Powell, N. P., Lochman, J. E., Boxmeyer, C. L., Barry, T. D., & Pardini, D. A. (2017). The coping power program for aggressive behavior in children. In J. R. Weisz & A. E. Kazdin (Eds.), *Evidence-based psychotherapies for children and adolescents* (3rd ed., pp. 159–176). New York: Guilford.

Pratt, D. S., Jandzio, M., Tomlinson, D., Kang, X., & Smith, E. (2006). The 5-10-25 challenge: An observational study of a Web-based wellness intervention for a global workforce. *Disease Management, 9,* 284–290.

Price, A. (2020). Online gambling in the midst of COVID-19: a nexus of mental health concerns, substance use and financial stress. *International Journal of Mental Health and Addiction,* 1–18.

Prins, S. J. (2014). Prevalence of mental illnesses in US state prisons: A systematic review. *Psychiatric Services, 65*(7), 862–872.

Prochaska, J. O., & Norcross, J. C. (2014). Systemic therapies. In J. O. Prochaska & J. C. Norcross (Eds.), *Systems of psychotherapy: A transtheoretical analysis* (9th ed., pp. 289–321). New York: Oxford University Press.

Proctor, A., Yairi, E., Duff, M. C., & Zhang, J. (2008). Prevalence of stuttering in African American preschoolers. *Journal of Speech, Language and Hearing Research, 51,* 1465–1479.

Procyshyn, R. M., Bezchlibnyk-Butler, K. Z., & Jeffries, J. J. (Eds.). (2017). *Clinical handbook of psychotropic drugs.* Boston: Hogrefe.

Project MATCH Research Group. (1998). Matching alcoholism treatments to client heterogeneity: Treatment main effects and matching effects on drinking during treatment. *Journal of Studies on Alcohol, 59,* 631–639.

Przeworski, A., Newman, M. G., Pincus, A. L., Kasoff, M. B., Yamasaki, A. S., Castonguay, L. G., & Berlin, K. S. (2011). Interpersonal pathoplasticity in individuals with generalized anxiety disorder. *Journal of Abnormal Psychology, 120,* 286–298.

Puglisi, G., Sciortino, T., Rossi, M., Leonetti, A., Fornia, L., Conti Nibali, M., . . . Bello, L. (2018). Preserving executive functions in nondominant frontal lobe glioma surgery: an intraoperative tool, *Journal of Neurosurgery JNS, 131*(2), 474–480. Retrieved Nov 1, 2020, from https://thejns.org/view/journals/j-neurosurg/131/2/article-p474.xml

Puolakanaho, A., Lappalainen, R., Lappalainen, P., Muotka, J. S., Hirvonen, R., Eklund, K. M., . . . Kiuru, N. (2019). Reducing stress and enhancing academic buoyancy among adolescents using a brief web-based program based on acceptance and commitment therapy: A randomized controlled trial. *Journal of Youth and Adolescence, 48*(2), 287–305. doi: http://dx.doi.org.mccc.idm.oclc.org/10.1007/s10964-018-0973-8

Putnam, F. W., Guroff, J. J., Silberman, E. K., & Barban, L. (1986). The clinical phenomenology of multiple personality disorder: Review of 100 recent cases. *Journal of Clinical Psychiatry, 47,* 285–293.

Putnam, F., Zahn, T., & Post, R. (1990). Differential autonomic nervous system activity in multiple personality disorder. *Physical Review, 31,* 251–260.

Q

Quidé, Y., Cohen-Woods, S., O'Reilly, N., Carr, V. J., Elzinga, B. M., & Green, M. J. (2018). Schizotypal personality traits and social cognition are associated with childhood trauma exposure. *British Journal of Clinical Psychology, 57*(4), 397–419.

Quinn, H. G. (2017). Self-deception in and out of illness: Are some subjects responsible for their delusions? *Palgrave Communications, 3*(1) doi: http://dx.doi.org.mccc.idm.oclc.org/10.1057/s41599-017-0017-0

R

Rabin, L. A., Smart, C. M., & Amariglio, R. E. (2017). Subjective cognitive decline in preclinical Alzheimer's disease. *Annual Review of Clinical Psychology, 13,* 369–396.

Rachman, S. (1993). Obsessions, responsibility and guilt. *Behaviour Research & Therapy, 31,* 149–154.

Racine, N., Cooke, J. E., Eirich, R., Korczak, D. J., McArthur, B., & Madigan, S. (2020). Child and adolescent mental illness during COVID-19: A rapid review. *Psychiatry research, 292,* 113307.

Radulovic, J., Lee, R. & Ortony, A. (2018). State-dependent memory: Neurobiological advances and prospects for translation to dissociative amnesia. *Frontiers in Behavioral Neuroscience, 12*:259. doi: 10.3389/fnbeh.2018.00259

Raikkonen, K., Matthews, K. A., Flory, J. D., Owens, J. F., & Gump, B. B. (1999). Effects of optimism, pessimism, and trait anxiety on ambulatory blood pressure and mood during everyday life. *Journal of Personality & Social Psychology, 76,* 104–113.

Raine, A. (2018). Antisocial personality as a neurodevelopmental disorder. *Annual Review of Clinical Psychology, 14,* 259–289

Raine, A., Lencz, T., Bihrle, S., LaCasse, L., & Colletti, P. (2000). Reduced prefrontal gray matter volume and reduced autonomic activity in antisocial personality disorder. *Archives of General Psychiatry, 57*(2), 119–127.

Raine, A., Yang, Y., Narr, K. L., & Toga, A. W. (2011). Sex differences in orbitofrontal gray as a partial explanation for sex differences in antisocial personality. *Molecular Psychiatry, 16,* 227–236.

Ramires, V. R. R., Godinho, L. B. R., & Goodman, G. (2017). The therapeutic process of a child diagnosed with disruptive mood dysregulation disorder. *Psychoanalytic Psychology, 34*(4), 488–498.

Rapee, R. M., Schniering, C. A., & Hudson, J. L. (2009). Anxiety disorders during childhood and adolescence: Origins and treatment. *Annual Review of Clinical Psychology, 5,* 311–341.

Rapoport, J. L. (1989). The biology of obsessions and compulsions. *Scientific American,* 83–89.

Rapoport, J. L., Jensen, P. S., Inoff-Germain, G., Weissman, M. M., Greenwald, S., Narrow, W. E., Lahey, B. B., & Canino, G. (2000). Childhood obsessive-compulsive disorder in the NIMH MECA study: Parent versus child identification of cases. *Journal of Anxiety Disorders, 14,* 535–548.

Rappaport, L. M., Sheerin, C., Savage, J. E., Hettema, J. M., & Roberson-Nay, R. (2017). Clinical characteristics of latent classes of CO_2 hypersensitivity in adolescents and young adults. *Behaviour research and therapy, 93,* 95–103. https://doi.org/10.1016/j.brat.2017.03.015

Rasmussen, H. N., Scheier, M. F., & Greenhouse, J. B. (2009). Optimism and physical health: A meta-analytic review. *Annals of Behavioral Medicine, 37*(3), 239–256.

Rastrelli, G., & Maggi, M. (2017). Erectile dysfunction in fit and healthy young men: Psychological or pathological?. *Translational Andrology and Urology, 6*(1), 79–90.

Ratcliffe, M., & Wilkinson, S. (2015). Thought Insertion Clarified. *Journal of Consciousness Studies: Controversies in Science & the Humanities, 22*(11–12), 246–269.

Rauch, S. L., Phillips, K. A., Segal, E., Makris, N., Shin, L. M., Whalen, P. J., . . . Kennedy, D. N. (2003). A preliminary morphometric magnetic resonance imaging study of regional brain volumes in body dysmorphic disorder. *Psychiatry Research: Neuroimaging, 122,* 13–19.

Razran, G. (1961). The observable unconscious and the inferable conscious in current Soviet psychophysiology: Interoceptive conditioning, semantic conditioning, and the orienting reflex. *Psychological Review, 68,* 81–150.

Ream G. L. (2019). What's Unique About Lesbian, Gay, Bisexual, and Transgender (LGBT) Youth and Young Adult Suicides? Findings From the National Violent Death Reporting System. *The Journal of Adolescent Health: Official Publication of the Society for Adolescent Medicine, 64*(5), 602–607. https://doi.org/10.1016/j.jadohealth.2018.10.303

Reardon, T., Harvey, K., Baranowska, M., O'Brien, D., Smith, L., & Creswell, C. (2017). What do parents perceive are the barriers and facilitators to accessing psychological treatment for mental health problems in children and adolescents? A systematic review of qualitative and quantitative studies. *European Child & Adolescent Psychiatry, 26,* 623–647.

Reas, D. L., & Grilo, C. M. (2008). Review and meta-analysis of pharmacotherapy for binge-eating disorder. *Obesity, 16,* 2024–2038.

Reay, R. E., Looi, J. C., & Keightley, P. (2020). Telehealth mental health services during COVID-19: summary of evidence and clinical practice. *Australasian Psychiatry: Bulletin of Royal Australian and New Zealand College of Psychiatrists, 28*(5), 514–516. https://doi.org/10.1177/1039856220943032

Redlich, A. D., Steadman, H. J., Monahan, J., Robbins, P. C., & Petrila, J. (2006). Patterns of practice in mental health courts: A national survey. *Law and Human Behavior, 30,* 347–362.

Reed, G. M., Kemeny, M. E., Taylor, S. E., & Visscher, B. R. (1999). Negative HIV-specific expectancies and AIDS-related bereavement as predictors of symptom onset in asymptomatic HIV-positive gay men. *Health Psychology, 18,* 354–363.

Regier, D. A., Kuhl, E. A., & Kupfer, D. J. (2013). The DSM-5: Classification and criteria changes. *World Psychiatry: Official Journal of the World Psychiatric Association (WPA), 12*(2), 92–98.

Rehan, M. A., Kuppa, A., Ahuja, A., Khalid, S., Patel, N., Budi Cardi, F. S., . . . Tohid, H. (2018). A strange case of dissociative identity disorder: Are there any triggers? *Cureus, 10*(7), e2957. https://doi.org/10.7759/cureus.2957

Rehm, J., Greenfield, T. K., & Rogers, J. D. (2001). Average volume of alcohol consumption, patterns of drinking, and all-cause mortality: Results from the U.S. National Alcohol Survey. *American Journal of Epidemiology, 153,* 64–71.

Rehm, J., Samokhvalov, A. V., Neuman, M. G., Room, R., Parry, C., Lönnroth, K., . . . Popova, S. (2009). The association between alcohol use, alcohol use disorders and tuberculosis (TB). A systematic review. *BMC Public Health, 9,* 450.

Rehm, L. P. (1977). A self-control model of depression. *Behavior Therapy, 8,* 787–804.

Reichow, B., Barton, E. E., Boyd, B. A., & Hume, K. (2012). Early intensive behavioral intervention (EIBI) for young children with autism spectrum disorders (ASD). *Cochrane Database of Systematic Reviews, 10,* CD009260.

Reid, R. C., Carpenter, B. N., Hook, J. N., Garos, S., Manning, J. C., Gilliland, R., . . . Fong, T. (2012). Report of findings in a *DSM-5* field trial for hypersexual disorder. *Journal of Sexual Medicine, 9,* 2868–2877.

Reinares, M., Bonnin, C. M., Hidalgo-Mazzei, D., Sánchez-Moreno, J., Colom, F., & Vieta, E. (2016). The role of family interventions in bipolar disorder: A systematic review. *Clinical Psychology Review, 43,* 47–57.

Reinders, A., Marquand, A. F., Schlumpf, Y. R., Chalavi, S., Vissia, E. M., Nijenhuis, E., . . . Veltman, D. J. (2019). Aiding the diagnosis of dissociative identity disorder: Pattern recognition study of brain biomarkers. *The British Journal of Psychiatry: The Journal of Mental Science, 215*(3), 536–544. Retrieved from https://doi.org/10.1192/bjp.2018.255

Reinders, A., Marquand, A., Schlumpf, Y., Chalavi, S., Vissia, E., Nijenhuis, E., . . . Veltman, D. (2019). Aiding the diagnosis of dissociative identity disorder: Pattern recognition study of brain biomarkers. *British Journal of Psychiatry, 215*(3), 536–544. doi: 10.1192/bjp.2018.255

Reitan, R. M., & Davidson, L. A. (1974). *Clinical neuropsychology: Current status and applications.* Washington, DC: V. H. Winston.

Resick, P. A., Wachen, J. S., Dondanville, K. A., Pruiksma, K. E., Yarvis, J. S., Peterson, A. L., . . . Young-McCaughan, S. (2017). Effect of group vs individual cognitive processing therapy in active-duty military seeking treatment for posttraumatic stress disorder: A randomized clinical trial. *JAMA Psychiatry, 74*(1), 28–36.

Resick, P. A., Williams, L. F., Suvak, M. K., Monson, C. M., & Gradus, J. L. (2012). Long-term outcomes of cognitive-behavioral treatments for posttraumatic stress disorder among female rape survivors. *Journal of Consulting and Clinical Psychology, 80*(2), 201–210.

Retzler, K. (2019). Erectile dysfunction: A review of comprehensive Treatment options for optimal outcome. *Journal of Restorative Medicine, 8*(1).

Reynolds, K., Pietrzak, R. H., El-Gabalawy, R., Mackenzie, C. S., & Sareen, J. (2015). Prevalence of psychiatric disorders in US older adults: Findings from a nationally representative survey. *World Psychiatry, 14*(1), 74–81.

Rhebergen, D., Beekman, A. T. F., de Graaf, R., Nolen, W. A., Spijker, J., Hoogendijk, W. J., & Pennix, B. W. J. H. (2010). Trajectories of recovery of social and physical functioning in major depression, dysthymic disorder, and double depression: A 3-year follow-up. *Journal of Affective Disorders, 124,* 148–156.

Rhee, S. J., Han, D., Lee, Y., Kim, H., Lee, J., Lee, K., . . . Ha, K. (2020). Comparison of serum protein profiles between major depressive disorder and bipolar disorder. *BMC Psychiatry, 20*(1), 145.

Rhoades, H., Rusow, J. A., Bond, D., Lanteigne, A., Fulginiti, A., & Goldbach, J. T. (2018). Homelessness, Mental Health and Suicidality Among LGBTQ Youth Accessing Crisis Services. *Child Psychiatry & Human Development, 49*(4), 643–651. doi: 10.1007/s10578-018-0780-1

Ridley, N. J., Draper, B., & Withall, A. (2013). Alcohol-related dementia: An update of the evidence. *Alzheimer's Research & Therapy, 5*(1), 3.

Rief, W., & Martin, A. (2014). How to use the new DSM-5 somatic symptom disorder diagnosis in research and practice: A critical evaluation and a proposal for modifications. *Annual Review of Clinical Psychology, 10,* 339–367.

Riemann, D., Nissen, C., Palagini, L., Otte, A., Perlis, M. L., & Spiegelhalder, K. (2015). The neurobiology, investigation, and treatment of chronic insomnia. *Lancet Neurology, 14*(5), 547–558.

Rienecke, R. D. (2017). Family-based treatment of eating disorders in adolescents: Current insights. *Adolescent Health, Medicine and Therapeutics, 8,* 69–79

Ripoll, L. H., Triebwasser, J., & Siever, L. J. (2011). Evidence-based pharmacotherapy for personality disorders. *International Journal of Neuropsychopharmacology, 14,* 1257–1288.

Risch, N., Herrell, R., Lehner, T., Liang, K. Y., Eaves, L., Hoh, J., . . . Merikangas, K. R. (2009). Interaction between the serotonin transporter gene (5-HTTLPR), stressful life events, and risk of depression: A meta-analysis. *Journal of the American Medical Association, 301,* 2462–2471.

Rivera, R. M., & Carballea, D. (2020). Coronavirus: A trigger for OCD and illness anxiety disorder? *Psychological Trauma: Theory, Research, Practice, and Policy, 12*(S1), S66. http://dx.doi.org/10.1037/tra0000725

Rizzo, A., Roy, M. J., Hartholt, A., Costanzo, M., Highland, K. B., & Jovanovic, T., . . . Difede, J. (2017). Virtual reality applications for the assessment and treatment of PTSD. In S. Bowles & P. Bartone. (Eds.), *Handbook of military psychology* (pp. 453–471). Cham: Springer.

Rizzo, M. D., Henriquez, J. E., Blevins, L. K., Bach, A., Crawford, R. B., & Kaminski, N. E. (2020). Targeting cannabinoid receptor 2 on peripheral leukocytes to attenuate inflammatory mechanisms implicated in HIV-associated neurocognitive disorder. *Journal of Neuroimmune Pharmacology*, 1–14.

Rizzo, R., Pellico, A., Silvestri, P. R., Chiarotti, F., & Cardona, F. (2018). A randomized controlled trial comparing behavioral, educational, and pharmacological treatments in youths with chronic tic disorder or Tourette syndrome. *Frontiers in psychiatry, 9*, 100.

Robbins, P. C., Monahan, J., & Silver, E. (2003). Mental disorder, violence, and gender. *Law and Human Behavior, 27*, 561–571.

Robbins, T. W., Vaghi, M. M., & Banca, P. (2019). Obsessive-compulsive disorder: Puzzles and prospects. *Neuron, 102*(1), 27–47.

Robert, L., Virpi, L., & John, L. (2019). Self sacrifice and kin psychology in war: threats to family predict decisions to volunteer for a women's paramilitary organization. *Evolution and Human Behavior, 40*(6), 543–550.

Roberts, A. L., Gilman, S. E., Breslau, J., Breslau, N., & Koenen, K. C. (2011). Race/ethnic differences in exposure to traumatic events, development of posttraumatic stress disorder, and treatment-seeking for posttraumatic stress disorder in the United States. *Psychological Medicine, 41*(1), 71–83.

Robinson & Adinoff (2018). The mixed message behind "Medication-Assisted Treatment" for substance use disorder. *The American journal of drug and alcohol abuse, 44*(2), 147–150.

Robles, T. F., & Kiecolt-Glaser, J. K. (2003). The physiology of marriage: Pathways to health. *Physiology & Behavior, 79*, 409–416.

Robles, T. F., Slatcher, R. B., Trombello, J. M., & McGinn, M. M. (2014). Marital quality and health: A meta-analytic review. *Psychological Bulletin, 140*, 140–187.

Rockloff, M., Browne, M., Greer, N., Armstrong, T., & Thorne, H. (2020). Mobile EGM games: Evidence that simulated games encourage real-money gambling. *Journal of Gambling Studies, 36*(4), 1253–1265.

Rockney, R. M., & Lemke, T. (1992). Casualties from a junior-senior high school during the Persian Gulf War: Toxic poisoning or mass hysteria? *Journal of Developmental & Behavioral Pediatrics, 13*, 339–342.

Rodin, J., Silberstein, L. R., & Striegel-Moore, R. H. (1984). Women and weight: A normative discontent. In T. B. Sonderegger (Ed.), *Nebraska symposium on motivation*. Lincoln: University of Nebraska Press.

Roehling, M. V., Pichler, S., & Bruce, T. A. (2013). Moderators of the effect of weight on job-related outcomes: A meta-analysis of experimental studies. *Journal of Applied Social Psychology, 43*(2), 237–252.

Roelofs, K., Hoogduin, K. A. L., Keijsers, G. P. J., Naring, G. W. B., Moene, F. C., & Sandijck, P. (2002). Hypnotic susceptibility in patients with conversion disorder. *Journal of Abnormal Psychology, 111*, 390–395.

Roessner, V., Hoekstra, P. J., & Rothenberger, A. (2011). Tourette's disorder and other tic disorders in *DSM-5*: A comment. *European Child and Adolescent Psychiatry, 20*, 71–74.

Roessner, V., Schoenefeld, K., Buse, J., Bender, S., Ehrlich, S., & Münchau, A. (2013). Pharmacological treatment of tic disorders and Tourette syndrome. *Neuropharmacology, 68*, 143–149.

Rogers, C. R. (1951). *Client-centered therapy, its current practice, implications, and theory*. Boston: Houghton Mifflin.

Rogler, L. H. (1989). The meaning of culturally sensitive research in mental health. *American Journal of Psychiatry, 146*, 296–303.

Rohan, K. J., Mahon, J. N., Evans, M., Ho, S. Y., Meyerhoff, J., Postolache, T. T., & Vacek, P. M. (2015). Randomized trial of cognitive-behavioral therapy versus light therapy for seasonal affective disorder: Acute outcomes. *American Journal of Psychiatry, 172*(9), 862–869.

Rohan, K. J., Roecklein, K. A., & Haaga, D. A. F. (2009). Biological and psychological mechanisms of seasonal affective disorder: A review and integration. *Current Psychiatry Reviews, 5*, 37–47.

Rohan, K. J., Roecklein, K. A., Lacy, T. J., & Vacek, P. M. (2009). Winter depression recurrence one year after cognitive-behavioral therapy, light therapy, or combination treatment. *Behavior Therapy, 40*, 225–238.

Rohan, K. J., Roecklein, K. A., Lindsey, K. T., Johnson, L. G., Lippy, R. D., Lacy, T. J., & Barton, F. B. (2007). A randomized controlled trial of cognitive-behavioral therapy, light therapy, and their combination for seasonal affective disorder. *Journal of Consulting and Clinical Psychology, 75*, 489–500.

Romanelli, R. J., Wu, F. M., Gamba, R., Mojtabai, R., & Segal, J. B. (2014). Behavioral therapy and serotonin reuptake inhibitor pharmacotherapy in the treatment of obsessive-compulsive disorder: A systematic review and meta-analysis of head-to-head randomized controlled trials. *Depression and Anxiety, 31*, 641–652.

Ronningstam, E. (2011a). Narcissistic personality disorder: A clinical perspective. *Journal of Psychiatric Practice, 17*, 89–99.

Ronningstam, E. (2011b). Narcissistic personality disorder in *DSM-V*—In support of retaining a significant diagnosis. *Journal of Personality Disorders, 25*, 248–259.

Rosell, D. R., Futterman, S. E., McMaster, A., & Siever, L. J. (2014). Schizotypal personality disorder: A current review. *Current Psychiatry Reports, 16*(7), 452.

Rosenbaum, M. (1980). The role of the term schizophrenia in the decline of the diagnoses of multiple personality. *Archives of General Psychiatry, 37*, 1383–1385.

Rosenblatt, P. C. (2008). Grief across cultures: A review and research agenda. In M. S. Stroebe, R. O. Hansson, H. Schut, & W. Stroebe (Eds.), *Handbook of bereavement research and practice: Advances in theory and intervention* (pp. 207–222). Washington, DC, US: American Psychological Association.

Rosen, G. (1968). *Madness in society: Chapters in the historical sociology of mental illness*. Chicago: University of Chicago Press.

Rosengren, A., Hawken, S., Ounpuu, S., Sliwa, K., Zubaid, M., Almahmeed, W. A., . . . INTERHEART investigators. (2004). Association of psychosocial risk factors with risk of acute myocardial infarction in 11,119 cases and 13,648 controls from 52 countries (the INTERHEART study): Case-control study. *Lancet, 364*, 953–962.

Rosenhan, D. L. (1973). On being sane in insane places. *Science, 179*, 250–258.

Rosenman, R. H., Brand, R. J., Jenkins, C. D., Friedman, M., Straus, R., & Wrum, M. (1976). Coronary heart disease in the Western Collaborative Group Study: Final follow-up experience of 8 years. *JAMA, 233*, 877–878.

Rosenstein, M. J., Milazzo-Sayre, L. J., & Manderscheid, R. W. (1989). Care of persons with schizophrenia: A statistical profile. *Schizophrenia Bulletin, 15*, 45–58.

Rosenström, T., Ystrom, E., Torvik, F. A., Czajkowski, N. O., Gillespie, N. A., Aggen, S. H., . . . Reichborn-Kjennerud, T. (2017). Genetic and environmental structure of DSM-IV criteria for antisocial personality disorder: A twin study. *Behavior Genetics, 47*(3), 265–277.

Rose, S. S. (2019). Neurocognitive Disorders and Neuropsychiatric Symptoms. In *Neurocognitive Behavioral Disorders* (pp. 39–69). Springer, Cham.

Ross, C. A. (1997). *Dissociative identity disorder: Diagnosis, clinical features, and treatment of multiple personality.* Toronto: Wiley.

Ross, C. A. (1999). Dissociative disorders. In T. Millon (Ed.), *Oxford textbook of psychopathology* (pp. 466–481). New York: Oxford University Press.

Ross, C. A. (2011). Possession experiences in dissociative identity disorder: A preliminary study. *Journal of Trauma and Dissociation, 12,* 393–400.

Ross, C. A., Aylward, E. H., Wild, E. J., Langbehn, D. R., Long, J. D., Warner, J. H., . . . Tabrizi, S. J. (2014). Huntington disease: Natural history, biomarkers and prospects for therapeutics. *Nature Reviews Neurology, 10*(4), 204.

Rosselló, J., & Bernal, G. (2005). New developments in cognitive-behavioral and interpersonal treatments for depressed Puerto Rican adolescents. In E. D. Hibbs & P. S. Jensen (Eds.), *Psychosocial treatments for child and adolescent disorders: Empirically based strategies for clinical practice* (2nd ed., pp. 187–217). Washington, DC: American Psychological Association.

Ross, L., Lepper, M. R., & Hubbard, M. (1975). Perseverance in self-perception and social perception: Biased attributional processes in the debriefing paradigm. *Journal of Personality and Social Psychology, 32*(5), 880–892.

Roth, A. (2018, March 31). *A 'hellish world': The mental health crisis in America's prisons.* Retrieved from https://www.theguardian.com/society/2018/mar/31/mental-health-care-crisis-overwhelming-prison-jail

Rothbaum, B. O., & Foa, E. B. (1991). Exposure treatment of PTSD concomitant with conversion mutism: A case study. *Behavior Therapy, 22,* 449–456.

Rothemund, Y., Preuschhof, C., Bohner, G., Bauknecht, H. C., Klingebiel, R., Flor, H., & Klapp, B. F. (2007). Differential activation of the dorsal striatum by high-calorie visual food stimuli in obese individuals. *NeuroImage, 37,* 410–421.

Rowe, R., Maughan, B., Worthman, C. M., Costello, E. J., & Angold, A. (2004). Testosterone, antisocial behavior, and social dominance in boys: Pubertal development and biosocial interaction. *Biological Psychiatry, 55,* 546–552.

Rowland, D. L., & Cooper, S. E. (2017). Treating men's orgasmic difficulties. In Z. D. Peterson (Ed.), *The Wiley handbook of sex therapy* (pp. 72–97). Oxford: Wiley.

Rudolph, K. D. (2008). The interpersonal context of adolescent depression. In S. Nolen-Hoeksema & L. M. Hilt (Eds.), *Handbook of depression in adolescents* (pp. 377–417). New York: Routledge.

Rudolph, K. D., & Conley, C. S. (2005). The socioeconomic costs and benefits of social-evaluative concerns: Do girls care too much? *Journal of Personality, 73,* 115–137.

Rueve, M. E., & Welton, R. S. (2008). Violence and mental illness. *Psychiatry (Edgmont), 5*(5), 34–48.

Ruffalo, M. (2019, June 25). The dire state of inpatient mental health. Retrieved from https://www.psychologytoday.com/us/blog/freud-fluoxetine/201906/the-dire-state-inpatient-mental-health

Ruhl, C. (2020). *Intelligence: Definition, theories and testing.* Retrieved November 13, 2020, from https://www.simplypsychology.org/intelligence.html

Ruiz, P., & Strain, E. C. (2014). *The substance abuse handbook.* Philadelphia: Lippincott Williams & Wilkins.

Runfola, C. D., Von Holle, A., Trace, S. E., Brownley, K. A., Hofmeier, S. M., Gagne, D. A., & Bulik, C. M. (2013). Body dissatisfaction in women across the lifespan: Results of the UNC-SELF and Gender and Body Image (GABI) studies. *European Eating Disorders Review: The Journal of the Eating Disorders Association, 21*(1), 52–59.

Ruocco, A. C., Amirthavasagam, S., & Zakzanis, K. K. (2012). Amygdala and hippocampal volume reductions as candidate endophenotypes for borderline personality disorder: A meta-analysis of magnetic resonance imaging studies. *Psychiatric Research: Neuroimaging, 201,* 245–252.

Ruscio A. M. (2019). Normal versus pathological mood: Implications for diagnosis. *Annual Review of Clinical Psychology, 15,* 179–205.

Ruscio, A. M., Gentes, E. L., Jones, J. D., Hallion, L. S., Coleman, E. S., & Swendsen, J. (2015). Rumination predicts heightened responding to stressful life events in major depressive disorder and generalized anxiety disorder. *Journal of Abnormal Psychology, 124,* 17–26.

Ruscio AM, Hallion LS, Lim CCW, et al. (2017). Cross-sectional Comparison of the Epidemiology of *DSM-5* Generalized Anxiety Disorder Across the Globe. *JAMA Psychiatry;* 74(5):465–475. doi: 10.1001/jamapsychiatry.2017.0056

Ruscio, A. M., Stein, D. J., Chiu, W. T., & Kessler, R. C. (2010). The epidemiology of obsessive-compulsive disorder in the National Comorbidity Survey Replication. *Molecular Psychiatry, 15*(1), 53–63.

Ruscio, A. M., Stein, D. J., Chiu, W. T., & Kessler, R. C. (2010). The epidemiology of obsessive-compulsive disorder in the National Comorbidity Survey Replication. *Molecular psychiatry, 15*(1), 53–63. https://doi.org/10.1038/mp.2008.94

Rush, S. E., & Sharma, M. (2017). Mindfulness-based stress reduction as a stress management intervention for cancer care: a systematic review. *Journal of Evidence-Based Complementary & Alternative Medicine, 22*(2), 348–360.

Russell, S. T., & Fish, J. N. (2016). Mental Health in Lesbian, Gay, Bisexual, and Transgender (LGBT) Youth. *Annual Review of Clinical Psychology, 12,* 465–487. https://doi.org/10.1146/annurev-clinpsy-021815-093153

Rutter, M., Caspi, A., Fergusson, D., Horwood, L. J., Goodman, R., Maughan, B., . . . Carroll, J. (2004). Sex differences in developmental reading disability: New findings from 4 epidemiological studies. *JAMA, 291,* 2007–2012.

Rutter, M., Silberg, J., O'Connor, T., & Simonoff, E. (1999). Genetics and child psychiatry: II. Empirical research findings. *Journal of Child Psychology & Psychiatry, 40,* 19–55.

Ryder, A. G., Yang, J., Zhu, X., Yao, S., Yi, J., Heine, S., & Bagby, R. M. (2008). The cultural shaping of depression: Somatic symptoms in China, psychological symptoms in North America? *Journal of Abnormal Psychology, 117,* 300–313.

Ryding, F. C., & Kuss, D. J. (2020). The use of social networking sites, body image dissatisfaction, and body dysmorphic disorder: A systematic review of psychological research. *Psychology of Popular Media, 9*(4), 412–435.

Rymarczyk, K., Turbacz, A., Strus, W., & Cieciuch, J. (2020). Type C personality: Conceptual refinement and preliminary operationalization. *Frontiers in Psychology, 11,* 552740. https://doi.org/10.3389/fpsyg.2020.552740

S

Sackeim, H. A., Prudic, J., Fuller, R., Keilp, J., Lavori, P. W., & Olfson, M. (2007). The cognitive effects of electroconvulsive therapy in community settings. *Neuropsychopharmacology, 32,* 244–254.

Sack, R. L., Auckley, D., Auger, R. R., Carskadon, M. A., Wright, K. P., Jr., Vitiello, M. V., & Zhdanova, I. V. (2007). Circadian rhythm sleep disorders: Part I, Basic principles, shift work and jet lag disorders. *Sleep, 30,* 1460–1483.

Safer, D. J. (2016). Recent trends in stimulant usage. *Journal of Attention Disorders, 20*(6), 471–477.

Safer, D. L., Telch, C. F., & Chen, E. Y. (2009). *Dialectical behavior therapy for binge eating and bulimia.* New York: Guilford Press.

Safran, J. D. (2012). *Psychoanalysis and psychoanalytic therapies.* Washington DC: American Psychological Association.

Saigal, C. S., Wessells, H., Pace, J., Schonlau, M., Wilt, T. J., & The Urologic Diseases in America Project. (2006). Predictors and prevalence of erectile dysfunction in a racially diverse population. *Archives of Internal Medicine, 166,* 207–212.

Sajadi, M., Goudarzi, K., Khosravi, S., Farmahini-Farahani, M., & Mohammadbeig, A. (2017). Benson's Relaxation Effect in Comparing to Systematic Desensitization on Anxiety of Female Nurses: A Randomized Clinical Trial. *Indian Journal of Medical and Paediatric Oncology: Official Journal of Indian Society of Medical & Paediatric Oncology, 38*(2), 111–115. https://doi.org/10.4103/ijmpo.ijmpo_183_16

Sajatovic, M., Madhusoodanan, S., & Fuller, M. A. (2008). Clozapine. In K. T. Mueser & D. V. Jeste (Eds.), *Clinical handbook of schizophrenia* (pp. 178–185). New York: Guilford Press.

Salkovskis, P. M. (1998). Psychological approaches to the understanding of obsessional problems. In R. Swinson (Ed.), *Obsessive-compulsive disorder: Theory, research, and treatment* (pp. 33–50). New York: Guilford Press.

Salkovskis, P. M., & Millar, J. F. (2016). Still cognitive after all these years? Perspectives for a cognitive behavioural theory of obsessions and where we are 30 years later. *Australian Psychologist, 51*(1), 3–13.

Sallinen, M., Harma, M., Akerstedt, T., Rosa, R., & Lillqvist, O. (1998). Promoting alertness with a short nap during a night shift. *Journal of Sleep Research, 7,* 240–247.

Saluja, G., Iachan, R., Scheidt, P. C., Overpeck, M. D., Sun, W., & Giedd, J. N. (2004). Prevalence of and risk factors for depressive symptoms among young adolescents. *Archives of Pediatrics & Adolescent Medicine, 158,* 760–765.

Salvatore, J. E., & Dick, D. M. (2016). Genetic influences on conduct disorder. *Neuroscience & Biobehavioral Reviews, 91,* 91–101.

Salvatore, S., Redaelli, A., Baini, I., & Candiani, M. (2016). Sexual function after delivery. In D. Riva & G. Minini (Eds.), *Childbirth-related pelvic floor dysfunction: Risk factors, prevention, evaluation, and treatment* (pp. 101–104). Springer: Cham.

Samara, M. T., Dold, M., Gianatsi, M., Nikolakopoulou, A., Helfer, B., Salanti, G., & Leucht, S. (2016). Efficacy, acceptability, and tolerability of antipsychotics in treatment-resistant schizophrenia: A network meta-analysis. *JAMA Psychiatry, 73*(3), 199–210.

Samara, M. T., Nikolakopoulou, A., Salanti, G., & Leucht, S. (2019). How many patients with schizophrenia do not respond to antipsychotic drugs in the short term? An analysis based on individual patient data from randomized controlled trials. *Schizophrenia Bulletin, 45*(3), 639–646. https://doi.org/10.1093/schbul/sby095

Samet, J. H., Botticelli, M., & Bharel, M. (2018). Methadone in primary care—one small step for Congress, one giant leap for addiction treatment. *New England Journal of Medicine, 379*(1), 7–8.

Sampson, R. J., & Laub, J. H. (1992). Crime and deviance in the life course. *Annual Review of Sociology, 18,* 63–84.

Samuels, E. A., Clark, S. A., Wunsch, C., Jordison Keeler, L. A., Reddy, N., Vanjani, R., & Wightman, R. S. (2020). Innovation during COVID-19: Improving addiction treatment access. *Journal of Addiction Medicine, 14*(4), e8–e9. https://doi.org/10.1097/ADM.0000000000000685

Samuels, J. F., Bienvenu, O. J., Grados, M. A., Cullen, B., Riddle, M. A., Liang, K. Y., . . . Nestadt, G. (2008). Prevalence and correlates of hoarding behavior in a community-based sample. *Behavior Research and Therapy, 46,* 836–844.

Sanchez-Roige, S., Gray, J. C., MacKillop, J., Chen, C. H., & Palmer, A. A. (2018). The genetics of human personality. *Genes, Brain and Behavior, 17*(3), e12439.

Sanchis-Gomar, F., Perez-Quilis, C., Leischik, R., & Lucia, A. (2016). Epidemiology of coronary heart disease and acute coronary syndrome. *Annals of Translational Medicine, 4*(13), 256.

Sanderson, W. C., Rapee, R. M., & Barlow, D. H. (1989). The influence of an illusion of control on panic attacks induced via inhalation of 5.5% carbon dioxide-enriched air. *Archives of General Psychiatry, 46*(2), 157–162.

Sand, M., & Fisher, W. A. (2007). Women's endorsement of models of female sexual response: The nurses' sexuality study. *Journal of Sexual Medicine, 4,* 708–719.

Sandnabba, N. K., Santtila, P., Alison, L., & Nordling, N. (2002). Demographics, sexual behaviour, family background and abuse experiences of practitioners of sadomasochistic sex: A review of recent research. *Sexual & Relationship Therapy, 17,* 39–55.

Sandstrom, A., Sahiti, Q., Pavlova, B., & Uher, R. (2019). Offspring of parents with schizophrenia, bipolar disorder, and depression: A review of familial high-risk and molecular genetics studies. *Psychiatric Genetics, 29*(5), 160–169.

Sanislow, C. A., da Cruz, K., Gianoli, M. O., & Reagan, E. (2012). Avoidant personality disorder, traits, and type. In T. A. Widiger (Ed.), *The Oxford handbook of personality disorders* (pp. 549–565). New York: Oxford University Press.

Sanislow, C. A., Pine, D. S., Quinn, K. J., Kozak, M. J., Garvey, M. A., Heinssen, R. K., . . . Cuthbert, B. N. (2011). Developing constructs for psychopathology research: Research domain criteria. *Journal of Abnormal Psychology, 119,* 631–639.

Santana, L. M., Perin, L., Lunelli, R., Inácio, J. F. S., Rodrigues, C. G., Eibel, B., & Goldmeier, S. (2019). Sexual dysfunction in women with hypertension: A systematic review and meta-analysis. *Current Hypertension Reports, 21*(3), 25.

Santarossa, S., & Woodruff, S. J. (2017). # SocialMedia: Exploring the relationship of social networking sites on body image, self-esteem, and eating disorders. *Social Media+ Society, 3*(2), 2056305117704407.

Sanz, J. A., & Aidy, S. E. (2019). Microbiota and gut neuropeptides: A dual action of antimicrobial activity and neuroimmune response. *Psychopharmacology, 236*(5), 1597–1609.

Sanz, J. A., & Aidy, S. E. (2019). Microbiota and gut neuropeptides: A dual action of antimicrobial activity and neuroimmune response. *Psychopharmacology, 236*(5), 1597–1609. doi: http://dx.doi.org.mccc.idm.oclc.org/10.1007/s00213-019-05224-0

Sapolsky, R. M. (2007). Why zebras don't get ulcers: Stress, metabolism, and liquidating your assets. In A. Monat, R. S. Lazarus, & G. Reevy (Eds.). *The Praeger handbook on stress and coping:* Vol. 1 (pp. 181–197). Westport, CT: Praeger.

Sarbin, T. R., & Juhasz, J. B. (1967). The historical background of the concept of hallucination. *Journal of the History of the Behavioral Sciences, 3,* 339–358.

Sariaslan, A., Fazel, S., D'Onofrio, B. M., Långström, N., Larsson, H., Bergen, S. E., . . . Lichtenstein, P. (2016). Schizophrenia and subsequent neighborhood deprivation: Revisiting the social drift hypothesis using population, twin and molecular genetic data. *Translational Psychiatry, 6*(5), e796.

Şar, V., Dorahy, M. J., & Krüger, C. (2017). Revisiting the etiological aspects of dissociative identity disorder: A biopsychosocial perspective. *Psychology Research and Behavior Management, 10,* 137–146. https://doi.org/10.2147/PRBM.S113743

Sar, V., Krüger, C., Martínez-Taboas, A., Middleton, W., & Dorahy, M. (2013). Sociocognitive and posttraumatic models of dissociation are not opposed. *The Journal of Nervous and Mental Disease, 201*(5), 439–440.

Sauer-Zavala, S., Cassiello-Robbins, C., Woods, B. K., Curreri, A., Wilner Tirpak, J., & Rassaby, M. (2020). Countering emotional behaviors in the treatment of borderline personality disorder. *Personality Disorders: Theory, Research, and Treatment, 11*(5), 328.

Saveanu, R. V., & Nemeroff, C. B. (2012). Etiology of depression: Genetic and environmental factors. *Psychiatric Clinics of North America, 35,* 51–71.

Savill, N. C., Buitelaar, J. K., Anand, E., Day, K. A., Treuer, T., Upadhyaya, H. P., & Coghill, D. (2015). The efficacy of atomoxetine for the treatment of children and adolescents with attention-deficit/hyperactivity disorder: A comprehensive review of over a decade of clinical research. *CNS Drugs, 29*(2), 131–151.

Savla, G. N., Moore, D. J., & Palmer, B. W. (2008). Cognitive functioning in K. T. Mueser & Dilip V. Jeste (Eds.), *Clinical handbook of schizophrenia* (pp. 91–99). New York: Guilford Press.

Saxena, S. (2008). Neurobiology and treatment of compulsive hoarding. *CNS Spectrums, 13* (9, Suppl. 14), 29–36.

Saxena, S., Brody, A. L., Ho, M. L., Zohrabi, N., Maidment, K. M., & Baxter, L. R., Jr. (2003). Differential brain metabolic predictors of response to paroxetine in obsessive-compulsive disorder versus major depression. *American Journal of Psychiatry, 160,* 522–532.

Saxena, S., Brody, A. L., Maidment, K. M., Dunkin, J. J., Colgan, M., Alborzian, S., Phelps, M. E., & Baxter, L. R. (1999). Localized orbitofrontal and subcortical metabolic changes and predictors of response to paroxetine treatment in obsessive-compulsive disorder. *Neuropsychopharmacology, 21,* 683–693.

Scaini, S., Belotti, R., & Ogliari, A. (2014). Genetic and environmental contributions to social anxiety across different ages: A meta-analytic approach to twin data. *Journal of Anxiety Disorders, 28*(7), 650–656.

Scammacca, N. K., Roberts, G. J., Cho, E., Williams, K. J., Roberts, G., Vaughn, S. R., & Carroll, M. (2016). A century of progress: Reading interventions for students in grades 4–12, 1914–2014. *Review of Educational Research, 86*(3), 756–800.

Scarella, T., Boland, R., Barsky, A. (2019). Illness anxiety disorder: Psychopathology, epidemiology, clinical characteristics, and treatment. *Psychosomatic Medicine, 81*(5) 398–407 doi: 10.1097/PSY.0000000000000691

Scarpa, A., & Wilson, L. (2017). Childhood mental disorders. *Encyclopedia of Human Behavior, 2012,* 467–475.

Schacter, D. L., Chiao, J. Y., & Mitchell, J. P. (2003). The seven sins of memory: Implications for the self. In J. LeDoux, J. Debiece, & H. Moss (Eds.), The self: From soul to brain. *Annals of the New York Academy of Sciences, 1001,* 226–239.

Schaefer, S. M., Morozink Boylan, J., van Reekum, C. M., Lapate, R. C., Norris, C. J., Ryff, C. D., & Davidson, R. J. (2013). Purpose in life predicts better emotional recovery from negative stimuli. *PloS One, 8*(11), e80329.

Schechter, D. S., Moser, D. A., Pointet, V. C., Aue, T., Stenz, L., Paoloni-Giacobino, A., . . . & Dayer, A. G. (2017). The association of serotonin receptor 3A methylation with maternal violence exposure, neural activity, and child aggression. *Behavioural Brain Research, 325,* 268–277.

Scheier, M. F., & Carver, C. S. (2018). Dispositional optimism and physical health: A long look back, a quick look forward. *American Psychologist, 73*(9), 1082.

Scheltens, P., Blennow, K., Breteler, M., de Strooper, B., Frisoni, G., Salloway, S., & der Flier, W. (2016). Alzheimer's disease. *Lancet, 388,* 505–517.

Schenck, C. H., & Mahowald, M. W. (2003). REM behavior disorder (RBD): Delayed emergence of Parkinsonism and/ or dementia in 65% of older men initially diagnosed with idiopathic RBD, and an analysis of the minimum & maximum tonic and/or phasic electromyographic abnormalities found during REM sleep. *Sleep, 26,* A316Abs.

Schienle, A., Hettema, J. M., Caceda, R., & Nemeroff, C. B. (2011). Neurobiology and genetics of generalized anxiety disorder. *Psychiatric Annals, 41*(2), 113–123.

Schildkraut, J. J. (1965). The catecholamine hypothesis of affective disorder: A review of supporting evidence. *American Journal of Psychiatry, 122,* 509–522.

Schilling, E. A., Lawless, M., Buchanan, L., & Aseltine, R. H. (2014). "Signs of Suicide" shows promise as a middle school suicide prevention program. *Suicide and Life-Threatening Behavior, 44*(6), 653–667.

Schimmenti, A., & Caretti, V. (2016). Linking the overwhelming with the unbearable: Developmental trauma, dissociation, and the disconnected self. *Psychoanalytic Psychology, 33*(1), 106–128.

Schlienz, N. J., Budney, A. J., Lee, D. C., & Vandrey, R. (2017). Cannabis withdrawal: A review of neurobiological mechanisms and sex differences. *Current Addiction Reports, 4,* 75–81.

Schlosser, D. A., Zinberg, J. L., Loewy, R. L., Casey-Cannon, S., O'Brien, M. P., Bearden, C. E., . . . Cannon, T. D. (2010). Predicting the longitudinal effects of the family environment on prodromal symptoms and functioning in patients at-risk for psychosis. *Schizophrenia Research, 118,* 69–75.

Schmidt-Kastner, R., Guloksuz, S., Kietzmann, T., Van Os, J., & Rutten, B. P. (2020). Analysis of GWAS-derived schizophrenia genes for links to ischemia-hypoxia response of the brain. *Frontiers in Psychiatry, 11.*

Schmidt, N. B., & Keough, M. E. (2010). Treatment of panic. *Annual Review of Clinical Psychology, 6,* 241–256.

Schneiderman, N., Ironson, G., & Siegel, S. D. (2005). Stress and health: Psychological, behavioral, and biological determinants. *Annual Review of Clinical Psychology, 1,* 607–628.

Scholten, M., Gather, J., & Vollmann, J. (2021, February). Equality in the informed consent process: Competence to consent, substitute decision-making, and discrimination of persons with mental disorders. In *The journal of medicine and philosophy: A forum for bioethics and philosophy of medicine, 46,*(1), 108–136). US: Oxford University Press.

Schonfeld, L., & Dupree, L. W. (2002). Age-specific cognitive-behavioral and self-management treatment approaches. In A. M. Gurnack, R. Atkinson, & N. J. Osgood (Eds.), *Treating alcohol and drug abuse in the elderly* (pp. 109–130). New York: Springer.

Schöttle, D., Schimmelmann, B. G., Ruppelt, F., Bussopulos, A., Frieling, M., Nika, E., . . . & Lambert, M. (2018). Effectiveness of integrated care including therapeutic assertive community treatment in severe schizophrenia-spectrum and bipolar I disorders: Four-year follow-up of the ACCESS II study. *PLoS One, 13*(2), e0192929.

Schuckit, M. A. (1995). *Drug and alcohol abuse: A clinical guide to diagnosis and treatment.* New York: Plenum Medical.

Schuckit, M. A. (1998). Biological, psychological, and environmental predictors of the alcoholism risk: A longitudinal study. *Journal of Studies on Alcohol, 59,* 485–494.

Schulkin, J., & Sterling, P. (2019). Allostasis: A brain-centered, predictive mode of physiological regulation. *Trends in Neurosciences, 42*(10), 740–752.

Schulte, E. M., Grilo, C. M., & Gearhardt, A. N. (2016). Shared and unique mechanisms underlying binge eating disorder and addictive disorders. *Clinical Psychology Review, 44,* 125–139.

Schultz, R. T. (2005). Developmental deficits in social perception in autism: The role of the amygdala and fusiform face area. *International Journal of Developmental Neuroscience, 23,* 125–141.

Schulz, R., Bookwala, J., Knapp, J. E., Scheier, M., & Williamson, G. M. (1996). Pessimism, age, and cancer mortality. *Psychology & Aging, 11,* 304–309.

Schumm, J. A., Dickstein, B. D., Walter, K. H., Owens, G. P., & Chard, K. M. (2015). Changes in posttraumatic cognitions predict changes in posttraumatic stress disorder symptoms during cognitive processing therapy. *Journal of Consulting and Clinical Psychology, 83,* 1161–1166.

Schwartz, J., Stoessel, P. W., Baxter, L. R., Martin, K. M., & Phelps, M. C. (1996). Systemic changes in cerebral glucose metabolic rate after successful behavior modification treatment of obsessive-compulsive disorder. *Archives of General Psychiatry, 53,* 109–113.

Schwartz, R. C., & Blankenship, D. M. (2014). Racial disparities in psychotic disorder diagnosis: A review of empirical literature. *World Journal of Psychiatry, 4*(4), 133–140.

Schwartz, S., Schultz, S., Rieder, A., & Saunders, E. (2016). Daily mood monitoring of symptoms using smartphones in bipolar disorder: A pilot study assessing the feasibility of ecological momentary assessment. *Journal of Affective Disorders, 191,* 88–93.

Sciberras, E., Mulraney, M., Silva, D., & Coghill, D. (2017). Prenatal risk factors and the etiology of ADHD: Review of existing evidence. *Current Psychiatry Reports, 19*(1), 1.

Scoboria, A., Wade, K. A., Lindsay, D. S., Azad, T., Strange, D., Ost, J., & Hyman, I. E. (2017). A mega-analysis of memory reports from eight peer-reviewed false memory implantation studies. *Memory, 25*(2), 146–163.

Scogin, F., Floyd, M., & Forde, J. (2000). Anxiety in older adults. In S. K. Whitbourne (Ed.), *Psychopathology in later adulthood* (pp. 117–140). New York: Wiley.

Scott, K. M., Hwang, I., Chiu, W.-T., Kessler, R. C., Sampson, N. A., Angermeyer, M., . . . Nock, M. K. (2010). Chronic physical conditions and their association with first onset of suicidal behavior in the World Mental Health Surveys. *Psychosomatic Medicine, 72,* 712–719.

Scott, K. M., Lim, C., Al-Hamzawi, A., Alonso, J., Bruffaerts, R., Caldas-de-Almeida, J. M., . . . Kessler, R. C. (2016). Association of mental disorders with subsequent chronic physical conditions: World mental health surveys from 17 countries. *JAMA Psychiatry, 73*(2), 150–158.

Scull, A. (1993). *The most solitary of afflictions.* New Haven: Yale University Press.

Searls, D. (2017). *The Inkblots: Hermann Rorschach, his iconic test, and the power of seeing.* Simon & Schuster.

Sears, C. S., Robinson, J. W., & Walker, L. M. (2018). A comprehensive review of sexual health concerns after cancer treatment and the biopsychosocial treatment options available to female patients. *European Journal of Cancer Care, 27*(2), e12738.

See, A. Y., Klimstra, T. A., Shiner, R. L., & Denissen, J. J. A. (2020). Linking narrative identity with schizotypal personality disorder features in adolescents. *Personality Disorders: Theory, Research, and Treatment, 12*(2), 182–192.

Seehuus, M., Stanton, A. M., & Handy, A. B. (2019). On the content of "real-world" sexual fantasy: Results from an analysis of 250,000+ anonymous text-based erotic fantasies. *Archives of Sexual Behavior, 48*(3), 725–737.

Seeman, M. V. (2008). Gender. In K. T. Mueser & Dilip V. Jeste (Eds.), *Clinical handbook of schizophrenia* (pp. 575–580). New York: Guilford Press.

Segal, S. P., Laurie, T. A., & Franskoviak, P. (2004). Ambivalence of PES patients toward hospitalization and factors in their disposition. *International Journal of Law & Psychiatry, 27,* 87–99.

Segerstrom, S. C., & Miller, G. E. (2004). Psychological stress and the human immune system: A meta-analytic study of 30 years of inquiry. *Psychological Bulletin, 130,* 601–630.

Segerstrom, S. C., Taylor, S. E., Kemeny, M. E., Reed, G. M., & Visscher, B. R. (1996). Causal attributions predict rate of immune decline in HIV seropositive gay men. *Health Psychology, 15,* 485–493.

Seidman, L. J., Faraone, S. V., Goldstein, J. M., Kremen, W. S., Horton, N. J., Makris, N., . . . Tsuang, M. T. (2002). Left hippocampal volume as a vulnerability indicator for schizophrenia. *Archives of General Psychiatry, 59,* 839–849.

Selby, E. A., Anestis, M., Bender, T., & Joiner, T. (2009). An exploration of the emotional cascade model in borderline personality disorder. *Journal of Abnormal Psychology, 118,* 375–387.

Seligman, M. E. (1970). On the generality of the laws of learning. *Psychological Review, 77,* 406–418.

Seligman, M. E. (1975). *Helplessness: On depression, development, and death.* San Francisco: Freeman, Cooper.

Seligman, M. E. (1993). *What you can change and what you can't: The complete guide to self-improvement.* New York: Knopf.

Seligman, M. E., & Maier, S. F. (1967). Failure to escape traumatic shock. *Journal of Experimental Psychology, 74,* 1–9.

Sellbom, M. (2019). The MMPI-2-restructured form (MMPI-2-RF): Assessment of personality and psychopathology in the twenty-first century. *Annual Review of Clinical Psychology, 15,* 149–177.

Sellers, R., Hammerton, G., Harold, G. T., Mahedy, L., Potter, R., Langley, K., . . . Collishaw, S. (2016). Examining whether offspring psychopathology influences illness course in mothers with recurrent depression using a high-risk longitudinal sample. *Journal of Abnormal Psychology, 125*(2), 256–266.

Selling, L. H. (1940). *Men against madness.* New York: Greenberg.

Semans, J. H. (1956). Premature ejaculation: A new approach. *Southern Medical Journal, 49,* 353–357.

Semler, C. N., & Harvey, A. G. (2007). An experimental investigation of daytime monitoring for sleep-related threat in primary insomnia. *Cognition and Emotion, 21,* 146–161.

Sempertegui, G. A., Karreman, A., Arntz, A., & Bekker, M. H. (2013). Schema therapy for borderline personality disorder: A comprehensive review of its empirical foundations, effectiveness and implementation possibilities. *Clinical Psychology Review, 33*(3), 426–447.

Semrau, M., Barley, E. A., Law, A., & Thornicroft, G. (2011). Lessons learned in developing community mental health care in Europe. *World Psychiatry, 10,* 217–225.

Senaratna, C. V., Perret, J. L., Lodge, C. J., Lowe, A. J., Campbell, B. E., Matheson, M. C., . . . Dharmage, S. C. (2017). Prevalence of obstructive sleep apnea in the general population: A systematic review. *Sleep Medicine Reviews, 34,* 70–81.

Sepede, G., Brunetti, M., & Di Giannantonio, M. (2020). Comorbid premenstrual dysphoric disorder in women with bipolar disorder: Management challenges. *Neuropsychiatric Disease and Treatment, 16,* 415–426.

Seto, M. C. (2008). Pedophilia: Psychopathology and theory. In D. R. Laws & W. T. O'Donohue (Eds.), *Sexual deviance: Theory, assessment, and treatment* (pp. 164–183). New York: Guilford Press.

Seto, M. C. (2009). Pedophilia. *Annual Review of Clinical Psychology, 5,* 391–407.

Shaffer, D., & Gould, M. S. (2000). Suicide prevention in the schools. In K. Hawton (Ed.), *The international handbook of suicide and attempted suicide* (pp. 585–724). New York: Wiley.

Shapiro, J. R., Berkman, N. D., Brownley, K. A., Sedway, J. A., Lohr, K. N., & Bulik, C. M. (2007). Bulimia nervosa treatment: A systematic review of randomized controlled trials. *International Journal of Eating Disorders, 40,* 321–336.

Sharf, A. J., Rogers, R., Williams, M. M., & Henry, S. A. (2017). The effectiveness of the MMPI-2-RF in detecting feigned mental disorders and cognitive deficits: A meta-analysis. *Journal of Psychopathology and Behavioral Assessment, 39*(3), 441–455.

Sharp, C., Kim, S., Herman, L., Pane, H., Reuter, T., & Strathearn, L. (2014). Major depression in mothers predicts reduced ventral striatum activation in adolescent female offspring with and without depression. *Journal of Abnormal Psychology, 123,* 298–309.

Sharp, C., Wright, A. G. C., Fowler, J. C., Frueh, B. C., Allen, J. G., Oldham, J., & Clark, L. A. (2015). The structure of personality pathology: Both general ('g') and specific ('s') factors? *Journal of Abnormal Psychology, 124,* 387–398.

Shaw, D. S., & Shelleby, E. C. (2014). Early-starting conduct problems: Intersection of conduct problems and poverty. *Annual Review of Clinical Psychology, 10,* 503–528.

Shaw, P., Lerch, J. P., Pruessner, J. C., Taylor, K. N., Rose, A. B., Greenstein, D., . . . Giedd, J. N. (2007). Cortical morphology in children and adolescents with different apolipoprotein E gene polymorphisms: An observational study. *Lancet Neurology, 6,* 494–500.

Shaywitz, B., Shaywitz, S., Blachman, B., Pugh, K., Fulbright, R., Skudlarski, P., . . . Gore, J. C. (2004). Development of left occipito-temporal systems for skilled reading in children after a phonologically-based intervention. *Biological Psychiatry, 55,* 926–933.

Shaywitz, S. (2003). *Overcoming dyslexia: A new and complete science-based program for reading problems at any level.* New York: Knopf.

Shaywitz, S. E., & Shaywitz, B. A. (2008). Paying attention to reading: The neurobiology of reading and dyslexia. *Development and Psychopathology, 20,* 1329–1349.

Shea, M. T., Stout, R., Gunderson, J., Morey, L. C., Grilo, C. M., McGlashan, T., . . . Keller, M. B. (2002). Short-term diagnostic stability of schizotypal, borderline, avoidant, and obsessive-compulsive personality disorders. *American Journal of Psychiatry, 159,* 2036–2041.

Shedler, J. (2010). The efficacy of psychodynamic psychotherapy. *American Psychologist, 65*(2), 98–109.

Sher, K. J., Grekin, E. R., & Williams, N. A. (2005). The development of alcohol use disorders. In S. Nolen-Hoeksema, T. D. Cannon, & T. A. Widiger (Eds.), *Annual review of clinical psychology* (Vol. 1, pp. 493–523). Palo Alto, CA: Annual Reviews.

Shimada-Sugimoto, M., Otowa, T., & Hettema, J. M. (2015). Genetics of anxiety disorders: Genetic epidemiological and molecular studies in humans. *Psychiatry and Clinical Neurosciences, 69*(7), 388–401.

Shin, L. M., Bush, G., Milad, M. R., Lasko, N. B., Brohawn, K. H., Hughes, K. C., . . . & Pitman, R. K. (2011). Exaggerated activation of dorsal anterior cingulate cortex during cognitive interference: A monozygotic twin study of posttraumatic stress disorder. *American Journal of Psychiatry, 168,* 979–985.

Shinn, A. K., Wolff, J. D., Hwang, M., Lebois, L., Robinson, M. A., Winternitz, S. R., . . . Kaufman, M. L. (2020). Assessing voice hearing in trauma spectrum disorders: A comparison of two measures and a review of the literature. *Frontiers in Psychiatry, 10,* 1011. https://doi.org/10.3389/fpsyt.2019.01011

Shirk, C. (2008). *Medicaid and mental health services.* Washington, DC: National Health Policy Forum.

Shortt, A. L., Barrett, P. M., & Fox, T. L. (2001). Evaluating the FRIENDS program: A cognitive-behavioral group treatment for anxious children and their parents. *Journal of Clinical Child Psychology, 30,* 525–535.

Sibrava, N. J., Beard, C., Bjornsson, A. S., Moitra, E., Weisberg, R. B., & Keller, M. B. (2013). Two-year course of generalized anxiety disorder, social anxiety disorder, and panic disorder in a longitudinal sample of African American adults. *Journal of Consulting and Clinical Psychology, 81,* 1052–1062.

Siever, L. J. (2008). Neurobiology of aggression and violence. *American Journal of Psychiatry, 165,* 429–442.

Siev, J., & Chambless, D. L. (2007). Specificity of treatment effects: Cognitive therapy and relaxation for generalized anxiety and panic disorders. *Journal of Consulting and Clinical Psychology, 75,* 513–522.

Sigman, M., Spence, S. J., & Wang, A. T. (2006). Autism from developmental and neuropsychological perspectives. *Annual Review of Clinical Psychology, 2,* 327–355.

Sigurdsson, E., Van Os, J., & Fombonne, E. (2002). Are impaired childhood motor skills a risk factor for adolescent anxiety? Results from the 1958 U.K. birth cohort and the National Child Development Study. *American Journal of Psychiatry, 159,* 1044–1046.

Silberg, J. L. (2014). Dissociative disorders in children and adolescents. *Handbook of Developmental Psychopathology* (pp. 761–775). Springer: Boston, MA.

Silberg, J. L., Maes, H., & Eaves, L. J. (2012). Unraveling the effect of genes and environment in the transmission of parental antisocial behavior to children's conduct disturbance, depression, and hyperactivity. *Journal of Child Psychology and Psychiatry, 53,* 668–677.

Silberg, J. L., Parr, T., Neale, M. C., Rutter, M., Angold, A., & Eaves, L. J. (2003). Maternal smoking during pregnancy and risk to boys' conduct disturbance: An examination of the causal hypothesis. *Biological Psychiatry, 53,* 130–135.

Silk, K. R., & Feurino, L., III (2012). Psychopharmacology of personality disorders. In T. A. Widiger (Ed.), *The Oxford handbook of personality disorders* (pp. 713–726). New York: Oxford University Press.

Silove, D., Alonso, J., Bromet, E., Gruber, M., Sampson, N., Scott, K., & Kessler, R.C. (2015). Pediatric-onset and adult-onset separation anxiety disorder across countries in the world. Mental Health Survey. *The American Journal of Psychiatry, 172,* 647–656.

Silva, C., & Van Orden, K. A. (2018). Suicide among Hispanics in the United States. *Current Opinion in Psychology, 22,* 44–49.

Silver, E., Cirincione, C., & Steadman, H. J. (1994). Demythologizing inaccurate perceptions of the insanity defense. *Law & Human Behavior, 18,* 63–70.

Silvers, J. A., Hubbard, A. D., Biggs, E., Shu, J., Fertuck, E., Chaudhury, S., . . . Stanley, B. (2016). Affective lability and difficulties with regulation are differentially associated with amygdala and prefrontal response in women with borderline personality disorder. *Psychiatry Research: Neuroimaging, 254,* 74–82.

Simeon, D., Guralnik, O., Schmeidler, J., Sirof, B., & Knutelska, M. (2001). The role of childhood interpersonal trauma in depersonalization disorder. *American Journal of Psychiatry, 158,* 1027–1033.

Simonelli, A., & Parolin, M. (2017). Dependent personality disorder. *Encyclopedia of Personality and Individual Differences* 10.1007/978-3-319-28099-8_578-1

Simpson, E. B., Yen, S., Costello, E., Rosen, K., Begin, A., Pistorello, J., & Pearlstein, T. (2004). Combined dialectical behavior therapy and fluoxetine in the treatment of borderline personality disorder. *Journal of Clinical Psychiatry, 65,* 379–385.

Singer, H. S. (2005). Tourette's syndrome: From behaviour to biology. *Lancet Neurology, 4,* 149–159.

Singh, M. K., & Gotlib, I. H. (2014). The neuroscience of depression: Implications for assessment and intervention. *Behaviour Research and Therapy, 62,* 60–73.

Singh, N. N. (2016). *Handbook of evidence-based practices in intellectual and developmental disabilities.* Cham: Springer.

Sing, L. (1995). Self-starvation in context: Towards a culturally sensitive understanding of anorexia nervosa. *Social Science & Medicine, 41,* 25–36.

Sinopoli, V. M., Erdman, L., Burton, C. L., Easter, P., Rajendram, R., Baldwin, G., . . . Arnold, P. D. (2020). Serotonin system gene variants and regional brain volume differences in pediatric OCD. *Brain Imaging & Behavior, 14*(5), 1612–1625.

Slavich, G. M., & Irwin, M. R. (2014). From stress to inflammation and major depressive disorder: A social signal transduction theory of depression. *Psychological Bulletin, 140*(3), 774.

Slotema, C. W., Blom, J. D., Hoek, H. W., & Sommer, I. E. (2010). Should we expand the toolbox of psychiatric treatment methods to include repetitive transcranial magnetic stimulation (rTMS)? A meta-analysis of the efficacy of rTMS in psychiatric disorders. *Journal of Clinical Psychiatry, 71,* 873–884.

Slotema, C. W., Blom, J. D., Niemantsverdriet, M., Deen, M., & Sommer, I. E. (2018). Comorbid diagnosis of psychotic disorders in borderline personality disorder: Prevalence and influence on outcome. *Frontiers in Psychiatry, 9,* 84.

Smart, C. M., Karr, J. E., Areshenkoff, C. N., Rabin, L. A., Hudon, C., Gates, N., . . . Subjective Cognitive Decline Initiative. (2017). Non-pharmacologic interventions for older adults with subjective cognitive decline: Systematic review, meta-analysis, and preliminary recommendations. *Neuropsychology Review, 27*(3), 245–257.

Smart, R., & Pacula, R. L. (2019). Early evidence of the impact of cannabis legalization on cannabis use, cannabis use disorder, and the use of other substances: Findings from state policy evaluations. *The American Journal of Drug and Alcohol Abuse, 45*(6), 644–663. https://doi.org/10.1080/00952990.2019.1669626

Smartt, C., Prince, M., Frissa, S., Eaton, J., Fekadu, A., & Hanlon, C. (2019). Homelessness and severe mental illness in low- and middle-income countries: scoping review. *BJPsych Open, 5*(4), e57.

Smink, F. R., van Hoeken, D., Donker, G. A., Susser, E. S., Oldehinkel, A. J., & Hoek, H. W. (2016). Three decades of eating disorders in Dutch primary care: Decreasing incidence of bulimia nervosa but not of anorexia nervosa. *Psychological Medicine, 46*(6), 1189–1196.

Smink, F. R., van Hoeken, D., & Hoek, H. W. (2013). Epidemiology, course, and outcome of eating disorders. *Current Opinion in Psychiatry, 26,* 543–548.

Smith, A., & Anderson, M. (2018). Social media use 2018: Demographics and statistics. Retrieved from http://www.pewinternet.org/2018/03/01/social-media-use-in-2018/

Smith, C. A., & Farrington, D. P. (2004). Continuities in antisocial behavior and parenting across three generations. *Journal of Child Psychology & Psychiatry, 45,* 230–247.

Smith, D. E., & Seymour, R. B. (1994). LSD: History and toxicity. *Psychiatric Annals, 24,* 145–147.

Smolak, L., Murnen, S. K., & Ruble, A. E. (2000). Female athletes and eating problems: A meta-analysis. *International Journal of Eating Disorders, 27,* 371–380.

Smolak, L., & Striegel-Moore, R. H. (2001). Challenging the myth of the golden girl: Ethnicity and eating disorders. In R. H. Striegel-Moore & L. Smolak (Eds.), *Eating disorders: Innovative directions in research and practice* (pp. 111–132). Washington, DC: American Psychological Association.

Smoller, J. (2016). The genetics of stress-related disorders: PTSD, depression, and anxiety disorders. *Neuropsychopharmacology, 41*(1), 297–319.

Smoller, J., Cerrato, F., & Weatherall, S. (2015). The genetics of anxiety disorders. In K. Ressler, D. S. Pine, & B. O. Rothbaum (Eds.), *Anxiety disorders: Translational perspectives on diagnosis and treatment (pp. 47–61).* Oxford: Oxford University Press.

Snipes, D. J., Calton, J. M., Green, B. A., Perrin, P. B., & Benotsch, E. G. (2017). Rape and posttraumatic stress disorder (PTSD): Examining the mediating role of explicit sex–power beliefs for men versus women. *Journal of Interpersonal Violence, 32*(16), 2453–2470.

Snitz, B. E., MacDonald, A. W., III, & Carter, C. S. (2006). Cognitive deficits in unaffected first-degree relatives of schizophrenia patients: A meta-analytic review of putative endophenotypes. *Schizophrenia Bulletin, 32,* 179–194.

Snowden, L. R. (2014). Poverty, safety net programs, and African Americans' mental health. *American Psychologist, 69*(8), 773–781.

Snowden, L. R., & Cheung, F. K. (1990). Use of inpatient mental health services by members of ethnic minority groups. *American Psychologist, 45,* 347–355.

Snowden, L. R., & Yamada, A. M. (2005). Cultural differences in access to care. *Annual Review of Clinical Psychology, 1,* 143–166.

Snowdon, D. A. (1997). Aging and Alzheimer's disease: Lessons from the Nun Study. *Gerontologist, 37,* 150–156.

Snowdon, D. A., Greiner, L. H., Mortimer, J. A., Riley, K. P., Greiner, P. A., & Markesbery, W. R. (1997). Brain infarction and the clinical expression of Alzheimer disease. The Nun Study. *JAMA, 277,* 813–817.

Snowdon, D. A., Kemper, S. J., Mortimer, J. A., Greiner, L. H., Wekstein, D. R., & Markesbery, W. R. (1996). Linguistic ability in early life and cognitive function and Alzheimer's disease in late life: Findings from the Nun Study. *JAMA, 275,* 528–532.

Soares Filho, L. C., Batista, R., Cardoso, V. C., Simões, V., Santos, A. M., Coelho, S., & Silva, A. (2020). Body image dissatisfaction and symptoms of depression disorder in adolescents. *Brazilian Journal of Medical and Biological Research = Revista brasileira de pesquisas medicas e biologicas, 54*(1), e10397.

Sobal, J., & Stunkard, A. J. (1989). Socioeconomic status and obesity: A review of the literature. *Psychological Bulletin, 105,* 260–275.

Sobell, M. B., & Sobell, L. C. (1978). *Behavioral treatment of alcohol problems.* New York: Plenum Press.

Sockol, L. E., Epperson, C. N., & Barber, J. P. (2013). Preventing postpartum depression: A meta-analytic review. *Clinical Psychology Review, 33,* 1205–1217.

Solmi, M., Murru, A., Pacchiarotti, I., Undurraga, J., Veronese, N., Fornaro, M., . . . Carvalho, A. F. (2017). Safety, tolerability, and risks associated with first- and second-generation antipsychotics: A state-of-the-art clinical review. *Therapeutics and Clinical Risk Management, 13,* 757–777. https://doi.org/10.2147/TCRM.S117321

Soloff, P. H., & Chiappetta, L. (2012). Prospective predictors of suicidal behavior in borderline personality disorder at 6-year follow-up. *American Journal of Psychiatry, 169,* 484–490.

Solomonov, N., Kuprian, N., Zilcha-Mano, S., Muran, J. C., & Barber, J. P. (2020). Comparing the interpersonal profiles of obsessive-compulsive personality disorder and avoidant personality disorder: Are there homogeneous profiles or interpersonal subtypes? *Personality Disorders: Theory, Research, and Treatment, 11*(5), 348–356. https://doi.org/10.1037/per0000391

Sophie Su, Y., Veeravagu, A., & Grant, G. (2016). Neuroplasticity after Traumatic Brain Injury. In D. Laskowitz (Eds.) et al., *Translational research in traumatic brain injury*. CRC Press/Taylor and Francis Group.

Soto, A., Smith, T. B., Griner, D., Rodríguez, M. D., & Bernal, G. (2018). Cultural adaptations and therapist multicultural competence: Two meta-analytic reviews. *Journal of Clinical Psychology, 74*(11), 1907-1923.

Southwick, S. M., Vythilingam, M., & Charney, D. S. (2005). The psychobiology of depression and resilience to stress: Implications for prevention and treatment. *Annual Review of Clinical Psychology, 1,* 255-292.

Sowell, E. R., Peterson, B. S., Thompson, P. M., Welcome, S. E., Henkenius, A., & Toga, A. W. (2003). Mapping cortical change across the human life span. *Nature Neuroscience, 6,* 309-315.

Spaan, P., van Luenen, S., Garnefski, N., & Kraaij, V. (2020). Psychosocial interventions enhance HIV medication adherence: A systematic review and meta-analysis. *Journal of Health psychology, 25*(10-11), 1326-1340.

Spanos, N. (1994). Multiple identity enactments and multiple personality disorder: A sociocognitive perspective. *Psychological Bulletin, 120,* 42-59.

Spanos, N. P. (1978). Witchcraft in histories of psychiatry: A critical analysis and an alternative conceptualization. *Psychological Bulletin, 85,* 417-439.

Spence, S. H., & Rapee, R. M. (2016). The etiology of social anxiety disorder: An evidence-based model. *Behaviour Research and Therapy, 86,* 50-67.

Spiegel, D. (2001). Mind matters—group therapy and survival in breast cancer. *New England Journal of Medicine, 345,* 1767-1768.

Spiegel, D., Bollm, J. R., Kraemer, H. C., & Gottheil, E. (1989). Psychological support for cancer patients. *Lancet, 2,* 1447.

Spiegel, D., Lewis-Fernández, R., Lanius, R., Vermetten, E., Simeon, D., & Friedman, M. (2013). Dissociative disorders in DSM-5. *Annual Review of Clinical Psychology, 9,* 299-326.

Spitzer, R. L. (1981). The diagnostic status of homosexuality in *DSM-III*: A reformulation of the issues. *American Journal of Psychiatry, 138,* 210-215.

Squires, A., Sadarangani, T., & Jones, S. (2020). Strategies for overcoming language barriers in research. *Journal of Advanced Nursing, 76*(2), 706-714. Retrieved from https://doi.org/10.1111/jan.14007

Ståhl, T., & Van Prooijen, J. W. (2018). Epistemic rationality: Skepticism toward unfounded beliefs requires sufficient cognitive ability and motivation to be rational. *Personality and Individual Differences, 122,* 155-163.

Stadler, C., Sterzer, P., Schmeck, K., Krebs, A., Kleinschmidt, A., & Poustka, F. (2007). Reduced anterior cingulate activation in aggressive children and adolescents during affective stimulation: Association with temperament traits. *Journal of Psychiatric Research, 41*(5), 410-417.

Stafford, K. P., & Sadoff, R. L. (2011). Competence to stand trial. In E. Y. Drogin, F. M. Dattilio, R. L. Sadoff, & T. G. Gutheil (Eds.), *Handbook of forensic assessment: Psychological and psychiatric perspectives* (pp. 3-23). New York: Wiley.

Stagl, J. M., Lechner, S. C., Carver, C. S., Bouchard, L. C., Gudenkauf, L. M., Jutagir, D. R., . . . Antoni, M. H. A randomized controlled trial of cognitive-behavioral stress management in breast cancer: Survival and recurrence at 11-year follow-up. *Breast Cancer Research and Treatment, 154,* 319-328.

Stan, I. (2020). Frotteuristic Disorder. *International Journal of Advanced Studies in Sexology, 2*(1), 15-19. DOI: 10.46388/ijass.2020.13.17

Staniloiu, A., & Markowitsch, H. J. (2014). Dissociative amnesia. *The Lancet Psychiatry, 1*(3), 226-241.

Staniloiu, A., & Markowitsch, H. J. (2014). Dissociative amnesia. *The Lancet Psychiatry, 1*(3), 226-241. https://doi.org/10.1016/S2215-0366(14)70279-2

Stanton, A. L., Danoff-Burg, S., Cameron, C. L., Bishop, M., Collins, C. A., Kirk, S. B., & Twillman, R. (2000). Emotionally expressive coping predicts psychological and physical adjustment to breast cancer. *Journal of Consulting and Clinical Psychology, 68,* 875-882.

Stanton, A. L., Luecken, L. J., MacKinnon, D. P., & Thompson, E. H. (2013). Mechanisms in psychosocial interventions for adults living with cancer: Opportunity for integration of theory, research, and practice. *Journal of Consulting and Clinical Psychology, 81,* 318-335.

Stanton, K., & Watson, D. (2020, September 24). *The temporal stability and construct validity of measures assessing mania symptoms and risk: A comparative analysis.* OSF Preprints. Retrieved from https://doi.org/10.31219/osf.io/a7e2g

Stanton, K., & Zimmerman, M. (2018). Clinician ratings of vulnerable and grandiose narcissistic features: Implications for an expanded narcissistic personality disorder diagnosis. *Personality Disorders: Theory, Research, and Treatment, 9*(3), 263.

Starcevic, V., & Castle, D. J. (2016). Stress: Concepts, cognition, emotion, and behavior. *Handbook of Stress, 1,* 203-211.

Starr, L. R., Hammen, C., Brennan, P. A., & Najman, J. M. (2012). Serotonin transporter gene as a predictor of stress generation in depression. *Journal of Abnormal Psychology, 121*(4), 810-818. https://doi.org/10.1037/a0027952

Staudt, M., Herring, E., Gao, K., Miller, J., & Sweet, J. (2019, January 29). Evolution in the Treatment of Psychiatric Disorders: From Psychosurgery to Psychopharmacology to Neuromodulation. Retrieved November 04, 2020, from https://www.frontiersin.org/articles/10.3389/fnins.2019.00108/full

Steadman, H. J., Mulvey, E. P., Monahan, J., Robbins, P. C., Appelbaum, P. S., Grisso, T., . . . Silver, E. (1998). Violence by people discharged from acute psychiatric inpatient facilities and by others in the same neighborhoods. *Archives of General Psychiatry, 55,* 393-401.

Steadman, H. J., Osher, F. C., Robbins, P. C., Case, B., & Samuels, S. (2009). Prevalence of serious mental illness among jail inmates. *Psychiatric Services, 60*(6), 761-765.

Steensma, T. D., McGuire, J. K., Kreukels, B. P., Beekman, A. J., & Cohen-Kettenis, P. T. (2013). Factors associated with desistence and persistence of childhood gender dysphoria: A quantitative follow-up study. *Journal of the American Academy of Child & Adolescent Psychiatry, 52*(6), 582-590.

Steensma, T. D., Van der Ende, J., Verhulst, F. C., & Cohen-Kettenis, P. T. (2013). Gender variance in childhood and sexual orientation in adulthood: A prospective study. *Journal of Sexual Medicine, 10*(11), 2723-2733.

Stefanska, E. B., Nitschke, J., Carter, A. J., & Mokros, A. (2019). Sadism among sexual homicide offenders: Validation of the Sexual Sadism Scale. *Psychological Assessment, 31*(1), 132-137.

Stein, A. (2016). Pelvic floor physical therapy in the treatment of sexual dysfunctions. In L. Lipshultz, A. Pastuszak, A. Goldstein, A. Giraldi, & M. Perelman (Eds.), *Management of sexual dysfunction in men and women* (pp. 189-195). New York: Springer.

Stein, A., Woolley, H., Cooper, S., Winterbottom, J., Fairburn, C. G., & Cortina-Borja, M. (2006). Eating habits and attitudes among 10-year-old children of mothers with eating disorders. *British Journal of Psychiatry, 189,* 324-329.

Steinberg, L. (2009). Adolescent development and juvenile justice. *Annual Review of Clinical Psychology, 5,* 459–486.

Stein, D. J., Chiu, W. T., Hwang, I., Kessler, R. C., Sampson, N., et al. (2010). Cross-national analysis of the associations between traumatic events and suicidal behavior: Findings from the WHO World Mental Health Surveys. *PLoS ONE, 5,* e10574.

Stein, D. J., Grant, J. E., Franklin, M. E., Keuthen, N., Lochner, C., Singer, H. S., & Woods, D. W. (2010). Trichotillomania (hair pulling disorder), skin picking disorder, and stereotypic movement disorder: Toward DSM-V. *Depression and Anxiety, 27*(6), 611–626.

Stein, D. J., Lim, C. C., Roest, A. M., de Jonge, P., Aguilar-Gaxiola, S., Al-Hamzawi, A., . . . WHO World Mental Health Survey Collaborators. (2017). The cross-national epidemiology of social anxiety disorder: Data from the World Mental Health Survey Initiative. *BMC Medicine, 15*(1), 143.

Steiner, M., Dunn, E., & Born, L. (2003). Hormones and mood: From menarche to menopause and beyond. *Journal of Affective Disorders, 74,* 67–83.

Stein, M. B., Jang, K. J., Taylor, S., Vernon, P. A., & Livesley, W. J. (2002). Genetic and environmental influences on trauma exposure and posttraumatic stress disorder: A twin study. *American Journal of Psychiatry, 159,* 1675–1681.

Stepanova, E., Dowling, S., Phelps, M., & Findling, R. L. (2017). Pharmacotherapy of emotional and behavioral symptoms associated with autism spectrum disorder in children and adolescents. *Dialogues in Clinical Neuroscience, 19*(4), 395–402.

Stephens, S., Kenny, R. A., Rowan, E., Allan, L., Kalaria, R. N., Bradbury, M., & Ballard, C. G. (2004). Neuropsychological characteristics of mild vascular cognitive impairment and dementia after stroke. *International Journal of Geriatric Psychiatry, 19,* 1053–1057.

Steptoe, A., & Kivimäki, M. (2013). Stress and cardiovascular disease: An update on current knowledge. *Annual Review of Public Health, 34,* 337–354.

Sternberg, R. J. (2015). Multiple intelligences in the new age of thinking. In S. Goldstein, D. Princiotta, & J. Naglieri (Eds.), *Handbook of intelligence.* New York: Springer.

Stern, S., Linker, S., Vadodaria, K. C., Marchetto, M. C., & Gage, F. H. (2018). Prediction of response to drug therapy in psychiatric disorders. *Open Biology, 8*(5), 180031.

Sterzer, P., Stadler, C., Krebs, A., Kleinschmidt, A., & Poustka, F. (2005). Abnormal neural responses to emotional visual stimuli in adolescents with conduct disorder. *Biological Psychiatry, 57,* 7–15.

Stevens, J. R., Prince, J. B., Prager, L. M., & Stern, T. A. (2014). Psychotic disorders in children and adolescents: A primer on contemporary evaluation and management. *The Primary Care Companion for CNS Disorders, 16*(2), PCC.13f01514. https://doi.org/10.4088/PCC.13f01514

Stevens, J. S., Almli, L. M., Fani, N., Gutman, D. A., Bradley, B., Norrholm, S. D., . . . Ressler, K. J. (2014). PACAP receptor gene polymorphism impacts fear responses in the amygdala and hippocampus. *Proceedings of the National Academy of Sciences, 111*(8), 3158–3163.

Stice, E. (2002). Risk and maintenance factors for eating pathology: A meta-analytic review. *Psychological Bulletin, 128,* 825–848.

Stice, E. (2016). Interactive and mediational etiologic models of eating disorder onset: Evidence from prospective studies. *Annual Review of Clinical Psychology, 12,* 359–381.

Stice, E., Bohon, C., Marti, C. N., & Fischer, K. (2008). Subtyping women with bulimia nervosa along dietary and negative affect dimensions: Further evidence of reliability and validity. *Journal of Counseling and Clinical Psychology, 76,* 1022–1033.

Stice, E., & Fairburn, C. G. (2003). Dietary and dietary-depressive subtypes of bulimia nervosa show differential symptom presentation, social impairment, comorbidity, and course of illness. *Journal of Consulting & Clinical Psychology, 71,* 1090–1094.

Stice, E., Marti, C. N., & Durant, S. (2011). Risk factors for onset of eating disorders: Evidence of multiple risk pathways from an 8-year prospective study. *Behavior Research and Therapy, 49,* 622–627.

Stice, E., Marti, C. N., & Rohde, P. (2013). Prevalence, incidence, impairment, and course of the proposed *DSM-5* eating disorder diagnoses in an 8-year prospective community study of young women. *Journal of Abnormal Psychology, 122*(2), 445–457.

Stice, E., Maxfield, J., & Wells, T. (2003). Adverse effects of social pressure to be thin on young women: An experimental investigation of the effects of "fat talk." *International Journal of Eating Disorders, 34,* 108–117.

Stice, E., Presnell, K., & Spangler, D. (2002). Risk factors for binge eating onset in adolescent girls: A 2-year prospective investigation. *Health Psychology, 21,* 131–138.

Stice, E., & Shaw, H. (2017). Eating disorders: Insights from imaging and behavioral approaches to treatment. *Journal of Psychopharmacology, 31*(11), 1485–1495.

Stice, E., & Shaw, H. E. (1994). Adverse effects of the media-portrayed thin-ideal on women and linkages to bulimic symptomatology. *Journal of Social & Clinical Psychology, 13,* 288–308.

Stice, E., Spangler, D., & Agras, W. S. (2001). Exposure to media-portrayed thin-ideal images adversely affects vulnerable girls: A longitudinal experiment. *Journal of Social & Clinical Psychology, 20,* 270–288.

Stice, E., Spoor, S., Bohon, C., Veldhuizen, M. G., & Small, D. M. (2008). Relation of reward from food intake and anticipated food intake to obesity: A functional magnetic resonance imaging study. *Journal of Abnormal Psychology, 117,* 924–935.

Stice, E., Spoor, S., Ng, J., & Zald, D. H. (2009). Relation of obesity to consummatory and anticipatory food reward. *Physiology & Behavior, 97*(5), 551–560.

Stice, E., Yokum, S., Bohon, C., Marti, N., & Smolen, A. (2010). Reward circuitry responsivity to food predicts future increases in body mass: Moderating effects of DRD2 and DRD4. *NeuroImage, 50,* 1618–1625.

Stilo, S. A., & Murray, R. M. (2019). Non-genetic factors in schizophrenia. *Current Psychiatry Reports, 21*(10), 100.

Stinson, F. S., Dawson, D. A., Goldstein, R. B., Chou, S. P., Huang, B., Smith, S. M., . . . Grant, B. F. (2008). Prevalence, correlates, disability, and comorbidity of *DSM-IV* narcissistic personality disorder: Results from the Wave 2 National Epidemiologic Survey on Alcohol and Related Conditions. *Journal of Clinical Psychiatry, 69,* 1033–1045.

Stoeckel, L. E., Weller, R. E., Cook, E. W., 3rd, Twieg, D. B., Knowlton, R. C., & Cox, J. E. (2008). Widespread reward-system activation in obese women in response to pictures of high-calorie foods. *NeuroImage, 41,* 636–647.

Stoffers, J. M., Ferriter, M., Vollm, B. A., Gibbon, S., Jones, H., Duggan, C., & Lieb, K. (2011). Pharmacological interventions for people with narcissistic personality disorder (protocol). *Cochrane Database Systematic Review, 2014*(3), 10:CD009399.

Stoffers, J. M., & Lieb, K. (2015). Pharmacotherapy for borderline personality disorder: Current evidence and recent trends. *Current Psychiatry Reports, 17*(1), 534.

Stolz, T., Schulz, A., Krieger, T., Vincent, A., Urech, A., Moser, C., . . . Berger, T. (2018). A mobile app for social anxiety disorder: A three-arm randomized controlled trial comparing mobile and PC-based guided self-help interventions. *Journal of Consulting and Clinical Psychology, 86*(6), 493–504.

Stone, J., LaFrance, W. C., Brown, R., Spiegel, D., Levenson, J. L., & Sharpe, M. (2011). Conversion disorder: Current problems and potential solutions for *DSM-5*. *Journal of Psychosomatic Research, 71,* 369–376.

Story, M., Nanney, M. S., & Schwartz, M. B. (2009). Schools and obesity prevention: Creating school environments and policies to promote healthy eating and physical activity. *Milbank Quarterly, 87,* 71–100.

Stouthamer-Loeber, M., Loeber, R., Homish, D. L., & Wei, E. (2001). Maltreatment of boys and the development of disruptive and delinquent behavior. *Development & Psychopathology, 13,* 941–955.

Stoving, R. K., Andries, A., Brixen, K., Bilenberg, N., & Horder, K. (2011). Gender differences in outcome of eating disorders: A retrospective cohort study. *Psychiatric Research, 186,* 362–366.

Stoving, R. K., Andries, A., Brixen, K. T., Bilenberg, N., Lichtenstein, M. B., & Horder, K. (2012). Purging behavior in anorexia nervosa and eating disorder not otherwise specified: A retrospective cohort study. *Psychiatry Research, 198,* 253–258.

St Pourcain, B., Robinson, E. B., Anttila, V., Sullivan, B. B., Maller, J., Golding, J., . . . & Fisher, S. E. (2018). ASD and schizophrenia show distinct developmental profiles in common genetic overlap with population-based social communication difficulties. *Molecular Psychiatry, 23*(2), 263–270.

Strauss, G. P., Harrow, M., Grossman, L. S., & Rosen, C. (2010). Periods of recovery in deficit syndrome schizophrenia: A 20-year multi-follow-up longitudinal study. *Schizophrenia Bulletin, 36,* 788–799.

Strauss, J. S. (1969). Hallucinations and delusions as points on continua function: Rating scale evidence. *Archives of General Psychiatry, 21,* 581–586.

Strauss, M., Mergl, R., Gürke, N., Kleinert, K., Sander, C., & Hegerl, U. (2018). Association between acute critical life events and the speed of onset of depressive episodes in male and female depressed patients. *BMC Psychiatry, 18*(1), 332.

Strawn, J. R., Welge, J. A., Wehry, A. M., Keeshin, B., & Rynn, M. A. (2015). Efficacy and tolerability of antidepressants in pediatric anxiety disorders: A systematic review and meta-analysis. *Depression and Anxiety, 32*(3), 149–157.

Striegel-Moore, R. H., Fairburn, C. G., Wilfley, D. E., Pike, K. M., Dohm, F.-A., & Kraemer, H. C. (2005). Toward an understanding of risk factors for binge-eating disorder in black and white women: A community-based case-control study. *Psychological Medicine, 35,* 907–917.

Striegel-Moore, R. H., & Franko, D. L. (2008). Should binge eating disorder be included in the *DSM-V*? A critical review of the state of the evidence. *Annual Review of Clinical Psychology, 4,* 305–324.

Stringaris, A., Cohen, P., Pine, D. S., & Leibenluft, E. (2009). Adult outcomes of youth irritability: A 20-year prospective community-based study. *American Journal of Psychiatry, 166*(9), 1048–1054.

Stroup, T. S., Gerhard, T., Crystal, S., Huang, C., & Olfson, M. (2016). Comparative effectiveness of clozapine and standard antipsychotic treatment in adults with schizophrenia. *American Journal of Psychiatry, 173*(2), 166–173.

Stunkard, A. J. (2003). A history of binge eating. In C. G. Fairburn & G. T. Wilson (Eds.), *Binge eating: Nature, assessment, and treatment.* New York: Guilford Press.

Stunkard, A. J. (2011). Eating disorders and obesity. *Psychiatric Clinic North America, 34,* 765–771.

Sturup, J., Monahan, J., & Kristiansson, M. (2013). Violent behavior and gender of Swedish psychiatric patients: A prospective clinical study. *Psychiatric Services, 64*(7), 688–693.

Substance Abuse and Mental Health Services Administration. (2019). Key substance use and mental health indicators in the United States: Results from the 2018 National Survey on Drug Use and Health (HHS Publication No. PEP19-5068, NSDUH Series H-54). Rockville, MD: Center for Behavioral Health Statistics and Quality, Substance Abuse and Mental Health Services Administration. Retrieved from https://www.samhsa.gov/data/

Substance Abuse and Mental Health Services Administration (SAMHSA). (2013). *Drug Abuse Warning Network, 2011: National Estimates of Drug-Related Emergency Department Visits.* HHS Publication No. (SMA) 13-4760, DAWN Series D-39. Rockville, MD.

Substance Abuse and Mental Health Services Administration (SAMHSA). (2017). *Key substance use and mental health indicators in the United States: Results from the 2016 National Survey on Drug Use and Health* (HHS Publication No. SMA 17-5044, NSDUH Series H-52). Rockville, MD: Center for Behavioral Health Statistics and Quality, Substance Abuse and Mental Health Services Administration. Retrieved from https://www.samhsa.gov/data/.

Substance Abuse and Mental Health Services Administration (SAMHSA). (2019). Key substance use and mental health indicators in the United States: Results from the 2018 National Survey on Drug Use and Health (HHS Publication No. PEP19-5068, NSDUH Series H-54). Rockville, MD: Center for Behavioral Health Statistics and Quality, Substance Abuse and Mental Health Services Administration. Retrieved from https://www.samhsa.gov/data/

Sue, D. W., & Sue, D. (2003). Counseling the culturally diverse: Theory and practice (4th ed.). New York: Wiley.

Sue, D. W., Sue, D., Neville, H. A., & Smith, L. L. (2019). *Counseling the culturally diverse: Theory and practice.* John Wiley et Sons.

Suhail, K., & Cochrane, R. (2002). Effect of culture and environment on the phenomenology of delusions and hallucinations. *International Journal of Social Psychiatry, 48,* 126–138.

Sullivan P. F. (2013). Questions about DISC1 as a genetic risk factor for schizophrenia. *Molecular psychiatry, 18*(10), 1050–1052. https://doi.org/10.1038/mp.2012.182

Sultzer, D. L., Davis, S. M., Tariot, P. N., Dagerman, K. S., Lebowitz, B. D., Lyketsos, C. G., . . . Schneider, L. S. (2008). Clinical symptom responses to atypical antipsychotic medications in Alzheimer's disease: Phase 1 outcomes from the CATIE-AD effectiveness trial. *American Journal of Psychiatry, 165,* 844–854.

Summers, B. J., & Cougle, J. R. (2018). An experimental test of the role of appearance-related safety behaviors in body dysmorphic disorder, social anxiety, and body dissatisfaction. *Journal of Abnormal Psychology, 127*(8), 770–780.

Sundgot-Borgen, J. (1994). Risk and trigger factors for the development of eating disorders in female elite athletes. *Medicine & Science in Sports & Exercise, 26,* 414–419.

Sundram, C. J. (2009). *Wyatt v. Stickney*–a long odyssey reaches an end. http://www.cqcapd.state.ny.us/pressreleases/wyattclarence.htm (accessed September 29, 2009).

Sun, D., Stuart, G. W., Jenkinson, M., Wood, S. J., McGorry, P. D., Velakoulis, D., . . . Pantelis, C. (2009). Brain surface contraction mapped in first-episode schizophrenia: A longitudinal magnetic resonance imaging study. *Molecular Psychiatry, 14,* 976–986.

Suneel, I., & Siddique, S. (2020). Impact of covert sensitization on recovery of alcoholics in Pakistan. *Rawal Medical Journal, 45*(3), 573–576.

Suomi, S. J. (1999). Developmental trajectories, early experiences, and community consequences: Lessons from studies with rhesus monkeys. In D. P. Keating (Ed.), *Developmental health and the wealth of nations: Social, biological, and educational dynamics* (pp. 185–200). New York: Guilford Press.

Susman, J., & Klee, B. (2005). The role of high-potency benzodiazepines in the treatment of panic disorder. *Primary Care Companion to the Journal of Clinical Psychiatry, 7(1),* 5–11.

Sutter, M., & Perrin, P. B. (2016). Discrimination, mental health, and suicidal ideation among LGBTQ people of color. *Journal of Counseling Psychology, 63*(1), 98–105. https://doi.org/10.1037/cou0000126

Suzuki, M., Zhou, S. Y., Takahashi, T., Hagino, H., Kawasaki, Y., Niu, L., et al. (2005). Differential contributions of prefrontal and temporolimbic pathology to mechanisms of psychosis. *Brain, 128,* 2109–2122.

Suzuki, T., Griffin, S. A., & Samuel, D. B. (2017). Capturing the *DSM-5* alternative personality disorder model traits in the five-factor model's nomological net. *Journal of Personality, 85*(2), 220–231.

Swaab, D. F., & Garcia-Falgueras, A. (2009). Sexual differentiation of the human brain in relation to gender identity and sexual orientation. *Functional Neurology, 24*(1), 17–28.

Swannell, S. V., Martin, G. E., Page, A., Hasking, P., & St. John, N. J. (2014). Prevalence of nonsuicidal self-injury in nonclinical samples: Systematic review, meta-analysis and meta-regression. *Suicide and Life-Threatening Behavior, 44*(3), 273–303.

Swanson, J., Arnold, L. E., Kraemer, H., Hechtman, L., Molina, B., Hinshaw, S., . . . Wigal, T. (2008). Evidence, interpretation, and qualification from multiple reports of long-term outcomes in the multimodal treatment study of children with ADHD (MTA): I. Executive Summary. *Journal of Attention Disorders, 12,* 4–14.

Swanson, J., Baler, R. D., & Volkow, N. D. (2011). Understanding the effects of stimulant medications on cognition in individuals with attention-deficit hyperactivity disorder: A decade of progress. *Neuropsychopharmacology, 36,* 207–226.

Swanson, J. M., Arnold, L. E., Molina, B. S., Sibley, M. H., Hechtman, L. T., Hinshaw, S. P., . . . Stern, K. (2017). Young adult outcomes in the follow-up of the multimodal treatment study of attention-deficit/hyperactivity disorder: Symptom persistence, source discrepancy, and height suppression. *Journal of Child Psychology and Psychiatry, 58*(6), 663–678.

Swanson, J. W., McGinty, E. E., Fazel, S., & Mays, V. M. (2015). Mental illness and reduction of gun violence and suicide: Bringing epidemiologic research to policy. *Annals of Epidemiology, 25*(5), 366–376.

Swanson, J. W., Tong, G., Robertson, A. G., & Swartz, M. S. (2020). Gun-related and other violent crime after involuntary commitment and short-term emergency holds. *J Am Acad Psychiatry Law, 48*(4).

Swanson, S. A., Crow, S. J., Le Grange, D., Swendsen, J., & Merikangas, K. R. (2011). Prevalence and correlates of eating disorders in adolescents. *Archive of General Psychiatry, 68,* 714–723.

Swartz, H. A., & Frank, E. (2001). Psychotherapy for bipolar depression: A phase-specific treatment strategy? *Bipolar Disorders, 3,* 11–12.

Swartz, M. S., Bhattacharya, S., Robertson, A. G., & Swanson, J. W. (2017). Involuntary outpatient commitment and the elusive pursuit of violence prevention: A view from the United States. *Canadian Journal of Psychiatry, 62*(2), 102–108.

Swartz, M. S., Swanson, J., Kim, M., & Petrila, J. (2006). Use of outpatient commitment or related civil court treatment orders in five U.S. communities. *Psychiatric Services, 57,* 343–349.

Swartz, M. S., Wilder, C. M., Swanson, J. W., Van Dorn, R. A., Robbins, P. C., Steadman, H. J., . . . Monahan, J. (2010). Assessing outcomes for consumers in New York's assisted outpatient treatment program. *Psychiatric Services, 61,* 976–981.

Swedo, S. E., Baird, G., Cook, E. H., Jr., Happé, F. G., Harris, J. C., Kaufmann, W. E., . . . Wright, H. H. (2012). Commentary from the *DSM-5* Workgroup on Neurodevelopmental Disorders. *Journal of the American Academy of Child and Adolescent Psychiatry, 51,* 347–349.

Sylvers, P., Brubaker, N., Alden, S. A., Brennan, P. A., & Lilienfeld, S. O. (2008). Differential endophenotypic markers of narcissistic and antisocial personality features: A psychophysiological investigation. *Journal of Research in Personality, 42,* 1260–1270.

Szasz, T. (1961). *The myth of mental illness.* New York: Hoeber-Harper.

Szasz, T. (2011). The myth of mental illness: 50 years later. *Psychiatrist, 35*(5), 179–182.

Szasz, T. S. (1963). *Law, liberty, and psychiatry: An inquiry into the social uses of mental health practice.* New York: Collier Books.

Szasz, T. S. (1977). *Psychiatric slavery.* New York: Free Press.

Szentkirályi, A., Völzke, H., Hoffmann, W., Trenkwalder, C., & Berger, K. (2014). Multimorbidity and the risk of restless legs syndrome in 2 prospective cohort studies. *Neurology, 82*(22), 2026–2033.

T

Takahashi, T., Zhou, S.-Y., Nakamura, K., Tanino, R., Furuichi, A., Kido, M., . . . Suzuki, M. (2011). A follow-up MRI study of the fusiform gyrus and middle and inferior temporal gyri in schizophrenia spectrum. *Progress in Neuro-Psychopharmacology & Biological Psychiatry, 35,* 1957–1964.

Tanay, E. (1992). The verdict with two names. *Psychiatric Annals, 22,* 571–573.

Tang, N. K. Y., Schmidt, D. A., & Harvey, A. G. (2007). Sleeping with the enemy: Clock monitoring in the maintenance of insomnia. *Journal of Behavior Therapy and Experimental Psychiatry, 38,* 40–55.

Tan, J. C. H. (2018). Cultural issues in the teaching of psychological disorders. In K. D. Keith (Ed.), *Culture and psychology. Culture across the curriculum: A psychology teacher's handbook* (p. 517–532). Cambridge University Press. https://doi.org/10.1017/9781316996706.028

Tanner, L. (2001). Nationwide survey shows bullying widespread among students. http://www.apbnews.com (accessed April 25, 2001).

Tannock, R. (2005). Mathematics disorder. In B. J. Sadock & V. A. Sadock (Eds.), *Kaplan & Sadock's comprehensive textbook of psychiatry* (pp. 3116–3123). Philadelphia: Lippincott Williams & Wilkins.

Tanofsky-Kraff, M., Schvey, N. A., & Grilo, C. M. (2020). A developmental framework of binge-eating disorder based on pediatric loss of control eating. *American Psychologist, 75*(2), 189.

Tan, P. Z., Forbes, E. E., Dahl, R. E., Ryan, N. D., Siegle, G. J., Ladouceur, C. D., & Silk, J. S. (2012). Emotional reactivity and regulation in anxious and nonanxious youth: A cell-phone ecological momentary assessment study. *Journal of Child Psychology & Psychiatry, 53,* 197–206.

Tasca, C., Rapetti, M., Carta, M. G., & Fadda, B. (2012). Women and hysteria in the history of mental health. *Clinical Practice and Epidemiology in Mental Health: CP & EMH, 8,* 110–119. https://doi.org/10.2174/1745017901208010110

Tatagiba, M., Ugarte, O. N., & Acioly, M. A. (2015). Neurosurgery: Past, present, and future. In J. Clausen & N. Levy (Eds.), *Handbook of neuroethics.* Dordrecht: Springer.

Tateyama, M., Asai, M., Kamisada, M., Hashimoto, M., Bartels, M., & Heimann, H. (1993). Comparison of schizophrenia delusions between Japan and Germany. *Psychopathology, 26,* 151–158.

Taylor, A., & Kim-Cohen, J. (2007). Meta-analysis of gene-environment interactions in developmental psychopathology. *Development and Psychopathology, 19,* 1029–1037.

Taylor, S., Asmundson, G. J. G., & Jang, K. L. (2011). Etiology of obsessive-compulsive symptoms and obsessive-compulsive personality traits: Common genes, mostly different environments. *Depression and Anxiety, 28,* 863–869.

Taylor, S. E., Eisenberger, N. I., Saxbe, D., Lehman, B. J., & Lieberman M. D. (2006). Neural responses to emotional stimuli are associated with childhood family stress. *Biological Psychiatry, 60,* 296–301.

Taylor, S. E., Klein, L. C., Lewis, B. P., Gruenwald, T. L., Gurung, R. A. R., & Updegraff, J. A. (2000). Biobehavioral responses to stress in females: Tend-and-befriend, not fight-or-flight. *Psychological Review, 3,* 411–429.

Taylor, S. E., & Master, S. L. (2011). Social responses to stress: The tend-and-befriend model. In A. Baum & R. Contrada (Eds.), *The handbook of stress science: Biology, psychology, and health* (pp. 101–109). New York: Springer

Taylor, S. E., & Stanton, A. L. (2007). Coping resources, coping processes and mental health. *Annual Review of Clinical Psychology, 3,* 377–401.

Telles, C., Karno, M., Mintz, J., Paz, G., Arias, M., Tucker, D., & Lopez, S. (1995). Immigrant families coping with schizophrenia. *British Journal of Psychiatry, 167,* 473–479.

Temple, E., Deutsch, G., Poldrack, R., Miller, S., Tallal, P., Merzenich, M., & Gabrieli, J. D. (2003). Neural deficits in children with dyslexia ameliorated by behavioral remediation: Evidence from fMRI. *Proceedings of the National Academy of Science of the United States of America, 100,* 2860–2865.

Templeman, T. N., & Stinnet, R. D. (1991). Patterns of sexual arousal and history in a "normal" sample of young men. *Archives of Sexual Behavior, 20,* 137–150.

Temple Newhook, J., Pyne, J., Winters, K., Feder, S., Holmes, C., Tosh, J., et al. (2018). A critical commentary on follow-up studies and "desistance" theories about transgender and gender-nonconforming children. *International Journal of Transgenderism, 19,* 212–224.

Teplin, L. A. (1990). The prevalence of severe mental disorder among male urban jail detainers: Comparison with the Epidemiologic Catchment Area program. *American Journal of Public Health, 80,* 663–669.

Teplin, L. A., Abram, K. M., & McClelland, G. M. (1996). Prevalence of psychiatric disorders among incarcerated women: I. Pretrial jail detainees. *Archives of General Psychiatry, 53,* 505–512.

Teplin, L. A., Abram, K. M., & McClelland, G. M. (1997). Mentally disordered women in jail: Who receives services? *American Journal of Public Health, 87,* 604–609.

Teplin, L. A., Abram, K. M., McClelland, G. M., Dulcan, M. K., & Mericle, A. A. (2002). Psychiatric disorders in youth in juvenile detention. *Archives of General Psychiatry, 59,* 1133–1143.

Teri, L., Gibbons, L. E., McCurry, S. M., Logsdon, R. G., Buchner, D. M., Barlow, W. E., . . . Larson, E. B. (2003).

Exercise plus behavioral management in patients with Alzheimer disease: A randomized controlled trial. *JAMA, 290,* 2015–2022.

Testa, M., & West, S. G. (2010). Civil commitment in the United States. *Psychiatry (Edgmont), 7*(10), 30–40.

Thase, M. E., Hahn, C.-G., & Berton, O. (2015). Neurobiological aspects of depression. In I. H. Gotlib & C. L. Hammen (Eds.), *Handbook of depression* (3rd ed., pp. 182–201). New York: Guilford.

Thase, M. E., Stanford, A. D., Memisoglu, A., Martin, W., Claxton, A., Bodkin, J. A. . . . Pathak, S. (2019). Results from a long-term open-label extension study of adjunctive buprenorphine/samidorphan combination in patients with major depressive disorder. *Neuropsychopharmacol, 44,* 2268–2276.

The State of Homelessness in America. (2019, September). Retrieved October 16, 2020, from https://www.nhipdata.org/local/upload/file/The-State-of-Homelessness-in-America.pdf

Thibaut, F., Cosyns, P., Fedoroff, J. P., Briken, P., Goethals, K., Bradford, J. M., & WFSBP Task Force on Paraphilias. (2020). The World Federation of Societies of Biological Psychiatry (WFSBP) 2020 guidelines for the pharmacological treatment of paraphilic disorders. *The World Journal of Biological Psychiatry, 21*(6), 412–490.

Thompson, P. M., Hayashi, K. M., De Zubicaray, G. I., Janke, A. L., Rose, S. E., Semple, J., . . . Toga, A. W. et al. (2004). Mapping hippocampal and ventricular change in Alzheimer disease. *NeuroImage, 22,* 1754–1766.

Thompson, R., Jones, N., Holman, & Silver, R. C. (2019). Media exposure to mass violence events can fuel a cycle of distress. *Science Advances, 5*(4), 1–6.

Thomson, P. A., Malavasi, E. L., Grünewald, E., Soares, D. C., Borkowska, M., & Millar, J. K. (2013). DISC1 genetics, biology and psychiatric illness. *Frontiers in Biology, 8*(1), 1–31. https://doi.org/10.1007/s11515-012-1254-7

Tienari, P., Wahlberg, K. E., & Wynne, L. C. (2006). Finnish Adoption Study of Schizophrenia: Implications for family interventions. *Families, Systems and Health, 24,* 442–451.

Tienari, P., Wynne, L. C., Läksy, K., Moring, J., Nieminen, P., Sorri, A., . . . Wahlberg, K. E. (2003). Genetic boundaries of the schizophrenia spectrum: Evidence from the Finnish Adoptive Family Study of Schizophrenia. *American Journal of Psychiatry, 160,* 1587–1594.

Tiet, Q. Q., Wasserman, G. A., Loeber, R., McReynolds, L. S., & Miller, L. S. (2001). Developmental and sex differences in types of conduct problems. *Journal of Child & Family Studies, 10,* 181–197.

Tiggemann, M., Martins, Y., & Kirkbride, A. (2007). Oh to be lean and muscular: Body image ideals in gay and heterosexual men. *Psychology of Men and Masculinity, 8,* 15–24.

Timmermans, I., Versteeg, H., Duijndam, S., Graafmans, C., Polak, P., & Denollet, J. (2019). Social inhibition and emotional distress in patients with coronary artery disease: The Type D personality construct. *Journal of Health Psychology, 24*(14), 1929–1944.

Tinland, A., Loubière, S., Boucekine, M., Boyer, L., Fond, G., Girard, V., & Auquier, P. (2020). Effectiveness of a housing support team intervention with a recovery-oriented approach on hospital and emergency department use by homeless people with severe mental illness: A randomised controlled trial. *Epidemiology and Psychiatric Sciences, 29.*

Todd, R. D., Lobos, E. A., Sun, L. W., & Neuman, R. J. (2003). Mutational analysis of the nicotinic acetylcholine receptor alpha 4 subunit gene in attention deficit/hyperactivity disorder: Evidence for association of an intronic polymorphism with attention problems. *Molecular Psychiatry, 8,* 103–108.

Tonigan, J. S., Pearson, M. R., Magill, M., & Hagler, K. J. (2018). AA attendance and abstinence for dually diagnosed patients: A meta-analytic review. *Addiction.*

Toogood S., Totsika V., Jones E., & Lowe K. (2016). Active support. In N. N. Singh (Ed.), *Handbook of evidence-based practices in intellectual and developmental disabilities* (pp. 537-560). Cham: Springer.

Torrey, E. F. (2013). *Surviving schizophrenia: A manual for families, patients, and providers* (6th ed.). New York: Harper Perennial.

Torti, F. M., Jr., Gwyther, L. P., Reed, S. D., Friedman, J. Y., & Schulman, K. A. (2004). A multinational review of recent trends and reports in dementia caregiver burden. *Alzheimer Disease & Associated Disorders, 18,* 99-109.

Torvik, F. A., Welander-Vatn, A., Ystrom, E., Knudsen, G. P., Czajkowski, N., . . . & Reichborn-Kjennerud, T. (2016). Longitudinal associations between social anxiety disorder and avoidant personality disorder: A twin study. *Journal of Abnormal Psychology, 125*(1), 114-124.

Toufexis, A., Blackman, A., & Drummond, T. (1996, April 29). Why Jennifer got sick. http://www.time.com/time/magazine/article/0,9171,984465,00.html (accessed October 29, 2009).

Trace, S. E., Baker, J. H., Peñas-Lledó, E., & Bulik, C. M. (2013). The genetics of eating disorders. *Annual Review of Clinical Psychology, 9,* 589-620.

Trauer, J. M., Qian, M. Y., Doyle, J. S., Rajaratnam, S. M., & Cunnington, D. (2015). Cognitive behavioral therapy for chronic insomnia: A systematic review and meta-analysis. *Annals of Internal Medicine, 163*(3), 191-204.

Treasure, J., & Cardi, V. (2017). Anorexia nervosa, theory and treatment: Where are we 35 years on from Hilde Bruch's foundation lecture? *European Eating Disorders Review, 25*(3), 139-147.

Trestman, R. L., Ford, J., Zhang, W., & Wiesbrock, V. (2007). Current and lifetime psychiatric illness among inmates not identified as acutely mentally ill at intake in Connecticut's jails. *Journal of the American Academy of Psychiatry and Law, 35,* 490-500.

Trifu, S. C., Kohn, B., Vlasie, A., & Patrichi, B. E. (2020). Genetics of schizophrenia. *Experimental and Therapeutic Medicine, 20*(4), 3462-3468.

Trindade, I. A., Mendes, A. L., & Ferreira, N. B. (2020). The moderating effect of psychological flexibility on the link between learned helplessness and depression symptomatology: A preliminary study. *Journal of Contextual Behavioral Science, 15,* 68-72.

Trotti, L. M., & Rye, D. B. (2011). Restless legs syndrome. *Handbook of Clinical Neurology, 100,* 661-673.

True, W. R., Rice, J., Eisen, S. A., Heath, A. C., Goldberg, J., Lyons, M. J., & Nowak, J. (1993). A twin study of genetic and environmental contributions to liability for posttraumatic stress symptoms. *Archives of General Psychiatry, 50,* 257-264.

Trull, T. J., Jahng, S., Tomko, R. L., Wood, P. K., & Sher, K. J. (2010). Revised NESARC personality disorder diagnoses: Gender, prevalence, and comorbidity with substance dependence disorders. *Journal of Personality Disorders, 24*(4), 412-426.

Trull, T. J., Solhan, M. B., Tragesser, S. L., Jahng, S., Wood, P. K., Paisecki, T. M., & Watson, D. (2008). Affective instability: Measuring a core feature of borderline personality disorder with ecological momentary assessment. *Journal of Abnormal Psychology, 117,* 647-661.

Tsanas, A., Saunders, A. C., Bilderbeck, N., Palmius, M., Osipov, G. D., Clifford, G. M., . . . De Vos, M. (2016). Daily longitudinal self-monitoring of mood variability in bipolar disorder and borderline personality disorder. *Journal of Affective Disorders, 205,* 225-233.

Tseng, W. (1973). The development of psychiatric concepts in traditional Chinese medicine. *Archives of General Psychiatry, 29,* 569-575.

Tsirigotis, K., Gruszczynski, W., & Tsirigotis, M. (2011). Gender differentiation in methods of suicide attempts. *Medical Science Monitor: International Medical Journal of Experimental and Clinical Research, 17*(8), PH65-PH70.

Ttofi, M. M., Farrington, D. P., & Lösel, F. (2012). School bullying as a predictor of violence later in life: A systematic review and meta-analysis of prospective longitudinal studies. *Aggression and Violent Behavior, 17*(5), 405-418.

Tucci, V., & Moukaddam, N. (2017). We are the hollow men: The worldwide epidemic of mental illness, psychiatric and behavioral emergencies, and its impact on patients and providers. *Journal of Emergencies, Trauma, and Shock, 10*(1), 4-6. https://doi.org/10.4103/0974-2700.199517

Tucker, J. A., Chandler, S. D., & Witkiewitz, K. (2020). Epidemiology of recovery from alcohol use disorder. *Alcohol Research: Current Reviews, 40*(3), 02. https://doi.org/10.35946/arcr.v40.3.02

Tummala-Narra, P., Claudius, M., Letendre, P. J., Sarbu, E., Teran, V., & Villalba, W. (2018). Psychoanalytic psychologists' conceptualizations of cultural competence in psychotherapy. *Psychoanalytic Psychology, 35*(1), 46-59. https://doi.org/10.1037/pap0000150

Turkheimer, E., & Parry, C. D. (1992). Why the gap? Practice and policy in civil commitment hearings. *American Psychologist, 47,* 646-655.

Turk, J. (2011). Fragile X syndrome: Lifespan developmental implications for those without as well as with intellectual disability. *Current Opinion in Psychiatry, 24,* 387-397.

Turner-Cobb, J. M., Sephton, S. E., Koopman, C., Blake-Mortimer, J., & Spiegel, D. (2000). Social support and salivary cortisol in women with metastatic breast cancer. *Psychosomatic Medicine, 62,* 337-345.

Turner, D. T., van der Gaag, M., Karyotaki, E., & Cuijpers, P. (2014). Psychological interventions for psychosis: A meta-analysis of comparative outcome studies. *American Journal of Psychiatry, 171*(5), 523-538.

Turolla, A., Venneri, A., Farina, D., Cagnin, A., and Cheung, V. C. K. (2018). Rehabilitation induced neural plasticity after acquired brain injury. *Neural Plast.* 2018:6565418. doi: 10.1155/2018/6565418

Tuvblad, C., & Baker, L. A. (2011). Human aggression across the lifespan: Genetic propensities and environmental moderators. *Advances in Genetics, 75,* 171-214. https://doi.org/10.1016/B978-0-12-380858-5.00007-1

Twenge, J. M., Joiner, T. E., Rogers, M. L., & Martin, G. N. (2018). Increases in depressive symptoms, suicide-related outcomes, and suicide rates among US adolescents after 2010 and links to increased new media screen time. *Clinical Psychological Science, 6*(1), 3-17.

Twenge, J. M., & Nolen-Hoeksema, S. (2002). Age, gender, race, SES, and birth cohort differences on the Children's Depression Inventory: A meta-analysis. *Journal of Abnormal Psychology, 111,* 578-588.

Tyrer, P., Cooper, S., Crawford, M., Dupont, S., Green, J., Murphy, D., . . . Tyrer, H. (2011). Prevalence of health anxiety problems in medical clinics. *Journal of Psychosomatic Research, 71,* 392-394.

U

Uchino, B. N. (2009). Understanding the links between social support and physical health: A life-span perspective with emphasis on the separability of perceived and received support. *Perspectives on Psychological Science, 4,* 236-255.

Udo, T., Bitley, S., & Grilo, C. M. (2019). Suicide attempts in US adults with lifetime DSM-5 eating disorders. *BMC Medicine, 17*(1), 1–13.

Ujike, H., Otani, K., Nakatsuka, M., Ishii, K., Sasaki, A., Oishi, T., Sato, T., Okahisa, Y., Matsumoto, Y., Namba, Y., Kimata, Y., & Kuroda, S. (2009). Association study of gender identity disorder and sex hormone–related genes. *Progress in Neuro-Psychopharmacology & Biological Psychiatry, 3,* 1241–1244.

UNAIDS. (2018). Fact sheet—Latest statistics on the status of the AIDS epidemic. http://www.unaids.org/en/resources/fact-sheet. Retrieved July 5, 2018.

Unwin, G. L., & Deb, S. (2011). Efficacy of atypical antipsychotic medication in the management of behaviour problems in children with intellectual disabilities and borderline intelligence: A systematic review. *Research in Developmental Disabilities, 32,* 2121–2133.

Upthegrove, R., Broome, M. R., Caldwell, K., Ives, J., Oyebode, F., & Wood, S. J. (2016). Understanding auditory verbal hallucinations: A systematic review of current evidence. *Acta Psychiatrica Scandinavica, 133*(5), 352–367.

Urbanoski, K. A., & Kelly, J. F. (2012). Understanding genetic risk for substance use and addiction: A guide for non-geneticists. *Clinical Psychology Review, 32,* 60–70.

U.S. Census Bureau. (2018). Older people projected to outnumber younger people for first time in U.S. history. https://www.census.gov/newsroom/press-releases/2018/cb18-41-population-projections.html. Retrieved July 4, 2018.

V

Vaishnav, M., Saha, G., Mukherji, A., & Vaishnav, P. (2020). Principles of marital therapies and behavior therapy of sexual dysfunction. *Indian Journal of Psychiatry, 62*(Suppl 2), S213–S222.

Valdez, J. N. (2014). Curanderismo: A complementary and alternative approach to Mexican American health psychology. In Gurung, R. A. R. (Ed.), *Multicultural approaches to health and wellness in America* (pp. 227–258). Santa Barbara, CA: Praeger.

Valenzuela, M. J. (2008). Brain reserve and the prevention of dementia. *Current Opinion in Psychiatry 21,* 296–302.

van Amsterdam, J., Pennings, E., & van den Brink, W. (2020). Fatal and non-fatal health incidents related to recreational ecstasy use. *Journal of Psychopharmacology, 34*(6), 591–599.

Vandelanotte, C., Kolt, G. S., Caperchione, C. M., Savage, T. N., Rosenkranz, R. R., et al. (2017). Effectiveness of a Web 2.0 intervention to increase physical activity in real-world settings: Randomized ecological trial. *Journal of Medical Internet Research, 19*(11): e390.

Vandelanotte, C., Müller, A. M., Short, C. E., Hingle, M., Nathan, N., Williams, S. L., . . . Maher, C. A. (2016). Past, present, and future of eHealth and mHealth research to improve physical activity and dietary behaviors. *Journal of Nutrition Education and Behavior, 48*(3), 219–228.

Vandelanotte, C., Spathonis, K. M., Eakin, E. G., & Owen, N. (2007). Website-delivered physical activity interventions: A review of the literature. *American Journal of Preventative Medicine, 33,* 54–64.

Van den Bosch, L. M. C., Rijckmans, M. J. N., Decoene, S., & Chapman, A. L. (2018). Treatment of antisocial personality disorder: Development of a practice focused framework. *International Journal of Law and Psychiatry, 58,* 72–78.

Van der Feltz-Cornelis, C., Allen, S., Van Eck van der Sluijs, J.F. (2020). Childhood sexual abuse predicts treatment outcome in conversion disorder/functional neurological disorder. An observational longitudinal study. *Brain and Behavior, 10*(3), 1–14. doi.org/10.1002/brb3.1558

VanderKruik, R., Barreix, M., Chou, D., Allen, T., Say, L., & Cohen, L. S. (2017). The global prevalence of postpartum psychosis: A systematic review. *BMC Psychiatry, 17*(1), 272.

van der Velden, P. G., van Loon, P., Benight, C. C., & Eckardt, T. (2012). Mental health problems among search and rescue workers deployed in the Haiti earthquake 2010: A pre-post comparison. *Psychiatry Research, 198,* 100–105.

Van Dijk, S., Jeffrey, J., & Katz, M. R. (2013). A randomized, controlled, pilot study of dialectical behavior therapy skills in a psychoeducational group for individuals with bipolar disorder. *Journal of Affective Disorders, 145,* 386–393.

Van Geel, M., Vedder, P., & Tanilon, J. (2014). Are overweight and obese youths more often bullied by their peers? A meta-analysis on the relation between weight status and bullying. *International Journal of Obesity, 38*(10), 1263–1267.

Van Meter, A. R., Youngstrom, E. A., Birmaher, B., Fristad, M. A., Horwitz, S. M., Frazier, T. W., Arnold, L. E., & Findling, R. L. (2017). Longitudinal course and characteristics of cyclothymic disorder in youth. *Journal of affective disorders, 215,* 314–322. https://doi.org/10.1016/j.jad.2017.03.019

van Ommeren, M., De Jong, J. T. V. M., Bhogendra, S., Komproe, I., Thapa, S. B., & Cardena, E. (2001). Psychiatric disorders among tortured Bhutanese refugees in Nepal. *Archives of General Psychiatry, 58,* 475–482.

Van Winkel, R., & Kuepper, R. (2014). Epidemiological, neurobiological, and genetic clues to the mechanisms linking cannabis use to risk for nonaffective psychosis. *Annual Review of Clinical Psychology, 10,* 767–791.

Vassos, E., Collier, D. A., & Fazel, S. (2014). Systematic meta-analyses and field synopsis of genetic association studies of violence and aggression. *Molecular Psychiatry, 19*(4), 471–477.

Vaughn, M. G., Fu, Q., Bender, K., DeLisi, M., Beaver, K. M., Perron, B. E., & Howard, M. O. (2010). Psychiatric correlates of bullying in the United States: Findings from a national sample. *Psychiatric Quarterly, 81*(3), 183–195.

Veasey, S. C., Guilleminault, C., Strohl, K. P., Sanders, M. H., Ballard, R. D., & Magalang, U. J. (2006). Medical therapy for obstructive sleep apnea: A review by the Medical Therapy for Obstructive Sleep Apnea Task Force of the Standards of Practice Committee of the American Academy of Sleep Medicine. *Sleep, 29,* 1036–1044.

Veith, I. (1965). *Hysteria: The history of a disease.* Chicago: University of Chicago Press.

Velikonja, T., Fisher, H. L., Mason, O., & Johnson, S. (2015). Childhood trauma and schizotypy: A systematic literature review. *Psychological Medicine, 45*(5), 947–963.

Velikonja, T., Velthorst, E., McClure, M. M., Rutter, S., Calabrese, W. R., Rosell, D., . . . & Perez-Rodriguez, M. M. (2019). Severe childhood trauma and clinical and neurocognitive features in schizotypal personality disorder. *Acta Psychiatrica Scandinavica, 140*(1), 50–64.

Velting, O. N., Setzer, N. J., & Albano, A. M. (2004). Update on and advances in assessment and cognitive-behavioral treatment of anxiety disorders in children and adolescents. *Professional Psychology: Research & Practice, 35,* 42–54.

Ventriglio, A., Bhat, P. S., Torales, J., & Bhugra, D. (2019). Sexuality in the 21st century: Leather or rubber? Fetishism explained. *Medical Journal, Armed Forces India, 75*(2), 121–124.

Ventriglio, A., Gentile, A., Bonfitto, I., Stella, E., Mari, M., Steardo, L., & Bellomo, A. (2016). Suicide in the early stage of schizophrenia. *Frontiers in Psychiatry, 7,* 116.

Ventura, J., Neuchterlein, K. H., Lukoff, D., & Hardesty, J. P. (1989). A prospective study of stressful life events and schizophrenic relapse. *Journal of Abnormal Psychology, 98,* 407–411.

Verduijn, J., Verhoeven, J. E., Milaneschi, Y., Schoevers, R. A., van Hemert, A. M., Beekman, A. T. F., & Penninx, B. W. J. H. (2017). Reconsidering the prognosis of major depressive disorder across diagnostic boundaries: Full recovery is the exception rather than the rule. *BMC Medicine, 15,* 215.

Verheul, R., & Widiger, T. A. (2004). A meta-analysis of the prevalence and usage of the personality disorder not otherwise specified (PDNOS) diagnosis. *Journal of Personality Disorders, 18,* 309–319.

Verma, K. K., Khaitan, B. K., & Singh, O. P. (1998). The frequency of sexual dysfunctions in patients attending a sex therapy clinic in north India. *Archives of Sexual Behavior, 27,* 309–314.

Vermeulen, J. M., van Rooijen, G., van de Kerkhof, M. P., Sutterland, A. L., Correll, C. U., & de Haan, L. (2019). Clozapine and long-term mortality risk in patients with schizophrenia: A systematic review and meta-analysis of studies lasting 1.1–12.5 years. *Schizophrenia Bulletin, 45*(2), 315–329.

Vervliet, B., Craske, M. G., & Hermans, D. (2013). Fear extinction and relapse: State of the art. *Annual Review of Clinical Psychology, 9,* 215–248.

Via, E., Radua, J., Cardoner, N., Happé, F., & Mataix-Cols, D. (2011). Meta-analysis of gray matter abnormalities in autism spectrum disorder: Should Asperger disorder be subsumed under a broader umbrella of autistic spectrum disorder? *Archive of General Psychiatry, 68,* 409–418.

Vigerland, S., Lenhard, F., Bonnert, M., Lalouni, M., Hedman, E., Ahlen, J., . . . Ljótsson, B. (2016). Internet-delivered cognitive behavior therapy for children and adolescents: A systematic review and meta-analysis. *Clinical Psychology Review, 50,* 1–10.

Viken, R. J., Treat, T. A., Nosofsky, R. M., McFall, R. M., & Palmeri, T. J. (2002). Modeling individual differences in perceptual and attentional processes. *Journal of Abnormal Psychology, 111,* 598–609.

Villadsen, A., Thorgaard, M. V., Hybel, K. A., Jensen, J. S., Thomsen, P. H., & Rask, C. U. (2017). Health anxiety symptoms in children and adolescents diagnosed with OCD. *European Child & Adolescent Psychiatry, 26*(2), 241–251. doi: http://dx.doi.org.mccc.idm.oclc.org/10.1007/s00787-016-0884-8

Villemagne, V. L., Doré, V., Burnham, S. C., Masters, C. L., & Rowe, C. C. (2018). Imaging tau and amyloid-β proteinopathies in Alzheimer disease and other conditions. *Nature Reviews Neurology, 14*(4), 225–236.

Visintainer, M. A., Volpicelli, J. R., & Seligman, M. E. (1982). Tumor rejection in rats after inescapable or escapable shock. *Science, 216,* 437–439.

Vismara, L. A., & Rogers, S. J. (2010). Behavioral treatments in autism spectrum disorder: What do we know? *Annual Review of Clinical Psychology, 6,* 447–468.

Visser, F. E., Aldenkamp, A. P., van Huffelen, A. C., Kuilman, M., Overweg, J., & van Wijk, J. (1997). Prospective study of the prevalence of Alzheimer-type dementia in institutionalized individuals with Down syndrome. *American Journal on Mental Retardation, 101,* 400–412.

Viswanath, B., & Chaturvedi, S. K. (2012). Cultural aspects of major mental disorders: a critical review from an Indian perspective. *Indian Journal of Psychological Medicine, 34*(4), 306–312. https://doi.org/10.4103/0253-7176.108193

Vogel, L. (2018). Growing consensus on link between strep and obsessive-compulsive disorder. *CMAJ: Canadian Medical Association Journal = journal de l'Association medicale canadienne, 190*(3), E86-E87.

Vohs, K. D., Voelz, Z. R., Pettit, J. W., Bardone, A. M., Katz, J., Abramson, L. Y., . . . Joiner, T. E. (2001). Perfectionism, body dissatisfaction, and self-esteem: An interactive model of bulimic symptom development. *Journal of Social & Clinical Psychology, 20,* 476–497.

Voitsidis, P., Gliatas, I., Bairachtari, V., Papadopoulou, K., Papageorgiou, G., Parlapani, E., . . . Diakogiannis, I. (2020). Insomnia during the COVID-19 pandemic in a Greek population. *Psychiatry Research, 289,* 113076. https://doi.org/10.1016/j.psychres.2020.113076

Volkert, J., Gablonski, T. C., & Rabung, S. (2018). Prevalence of personality disorders in the general adult population in Western countries: Systematic review and meta-analysis. *The British Journal of Psychiatry, 213*(6), 709–715.

Volkmar, F. R., State, M., & Klin, A. (2009). Autism and autism spectrum disorders: Diagnostic issues for the coming decade. *Journal of Child Psychology and Psychiatry, 50,* 108–115.

Volkow, N. D., & Boyle, M. (2018). Neuroscience of addiction: Relevance to prevention and treatment. *American Journal of Psychiatry.* Doi: 10.1176/appi.ajp.2018.17101174.

Volkow, N. D., Wise, R. A., & Baler, R. (2017). The dopamine motive system: Implications for drug and food addiction. *Nature Reviews Neuroscience, 18*(12), 741.

von Bernhardi, R., Bernhardi, L. E., & Eugenín, J. (2017). What is neural plasticity?. *Advances in Experimental Medicine and Biology, 1015,* 1–15.

Vonderlin, R., Kleindienst, N., Alpers, G. W., Bohus, M., Lyssenko, L., & Schmahl, C. (2018). Dissociation in victims of childhood abuse or neglect: A meta-analytic review. *Psychological Medicine,* 1–10.

Voort, J. L. V., He, J. P., Jameson, N. D., & Merikangas, K. R. (2014). Impact of the DSM-5 attention-deficit/hyperactivity disorder age-of-onset criterion in the US adolescent population. *Journal of the American Academy of Child & Adolescent Psychiatry, 53*(7), 736–744.

Vriends, N., Pfaltz, M. C., Novianti, P., & Hadiyono, J. (2013). Taijin kyofusho and social anxiety and their clinical relevance in indonesia and Switzerland. *Frontiers in psychology, 4,* 3. https://doi.org/10.3389/fpsyg.2013.00003

Vukasović, T., & Bratko, D. (2015). Heritability of personality: A meta-analysis of behavior genetic studies. *Psychological Bulletin, 141*(4), 769–785.

Vyskocilova, J., & Prasko, J. (2014). EPA-1344 – Countertransference, schema modes and ethical considerations in cognitive behavioral therapy. *European Psychiatry, 55* (1–2), 33–39. doi: 10.1016/S0924-9338(14)78559-1

Vythilingam, M., Heim, C., Newport, J., Miller, A. H., Anderson, E., Bronen, R., . . . Bremner, J. D. (2002). Childhood trauma associated with smaller hippocampal volume in women with major depression. *American Journal of Psychiatry, 159,* 2072–2080.

W

Wadden, T. A., Neiberg, R. H., Wing, R. R., Clark, J. M., Delahanty, L. M., Hill, J. O., . . . Vitolins, M. Z. (2011). Four-year weight losses in the Look AHEAD study: Factors associated with long-term success. *Obesity, 19,* 1987–1998.

Wadden, T. A., Wilson, G. T., Stunkard, A. J., & Berkowitz, R. I. (2011). Obesity and associated eating disorders: A guide for mental health professionals. *Psychiatric Clinics of North America, 34,* xiii-xvi.

Wade, T. D., Gillespie, N., & Martin, N. G. (2007). A comparison of early family life events amongst monozygotic twin women with lifetime anorexia nervosa, bulimia nervosa, or major depression. *International Journal of Eating Disorders, 40,* 679–686.

Wade, T. D., Tiggemann, M., Bulik, C. M., Fairburn, C. G., Wray, N. R., & Martin, N. G. (2008). Shared temperament risk factors for anorexia nervosa: A twin study. *Psychosomatic Medicine, 70,* 239–244.

Wade, T. D., & Watson, H. J. (2012). Psychotherapies in eating disorders. In J. Alexander & J. Treasure (Eds.), *A collaborative approach to eating disorders* (pp. 125-135). New York: Routledge/Taylor & Francis Group.

Wakschlag, L. S., Pickett, K. E., Kasza, K. E., & Loeber, R. (2006). Is prenatal smoking associated with a developmental pattern of conduct problems in young boys? *Journal of the American Academy of Child and Adolescent Psychiatry, 45,* 461-467.

Walderhaug, E., Krystal, J. H., & Neumeister, A. (2011). In D. M. Benedek & G. H. Wynn (Eds.), *Clinical manual for management of PTSD* (pp. 45-68). Arlington, VA: American Psychiatric Publishing.

Waldinger, M. D. (2015). Psychiatric disorders and sexual dysfunction. *Handbook of Clinical Neurology, 130,* 469-489.

Walker, E. F., Cornblatt, B. A., Addington, J., Cadenhead, K. S., Cannon, T. D., McGlashan, T. H., . . . Heinssen, R. (2009). The relation of antipsychotic and antidepressant medication with baseline symptoms and symptom progression: A naturalistic study of the North American Prodrome Longitudinal Sample. *Schizophrenia Research, 115,* 50-57.

Walker, E. R., Cummings, J. R., Hockenberry, J. M., & Druss, B. G. (2015). Insurance status, use of mental health services, and unmet need for mental health care in the United States. *Psychiatric services (Washington, D.C.), 66*(6), 578-584.

Walkup, J. T., Albano, A. M., Piacentini, J., Birmaher, B., Compton, S. N., Sherrill, J. T., . . . Kendall, P. C. (2008). Cognitive behavioral therapy, sertraline, or a combination in childhood anxiety. *New England Journal of Medicine, 359*(26), 2753-2766.

Walkup, J. T., Ferraõ, Y., Leckman, J. F., Stein, D. J., & Singer, H. (2010). Tic disorders: Some key issues for *DSM-V. Depression and Anxiety, 27,* 600-610.

Wallace, E. R., IV, & Gach, J. (Eds.). (2008). *History of psychiatry and medical psychology: With an epilogue on psychiatry and the mind-body relation.* New York: Springer Science.

Walsh, A. E., Browning, M., Drevets, W. C., Furey, M., & Harmer, C. J. (2018). Dissociable temporal effects of bupropion on behavioural measures of emotional and reward processing in depression. *Philosophical Transactions of the Royal Society B: Biological Sciences, 373*(1742), 20170030.

Wampold, B. E. (2015). How important are the common factors in psychotherapy? An update. *World Psychiatry, 14*(3), 270-277.

Wang, C., Shao, X., Jia, Y., Zhang, B., Shen, C., & Wang, W. (2020). Inhibitory brainstem reflexes under external emotional-stimuli in schizoid and histrionic personality disorders. *Personality and Individual Differences, 158,* 109843.

Wang, P. S., Aguilar-Gaxiola, S., Alonso, J., Angermeyer, M. C., Borges, G., & Bromet E. J. (2007). Use of mental health services for anxiety, mood, and substance disorders in 17 countries in the WHO World Mental Health surveys. *Lancet, 370,* 841-850.

Wang, S., & Blazer, D. G. (2015). Depression and cognition in the elderly. *Annual Review of Clinical Psychology, 11,* 331-360.

Wang, X., Chen, Q., & Yang, M. (2017). Effect of caregivers' expressed emotion on the care burden and rehospitalization rate of schizophrenia. *Patient Preference and Adherence, 11,* 1505-1511. https://doi.org/10.2147/PPA.S143873

Wang, X., Sirianni, A. D., Tang, S., Zheng, Z., & Fu, F. (2020). Public discourse and social network echo chambers driven by socio-cognitive biases. *Physical Review X, 10*(4), 041042.

Wanic, R., & Kulik, J. (2011). Toward an understanding of gender differences in the impact of marital conflict on health. *Sex Roles, 65*(5-6), 297-312.

Warren, J. I., Burnette, M., South, S. C., Chauhan, P., Bale, R., & Friend, R. (2002). Personality disorders and violence among female prison inmates. *Journal of the American Academy of Psychiatry and the Law, 30*(4), 502-509.

Warren, J. I., Murrie, D. C., Chauhan, P., Dietz, P. E., & Morris, J. (2004). Opinion formation in evaluating sanity at the time of the offense: An examination of 5175 pre-trial evaluations. *Behavioral Sciences and the Law, 22,* 171-186.

Wassertheil-Smoller, S., Arredondo, E. M., Cai, J., Castaneda, S. F., Choca, J. P., Gallo, L. C., . . . Zee, P. C. (2014). Depression, anxiety, antidepressant use, and cardiovascular disease among Hispanic men and women of different national backgrounds: Results from the Hispanic Community Health Study/Study of Latinos. *Annals of Epidemiology, 24*(11), 822-830.

Waszczuk, M., Coulson, A., Gregory, A., & Eley, T. (2016). A longitudinal twin and sibling study of the hopelessness theory of depression in adolescence and young adulthood. *Psychological Medicine, 46*(9), 1935-1949.

Waters, F., & Fernyhough, C. (2017). Hallucinations: A systematic review of points of similarity and difference across diagnostic classes. *Schizophrenia Bulletin, 43*(1), 32-43.

Watson, D. (2009). Differentiating the mood and anxiety disorders: A quadripartite model. *Annual Review of Clinical Psychology, 5,* 221-247.

Watson, D., Clark, L. A., & Chmielewski, M. (2008). Structures of personality and their relevance to psychopathology: II. Further articulation of a comprehensive unified trait structure. *Journal of Personality, 76,* 1545-1585.

Watson, J. B. (1930). *Behaviorism.* Chicago: University of Chicago Press.

Watson, J. B., & Raynor, R. (1920). Conditioned emotional reactions. *Journal of Experimental Psychology, 3,* 1-14.

Watson, M., Haviland, J. S., Greer, S., Davidson, J., & Bliss, J. M. (1999). Influence of psychological response on survival in breast cancer: A population-based cohort study. *Lancet, 354,* 1331-1336.

Waugh, M. H., Hopwood, C. J., Krueger, R. F., Morey, L. C., Pincus, A. L., & Wright, A. G. (2017). Psychological assessment with the DSM-5 Alternative Model for Personality Disorders: Tradition and innovation. *Professional Psychology: Research and Practice, 48*(2), 79-89.

Webb, R. L., & Murphy, M. P. (2012). ß-Secretases, Alzheimer's disease, and Down syndrome. *Current Gerontology and Geriatrics Research, 2012,* 362839.

Webster-Stratton, C., & Reid, M. J. (2017). The Incredible Years Parents, Teachers, and Children Training Series: A multifaceted treatment approach for young children with conduct problems. In J. R. Weisz & A. E. Kazdin (Eds.), *Evidence-based psychotherapies for children and adolescents* (3rd ed., pp. 122-141). New York: Guilford.

Wechsler, H., Lee, J. E., Kuo, M., Seibring, M., Nelson, T. F., & Lee, H. (2002). Trends in alcohol use, related problems and experience of prevention efforts among U.S. college students 1993 to 2001: Results from the 2001 Harvard School of Public Health College Alcohol Study. *Journal of American College Health, 50,* 203-217.

Weems, C. F., Pina, A. A., Costa, N. M., Watts, S. E., Taylor, L. K., & Cannon, M. F. (2007). Predisaster trait anxiety and negative affect predict posttraumatic stress in youths after Hurricane Katrina. *Journal of Counseling and Clinical Psychology, 75,* 154-159.

Wei, M., Guo, L., Zhu, Y., Guo, Y., Yv, S., Namassevayam, G., . . . Chen, F. (2019). Type C personality and depression among newly diagnosed breast cancer patients: The mediating role of sense of coherence. *Neuropsychiatric*

Disease and Treatment, 15, 3519–3529. https://doi.org/10.2147/NDT.S230278

Weinberg, A., & Klonsky, E. D. (2012). The effects of self-injury on acute negative arousal: A laboratory simulation. *Motivation and Emotion, 36,* 242–254.

Weiner, B. A., & Wettstein, R. M. (1993). *Legal issues in mental health care.* New York: Plenum Press.

Weiner, L., & Avery-Clark, C. (2017). *Sensate focus in sex therapy: The illustrated manual.* Taylor & Francis.

Weintraub, E., Greenblatt, A. D., Chang, J., Welsh, C. J., Berthiaume, A. P., Goodwin, S. R., . . . Belcher, A. M. (2021). Outcomes for patients receiving telemedicine-delivered medication-based treatment for Opioid Use Disorder: A retrospective chart review. *Heroin Addiction and Related Clinical Problems, 23*(2), 5–12.

Wei, Q., Bai, T., Chen, Y., Ji, G., Hu, X., Xie, W., . . . & Yu, Y. (2018). The changes of functional connectivity strength in electroconvulsive therapy for depression: A longitudinal study. *Frontiers in Neuroscience, 12,* 661.

Weissman, M., & Cuijpers, P. (2017). Psychotherapy over the last four decades. *Harvard Review of Psychiatry, 25*(4), 155–158.

Weissman, M. M., Markowitz, J. C., & Klerman, G. J. (2017). *The guide to interpersonal psychotherapy: Updated and expanded edition.* New York: Oxford University Press.

Weissman, M. M., & Verdeli, H. (2013). Interpersonal psychotherapy: Evaluation, support, triage. *Clinical Psychology & Psychotherapy, 19,* 106–112.

Weller, J., & Budson, A. (2018). Current understanding of Alzheimer's disease diagnosis and treatment. *F1000Research, 7,* F1000 Faculty Rev-1161. https://doi.org/10.12688/f1000research.14506.1

Werner, K. B., Few, L. R., & Bucholz, K. K. (2015). Epidemiology, comorbidity, and behavioral genetics of antisocial personality disorder and psychopathy. *Psychiatric Annals, 45*(4), 195–199.

Wersebe, H., Sijbrandij, M., & Cuijpers, P. (2013). Psychological group-treatments of social anxiety disorder: A meta-analysis. *PLoS ONE, 8,* e79034.

Westefeld, J. S., Gann, L. C., Lustgarten, S. D., & Yeates, K. J. (2016). Relationships between firearm availability and suicide: The role of psychology. *Professional Psychology: Research and Practice, 47*(4), 271–277.

Westen, D. (1998). The scientific legacy of Sigmund Freud: Toward a psychodynamically informed psychological science. *Psychological Bulletin, 124,* 333–371.

Westhoff-Bleck, M., Winter, L., Davila, L. A., Herrmann-Lingen, C., Treptau, J., Bauersachs, J., . . . Kahl, K. G. (2019). Diagnostic evaluation of the hospital depression scale (HADS) and the Beck depression inventory II (BDI-II) in adults with congenital heart disease using a structured clinical interview: Impact of depression severity. *European Journal of Preventive Cardiology, 27*(4), 381–390.

Wetherell, J. L., Lenze, E. J., & Stanley, M. A. (2005). Evidence-based treatment of geriatric anxiety disorders. *Psychiatric Clinics of North America, 28,* 871–896.

Wetzel, E., Brown, A., Hill, P. L., Chung, J. M., Robins, R. W., & Roberts, B. W. (2017). The narcissism epidemic is dead; long live the narcissism epidemic. *Psychological Science, 28*(12), 1833–1847.

Wexler, L., Chandler, M., Gone, J. P., Cwik, M., Kirmayer, L. J., LaFromboise, T., . . . Allen, J. (2015). Advancing suicide prevention research with rural American Indian and Alaska Native populations. *American Journal of Public Health, 105*(5), 891–899.

Whalley, B., Thompson, D. R., & Taylor, R. S. (2014). Psychological interventions for coronary heart disease: Cochrane systematic review and meta-analysis. *International Journal of Behavioral Medicine, 21*(1), 109–121.

Wheaton, M. G., Pinto, A., Fontenelle, L. F., & Yücel, M. (2019). Transdiagnostic factors in obsessive-compulsive personality disorder. *L., Fontenelle, M. Yucel,(Eds.), A transdiagnostic diagnostic approach to obsessions, compulsions and related phenomena,* 345–356.

Wheaton, M. G., & Ward, H. E. (2020). Intolerance of uncertainty and obsessive-compulsive personality disorder. *Personality Disorders: Theory, Research, and Treatment, 11*(5), 357–364. https://doi.org/10.1037/per0000396

Wheeler, J., Newring, K. A. B., and Draper, C. (2008). Transvestic fetishism: Psychopathology and theory. In D. R. Laws & W. T. O'Donohue (Eds.), *Sexual deviance: Theory, assessment, and treatment* (pp. 272–284). New York: Guilford Press.

Whelan, E., Laato, S., Islam, A. N., & Billieux, J. (2021). A casino in my pocket: Gratifications associated with obsessive and harmonious passion for mobile gambling. *PloS one, 16*(2), e0246432.

White A. M. (2020). Gender differences in the epidemiology of alcohol use and related harms in the United States. *Alcohol Research: Current Reviews, 40*(2), 01. https://doi.org/10.35946/arcr.v40.2.01

White, H. R., Xie, M., & Thompson, W. (2001). Psychopathology as a predictor of adolescent drug use trajectories. *Psychology of Addictive Behaviors, 15,* 210–218.

Whooley, M. A., de Jonge, P., Vittinghoff, E., Otte, C., Moos, R., Carney, R. M., . . . Browner, W. S. (2008). Depressive symptoms, health behaviors, and risk of cardiovascular events in patients with coronary heart disease. *JAMA, 300,* 2379–2388.

Whooley, M. A., & Wong, J. M. (2013). Depression and cardiovascular disorders. *Annual Review of Clinical Psychology, 9,* 327–354.

WHO World Mental Health Survey Consortium. (2004). Prevalence, severity, and unmet need for treatment of mental disorders in the World Health Organization World Mental Health Surveys. *Journal of the American Medical Association, 291,* 2581–2590.

Widiger, T. A., & Costa, P. T. C., Jr. (2013). *Personality disorders and the five-factor model of personality* (3rd ed.). Washington, DC: American Psychological Association.

Widiger, T. A., & Mullins-Sweatt, S. N. (2009). Five-factor model of personality disorder: A proposal for *DSM-V. Annual Review of Clinical Psychology, 5,* 197–220.

Widom, C. S., DuMont, K., & Czaja, S. J. (2007). A prospective investigation of major depressive disorder and comorbidity in abused and neglected children grown up. *Archives of General Psychiatry, 64,* 49–56.

Wiewel, E. W., Torian, L. V., Merchant, P., Braunstein, S. L., & Shepard, C. W. (2016). HIV diagnoses and care among transgender persons and comparison with men who have sex with men: New York City, 2006-2011. *American Journal of Public Health, 106*(3), 497–502.

Wilens, T. E., Biederman, J., & Spencer, T. J. (2002). Attention deficit/hyperactivity disorder across the lifespan. *Annual Review of Medicine, 53,* 113–131.

Wilfley, D. E., Pike, K. M., & Striegel-Moore, R. H. (1997). Toward an integrated model of risk for binge-eating disorder. *Journal of Gender, Culture, & Health, 2,* 1–32.

Williams, A. R., Santaella-Tenorio, J., Mauro, C. M., Levin, F. R., & Martins, S. S. (2017). Loose regulation of medical marijuana programs associated with higher rates of adult marijuana use but not cannabis use disorder. *Addiction (Abingdon, England), 112*(11), 1985–1991. https://doi.org/10.1111/add.13904

Williams, D. H., IV, & Johnson, B. A. (2016). Clinical evaluation and treatment of disorders of ejaculation. In L. Lipshultz, A. Pastuszak, A. Goldstein, A. Giraldi, & M. Perelman (Eds.), *Management of sexual dysfunction in men and women* (pp. 139–157). New York: Springer.

Williams, D. L. (2010). *Developmental language disorders: Learning, language, and the brain.* San Diego, CA: Plural.

Williams, J. M. G., Barnhofer, T., Crane, C., Hermans, D., Raes, F., Watkins, E., & Dalgleish, T. (2007). Autobiographical memory specificity and emotional disorder. *Psychological Bulletin, 133,* 122–148.

Williams, M., Baskin-Sommers, A. R., Xian, H., Wirth, L., Scherrer, J. F., Volberg, R. A., . . . & Potenza, M. N. (2020). Examining relations between obsessive-compulsive features, substance-use disorders, and antisocial personality disorder in the Vietnam era twin cohort. *International Journal of Mental Health and Addiction,* 1–11.

Williams, M., Chapman, L., Wong, J., Turkheimer, E. (2012). The role of ethnic identity in symptoms of anxiety and depression in African Americans. *Psychiatry Research, 199*(1); 31–36.

Williams, R. B. (2008). Psychosocial and biobehavioral factors and their interplay in coronary heart disease. *Annual Review of Clinical Psychology, 4,* 349–365.

Williams, R. B., Barefoot, J. C., Haney, T. L., & Harrell, F. E. (1988). Type A behavior and angiographically documented coronary atherosclerosis in a sample of 2,289 patients. *Psychosomatic Medicine, 50,* 139–152.

Wilps, R. F., Jr. (1990). Male bulimia nervosa: An autobiographical case study. In A. E. Andersen (Ed.), *Males with eating disorders* (pp. 9–29). New York: Brunner/Mazel.

Wilson, A. D., Roos, C. R., Robinson, C. S., Stein, E. R., Manuel, J. A., Enkema, M. C., . . . Witkiewitz, K. (2017). Mindfulness-based interventions for addictive behaviors: Implementation issues on the road ahead. *Psychology of Addictive Behaviors, 31*(8), 888–896.

Wilson, G. T., Fairburn, C. C., Agras, W. S., Walsh, B. T., & Kraemer, H. (2002). Cognitive-behavioral therapy for bulimia nervosa: Time course and mechanisms of change. *Journal of Consulting & Clinical Psychology, 70,* 267–274.

Wilson, K. A., & Hayward, C. (2005). A prospective evaluation of agoraphobia and depression symptoms following panic attacks in a community sample of adolescents. *Journal of Anxiety Disorders, 19,* 87–103.

Wilver, N. L., Summers, B. J., & Cougle, J. R. (2020). Effects of safety behavior fading on appearance concerns and related symptoms. *Journal of Consulting and Clinical Psychology, 88*(1), 65–74.

Wimberley, T., MacCabe, J. H., Laursen, T. M., Sørensen, H. J., Astrup, A., Horsdal, H. T., . . . & Støvring, H. (2017). Mortality and self-harm in association with clozapine in treatment-resistant schizophrenia. *American Journal of Psychiatry, 174*(10), 990–998.

Wincze, J. P., Bach, A. K., & Barlow, D. H. (2008). Sexual dysfunction. In D. H. Barlow (Ed.), *Clinical handbook of psychological disorders* (4th ed., pp. 615–661). New York: Guilford Press.

Wincze, J. P., & Weinberg, R. B. (2015). *Sexual dysfunction: A guide for assessment and treatment* (3rd ed.). New York: Guilford Press.

Winger, G., Hofmann, F. G., & Woods, J. H. (2004). *Handbook on drug and alcohol abuse: The biomedical aspects* (4th ed.). New York: Oxford University Press.

Winkelmann, J., Schormair, B., Lichtner, P., Ripke, S., Xiong, L., Jalilzadeh, S., . . . & Meitinger, T. (2007). Genome-wide association study of restless legs syndrome identifies common variants in three genomic regions. *Nature Genetics, 39,* 1000–1006.

Winter, G., Hart, R. A., Charlesworth, R. P., & Sharpley, C. F. (2018). Gut microbiome and depression: What we know and what we need to know. *Reviews in the Neurosciences, 29*(6), 629–643.

Wintersteen, M. B., Mensinger, J. L., & Diamond, G. S. (2005). Do gender and racial differences between patient and therapist affect therapeutic alliance and treatment retention in adolescents? *Professional Psychology: Research and Practice, 36,* 400–408.

Witkiewitz, K., Van der Maas, H. L. J., Hufford, M. R., & Marlatt, G. A. (2007). Nonnormality and divergence in posttreatment alcohol use: Reexamining the project MATCH data "another way." *Journal of Abnormal Psychology, 116,* 378–394.

Wittchen, H.-U., Gloster, A. T., Beesdo-Baum, K., Fava, G., & Craske, M. G. (2010). Agoraphobia: A review of the diagnostic classificatory position and criteria. *Depression and Anxiety, 27,* 113–133.

Witthöft, M., Kerstner, T., Ofer, J., Mier, D., Rist, F., Diener, C., & Bailer, J. (2016). Cognitive biases in pathological health anxiety: The contribution of attention, memory, and evaluation processes. *Clinical Psychological Science, 4*(3), 464–479.

Wolfe, B. E., Baker, C. W., Smith, A. T., & Kelly-Weeder, S. (2009). Validity and utility of the current definition of binge eating. *International Journal of Eating Disorders, 42,* 674–686.

Wolfson, A. R. (2010). Adolescents and emerging adults' sleep patterns: New developments. *Journal of Adolescent Health, 46,* 97–99.

Wollert, R., & Cramer, E. (2011). Sampling extreme groups invalidates research on the paraphilias: Implications for *DSM-5* and sex offender risk assessments. *Behavioral Sciences & the Law, 29,* 554–565.

Wonderlich, S. A., Gordon, K. H., Mitchell, J. E., Crosby, R. D., & Engel, S. G. (2009). The validity and clinical utility of binge eating disorder. *International Journal of Eating Disorders, 42,* 687–705.

Won, E., & Kim, Y. K. (2017). An oldie but goodie: Lithium in the treatment of bipolar disorder through neuroprotective and neurotrophic mechanisms. *International Journal of Molecular Sciences, 18*(12), 2679.

Wong, C., Odom, S. L., Hume, K. A., Cox, A. W., Fettig, A., Kucharczyk, S., . . . Schultz, T. R. (2015). Evidence-based practices for children, youth, and young adults with autism spectrum disorder: A comprehensive review. *Journal of Autism and Developmental Disorders, 45*(7), 1951–1966.

Wong, J. M., Na, B., Regan, M. C., & Whooley, M. A. (2013). Hostility, health behaviors, and risk of recurrent events in patients with stable coronary heart disease: Findings from the Heart and Soul Study. *Journal of the American Heart Association, 2*(5), e000052.

Wong, Q. J., & Rapee, R. M. (2016). The aetiology and maintenance of social anxiety disorder: A synthesis of complementary theoretical models and formulation of a new integrated model. *Journal of Affective Disorders, 203,* 84–100.

Wong Sarver, N., & Gros, D. F. (2014). A modern behavioral treatment to address fetishism and associated functional impairment. *Clinical Case Studies, 13*(4), 336–351.

Woodford, M. R., Weber, G., Nicolazzo, Z., Hunt, R., Kulick, A., Coleman, T., . . . Renn, K. A. (2018). Depression and attempted suicide among LGBTQ college students: Fostering resilience to the effects of heterosexism and cisgenderism on campus. *Journal of College Student Development, 59*(4), 421–438.

Wood, R. & Worthington, A. (2017). Neurobehavioral abnormalities associated with executive dysfunction after traumatic brain injury. *Frontiers in Behavioral Neuroscience, 11,* 195. https://doi.org/10.3389/fnbeh.2017.00195

Woods, D. W., & Houghton, D. C. (2014). Diagnosis, evaluation, and management of trichotillomania. *The Psychiatric Clinics of North America, 37*(3), 301–317.

Woody, M. L., McGeary, J. E., & Gibb, B. E. (2014). Brooding rumination and heart rate variability in women at high and low risk for depression: Group differences and moderation by COMT genotype. *Journal of Abnormal Psychology, 123,* 61–67.

World Health Organization (WHO). (2014). *Global status report on alcohol and health.* Geneva, Switzerland: Author.

World Health Organization (WHO). (2017). Suicide prevention. Retrieved May 14, 2018, from http://www.who.int/mental_ health/suicide-prevention/en/

World Health Organization (WHO). (2018a). Cardiovascular diseases (CVDs). http://www.who.int/en/news-room/fact-sheets/detail/cardiovascular-diseases-(cvds). Retrieved July 5, 2018.

World Health Organization (WHO). (2018b). HIV/AIDS. http://www.who.int/en/news-room/fact-sheets/detail/hiv-aids. Retrieved July 5, 2018.

World Health Organization (WHO). (2018c). Obesity. Retrieved June 21, 2018, from http://www.who.int/topics/obesity

World Health Organization (WHO). (2018d). WHO releases new international classification of diseases (ICD 11). http://www.who.int/news-room/detail/18-06-2018-who-releases-new-international-classification-of-diseases-(icd-11). Retrieved July 4, 2018.

World Health Organization (WHO). Global status report on alcohol and health 2018. Geneva: World Health Organization, 2019. https://www.who.int/ substance_abuse/publications/ global_alcohol_ report/en/ (accessed February 21, 2021).

Worthman, C. M., & Panter-Brick, C. (2008). Homeless street children in Nepal: Use of allostatic load to assess the burden of childhood adversity. *Development and Psychopathology, 20,* 233–255.

Wren, Y., Harding, S., Goldbart, J., & Roulstone, S. (2018). A systematic review and classification of interventions for speech-sound disorder in preschool children. *International Journal of Language & Communication Disorders, 53*(3), 446–467.

Wright, A. G. C., Calabrese, W. R., Rudick, M. M., Yam, W. H., Zelazny, K., Williams, T. F., . . . Simms, L. J. (2015). Stability of the DSM-5 Section III pathological personality traits and their longitudinal associations with psychosocial functioning in personality disordered individuals. *Journal of Abnormal Psychology, 124,* 199–207.

Wright, A. G. C., Thomas, K. M., Hopwood, C. J., Markon, K. E., Pincus, A. L., & Krueger, R. F. (2012). The hierarchical structure of DSM-5 pathological personality traits. *Journal of Abnormal Psychology, 121,* 951–957.

Wurtzel, E. (1995). *Prozac nation.* New York: Berkley.

Wyatt, R. B., de Jong, D. C., & Holden, C. J. (2019). Spectatoring mediates the association between penis appearance concerns and sexual dysfunction. *Journal of Sex & Marital Therapy, 45*(4), 328–338.

Wyse, J. J., Pogoda, T. K., Mastarone, G. L., Gilbert, T., & Carlson, K. F. (2020). Employment and vocational rehabilitation experiences among veterans with polytrauma/ traumatic brain injury history. *Psychological Services, 17*(1), 65–74. https://doi.org/10.1037/ser0000283

X

Xie, W., & Zhang, W. (2018). Mood-dependent retrieval in visual long-term memory: Dissociable effects on retrieval probability and mnemonic precision. *Cognition and Emotion, 32*(4), 674–690.

Xu, G., Stratharn, L., Liu, B., O'Brien, M., Kopelman, T. G., Zhu, J., . . . & Bao, W. (2019). Prevalence and treatment patterns of autism spectrum disorder in the United States, 2016. *JAMA pediatrics, 173*(2), 153–159.

Xu, Y., Schneier, F., Heimberg, R. G., Princisvalle, K., Liebowitz, M. R., Wang, S., & Blanco, C. (2012). Gender differences in social anxiety disorder: Results from the national epidemiologic sample on alcohol and related conditions. *Journal of Anxiety Disorders, 26*(1), 12–19.

Y

Yıldız, M., Orak, U., Walker, M. H., & Solakoglu, O. (2019). Suicide contagion, gender, and suicide attempts among adolescents. *Death Studies, 43*(6), 365–371.

Yadav, T., Balhara, Y. P., & Kataria, D. K. (2012). Pseudocyesis versus delusion of pregnancy: Differential diagnoses to be kept in mind. *Indian Journal of Psychological Medicine, 34*(1), 82–84. https://doi.org/10.4103/0253-7176.96167

Yaffe, Y. (2018). Establishing specific links between parenting styles and the S-anxieties in children: Separation, social, and school. *Journal of Family Issues, 39*(5), 1419–1437.

Yakeley, J. (2018). Current understanding of narcissism and narcissistic personality disorder. *BJPsych Advances, 24*(5), 305–315.

Yang, J., Dai, X., Yao, S., Cai, T., Gao, B., McCrae, R. R., & Costa, P. T. (2002). Personality disorders and the five-factor model of personality in Chinese psychiatric patients. In P. T. Costa & T. A. Widiger (Eds.), *Personality disorders and the five-factor model of personality* (2nd ed., pp. 215–221). Washington, DC: American Psychological Association.

Yanovski, S. Z., & Yanovski, J. A. (2014). Long-term drug treatment for obesity: A systematic and clinical review. *Journal of the American Medical Association, 311*(1), 74–86.

Yao, S., Larson, H., Norring, C., Birgegard, A., Lichtenstein, P., D'Onofrio, B. M., . . . Kuja-Alkola, R. (2021). Genetic and environmental contributions to diagnostic fluctuation in anorexia nervosa and bulimia nervosa. *Psychological Medicine, 51,* 62–69.

Yarbrough, E. (2018). *Transgender mental health.* Washington, DC: American Psychiatric Association.

Yatham, L. N., Kennedy, S. H., Parikh, S. V., Schaffer, A., Bond, D. J., Frey, B. N., ... Berk, M. (2018). Canadian Network for Mood and Anxiety Treatments (CANMAT) and International Society for Bipolar Disorders (ISBD) 2018 guidelines for the management of patients with bipolar disorder. *Bipolar disorders, 20*(2), 97–170.

Yazigi, L., Semer, N. L., Fiore, M. L. d. M., Abela, R. K., Lerman, T. G., & Marques, T. C. (2016). Form quality in rorschach comprehensive system and R-PAS: Sample of psychiatric cases. *Paideía, 26*(63), 53–62.

Yeh, M., & Weisz, J. R. (2001). Why are we here at the clinic? Parent-child (dis)agreement on referral problems at outpatient treatment entry. *Journal of Consulting & Clinical Psychology, 69,* 1019–1025.

Yehuda, R., Blair, W., Labinsky, E., & Bierer, L. M. (2007). Effects of parental PTSD on the cortisol response to dexamethasone administration in their adult offspring. *American Journal of Psychiatry, 164,* 163–166.

Yehuda, R., Pratchett, L., & Pelcovitz, M. (2012). Biological contributions to PTSD: Differentiating normative from pathological response. In J. G. Beck & D. M. Sloan (Eds.), *The Oxford handbook of traumatic stress disorders* (pp. 159–174). New York: Oxford University Press.

Yim, I. S., Tanner Stapleton, L. R., Guardino, C. M., Hahn-Holbrook, J., & Dunkel Schetter, C. (2015). Biological and psychosocial predictors of postpartum depression: Systematic review and call for integration. *Annual Review of Clinical Psychology, 11,* 99–137.

Yip, S. W. & Potenza, M. N. (2014). Treatment of gambling disorders. *Current Treatment Options in Psychiatry, 1,* 189–203.

Yi, S., Chang, E. C., Chang, O. D., Seward, N. J., McAvoy, L. B., Krause, E. R., . . . & Hirsch, J. K. (2020). Coping and suicide in college students. *Crisis, 42*(1), 5–12.

Yli-Länttä, H. (2020). Young people's experiences of social fears. *International Journal of Adolescence and Youth, 25*(1), 1022–1035.

Yolken, R., Stallings, C., Origoni, A., Katsafanas, E., Sweeney, K., Squire, A., & Dickerson, F. (2019). Exposure to household pet cats and dogs in childhood and risk of subsequent diagnosis of schizophrenia or bipolar disorder. *PloS One, 14*(12), e0225320.

Yonkers, K., & Caser, R. (2019). *Epidemiology and pathogenesis of premenstrual syndrome and premenstrual dysphoric disorder.* Retrieved December 15, 2020, from https://www.uptodate.com/contents/epidemiology-and-pathogenesis-of-premenstrual-syndrome-and-premenstrual-dysphoric-disorder

Yoshikawa, H., Aber, J. L., & Beardslee, W. R. (2012). The effects of poverty on the mental, emotional, and behavioral health of children and youth: Implications for prevention. *American Psychologist, 67*(4), 272–284.

Young, E., & Korzun, A. (1999). Psychoneuroendocrinology of depression: Hypothalamic-pituitary-gonadal axis. *Psychiatric Clinics of North America, 21,* 309–323.

Young-Wolff, K. C., Kendler, K. S., Ericson, M. L., & Prescott, C. A. (2011). Accounting for the association between childhood maltreatment and alcohol-use disorders in males: A twin study. *Psychological Medicine, 41,* 59–70.

Yu-Ru, L., & Wen-Ting, C. (2020). The dynamics of twitter users' gun narratives across major mass shooting events. *Palgrave Communications, 7*(1).

Yusuf, S., Hawken, S., Ounpuu, S., Dans, T., Avezum, A., Lanas, F., . . . Lisheng, L. (2004). Effect of potentially modifiable risk factors associated with myocardial infarction in 52 countries (the INTERHEART study): Case-control study. *Lancet, 364,* 937–952.

Z

Zadra, A., Desautels, A., Petit, D., & Montplaisir, J. (2013). Somnambulism: Clinical aspects and pathophysiological hypotheses. *Lancet Neurology, 12*(3), 285–294.

Zalta, A. K., Gillihan, S. J., Fisher, A. J., Mintz, J., McLean, C. P., Yehuda, R., & Foa, E. B. (2014). Change in negative cognitions associated with PTSD predicts symptom reduction in prolonged exposure. *Journal of Consulting and Clinical Psychology, 82,* 171–175.

Zanarini, M. C., Frankenburg, F. R., Reich, D. B., & Fitzmaurice, G. (2012). Attainment and stability of sustained symptomatic remission and recovery among patients with borderline personality disorder and axis II comparison subjects: A 16-year prospective follow-up study. *American Journal of Psychiatry, 169,* 476–483.

Zanarini, M. C., Schulz, S. C., Detke, H., Zhao, F., Lin, D., Pritchard, M., . . . Corya, S. (2012). Open-label treatment with olanzapine for patients with borderline personality disorder. *Journal of Clinical Psychopharmacology, 32,* 398–402.

Zanarini, M. C., Skodol, A.-E., Bender, D., Dolan, R., Sanislow, C., Schaefer, E., . . . Gunderson, G. (2000). The collaborative longitudinal personality disorders study: Reliability of axis I and II diagnoses. *Journal of Personality Disorder, 14,* 291–299.

Zayas, L. H., Lester, R. J., Cabassa, L. J., & Fortuna, L. R. (2005). Why do so many Latina teens attempt suicide? A conceptual model for research. *American Journal of Orthopsychiatry, 75,* 275–287.

Zdanys, K. F., & Steffens, D. C. (2015). Sleep disturbances in the elderly. *Psychiatric Clinics, 38*(4), 723–741.

Zhang, B., & Wing, Y.-K. (2006). Sex differences in insomnia: A meta-analysis. *Sleep, 29,* 85–93.

Zhang, C., Yang, L., Liu, S., Ma, S., Wang, Y., Cai, Z., . . . & Zhang, B. (2020). Survey of insomnia and related social psychological factors among medical staff involved in the 2019 novel coronavirus disease outbreak. *Frontiers in Psychiatry, 11,* 306.

Zhang, L., Pan, J., Chen, W., Jiang, J., & Huang, J. (2020). Chronic stress-induced immune dysregulation in cancer: Implications for initiation, progression, metastasis, and treatment. *American journal of cancer research, 10*(5), 1294–1307.

Zhang, X., Beaulieu, J. M., Sotnikova, T. D., Gainetdinov, R. R., & Caron, M. G. (2004). Tryptophan hydroxylase-2 controls brain serotonin. *Science, 305,* 217.

Zhou, Z., Shek, D.T., Zhu, X., Dou, D. (2020). Positive Youth Development and Adolescent Depression: A Longitudinal Study Based on Mainland Chinese High School Students. *International Journal of Environmental Research and Public Health, 17,* 4457. Retrieved from http://dx.doi.org/10.3390/ijerph17124457

Zhu, B., Chen, C., Loftus, E. F., He, Q., Chen, C., Lei, X., . . . Dong, Q. (2012). Brief exposure to misinformation can lead to long-term false memories. *Applied Cognitive Psychology, 26,* 301–307.

Ziegelstein, R. C., Fauerbach, J. A., Stevens, S. S., Romanelli, J., Richter, D. P., & Bush, D. E. (2000). Patients with depression are less likely to follow recommendations to reduce cardiac risk during recovery from a myocardial infarction. *Archives of Internal Medicine, 160,* 1818–1823.

Zigler, E., Gilliam, W. S., & Jones, S. M. (2006). *A vision for universal preschool education.* New York: Cambridge University Press.

Zigler, E., & Styfco, S. J. (2004). Applying the findings of developmental psychology to improve early childhood intervention. In M. A. Feldman (Ed.), *Early intervention: The essential readings* (pp. 54–72). Malden, UK: Blackwell.

Zigler, E., & Styfco, S. J. (2008). America's Head Start program: An effort for social justice. In C. Wainryb, J. Smetana, & E. Turiel (Eds.), *Social development, social inequalities, and social justice* (pp. 53–80). New York: Taylor & Francis Group/Lawrence Erlbaum.

Zilboorg, G., & Henry, G. W. (1941). *A history of medical psychology.* New York: W. W. Norton.

Zimmer, A., Youngblood, A., Adnane, A., Miller, B. J., & Goldsmith, D. R. (2021). Prenatal exposure to viral infection and neuropsychiatric disorders in offspring: A review of the literature and recommendations for the COVID-19 pandemic. *Brain, Behavior, and Immunity.*

Zimmer-Gembeck, M. J., Hawes, T., & Pariz, J. (2020). A closer look at appearance and social media: Measuring activity, self-presentation, and social comparison and their associations with emotional adjustment. *Psychology of Popular Media.* Retrieved from https://doi-org.mccc.idm.oclc.org/10.1037/ppm0000277

Zimmerman, M., Rothschild, L., & Chelminski, I. (2005). The prevalence of *DSM-IV* personality disorders in psychiatric outpatients. *American Journal of Psychiatry, 162,* 1911–1918.

Zintzaras, E., Kitsios, G. D., Papathanasiou, A. A., Konitsiotis, S., Miligkos, M., Rodopoulou, P., & Hadjigeorgiou, G. M. (2010). Randomized trials of dopamine agonists in restless legs syndrome: A systematic review, quality assessment, and meta-analysis. *Clinical Therapeutics, 32,* 221–237.

Zinzow, H. M., Resnick, H. S., McCauley, J. L., Amstadter, A. B., Ruggiero, K. J., & Kilpatrick, D. G. (2012). Prevalence and risk of psychiatric disorders as a function of variant rape histories: Results from a national survey of women. *Social Psychiatry and Psychiatric Epidemiology, 47,* 893–902.

Zipursky, R. B., & Agid, O. (2015). Recovery, not progressive deterioration, should be the expectation in schizophrenia. *World Psychiatry: Official Journal of the World Psychiatric Association (WPA), 14*(1), 94–96. https://doi.org/10.1002/wps.20194

Zucker, K. J. (2018). The myth of persistence: Response to "A critical commentary on follow-up studies and 'desistance' theories about transgender and gender non-conforming children" by Temple Newhook et al. (2018). *International Journal of Transgenderism, 19,* 231–235.

Zucker, K. J., & Cohen-Kettenis, P. T. (2008). Gender identity disorder in children and adolescents. In D. L. Rowland & L. Incrocci (Eds.), *Handbook of sexual and gender identity disorders* (pp. 376–422). Hoboken, NJ: Wiley.

Zucker, K. J., & Duschinsky, R. (2016). Dilemmas encountered by the Sexual and Gender Identity Disorders Work Group for DSM-5: An interview with Kenneth J. Zucker. *Psychology & Sexuality, 7*(1), 23–33.

Zucker, K. J., Lawrence, A. A., & Kreukels, B. P. (2016). Gender dysphoria in adults. *Annual Review of Clinical Psychology, 12,* 217–247.

Zucker, K. J., & Wood, H. (2011). Assessment of gender variance in children. *Child and Adolescent Psychiatric Clinics of North America, 20,* 665–680.

Zucker, R. A., Heitzeg, M. M., & Nigg, J. T. (2011). Parsing the undercontrol-disinhibition pathway to substance use disorders: A multilevel developmental problem. *Child Development Perspectives, 5*(4), 248–255.

Zucker, R. A., Kincaid, S. B., Fitzgerald, H. E., & Bingham, C. R. (1995). Alcohol schema acquisition in preschoolers: Differences between children of alcoholics and children of nonalcoholics. *Alcoholism: Clinical & Experimental Research, 19,* 1011–1017.

Zuvekas, S. H., & Vitiello, B. (2012). Stimulant medication use in children: A 12-year perspective. *American Journal of Psychiatry, 169,* 160–166.

Zvolensky, M. J., & Smits, J. A. J. (Eds.). (2008). *Anxiety in health behaviors and physical illness.* New York: Springer Science & Business Media.

Zwerdling, D. (2009, November 11). Walter Reed officials asked: Was Hasan psychotic? http://www.npr.org/templates/story/story.php?storyId=120313570.

Marques, T. R., 212
Marques-Portella, C., 148
Marrocco, F., 233
Marroquin, B., 209, 476, 477
Marshall, G. N., 175
Marshall, L. E., 427
Marshall, R. D., 151, 152, 153
Marshall, S., 489
Marshall, W. L., 427
Martell, C., 218
Marti, C. N., 380, 381, 382, 393
Marti, H. H., 262
Marti, N., 386
Martin, A., 164, 165
Martin, C., 250
Martin, G. E., 228
Martin, G. N., 230
Martin, J. K., 361, 511
Martin, K. M., 140
Martin, L. R., 476
Martin, N. G., 298, 392, 394
Martin, W., 191
Martin-Blanco, A., 297
Martinez, D., 292
Martinez, K. B., 204, 263
Martinez-Aran, A., 197
Martinez-Taboas, A., 172, 173, 174, 175, 176, 177
Martin-Mittag, B., 164
Martino, S., 463
Martins, C. M. S., 297
Martins, S. S., 443, 453
Martins, Y., 375
Martin-Soelch, C., 165
Martland, N., 266
Martland, R., 266
Martorana, A., 347
Martorella, S. R., 181
Marzilli, E., 384
Masheb, R. M., 383
Masland, S. R., 298, 299
Mason, E., 166
Mason, O., 293
Masoud, S., 200, 201, 202
Massimetti, E., 116
Masson P., 412, 413
Mastarone, G. L., 346
Masten, A. S., 475
Master, S. L., 477
Masters, C. L., 342
Masters, G. A., 211
Masters, K. S., 478
Masters, W. H., 402, 403, 409, 410, 415, 416
Masuda, A., 49
Mataix-Cols, D., 135, 136, 140, 141, 328
Matarazzo, J. D., 15

Mather, A., 297, 302, 304, 309, 312, 369
Matheson, B. E., 73
Matheson, M. C., 497
Mathew, S. J., 122
Mathews, A., 121
Mathews, C. A., 132
Mathis, A., 266
Matroos, G. E., 380
Matson, J. L., 334
Matsumoto, Y., 430
Matt, G. E., 208
Matthews, J. C., 205
Matthews, K. A., 476, 486
Matthiasdottir, E., 375
Matthys, W., 361, 362
Mattick, R. P., 461
Mattila, M.-L., 326, 327
Mattila, T., 249
Maughan, B., 327, 335, 360
Maurer, D. M., 85
Mauri, M., 37, 219
Mauro, C. M., 453
Mausbach, B. T., 347
Mauss, I. B., 228, 478
Maussion, G., 368
Mavranezouli, I., 126, 127
Mawlawi, O., 292
Maxfield, J., 391
May, A. M., 228, 229, 231
May, T., 326, 327, 431
Mayberg, H. S., 217
Mayes, L. C., 210
Mayes, S. D., 191
Maynard, H., 274, 275
Mayo, D., 266
Mayou, R., 149
Mayo-Wilson, E., 126, 127
Mays, V. M., 145, 512
Mazzoli, F., 417
Mazzoni, G., 181
McAloon, J., 51, 73, 468
McArthur, B., 193
McArthur, J., 345
McAvoy, L. B., 227
McCabe, J. E., 189, 204
McCabe, M. P., 405, 406, 407
McCabe, R., 125
McCabe, S. E., 446, 458
McCaffery, J. M., 479
McCarthy, B. W., 410, 413, 414, 415, 416
McCarthy, M., 389
McCarthy-Jones, R., 245
McCarthy-Jones, S., 245
McCarton, C., 334
McCartoon, C., 334
McCauley, J. L., 147, 149
McClay, J, 361

McClelland, G. M., 521, 522
McCloskey, M. S., 370, 371
McClure, M. M., 247, 287, 293
McCormick, B., 298
McCormick, D., 479
McCormick, M. C., 334
McCourt, A. D., 233
McCrady, B. S., 459, 461, 462
McCrae, N., 208, 209
McCrae, R. R., 282, 310
McCurry, S. M., 347, 348
McCutchan, A. J., 483
McCutcheon, R., 259, 261, 263, 264, 266, 276
McEwen, B. S., 473, 479
McFall, R. M., 392
McFarlane, A. C., 151
McFarlane, T. L., 395
McFarlane, W. R., 273
McGeary, J. E., 208
McGinn, M. M., 477, 478, 481
McGinty, E. E., 512
McGlashan, T. H., 271, 292, 296, 297, 298, 310
McGorry, P. D., 260
McGovern, C. M., 13
McGreevy, M. A., 517
McGue, M., 458
McGuffin, P., 202, 211
McGuire, J. F., 340
McGuire, J. K., 430
McGuire, T. G., 50
McGurk, D., 149
McGurk, S. R., 287
McHugh, R. K., 462
McIntosh, A. M., 200, 201, 202, 260, 261
McIntosh, J. L., 228
McIntyre, L. L., 334, 335
McKay, R., 252
McKenna, P. J., 273
McKenzie, S. K., 230
McKinnon, D. H., 337
McKlveen, J. M., 202, 203
McKnight, P., 467
McLaughlin, J., 229
McLaughlin, K. A., 27, 142
McLean, C. P., 42, 141, 142, 153
McLeod, J. D., 511
McLeod, S., 337
McLoughlin, D. M., 216
McMahon, C. A., 362
McMahon, F. J., 210
McMahon, P., 169
McManus, F., 153
McMaster, A., 290, 291, 292, 293
McMillan, T. M., 369

McNally, R. J., 112, 180, 181
McNary, S. W., 174
McNeill, A., 448–449
McNiel, D. E., 513
McPartland, J., 327
McRae, K., 228
McRae, T. D., 460
McReynolds, L. S., 360, 361
McRobbie, H., 450
McVary, K. T., 413
McWhirter, L., 168
McWilliams, N., 44
Meador-Woodruff, J., 261
Meagher, S., 288, 302, 306, 308, 309, 312, 367, 369
Mechanic, D., 19
Mechelli, A., 31
Medda, P., 37, 219
Medford, N., 179
Mednick, B., 368
Medrano, L. A., 66
Meehl, P. E., 63
Mehler, P. S., 377, 378
Mehrotra, A., 463
Mehta, K. M., 346
Meier, S., 56
Meijer, C. J., 272, 273
Meinlschmidt, G., 152
Meitinger, T., 502
Melchiorre, M. G., 165
Melton, G. B., 509, 517, 520
Meltzer, S., 165
Memisoglu, A., 191
Mendelson, M., 75
Mendes, A. L., 206
Mendlowicz, M. V., 148
Mendrek, A., 246, 252
Menezes, N. M., 249, 251
Mennes, M., 322
Mennin, D. S., 121, 123
Mensah, G., 444
Mensinger, J. L., 53
Mento, C., 191
Menvielle, E., 430, 431
Menzel, J. E., 390
Merai, R., 484
Mercado, C. C., 522
Mercer-Lynn, K. B., 395
Merchant, P., 428
Merckelbach, H., 169, 171, 176, 180
Mergl, R., 205
Mericle, A. A., 521
Merikangas, K. R., 130, 192, 197, 198, 199, 200, 212, 229, 320, 380, 382
Merikangas, M. R., 78, 111, 125, 127, 135, 144
Merkouris, S. S., 329, 468